# HANDBUCH DER SPEZIELLEN PATHOLOGISCHEN ANATOMIE UND HISTOLOGIE

BEGRÜNDET VON

O. LUBARSCH UND F. HENKE

FORTGEFÜHRT VON

R. RÖSSLE

HERAUSGEGEBEN VON

E. UEHLINGER

ZÜRICH

ERSTER BAND

## BLUT · KNOCHENMARK · LYMPHKNOTEN · MILZ

DRITTER TEIL

## LYMPHKNOTEN/LYMPH NODES

BANDTEIL B

## MALIGNANT LYMPHOMAS

OTHER THAN HODGKIN'S DISEASE

SPRINGER-VERLAG

BERLIN · HEIDELBERG · NEW YORK

1978

# MALIGNANT LYMPHOMAS
## OTHER THAN HODGKIN'S DISEASE

HISTOLOGY · CYTOLOGY · ULTRASTRUCTURE · IMMUNOLOGY

BY

KARL LENNERT

IN COLLABORATION WITH

NOBORU MOHRI · HARALD STEIN

EDWIN KAISERLING · HANS KONRAD MÜLLER-HERMELINK

TRANSLATED BY

FREDERICK D. DALLENBACH AND MARTHA SOEHRING

WITH 287 FIGURES, 47 IN COLOR

425 SEPARATE ILLUSTRATIONS

SPRINGER-VERLAG

BERLIN · HEIDELBERG · NEW YORK

1978

Prof. Dr. med. K. LENNERT
Dr. med. habil. H. STEIN
Dr. med. habil. E. KAISERLING
Dr. med. habil. HANS KONRAD MÜLLER-HERMELINK

Pathologisches Institut der Universität, Hospitalstraße 42, D-2300 Kiel

Prof. Dr. med. N. MOHRI

Tokyo University Branch Hospital, Bunkyoku, Mejirodai 3-28-6, 112 Tokyo (Japan)

ISBN-13: 978-3-642-81094-7 e-ISBN-13: 978-3-642-81092-3
DOI: 10.1007/978-3-642-81092-3

Library of Congress Cataloging in Publication Data (Revised). Henke, Friedrich, 1868–1943, ed. Handbuch der speziellen pathologischen Anatomie und Histologie. Each vol. has also special t.p. Edited 1934– by O. Lubarsch, F. Henke, and R. Rössle; 1969– by E. Uehlinger. Includes bibliographies. On t.p. of vols. issued from 1969– : Begründet von O. Lubarsch und F. Henke. Fortgeführt von R. Rössle. Hrsg. von E. Uehlinger. Vol. 3, pt. 5 entirely in English. Contents: 1. Bd. Blut. Knochenmark. Lymphknoten. Milz. 3. Bd. Atmungswege und Lungen. [etc.] Anatomy, Pathological. 2. Histology, Pathological. I. Lubarsch, Otto, 1860–1933, joint ed. II. Rössle, Robert, 1876–1956, ed. III. Uehlinger, Erwin A., ed. IV. Title.
RB25.H4 616.07 25-11247


Softcover reprint of the hardcover 1st edition 1978

2122/3120-543210

*To*
*my wife Amanda*
*and*
*my daughters Monika and Claudia*

*ὡς κινδυνεύω ἔγωγε ἐν τῷ παρόντι περὶ αὐτοῦ τούτου οὐ φιλοσόφως ἔχειν ἀλλ' ὥσπερ οἱ πάνυ ἀπαίδευτοι φιλονίκως. καὶ γὰρ ἐκεῖνοι ὅταν περί του ἀμφισβητῶσιν, ὅπῃ μὲν ἔχει περὶ ὧν ἂν ὁ λόγος ἦ οὐ φροντίζουσιν, ὅπως δὲ ἃ αὐτοὶ ἔθεντο ταῦτα δόξει τοῖς παροῦσιν, τοῦτο προθυμοῦνται.*

... since that very issue is one that I may not be facing as a philosopher should, but rather as one bent on victory, like those quite devoid of education. They too, when they dispute about something, care nothing for the truth of the matter under discussion, but are eager only that those present shall accept their own thesis.
SOCRATES in PLATO's *Phaedo* (91 a).

# Preface

The first review of malignant lymphomas, other than Hodgkin's disease, in this Handbook series was given by C. STERNBERG in 1926. It comprised seven pages. The magnitude of this second presentation of the same subject reflects the enormous increase in knowledge gathered over the past 50 years. Experimental immunology and lymphocyte research of the past two decades are especially to blame. They forced us to reconsider lymphocytic reactions and neoplasms and to correlate these with new experimental data. In order to make such correlations, it was necessary to apply the tools of experimental immunology to the definition of the cells involved. In this way, it was possible not only to redefine the normal and reactive cells of lymphatic tissue, but also to come to a better understanding of the malignant neoplasms of these cells.

In collaboration with E. KAISERLING, N. MOHRI, H.K. MÜLLER-HERMELINK, and H. STEIN, I have endeavored since 1970 to study and to classify the malignant lymphomas in the light of modern lymphocyte research. Our investigations made use of both special morphologic methods (Giemsa staining in sections, imprints, cytochemistry, and electron microscopy) and immunologic techniques. The major morphologic groundwork for our lymphoma studies was laid by the experimental work of F.J. KEUNING and his school. With the help of the methods we applied, particularly the immunologic techniques, it was possible to confirm some of our earlier, morphologically defined concepts, e.g., the morphologic identity of germinal-center cells and the tumors of these cells. It was also possible, however, to eliminate certain errors made in the past. It was shown, for instance, that most cases of "reticulosarcoma" are actually immunoblastic lymphomas. Furthermore, some new entities were discovered, e.g., lymphoplasmacytoid immunocytoma.

These and other data encouraged us to make an attempt to draft and pursue a new concept of the malignant lymphomas other than Hodgkin's disease, which are now generally known as "non-Hodgkin's lymphomas". We were honored to have our concept accepted in principle by the other members of the European Lymphoma Club, R. GÉRARD-MARCHANT, IRIS HAMLIN, F. RILKE,

A.G. STANSFELD, and J.A.M. VAN UNNIK. In joint discussions in 1974, the Club worked out a new terminology that was acceptable to all members and will hopefully be acceptable to other pathologists. Since then, it has been called the Kiel Classification. We are also pleased that the clinicians belonging to the Kiel Lymphoma Study Group – foremost A. STACHER and G. BRITTINGER – have been able to present preliminary data on the clinical relevance of the new classification. Finally, our optimism was fortified by the findings of R.J. LUKES and R.D. COLLINS, which largely concur with ours in both concept and practical significance.

This book is divided into six main sections. First, there is a chapter on normal cytology that supplements and, in some respects, revises the presentation given in Part A of this Handbook (1961). H.K. MÜLLER-HERMELINK played a major role in the writing of the first chapter. The second chapter is a brief description of the light-microscopic techniques that are used in our laboratories and have proved to be suitable for a precise diagnosis of lymph-node diseases. In the third chapter, a number of basic considerations are presented in relation to malignant lymphomas and their classification. Part Four is the focus of this book. In separate chapters on each type of lymphoma, it describes the histologic, cytologic, and cytochemical features of each one. Furthermore, in conformity with Part A, it provides data on the occurrence, localization, diagnosis, differential diagnosis, and prognosis of the various types of lymphomas. N. MOHRI of Tokyo had a major part in the preparation of the histologic and statistical data. In Part Five, E. KAISERLING presents the ultrastructure of the malignant lymphomas. Part Six was written by H. STEIN and describes immunologic techniques and the results of their application to lymphomas.

Hodgkin's disease and the malignant neoplasms of reticulum cells have been left out of this book on purpose. Although much is known about Hodgkin's disease, we are still looking for answers to fundamental questions, e.g., the origin of Sternberg-Reed cells. The whole concept of reticulosarcoma and malignant reticulosis (histiocytosis) was upset by the separation of immunoblastic lymphoma and will have to be reconsidered and studied with new methods.

The magnitude of this book may be appalling at first. Nevertheless, it is incomplete in many respects. For instance, the historical review of some of the lymphomas is unjustly confined to the literature written in English, French, and German. Readers who are familiar with other languages are asked to forgive this selection. I recommend the reader who is in a hurry, i.e., the pathologist who is looking for quick information under the pressure of daily routine, to concentrate on the sections Definition and Diagnosis in each chapter of Part Four and on the illustrations. The most important diagnostic criteria are summarized in tabular form.

Since the publishers gave us no other choice but to publish this book in English, we were at a loss for a good translation. So we were all the more thankful that F.D. DALLENBACH, Deutsches Krebsforschungszentrum, Heidelberg, spontaneously offered to translate the manuscript – truly a great sacrifice for an active scientist. He translated about half of the book. The other half was translated with help of Mrs. M. SOEHRING, our secretary from Boston. A.G. STANSFELD, Department of Pathology, St. Bartholomew's Hospital, London, was then kind enough to read most of the English manuscript from the viewpoint of a lymphoma expert and to make helpful suggestions.

The original manuscript of Parts Two, Three, and Four was delivered to the translator in May 1975. Later, we were able to include references that appeared up to July 1, 1976. More recent references could merely be mentioned here and there or added to the footnotes. Parts One and Five were completed in June 1976; again, more recent literature could not be taken into full consideration. Part Six was not ready until January 1977; the literature cited in that chapter is, understandably, the most up-to-date. It is evident from the text of the chapters written in 1975, however, that the investigations of the past two years have not necessitated any significant changes.

We are aware that our concept will not be the last word. The future will have to show how far it fulfills the ultimate criterion of scientific truth, viz.: the ability to forecast events. Nevertheless, we believe that it is time to abandon all the old lymphoma concepts that pathologists have become so fond of, and to embark on a new one that takes account of both the structure and the function of the tumor cells. One should no longer cling to old, scientifically incorrect classifications, even if they have so far been clinically useful—there are no arguments indicating that our new classification is not just as clinically useful.

In London in 1973, H. RAPPAPORT quoted an old saying, which is symbolically inscribed on a bridge: "*Alles ist nur ein Übergang*"—everything is merely a transition. Our classification may be seen as such a transition. Its purpose is to help the sufferers from lymphoma without hindering scientific progress.

Kiel, February 1978 KARL LENNERT

# Acknowledgements

This book is not the work of just one or five persons—it is the fruit of manifold cooperation, friendship, and criticism. We are therefore indebted to many people for their assistance and guidance.

A decisive role in the genesis of this book was played by our clinical partners, particularly those who belong to the Kiel Lymphoma Study Group, which was originally initiated by Professor Dr. A. STACHER, Vienna, and is thriving under the leadership of Professor Dr. G. BRITTINGER, Essen. The groups working in the fields of leukemia and oncology in childhood led by Professor Dr. G. LANDBECK, Hamburg, and Professor Dr. B. KORNHUBER, Frankfurt, made a similar contribution to the lymphomas of childhood. Finally, there were surgeons and otolaryngologists at the University of Kiel (under the leadership of Professor Dr. B. LÖHR and Professor Dr. E. MÜLLER, respectively) and at several other German hospitals who were willing to cooperate with us. All the mentioned clinicians cooperated by sending us fresh tissue, imprints, and tumor tissue specially fixed for electron microscopy. This was the crucial reason why we were able to work out a classification based on morphologic (histologic, cytologic, and ultrastructural), cytochemical, and immunologic studies.

The hours invested by our clinical colleagues were innumerable. The time spent per case often amounted to several hours. This book is a commemorative to such unique, selfless cooperation. Not to be forgotten are the pathologists who normally work with the cooperating clinicians—they willingly agreed to our receiving material from the clinicians and were contented with a copy of our diagnosis. Especially helpful colleagues from the very first were Professor Dr. ALEXANDRA PIRINGER-KUCHINKA, Vienna; Professor Dr. H.-W. ALTMANN, Würzburg; Professor Dr. H. BREDT, Mainz; Professor Dr. E. LANGER, Munich; and Professor Dr. W. MÜLLER, Essen.

A second group of colleagues who played a crucial role in the genesis of this book was the so-called European Lymphoma Club, which is made up of Professor Dr. N. CHELLOUL†, Paris; Dr. R. GÉRARD-MARCHANT, Villejuif; Dr. IRIS M.E. HAMLIN, London; Professor Dr. F. RILKE, Milan; Dr. A.G. STANSFELD, London; Professor Dr. J.A.M. VAN UNNIK, Utrecht; and the author (K.L.). All members of the Club have advocated the jointly created Kiel Classification in their own countries and elsewhere. This scientific and amicable solidarity among lymphoma experts from five different European countries also set an example for cooperation in Europe, i.e., irrespective of national borders. The many suggestions, corrections, and comments made by our Club colleagues are reflected in this book. Their constant support as friends encouraged us to stay on the path and to present this publication.

The writer is also indebted to all the people who work at our Institute for the loyalty they showed, either directly or indirectly, during the whole project—directly by being actively involved in the project; indirectly by doing more than their normal share of work to give us time to prepare this book. The indirect helpers are too numerous to mention by name; but they are represented by my head assistants Professor Dr. L.-D. LEDER and Professor Dr. H.-J. STUTTE; Professor Dr. D. HARMS, Head of the Department of Paidopathology; Professor Dr. M.R. PARWARESCH, who introduced us to polyacrylamide-gel electrophoresis; and Dr. E.-W. SCHWARZE, who offered me constant assistance in the work of the Lymph Node Registry.

Directly involved in the preparation of this book were:

Mrs. M. SOEHRING, who not only helped to translate, but also prepared the English manuscript for publication with a critical eye and good judgment. She also read and corrected all of the proofs with perfection.

Miss K. SOHRWEIDE, who typed the German manuscript, and Mrs. S. SOOTER, who typed parts of the English manuscript.

Professor Dr. H. UHLIG, who helped us prepare the color photomicrographs with a Zeiss Ultraphot II (photomicroscope).

Mrs. H. BLESSMANN, who developed and enlarged the photomicrographs.

Mrs. R. KÖPKE, who was responsible for enlarging the electron micrographs.

Mr. W. VATER, who did all of the graphic work with utmost precision and competence.

Mrs. A. ROHDE and Mrs. D. SCHMIDT, who were responsible for the precise preparation of the references. Mrs. SCHMIDT also read and corrected the proofs of the references and footnotes.

Mrs. A. LURZ and Mr. W. GLÜCK, who prepared the histologic sections of excellent technical quality.

Mrs. B. PETERSEN, who assisted with the cytochemical reactions.

Mrs. I. HORN, Mrs. K. KÖNIG, Miss C. MÄDER, Miss P. MICHEELS, and Mr. E. GROSSKOPF, who assisted with the immunologic investigations.

Miss D. AECKERLE, Miss O. BRACKER, Miss F. KHUEN, Miss F. MARTEN, Miss M. NEUBERT, and Miss A. VOGLER, who provided excellent technical assistance in our electron-microscopic laboratory.

The preparation of the statistical data was possible only through the effort of the secretarial and technical assistants at our Lymph Node Registry, Mrs. C. BANNER and Mrs. I. KIEKBUSCH. Professor Dr. G. GRIESSER and his assistant Mr. J.D. VOSS from the Department of Medical Statistics and Documentation helped us in every way with the computerization and storage of our data.

Dr. R. SATODATE, Dr. R. SUGIYAMA, Dr. E.-W. SCHWARZE, Mrs. D. HELBRON, and Mrs. U. MÜLLER-HERMELINK made contributions to certain chapters and the application of certain special techniques. These are mentioned in the text.

The loyal support of those who work at our Institute never faltered, from the time we started to write this book in 1974 until its completion. In addition, however, I received much help, stimulation, and criticism from colleagues both in and outside Germany. I can name only a few of the many colleagues who gave us substantial support:

Professor Dr. Dr. E. UEHLINGER, the Editor of this Handbook, has not only encouraged me with constant sympathy for two decades, but also read this book with a critical eye and made valuable suggestions.

Professor W.ST.C. SYMMERS, London, pointed out important matters of style and terminology.

Professor Dr. H. ZUR HAUSEN, Erlangen, made a significant contribution to the serology of EBV infection in Burkitt's tumor and lymphoepithelial carcinoma.

Dr. W. HIJMANS, Rijswijk, and Dr. P. LOPES CARDOZO, Leiden, an inimitable pioneer in cytology, were a source of stimulation in fruitful discussions.

Dr. F.C. COLLIER, Rutherford, Professor L. FIORE-DONATI, Verona, and Dr. RENATE REIF, Zrifin, read various parts of this book. We are grateful for their comments and suggestions.

Finally, we wish to thank all skeptics for often questioning us and forcing us to exercise self-scrutiny.

Many of the studies behind this book, especially those of our immunologic laboratory, would not have been possible without the generous financial support of the Deutsche Forschungsgemeinschaft (Sonderforschungsbereich 111) and the Kind-Philipp-Stiftung.

The publishers also contributed all they could to the success of this book. Dr. H. GÖTZE accepted and encouraged its publication even before it was written—an expression of unearned trust and his own optimism. Mr. W. BERGSTEDT and Mr. K. TEICHMANN were always willing to help, even when adverse circumstances might have earned their resentment. The color illustrations are worthy of praise, and we thank the Graph. Kunstanstalt Gustav Dreher GmbH, Stuttgart, for their effort.

We are much indebted to all the many people who contributed to the success of this book. They all have given more than the actual writers, whose main task was to interpret and verbalize the results of much hard work.

# Contents

## Part Six

## The Immunologic and Immunochemical Basis for the Kiel Classification

# Abbreviations

| | |
|---|---|
| AET | 2-amino-ethylisothiouronium-bromide |
| ALL | acute lymphoblastic leukemia |
| AML | acute myeloid leukemia |
| ATPase | adenosine triphosphatase |
| B-ALL | acute lymphoblastic leukemia of the B-cell type |
| BCG | bacillus Calmette-Guérin |
| B-CLL | chronic lymphocytic leukemia of the B-cell type |
| C3 | third component of complement |
| C3b | large fragment of C3 that generates from C3 through cleavage and liberation of the small fragment, C3a, by C3 convertase, nonspecific proteases, or activation *via* the alternative pathway |
| C3d | fragment of C3 that generates from C3b through cleavage and liberation of the C3c fragment by C3b inactivator |
| CIg | (intra)cytoplasmic immunoglobulin |
| CLL | chronic lymphocytic leukemia |
| CLL-THYA | CLL/thymus antigen |
| CML | chronic myeloid leukemia |
| common ALL | acute lymphoblastic leukemia devoid of T- and B-cell markers, but expressing common-ALL antigen (Greaves antigen) |
| Con A | concanavalin A |
| DOC | sodium desoxycholate |
| E | erythrocyte |
| EA | erythrocyte-antibody complex |
| EAC | erythrocyte-antibody-complement complex |
| EAC3b | EAC composed of erythrocytes coated with IgM antibodies and purified human C3b |
| EAC3d | EAC3b cleaved by C3 inactivator and after liberation of C3c |
| EAChuman | EAC prepared with human complement |
| EACmouse | EAC prepared with mouse complement |
| EA test | early-antigen test |
| EBNA | Epstein-Barr nuclear antigen |
| EBV | Epstein-Barr virus |
| EBV-DNA | Epstein-Barr-virus deoxyribonucleic acid |
| ESR | erythrocyte sedimentation rate |
| Fab | antigen-binding fraction of antibody |
| Fc | constant region of antibody |
| FCC | follicular-center cell |
| HCL | hairy-cell leukemia |
| hexosaminidase I | isoenzyme I of α-N-acetyl-hexosaminidase |

| | |
|---|---|
| HP | hemagglutinin A from the snail *Helix pomatia* |
| H rosette | rosette with homologous (human) group-0 Rh-negative erythrocytes |
| HTHY-L | human thymus/leukemia-associated antigen |
| HTLA | human T-lymphocyte antigen |
| Ia-like antigen | human glycoprotein complex resembling murine Ia-antigen |
| Ig | immunoglobulin |
| IgGEA | antigen-antibody complex composed of erythrocytes coated with anti-erythrocyte antibodies of the IgG type |
| IgG-Fc receptor | receptor for the Fc fragment (constant region) of the IgG molecule |
| IgG-humanEA | IgGEA prepared with human erythrocytes |
| IgG-oxEA | IgGEA prepared with ox erythrocytes |
| IgG-sheepEA | IgGEA prepared with sheep erythrocytes |
| IgMEA | antigen-antibody complex composed of erythrocytes coated with anti-erythrocyte antibodies of the IgM type |
| IgMEAC | EAC composed of erythrocytes coated with IgM antibodies and complement |
| IgM-EAC3b | =EAC3b |
| IgM-EAC3d | =EAC3d |
| IgM-Fc receptor | receptor for the Fc fragment (constant region) of the IgM molecule |
| Lit. | literature (used in footnotes to indicate where a more complete list of references may be found) |
| LP immunocytoma | malignant lymphoma, lymphoplasmacytic/lymphoplasmacytoid |
| LPS | lipopolysaccharides from *Escherichia coli* |
| MA test | membrane-antigen test |
| M.F. | mycosis fungoides |
| MIF | migration-inhibitory factor |
| MGP | methyl-green pyronine |
| M.L. | malignant lymphoma |
| MPS | mononuclear phagocyte system |
| nullALL | acute lymphoblastic leukemia devoid of T- and B-cell markers |
| PAP | peroxidase-antiperoxidase |
| PAS | periodic-acid Schiff |
| PHA | phytohemagglutinin |
| RES | reticuloendothelial system |
| RHS | reticulohistiocytic system |
| SIg | surface immunoglobulin |
| T-ALL | acute lymphoblastic leukemia of the T-cell type |
| T-CLL | chronic lymphocytic leukemia of the T-cell type |
| Tdt | terminal deoxynucleotidyl transferase |
| THYSA | thymocyte-specific antigen |
| VCA | viral-capsid antigen |

Part One

# The Cytologic, Histologic, and Functional Bases for a Modern Classification of Lymphomas

H.-K. MÜLLER-HERMELINK and K. LENNERT

Since 1961, when Part A of this Handbook appeared, experimental lymphocyte research and immunology have provided so many revolutionary data that it is necessary to reassess our cytologic and histologic bases of classification. Therefore, some of the most important data will be presented here. This will lead to a substantial widening of our horizons of 1961 and also to certain corrections. These cannot affect the morphology itself, of course, but rather its interpretation, in particular that of the cytogenetic derivation of the cells and their different morphologic appearances. Above all, it has become evident that lymphocytes and plasma cells are not derived from reticulum cells. Instead, stimulation and transformation of small lymphocytes result in the development of large blast cells (immunoblasts, centroblasts), which serve as the precursors of lymphocytes and plasma cells. Some other variants (stimulated lymphocytes, "immature sinus histiocytes") that have been separated morphologically are probably such transformed or activated lymphocytes. Furthermore, it has been shown that most macrophages and one of their specific functional forms, namely, epithelioid cells, are of monocytic origin.

Although an "undifferentiated" reticulum cell may no longer be considered to be the mother cell of all lymphocytic and plasmacytic cells, the structural cells of lymphatic and hemopoietic tissue are still of great importance. New findings indicate that one can no longer speak of *the* reticulum cell, but instead must distinguish at least four different types with different morphologies, localizations, enzyme contents, and functions.

In addition, the concepts RES and RHS have been criticized and replaced by the concept "MPS" (mononuclear phagocyte system).[1] The following cells are included in the MPS: monocyte precursors in the bone marrow, blood monocytes, and tissue macrophages derived from monocytes. The latter include histiocytes of the connective tissue, Kupffer cells of the liver, alveolar macrophages of the lung, free and fixed macrophages in the spleen and lymph nodes, macrophages in bone marrow, pleural and peritoneal macrophages, osteoclasts (?), and microglial cells (?). The basis for inclusion in the MPS is similarity in the origin, cytogenetics, function, and morphology of the phagocytes. Using

[1] VAN FURTH, COHN, HIRSCH, HUMPHREY *et al.*, 1972.

Table 1. Comparison of our nomenclature used for lymph-node cells in 1961 and at present

| 1961 | 1976 |
|---|---|
| Reticulum cell, medium-sized and large | Same, but 4 types: histiocytic, fibroblastic, dendritic, interdigitating |
| Small reticulum cell | ? (Monocyte?) |
| Histiocyte | Monocyte |
| Immature histiocyte of sinuses | Stimulated lymphocyte |
| Epithelioid cell | Same |
| *Retikuläre Reizzellen* | *Lymphatische Reizformen* (stimulated lymphocytes) |
| Basophilic stem cell | Immunoblast (B and T) |
| Lymphoblast | T-associated plasma cell |
| Germinoblast | Centroblast |
| Germinocyte[a] | Centrocyte |
| Plasmablast | Same |
| Proplasmacyte | Same |
| Lymphatic plasma cell | Same (lymphoplasmacytoid cell) |
| Reticular plasma cell | Same (Marschalkó type) |
| Tissue mast cell | Mast cell |
| Blood mast cell | Basophil granulocyte |

[a] First defined in 1964 (not in 1961)

these criteria, reticular cells, dendritic cells, endothelial cells, and fibroblasts (fibrocytes) are excluded from the MPS. In contrast, DAEMS[1a] and other authors have presented morphologic and functional evidence that there are two types of macrophages in animal tissue. One type was said to be monocytogenic and the other histiogenic. They have been differentiated by ultrastructural demonstration of different patterns of peroxidase activity.

The new knowledge gained has also led to new terms. Therefore, we present a table comparing our terms of 1961 with those used today (Table 1).

# I. Lymphocytes

## A. A New Understanding of Lymphocyte Physiology

Before we turn to the morphology of the various structures of the lymphatic tissue, we must heed three established facts about the physiology of lymphocytes:

[1a] DAEMS and BREDEROO, 1971; DAEMS, KOERTEN and SORANZO, 1976.

(1) lymphocytes are not obligate end cells; (2) lymphocytes are a heterogeneous group of cells with different origins and functions; (3) lymphocytes are destined to migrate—they are found only temporarily in lymphatic tissue.

## *1. Lymphocytes Are Not Obligate End Cells*

NOWELL[2] showed that an extract of the green bean (*Phaseolus vulgaris*), phytohemagglutinin (PHA), otherwise used to induce hemagglutination, can also stimulate lymphocytes to divide by mitosis. In light-[3] and electron-microscopic[4] studies, it could be shown that the lymphocytes transform into large blast cells. This takes only 48–72 hours. Since these reports appeared, a number of other lectins have been described as mitogenic substances. One of these substances, pokeweed mitogen (*Phytolacca americana*),[5] has acquired a certain significance for humans, since it was the first lectin observed to stimulate not only transformation into blast cells, but also further development into plasma cells.[6] It has been shown that differences in the effects induced by various lectins are caused by the activation of different lymphocyte subpopulations, e.g., the activation of T-lymphocytes by PHA and of T- and B-lymphocytes by pokeweed mitogen (see Part Six). Antigens may also effect *in-vitro* transformation of lymphocytes. In that case, however, only the specifically reacting lymphocyte clone becomes stimulated. In contrast, under the influence of mitogen a large number of different lymphocyte clones are stimulated nonspecifically (independent of antigen). Therefore, this process has been called polyclonal activation.[7] At the individual cellular level the transformation of lymphocytes through stimulation by mitogen or antigen leads to the same result; thus, the plasma cells that arise after activation with pokeweed mitogen actually produce considerable amounts of IgM.[8]

These and numerous other experiments have shown that the small lymphocytes are not end cells, since they can be stimulated to transform into large blast cells. That is the process by which lymphocytes enter the cell cycle. The blast cells show very active mitotic division. Some generate specific effector cells such as plasma cells, while others produce lymphocytes that enlarge the respective clone of specifically reacting immunocompetent cells (clonal expansion, memory cells).

"Lymphopoiesis" in the lymph node appears to be the result of such transformations of specifically sensitive lymphocyte clones, which are furnished by the bone marrow or thymus. It has not been determined whether there is another lymphopoiesis in the lymph node that serves to provide lymphocytes of various specificities (clonal diversification). KEUNING[9] attributes such a function to ger-

[2] 1960.

[3] NOWELL, 1960; COOPER, BARKHAN and HALE, 1963; YOFFEY, WINTER, OSMOND and MEEK, 1965.

[4] INMAN and COOPER, 1963, 1965; MARSHALL and ROBERTS, 1963; TANAKA, EPSTEIN, BRECHER and STOHLMAN, 1963.

[5] FARNES, BARKER, BROWNHILL and FANGER, 1964.

[6] CHESSIN, BÖRJESON, WELSH, DOUGLAS *et al.*, 1966; DOUGLAS, HOFFMAN, BÖRJESON and CHESSIN, 1967.

[7] GREAVES and JANOSSY, 1972.

[8] PARKHOUSE, JANOSSY and GREAVES, 1972.

[9] 1972.

minal centers. Morphologically, the process would probably be equivalent to the specific transformation. Therefore, it has become improbable that an independent, morphologically separable "lymphoblast" exists besides the transformed T-lymphocytes (=T-immunoblasts) and the transformed B-lymphocytes (=centroblasts) in the peripheral lymphatic tissue of the adult organism.

Lymphopoiesis is fundamentally different from granulopoiesis. In granulopoiesis billions of granulocytes develop from precursors every day and perish in the fulfillment of their function, i.e., they are end cells. The formation and maturation of cells in the central lymphatic organs, namely, the bone marrow and thymus, lead on the one hand to lymphocytes that transform into effector cells after contact with the corresponding antigen and then die in the fulfillment of their function. On the other hand, under antigenic stimulation, new lymphocytes that can react to the appropriate antigens are formed *via* a blast-cell stage. Therefore, the lymphocytes produced in the central organs represent the end of lymphopoiesis in these organs and the beginning of renewed lymphocyte formation in response to the appropriate antigens. Thus, they possess fundamental properties of stem cells. Nevertheless, a certain renewal of cells is necessary. Even in adults, it comes from the central lymphatic organs, i.e., the bone marrow and thymus.[10] Earlier experimental data and morphologic findings appeared to contradict this fact. The great atrophy of the thymus in adults seemed difficult to reconcile with a considerable cytopoietic activity. In addition, although severe immune defects appeared after neonatal thymectomy of mice, they did not arise after thymectomy in adult mice. A more thorough study of the effects of thymectomy on young adult animals showed, however, that within weeks or months considerable lymphopenia developed, with peripheral lymphocyte counts that lay 30–50% below control values.[11] These results also hold true for humans. At reexamination after 20 years, patients who had been subjected to thymectomy for various reasons showed a decrease in the peripheral T-lymphocyte counts of about 50% and a clear depression of cellular immune reactions.[12] To be sure, deficiencies as severe as those observed after neonatal or prenatal thymectomy do not result. Therefore, the possibility that an antigen-independent lymphopoiesis also takes place in the peripheral lymphatic organs of the adult organism cannot be ruled out.

## *2. Lymphocytes Are a Heterogeneous Group of Cells with Different Origins and Functions*

In the embryo the first lymphocyte precursors ("macrolymphocytes" according to MAXIMOW[13]) develop in the hemopoietic tissue of the yolk sac and somewhat later in the liver and bone marrow. Some of the lymphocyte precursors migrate from these sites into the epithelial thymus *via* the blood. In the microecologic milieu of the thymus they mature into small lymphocytes.[14] Other

[10] METCALF and MOORE, 1971; STUTMAN, YUNIS and GOOD, 1972; MICKLEM, OGDEN and PAYNE, 1973.

[11] Review: METCALF, 1966.

[12] BJÖRKHOLM, HOLM, JOHANSSON and MELLSTEDT, 1975.

[13] 1909.

[14] OWEN and RITTER, 1969.

lymphocyte precursors transform into small lymphocytes without any apparent assistance from the thymus. In mammals, and probably in humans as well, thymus-independent lymphopoiesis takes place first in the fetal liver[15] and later in the bone marrow.[16] The cells belonging to the lymphocyte population that matures in the thymus are now called T-lymphocytes. The cells of the lymphocyte population that matures in the bone marrow are known as B-lymphocytes. The now generally accepted distinction of B- and T-lymphocytes is based on a number of experimental data and observations in human pathology. The core of these data is made up of differences in (1) the immune reactions, (2) the phylogeny and ontogeny, (3) the cell surface receptors, (4) the response to mitogenic stimulation, and (5) the pathways of differentiation of the lymphocytes.

(1) It is well known that, since the report of LANDSTEINER and CHASE,[17] we distinguish humoral and cellular immunity. In *humoral* immunity the changed immune status of one animal can be transferred to another by giving serum from the first animal to the second, i.e., through the antibodies contained in the serum. In *cellular* immunity living cells or extracts of them are necessary. Humoral immunity is of particular importance in infections with gram-positive bacteria. Cellular immunity plays the leading role in infections with facultative intracellular parasites (e.g., mycobacteria), fungi, and viruses, and in transplant rejection and contact dermatitis. Lymphocytes or their derivatives are responsible for both types of immune reaction. Therefore, these cells are the carriers of immunologic competence.

(2) MILLER[18] recognized that the thymus is of particular importance for cellular immune reactions in transplant rejection. He found that mice tolerated allogeneic skin transplants after neonatal thymectomy. Similar studies of rabbits, mice, and rats were performed by ARCHER and PIERCE,[19] GOOD *et al.*,[20] and WAKSMAN and his group.[21] WARNER *et al.*[22] investigated both types of immune reaction in newborn chicks after thymectomy or destruction of the bursa of Fabricius with testosterone ("hormonal bursectomy"). They found a dichotomous behavior of the humoral and cellular immune reactions. Humoral immunity was absent after bursectomy (as reported earlier by GLICK *et al.*[23]) and cellular immunity after thymectomy. COOPER *et al.*[24] refined these studies further and correlated the results with the pathologic equivalents in humans, the various immune-deficiency diseases. They showed that there is complete fundamental agreement. There was still no answer to the question about the structural equivalent of the bursa of Fabricius in mammals and humans, or, in other words, whether the maturation of humoral immunity (now attributed to B-lymphocytes) in the mammalian organism also requires a structurally adequate organ like the bursa of Fabricius. Some authors have suggested the lymphoepithelial tissue

---

[15] OWEN, COOPER and RAFF, 1974.
[16] EVERETT and CAFFREY, 1967.
[17] 1942.
[18] 1961.
[19] 1961.
[20] GOOD, DALMASSO, MARTINEZ, ARCHER *et al.*, 1962.
[21] ARNASON, JANKOVIĆ, WAKSMAN and WENNERSTEN, 1962; JANKOVIĆ, WAKSMAN and ARNASON, 1962; WAKSMAN, ARNASON and JANKOVIĆ, 1962.
[22] WARNER, SZENBERG and BURNET, 1962.
[23] GLICK, CHANG and JAAP, 1956.
[24] COOPER, PETERSON and GOOD, 1965 and later.

of the alimentary canal (appendix,[25] tonsils,[26] Peyer's patches,[27] all lymphoepithelial organs[28]). Findings in larger animals, such as sheep,[29] and the behavior of lymphoepithelial tissue in antigenic deprivation (germ-free animals)[30] and in kinetic studies,[31] however, were not consistent with this interpretation. More recently, NOSSAL and PIKE[32] showed that the maturation of B-cells in mice does not occur in a specific, defined organ, but, corresponding to hemopoiesis, at various sites in the (mammalian) organism. They are called B-lymphocytes, no matter whether *b*one marrow or *b*ursa is meant. One could also speak of "non-T"-lymphocytes.

(3-5) Differences in the surface properties, the responses to mitogenic stimulation, and the pathways of differentiation of B- and T-lymphocytes will be discussed below. These properties are now used to distinguish between the two types of lymphocytes. Study of the morphology and function of the different cells is therefore possible.

B- and T-lymphocytes cannot be directly compared to the two types of lymphocytes distinguished by GRUNDMANN,[33] which he called follicle and sinus (pulp) lymphocytes. We were not able to differentiate two types of lymphocytes in humans according to the nucleolus content. With the electron microscope, we usually found only one, occasionally two nucleoli in the lymphocyte nucleus.

### *3. Lymphocytes Are Destined to Migrate*

Lymphocytes are only temporarily found in the tissue. After staying in the lymphatic tissue for several hours to days, they migrate into the blood *via* the efferent lymphatics. In general, they circulate in the blood for only a few hours—14 hours on average in mice[34]—and then usually return to the lymphatic tissue *via* the epithelioid venules.[35] After emigrating to other tissues, a few of the lymphocytes reenter the lymph node *via* afferent lymphatics. In healthy organisms the immigrating and emigrating populations remain in equilibrium. That is true for both the lymph nodes and the blood. *Recirculation* is substantial. It has been estimated that the number of recirculating cells is as large as that of nonrecirculating cells.[36]

GOWANS and KNIGHT[35] showed that the "postcapillary"[37] venules of the paracortical area are of particular importance for recirculation. At this site the lymphocytes penetrate the vascular wall and enter the lymphatic parenchyma. Recent scanning electron-microscopic findings[38] disprove the original view that the lymphocytes immigrate to the lymphatic parenchyma through endothelial cells.[39] These findings show that the lymphocytes instead penetrate the intercel-

[25] ARCHER, SUTHERLAND and GOOD, 1964; SUTHERLAND, ARCHER and GOOD, 1964.
[26] PETERSON, COOPER and GOOD, 1965.
[27] COOPER, PEREY, MCKNEALLY, GABRIELSEN *et al.*, 1966; PEREY, FINSTAD, POLLARA and GOOD, 1968.
[28] FICHTELIUS, 1968; FICHTELIUS, GROTH and LIDÉN, 1970.
[29] SILVERSTEIN and PRENDERGAST, 1971.
[30] MIYAKAWA, 1959; POLLARD, 1970.
[31] MICHALKE, HESS, RIEDWYL, STONER *et al.*, 1969; JOEL, HESS and COTTIER, 1972.
[32] 1973.
[33] 1959.
[34] FORD and MARCHESI, 1971.
[35] GOWANS and KNIGHT, 1964.
[36] TREPEL, 1973, 1974.
[37] SCHULZE, 1925.
[38] VAN EWIJK, BRONS and ROZING, 1975.
[39] MARCHESI and GOWANS, 1964.

lular junctions and pass between the endothelial cells. Consistent changes in these prismatic "epithelioid" endothelial cells occur as a consequence of lymphocyte emigration. When recirculation does not occur (e.g., after lethal irradiation of experimental animals, in immune deficiencies in humans), the endothelial cells are flat, whereas they are thick when lymphocytes are actively emigrating to lymphatic tissue. In chronic inflammations this type of blood vessel may even be found in other tissues, e.g., in skin lesions of *lichen planus*. The cytoplasm of the endothelial cells contains abundant lysosomes (Fig. 1). Enzyme histochemical studies show that the nonspecific esterase and adenosine triphosphatase (ATPase) reactions are clearly positive in these cells, whereas in capillaries and arterioles the alkaline phosphatase reaction is positive. Migrating lymphocytes can be seen in the splintered basement membrane. Most of the recirculating lymphocytes are probably T-lymphocytes. B-lymphocytes,[40] however, – in infections together with monocytes and granulocytes[41] – also reach the lymphatic tissue through these venules. Since every venule is actually postcapillary and on account of the high epithelial cell-like endothelial cells, we prefer the term epithelioid venule to postcapillary venule.

The mechanism of recirculation is not yet fully understood. Pretreatment of lymphocytes with neuraminidase or proteolytic enzymes prevents recirculation of these cells,[42] indicating that the glycocalyx on the surface of lymphocytes has a considerable influence on their recirculatory behavior. Immunoglobulins that are present in the walls of epithelioid venules might, however, also affect the recirculatory behavior of lymphocytes.[43]

At least the B-lymphocytes show a certain affinity for resettling at specific sites. For instance, they preferably return to Peyer's patches or mesenteric lymph nodes when cell suspensions of Peyer's patches and mesenteric lymph nodes are injected into syngeneic recipients.[44] Antigens may play a crucial role in determining the direction of migration and the number of lymphocytes settling in a particular lymph node.[45] In addition, cell interaction may control lymphocyte traffic.[46]

If half the lymphocytes present in the body recirculate and the other half are stationary, then the number of lymphocytes in the blood must be crucially determined by factors that interfere with the circulatory behavior of the cells. We know of diseases, such as pertussis, that are characterized by extreme lymphocytosis of the blood that is not caused by an increase in lymphocyte production, but by a block in the recirculation.[47] Furthermore, several factors are known to influence the resting time of lymphocytes in tissues (e.g., doses of heparin[48]) or the distribution of lymphocytes in the various lymphatic organs, in particular their migration out of the bone marrow (corticosteroids).[49] Such factors therefore directly affect the number of lymphocytes in the blood and/or lymphatic tissue.

[40] Kotani, Nawa, Fujii, Fukumoto *et al.*, 1974.
[41] Racz, Kaiserling, Tenner and Wuthe, 1974.
[42] Woodruff and Gesner, 1968, 1969.
[43] Sordat, Hess and Cottier, 1971.
[44] DeKruyff, Durkin, Gilmour and Thorbecke, 1975; Durkin, Caporale and Thorbecke, 1975.
[45] Durkin and Thorbecke, 1973.
[46] Freitas and de Sousa, 1976.
[47] Morse, 1965; Morse and Barron, 1970.
[48] Ford and Gowans, 1969.
[49] Van den Broek, 1971a, b.

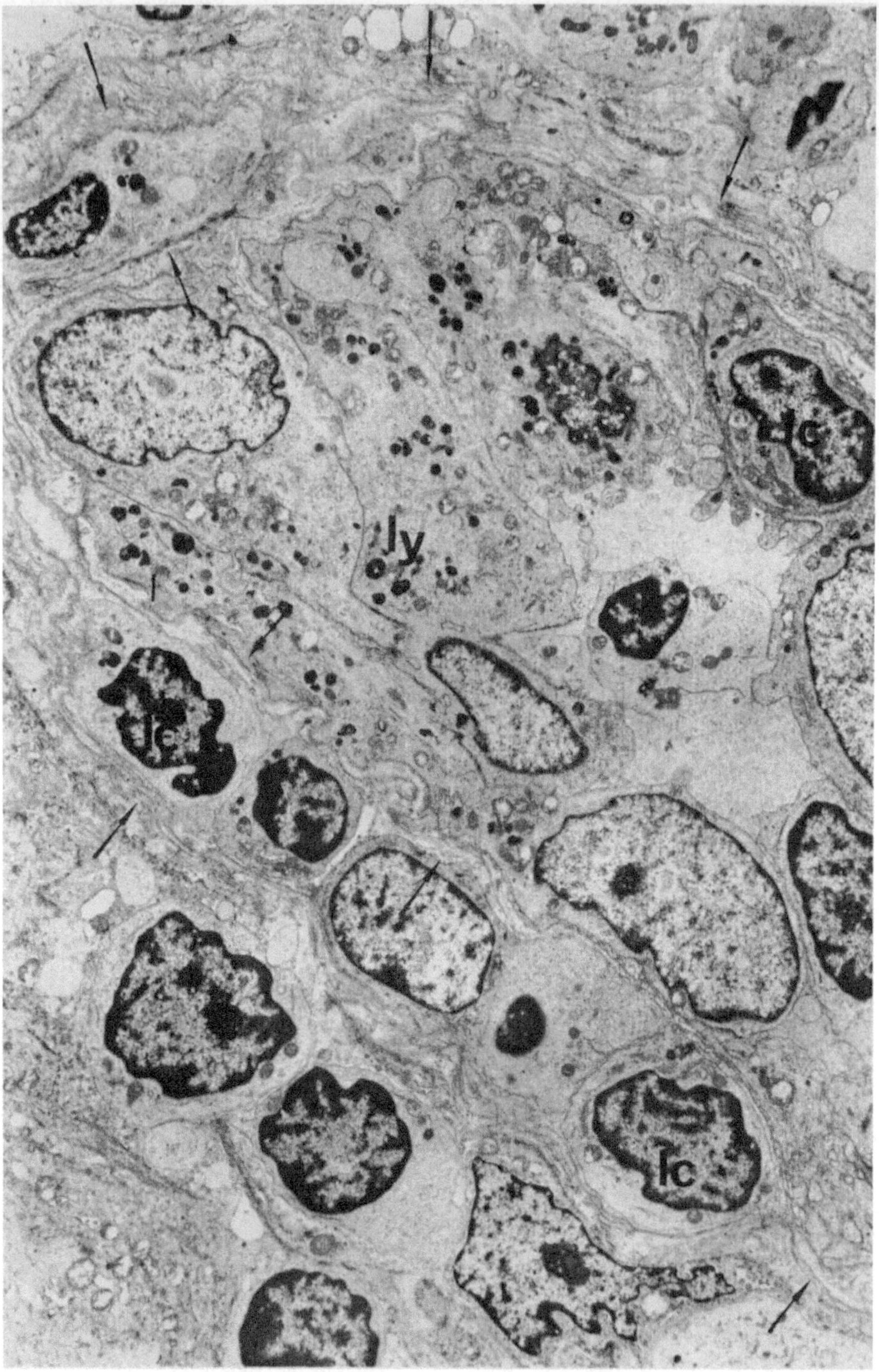


Fig. 1. Epithelioid venule. The cytoplasm of endothelial cells contains numerous lysosomes (*ly*). Some lymphocytes (*lc*) are passing through the endothelium and some are lying in the splintered basement membrane (arrows). ×6,800

Even in healthy persons, however, the lymphocyte content of the blood fluctuates considerably. These variations may reach more than 100% of the initial value within a few hours, even though a clear circadian rhythm may not be demonstrable. The fluctuations in the absolute blood lymphocyte counts depend mainly on fluctuations in the number of T-lymphocytes alone, but small variations in the number of peripheral blood lymphocytes can also be caused by B-lymphocytes.[50]

The virtually unlimited capacity of lymphocytes to transform and their ability to recirculate make the question about the actual *life span* of the cells difficult to answer. Long-lived and short-lived lymphocytes have been separated in experiments using labeling with $^3$H-thymidine.[51] This distinction also has a certain validity for humans. SCHICK[52] distinguished a short-lived population of blood lymphocytes in humans that could be demonstrated for up to about 12 days, and a long-lived one with an average life expectancy of 500 days. The initially assumed functional correlation to B- or T-lymphocytes is no longer claimed. The average life span of T-lymphocytes in the blood appears to be longer; but there are also extremely long-lived populations of B-lymphocytes, for example, in the outer cortex of the lymph node.[53] The life span, defined through the demonstration of radioactive labeling, is dependent on various factors: (1) some of the lymphocytes die in the fulfillment of their function or because of aging; (2) some migrate to mucous membranes of various organs and are eliminated; (3) some transform into plasma cells after a blast-cell phase and perish within a few weeks; (4) a significant number transform into blast cells that are then the origin of new lymphocytes. All of these factors lead to loss of labeling. Chromosome studies performed years after radiotherapy demonstrated that at least a few extremely long-lived lymphocytes circulate in human blood. From characteristic chromosome alterations, it could be determined that a few lymphocytes that transformed after stimulation by PHA did not enter mitosis until more than 10 years later.[54]

## B. Identification of B- and T-Lymphocytes

The usual light- and electron-microscopic techniques have not allowed a clear distinction between B- and T-lymphocytes. By applying morphometric, cytochemical, and electron-microscopic methods, it is certainly possible to define lymphocyte subpopulations in the blood or lymphatic tissue that differ on the basis of some criterion.[55] So far, however, only a few attempts have been made to clearly correlate such criteria with the T- or B-cell nature of the lymphocyte population in humans.[56] WATANABE *et al.*[56] mentioned a characteristic lysosome formation by human T-lymphocytes, which represented the

[50] MÜLLER, MÜLLER-HERMELINK and SCHLAAK, unpublished.
[51] EVERETT, CAFFREY and RIEKE, 1964.
[52] 1973.
[53] Cited by COTTIER, HESS, SCHÄDELI and BÜRKI, 1973.
[54] BUCKTON, COURT BROWN and SMITH, 1967.
[55] Review: ACKERMAN, 1970.
[56] WATANABE, TAMAOKI, HABU, TASHIRO *et al.*, 1974.

first indication of a morphologic distinction between T- and B-lymphocytes of the peripheral blood in humans. Furthermore, the validity of the specific morphologic features would have to be proved not only for small lymphocytes, but also for their functional stages, the blast cells, etc. That is usually not possible. The degree of activation of the lymphocytes can be defined by means of common morphologic techniques. One cannot say to which type of lymphocyte subpopulation a blast cell belongs, though. Somewhat clearer morphologic differences seem to exist in mice, in which structural, qualitatively measurable differences have been demonstrated by electron microscopy.[57] Although these results cannot be applied directly to humans, cytochemical and scanning electron-microscopic studies have provided certain findings suggesting that there are also recognizable differences between the B- and T-cell systems in humans.

Some caution is necessary when simply relating the results of cytochemical studies[58] on laboratory animals to humans. According to our findings, the surface of most B-lymphocytes in peripheral blood seems to reveal a positive ATPase reaction, whereas only a few show 5-nucleotidase activity.[58] Most of the T-lymphocytes (like those of rats) show a solitary, coarse deposit in the demonstration of acid phosphatase and also $\beta$-glucuronidase (Fig. 2).[59] A similar reaction was recently reported for $\alpha$-naphthyl acetate esterase at pH 5.6.[60] It remains to be determined whether these enzyme reactions are valid for all B- and T-lymphocytes or for only certain subgroups. The pattern of acid phosphatase activity changes considerably during lymphocyte activation, independent of whether the activation is polyclonal (PHA) or specific (tuberculin).[61] Changes in the characteristic cytochemical patterns of acid phosphatase and acid nonspecific esterase are also observed during ontogeny of T-lymphocytes. It may be concluded that the focal coarse activity of both enzymes is lysosomal and related to mature peripheral T-lymphocytes. In contrast, fetal thymocytes show acid phosphatase activity localized in the Golgi complex. They are negative or only very weakly positive for acid nonspecific esterase.

With the scanning electron microscope, POLLIACK *et al.*[62] showed that the surface of B-lymphocytes reveals more numerous and longer cytoplasmic projections than that of T-lymphocytes. The difference is therefore only quantitative. According to LIN *et al.*,[63] it is also dependent on several variables, such as temperature, and generally also on the conditions under which the cells are prepared. Exact comparison of transmission and scanning electron-microscopic analyses of T- and B-lymphocytes using specific surface antigens or surface-immunoglobulin markers also suggested that there are B-lymphocytes with many surface villi as well as those with only a few or none at all.[64] Recently, it was

---

[57] MATTER, LISOWSKA-BERNSTEIN, RYSER, LAMELIN *et al.*, 1972; LE BOUTEILLER, VUJANOVIC, DUC, KINSKY *et al.*, 1974.

[58] MÜLLER-HERMELINK, 1974; MÜLLER-HERMELINK and TAUTZ, unpublished.

[59] TAMAOKI and ESSNER, 1969; BARR and PERRY, 1976.

[60] COTTIER, 1975, personal communication; MUELLER, BRUN DEL RE, BUERKI, KELLER *et al.*, 1975.

[61] DRESCHER and RÜSSLER, 1974; MERK, 1976.

[62] POLLIACK, LAMPEN, CLARKSON, DE HARVEN *et al.*, 1973.

[63] LIN, WALLACH and TSAI, 1973.

[64] LIN, COOPER and WORTIS, 1973; SULLIVAN, ADAMS, SILKE and JERRY, 1974; HÄMMERLING, POLLIACK, LAMPEN, SABETY *et al.*, 1975; REYES, LEJONC, GOURDIN, MANNONI *et al.*, 1975.

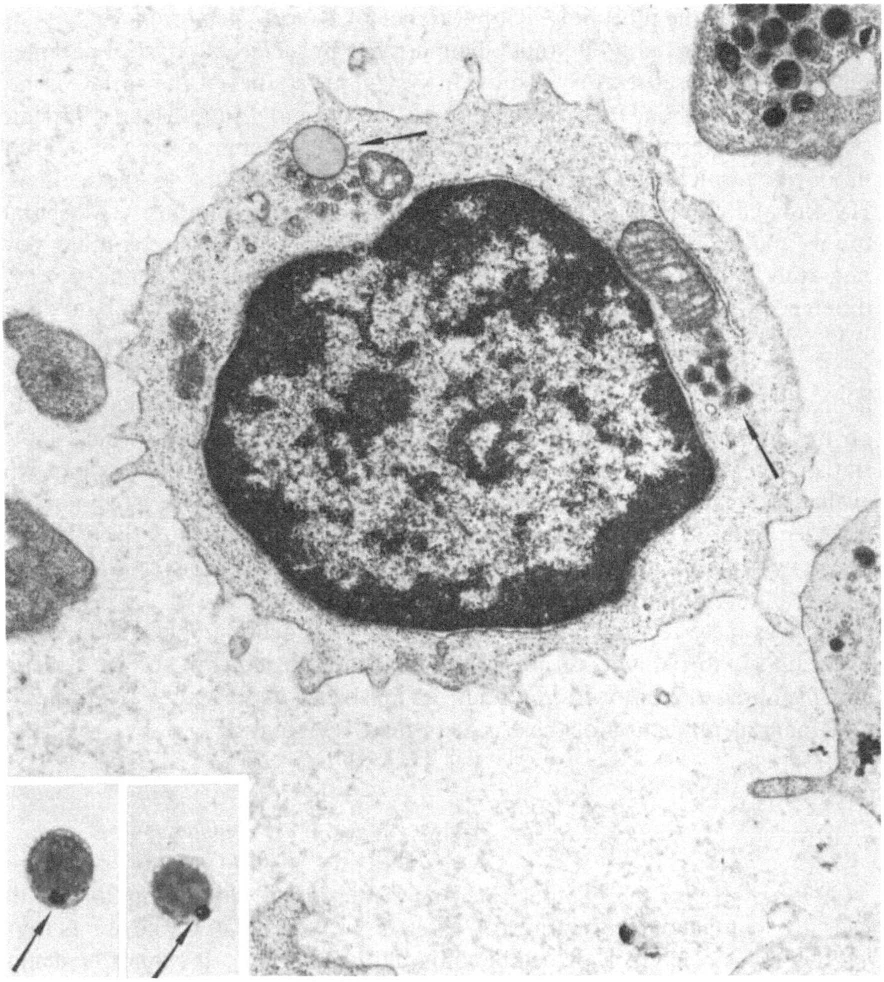

Fig. 2. T-lymphocytes of peripheral blood. Insets: coarse, localized acid nonspecific esterase activity in two lymphocytes. In the one on the right the activity is ring-like. ×880. Electron microscopy: the esterase activity is equivalent to aggregated lysosomes (arrows), the ring-like activity to lipid droplets demonstrated in one of the lysosomes (top arrow). ×12,500

demonstrated that differences in the surfaces of normal peripheral blood lymphocytes in humans are mainly of technical origin.[65]

Differences in the surface structure of lymphocytes are also dependent on whether the cells are studied in suspension or in a tissue matrix.[66] VAN EWIJK *et al.*[67] recently found that lymphocytes within vessels in mouse lymph nodes possess surface villi, whereas they are smooth after passage through the vascular wall and do not have surface villi again until they appear in the sinuses. These

[65] ALEXANDER and WETZEL, 1975; ALEXANDER, SANDERS and BRAYLAN, 1976; NEWELL, ROATH and SMITH, 1976.

[66] REYES, LEJONC, GOURDIN, MANNONI *et al.*, 1975.

[67] VAN EWIJK, BRONS and ROZING, 1975.

findings show that mistakes may be expected when one starts with overly fixed conceptions of the morphologic appearance of the cell membrane.

Attempts to separate B- and T-lymphocytes by means of physical parameters have also had unsatisfactory results. In systematic studies of the surface charges of lymphocytes from rats, RUHENSTROTH-BAUER and LÜCKE-HUHLE[68] demonstrated two different lymphocyte populations with different speeds of migration in an electric field. In carrier-free electrophoresis according to the method of HANNIG and ZEILLER,[69] these populations could be semiquantitatively separated in rats and mice. A fast-migrating T-lymphocyte population and a more slowly migrating B-lymphocyte population could be distinguished. Semiquantitative differences in the surface charges have also been used to differentiate T- and B-lymphocytes in humans. The overlapping between the two populations was relatively great, however, and could not be reliably reproduced in reactive or neoplastic tissue.[70] The negative surface charge of lymphocytes depends partly on the amount of acid mucopolysaccharide of the glycocalyx, which showed statistically significant differences among the lymphocytes of guinea pigs when evaluated quantitatively.[71] Unequivocal results for humans have not been reported so far. T- and B-lymphocytes could also be semiquantitatively differentiated by separating human blood lymphocytes on the basis of their specific density in discontinuous albumin gradients.[72]

Besides these few attempts to distinguish T- and B-lymphocytes in humans by means of morphologic or physical parameters, a number of surface structures and membrane receptors have been demonstrated in recent years that allow functional identification of these cells in mixed populations.

### *1. Functional Identification of Human T-Lymphocytes*

A receptor has been demonstrated on a number of blood lymphocytes that leads to spontaneous formation of rosettes with sheep erythrocytes (sheep-E rosettes). This receptor is detectable only on living cells.[73] It cannot be demonstrated after treatment of the lymphocytes with anti-lymphocyte serum, but it is not influenced by anti-immunoglobulin serum. The nature of the sheep-E receptor is not understood. It has also been demonstrated on human thymocytes[74] and may be considered to be a characteristic marker of human T-lymphocytes.[75] Treatment of the sheep erythrocytes with neuraminidase[76] or AET[77] (see Part Six) increases the rosette yield considerably. BENTWICH *et al.*,[78] however, observed that some B-cells also formed rosettes with treated sheep erythrocytes.

[68] 1968.
[69] 1969.
[70] STEIN, FLAD, PABST and TREPEL, 1973; WIIG and THUNOLD, 1973; WIIG, 1975; VASSAR, LEVY and BROOKS, 1976.
[71] GIACOMELLI, WIENER, KRUSKAL, POMERANZ *et al.*, 1971.
[72] RIETHMÜLLER, RIEBER and RIETHMÜLLER, 1970.
[73] BRAIN, GORDON and WILLETTS, 1970; COOMBS, GURNER, WILSON, HOLM *et al.*, 1970; JONDAL, HOLM and WIGZELL, 1972.
[74] WHITTINGHAM and MACKAY, 1973.
[75] JONDAL, HOLM and WIGZELL, 1972.
[76] SEILER, SEDLACEK, KANZY and LANG, 1972; WEINER, BIANCO and NUSSENZWEIG, 1973.
[77] KAPLAN and CLARK, 1974.
[78] BENTWICH, DOUGLAS, SKUTELSKY and KUNKEL, 1973.

This finding was not confirmed by STEIN and PETERSEN[79] of our group. The number of T-lymphocytes that not only form spontaneous rosettes, but also bear receptors for C 3 (third component of complement) and the Fc fragment of IgG in simultaneous assays did not increase after treatment of the sheep erythrocytes with neuraminidase.

Lymphocytes with "double markers," i.e., those bearing both the C 3 receptor and the sheep-E receptor, are now of great interest. GATIEN *et al.*[80] showed that the cells with great proliferative capacities and bearing the C 3 receptor are found in human peripheral blood; these cells are able to differentiate *in vitro* into lymphoid cells bearing the sheep-E receptor. The same type of cell is found in early embryonic thymuses, whereas later only sheep-E receptor-bearing thymocytes are found. In addition, our own studies[81] have shown that cells with receptors for both C 3 and sheep erythrocytes exist in fetal thymuses. Thus, these double-marker lymphocytes probably represent early stages of T-lymphocyte differentiation. Morphologic identification of the cells is possible, since they exhibit a strong, focal, paranuclear acid phosphatase reaction. This is of importance, as we shall meet this type of cell again when considering lymphoblastic lymphoma.

WYBRAN and FUDENBERG[82] and FUDENBERG *et al.*[83] found that a subgroup of the spontaneous rosette-forming T-lymphocytes occupied a special position in the evaluation of immunologic reactivity. The cells of this subgroup formed rosettes after only a short incubation period, even at 37° C, and normally made up one third of the T-lymphocytes. They were called "active T-cells." A small percentage of T-lymphocytes form rosettes with homologous (human) group-0 Rh-negative erythrocytes (H rosettes). These cells may represent another subgroup of T-lymphocytes.[83a]

Specific antisera that are directed only at human T-lymphocytes in test assays can be obtained from animals after heterologous immunization with human thymus lymphocytes or with blood lymphocytes from children with Bruton's agammaglobulinemia, and then suitable exhaustive absorptions with lymphocytes from patients with chronic lymphocytic leukemia.[84] Moreover, receptors for certain hemagglutinins of snail lymph (*Helix pomatia* A-hemagglutinin) have been found on human T-lymphocytes.[85] T-lymphocytes of humans, monkeys, dogs, and cows also bear a specific receptor for measles virus. This receptor is not found on B-lymphocytes.[86]

The semiquantitative separation of the lymphocyte fraction in a mixed cell population is also possible on the basis of the degree of transformation of the cells after stimulation by various mitogens. In particular, PHA and concanavalin A (Con A) lead, under certain conditions, to a selective transformation

---

79 1975, unpublished data.

80 GATIEN, SCHNEEBERGER and MERLER, 1975; GATIEN, SCHNEEBERGER, PARKMAN and MERLER, 1975.

81 STEIN and MÜLLER-HERMELINK, 1977.

82 1973.

83 FUDENBERG, WYBRAN and ROBBINS, 1975.

83a SHELDON and HOLBOROW, 1975.

84 AIUTI and WIGZELL, 1973; YATA, TSUKIMOTO and TACHIBANA, 1973.

85 HAMMARSTRÖM, HELLSTRÖM, PERLMANN and DILLNER, 1973; UHLENBRUCK, WERNET and SCHUMACHER, 1973.

86 AGNARSDOTTIR and VALDIMARSSON, 1975; VALDIMARSSON, AGNARSDOTTIR and LACHMANN, 1975.

of T-lymphocytes during the first days,[87] although both mitogens bind equally well to the membranes of T- and B-cells.[88]

### 2. Functional Identification of Human B-Lymphocytes

The detection of immunoglobulin on the surface of lymphocytes is of practical importance for the identification of B-cells. This characteristic feature was demonstrated on about 20% of the blood lymphocytes in studies of mice and rabbits.[89] In studies of human blood lymphocytes, equal numbers of cells with surface immunoglobulin were found, in addition to those that revealed no, or at least no detectable, immunoglobulin.[90] In the simultaneous demonstration of surface immunoglobulin and spontaneous rosette formation with sheep erythrocytes, only a slight overlapping of 0.5%[91] to 3%[92] was found with the sheep-E rosette-forming lymphocytes.

Another feature of B-lymphocytes is their C 3 receptor (Fig. 3).[93] The detection of this receptor was particularly important for our subsequent studies, since it can be demonstrated not only on living lymphocytes, but also on cryostat sections of lymphatic tissue.[94] The B-cell regions of the peripheral lymphatic organs are selectively demonstrated by this method. The receptor can be found on about 15% of human blood lymphocytes. In the simultaneous demonstration of C 3 receptors and spontaneous rosette formation, there was a slight overlapping of about 2% of the spontaneous rosette-forming lymphocytes.[95]

Furthermore, a receptor for the Fc fragment of IgG has been detected on B-lymphocytes.[96] More recent findings, however, indicate that a subpopulation of T-lymphocytes, primarily T-immunoblasts, also bears this receptor. That was demonstrated in mice[97] and guinea pigs.[98] According to STEIN and PETERSEN,[99] in human blood 1–3% of the spontaneous rosette-forming lymphocytes also bear the IgG-Fc receptor. Using other methods, FERRARINI *et al.*[100] demonstrated IgG-Fc receptors on up to 20% of the T-lymphocytes.

These surface markers have found the widest use for identifying human B-lymphocytes. Several other receptors have also been found. For instance, human B-lymphocytes have a specific receptor for Epstein-Barr virus that is not found on T-lymphocytes.[101] It is closely associated or identical with the C 3 recep-

---

[87] GREAVES, JANOSSY and DOENHOFF, 1974.
[88] GREAVES, BAUMINGER and JANOSSY, 1972.
[89] PERNIS, FORNI and AMANTE, 1970; RABELLINO, COLON, GREY and UNANUE, 1971.
[90] FRÖLAND, NATVIG and BERDAL, 1971; WILSON and NOSSAL, 1971.
[91] BENTWICH, DOUGLAS, SKUTELSKY and KUNKEL, 1973.
[92] DICKLER, ADKINSON and TERRY, 1974.
[93] LAY and NUSSENZWEIG, 1968; BIANCO, PATRICK and NUSSENZWEIG, 1970.
[94] DUKOR, BIANCO and NUSSENZWEIG, 1970; SILVEIRA, MENDES and TOLNAI, 1972; SHEVACH, JAFFE and GREEN, 1973.
[95] CHIAO, PANTIC and GOOD, 1974; SANDILANDS, GRAY, COONEY, BROWNING *et al.*, 1974; SHEVACH, EDELSON, FRANK, LUTZNER *et al.*, 1974; STEIN and PETERSEN, 1975, unpublished data.
[96] BASTEN, MILLER, SPRENT and PYE, 1972; BASTEN, WARNER and MANDEL, 1972; DICKLER and KUNKEL, 1972.
[97] GREY, KUBO and CEROTTINI, 1972; MODABBER and COONS, 1972; PARASKEVAS, LEE, ORR and ISRAELS, 1972; YOSHIDA and ANDERSSON, 1972.
[98] VAN BOXEL and ROSENSTREICH, 1974.
[99] 1975, unpublished data.
[100] FERRARINI, MORETTA, ABRILE and DURANTE, 1975.
[101] JONDAL and KLEIN, 1973.

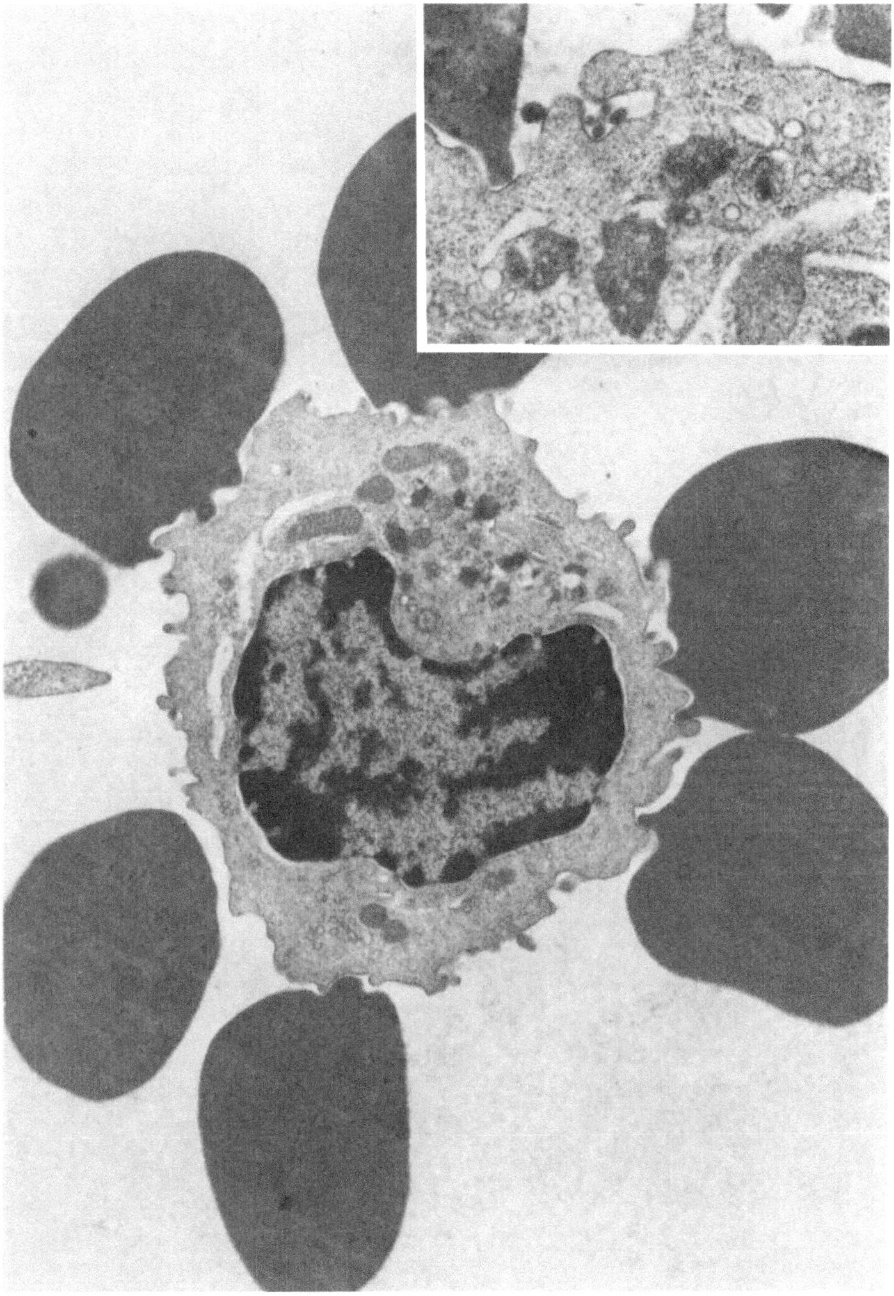

Fig. 3. EAC-rosetting lymphocyte from peripheral blood (probably a B-lymphocyte). Electron-dense lysosomal organelles are seen around the Golgi region near the nuclear indentation. ×12,500. Inset: at higher magnification, similar EAC-rosetting cells contain interwoven tubular structures. ×32,500

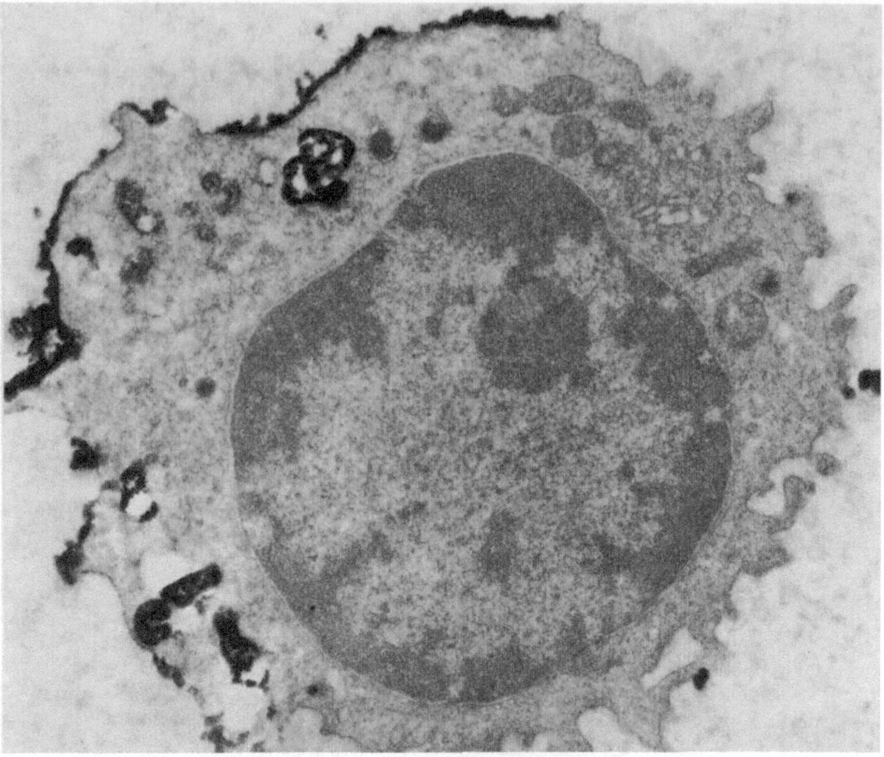

(a)

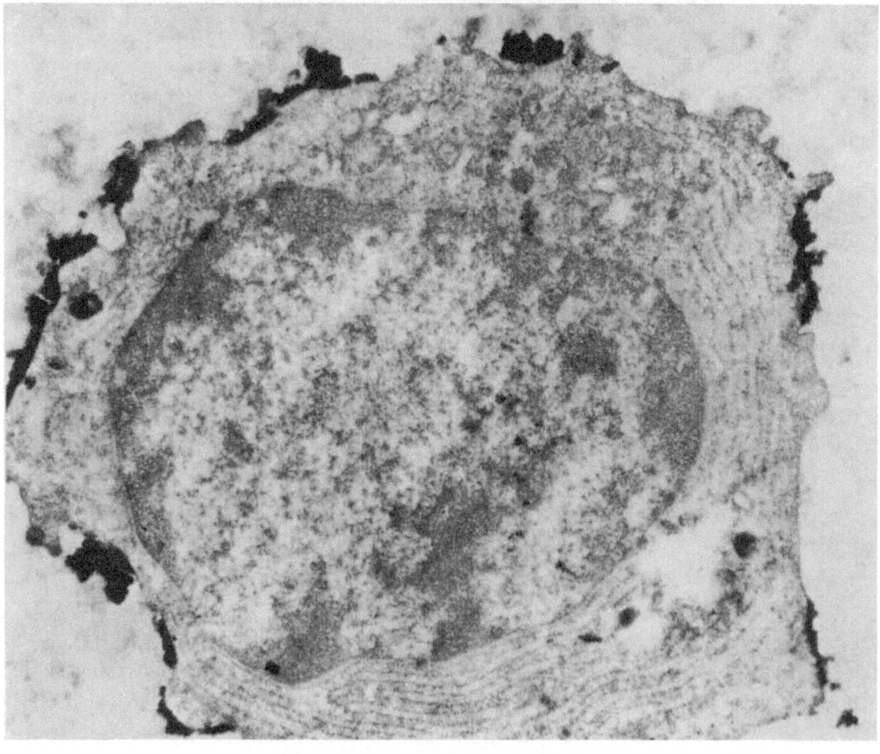

(b)

tor. In addition, one or several B-cell antigens can be demonstrated after heterologous immunization with cells from patients with chronic lymphocytic leukemia and suitable exhaustive absorptions with thymus lymphocytes and other cells.[102] Recently, a receptor for mouse erythrocytes was found on some normal human B-cells[103] and in lymphocytic leukemia of B-cell origin.[104]

With the maturation into plasma cells, the lymphocytes finally lose their surface receptors, at least the surface immunoglobulin and the IgG-Fc and C 3 receptors.

While various mitogenic substances are known to selectively activate B-lymphocytes in rodents, it appears that such substances rarely have a similar effect in humans. Pokeweed mitogen[105] stimulates both B- and T-lymphocytes, but leads to preponderant transformation of B-lymphocytes[106] and maturation into typical plasma cells.[107] Human peripheral B-lymphocytes apparently can be specifically stimulated by anti-$\beta_2$ microglobulin.[108] Various B-cell mitogens have an affinity for different stages of maturity of the B-lymphocytes. During activation, further differentiation of the cells occurs, although it does not necessarily reach the plasma-cell stage.[109] Two pathways of differentiation were observed when cells from murine spleens were activated by LPS, a B-lymphocyte mitogen. One led to small lymphocytes and the other to plasma cells.[109a] A systematic study showed that various endotoxins and lectins have very different stimulative effects on B-lymphocytes in humans that depend on the origin of the cell suspension.[110]

### 3. *Lymphocytes of Cell-Mediated, Antibody-Dependent Cytotoxicity (K-Cells)*

A further lymphocyte subpopulation has been differentiated on the basis of the surface receptors and especially of the function of the cells: the effector cells of antibody-induced, cell-mediated cytotoxicity.[111] Their function can be observed in complement-independent cytolysis, in which these lymphocytes, in contrast to cytotoxic T-lymphocytes, do not react specifically to cell-wall antigens, but display their effect *via* the specific antibodies already bound to the cell wall of the target cells. It has not yet been proved whether this function, which was demonstrated *in vitro*, is also of importance in addition to the known complement-dependent and -independent effector mechanisms of immunologic reactivity *in vivo*. The physiopathologic role of antibody-induced, cell-mediated

[102] Aiuti and Wigzell, 1973.
[103] Gupta and Grieco, 1975; Dobozy, Husz, Hunyadi and Simon, 1976.
[104] Catovsky, Cherchi, Okos, Hegde *et al.*, 1976.
[105] Farnes, Barker, Brownhill and Fanger, 1964.
[106] Greaves, Janossy and Doenhoff, 1974.
[107] Douglas, Hoffman, Börjeson and Chessin, 1967.
[108] Möller and Rubin, 1975.
[109] Möller, 1974.
[109a] Askonas, Roelants, Mayor-Withey and Welstead, 1976.
[110] Ivanyi and Lehner, 1974.
[111] Möller, 1965; MacLennan and Loewi, 1968; Perlmann and Holm, 1969; Perlmann and Perlmann, 1970; MacLennan, 1972; Möller and Svehag, 1972; Perlmann, Perlmann and Wigzell, 1972.

◁ Fig. 4. (a) B-lymphocyte (peripheral blood) with surface IgM. (b) Lymphatic plasma cell (peripheral blood) with surface IgM. Indirect immunoperoxidase technique. × 19,200 cytotoxicity is suggested chiefly in connection with reactions against viruses, in tumor immunology, and in autoimmune diseases, such as Hashimoto's disease and ulcerative colitis.

The morphologic identity of the cells responsible for this reaction was disputed for a time. Whereas PERLMANN and HOLM[112] called them lymphocytes and BIBERFELD and PERLMANN[113] morphologically identified them as lymphocytes in a study using human blood cells, other authors[114] described them as nonphagocytic or phagocytic monocytes. The problem now appears to have been solved insofar as antibody-induced, cell-mediated cytolysis can be attained with different cells under experimental conditions *in vitro*.[115] The various types of cells can be distinguished functionally, however, on the basis of their surface receptors.[116]

At first, the lymphocytes that were observed as the effector cells in antibody-induced, cell-mediated cytotoxicity could not be clearly identified as B- or T-lymphocytes. As on T-lymphocytes, no immunoglobulin can be found on the cell surface. On the other hand, receptors for the Fc fragment of IgG and for C 3 can be observed, as on B-lymphocytes. The cells could be distinguished from macrophages, which also reveal both receptors, through affinity of the IgG-Fc receptor for certain subgroups of IgG.[117] In addition, cell-mediated, antibody-induced cytotoxicity is activated by anti-immunoglobulin sera at certain concentrations when lymphocytes act as effector cells, whereas macrophages are inhibited.[118] Specific inactivation of macrophages did not significantly reduce antibody-dependent cytotoxicity.[119] The finding that the lymphocytes demonstrated in antibody-induced, cell-mediated cytolysis in mice were negative for $\theta$ antigen[120] makes it unlikely that they are T-lymphocytes. That is the basis for the view that these lymphocytes must belong to the B-lymphocyte population, even though surface immunoglobulin cannot be demonstrated.

*"Null cells,"* i.e., lymphocytes with no surface markers,[121] are extremely rare in normal blood. This population, which was originally thought to represent one certain functional class of lymphocytes, seems to be extremely heterogeneous. Immature B- and T-cells, plasma cells, stem cells, and cells of several functional activities, namely, cell-mediated cytotoxicity and cell-mediated, antibody-dependent cytotoxicity, are found in this cell fraction. Therefore, the common term "null" cell should be avoided. Furthermore, the percentage of lymphocytes that neither form spontaneous rosettes with sheep erythrocytes nor bear the C 3 receptor seems to be largely dependent on the technical conditions of lymphocyte preparation and the assay.

Even an approximately comprehensive review and discussion of the papers dealing with the surface structures of T- and B-lymphocytes would be beyond the scope of this chapter. Although there is an increasing amount of literature

---

[112] 1969.
[113] 1970.
[114] DENNERT and LENNOX, 1973; GREENBERG, HUDSON, SHEN and ROITT, 1973.
[115] PENFOLD, GREENBERG and ROITT, 1976.
[116] ZIGHELBOIM, BONAVIDA and FAHEY, 1973; RESCH, GELFAND and PRESTER, 1974.
[117] CEROTTINI and BRUNNER, 1974.
[118] RESCH, GELFAND and PRESTER, 1974.
[119] SANDERSON and TAYLOR, 1976.
[120] VAN BOXEL, STOBO, PAUL and GREEN, 1972.
[121] GREENBERG, HUDSON, SHEN and ROITT, 1973; WILLIAMS, DEBOARD, MELLBYE, MESSNER *et al.*, 1973; JØNSSON, 1974.

on this subject, the reader is asked to refer to the reviews by GREAVES *et al.*,[122] NUSSENZWEIG,[123] SERCARZ *et al.*,[124] and WARNER,[125] and to *Transplantation Review*, Vol. 16, 1973.

## C. Cooperation of B- and T-Lymphocytes

The now well-established distinction of B- and T-lymphocytes and their different localizations in the lymphatic tissue (see below) might lead to the conclusion that these cells function independently. During induction of an immunologic response to most antigens, however, several mechanisms of cellular cooperation are necessary.

The whole meaning of cellular cooperation and of its molecular mechanisms is not yet fully understood. Hypothetically, activating and suppressive phenomena due to cellular cooperation are interpreted as a lattice of feedback regulations.[126] As a rule, *antibody production* in response to most antigens (so-called T-cell-dependent antigens) can be induced *in vitro* and *in vivo* only through cooperation between T-lymphocytes, B-lymphocytes, and macrophages.[127] Whereas T- and B-lymphocytes usually act antigen-specifically, the role of macrophages is seen more as a regulatory one. Recently, the specific interaction between T- and B-cells in antibody production was elucidated on a genetic and molecular basis.[128] Findings in immune-deficiency diseases indicate that the effect of T-cells is also necessary for antibody production in man.

In addition to the antigen-specific action of T-cells during the cooperation process, they may also act antigen-nonspecifically. A soluble factor produced by activated T-cells can induce antigen-specific stimulation of B-cells *in vitro*. This is of importance in bacterial infections, in which endotoxins can induce antigen-independent activation of T-cells and thus mediate T-cell-dependent activation of B-cells ("helper effect").[129] That may explain why various experiments *in vivo* produced results that contradicted *in-vitro* findings.

*In vivo*, T-cell cooperation is important for the formation of germinal centers and for IgG and IgA production. It is therefore interesting that a percentage of up to 20% T-cells may be found in germinal centers, which are the main B-territory in the lymph node.[130]

Cooperative phenomena are also observed in *T-cell-dependent immune reactions*.[131] Most of the findings were obtained through analysis of *in-vitro* systems using purified cell suspensions. The fundamental significance of these findings also appears to be valid for the *in-vivo* situation, as may be concluded from

[122] GREAVES, OWEN and RAFF, 1973.
[123] 1974.
[124] SERCARZ, WILLIAMSON and FOX, 1974.
[125] 1974.
[126] JERNE, 1975.
[127] Review: PLAYFAIR, 1971; GREAVES, OWEN and RAFF, 1973.
[128] MUNRO and TAUSSIG, 1975; WALDMANN and MUNRO, 1975; TAUSSIG, 1976.
[129] ARMERDING and KATZ, 1974; COUTINHO, GRONOWICZ, BULLOCK and MÖLLER, 1974; KOLB, DI PAULI and WEILER, 1974.
[130] WEISSMAN, GUTMAN, FRIEDBERG and JERABEK, 1976.
[131] CANTOR and ASOFSKY, 1972; COHEN and HOWE, 1973; TITTOR and WALFORD, 1974.

the clinical manifestation of immune-deficiency diseases. The degree and the type of cooperation in the various immune reactions *in vivo*, however, remain to be explored in detail.[132]

## D. Derivation of Lymphocytes from the Hemopoietic Stem Cell

Until a few years ago, there was considerable discussion over whether the stem cell that leads to the formation of erythrocytes, granulocytes, monocytes, and thrombocytes (united under the term hemopoiesis) should be distinguished from the stem cell that leads to the formation of lymphocytes. Since then, it has been shown that hemopoiesis and lymphopoiesis definitely have a common precursor cell. This cell could be demonstrated only functionally.

The first systematic studies of radiation chimera (lethally irradiated animals whose hemopoietic tissue was repopulated through bone-marrow transplants from other animals) showed that the bone marrow possesses the ability to regenerate the thymus and later the peripheral lymphatic tissues.[133] Repopulation of the thymic parenchyma is successful practically only when bone-marrow cells, but not thymus cells or peripheral lymph-node cells, are transplanted.[134] When bone-marrow cells are given to lethally irradiated recipient animals, the cells of the donor then predominate in the thymus.[135] By transferring splenic colonies (clonal proliferations of hemopoietic stem cells and blood cells derived from these cells in the spleens of lethally irradiated recipient animals after bone-marrow transplantation), it was also shown that repopulation of the hemopoietic and lymphatic tissues occurs through a common precursor cell.[136]

Thus, the pluripotent hemopoietic stem cell of the bone marrow is also the cellular origin of the free cells of lymphatic tissue. Complete restitution of peripheral lymphatic tissues (lymph nodes, spleen, and lymphatic tissue of the gastrointestinal tract) and of immunologic reactivity is successful, however, only when a thymus or a thymic stroma is present in the lethally irradiated recipient animal.[137] Experimentally, when lethally irradiated animals received bone-marrow transplants, the bone-marrow cells lost their pluripotency after they entered the thymus. Subsequently, the cells possessed only the ability to mature into lymphoid cells.[138] Differentiation of the pluripotent stem cell into the determined prethymic precursor cell seems to occur in the bone marrow. Merely a few, perhaps only one or two, precursor cells repopulated the whole thymus under such experimental conditions.[139] Extreme reduction in the number of transplanted bone-marrow cells finally results in the thymus not being populated at all, even though hemopoiesis may still occur.[140]

---

[132] Review of cellular cooperative phenomena: GREAVES, OWEN and RAFF, 1973.

[133] KAPLAN, BROWN and PAULL, 1953; HIRSCH, BROWN, NAGAREDA and KAPLAN, 1956; GENGOZIAN, URSO, CONGDON, CONGER *et al.*, 1957.

[134] MICKLEM and FORD, 1960.

[135] POPP, 1961.

[136] TRENTIN and FAHLBERG, 1963; JURÁŠKOVÁ and TKADLEČEK, 1965; WU, TILL, SIMINOVITCH and MCCULLOCH, 1967, 1968; NOWELL, HIRSCH, FOX and WILSON, 1970.

[137] CROSS, LEUCHARS and MILLER, 1964.

[138] ORDER and WAKSMAN, 1969.

[139] WALLIS, LEUCHARS, CHWALINSKI and DAVIES, 1975.

[140] URSO and CONGDON, 1957.

The studies discussed here show that the pluripotent hemopoietic stem cell is also the stem cell of lymphoid cells. They indicate that specific histogenetic effects of a micromilieu that lead to maturation and differentiation of the lymphocytes are necessary, as in the differentiation of hemopoietic cells. It is possible that the determination of lymphatic differentiation, or at least certain early developmental phases of lymphocytes, occurs outside the bone marrow, namely, in the thymus, perhaps also in peripheral lymphatic organs, and can be initiated only through the tissue milieu of these organs.

Even if the ability to populate lymphatic and hemopoietic tissues is attributed to the pluripotent hemopoietic stem cell, that does not exclude the possibility that lymphocytes themselves or one of their subpopulations are identical with this cell. In order to shed more light on this problem, we must examine the function and morphology of bone-marrow lymphocytes more closely and compare them with new findings on stem cells.

Whereas bone-marrow lymphocytes were spoken of as one cell class until a few years ago, there are now many indications that they are functionally heterogeneous. The possibility of separating various lymphocyte populations into T- and B-lymphocytes on the basis of their surface characteristics and functions also enabled a detailed analysis of the functions of bone-marrow lymphocytes in laboratory animals and humans.[141] In particular, the following types of lymphocytes were found: (1) immature and mature B-lymphocytes,[142] (2) various B-lymphocyte subpopulations with a long or short life expectancy,[143] (3) T-lymphocytes,[144] and (4) cells with questionable stem-cell function. In addition to these functionally identifiable groups of small lymphocytes, activated or transitional stages ("transitional cells") are seen as larger cell forms in immune reactions and in normal animals as well.[145]

Most radioautographic investigations have shown that an overwhelming majority of the small bone-marrow lymphocytes reveal a high turnover, living for no more than 5–6 days.[146] The bone-marrow lymphocytes are usually formed in the bone marrow itself.[147] Precursor cells of small lymphocytes that are functionally inactive, but capable of proliferation, can be demonstrated in bone marrow-cell suspensions.[148] Besides the rapidly proliferating bone-marrow lymphocytes, a long-lived type of lymphocyte also exists in the bone marrow.[149]

In the search for the morphologic equivalent of the hemopoietic stem cell, many authors considered the lymphatic or lymphoid cells of the bone marrow to be candidates.[150] Usually the only thing that could be concluded from

---

[141] BORELLA and SEN, 1974.

[142] LAFLEUR, MILLER and PHILLIPS, 1972, 1973; NOSSAL and PIKE, 1973; OSMOND and NOSSAL, 1974a, b.

[143] HOWARD, 1972.

[144] BURLESON and LEVEY, 1972; HOWARD and SCOTT, 1972.

[145] YOFFEY, HUDSON and OSMOND, 1965; SHARP, THOMAS and BRISCOE, 1971.

[146] EVERETT, CAFFREY and RIEKE, 1964; OSMOND and EVERETT, 1964; CRADDOCK, 1965; EVERETT and CAFFREY, 1967; ROSSE, 1971.

[147] EVERETT and CAFFREY, 1967.

[148] YOSHIDA and OSMOND, 1971; LAFLEUR, MILLER and PHILLIPS, 1972.

[149] CRADDOCK, 1965; HAAS, BOHNE and FLIEDNER, 1969; IVERSEN and BENESTAD, 1970; ROSSE, 1971; HOWARD and SCOTT, 1972.

[150] CUDKOWICZ, UPTON, SMITH, GOSSLEE *et al.*, 1964; THOMAS, FLIEDNER, THOMAS and CRONKITE, 1965; BENNETT and CUDKOWICZ, 1967, 1968; FREY-WETTSTEIN and CRADDOCK, 1970; HAAS, FLAD, FLIEDNER and FACHE, 1973.

their morphologic descriptions was that the cells in question were small and had a round, dense nucleus like that of lymphocytes. Other authors attributed stem-cell potency to other morphologically identifiable cell forms: monocytoid cells[151] or so-called transitional cells.[152] The latter were defined as a larger group of various cells whose common characteristics were a light leptochromatic nucleus and a moderately broad rim of usually weakly basophilic cytoplasm. The experimental evidence at the root of these studies was as a rule indirect. It was provided by the analysis of cell populations that appeared or disappeared after bone-marrow transplantation.

More recent experiments have approached a direct morphologic identification of these cells through considerable enrichment of the hemopoietic stem cells (demonstrated in various test systems). A relative increase in stem cells by a factor of 70–100 could be attained after biologic enrichment by means of treatment with vinblastine nitrogen mustard for 3 days and subsequent density gradient centrifugation of the bone marrow in discontinuous albumin gradients.[153] The cell form described electron microscopically as the stem-cell candidate had a diameter of 8–10 μm and a very loosely structured, sparse, light, irregularly defined nucleus with one or two large nucleoli. The cytoplasm did not contain a Golgi complex, multivesicular bodies or lysosomes, or polyribosomes. This cell form was found not only in murine, but also in human and primatial bone marrow. NIEWISCH *et al.*[154] enriched stem cells by means of a linear Ficoll gradient. According to their criteria, the stem cell has a diameter of 14–17 μm, a strongly basophilic cytoplasm, and a nucleus with a diameter of 13–16 μm and a loose chromatin structure. RUBINSTEIN and TROBAUGH[155] observed that only one characteristic type of cell remained morphologically intact after freezing murine bone-marrow cells in glycerin to −70° C. The number of these cells correlated with the number of splenic colonies after transplantation to lethally irradiated syngeneic recipient mice. This type of cell is clearly different from lymphocytes treated in the same way. It is 8–10 μm in diameter and has a round or oval, central nucleus. The cytoplasm contains vesicles and a few multivesicular bodies. In the narrow rim of cytoplasm there are also numerous, regularly distributed ribosomes, a few small, round or oval mitochondria, short profiles of rough endoplasmic reticulum, and occasionally a Golgi apparatus. ZUCKER-FRANKLIN *et al.*[156] found the hemopoietic stem cells that circulate in the peripheral blood in a purified lymphocyte fraction, whereas BARR and WHANG-PENG[157] were able to separate human stem cells from most of the circulating lymphocytes by velocity sedimentation.

The diversity in the morphologic descriptions, which include contradictions, reflects the difficulties with a morphologic definition of hemopoietic stem cells. It must remain undecided which description is the correct one. In functional experiments using highly purified heterologous anti-lymphocyte sera, we demon-

---

[151] CAFFREY TYLER and EVERETT, 1966.
[152] MOFFAT, ROSSE and YOFFEY, 1967; THOMAS, 1973; YOFFEY, 1973.
[153] VAN BEKKUM, VAN NOORD, MAAT and DICKE, 1971; DICKE, VAN NOORD and VAN BEKKUM, 1973.
[154] NIEWISCH, VOGEL and MATIOLI, 1967.
[155] 1973.
[156] ZUCKER-FRANKLIN, GRUSKY and L'ESPERANCE, 1973.
[157] 1975.

strated that hemopoietic stem cells can be distinguished from all other lymphoid cells of the bone marrow.[158] Therefore, they are not functionally identical with lymphoid cells.

In order to trace the early stages of lymphocytic differentiation, cell-surface receptors have been investigated. The results of these studies are not yet fully conclusive. Nevertheless, certain steps in the development of T- and B-lymphocytes can be identified.

At present, it is not clear whether there is a common determined precursor cell for the T- and B-lymphocytes, or whether separate independent precursors are formed after the stage of the pluripotent hemopoietic stem cell. The earliest cell identified in B- and in T-cell differentiation bears the C 3 receptor and a small amount of surface immunoglobulin. In embryogenesis it is localized among the yolk-sac cells of mice[159] and also in the early fetal thymus of humans.[160] Recent findings suggest that T-lymphopoiesis also starts in the bone marrow in humans. Terminal deoxynucleotidyl transferase (Tdt) is found in some bone-marrow lymphocytes.[161] This enzyme has been shown to be specific to the early thymocyte population in a wide variety of species. Normally, it is found only in the thymus and in some bone-marrow lymphocytes, which are therefore considered to be a prothymocyte population. Pathologically, it is found in blast cells of acute lymphoblastic leukemia of children[162] and during the blast crisis in a number of cases of adult granulocytic leukemia.[163]

T-lymphopoiesis in the human fetus and in the adult starts with the cell bearing the C 3 receptor and surface immunobglobulin. During differentiation, a cell without demonstrable surface immunoglobulin, but with the C 3 and sheep-E receptors can be identified.[164] After this stage, only the sheep-E receptor is found. The behavior of other receptors and surface properties during this differentiation process and further steps (from thymocyte to T-lymphocyte) have not been identified in humans. Rather precise information is available for mice.[165] The transformation of a prethymic lymphocyte in the bone marrow into lymphocytes bearing surface characteristics of T-lymphocytes seems to occur under the influence of a thymic hormone.[166]

In B-lymphopoiesis the C 3 receptor is apparently retained. During differentiation the amount of surface immunoglobulin increases.[167] In embryogenesis the first immunoglobulin classes present on the cells are IgM, IgG, and IgA, in that order.[168] IgD, which is present in a large population of lymphocytes in cord blood,[169] is formed earlier than IgM in the human fetus.

---

[158] Müller-Hermelink, Wottge and Müller-Ruchholtz, 1973; Müller-Ruchholtz, Müller-Hermelink and Sonntag, 1973; Müller-Hermelink, 1975; Müller-Ruchholtz, Wottge and Müller-Hermelink, 1975.

[159] Globerson, Kirov and Parish, 1976.

[160] Gatien, Schneeberger and Merler, 1975; Gatien, Schneeberger, Parkman and Merler, 1975.

[161] Barr, Sarin and Perry, 1976.

[162] McCaffrey, Harrison, Parkman and Baltimore, 1975.

[163] Sarin and Gallo, 1974.

[164] Stein and Müller-Hermelink, 1977.

[165] Roelants, Mayor, Hägg and Loor, 1976.

[166] Goldstein, Guha, Zatz, Hardy *et al.*, 1972; Aiuti, Schirrmacher, Ammirati and Fiorilli, 1975; Kook, Yakir and Trainin, 1975; Potworowski, Lefebvre, Lussier and Teodorczyk, 1975.

[167] Osmond and Nossal, 1974a, b; Osmond, 1975; Abdou, Alavi and Abdou, 1976.

[168] Lawton, Self, Royal and Cooper, 1972; Gupta, Pahwa, O'Reilly, Good *et al.*, 1976.

[169] Rowe, Hug, Forni and Pernis, 1973.

## II. Immunoblasts (Basophilic Stem Cells)

B- and T-lymphocytes can be stimulated by certain mitogenic substances or antigens to transform into large blast cells that are capable of dividing. These cells are now called immunoblasts—a term proposed by DAMESHEK[169a] for plasma-cell precursors. We follow a suggestion made by REBUCK[170] and distinguish B- and T-immunoblasts. B-immunoblasts differentiate further into plasma cells, whereas T-immunoblasts are the origin of ("committed") T-lymphocytes and T-effector lymphocytes, e.g., the cytotoxic T-cell.

A distinction between the two types of immunoblasts is still impossible by means of morphologic, cytochemical, and electron-microscopic techniques. Light microscopically, immunoblasts have large light nuclei with very large nucleoli. The latter are often solitary and are found in the middle of the nucleus or at an indentation of the nuclear membrane. The rim of cytoplasm is moderately broad to broad and strongly basophilic with Giemsa staining, or strongly pyroninophilic with methyl-green pyronine staining. Therefore, the immunoblast is also called a "large pyroninophilic cell."[171] Cytochemically, the nonspecific esterase and numerous other enzyme reactions are negative, whereas the acid phosphatase reaction shows a moderately strong, chiefly granular positivity. The PAS reaction occasionally reveals small glycogen granules.

Electron microscopically, the nucleus is irregularly defined and contains moderately coarse chromatin (Fig. 5). There are narrow chromatin condensations along the nuclear membrane. The nucleoli are markedly large and band-shaped. They frequently extend beyond the middle of the nucleus together with interwoven nucleolonemata. The broad rim of cytoplasm is filled with polysomes, which consist of 5—15 monoribosomes. There are only a few or no profiles of ergastoplasm. The medium-sized Golgi apparatus and the centrioles are found in a flat nuclear indentation. The mitochondria are large and often swollen. Occasionally, spotty accumulations of glycogen are seen. The cytoplasm is usually transparent. There are differences, however, so that "light" and "dark" immunoblasts can be discriminated. Both types of immunoblasts appear at the same time in experimental immune reactions of rabbits.[172] In the human tuberculin reaction they also appear together up to 48—72 hours after tuberculin injection.[173] Immunoblasts of germinal centers show the same morphology as immunoblasts of the paracortical area and as those in the course of a tuberculin reaction. Functionally, immunoblasts represent the most active proliferation stages of T- and B-cells. More than 50% of the immunoblasts reveal active DNA synthesis after a short incubation with $^{3}$H-thymidine. Most of them are tetraploid.[174]

B-immunoblasts are the most immature cells in plasmacytopoiesis and are capable of producing secretory immunoglobulin.[175] T-immunoblasts produce

[169a] 1964.

[170] 1973, personal communication.

[171] SCOTHORNE and MCGREGOR, 1955.

[172] VELDMAN, 1970.

[173] DESAGA, MÜLLER-HERMELINK and LENNERT, unpublished data.

[174] QUEISSER, NOESKE, SANDRITTER and LENNERT, 1967.

[175] HARRIS, HUMMELER and HARRIS, 1966; LEDUC, AVRAMEAS and BOUTEILLE, 1968; GUDAT, HARRIS, HARRIS and HUMMELER, 1970; HUMMELER, HARRIS, HARRIS and FARBER, 1972.

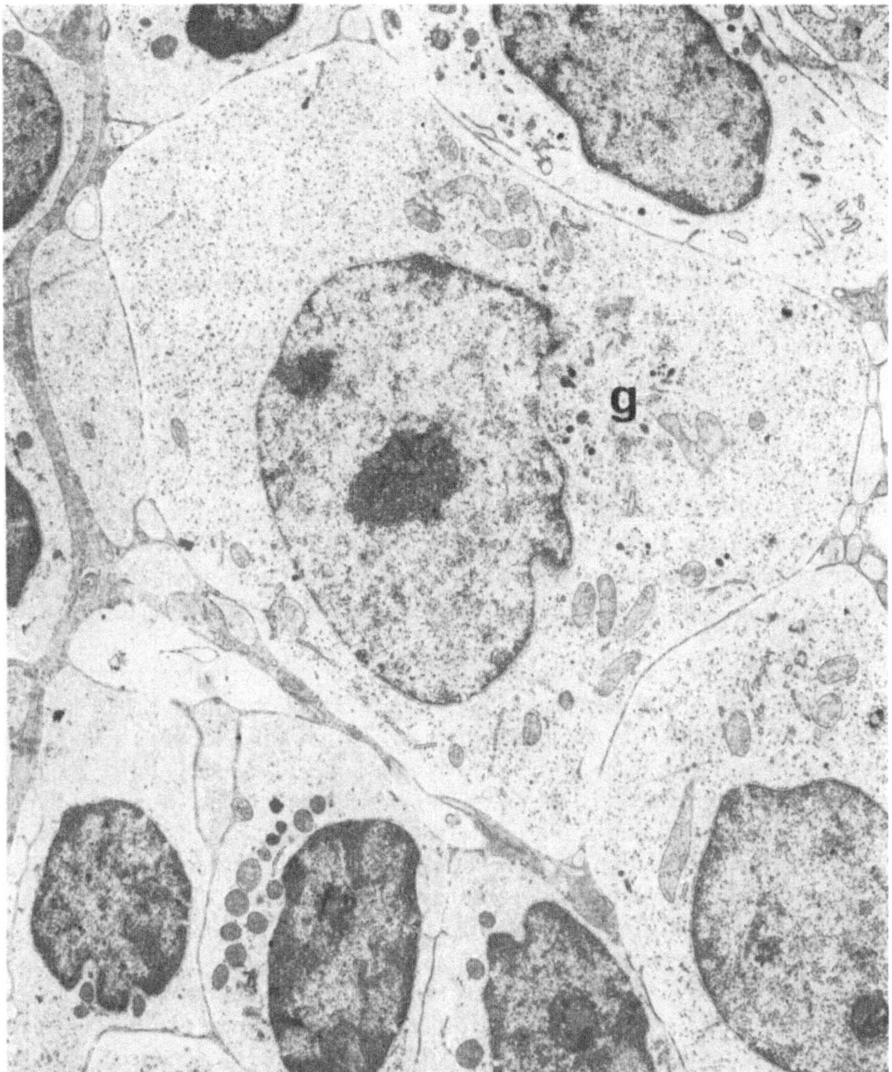


Fig. 5. Immunoblast in immunoblastic hyperplasia of the pulp. The large central nucleolus consists of interwoven nucleolonemata. Another small part of a nucleolus is found at the nuclear membrane. The abundant cytoplasm is filled with polysomes. There are only a few strands of rough endoplasmic reticulum. Some small electron-dense lysosomes are seen around the Golgi region (*g*). Note the size of the cell in comparison with adjacent lymphocytes. × 7,500

mediator molecules, such as migration-inhibitory factors (MIF), mitogenic factors, cytotoxins, etc., as shown in nonspecific T-cell activation induced by PHA and Con A. The mean proliferation time of T-immunoblasts in mice seems to be somewhat longer than that of blast cells of germinal centers (9 as against 6 hours).[176]

[176] HANNA, 1964.

# III. Plasma Cells

Whereas B-lymphocytes are typically located in the outer cortex of lymph nodes and the first changes in response to antigenic stimulation are also found there, the effector cells of B-lymphocytes, plasma cells, are found elsewhere in the lymph node. Maturation from basophilic blastic precursors, i.e., immunoblasts (basophilic stem cells), to plasma cells takes place as they migrate from the outer cortex to the lymph-node medulla. Thereby the cells move through the paracortical pulp, particularly along the intermediary sinuses and the venous and arterial vessels, as shown by VELDMAN.[177]

FAGRAEUS[178] established that plasma cells probably produce the antibodies (immunoglobulins) of the blood serum. This finding has been substantiated many times. Numerous experimental studies on the origin and morphology of plasma cells in immune reactions indicate that plasma cells develop from immunoblasts *via* plasmablasts and proplasmacytes (see Part A of this Handbook.) In several mitotic phases these cells mature to plasma cells with increasing amounts of rough endoplasmic reticulum.[179] Notwithstanding these experimentally based facts, human plasma cells differ somewhat in their morphology; thus, our knowledge may be incomplete regarding their respective significance.

In the secondary reaction to antigens, plasma cells originate from specific $B_2$-lymphocytes of the germinal centers (see p. 35ff.). Normally, these plasma cells are responsible for the production of 7 S immunoglobulin. Plasma-cell maturation may take place in the same lymph node, particularly in the medulla or even in germinal centers, as well as in other parts of the lymphatic tissue, at the site of inflammation, and in the bone marrow.

In the primary reaction, IgM (19 S immunoglobulin) production by plasma cells is normally found without germinal-center formation. Then, $B_1$-lymphocytes serve as precursors of immunoblasts. Their surface IgM (8 S) acts as the recognition site for the antigens.

In most primary immune responses, germinal centers develop in later phases. During the response, a switch from IgM to IgG production can be observed, whereas in the secondary immune response mainly IgG is produced. NOSSAL *et al.*[180] examined the class of surface immunoglobulin on isolated lymphocytes. They found that some cells bore both IgM and IgG immunoglobulin. That means that the switch of immunoglobulin class is not necessarily caused by the separate development of two cell lines. This fact has been substantiated in embryologic experiments[181] and in labeling studies on isolated cells.[182] It is still unclear, however, in which morphologic type of cell this switch of immunoglobulin class takes place: in lymphocytes (e.g., between $B_1$- and $B_2$-

[177] 1970.
[178] 1948.
[179] E.g., DE PETRIS, KARLSBAD and PERNIS, 1963; MOVAT and FERNANDO, 1965; VELDMAN, 1970.
[180] NOSSAL, SZENBERG, ADA and AUSTIN, 1964; NOSSAL, WARNER, LEWIS and SPRENT, 1972.
[181] KINCADE, LAWTON, BOCKMAN and COOPER, 1970.
[182] GREAVES and HOGG, 1971.

lymphocytes) or during maturation to the plasma cell. It was recently shown in functional studies that the memory cells of IgG-producing plasma cells bear surface IgM.[183]

The so-called *marginal-zone cell*[183a] represents an intermediate morphologic form between $B_1$-lymphocytes and plasmablasts. It was demonstrated particularly in the outer follicular zone of the spleen and in the submarginal B-cell region of the lymph node in rabbits. Studies of humans also revealed these somewhat larger lymphoid cells with active nucleoli, a few strands of ergastoplasm, a relatively well-developed Golgi field, and small electron-dense lysosomes. Their typical localization at the margins of the B-cell region in the spleen and lymph nodes indicates that these cells also belong to the B-cell system.

The typical plasma cell is also known as the *Marschalkó type* or as the *reticular plasma cell.* Light microscopically, it is characterized by a round nucleus that exhibits the often-quoted "spoke" pattern, especially in autolysed autopsy material. It is eccentrically located in the cytoplasm. With the exception of a perinuclear lighter-staining area corresponding to the Golgi body, the broad rim of cytoplasm is strongly basophilic. A large solitary vacuole is often found in the cytoplasm. This vacuole is sometimes referred to as a lipochondrion or lipid globule.[184] Electron microscopically, all plasma cells show the typical large amount of rough endoplasmic reticulum around the nucleus (Fig. 6). In the Marschalkó type of plasma cell, the Golgi apparatus is exceptionally large. Electron-dense lysosomes are found in this area. Both the Golgi apparatus and the lysosomes show comparatively strong acid phosphatase activity and moderate nonspecific esterase activity. In addition, the cells reveal strong $Mg^{++}$-dependent membrane ATPase activity, as does the following type of plasma cell.[185]

The second type of plasma cell, which we call the *lymphatic plasma cell* (in accordance with MOESCHLIN)—also referred to as "lymphoplasmacytoid" in Anglo-American publications—often appears in virus infections (e.g., rubella). They can also be found in larger numbers in (perhaps virus-induced) nonspecific mesenteric lymphadenitis. These cells are smaller than the reticular plasma cells. Their Golgi apparatus is not defined to the same extent, and the nucleus is not as eccentrically located in the much smaller rim of cytoplasm. The nuclear chromatin is not as coarse as that of reticular plasma cells and gives the impression of being "lymphoid." Electron microscopically (see Fig. 7), there does not seem to be a significant difference between the cytoplasmic organelles of these two types of cells; both show perinuclear formation of rough endoplasmic reticulum. Lymphatic plasma cells just seem to be smaller. Semiquantitative morphologic dissimilarities in the two cell types, which have led to their distinction, also seem to be verified by immunologic differences in the cell surfaces: in some cases surface immunoglobulin, usually IgM,[186]

---

[183] ABNEY, KEELER, PARKHOUSE and WILLCOX, 1976.
[183a] KEUNING and BOS, 1967; VELDMAN, 1970.
[184] RIND, 1955; LENNERT, 1961; MORI and LENNERT, 1969.
[185] RINNEBERG, 1961; LENNERT and RINNEBERG, 1961.
[186] KAISERLING and STEIN, personal communication.

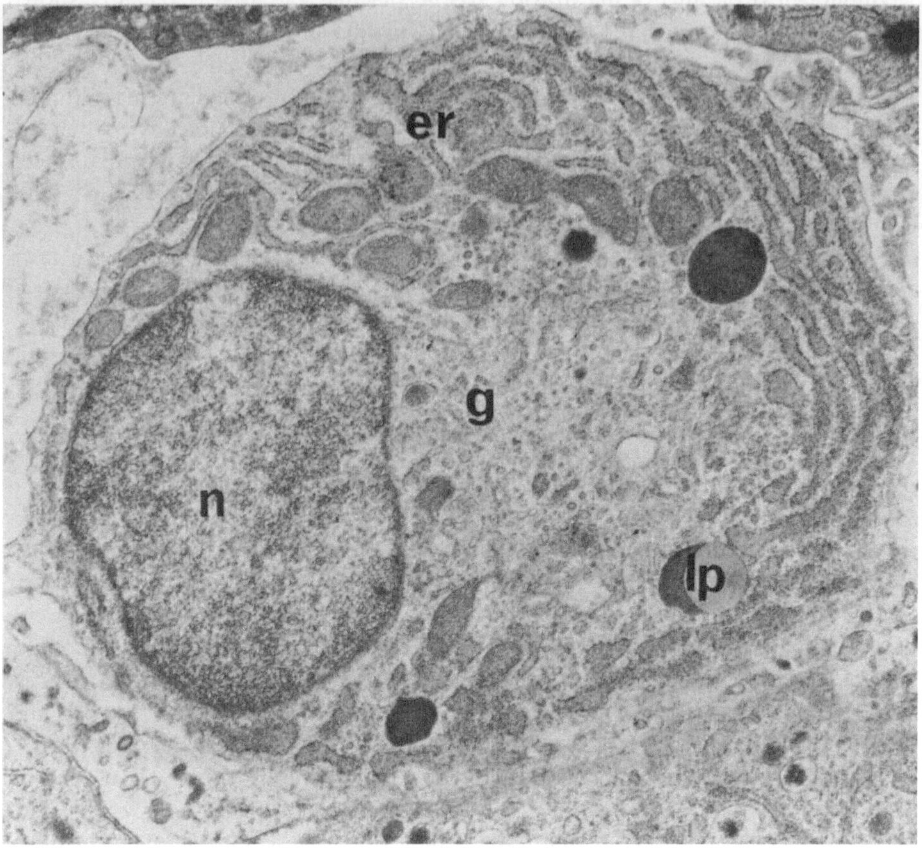


Fig. 6. Marschalkó type of plasma cell (reticular plasma cell) from human bone marrow. Nucleus (*n*). Golgi complex (*g*). Rough endoplasmic reticulum (*er*). Lysosomes with lipid droplets (*lp*), which used to be known as lipochondria. × 15,500

could be found on the circulating lymphatic plasma cells (see Fig. 4b), whereas reticular plasma cells are usually negative for immunoglobulin.

It would be tempting to attribute specific behaviors to these two types of plasma cells during antibody production. Although there is no proof, the following working hypothesis appears to us to be justifiable: lymphatic plasma cells (lymphoplasmacytoid cells) originate (even without germinal centers and perhaps even without T-cell cooperation) directly from IgM-bearing $B_1$-lymphocytes (*via* corresponding blast cells). They are mainly responsible for the initial production of low-affinity IgM. As a rule, reticular plasma cells are formed after the development of germinal centers and with the cooperation of T-cells. They are mainly responsible for the production of IgG and IgA.

The fate of lymphatic plasma cells has not been clarified beyond doubt. Labeling studies have shown that the average survival time of plasma cells in regional lymph nodes is 2–8 days.[187] It could well be, however, that they

[187] Nossal, 1962.

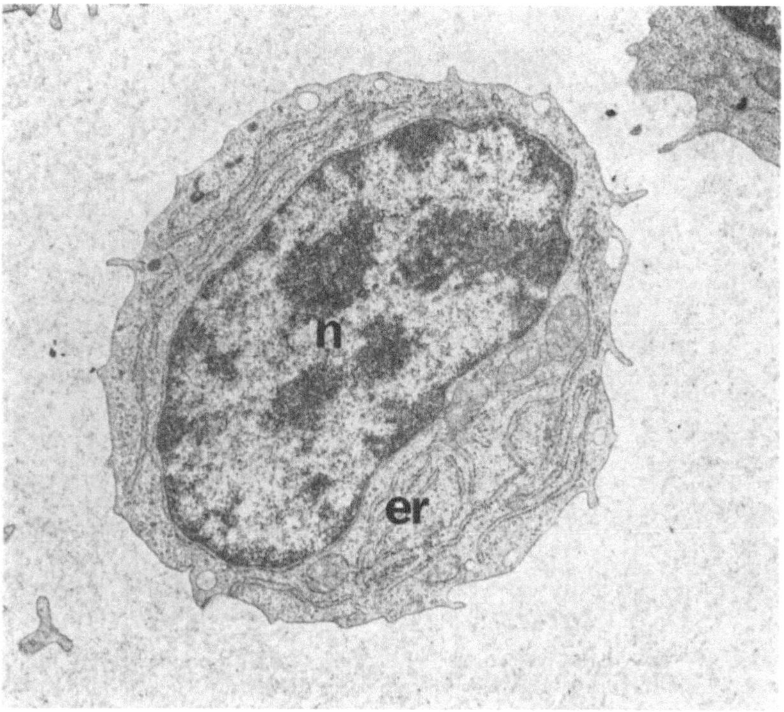


Fig. 7. Lymphoplasmacytoid cell (lymphatic plasma cell) of peripheral blood. Nucleus (*n*). Rough endoplasmic reticulum (*er*). Compare size with Fig. 6 (same magnification). × 15,500

continue to develop into larger reticular plasma cells in other tissue localizations, such as the bone marrow,[188] after circulating in the blood. That might explain why lymphatic plasma cells are regularly found in the blood. There is another possible origin of plasma cells in the bone marrow, however: reticular plasma cells might be formed from lymphoid precursors. Results of experiments on the distribution of antibody-production capacity in the body after primary or secondary subcutaneous antigen injection showed that the production of antibodies is found initially in regional lymph nodes and the spleen. Even in the primary antibody reaction, however, a small peak was evident in the bone marrow after 20 – 30 days. In a secondary reaction to the same antigen, considerable production of antibodies took place only in the spleen and bone marrow, not in the lymph nodes. After splenectomy there was no decrease in antibody production by bone-marrow plasma cells in a specific secondary reaction. These findings support the assumption that the precursors of plasma cells (memory cells) are stored in the bone marrow in the late primary reaction and are then in a position to show a specific immune reaction in the secondary antibody reaction.[189] That explains why, morphologically, practically no precursors or mitosis

[188] Chaperon, Selner and Claman, 1968; Hijmans and Schuit, 1972.

[189] Benner, Meima, van der Meulen and van Ewijk, 1974; Benner, Meima, van der Meulen and van Muiswinkel, 1974.

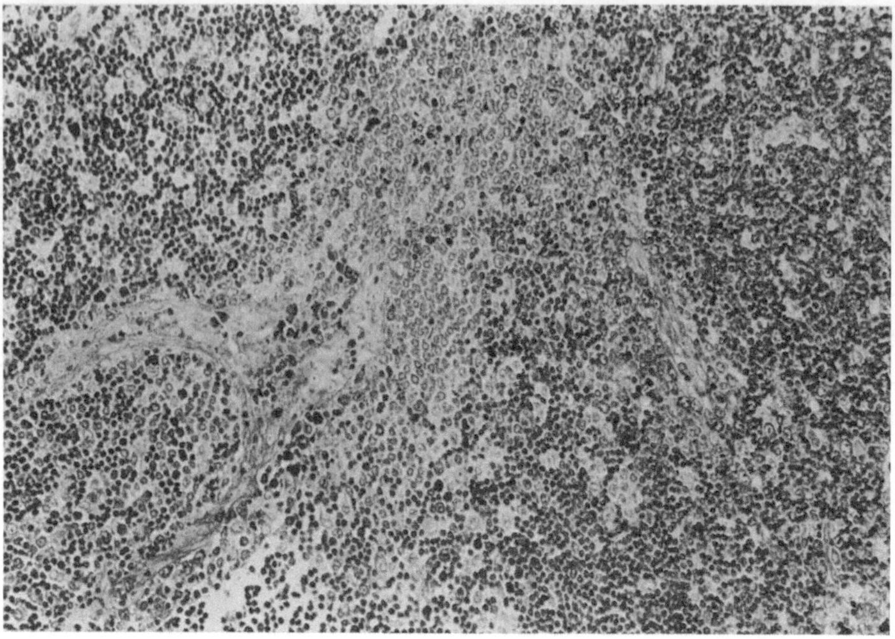

Fig. 8. Nest of "T-associated plasma cells" (*Lymphoblastennest*). In the center and central upper part of the figure there is a sheet of medium-sized, uniform cells that stain more weakly than the surrounding lymphocytes in this T-region. Many immunoblasts are seen among the lymphocytes. An epithelioid venule is evident at center left. Lymphadenitis in herpes zoster. ♂, 47 years. Axillary node. Giemsa. ×175

of plasma cells can be found in the bone marrow, whereas they are seen in lymph nodes.[190] At present we cannot morphologically identify the plasma-cell precursors in the bone marrow. Studies of bone-marrow cytology suggest that these precursors are lymphocyte-like cells ("lymphoid reticulum cells" of ROHR[190a]) that transform without a blast stage into plasma cells. Comparable transformation may be seen in germinal centers. Electron microscopy reveals that germinal centers may contain some centrocytes with a large amount of ergastoplasm that might be such transitional forms.

According to studies by HIJMANS *et al.*[191] and MCMILLAN *et al.*,[192] more than 90% of serum immunoglobulin is produced by plasma cells of the bone marrow. The distribution of IgM-, IgG-, and IgA-producing plasma cells in the bone marrow parallels the distribution of serum immunoglobulin, whereas this does not apply to plasma cells of the blood.[193]

In summary, we may speculate that the lymphatic plasma cells (lymphoplasmacytoid cells) formed in the primary immune reaction are transferred *via* peripheral blood to other tissue localizations and to the bone marrow, where they perish after a yet undetermined survival time. Lymphoid precursors of mainly IgG- or IgA-producing cells are formed in the late primary reaction

[190] AMANO, 1958.
[190a] 1960.
[191] HIJMANS, SCHUIT and HULSING-HESSELINK, 1971.
[192] MCMILLAN, LONGMIRE, YELENOSKY and CRADDOCK, 1972.
[193] HIJMANS and SCHUIT, 1972.

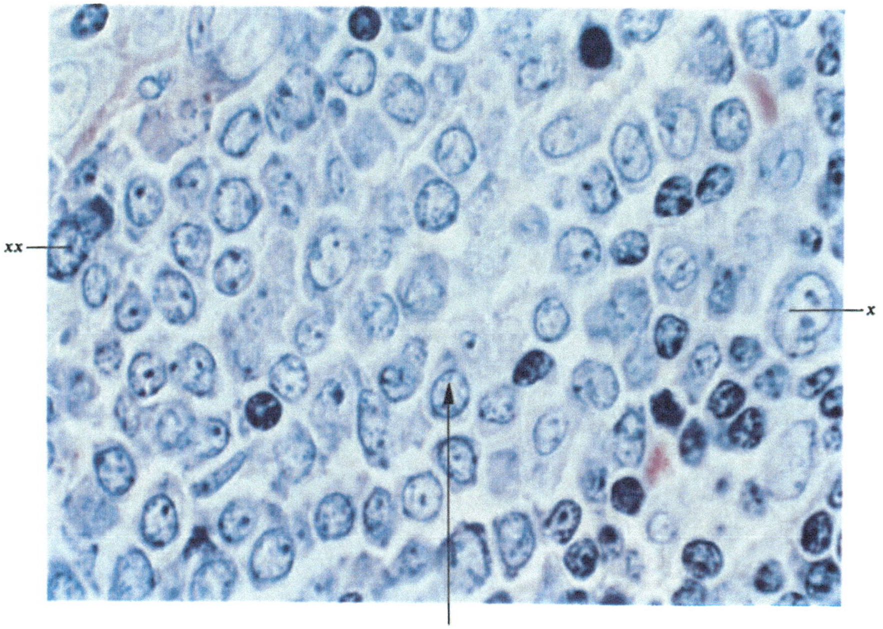


Fig. 9. Nest of "T-associated plasma cells" (*Lymphoblastennest*), which are relatively uniform and medium-sized (↑). They have grayish blue cytoplasm. On the right (*x*) there is a large, moderately basophilic cell (precursor of T-associated plasma cells?). On the left (*xx*) there is a hyperbasophilic cell (plasmablast) with no relationship to the T-associated plasma cells(?). Scattered pyknotic cells are also seen. Some lymphocytes of adjacent lymphatic tissue are evident at the lower right. Same node as Fig. 8. Giemsa. ×1,500

and are also transferred to the bone marrow, where they transform into typical plasma cells in the secondary reaction to antigen. The production of these precursor cells is attributed to the germinal centers (see p. 43ff.).

The assumption that lymphatic plasma cells (lymphoplasmacytoid cells) produce mainly IgM and that reticular plasma cells (Marschalkó plasma cells) synthesize chiefly IgG and IgA, is paralleled to a certain extent in the morphology of IgM-, IgG-, and IgA-producing malignant tumors: IgM-producing lymphoma contains primarily lymphoplasmacytoid cells; IgG- and IgA-producing tumors represent mainly neoplasms of the reticular plasma cells of bone marrow. There are exceptions, however, e.g., IgM-producing lymphoma with typical plasma cells and IgG- or IgA-producing lymphomas with lymphoplasmacytoid cells.

## *Addendum*
## *The So-Called T-Associated Plasma Cell*

Besides these well-known types of plasma cells, there is yet another morphologically definable cell in human lymph nodes, which we called "lymphoblasts"[194] in earlier publications (Fig. 8). Our recent electron-microscopic studies[195] suggested, however, that they might be a special type of plasma cell. This

[194] Lennert and Remmele, 1958; Lennert, 1961.

[195] Müller-Hermelink, Kaiserling and Lennert, 1973.

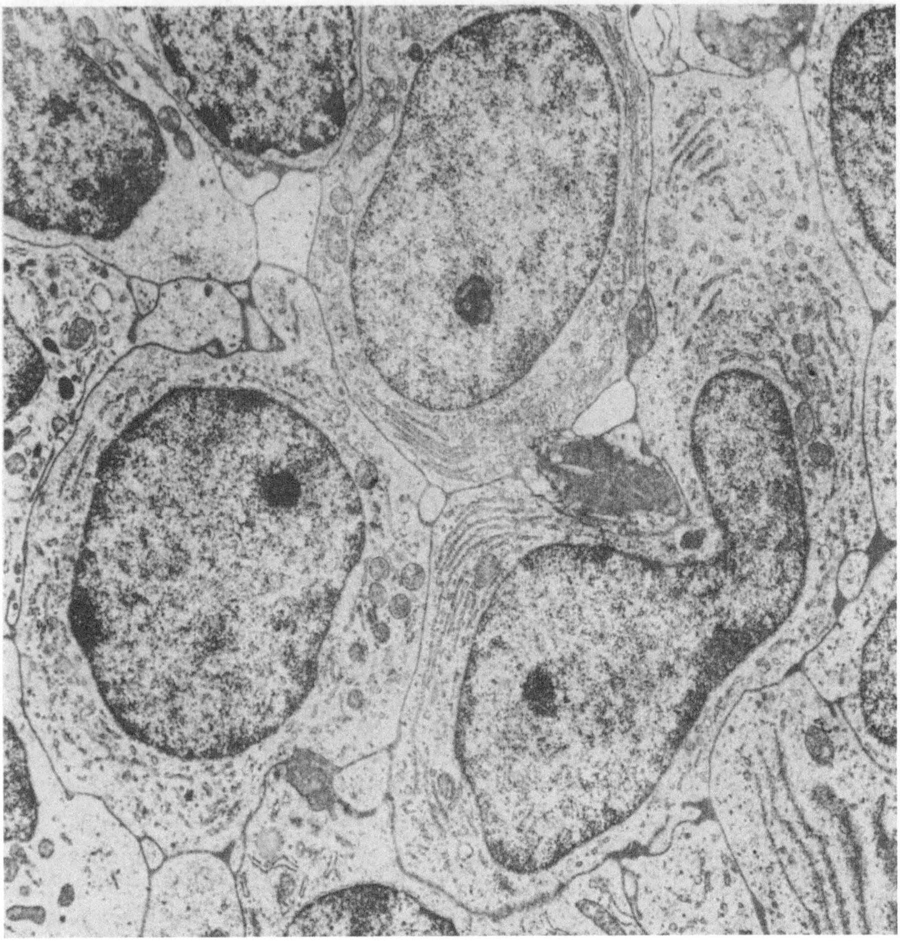

Fig. 10. Nest of "T-associated plasma cells" (*Lymphoblastennest*). The cells contain merely a moderate number of long strands of rough endoplasmic reticulum and a few scattered free ribosomes. Small central nucleoli are evident. × 8,400

cell type has two peculiarities: (1) instead of the blue-violet color shown by all other plasma cells with Giemsa staining, these cells stain gray-blue (Fig. 9), and (2) they are always located in the paracortical pulp of the lymph nodes, especially near epithelioid venules. Electron microscopically, compared with the other types of plasma cells, they show a less developed rough endoplasmic reticulum and only a few free ribosomes (Fig. 10). Such cells have also been found in the thymus of children.[196] We called them *T-associated plasma cells.*[196a]

These cells occur quite frequently. We found them in one out of every 10 cases of nonspecific lymphadenitis, in which there was hyperplasia of the

[196] Kaiserling, Stein and Müller-Hermelink, 1974.

[196a] Lennert, Kaiserling and Müller-Hermelink, 1975.

paracortical area even when germinal centers were absent. They have also been found in benign lymphoma of Castleman and even in dermal infiltrates of mycosis fungoides,[197] which is known to be a T-lymphocytic lesion (see p. 166). Morphologic investigation of localized accumulations of T-associated plasma cells suggest that they are derived from blast cells that have strong paranuclear acid phosphatase activity.[198] Because PAPADIMITRIOU[199] was unable to demonstrate immunoglobulin in the cytoplasm of T-associated plasma cells in paraffin sections, however, we have no final proof that these cells are actually of plasmacytic nature. We also have not been able to establish anything about their function.

# IV. Histomorphology of the B-Cell Region

Abundant experimental data show that the dichotomy of the immune system is not only cellular, but also histologic, i.e., definite B- and T-cell regions can be distinguished in the complicated structure of lymphatic organs.[200] Evidence supporting the B/T-dichotomy of the lymphatic tissue has been provided by experiments using (1) repopulation of the lymphatic tissue or of certain regions with cells of known origin and differentiation after experimental depopulation of the lymphatic tissue,[201] (2) histologic findings in immune-deficiency diseases before and after thymus transplantation,[202] (3) demonstration of specific lymphocyte surface receptors in the lymphatic tissue,[203] (4) histologic changes in lymphatic tissue in relation to cellular and humoral immune reactions,[204] and (5) demonstration of the B- and T-cell regions with histochemical methods.[205]

B-lymphocytes are chiefly located in the follicles of all lymphatic tissues. Therefore, these follicles correspond to the B-cell region of the peripheral lymphatic tissue. They are commonly located in the outer cortex of lymph nodes. Within these follicles, germinal centers are formed as a reaction to antigenic stimulation.

## A. Cytology of Germinal Centers

Since 1957, we have held to our concept that the cells of germinal centers, which we called germinoblasts[206] and germinocytes,[207] are cytologically distinc-

[197] GOOS, unpublished data.
[198] KAISERLING, unpublished data.
[199] Unpublished data.
[200] Review: PARROTT and DE SOUSA, 1971.
[201] GOWANS and KNIGHT, 1964; PARROTT and DE SOUSA, 1966, 1967, 1969; PARROTT, DE SOUSA and EAST, 1966; DE SOUSA, 1971.
[202] CLEVELAND, FOGEL, BROWN and KAY, 1968.
[203] DUKOR, BIANCO and NUSSENZWEIG, 1970; SILVEIRA, MENDES and TOLNAI, 1972; SHEVACH, JAFFE and GREEN, 1973.
[204] TURK, 1967; VELDMAN, 1970.
[205] MÜLLER-HERMELINK, 1974; MÜLLER-HERMELINK, HEUSERMANN and STUTTE, 1974.
[206] LENNERT, 1957, 1961.
[207] LENNERT, 1964.

tive. They were renamed centroblasts and centrocytes at a lymphoma meeting in Kiel in May 1974, to avoid confusion with cells of the germinal layer of the gonads. Mature plasma cells and their precursors usually appear in smaller numbers in germinal centers. According to the immunologic and morphologic studies of MITCHELL and ABBOT[208] and NOSSAL *et al.*,[209] and to the electron-microscopic studies of MILANESI[210] and others, there is another cell specific to the B-cell region. This third cell, called the dendritic reticulum cell, is also found in human lymph nodes[211] and tonsils.[212] Histiocytic reticulum cells (macrophages), which often contain abundant debris of germinal-center cells, including plasma cells,[213] are also found in germinal centers. The pyknotic nuclei and cellular debris found in macrophages are still referred to as tingible bodies according to FLEMMING.[214] FLIEDNER[215] and ODARTCHENKO *et al.*[216] showed that some of the phagocytosed cells had incorporated $^3$H-thymidine, thus appearing to have been in the process of DNA synthesis.

*Centroblasts* (germinoblasts) vary in size and have a round nucleus. The rim of cytoplasm is narrow and strongly basophilic (Fig. 11). The nuclear chromatin is fine and dispersed. Several medium-sized nucleoli are often found at the inner nuclear membrane. Frequently, there are vacuoles in the cytoplasm. Electron-microscopic studies revealed that centroblasts have abundant polyribosomes and a small amount of rough and smooth endoplasmic reticulum (Figs. 12 and 13).[217] In cytochemical analyses one finds little granular acid phosphatase activity.[218] All other enzyme reactions and fat reactions are negative. Centroblasts are occasionally PAS-positive in imprints.

*Centrocytes* (germinocytes) are small or medium-sized and conspicuous chiefly because of their notched, often indented or deformed nuclei (Fig. 11). The nuclei reveal small nucleoli, which are usually central, but occasionally located at the nuclear membrane. The cytoplasm is weak gray-blue with Giemsa staining. Centrocytes can be distinguished from centroblasts by their nuclear form and weak basophilia. They differ from lymphocytes of the mantle zone in their light nucleus, i.e., the nucleus is poor in heterochromatin. Electron microscopically, centrocytes frequently possess monoribosomes, whereas centroblasts contain polyribosomes (Fig. 12). Furthermore, there is a somewhat larger amount of smooth endoplasmic reticulum. Coated vesicles appear more frequently in centrocytes than in centroblasts. No cytochemical differences could be established.

Besides typical centroblasts and centrocytes, blast cells apparently occur in actively proliferating germinal centers. They have round, noncleaved nuclei and several medium-sized, central nucleoli. This type of cell will be described and illustrated in detail in the chapter on Burkitt's lymphoma (p. 366, Fig. 180).

---

[208] 1965.

[209] NOSSAL, ABBOT, MITCHELL and LUMMUS, 1968.

[210] 1965.

[211] LENNERT and NIEDORF, 1969; MORI and LENNERT, 1969.

[212] MÜLLER-HERMELINK and CAESAR, 1969.

[213] LENNERT, CAESAR and MÜLLER, 1967; MÜLLER-HERMELINK and CAESAR, 1969.

[214] 1885.

[215] 1967.

[216] ODARTCHENKO, LEWERENZ, SORDAT, ROOS *et al.*, 1967.

[217] LENNERT, CAESAR and MÜLLER, 1967; MORI and LENNERT, 1969; MÜLLER-HERMELINK and CAESAR, 1969.

[218] STEPHAN and BLÜMCKE, 1971.

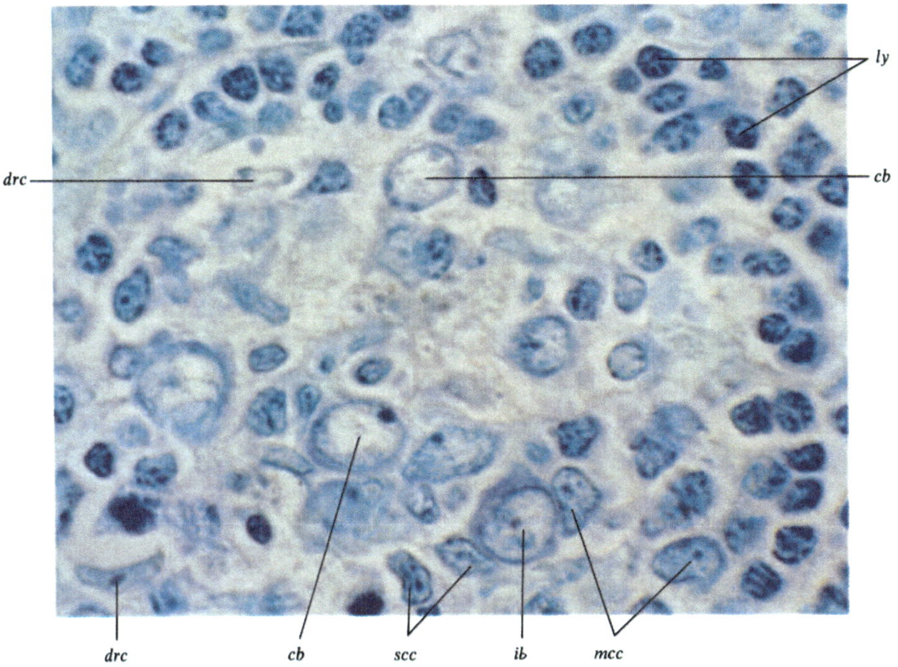


Fig. 11. Germinal center of moderate activity. On the right, lymphocytes (*ly*) in the mantle zone. Large centroblasts (*cb*). Immunoblast (*ib*) whose nucleolus is only partly visible. Medium-sized centrocytes (*mcc*) and small centrocytes (*scc*). Dendritic reticulum cells (*drc*). Chronic nonspecific lymphadenitis in chronic ulcus cruris. ♂, 54 years. Inguinal node. Giemsa. × 1,550

*Dendritic reticulum cells* were first defined according to electron-microscopic findings.[219] They have long-branching, desmosome-connected cytoplasmic processes (see Figs. 28 and 29). The fine cell branches weave together, forming a network that contains electron-dense material in between the cellular processes. The nuclear chromatin is somewhat coarser than that of histiocytic reticulum cells. They develop mainly in the light zone of the germinal center (see p. 38).

*Histiocytic reticulum cells* (macrophages) can be recognized by their light, usually round nucleus, which has a central nucleolus. In the broad rim of cytoplasm one may find so-called tingible bodies; electron-microscopic studies reveal that they are debris of various cells (centroblasts, centrocytes, lymphocytes, and plasma cells[220]).

VON GAUDECKER and HINRICHSEN,[221] our group[222] and others have reported the presence of plasma cells and their precursors in germinal centers. All morphologically defined phases of plasma-cell maturation can be seen in germinal centers.[223] The sequence of development, however, is difficult to reconstruct from static pictures. In principle, there are two possibilities. The first

[219] MILANESI, 1965; SWARTZENDRUBER, 1965, 1967; NOSSAL, ABBOT, MITCHELL and LUMMUS, 1968.

[220] LENNERT, CAESAR and MÜLLER, 1967; MÜLLER-HERMELINK and CAESAR, 1969.

[221] 1965.

[222] LENNERT, CAESAR and MÜLLER, 1967.

[223] KOJIMA and IMAI, 1973.

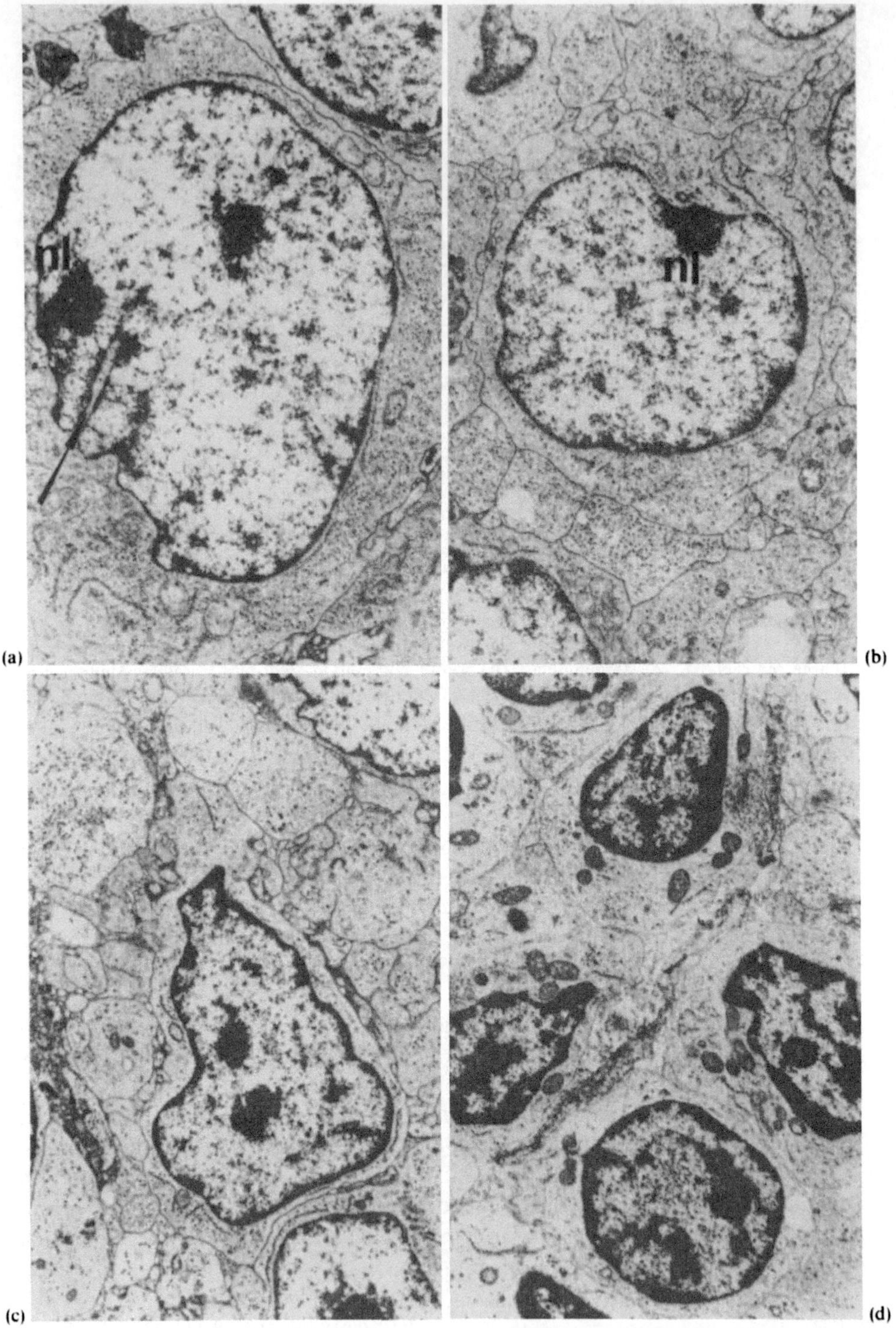
nl
nl
(a)
(b)
(c)
(d)

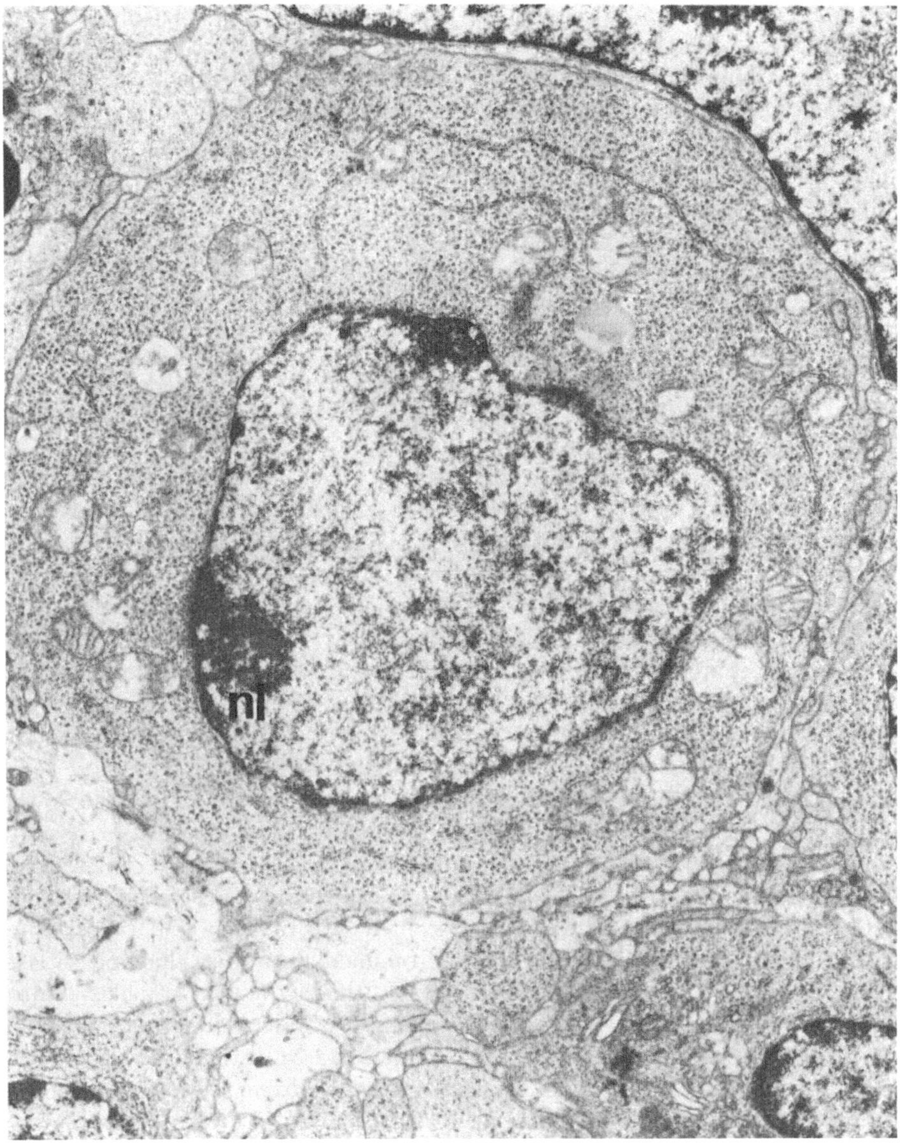


Fig. 13. Transitional stage between large centroblast and immunoblast of a germinal center. The broad rim of cytoplasm is filled with polyribosomes. There are only a few strands of rough endoplasmic reticulum. Two nucleoli (*nl*) are found at the nuclear membrane. ×10,400

---

◁ Fig. 12a–d. Germinal-center cells of a lymph node in nonspecific lymphadenitis. (a) Large centroblast. Its nucleus is deeply indented (arrow) and the nucleolus (*nl*) is found at the nuclear membrane. The cytoplasm contains abundant polyribosomes. (b) Small centroblast. It reveals fundamentally the same morphology as the cell in (a). (c) Centrocyte. The nucleus has an irregular contour and a more condensed chromatin pattern than the centroblast. The cytoplasm contains free ribosomes and only a few polyribosomes. (d) Lymphocytes of the mantle zone. They show an even more condensed chromatin pattern. The nuclei are round or oval. The cytoplasm contains some mitochondria with electron-dense matrices. ×6,500 is that large centroblasts transform into *immunoblasts* with a broad rim of strongly basophilic cytoplasm and very large nucleoli. Plasmablasts and proplasmacytes are then formed from these cells. Conversely, functional data indicate that centrocytes may also enter the plasma-cell series after transformation into blast cells.[224] Some centrocytes exhibit active formation of ergastoplasm and are therefore likely candidates for the transformation process, which might also take place without an intermediate plasmablastic stage (see p. 245). The plasma cells are found chiefly in the middle parts of germinal centers, and they may form Russell bodies.

## B. Phases of Germinal-Center Development

EHRICH[225] and CONWAY[226] referred to cyclic changes in germinal-center development after antigenic stimulation. Studies by VAN BUCHEM[227] and VELDMAN[228] have provided a precise analysis of these phenomena in rabbits. The conditions are probably similar in humans. Four days after antigen injection, foci with numerous centroblasts can be found in the primary follicles. This *first phase* lasts only about 24 hours. No "starry-sky" cells are seen at this time, and there are only medium-sized centroblasts with increased mitotic activity (Fig. 14). In the *second phase* one finds the typical "starry-sky" pattern. Cytologically, however, the germinal center still consists mostly of centroblasts (Fig. 15). This phase continues over a period of 1–3 weeks. The *third phase* reveals a zonal structure of the germinal center (Fig. 16).[229] In the lower, dark side of the germinal center there are densely packed centroblasts with abundant mitotic figures. In the upper, light zone of the germinal center facing toward the marginal sinus, one sees mostly centrocytes, a few immunoblasts, and some plasma cells. Between these cells a web of small cell processes of dendritic reticulum cells is found on electron microscopy. The third phase lasts for a longer period–sometimes for months. In the *fourth* and last phase centroblasts are no longer seen; only centrocytes and dendritic reticulum cells remain.

Two pathologic variants of germinal centers can be distinguished in nonspecific lymphadenitis of humans. *Regressively transformed germinal centers* can be found, for instance, as a consequence of corticosteroid therapy. In these very small germinal centers one sees practically no lymphoid cells. In addition to hyalinized, PAS-positive intercellular material, only onion skin-like dendritic reticulum cells and vascular endothelial cells may be found. *Progressive transformation* of the germinal centers is occasionally observed in follicular hyperplasia. Thereby the secondary follicles become larger, and the borderline between the germinal center and the lymphocytes of the mantle zone becomes indefinable. The germinal-center cells (centrocytes, centroblasts, dendritic reticulum cells, plasma cells, "starry-sky" cells) are lost in a mass of lymphocytes. Finally, a large nodule with abundant lymphocytes results; then its origin from the germinal center cannot be easily discerned (Fig. 17).

[224] See LENNERT, CAESAR and MÜLLER, 1967; MÜLLER-HERMELINK and CAESAR, 1969.
[225] 1929.
[226] 1937.
[227] 1962.
[228] 1970.
[229] RÖHLICH, 1930.

(a) 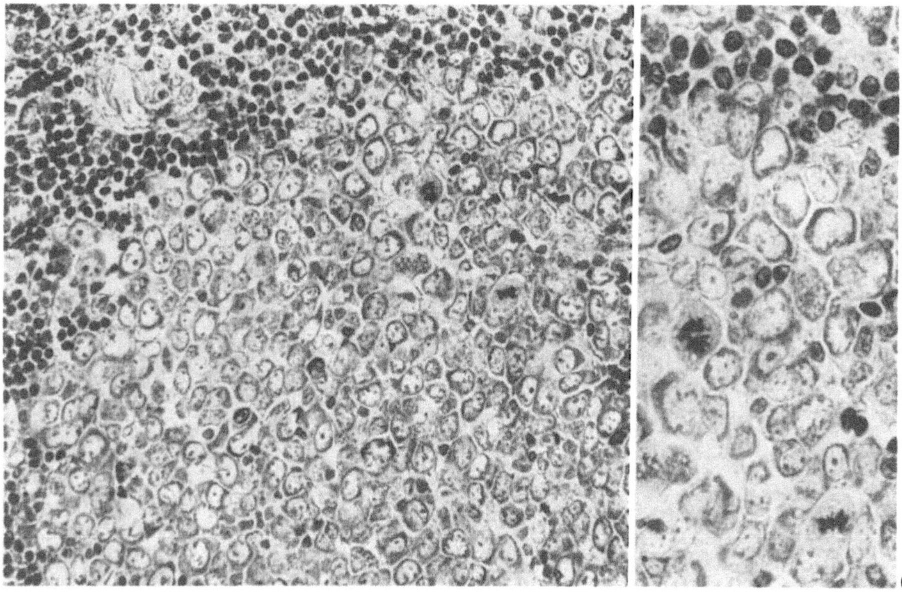 (b)

Fig. 14a and b. Germinal center at an early stage of formation (phase I). Large centroblasts are uniformly distributed in the germinal center. Many mitotic figures are evident. The germinal center is poorly demarcated from the surrounding mantle zone. Giemsa. (a) ×140, (b) ×560

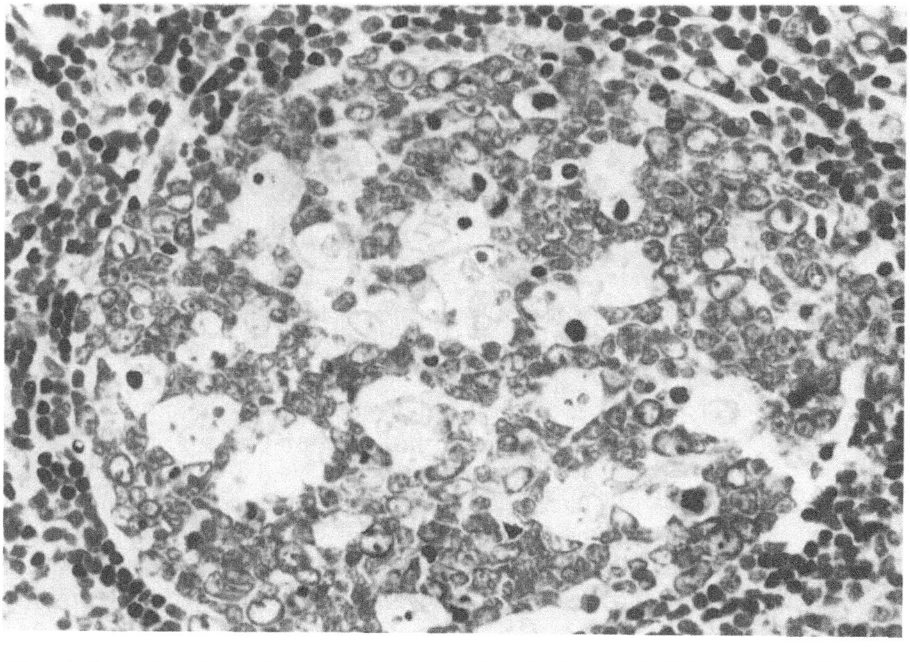

Fig. 15. Starry-sky pattern of a germinal center in phase II. One sees both large and small centroblasts, and large histiocytic reticulum cells containing phagocytosed cells with pyknotic nuclei. The germinal center is sharply demarcated from surrounding lymphocytes. Giemsa. ×140

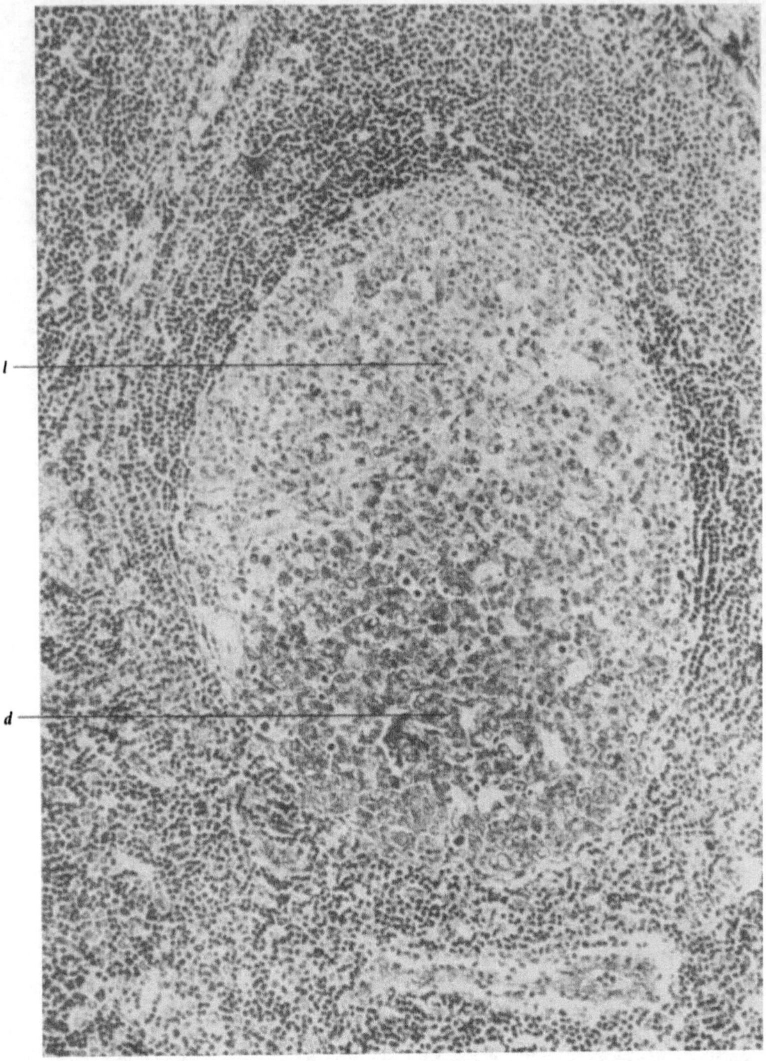


Fig. 16. Typical zonal pattern of a germinal center in phase III. The dark zone at the bottom (*d*) contains chiefly centroblasts. The light zone at the top (*l*) contains chiefly centrocytes and dendritic reticulum cells. Giemsa. ×56

## C. Kinetics of Germinal-Center Cells

In healthy persons cell immigration, cell production, cell emigration, and cell death are in balance in the germinal center.[230] Cell turnover is high. Thirty minutes after a single injection of $^3$H-thymidine, 20–50% of the centroblasts are radioactively labeled.[231] Corresponding results were observed in short-term

[230] Fliedner, Kesse, Cronkite and Robertson, 1964; Hanna, 1964; Hanna, Szakal and Walburg, 1969; van den Broek, 1971a.

[231] Fliedner, Kesse, Cronkite and Robertson, 1964.

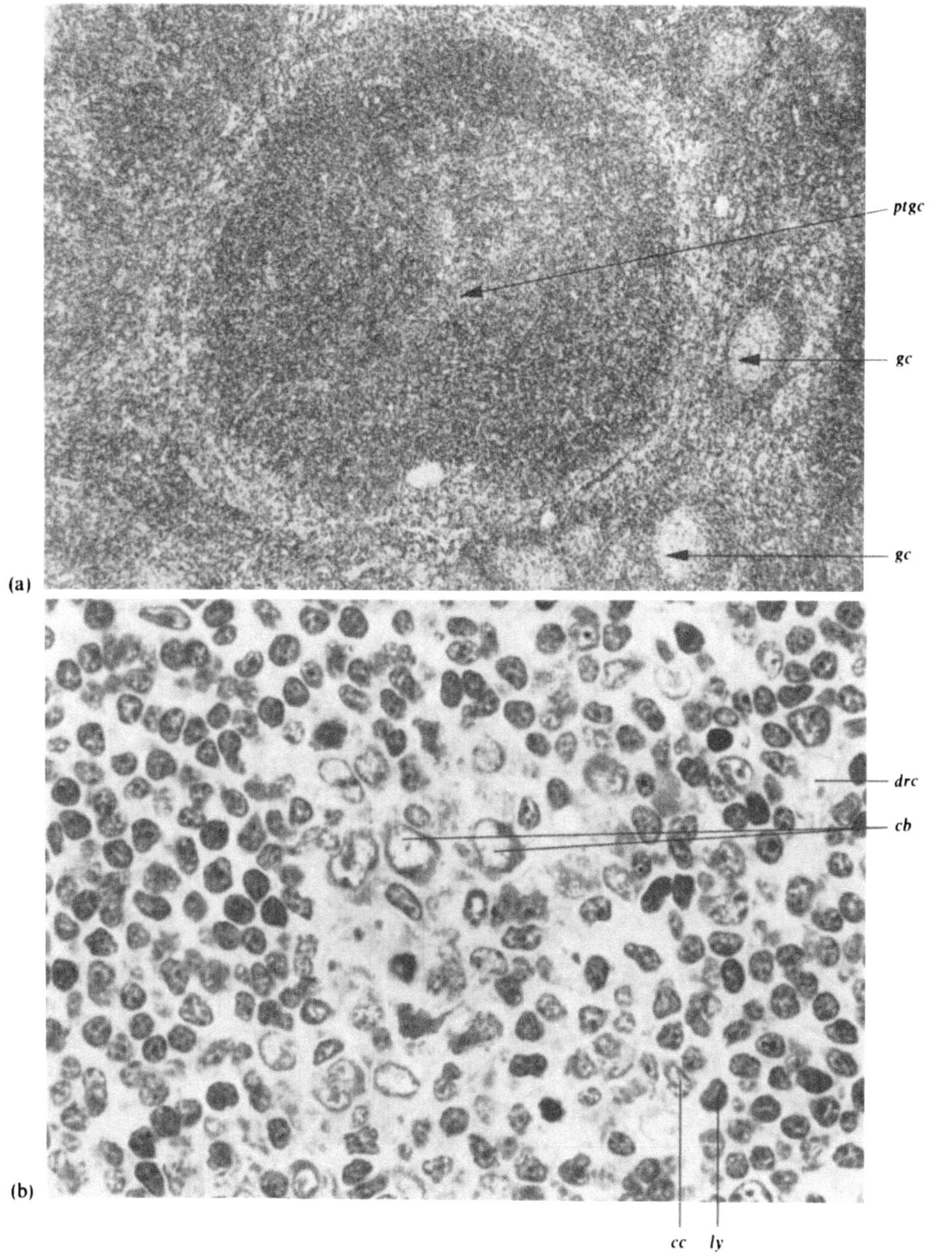


Fig. 17a and b. Progressively transformed germinal center in chronic nonspecific lymphadenitis. ♀, 56 years. Cervical node. (a) In the middle, a large, progressively transformed germinal center (*ptgc*) surrounded by some follicles with small germinal centers (*gc*). Note the difference in size between progressively transformed and resting germinal centers. Gomori. ×35. (b) The same progressively transformed germinal center at a higher magnification. Germinal-center cells (centroblasts = *cb*, centrocyte = *cc*) are seen among lymphocytes (*ly*). Dendritic reticulum cell (*drc*). Giemsa. ×880

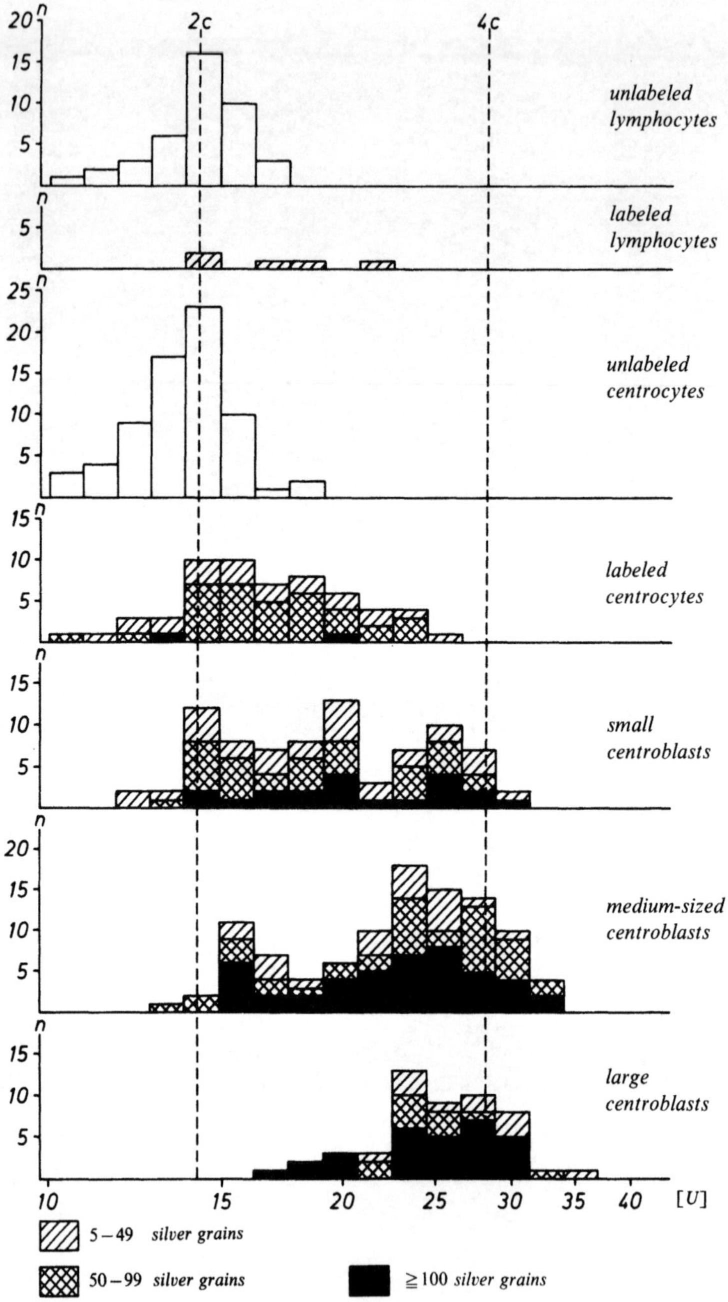


Fig. 18. Simultaneous demonstration of DNA content (Feulgen cytophotometry, expressed in working units [*U*]) and $^{3}H$-thymidine-incorporation after short-term incubation for 1 hour (autoradiography). Labeling index of centrocytes: 8.3%, of centroblasts: 49%. The vertical dashed lines represent the diploid (*2c*) and tetraploid (*4c*) values. Logarithmic scale. The blank columns stand for *no silver grains*. (From Mitrou, Queisser, Lennert and Sandritter, 1969)

cultures of human germinal-center cells (Fig. 18).[232] Quantitative cytophotometric studies, combined with autoradiographic studies of short-term cultures of 30 min, revealed a higher total protein content and greater $^3$H-leucine incorporation in centrocytes than in lymphocytes. Of the centrocytes, 91.7% remained unlabeled with $^3$H-thymidine, while 8.3% showed $^3$H-thymidine incorporation. Of the centroblasts, 49% were labeled with $^3$H-thymidine. When a distinction was made between small, medium-sized, and large centroblasts, the labeled small forms showed diploid to tetraploid DNA values, whereas the medium-sized and large forms revealed mostly tetraploid and hypotetraploid values. The labeled large centroblasts were never diploid.

The results of our studies of short-term cultures might indicate the following interpretation. B-lymphocytes flow into the germinal center, where they transform into small centroblasts. An intermediate stage may be morphologically indistinguishable from centrocytes. With additional DNA and RNA synthesis, the rim of cytoplasm of the centroblasts increases in width and basophilia. Most centroblasts do not divide as small cells, but rather increase in volume and then give rise to smaller forms. For this reason, large centroblasts do not reveal diploid DNA values. Centrocytes originate from small centroblasts and may end up as small lymphocytes ($B_2$-lymphocytes). Locally formed centrocytes as well as newly arrived B-lymphocytes may also "retransform" into centroblasts before leaving the germinal center. Thus, the 8.3% of the centrocytes that are labeled may be precursors of small centroblasts, regardless of whether they originate from immigrated B-lymphocytes, which appears probable from experiments by DURKIN *et al.*,[233] or from newly formed centrocytes that enter the cycle again. LUKES and COLLINS[233a] concluded from our experiments and from their own PHA studies that all centroblasts are derived from centrocytes. That does not agree with our interpretation.

## D. The Function of Germinal Centers

The discussion about the functional meaning of germinal centers has not ceased since the early controversy between FLEMMING and HELLMAN. One of the main questions in the recent discussion has been whether germinal centers are of principal qualitative importance or whether their formation has to be regarded as an auxiliary reaction secondary to the (indefinable) "normal" reaction. Another question concerned the type of reaction in which germinal-center formation is involved.

The finding of immunoglobulin in germinal centers[234] first suggested their involvement in immunoglobulin synthesis. KEUNING *et al.*[235] and DIENER and NOSSAL[236] demonstrated, however, that immunoglobulin production can occur

---

[232] LENNERT, MITROU and MÜLLER-HERMELINK, 1969; MITROU, QUEISSER, LENNERT and SANDRITTER, 1969.

[233] DURKIN and THORBECKE, 1973; DURKIN, CAPORALE and THORBECKE, 1975.

[233a] 1973.

[234] ORTEGA and MELLORS, 1957; WHITE, 1960.

[235] KEUNING, VAN DER MEER, NIEUWENHUIS and OUDENDIJK, 1963.

[236] 1966.

without germinal-center formation. BALFOUR and HUMPHREY[237] showed that immunoglobulin is essential for the localization of antigens within germinal centers. Immunoglobulins are bound with their Fc fragments to the surface of long branching cytoplasmic processes of dendritic reticulum cells.[238] Thus, antigens may also be found here, attached at the antigen-binding sites on the Fab fragment of the immunoglobulins. This antigen localization is seen mainly in the late primary and in the secondary immune response to antigens, after the first antibodies, for the most part IgM, have already formed. Antigens on the cellular processes are not ingested, but instead remain at this site for a long time and are thus in a position to restimulate specifically reacting lymphocytes.

The destiny of the rapidly dividing lymphatic germinal-center cells, the centroblasts, remained obscure for many years. Results of cytokinetic studies using $^{3}$H-thymidine labeling suggest that germinal centers might be the "graveyards" for lymphocytes.[239] Premitotically labeled centroblasts are apparently ingested by germinal-center macrophages and digested in less than an hour. The functional significance of this phenomenon is not clear. In connection with the functional behavior of germinal-center cells, the results of labeling studies indicated that lymphoid cells leave the germinal centers and colonize other lymphatic organs or the bone marrow.[239a]

COOPER and WELLER[240] found that germinal centers are especially important for 7 S immunoglobulin production. COTTIER and SORDAT[241] pointed out that this effect might be more of a quantitative one, since investigations by their group and by others showed that small amounts of 7 S immunoglobulin may be produced in a real primary reaction without germinal-center formation.

The formation of germinal centers in mammals depends on the integrity of the T lymphocyte system. JACOBSON *et al.*[242] showed that active germinal-center formation in nude mice that do not have a thymus is possible only after transfer of living or 3000 rad-irradiated syngeneic thymus cells. In this context, it is interesting that WEISSMAN *et al.*[243] found up to 20% of the cells in the upper germinal-center region to be T-lymphocytes, using a specific anti-T-lymphocyte serum in mice.

The present views on germinal-center function may be summarized as follows. At least in the early stages, germinal centers are the site of transformation and multiplication of specifically reacting clones of lymphocytes after antigenic stimulation. These processes take place particularly in the secondary immune reaction. Then, specifically reacting B-lymphocytes are arrested and stimulated to proliferate by the antigen on the cytoplasmic projections of dendritic reticulum cells. In an animal system, that has been most clearly demonstrated in the so-called milky spots of the omentum of mice.[244] The most important function of germinal centers is the formation of precursors of immunoglobulin-secreting cells, whereas immunoglobulin production seems to be of minor importance.[245]

[237] 1967.
[238] PERNIS, 1967.
[239] FLIEDNER, 1967.
[239a] NIEUWENHUIS and KEUNING, 1974; NIEUWENHUIS, VAN NOUHUIJS, EGGENS and KEUNING, 1974.
[240] 1969.
[241] 1971.
[242] JACOBSON, CAPORALE and THORBECKE, 1974.
[243] WEISSMAN, GUTMAN, FRIEDBERG and JERABEK, 1976.
[244] MATTHES, AX and FISCHER, 1971.
[245] GROBLER, BUERKI, COTTIER, HESS *et al.*, 1974.

This process results in the important increase in antigen-reactive and immunoglobulin-secreting cells in the late primary and the secondary immune reactions. The antigen-reactive small lymphocytes formed in the germinal-center reaction probably represent the cellular basis of immunologic memory of the humoral immune reaction ("memory cells").[245a] They are long-lived and able to recirculate *via* the blood stream. In any immune reaction to the same antigens occurring later, these cells are capable of more intense antibody production, owing to the greater number of initially reacting and the selection of "best-fitting" antibody-producing cells.[246]

NIEUWENHUIS[247] and KEUNING[248] found evidence of formation of $B_1$-lymphocytes whose antigenic specificity was unrelated to the eliciting antigen. This finding may indicate that germinal centers are the main cell-renewal system for B-lymphocytes and therefore have some functional resemblance to the avian bursa of Fabricius. Accordingly, germinal centers are real *germinal* centers, i.e., they produce lymphocytes. Hence, there is no reason to object to the term germinal center as originally applied by FLEMMING. On the other hand, HELLMAN's interpretation is also correct, namely, that germinal centers are formed only in response to – under normal conditions inevitable – antigenic stimulation. Therefore, it is futile to argue over terminology. We are certainly not making an error by continuing to use the old term germinal center conceived by FLEMMING.

# V. Histomorphology of the T-Cell Region

Histologic investigations of lymphatic tissue from neonatally thymectomized mice,[249] rats,[250] rabbits,[251] and chickens,[252] and from children with thymic aplasia[253] showed that absence of the thymus leads to selective deficiency of lymphocytes in certain areas of the lymphatic tissue. Normally, these regions are mainly populated with T-lymphocytes.[254] In the lymph node, however, B-lymphocytes may also be found there, especially under pathologic conditions, since the flow of lymphocytes from the outer cortex to the medulla passes through this region. The most significant alterations of these areas are found in cellular immune reactions.

The thymus-dependent region (T-zone) of the lymph node is localized in the cortical lymphoid tissue, beneath the follicles (Fig. 19). It may extend as far as the marginal sinus, even in normal tissue, thus appearing "cortical"

[245a] WAKEFIELD and THORBECKE, 1968a, b.
[246] MITCHELL, 1972; DURKIN and THORBECKE, 1973.
[247] 1973; NIEUWENHUIS and KEUNING, 1974; NIEUWENHUIS, VAN NOUHUIJS, EGGENS and KEUNING, 1974.
[248] 1972.
[249] PARROTT, DE SOUSA and EAST, 1966.
[250] WAKSMAN, ARNASON and JANKOVIĆ, 1962.
[251] GOOD, DALMASSO, MARTINEZ, ARCHER *et al.*, 1962.
[252] WARNER, SZENBERG and BURNET, 1962.
[253] CLEVELAND, FOGEL, BROWN and KAY, 1968.
[254] Review: Parrott and DE SOUSA, 1971; DE SOUSA, 1973.

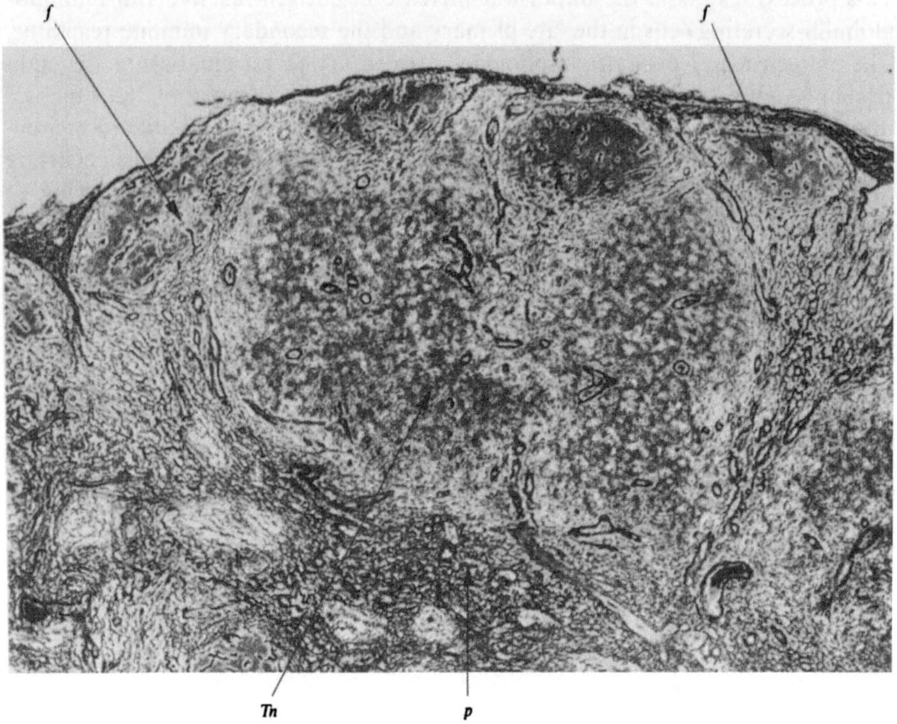


Fig. 19. T-nodule (*Tn*). At the top, four smaller follicles (*f*; B-cell region) are sharply demarcated from the large T-nodule. Epithelioid venules are seen in the T-nodule and in the surrounding pulp (*p*). Nonspecific lymphadenitis. Inguinal node. Gomori. ×35

and not "paracortical" as this area was originally designated. The presence of epithelioid venules in the T-cell region, especially at the margins, is very typical. The venules are seen most clearly with PAS staining. In superficial lymph nodes, more often than in deeper ones, the T-cell region acquires a nodular appearance. The nodular structures used to be called tertiary nodules or tertiary follicles.[255] They represent constant, well-defined structures of the T-zone and are comparable to the follicles with and without germinal centers seen in the B-cell region. We therefore prefer the term T-nodule.

T-nodules are greatly enlarged in itching skin diseases. The enlargement is mainly due to an increase in histiocytic and interdigitating reticulum cells. The lesion is called dermatopathic lymphadenitis or lipomelanic reticulocytosis.

Other diseases, such as viral infections, lead to a more diffuse type of hyperplasia. The T-zones then contain numerous stimulated lymphocytes and immunoblasts, but no discernible nodules. The dominant histologic impression, namely, the typical mixture of small lymphocytes and activated lymphocytes of different sizes and variable cytoplasmic basophilia, led to the name of this condition: polymorphic hyperplasia of the pulp (*bunte Pulpahyperplasie*; Fig. 20).

[255] Ehrich, 1946; Scothorne and McGregor, 1955.

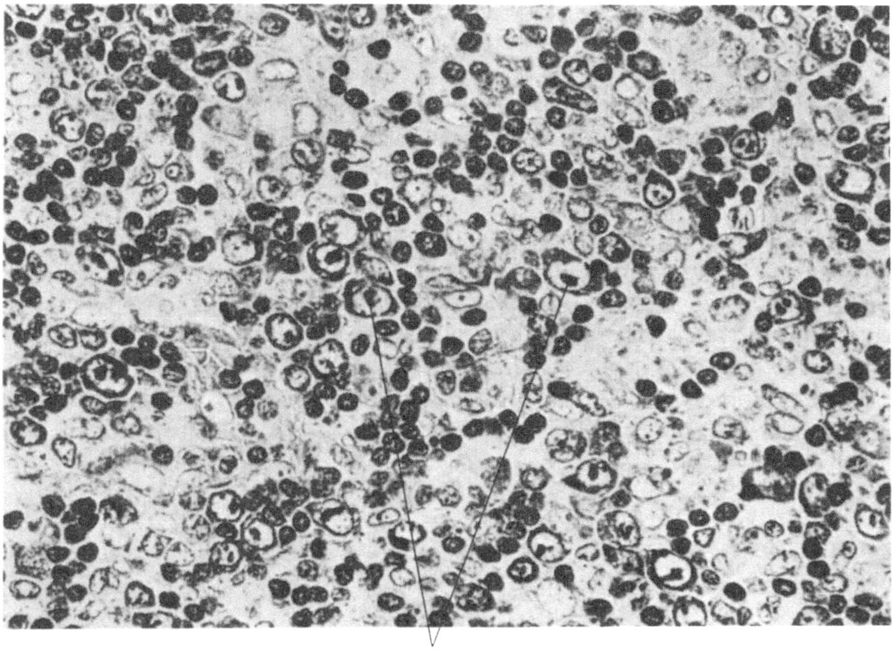


Fig. 20. Polymorphic hyperplasia (*bunte Pulpahyperplasie*) of the pulp. Numerous large immunoblasts (*ibl*) are found among small and activated lymphocytes. Lymph node in infectious mononucleosis. Giemsa. ×350

Both dermatopathic lymphadenitis and polymorphic hyperplasia of the pulp are sequelae of cellular immune reactions.

When we use the term pulp, we mean the diffuse part of lymphatic tissue that is identifiable as neither B- nor T-zone. It is, so to speak, a neutral area of lymphatic tissue. The pulp is composed chiefly of lymphocytes and cells of the plasma-cell series, which are found in perivascular and perisinusoidal areas, i.e., the main traffic routes from the outer cortex to the medulla. The lymphocyte population seen here is thought to comprise a mixture of T- and B-lymphocytes. In so-called polymorphic hyperplasia of the pulp, the infiltrating cells are found in the pulp, including the T-areas, which in this instance are indistinguishable from other parts of the pulp.

Like the B-cell region, T-zones also contain a specific type of reticulum cell in addition to histiocytic and fibroblastic reticulum cells. This cell was first described in rabbits by VELDMAN.[256] Since then, it has also been found in human lymph nodes, spleen, tonsils, and thymic medulla. It is confined to the T-cell regions (see Figs. 23 and 30–32). VELDMAN called this type of reticulum cell the "interdigitating cell" because of the broad villous cell-surface projections that interdigitate with each other. This cytologic feature is most prominent in dermatopathic lymphadenitis.

Whereas different stages of cellular evolution and differentiation can be clearly characterized in B-lymphocytes, this is not possible for T-lymphocytes, at least in man. Many experimental data suggest, however, that similar stages with different functional activities can also be distinguished in T-lymphocytes.

[256] 1970.

# VI. Histochemistry of B- and T-Cell Regions

Different functional compartments in the lymphatic tissue of man can be easily identified by means of cytochemical techniques.[257] The most useful histochemical reactions, which we apply singly or in combination, are the following: (1) nonspecific esterase (α-naphthyl acetate esterase[258]), (2) acid phosphatase,[258] (3) $Mg^{++}$-dependent membrane adenosine triphosphatase (ATPase),[259] (4) 5-nucleotidase,[259] and (5) alkaline phosphatase.

In *B-cell regions* both lymphoid cells and the stationary reticulum cells can be identified cytochemically. The histiocytic reticulum cells of follicles with and without germinal centers are clearly demonstrated by the nonspecific esterase reaction, since they are strongly positive. Dendritic reticulum cells are only moderately positive (Fig. 21). With the acid phosphatase reaction only

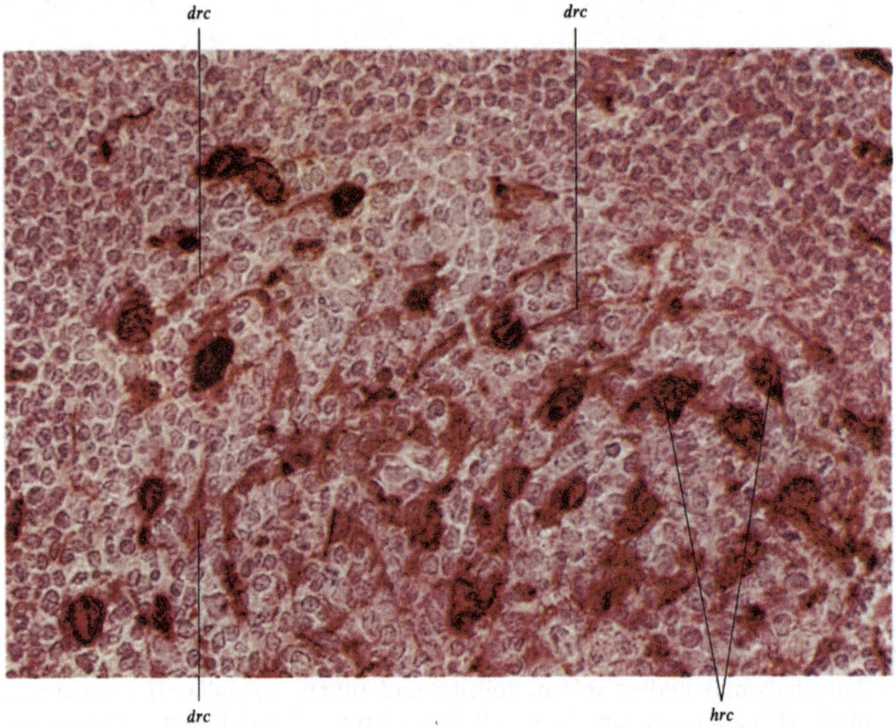


Fig. 21. Germinal center and mantle zone with nonspecific esterase reaction. Note the long cytoplasmic projections of dendritic reticulum cells (*drc*), which reveal moderate enzyme activity. There are some large histiocytic reticulum cells (*hrc*; starry-sky cells) among them that exhibit strong enzyme activity. Nonspecific lymphadenitis. Iliac node. Neutral α-naphthyl acetate esterase reaction. ×340

---

[257] Müller-Hermelink, 1974; Müller-Hermelink, Heusermann and Stutte, 1974; Müller-Hermelink and Kaiserling, 1975.
[258] Leder, 1967.
[259] Lennert and Rinneberg, 1961; Rinneberg, 1961; Müller-Hermelink, 1974; Müller-Hermelink, Heusermann and Stutte, 1974.

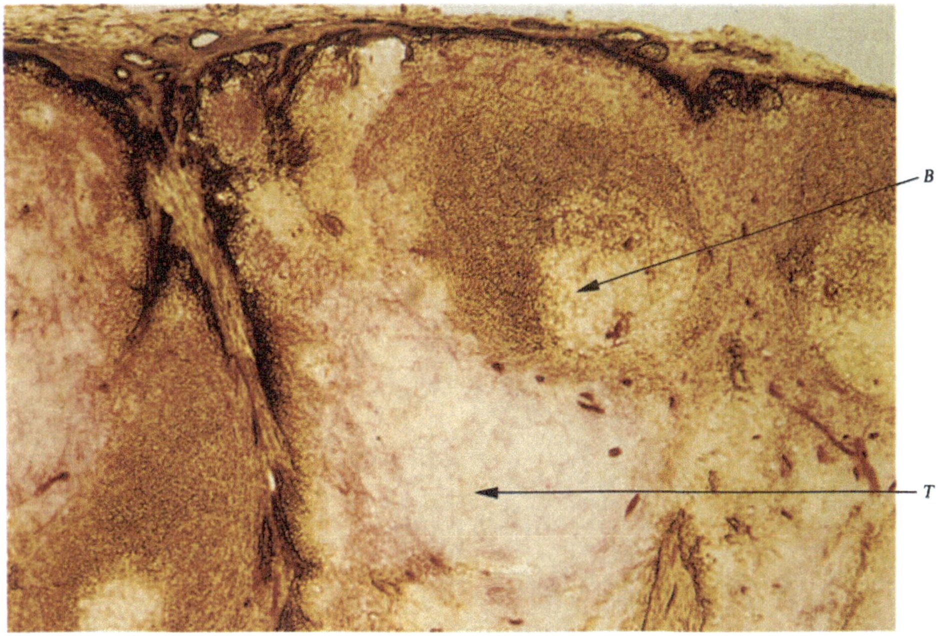


Fig. 22. B- and T-regions of a lymph node in the simultaneous demonstration of alkaline phosphatase (red) and 5-nucleotidase (brown) activity. Germinal centers are weakly positive and lymphocytes in the B-region (*B*) are strongly positive for 5-nucleotidase. The T-region (*T*) is negative for 5-nucleotidase and weakly positive for alkaline phosphatase. Nonspecific lymphadenitis. ♂, 48 years. Cervical node. ×64

histiocytic reticulum cells are strongly positive, whereas dendritic reticulum cells are negative. A positive reaction for acid phosphatase has been reported on the cell surface only at pH values higher than 5.6,[260] which is not comparable to the usual reaction found at pH values below 5.0.

Dendritic reticulum cells exhibit a strong 5-nucleotidase reaction (Fig. 27). The lymphocytes of the follicular mantle zone also react positively (Fig. 22), whereas T-lymphocytes and reticulum cells of the T-nodules remain negative for this enzyme. The histochemical demonstration of ATPase reveals a positive reaction in follicle-mantle lymphocytes and in plasma cells, whereas germinal-center cells (centroblasts and centrocytes) and lymphocytes of T-cell regions are negative. Since B-cell regions are positive for ATPase und 5-nucleotidase, these methods make it easy, at least in cryostat sections of lymphatic tissue, to distinguish positive B-cell regions from negative T-cell regions.

In the *T-cell regions* the specific interdigitating reticulum cells can be recognized by means of histochemical methods. These reticulum cells exhibit a positive ATPase reaction, whereas lymphocytes, as mentioned previously, react negatively (Fig. 23a). In addition, interdigitating reticulum cells show a weak paranuclear reaction for acid phosphatase (Fig. 23b) and a very faint reaction for nonspecific

[260] STEPHAN and BLÜMCKE, 1971.

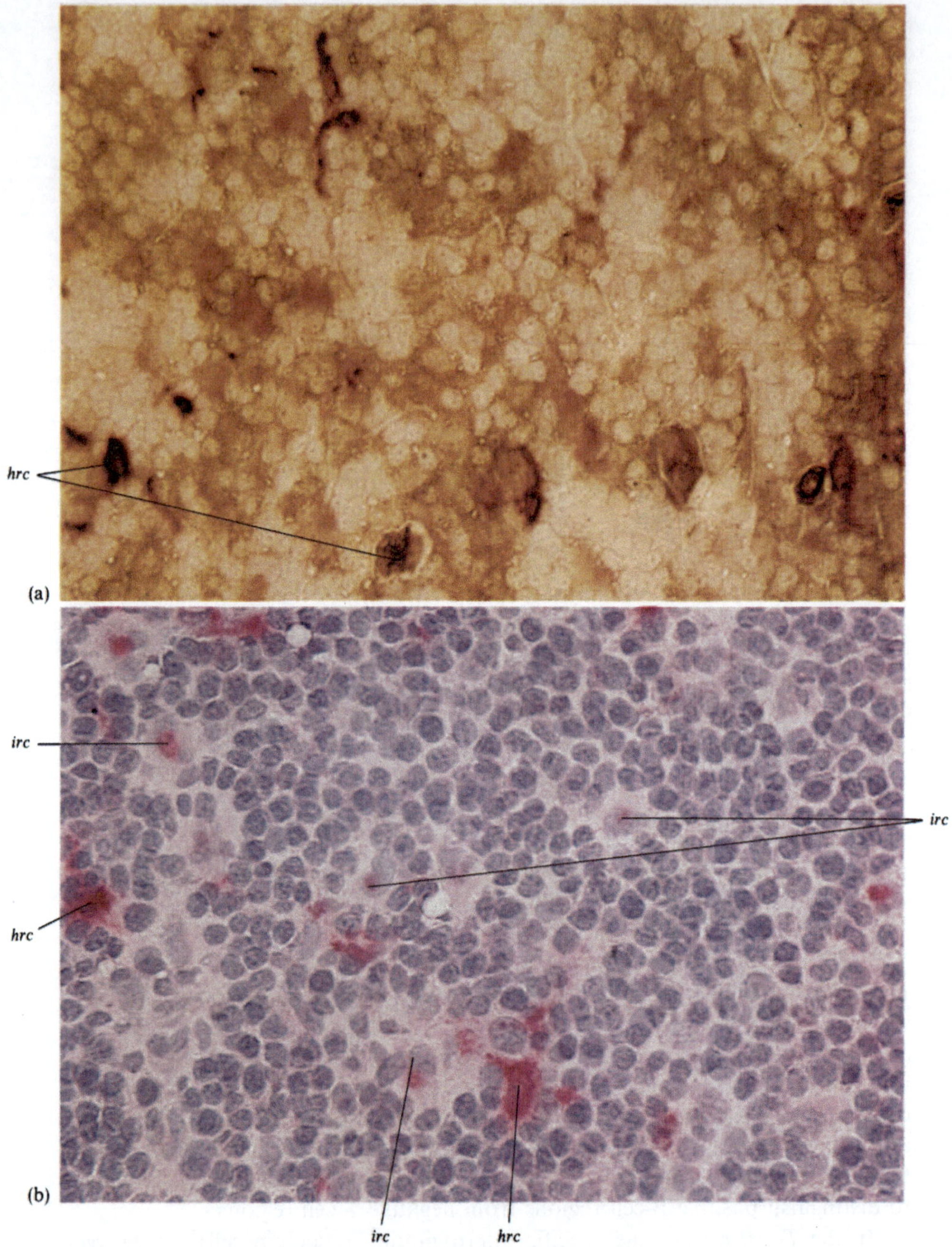


Fig. 23a and b. T-zone with various enzyme reactions. (a) Simultaneous demonstration of ATPase (brown) and α-naphthyl acetate esterase (red) activity. Epithelioid venules and histiocytic reticulum cells (*hrc*) are strongly positive for nonspecific esterase. Interdigitating reticulum cells are moderately positive for ATPase. They form a brown network among the negative lymphocytes. Nonspecific lymphadenitis. ♂, 19 years. Iliac node. × 540. (b) Acid phosphatase reaction. There is weak focal positivity in interdigitating reticulum cells (*irc*). Histiocytic reticulum cells (*hrc*) are strongly positive. Same node as in (a). × 540 esterase. The boundary of the T-nodule is frequently well defined by fibroblastic reticulum cells, which show positive alkaline phosphatase activity.

With the combined demonstration of alkaline phosphatase and 5-nucleotidase activity or of ATPase and acid phosphatase activity, B-cell and T-cell regions are clearly distinguishable in all peripheral lymphatic tissues in man. So far, the enzyme reactivity of the cells has been used only for their cytologic identification. The functional interpretation of these activities, which for the most part represent surface enzymes, has not yet been clarified.

# VII. Stationary Elements of the Lymph Node

## A. Reticulum Cells

The terminology for the stationary elements of the lymph node used to be confusing, because when someone spoke of reticulum cells, he usually presented a table of synonyms for the cells he meant.[261] Even today there is no general agreement on the identity of these cells. As a general morphologic definition, reticulum cells have been considered to be stellate cells with slender cell processes and a light, oval or polymorphic, leptochromatic nucleus. The nucleus has a distinct nuclear membrane and a small or medium-sized nucleolus when observed in hematoxylin and eosin- or Giemsa-stained sections. The cytoplasm is only slightly stained and not basophilic. It is obvious that this definition applies to a variety of cells with different functions. They can be clearly distinguished from each other by means of other techniques.

Some new attempts at classifying reticulum cells have been made. CARR[262] speaks of "reticul*ar* cells," meaning only the antigen-retaining dendritic cells described by NOSSAL *et al.*,[263] and of reticul*um* cells, which include a variety of cells showing transitions to macrophage morphology. STUART[264] interpreted reticulum cells as fiber-associated structural cells, which he studied *in vivo* and *in vitro*. In their proposal for an improved classification of mononuclear phagocytes, VAN FURTH *et al.*[265] agree that the terms reticulum cell and reticular cell may be used synonymously. These authors include the following cells in the common group of mesenchymal cells, which is different from the monocyte-derived MPS: "reticulum cell, dendritic cell, fibroblast, and endothelial cell." The results of our own studies[266] on the structural cells of the human lymphatic system strongly favor the classification of VELDMAN.[267] Among the structural

---

[261] Cf., LENNERT, 1961; HOEFSMIT, 1975.
[262] 1973.
[263] NOSSAL, ABBOT, MITCHELL and LUMMUS, 1968.
[264] 1970, 1975.
[265] VAN FURTH, LANGEVOORT and SCHABERG, 1975.
[266] HEUSERMANN, STUTTE and MÜLLER-HERMELINK, 1974; KAISERLING and LENNERT, 1974; KAISERLING, STEIN and MÜLLER-HERMELINK, 1974; MÜLLER-HERMELINK, 1974; MÜLLER-HERMELINK, HEUSERMANN and STUTTE, 1974; LENNERT and MÜLLER-HERMELINK, 1975; MÜLLER-HERMELINK, 1975; MÜLLER-HERMELINK, HEUSERMANN, KAISERLING and STUTTE, 1976.
[267] 1970.

cells in lymphatic tissue of rabbits, he distinguished dendritic cells, interdigitating cells, fiber-associated reticulum cells, and phagocytic reticulum cells (macrophages). HOEFSMIT[268] includes interdigitating cells in the mononuclear phagocyte system; but she also distinguished four types of reticulum cells. We do not yet know the exact interrelationships between these different cell types. There is practically no information about their cytogenetic derivation and proliferation capacities.

Despite the doubts and myths surrounding the term reticulum cell, we continue to use it. Substituting the word "histiocyte" has only led to further confusion; thus, it is now as surrounded by myths as the term reticulum cell is. The word "macrophage" (free and fixed[269]) does not solve the problem, either, since "macrophage" covers only one variety of reticulum cell of the lymphatic system.

One of the reasons for continuing to use the term reticulum cell is a traditional one. Thousands of pathologists, hematologists, and students of medicine are familiar with its proper sense. That is the sense in which we use it, namely, that reticulum cells are the stationary, structural cells of lympho*reticular* tissue. A more sophisticated distinction of different types of structural cells involved in different functions should not interfere with this general interpretation. We wish to emphasize, however, that the common term does not at all imply a common origin or function. In the following, the term reticulum cell will be applied to a group of at least four different cell types. They are very similar and not every cell can be clearly identified on ordinary light microscopy, but may be differentiated by means of other methods. None of the reticulum cells has a stem-cell function, as we and nearly all hematologists used to believe.

On the basis of our morphologic, cytochemical, and electron-microscopic findings and the function of reticulum cells, we distinguish the following four main types:

1. Histiocytic reticulum cell.
2. Fibroblastic reticulum cell.
3. Dendritic reticulum cell.
4. Interdigitating reticulum cell.

Even the broad interpretation applied here is not without difficulties. We wish to mention two main reasons for confusion:

1. We include the term "histiocytic" reticulum cell, although most investigators agree that these cells are derived from monocytes and belong to the MPS. Even today, though, there is no general agreement on whether all macrophages of the tissue are monocytogenic. Another reason for using this term is one of tradition, namely, that this type of cell has always been called reticulum cell. When the cells do not contain ingested material, they cannot be distinguished from other types of reticulum cells on ordinary light microscopy.

2. We use the term "fibroblastic" reticulum cell for the reticulum cells that are closely associated with reticulin fibers and that are positive for alkaline phosphatase. These cells differ from fibroblasts and fibrocytes of the connective tissue in two morphologic features: (1) they exhibit a close hemidesmosome-

[268] 1975.

[269] VAN FURTH, COHN, HIRSCH, HUMPHREY *et al.*, 1972.

like junction to the accompanying fibers, and (2) the fibers are of the reticular type with a large amount of basement membrane-like, amorphous or fibrillar substance. Fiber production by fibroblastic reticulum cells cannot be proved morphologically. The strong alkaline phosphatase activity seen along the cells, however, points to some function in fiber formation.

When we say that reticulum cells belong to the stationary parts of the lymph node, we do not mean that additional cells cannot come from the blood or that an increase in reticulum cells is not possible. The term stationary is used to express the fact that these parts represent the relatively stable structural elements of the lymph node that offer the emigrating and immigrating lymphocytes a "home," making it possible for these cells to reside in the lymph node for a certain time. The specific reticulum cells of the B- and T-cell regions might have some sort of guiding function: they might provide the ecologic milieu that attracts the B- or T-lymphocytes and motivates their functional cooperation. Therefore, reticulum cells probably have not only a supporting function; i.e., they not only form the stroma of lymphatic tissue, but also probably interact with the lymphocytes in a relatively specific manner. It is likely that a very finely tuned synergy is realized, although we do not yet understand the details.

### *1. Histiocytic Reticulum Cell*

The histiocytic reticulum cell corresponds chiefly to the cell that has been called "histiocyte" since the time of KIYONO.[270] We avoid using the term histiocyte. One reason is that, like BESSIS,[271] we applied it to a medium-sized cell of the lymph node that was able to phagocytose and that we now regard as an immigrant monocyte. Our histiocytic reticulum cell is equivalent to the fixed macrophage defined in the new classification of the MPS.[269]

The histiocytic reticulum cell is large and has plump, moderately long processes that extend between the cells of the lymphatic parenchyma. Sometimes the cell is rounded, particularly in the sinus. Histiocytic reticulum cells are found in all areas of the lymph node, even in germinal centers, where they are distributed like stars in the sky (starry-sky cells). They are often densely concentrated in the sinus (so-called sinus histiocytosis). Otherwise, they show a relatively uniform distribution in the pulp and follicles.

**Cytochemistry.** Histiocytic reticulum cells contain the greatest amount of acid phosphatase and nonspecific esterase known in lymphatic tissue. The PAS reaction is generally negative, but after phagocytosis of lymphocytes, for example, histiocytic reticulum cells frequently show globular or uncharacteristic PAS-positive intracytoplasmic deposits. They may also contain Sudan-positive lipoids, hemosiderin, and other substances. Furthermore, they are metallophilic.

**Ultrastructure.** The nucleus is round or oval. In its center there is a medium-sized nucleolus with coarse nucleolonemata (Fig. 24). The chromatin is slightly

[270] 1914. [271] 1954.

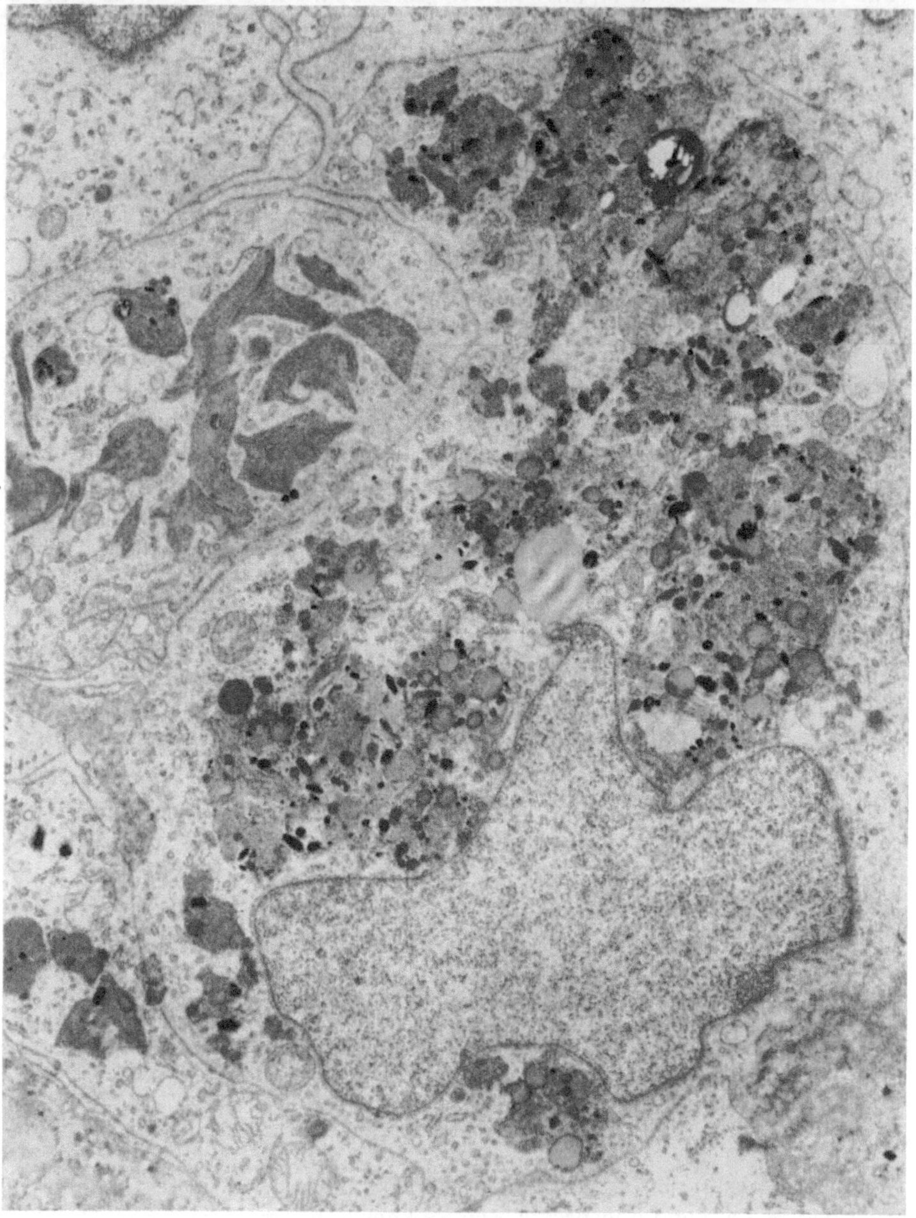


Fig. 24. Histiocytic reticulum cell in the pulp in a case of dermatopathic lymphadenitis. The large phagosomes contain amorphous material, melanin, and lipofuscin (*x*). At the upper left, part of another histiocytic reticulum cell with phagosomes containing ceroid (*xx*). × 10,000

electron-dense and fine; it reveals slight condensation along the nuclear membrane. The rim of cytoplasm is usually broad. Wide cell processes extend between the lymphoid cells. The cytoplasm reveals one or more large, well-developed Golgi fields. In the rest of the cytoplasm one sees short, sometimes branched membranes of smooth endoplasmic reticulum and a variable amount of rough endoplasmic reticulum. Most characteristic are the often large phagolysosomes containing still-recognizable cell and membrane remnants. There are also smaller electron-dense lysosomes. The relatively large number of mitochondria indicates high metabolic activity.

In the lymph node histiocytic reticulum cells differ especially in the type of inclusions. For example, in germinal centers one finds practically only starry-sky cells, i.e., macrophages that have phagocytosed cells and whose phagolysosomes contain cells in various stages of degradation or cell fragments. Characteristically, these starry-sky cells have a light, round or oval nucleus and a light, translucent cytoplasm with relatively little ergastoplasm. The paracortical area reveals histiocytic reticulum cells that as a rule contain other products. In the phagolysosomes of these cells one often sees particularly abundant ceroid, melanin, or hemosiderin and other substances that cannot be clearly defined.

**Function.** Histiocytic reticulum cells phagocytose endogenous cells and every type of foreign substance, and digest them when possible. When that is not possible, the foreign substances are stored. When phagocytosis is pronounced, the histiocytic reticulum cells become rounded; they are then also called macrophages. Such macrophages also develop from immigrant monocytes. These cells are at first much smaller and contain only moderate acid phosphatase and nonspecific esterase activity. Within 24 hours they may be strongly activated. They then attain the size and enzyme activity of stationary histiocytic reticulum cells ("activated macrophages" of MACKANESS[272]). Histiocytic reticulum cells do not form reticulin fibers.

## *Addendum*

### *Epithelioid Cell*

We understand the epithelioid cell as a special monocyte-derived, evolutionary form of macrophages. It is found chiefly in the T-cell region, but may also be observed in germinal centers and sinuses.

**Cytochemistry.** The nonspecific esterase and acid phosphatase reactions are weakly to strongly positive, but not as strongly positive as in macrophages. A granular PAS reaction is always seen in imprints. Furthermore, one finds very strong ATPase activity. Recent histochemical investigation of epithelioid-cell granulomas showed that acid phosphatase activity was high in early stages, but that it decreased in later stages. Nonspecific esterase and ATPase activity did not change, whereas aminopeptidase activity increased.[273] Epithelioid cells exhibit high metabolic activity, as suggested by the high enzymatic activities of the pentose cycle, the Krebs cycle, anaerobic glycolysis, enzymes of the respiratory chain, and hydrolytic enzymes.[274]

---

[272] 1969, 1970, 1971; LEDER, 1967; RABENHORST, 1972.

[273] ECKERT, ZAUMSEIL and SEHRT, 1976, personal communication.

[274] WILLIAMS, WILLIAMS and WILLIAMS, 1969; PALVA, DAMMERT and PALVA, 1973; ECKERT, ZAUMSEIL and SEHRT, 1976, personal communication.

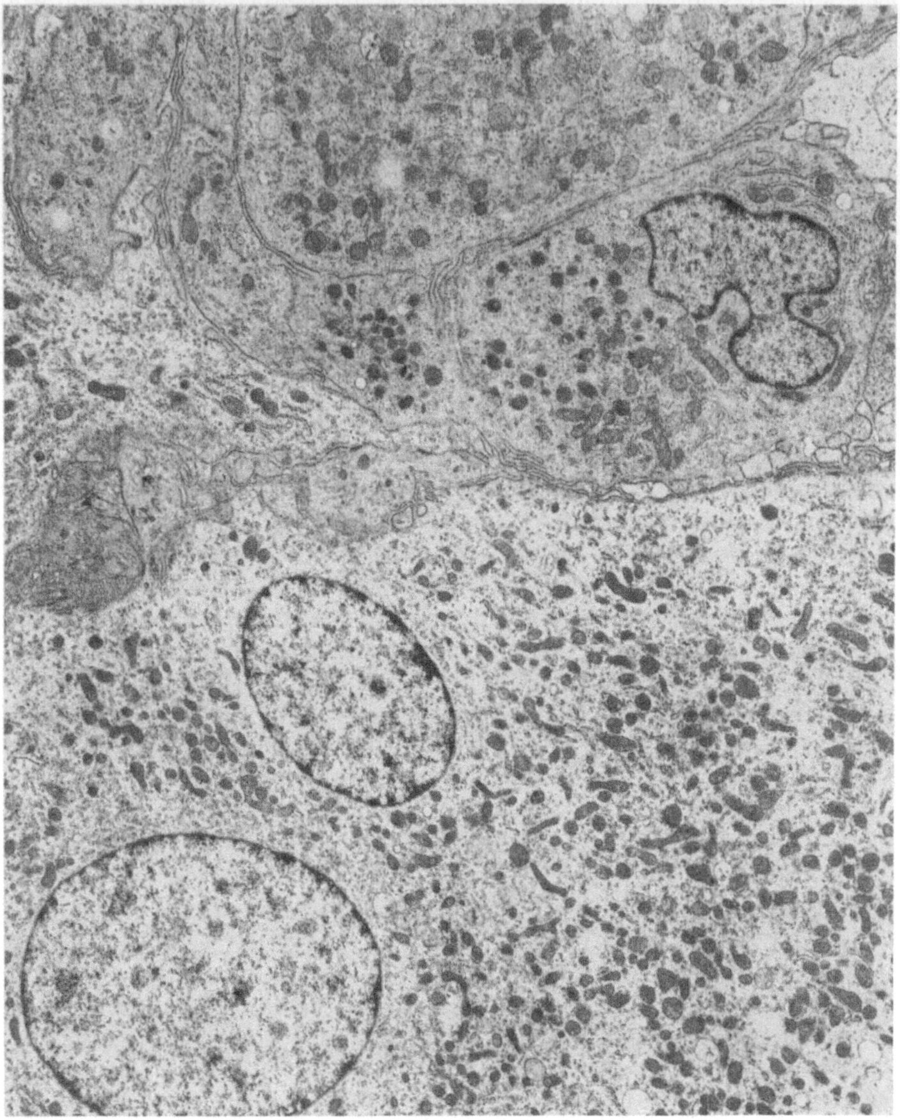

Fig. 25. Epithelioid cells (top) and Langhans' giant cell (bottom) in sarcoidosis. They are interconnected by interdigitating surface projections. The epithelioid cells and the giant cell contain abundant electron-dense vesicles and ergastoplasm. × 8,500

**Ultrastructure.**[275] The epithelioid cell (Fig. 25) ranges up to 20 μm or more in diameter. Its cytoplasmic membrane displays irregular projections. At points of contact between neighboring cells the invaginations of one cell often interdigitate closely with evaginations of another. The nucleus is situated eccentrically and measures about 10 μm in diameter. For the most part, the nuclear membrane exhibits irregular indentations, and the nuclear chromatin is uniformly dispersed.

[275] Mori and Lennert, 1969.

One or two medium-sized nucleoli may be visible. Numerous mitochondria and a large amount of smooth endoplasmic reticulum fill a large portion of the cytoplasm. The mitochondria display denser matrices than the cytoplasm and contain cristae in an orderly array. Many endoplasmic vesicles may be encountered in the center of the cells. In typical epithelioid cells the vesicles contain electron-lucent material. In some cells, however, presumed to be somewhat younger epithelioid cells, electron-opaque material is enclosed within the vesicles. A small amount of rough endoplasmic reticulum tends to concentrate at the periphery of the cell. Several Golgi bodies occupy central positions. They consist of lamellar, vacuolar, and vesicular components. YAMORI[276] has divided epithelioid cells into two groups: typical epithelioid cells and "pre-epithelioid cells." The latter do not yet reveal distinct interdigitations, and they have a paucity of rough endoplasmic reticulum. Ribosomes are greatly reduced in number, and large phagosomes are absent.

**Function.** *Macrophages* are not, or are only insufficiently, capable of killing facultative intracellular parasites such as BCG, listeria, or toxoplasmas. Subtle quantitative electron-microscopic studies revealed that dead BCG and toxoplasmas can be digested immediately by macrophages, but that living pathogens can proliferate in the cytoplasm.[277] Furthermore, electron-microscopic analysis showed that when living pathogens are present, the primary lysosomes do not empty into the phagosome to provide the necessary digestive enzymes.[277] The ability to kill bacteria intracellularly is transferred to macrophages through sensitized lymphocytes,[278] especially T-lymphocytes,[279] or lymphocyte mediators.[280] There is a fundamental change in the metabolism of the macrophages; they are then called activated macrophages.[281] The decisive substance effecting the intracellular killing of bacteria under these conditions has not yet been clearly identified; but mechanisms similar to the ones in extracellular killing of bacteria may be involved.[282] The killing of intracellular bacteria does not occur specifically: macrophages activated by BCG are also able to decompose and kill listeria more quickly.[281]

Immunologically activated macrophages are able not only to decompose intracellular pathogens more quickly, but also to secrete a product that is able to kill extracellular listeria.[283] The secretion of acid phosphatase,[284] collagenase, elastase,[285] lysozyme, and plasminogen activator[286] has also been observed.[287]

In contrast to activated macrophages with increased phagocytic capacities, *epithelioid cells* do not phagocytose to any considerable degree. They show instead high secretory activity owing to a large amount of rough endoplasmic reticulum, multiple large Golgi bodies, and a large number of intracytoplasmic vesicles. This change in function was demonstrated by GORDON,[286] who found that cultured macrophages show increased secretory activity with time, i.e., that

[276] 1964.
[277] ARMSTRONG and D'ARCY HART, 1971; JONES and HIRSCH, 1972.
[278] MACKANESS, 1969.
[279] LANE and UNANUE, 1972.
[280] NATH, POULTER and TURK, 1973.
[281] MACKANESS, 1970.
[282] KLEBANOFF and HAMON, 1975.
[283] BAST, CLEVELAND, LITTMAN, ZBAR *et al.*, 1974.
[284] KALINA, KLETTER, SHAHAR and ARONSON, 1971.
[285] WERB and GORDON, 1975a, b.
[286] GORDON, 1975.
[287] UNANUE, 1976.

during the maturation process the function of macrophages turns from ingestion to secretion. One of the most important factors in the formation of epithelioid cells is time,[288] which would also fit into this concept.

Although formation of epithelioid cells also occurs in chronic foreign-body granulomas and in other chronic nonspecific inflammatory reactions, it usually seems to be conditioned immunologically. It may be effected either through increased local immobilization of macrophages by T-lymphocyte products, or through direct stimulation of macrophages by certain lymphocyte mediators, as suggested by the work of SCHMIDT *et al.*[288a] Thus, an epithelioid-cell granuloma may be considered to be a second-line barrier that acts when the defense mechanism of phagocytosis is not capable of eliminating invading microorganisms. This interpretation is given further support by the finding that epithelioid-cell granulomas are found in infections with pus-forming, gram-positive bacteria when the phagocytosis mechanism is defect, e.g., in chronic septic granulomatosis.

Our findings on BCG histiocytosis[289] and similar changes in lepromatous leprosy[290] show that a great increase in macrophages occurs in both lesions. The macrophages contain massive numbers of bacteria that evidently cannot be killed. On the other hand, the formation of epithelioid-cell tubercles is not possible in either lesion, in contrast to typical tuberculosis and tuberculoid leprosy. The main reason for that is probably insufficiency of the cellular immune apparatus. The lack of T-lymphocytes or of certain clones of T-lymphocytes prevents the formation of epithelioid cells. A second prerequisite for the development of BCG histiocytosis is evidently the kind of pathogen. It must not be too toxic. Mycobacterial histiocytosis is induced by BCG, *Mycobacterium avium,* and photochromogenic mycobacteria. These mild infections affect individuals with a defective immune system, e.g., with Swiss-type agammaglobulinemia.

In conclusion, the epitheloid cell is not simply a histiocyte, as is often maintained. Instead, it is, as a rule, a monocyto*genic* cell that no longer phagocytoses. Its development is complicated and, at least in bacterial infections, immunologically conditioned.

### *2. Fibroblastic Reticulum Cell ("Dictyocyte")*

Fibroblastic reticulum cells are found chiefly in the neighborhood of capillaries and venous and arterial vessels. A characteristic pattern of fibroblastic reticulum cells is found at the margins of the T-zones in the various peripheral lymphatic tissues. In principle, however, single fibroblastic reticulum cells can be found in all regions of the lymph node. We cannot yet identify them on light microscopy.

**Cytochemistry.** Fibroblastic reticulum cells contain only small amounts of nonspecific esterase and acid phosphatase. The latter can hardly be identified in sections. Instead, they reveal large amounts of the surface enzyme alkaline

---

[288] SPECTOR and MARIANO, 1975.
[288a] SCHMIDT, DOUGLAS and RUBIN, 1973.
[289] KAISERLING, LENNERT, NITSCH and DRESCHER, 1972.
[290] TURK and WATERS, 1971.

phosphatase, which can be demonstrated by light and electron microscopy. The demonstration of alkaline phosphatase on fibroblastic reticulum cells represents a criterion of activity. One always finds alkaline phosphatase when fresh formation of collagenous fibers can be suspected. On the other hand, fibrocytes, i.e., inactive fiber-producers, of the lymph-node capsule and in older scarred areas are negative for alkaline phosphatase.

**Ultrastructure.** Fibroblastic reticulum cells are often extremely electron-dense. Many of these cells might be equivalent to the so-called dark reticulum cells that have been described in animals and man.[291] In earlier papers,[292] we expressed the opinion that the increased electron density of these reticulum cells can be attributed to intravital damage and therefore represents a manifestation of degeneration. The fibroblastic reticulum cells of lower electron density show the slightly dilated rough endoplasmic reticulum typical of fibroblasts. In addition, the cytoplasm contains a few free ribosomes, a little smooth endoplasmic reticulum, and occasionally a small Golgi apparatus. The nucleus is oblong, sometimes with indentations similar to the teeth of a saw. It contains a central or marginal nucleolus, occasionally layered in rings like that of lymphocytes. Nucleospheroids have been seen several times. A special characteristic is the relationship of the cells to reticulin fibers. This relationship is often seen as hemidesmosomes (Fig. 26). The cytoplasmic side of the unit membrane is condensed, and on this side one sees converging tonofibrils, whereas the side of the cytomembrane lying against the fibers is smooth. Occasionally, tonofibrils appear to break through the membrane and to penetrate the adjacent fibers. In addition to rough endoplasmic reticulum, the cytoplasm may contain bundles of tonofibrils. The adventitia cells of vessels often cannot be distinguished from fibroblastic reticulum cells. They are identical according to morphologic criteria. In contrast, fibroblasts of connective tissue usually do not show a close relationship to adjacent fibers. Furthermore, the type of fiber differs. In connective tissue the fibers are collagenous and there is little interfibrillar substance, whereas lymphatic tissue contains mostly basement membrane-like substances and little collagen.

**Function.** By definition, the cells are thought to form the reticulin fibers of the lymph node, whereas they do not phagocytose, or at least not to any significant degree.

### *3. Dendritic Reticulum Cell (Long-Branching Nonphagocytosing Reticulum Cell)*

Dendritic reticulum cells are specific to the B-cell region and, accordingly, are found in large numbers in germinal centers (see p. 34ff.), where they are difficult to distinguish from starry-sky cells on light microscopy. With some practice, however, a distinction is often possible (see Table 2). The nuclei of dendritic reticulum cells are elongate, often irregularly cornered or angular.

[291] Izard and DeHarven, 1968; Mollo, Monga and Stramignoni, 1969.

[292] Müller-Hermelink and Caesar, 1969; Müller-Hermelink, Kaiserling and Lennert, 1973.

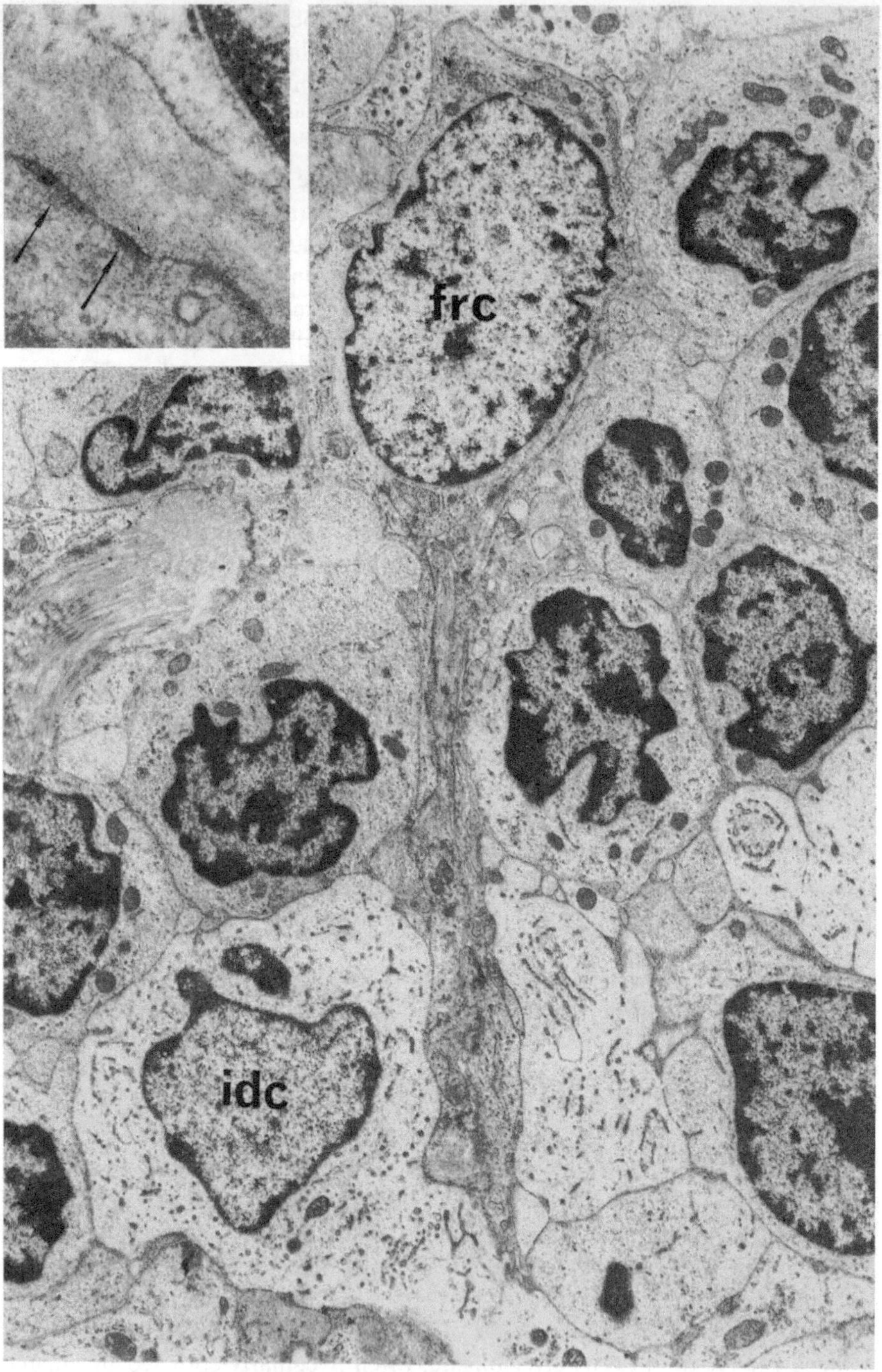


Fig. 26. Fibroblastic reticulum cell (*frc*) and interdigitating reticulum cell (*idc*) in the T-zone. × 8,500. Inset: the fibroblastic reticulum cell shows hemidesmosomal junctions (arrows) to adjacent reticulin fibers. × 48,000

Table 2. Light-microscopic and cytochemical differences between dendritic reticulum cells and starry-sky cells (histiocytic reticulum cells) of germinal centers

| | Dendritic reticulum cell | Starry-sky cell |
|---|---|---|
| Nucleus | | |
| Shape | Elongate, occasionally angular | Round |
| Nucleolus | Single, medium-sized, moderately basophilic (gray) | Single, medium-sized, slightly basophilic (gray-reddish) |
| Membrane | Clearly discernible | Weaker-staining |
| Cytoplasm | | |
| Staining | Light gray, hardly visible | Gray-reddish, clearly visible |
| Amount | Very small | Large |
| Phagocytosis | – | +++ |
| Localization | Especially in light part of germinal center and in marginal zone | Either uniformly distributed in germinal center or in dark part |
| Cytochemistry | | |
| Nonspecific esterase | + | +++ |
| Acid phosphatase | – | +++ |
| 5-nucleotidase | + | – |
| PAS | – | Occasional positive cytoplasmic inclusions |

The nuclear membrane is clearly defined. In the middle of the nucleus there is a medium-sized, moderately basophilic nucleolus. With Giemsa staining the rim of cytoplasm around the nucleus is narrow and very weakly stained light gray. The long thin cytoplasmic processes cannot be made out.

In contrast, the histiocytic reticulum cells of germinal centers (starry-sky cells) show large round bright nuclei with a fainter nuclear membrane with Giemsa staining. There are likewise large reddish violet (i.e., very slightly basophilic) nucleoli in the middle of the cell. The rim of cytoplasm is wide and weakly stained gray-reddish. It usually contains cell debris and vacuoles. The outer margin of the cells is usually identifiable.

The distribution of both types of reticulum cells in the germinal center makes their identification easier. Dendritic reticulum cells are found chiefly in the light (upper) part of the germinal center, whereas the histiocytic forms (starry-sky cells) are uniformly distributed throughout the germinal center, or they are situated in the dark lower part.

**Cytochemistry.** Dendritic reticulum cells contain moderately abundant nonspecific esterase, which can be followed right out into the processes. This esterase activity is much weaker than that of histiocytic reticulum cells or macrophages. In contrast to these cells, dendritic reticulum cells do not reveal any acid phos-

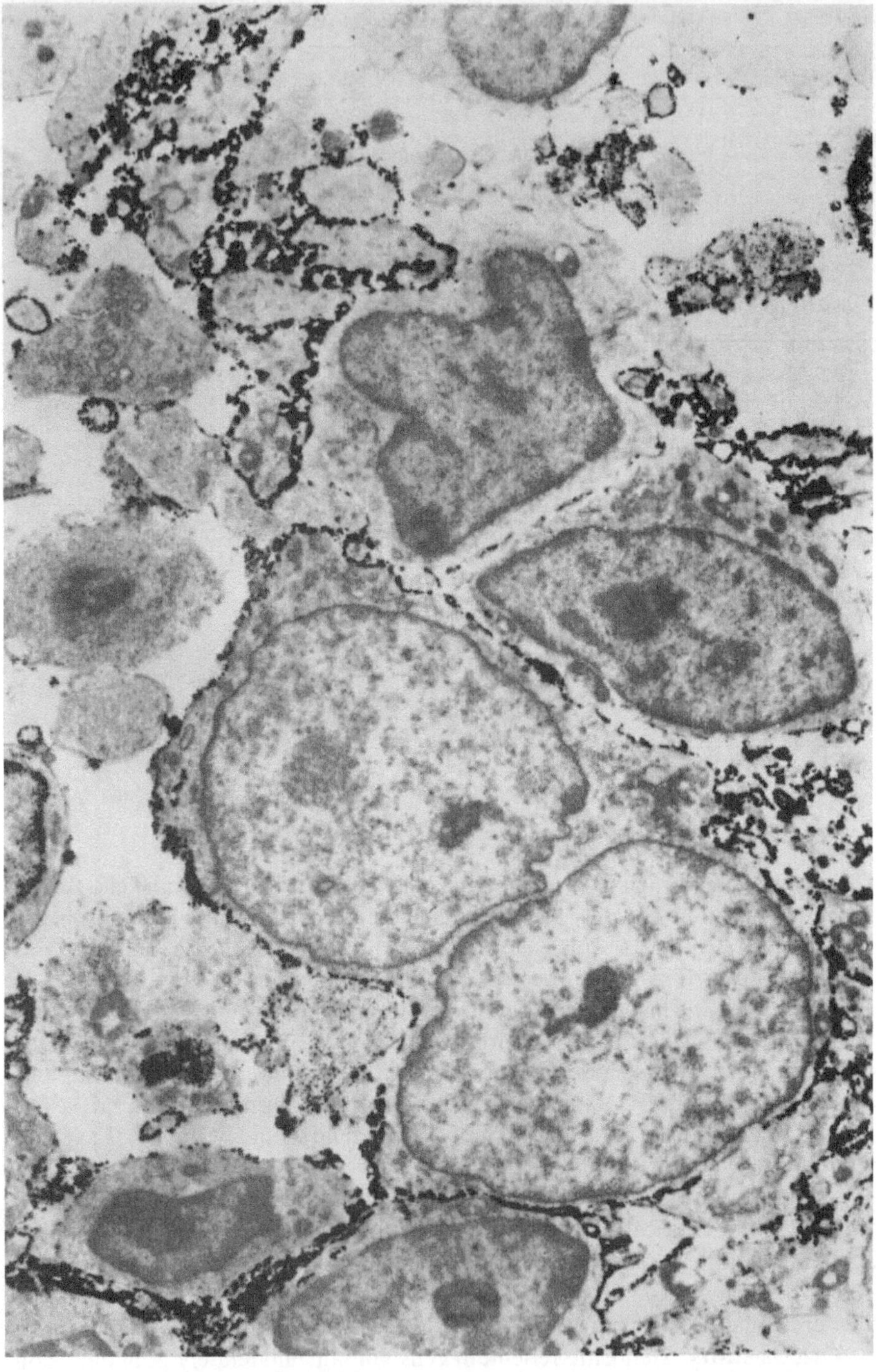

Fig. 27. 5-nucleotidase reaction of a binucleate dendritic reticulum cell (lower half of the picture). There is strong surface activity. Adjacent centrocytes are negative. The lymphocyte at the bottom (mantle zone) is positive. ×9,200

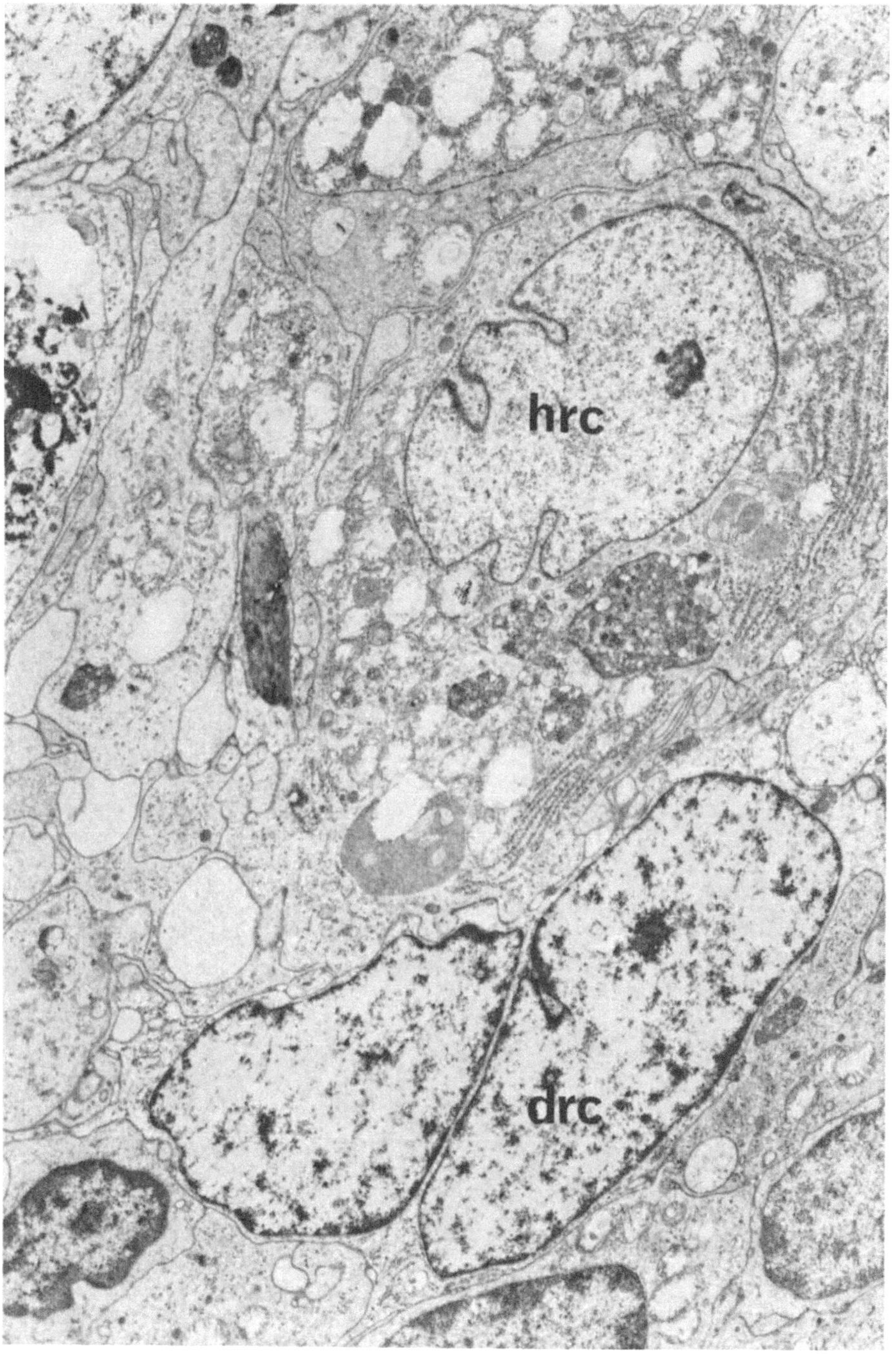


Fig. 28. Histiocytic reticulum cell (*hrc*) and binucleate dendritic reticulum cell (*drc*) in a germinal center. Note the difference in the chromatin patterns of the nuclei. The broad rim of cytoplasm of the histiocytic reticulum cell contains remnants of phagocytosed and degraded cells. ×8,500

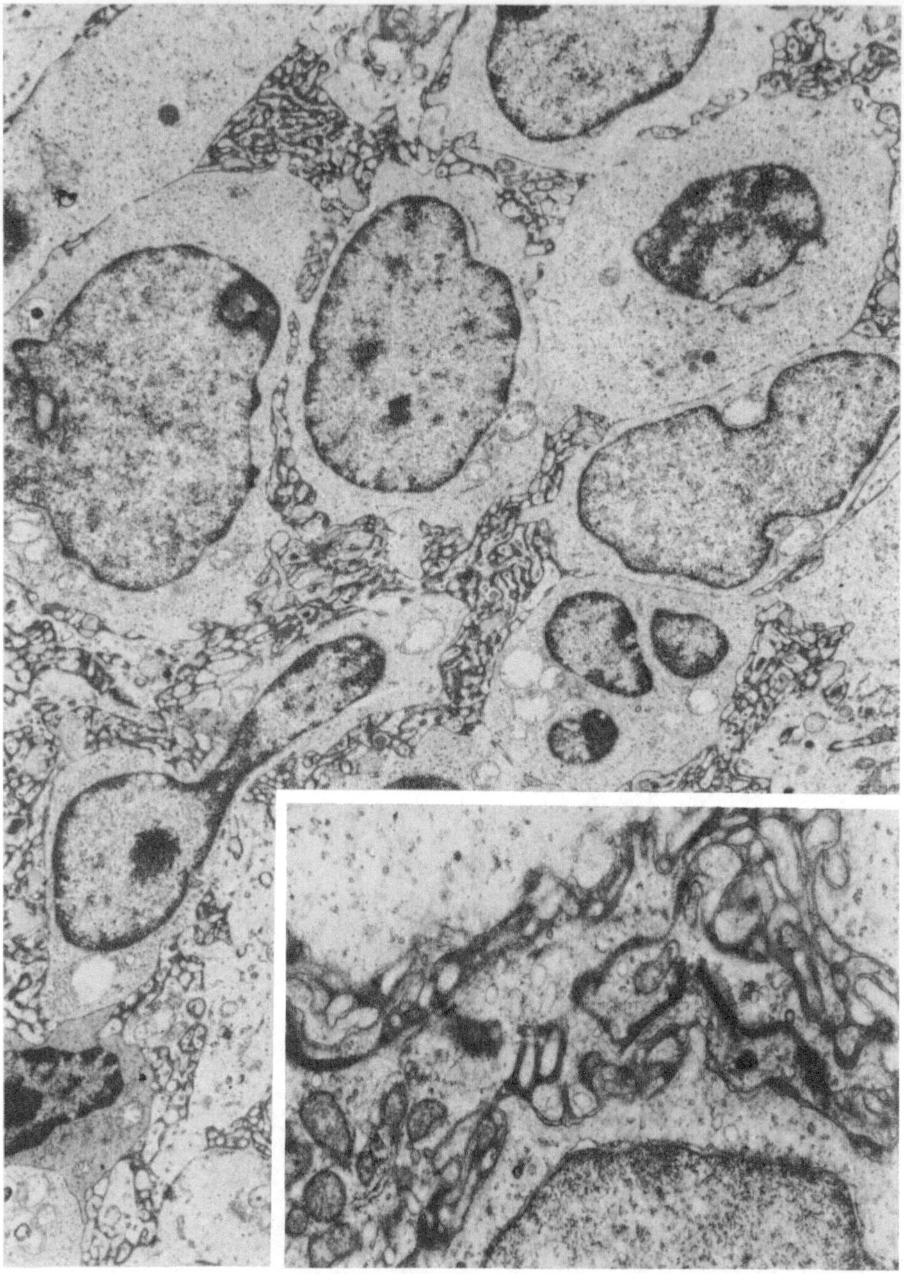

Fig. 29. Part of the light zone of a germinal center revealing interwoven cellular projections of dendritic reticulum cells lying among centroblasts and centrocytes. The surface projections are connected by desmosomes (inset). × 4,600, inset: × 22,000

phatase on light microscopy. The 5-nucleotidase reaction is strongly positive in dendritic reticulum cells (Fig. 27). The PAS reaction is negative.

**Ultrastructure.** Dendritic reticulum cells of germinal centers usually have an oval nucleus. Sometimes it has three or more corners. As a rule, the nuclear chromatin is coarser than that of histiocytic reticulum cells, and it is clearly condensed in a narrow zone along the inner nuclear membrane. The central solitary nucleolus shows coarsely interwoven nucleolonemata. Nucleospheroids are frequently seen. The rim of cytoplasm is extremely narrow around the nucleus and is often only a fraction of a micron wide. In the cytoplasm one recognizes profiles of well-developed smooth endoplasmic reticulum, but no acid phosphatase-positive lysosomes and certainly no phagosomes. The cytoplasm pushes itself between the centrocytes and centroblasts as very fine interwoven processes and forms a rootlike network with other dendritic reticulum cells and with adjacent centroblasts. The cell projections of the dendritic reticulum cells are often connected with each other by desmosomes. KOJIMA and IMAI[293] also found desmosomal junctions with lymphoid cells. We could not confirm this finding. Between the cell processes one sees electron-dense granular material, which corresponds to the antigen-antibody complexes demonstrated there. In later stages of germinal-center formation, fibrin and collagen fibrils are also seen between the processes. The relationship of the cell membrane to the adjacent collagenous fibers is, however, different from that of the fibroblastic reticulum cells in that no hemidesmosomal junctions are formed.

### *4. Interdigitating Reticulum Cell*

Interdigitating reticulum cells are found only in T-cell regions. It is easiest to study this type of reticulum cell in dermatopathic lymphadenitis. The nuclei are polymorphic, often indented on one side or oddly "crumpled" with several folds and depressions (Fig. 30). The nucleoli are small and lie either at the nuclear membrane or in the middle of the nucleus. The nuclear membrane is clearly defined. The rim of cytoplasm is broad and weak grayish blue with Giemsa staining.

**Cytochemistry.** In contrast to histiocytic reticulum cells, interdigitating reticulum cells contain almost no nonspecific esterase. The α-naphthyl acetate esterase reaction reveals only a fine reddish sheen over the cytoplasm. The acid phosphatase reaction is also weakly positive, namely, in a circumscribed cytoplasmic area at the site of nuclear indentations, probably in and near the Golgi zone. On the other hand, interdigitating reticulum cells show a moderately strong ATPase reaction (Fig. 31),[294] which is not found in histiocytic reticulum cells. The alkaline phosphatase reaction is negative. The PAS reaction usually reveals *very* fine granules. These granules can be demonstrated better by means of the silver methenamine method on electron microscopy.[295]

**Ultrastructure.** The nucleus is markedly lobed and indented (Fig. 32). The chromatin is finely dispersed and condensed at the inner nuclear membrane.

[293] 1973.

[294] MÜLLER-HERMELINK, 1974.

[295] VELDMAN, 1970; KAISERLING and LENNERT, 1974.

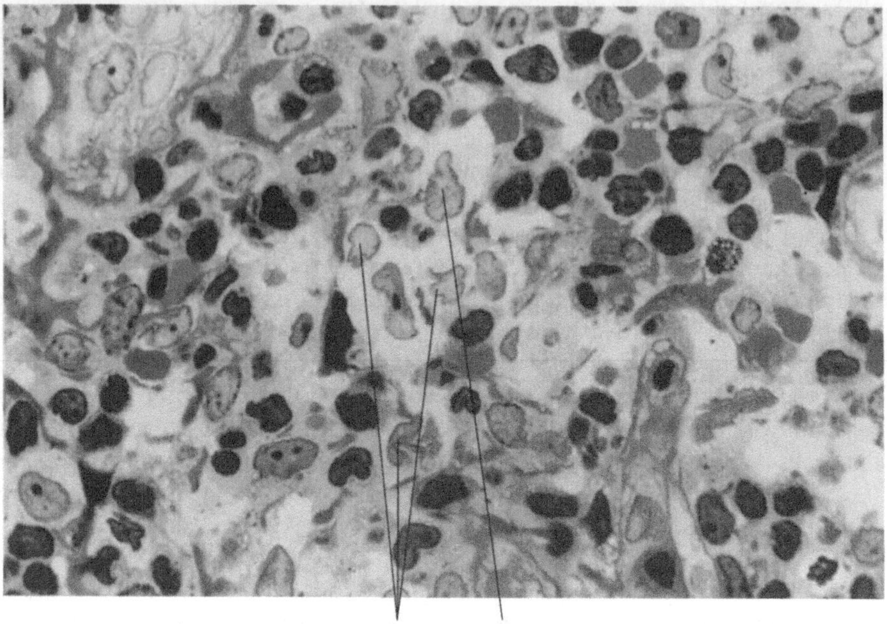


Fig. 30. Interdigitating reticulum cells (*irc*) in dermatopathic lymphadenitis. Note the irregular nuclear contours and the clear cytoplasm. Semithin section, azure II methylene blue. ×480

There is usually a marginal nucleolus. The rim of cytoplasm contains numerous short narrow vesicles and profiles of rough and smooth endoplasmic reticulum. Near the nucleus one finds a medium-sized or large Golgi apparatus. In the cytoplasm there are sometimes larger vesicles surrounded by a unit membrane. The cell surface is especially characteristic. It has numerous processes that are interwoven with neighboring interdigitating cells and lymphocytes, thus forming a system of interdigitating cell projections and membrane invaginations. The tubules and vesicles of endoplasmic reticulum are positive with silver methenamine staining. In the cytoplasm one also finds a moderate number of ribosomes, free ribosomes, a few polyribosomes, and moderately abundant mitochondria.

**Function.** The exact function of interdigitating reticulum cells is still unknown. They have been found in all peripheral lymphatic tissues in man.[296] VEERMAN[297] presented some evidence that they are derived from monocytes. Phagocytosis, however, is not a major function of interdigitating reticulum cells. A few small electron-dense inclusions have been found in these cells only in severe dermatopathic lymphadenitis. The sometimes large Golgi apparatus may indicate morphologically that interdigitating reticulum cells have a secretory function.

[296] HEUSERMANN, STUTTE and MÜLLER-HERMELINK, 1974; KAISERLING and LENNERT, 1974; MÜLLER-HERMELINK, 1974, 1975; MÜLLER-HERMELINK, HEUSERMANN, KAISERLING and STUTTE, 1976.

[297] 1974.

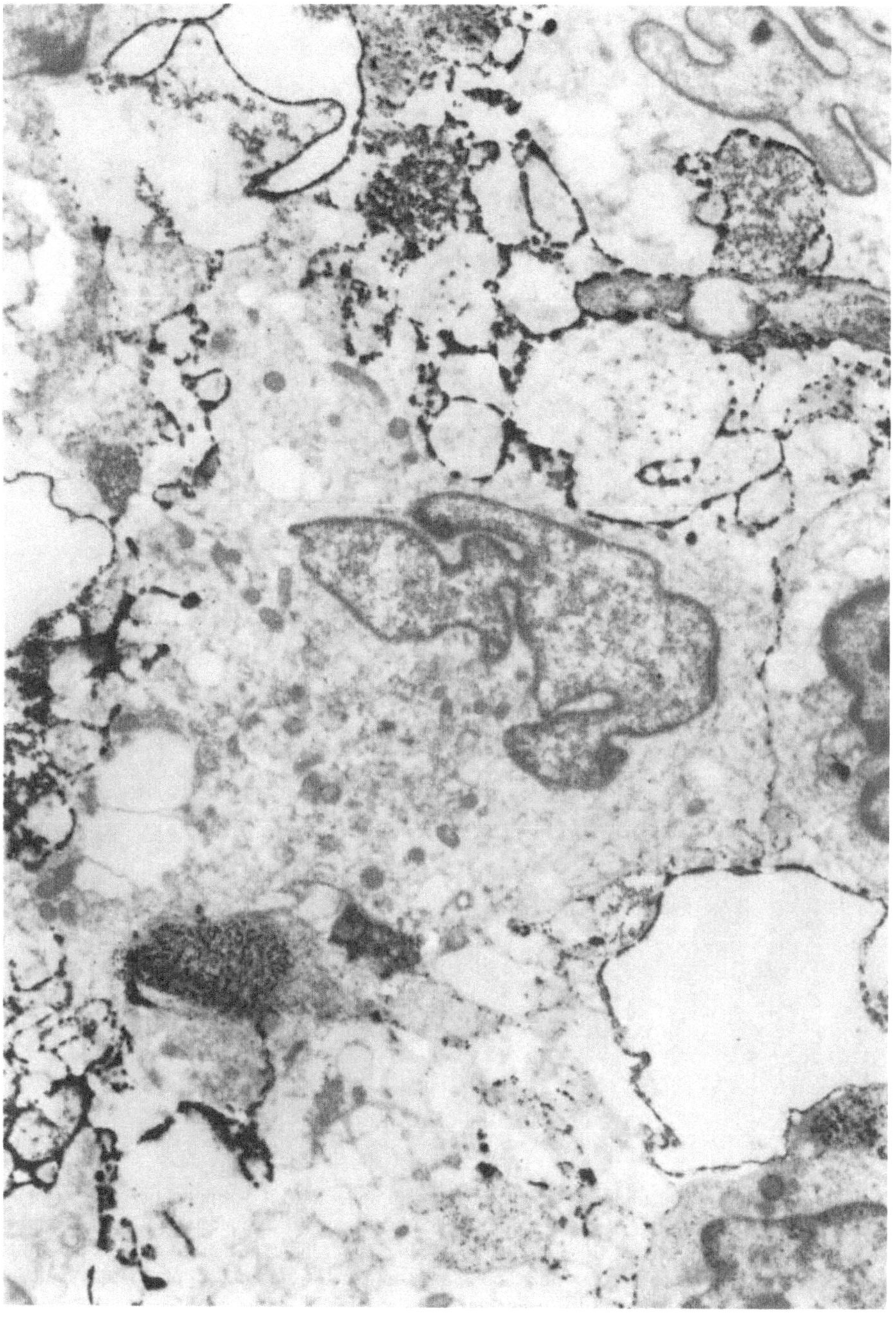

Fig. 31. Demonstration of $Mg^{++}$-dependent ATPase activity in an interdigitating reticulum cell. All of the broad surface projections reveal enzyme activity. × 15,000

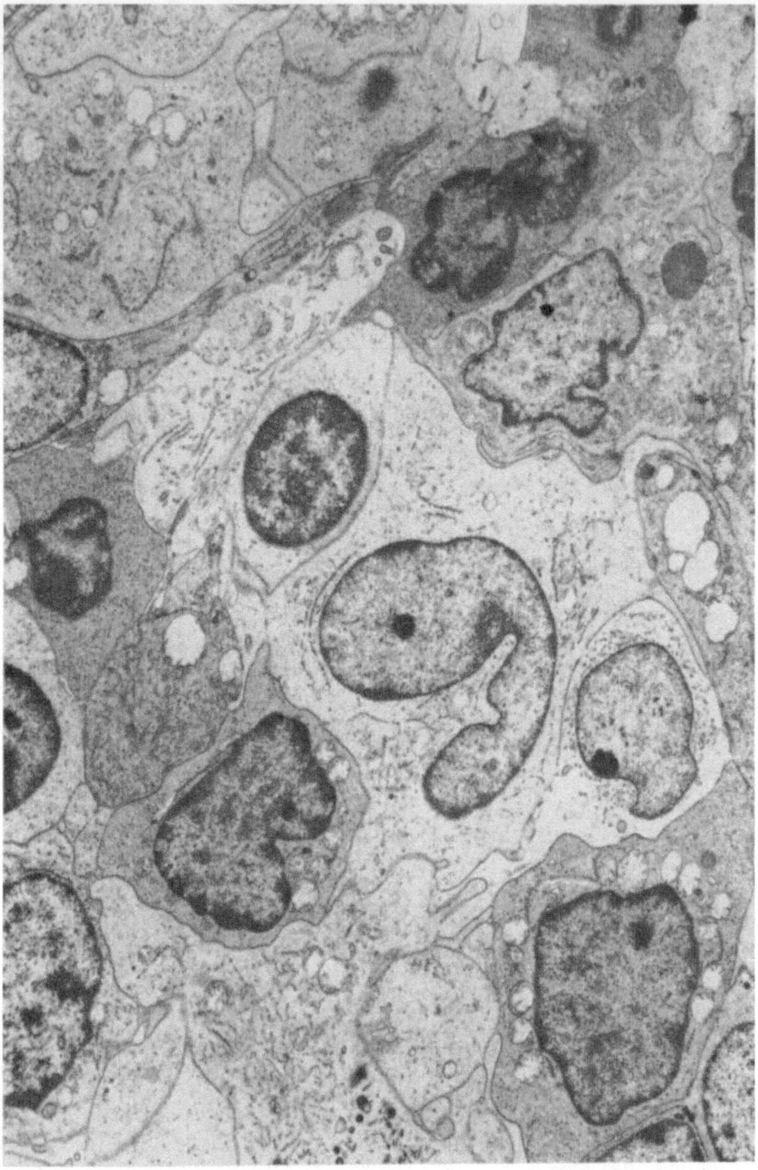


Fig. 32. Interdigitating reticulum cells in a human lymph node. Part of an epithelioid venule (*epv*) is seen at the upper left margin. At upper right there is a histiocytic reticulum cell (*hrc*) that has a more electron-dense cytoplasm than the interdigitating reticulum cells. The latter (central and lower part of the picture) have irregular nuclear contours and a translucent cytoplasm that contains characteristic tubulovesicular endoplasmic reticulum. ×7,500

It is tempting to presume that they build a microenvironment that is necessary for the differentiation and proliferation of T-cells. This has also been stressed by VELDMAN[298] and KAISERLING *et al.*[299]

[298] 1970.

[299] KAISERLING, STEIN and MÜLLER-HERMELINK, 1974.

# B. Sinus Endothelial Cells

Since the publication of Part A of this Handbook, there have been no significant new light-microscopic findings on sinus endothelial cells. Progress in the fields of cytochemistry and electron microscopy has also been modest.

**Cytochemistry.** The acid phosphatase reaction is weakly positive. The nonspecific esterase reaction is strongly positive. The alkaline phosphatase reaction is negative. Under the marginal sinus, however, there is weak alkaline phosphatase activity, which might be connected with the fibroblastic reticulum cells found there. The PAS reaction is negative.

**Ultrastructure.**[300] The ultrastructure of the sinus wall is dealt with separately owing to structural variations in different areas (marginal, intermediate, and medullary) of the lymph node. Sinus endothelial cells, which have also been called retothelial cells,[300] exhibit variations in fine structures depending on their location.

## *1. Endothelial Cells of the Marginal Sinus*

On the *capsular side* of the marginal sinus these cells have a relatively simple structure. Their cytoplasm covers the connective tissue of the capsule, which is limited by a typical basement membrane that consists of amorphous or finely filamentous, moderately electron-dense material. The cells are united by desmosomes and are usually flat, except in the region of the nucleus. The nucleus shows moderate electron opacity with widespread nucleoplasm. Sometimes a small nucleolus and one or two nuclear dense bodies (*Sphaeridien*[301]) are encountered. In the cytoplasm a finely vesicular smooth endoplasmic reticulum is fairly well developed, and large numbers of pinocytotic vesicles may gather at the cytoplasmic periphery. The mitochondria are small and ovoid or long and rod-shaped. Scanty rough endoplasmic reticulum is observed only if the lymph nodes take up and process increased amounts of material.

The cells on the *inner side* of the marginal sinus are attached to a structure that corresponds to argyrophilic fibers as seen with the light microscope. It is composed of collagenous fibers and amorphous or finely filamentous, moderately electron-dense material. It is thought to be equivalent to the basement membrane mentioned previously, but does not represent a real basement membrane by itself. The nucleus of these cells is identical to the nucleus of the cells on the capsular side, although the latter cells are somewhat flatter. Intracytoplasmic organelles are fairly prominent. They consist of finely vesicular or vacuolar smooth endoplasmic reticulum, rough endoplasmic reticulum, and some lysosomes. Occasionally, the tubules of rough endoplasmic reticulum are found to have saccular distensions. The mitochondria are small, round, or ovoid. Most of the sinus endothelial cells contain fine filamentous elements in the cytoplasm arranged along the longitudinal axis. The cells are also attached to neighboring cells by desmosomes.

---

[300] MORI and LENNERT, 1969. [301] BÜTTNER and HORSTMANN, 1967.

Histiocytic reticulum cells are regularly found beneath the marginal sinus. They are referred to as submarginal macrophages. These cells probably represent a first line of defense against exogenous material penetrating the lymphatic tissue, as indicated by very early and active phagocytosis of subcutaneously injected flaggellin,[302] carbon,[303] or bacteria such as *L. monocytogenes.*[304]

The *intraluminal cells* of the marginal sinus were previously referred to as intrasinusoidal reticulum cells. We could not distinguish these cells, however, from the retothelial cells bordering the sinus lumen. The difference is noteworthy only as far as the relationship between cells and basement-membrane structures is concerned. In contrast to the retothelium lining the wall of the sinus, the intraluminal cells encase parts of the described basement membrane-like material in infoldings of the cytoplasmic membrane. The distinction is made on the basis of the fact that the cells are associated with the filamentous framework in the lumen, whereas the retothelium of the sinus wall covers both the inner and outer surfaces, only the latter representing a true basement membrane.

### 2. *Endothelial Cells of the Intermediate and Medullary Sinuses*

In contrast to the retothelium of the marginal sinus, intracytoplasmic organelles are most abundant in the cells of the medullary sinus. A large amount of vesicular smooth endoplasmic reticulum and also fairly long channels of rough endoplasmic reticulum are seen.

In the authors' opinion, all sinus endothelial cells are of the same basic type. Variations noted in fine structure appear to be related to the degree of activity, which depends on the location of the cell in question.

**Function.** Sinus endothelial cells line the lymph vessels of the lymph node and therefore first of all fulfill a true endothelial function. The sinus wall is not continuous, however, so that the passage of substances and cells is always possible. Endothelial cells show only slight ability to phagocytose. The formation of basement membrane-like structures is very probable.

## C. Mast Cells

One may argue whether mast cells belong to the stationary cells of the lymph node. They can definitely leave the lymph node *via* lymph vessels. We do not yet know whether this is an active, functionally significant process, or whether the cells die in the blood. It is probable, however, that most mast cells remain stationary in the lymphatic tissue.

There are two new important findings supplementing our earlier cytologic description of mast cells in Part A of this Handbook:

---

[302] ADA, NOSSAL and AUSTIN, 1964.
[303] NOPAJAROONSRI and SIMON, 1971.
[304] RACZ, KAISERLING, TENNER and WUTHE, 1974.

1. Mast cells can be demonstrated excellently in paraffin sections with the chloroacetate-esterase method,[305] even when they are extremely immature, e.g., in highly anaplastic malignant mastocytosis (mast-cell reticulosis).

2. Homoplastic proliferation of mast cells is possible. We have found occasional tetraploid nuclei.[306] Cytochemical, ultrastructural, and immunologic findings indicate, however, that heteroplastic development from blood monocytes or common precursors in the bone marrow is also possible.[307] One sees all morphologic and cytochemical transitions between a small monocytoid form [peroxidase (+), chloroacetate esterase (+)] and the large form with abundant granules, a wide rim of cytoplasm, and a round nucleus (peroxidase −, chloroacetate esterase + +).

---

[305] LEDER, 1964.

[306] QUEISSER, NOESKE, SANDRITTER and LENNERT, 1967.

[307] DESAGA, PARWARESCH and MÜLLER-HERMELINK, 1971; MÜLLER-HERMELINK, THIEDE, SONNTAG, MÜLLER-RUCHHOLTZ *et al.*, 1971; PARWARESCH, MÜLLER-HERMELINK, DESAGA, ZAKARI *et al.*, 1971; THIEDE, MÜLLER-HERMELINK, SONNTAG, MÜLLER-RUCHHOLTZ *et al.*, 1971.

Part Two

# Methodologic Prerequisites for a Differential Diagnosis of Lymphomas

K. LENNERT

Although the methods for studying lymph nodes have already been discussed in detail in Part A of this Handbook, we would like now to consider the subject again in greater detail. For, not only have our methods been subject to improvement and further development, but the diagnosis of lymphomas requires a few additional techniques that are unimportant for the study of lymphadenitis.

Since the diagnosis of lymphomas is based most of all on cytologic study, we must use all methods that enable us to obtain maximum detail and optimal reproducibility. In general, for routine diagnostic work only methods applicable to light microscopy can be considered. Every laboratory should be able to apply them, although some of them go beyond the "mass production" techniques of daily work and are somewhat more time-consuming and more complicated. In principle, however, even these methods can be applied in almost any laboratory.

Actually, factors influencing the diagnosis of lymphomas begin as early as the excision and depend on the surgeon's skill. He must avoid squeezing the tissue specimen with forceps or similar instruments.

Before fixation, the lymph node should be sectioned in half. It is then easy to prepare imprints from the fresh surfaces. Imprints are very useful for differentiation, in particular of immature-cell lymphomas and leukemias. They also reveal some morphologic details better than sections do.

The lymph node can be fixed in formalin, diluted 1:9 or 1:4. One should use buffered neutral formalin. Fixation in Zenker's or Maximow's solution provides better cytologic results. The advantage of fixation in formalin, however, is that the material can be embedded later for electron microscopy. When Bouin's fixative is used, the sections must be hydrated for 2–5 hours before being placed in Giemsa solution.[1]

One half of the lymph node is embedded in paraffin or, even better, in Paraplast®. In our laboratory, an Ultratechnicon® is the machine used for the embedding process, with the following solutions and times, as worked out and recommended by our technician, W. GLÜCK:

---

[1] GÉRARD-MARCHANT, 1975, personal communication.

| Solution | Time (in hours) |
|---|---|
| 1. 50% alcohol | 1 |
| 2. 60% alcohol | 1 |
| 3. 70% alcohol | 1 |
| 4. 80% alcohol | 1 |
| 5. 96% alcohol | 2 |
| 6. 100% alcohol | 1 |
| 7. 100% alcohol | 2 |
| 8. Methyl benzoate | 2 |
| 9. Methyl benzoate | 1 |
| 10. Benzol | 1/2 |
| 11. Paraffin or Paraplast® | 1 |
| 12. Paraffin or Paraplast® | 2 (−6) |

Proper embedding in paraffin is an essential prerequisite for the subsequent cytologic analysis of the slides. If the embedding is only moderately good or poor, then even the greatest skill in staining will be of no help in correcting the damage caused by inadequate embedding.

In recent years, embedding in synthetics has been recommended. We have convinced ourselves time and again just how excellent the sections of such material are. The slides are a delight for the eye, but certainly not necessary for a histologic diagnosis. We even venture to doubt whether they are really better for histologic study. In any event, we find it easier to make diagnoses with paraffin sections that are 2–3 μm thick, with their recurrent artifacts, than with methacrylate sections only 0.5–1 μm thick. Because they are so thin, the latter also provide less information per cell. Thus, the evaluation of such a slide requires considerably more time than that of a paraffin section. In our opinion, embedding in synthetics is therefore not worth the trouble, unless the slides are intended for special scientific purposes.

The second half of the lymph node is left unfixed and kept for possible histochemical analysis, in particular enzyme histochemical reactions (acid and alkaline phosphatase, nonspecific esterase, ATPase, and 5-nucleotidase) and the PAS reaction. This measure is also a valuable safeguard against accidents during embedding of the first half.

The paraffin sections should not be cut thicker than 3–4 μm, which is readily attained if the embedding has been performed properly. Drying of the sections at too high temperatures must be avoided to prevent certain particularly sensitive tissues (chronic lymphocytic leukemia, centroblastic/centrocytic lymphoma, lymphoblastic lymphoma) from developing cracks.

For the diagnosis of lymphomas we always use four standard staining methods: (1) Giemsa stain, (2) hematoxylin and eosin, (3) PAS reaction according to Hotchkiss, and (4) silver impregnation according to Gomori. We include the naphthol-AS-D-chloroacetate esterase reaction when necessary.

To supplement or replace the Giemsa stain, some investigators[2] have for many decades employed the methyl-green pyronine (MGP) stain to demonstrate

[2] E.g., Ghon and Roman, 1916.

Table 3. Histologic and cytologic methods for diagnosing lymph nodes

| Method | Results | Indications |
|---|---|---|
| **I. Obligatory histologic methods for paraffin sections** | | |
| 1. *Giemsa staining* | RNA, DNA: blue<br>Acidophilic substances: eosin red<br>Acid mucopolysaccharides: red-violet | Cytologic analysis of *all* lymphomas<br>Comparison with imprints and blood smears |
| 2. *Hematoxylin and eosin* | Nuclei: blue<br>Cytoplasm: reddish to "amphophilic" | Poor fixation and embedding<br>Autopsy material<br>Nuclear structure (epithelioid cells, etc.) |
| 3. *PAS reaction* | | |
| a) diastase-sensitive | Glycogen: diffuse | Metastases of seminoma, hypernephroma, squamous epithelial carcinoma, juvenile rhabdomyosarcoma, Ewing's sarcoma |
| | Glycogen: granular | Very rare in lymphoblastic lymphoma (well preserved in cryostat sections) |
| b) diastase-resistant | Immunoglobulin:<br>globular<br>intracytoplasmic<br>intranuclear<br>diffuse | Ig-producing lymphomas (LP immunocytoma, immunoblastic sarcoma, etc.) |
| | Proteoglycan | Mast cells and mast-cell neoplasms<br>Metastases of adenocarcinoma |
| 4. *Silver staining* | "Reticulin" fibers: black<br>"Collagenous" fibers: brown<br>→ abundance and arrangement of fibers, basic structure of lymph node or tumor | Architecture<br>Differentiation of diffuse and nodular/follicular growth<br>Differentiation of lymphomas and metastases |
| **II. Optional histologic methods for paraffin sections** | | |
| 5. *Chloroacetate esterase* | Promyelocytes and neutrophilic myelopoietic cells: +<br>Mast cells: + | Myeloid leukemia, myelosarcoma, monocytic leukemia, extramedullary hematopoiesis<br>Normal and neoplastic mast cells |
| 6. *Methyl-green pyronine* | RNA: red | Degree of cytoplasmic basophilia (↑ in plasma cells, immunoblasts, centroblasts, etc.) |

Table 3 (continued)

| Method | Results | Indications |
|---|---|---|
| 7. *Ladewig's modification of Mallory staining* | Collagen, IgM, amyloid: gray-blue to blue<br>Fibrin, IgG, IgA: orange-red to red | Ig-producing (PAS +) lymphomas |
| 8. *Goldner's modification of Masson trichrome staining* | Collagen, IgM: green<br>Fibrin, IgG, IgA: orange-red | Ig-producing (PAS +) lymphomas |
| 9. *van Gieson* | Collagen: red<br>Amyloid, Ig, fibrin: yellow<br>Hyalin: yellow or red | Amyloid suspected |
| 10. *Congo red* | Amyloid under polarization: greenish shine | Amyloid suspected |
| 11. *Prussian blue reaction* | Hemosiderin: +<br>Melanin: – | Melanoma suspected |
| | III. Obligatory methods for imprints | |
| 1. *Pappenheim or Giemsa staining* | Finest nuclear and cytoplasmic details (granules, degree of basophilia) | All lymphomas |
| 2. *PAS reaction* | Nucleoli especially well demonstrated | |
| a) diastase-sensitive | Glycogen | Lymphoblastic lymphomas |
| b) diastase-resistant | Immunoglobulin<br>globular<br>diffuse | Ig-producing lymphomas |
| 3. *Acid phosphatase* | | |
| a) tartrate-sensitive | Diffusely granular to clumpy + | Lymphomas of the plasma-cell series |
| | Diffusely granular to clumpy + + | Monocytes, reticulum cells |
| | Paranuclear, solitary "blotches" | Lymphoblastic lymphoma of convoluted-cell (acid phosphatase) type |
| b) tartrate-resistant | Granular | Hairy-cell leukemia |
| 4. *α-Naphthyl acetate esterase (neutral)* | Monocytes: diffuse + | Monocytic leukemia |
| | Histiocytic reticulum cells: diffuse + + + | True (histiocytic) reticulosarcoma |
| | IV. Optional methods for imprints | |
| 5. *Chloroacetate esterase* | As in sections | As in sections |
| 6. *Peroxidase* | Neutrophilic, eosinophilic, and basophilic myelopoietic cells: +<br>Monocytes: (+)<br>More sensitive than chloroacetate esterase | All myeloid neoplasms including monocytic leukemia |

the cytoplasmic basophilia in bright red. It is actually a highly valuable stain, but it does not allow comparison with imprints. MGP staining is good for demonstrating RNA content. Thus, it reveals only basophilic components of a cell and not eosinophilic or metachromatic structures.

In addition, the following staining methods should be available on a routine basis when needed: van Gieson, Congo red, Ladewig's modification of the Mallory stain, Goldner's modification of the Masson trichrome stain, and the Prussian blue reaction.

On *imprints* we carry out the following stains or reactions: Pappenheim or Giemsa stain, PAS reaction with or without pretreatment with diastase, acid phosphatase reaction with or without pretreatment with tartrate, acid or neutral α-naphthyl acetate esterase reaction, naphthol-AS-D-chloroacetate esterase reaction, and the peroxidase reaction. We always employ the first four methods, the last two only when needed.

The directions for carrying out the most important stainings and reactions are given in the Appendix. Table 3 summarizes what they demonstrate (results) and when they should be used (indications).

In the vast majority of cases the methods listed for studies with the light microscope suffice for making precise diagnoses of lymphomas. In a small percentage of cases, however, *electron-microscopic* studies are helpful or even indispensable. In particular, the demonstration of rough endoplasmic reticulum on electron microscopy has proved of great value in interpreting tumors that produce immunoglobulin (see Part Five).

In addition to the morphologic techniques mentioned, and depending on the circumstances, we also utilize *immunologic methods* (rosette techniques, determination of surface immunoglobulin, demonstration of immunoglobulin in tissue homogenates, etc.). This subject is discussed in detail in Part Six.

*Appendix:*

# Some Stainings and Cytochemical Reactions Used in Our Laboratories

### *Giemsa staining (modification of* LENNERT, *1952a, 1961)*

1. The deparaffinized sections are removed from distilled water and put into the following solution:

   80 ml distilled water
   20 ml Giemsa solution (Merck, Darmstadt, Fed. Rep. Germany).

   They remain in the solution for 1 hour.

2. The sections are removed from the Giemsa solution and put into 100 ml distilled water, to which 3–4 drops of undiluted glacial acetic acid have been added. The sections are agitated lightly in this solution for a few seconds, slightly differentiated (2–3 sec), and then immediately put into:
3. 96% alcohol, in which they are differentiated further until the desired staining is reached (microscopic control).

4.5.6. Differentiation is stopped and, at the same time, dehydration is achieved by dipping 3 times in isopropanol for 2 min each, and

7.8.9. three times in xylene for 2 min each.

*Results:*

RNA, DNA: blue ("basophilic").
Acidophilic substances: orange-red.
Acid mucopolysaccharides: red-violet.

*Modification of the Mallory-Heidenhain technique according to* LADEWIG *(1938), but slightly changed*

1. Nuclear staining with Weigert's hematoxylin for approx. 10 min.
2. 5% phosphotungstic acid for 1–3 min (connective tissue turns light red to pink).
3. Quick rinsing in distilled water.
4. Aniline blue–acid fuchsin–gold orange solution for 4 min.
5. Quick rinsing in distilled water.
6. 96% alcohol for 1 min (agitate the slides a little).
7. Absolute alcohol.
8. Xylene.

*Results:* Nuclei are dark brown; connective tissue is blue, blue-violet, red-violet, or carmine (vivid) red (depending on nature and structure of the tissue); erythrocytes are light orange; fibrin is bright scarlet red; mucus and secretions are blue; amyloid is light vitreous blue.

*Staining solution:*

Combine, boil, cool, and filter:

0.5 g water-soluble aniline blue
2 g gold orange
1 g acid fuchsin
100 ml distilled water

Add:

8 ml glacial acetic acid.

### *Modification of Masson's trichrome stain according to* GOLDNER *(1938)*

1. Deparaffin.
2. Remove from 50% alcohol after 2 min.
3. Nuclear staining with Weigert's hematoxylin for 5—10 min.
4. Differentiation in 1% HCl/alcohol.
5. Rinse in distilled water.
6. Rinse for 10 min under running water, then put into distilled water.
7. Stain in acid fuchsin Ponceau for 10 min.
8. Rinse twice in 1% acetic acid.
9. Differentiation with phosphomolybdic acid orange G (decoloration of the connective tissue). Observe under the microscope after at most 5 min.
10. Rinse quickly in 1% acetic acid twice.
11. Differential staining of the connective tissue with 0.1% light green for 5 min.
12. Wash in 1% acetic acid for 5 min.
13. 96% alcohol twice.
14. 100% alcohol three times.
15. Xylene.

*Results:* Nuclei: brown-black; cytoplasm: brick red; erythrocytes: orange-yellow; connective tissue and mucus: green.

The staining is particularly successful after Bouin and Susa fixation, but it is also applicable after formalin or Carnoy fixation.

*Staining solutions:*

1. Acid fuchsin Ponceau:
   0.2 g Ponceau de xylidine
   0.1 g acid fuchsin
   300 ml distilled water
   0.6 ml glacial acetic acid

2. Mordant:
   4 g phosphomolybdic acid
   100 ml distilled water
   2 g orange G

3. Light green:
   2 g light green
   100 ml distilled water
   0.2 ml acetic acid

### *Acid phosphatase*

(GOLDBERG and BARKA, 1962; LEDER, 1967a; LEDER and STUTTE, 1975)

Fixation: none.

Stock solution A ("hexazonium pararosaniline" according to DAVIS and ORNSTEIN, 1959):

Mix well:

6 drops of 4% solution of pararosaniline and
6 drops of 4% solution of sodium nitrite.

After about 60 sec dilute with

30 ml veronal-acetate buffer, pH 7.62
(if the mixture turns red, then pararosaniline was not sufficiently "hexazotized").

Adjust pH of the mixture to 5.0–5.1 with 2*N* HCl.

Stock solution B:

Dissolve 10 mg naphthol-AS-BI phosphate (Sigma, Munich, Fed. Rep. of Germany) in
1 ml dimethyl formamide or 2 ml dimethyl sulfoxide.

Stir solution A into solution B, mixing well, and then filter.

Incubation for 4(–10) hours. Then rinse the slides in tap water.

Nuclear staining with hemalum (Merck, Darmstadt, Fed. Rep. of Germany) for 10 min. Then blue in tap water.

Mount with glycerin-gelatin.

*Result:* red reaction indicates enzyme activity.

*Tartrate-resistant acid phosphatase*
(YAM, LI and LAM, 1971; LEDER and STUTTE, 1975)

Fixation: none.

Stock solution A:

Mix well:

6 drops of 4% solution of pararosaniline and
6 drops of 4% solution of sodium nitrite.

After about 60 sec dilute with

30 ml veronal-acetate buffer, pH 7.62.

Add 225 mg tartaric acid and mix well.
Adjust pH of the mixture to 5.0–5.1 with 1*N* NaOH.

Stock solution B:

Dissolve 10 mg naphthol-AS-BI phosphate (Sigma, Munich, Fed. Rep. of Germany) in
1 ml dimethyl formamide or 2 ml dimethyl sulfoxide.

Stir solution A into solution B, mixing well, and then filter.

Rest of the procedure as for acid phosphatase.

*Result:* Tartrate-resistant acid phosphatase (e.g., in cells of hairy-cell leukemia) is represented by a bright red reaction.

### *Naphthol-AS-D-chloroacetate esterase*
### (Leder, 1964; Leder and Stutte, 1975)

Fixation:

1. Smears:

30 sec in a mixture of absolute methanol and 4% formalin (9:1 vol/vol) at 4° C, rinse in tap water, and air-dry.

2. Sections:

Thoroughly deparaffinized sections of formalin- or Maximow-fixed tissue embedded in paraffin in the usual manner.

Stock solution A ("hexazonium pararosaniline" according to Davis and Ornstein, 1959):

Mix well:

1 drop of 4% solution of pararosaniline and
1 drop of 4% solution of sodium nitrite.

After about 60 sec dilute with:

30 ml veronal-acetate buffer, pH 7.62
(if the mixture turns red, then pararosaniline was not sufficiently "hexazotized").

Adjust pH of the mixture to 6.3 with 2*N* HCl.

Stock solution B:

Dissolve 10 mg naphthol-AS-D chloroacetate (Sigma, Munich, Fed. Rep. of Germany) in
1 ml dimethyl formamide.

Stir solution A into solution B, mixing well, and then filter.

Incubate for 30 min or 2 × 30 min, agitating constantly. Then rinse the slides in tap water.

Nuclear staining with hemalum (Merck, Darmstadt, Fed. Rep. of Germany) for 10 min. Then blue in tap water.

Mount with glycerin-gelatin.

*Result:* enzyme activity is represented by a bright red reaction.

### *Nonspecific esterase (α-naphthyl acetate esterase)*

#### *a) Neutral nonspecific esterase (method of* Leder, *1967a)* [3]

Material: fresh cryostat sections or air-dried smears.

Fixation: none.

[3] The amounts and times given in parentheses are for structures with high enzyme activity and for sections. The others are for structures with low activity and for imprints.

Stock solution A:

Mix well:
1 (4) drops of 4% solution of pararosaniline and
1 (4) drops of 4% solution of sodium nitrite.

After about 60 sec dilute with:
25 (40) ml phosphate buffer, pH 7.5 (7.0)
(if the mixture turns red, then pararosaniline was not sufficiently "hexazotized").

Stock solution B:
Dissolve 10 mg α-naphthyl acetate in 0.8 ml acetone.

Stir solution A into solution B, mixing well, and filter.

Incubate for 30 (5–30) min. Then rinse the slides well, since a flaky precipitate forms quickly in the solution.

Nuclear staining with hemalum (Merck, Darmstadt, Fed. Rep. of Germany) for 10 min. Then blue in tap water.

Mount with glycerin-gelatin.

*Results:* enzyme activity is represented by a red-brown reaction. Monocytes are diffusely positive. Histiocytic reticulum cells also show a diffuse, but stronger reaction.

### *b) Acid nonspecific esterase (method of* MUELLER *et al., 1975)*

Material: air-dried smears or imprints.

Fixation:
4 min in buffered (0.1 M Na-cacodylate, pH 7.2) 4% formalin.
Dry at room temperature.

Solution A:
Dissolve 2 g pararosaniline, acridine-free, C.I. No. 42500 (Chroma, Stuttgart-Untertürkheim, Fed. Rep. of Germany), in 50 ml 2*N* HCl. Mix thoroughly. This solution can be stored in the dark at 4° C.

Solution B:
Freshly prepared 4% aqueous solution of Na-nitrite.

Mix equal parts (1.2 ml each) of solutions A and B until the color of the mixture becomes amber.

Dissolve substrate (10 mg α-naphthyl acetate; Sigma, St. Louis, Missouri, USA) in 0.4 ml acetone in a second vessel.

Add the mixture of hexazotized pararosaniline and buffer to substrate. Adjust to pH 5.8 with 2*N* NaOH.

Incubation for 2 hours at room temperature.

Counterstain with hemalum.

*Results:* enzyme activity is represented by a red-brown reaction. T-lymphocytes show localized coarse paranuclear activity. Monocytes and histiocytic reticulum cells show diffuse activity.

Part Three

# Classification of Non-Hodgkin's Lymphomas

K. LENNERT

## I. Historical Review of the Classifications of Lymphomas

Since ROSENBERG *et al.*[1] and KAPLAN[2] have already presented comprehensive reviews of the history of malignant lymphoma (M.L.), we may forego repeating them in detail. A few especially important milestones, however, should be pointed out.

| | |
|---|---|
| 1832 HODGKIN: | identified malignant tumors of lymph nodes; among these were the entity that we now refer to as Hodgkin's disease as well as some "non-Hodgkin's lymphomas." |
| 1845 VIRCHOW: | conceived of and clearly defined leukemia. |
| 1863 VIRCHOW: | defined the concepts of lymphosarcoma and lymphoma. |
| 1865 COHNHEIM: | proposed "pseudoleukemia" in place of VIRCHOW'S aleukemic leukemia. |
| 1892 DRESCHFELD: | separated lymphosarcoma from pseudoleukemia. |
| 1893 KUNDRAT<br>1897 PALTAUF | distinguished lymphosarcoma from pseudoleukemia and Hodgkin's disease (granuloma malignum). |
| 1898 STERNBERG<br>1902 REED | histologically defined Hodgkin's disease, emphasizing thereby the characteristic giant cells. |
| 1925 BRILL *et al.*<br>1927 D. SYMMERS | described tumors of germinal centers, later called follicular lymphoblastoma (Brill-Symmers disease). |
| 1930 ROULET: | distinguished reticulum-cell sarcoma ("retothelsarcoma") from lymphosarcoma. |
| 1958 BURKITT<br>1960 O'CONOR and DAVIES | described African lymphoma (Burkitt's tumor). |

The last chapter in the story of Hodgkin's lymphoma ended for the time being at the Rye Conference. That was only true, however, for the pragmatic

[1] ROSENBERG, DIAMOND, JASLOWITZ and CRAVER, 1961.

[2] 1972.

activities of clinicians and pathologists. In our opinion, the leveling process of the Rye Conference contrived to obscure or cover up important scientific problems that remain to be solved. Nonetheless, for those treating patients with Hodgkin's disease, the Rye Conference represented a good end to a multicentric development and a notable start for joint clinicotherapeutic efforts.

A conference like the one at Rye for discussing non-Hodgkin's lymphomas has yet to be held, although attempts have been made since 1973 to arrange one. Therefore, the present state of the various efforts to establish a uniform classification will be presented here.

Until recently, there were essentially two different concepts for classifying non-Hodgkin's lymphoma. Both were presented in 1966 at the first International Symposium on Lymphology in Zurich—the "American concept" by LUKES[3] and the "European concept" by the author.[4] The fundamental studies of RAPPAPORT[5] served as the chief basis for the American concept, whereas the so-called European concept, as it was presented at the time, rested on the fundamental investigations of ROBB-SMITH[6] and on the more cytologically oriented observations of the author.[7] We realize that it is an oversimplification and a presumptuous act to speak of the American and European concepts and to mention only four names (RAPPAPORT, LUKES, ROBB-SMITH, and the author). We of course have no right to simply pass over other European concepts and not take them seriously. The comparison of the "American" and "European" concepts, which was initiated by the leaders of the symposium in Zurich, does, however, underline the difference between two fundamentally different viewpoints.

The two principal differences distinguishing the American and European concepts were as follows:

1. RAPPAPORT maintained that all cytologic types of malignant lymphomas can be either nodular or diffuse, whereas we distinguished follicular lymphoma as a cytologically defined entity from lymphocytic and reticular neoplasms.

2. ROBB-SMITH and the author agreed that two degrees of malignancy of lymphomas could be distinguished—"irreversible progressive hyperplasias" (previously referred to as "reticuloses" by ROBB-SMITH) and "sarcomas." RAPPAPORT did not distinguish corresponding main groups of lymphomas.

RAPPAPORT's classification (Table 4) was adopted by more and more investigators in the USA[8] and outside America. The author, on the other hand, held to his concept, which was based on increasingly refined cytologic studies, later amplified by electron-microscopic techniques[9] and other methods. The classification that resulted from these studies is given in the first column of the table below (Table 5).

In 1970, we (LENNERT, STEIN and KAISERLING) began a new approach to the classification of lymphomas. We attempted to apply recent results of lymphocyte research to the study of lymphomas and to distinguish between malignant

[3] 1967.

[4] LENNERT, 1967.

[5] RAPPAPORT, WINTER and HICKS, 1956; RAPPAPORT, 1964a, b, 1966.

[6] 1938, 1947, 1964.

[7] LENNERT, 1964a, 1967.

[8] LUKES, 1964, 1967; BERARD, 1972, 1975; BERARD and DORFMAN, 1974; DORFMAN, 1975.

[9] MORI and LENNERT, 1969.

Table 4. Classification of non-Hodgkin's lymphomas (RAPPAPORT, 1966)

| Nodular | Diffuse |
|---|---|
| Lymphocytic, well differentiated | |
| Lymphocytic, poorly differentiated | |
| Mixed (lymphocytic-histiocytic) | |
| Histiocytic | |
| Undifferentiated | |

lymphomas derived from the B- and T-lymphocyte series. At first we tried analyzing the immunoglobulins (Ig) in tumor homogenates and soon after utilized numerous other methods (immunoperoxidase technique for demonstrating Ig on cell surfaces and various techniques for demonstrating rosette formation on light and electron microscopy). These investigations were combined with cytochemical analyses of imprints, electron-microscopic studies of each tumor, and examinations of peripheral blood smears.

In 1971, at a meeting in Nagoya, Japan, we reported that we had studied four "reticulosarcomas," all of which showed high concentrations of IgM in the tumor homogenate. Consequently, we proposed that at least most cases of reticulosarcoma are actually immunoblastic sarcomas, a suggestion we had already made in 1967[10] on the basis of our electron-microscopic studies of a tumor that revealed a large amount of rough endoplasmic reticulum.

We presented our first large series of B-cell lymphomas at a symposium on leukemia in Vienna in March, 1972.[11] That presentation stimulated a number of clinicians (particularly STACHER), who are now members of the Kiel Lymphoma Study Group, to collaborate with us in a larger lymphoma program. Results of this cooperation have been presented on several occasions.[12]

In essence, the results were as follows:

1. Most so-called reticulosarcomas are actually immunoblastic sarcomas of the B-cell type.

2. The histologic picture regarded until now as being so characteristic of macroglobulinemia of Waldenström occurs twice as often without macroglobulinemia, although homogenates of the lymphomatous tissue usually contain increased amounts of IgM. Moreover, the condition may develop with an increase in the levels of IgG or IgA in the serum or neoplastic tissue. Since the morphologic substrate consists of lymphocytes and plasmacytoid cells, as has been known for macroglobulinemia of Waldenström for a long time, we suggested naming it lymphoplasmacytoid immunocytoma. In addition, we recommended that the term macroglobulinemia of Waldenström be abandoned, above all because other malignant lymphomas, for example, immunoblastic lymphoma, can produce a monoclonal increase in IgM in the blood.

---

[10] LENNERT, 1967.

[11] LENNERT, 1973c; STEIN, KAISERLING and LENNERT, 1973.

[12] STEIN, LENNERT and PARWARESCH, 1972; LENNERT, 1973b, 1973c; LENNERT, STEIN and KAISERLING, 1974; LENNERT, STEIN and KAISERLING, 1975; LENNERT, 1975; BRITTINGER, BARTELS, BREMER, DÜHMKE *et al.*, 1976; KAISERLING, 1976; LENNERT, 1976; STACHER, WALDNER and THEML, 1976; STEIN, 1976.

Table 5. Comparison of five classifications

| Former German Classification[a] | New Classification of LENNERT *et al.*, 1974[b] | LUKES and COLLINS, 1974 | Kiel Classification 1974[d] | RAPPAPORT's Classification, 1966 |
|---|---|---|---|---|
| | *Low-grade malignant lymphomas* | | *Low-grade malignant lymphomas* | |
| | *"Lymphocytoma"* | | *Lymphocytic* | M.L. lymphocytic, well differentiated, diffuse |
| | B-cell types: | B-cell: | | |
| *CLL* | CLL | small lymphocyte (CLL) | CLL and others | |
| *Lymphoide Retikulose* | hairy-cell leukemia | | | |
| | T-cell types: | T-cell: | | |
| *Sézary-Syndrom* | Sézary syndrome (and mycosis fungoides?) | Sézary's syndrome (and mycosis fungoides) | | |
| | Others | | | |
| Some = *Makroglobulinämie Waldenström* | *Immunocytoma* (lymphoplasmacytoid) | B-cell: plasmacytoid lymphocyte | *Lymphoplasmacytoid* (immunocytic) | M.L. lymphocytic with dysproteinemia |
| | lymphoplasmacytic | | | |
| | lymphoplasmacytoid | | | |
| | polymorphic | | | |
| *Lymphocytäres Lymphosarkom* | *Germinocytoma* (diffuse) | B-cell: small cleaved FCC[c] large cleaved FCC | *Centrocytic* | M.L. lymphocytic, well and poorly differentiated, nodular or diffuse |
| *Großfollikuläres Lymphoblastom (Brill-Symmers)* | *Germinoblastoma* | | *Centroblastic/centrocytic* | M.L. lymphocytic, well differentiated (nodular or diffuse) |
| | follicular | follicular | follicular | M.L. lymphocytic, poorly differentiated (nodular or diffuse) |
| | follicular and diffuse | follicular and diffuse | follicular and diffuse | M.L. lymphocytic-histiocytic (nodular or diffuse) |
| | diffuse | diffuse | diffuse | M.L. histiocytic (nodular or diffuse) |
| | nonsclerotic | with or without sclerosis | with or without sclerosis | |
| | sclerotic (Bennett's type) | | | |

| | | | | |
|---|---|---|---|---|
| | *High-grade malignant lymphomas* | | *High-grade malignant lymphomas* | |
| *Retikulosarkom* | *Germinoblastic sarcoma* | B-cell: large noncleaved FCC | *Centroblastic* | M.L. histiocytic, M.L. undifferentiated } nodular or diffuse |
| *Lymphoblastisches Lymphosarkom u. Lymphoblasten- (Paraleukoblasten-) leukämie* | *Lymphoblastic sarcoma,* including ALL | B-cell: small noncleaved FCC | *Lymphoblastic* | M.L. undifferentiated, diffuse; M.L. lymphocytic, poorly differentiated, diffuse |
| | B-cell types: Burkitt's tumor | Burkitt type | Burkitt type | |
| | non-Burkitt's tumor | | | |
| | T-cell type: convoluted type of Lukes | T-cell: convoluted lymphocyte | convoluted-cell type | |
| | undefined | U-cell (undefined) | others | |
| | unclassifiable | Unclassifiable | | |
| *Retikulosarkom (Retothelsarkom)* | *Immunoblastic sarcoma* | B-cell: immunoblastic sarcoma | *Immunoblastic* | M.L. histiocytic, diffuse |
| | | T-cell: immunoblastic sarcoma | | |

[a] Cf., LENNERT, 1969a.

[b] Presented at meeting in Kiel, May 16–18, 1974, on the basis of studies done together with KAISERLING, MOHRI and STEIN (cf., LENNERT, STEIN and KAISERLING, 1975).

[c] FCC = follicular-center cell.

[d] GÉRARD-MARCHANT, HAMLIN, LENNERT, RILKE, STANSFELD and VAN UNNIK, 1974.

3. We distinguished two main types of germinal-center tumors. The first type was composed only of polymorphic germinocytes; it was first called germinocytic sarcoma or germinocytoma. The second type was composed of germinocytes *and* germinoblasts and was referred to as germinoblastoma (follicular lymphoma).

4. Most of the lymphomas we have studied belonged to the B-cell system. Only lymphoblastic sarcoma and lymphoblastic leukemia of the acid phosphatase type proved in many cases to be free of immunoglobulins and to form sheep-E rosettes. Thus, we classed them in the T-cell system. [13]

During approximately the same period of time, LUKES and COLLINS were studying non-Hodgkin's lymphomas by means of a simple objective method. With the aid of a camera lucida they sketched the nuclei of the tumor cells and found that most of the non-Hodgkin's lymphomas seemed to arise from germinal centers. The cell we called a germinocyte they named a cleaved follicular-center cell, and our germinoblast for them was a noncleaved follicular-center cell.[14]

From the results of their studies they proposed a new classification, which they presented for discussion at a lymphoma meeting in Freiburg in September, 1972. Their ideas for a new classification [15] agreed well with ours. Accordingly, LUKES introduced the following table (Table 6) at the CRC Symposium on Non-Hodgkin's Lymphomata in London in October, 1973.[16] At the same symposium, BUTLER *et al.*[16a] presented the initial results of studies using the classification of LUKES and COLLINS. Following the symposium, ROBB-SMITH[17] published a Letter to the Editor in *Lancet* in which he solicited support for utilizing the latest information about B- and T-cell regions for the classification of lymphomas. A subsequent editorial in the same journal[18] recommended, as LUKES, KOJIMA, and the author had already done, that a distinction be made between tumors arising from follicular centers and those that do not. In addition, GÉRARD-MARCHANT [19] published two papers in which he warmly supported the concepts presented by LUKES and by the author.

The situation soon became embarrassing, however, after BERARD and SELIGMANN dismissed the classifications suggested by LUKES and the author at the meeting in London as "premature." Consequently, at the end of the symposium, a group of European pathologists (BENNETT, GÉRARD-MARCHANT, HAMLIN, RILKE, STANSFELD, VAN UNNIK, and the author) were asked to get together to work out a useful classification and terminology. That led to the formation of the European Lymphoma Club. As a first step, they studied under the expert guidance of LUKES the classification of lymphomas that he and COLLINS had recommended. In May, 1974, the Club met for the second time in Kiel and discussed the classification proposed by the author and his co-workers (STEIN and KAISERLING), using model cases as examples. The members of the Club approved this classification and agreed on a provisional terminology, which was

---

[13] LENNERT, 1975.
[14] LUKES and COLLINS, Nagoya, 1971, published 1973.
[15] LUKES and COLLINS, 1974a, b.
[16] See HANSEN and GOOD, 1974.
[16a] BUTLER, STRYKER and SHULLENBERGER, 1975.
[17] ROBB-SMITH, 1974.
[18] June 1, 1974.
[19] 1974a, b.

Table 6. Comparison of the classifications of LENNERT *et al.* and LUKES and COLLINS, presented in London, October, 1973

| LENNERT *et al.* | LUKES and COLLINS |
|---|---|
| *I. Undefined (not B or T)* | |
| *II. B-Cell (Lymphocytic) Types* | |
| 1. CLL | 1. Small lymphocytic type (CLL) |
| 2. Immunocytoma, lymphoplasmacytoid | 2. Plasmacytoid lymphocytic |
| 3. Germinal center cell tumors | 3. Follicle center cell (FCC) tumors<br>follicular, follicular and diffuse, diffuse, sclerotic |
| a) Germinocytoma (gc)<br>diffuse<br>b) Germinoblastoma (gc+gbl)<br>follicular, follicular and diffuse, diffuse, sclerotic | ↔ a) cleaved FCC<br>1. small<br>2. small and large |
| c) Germinoblastic sarcoma (gbl)<br>usually diffuse<br>? Paraleukoblastic (lymphoblastic B) sarcoma incl. Burkitt's | ↔ b) noncleaved FCC<br>1. small (Burkitt's)<br>2. large |
| 4. Immunoblastic sarcoma, B-cell type | 4. Immunoblastic sarcoma, B-cell type |
| *III. T-Cell (Lymphocytic) Types* | |
| 1. Mycosis fungoides (including Sézary syndrome) | 1. Mycosis fungoides (including Sézary syndrome) |
| 2. ? Lymphoblastic sarcoma, T-cell type | 2. Convoluted lymphocyte |
| 3. ? Immunoblastic sarcoma, T-cell type | 3. ? Immunoblastic sarcoma, T-cell type |
| *IV. Reticulo-histiocytic* | |
| Reticulosarcoma | Histiocytic |
| *V. Unclassified* | |

accepted as final at a meeting in Amsterdam on July 7, 1974. It was published as a Letter to the Editor in *Lancet*[20] and called the Kiel Classification (Table 7).

Shortly before the Kiel Classification appeared in print, however, DORFMAN[21] presented in the same journal a "working classification," which was a compromise between the classification of RAPPAPORT and those suggested by LUKES and the author (Table 8). The issue of *Lancet* with the letter of GÉRARD-MARCHANT *et al.*[20] also contained the classification of BENNETT *et al.*[22] (Table 9). Again, their proposal represented a compromise of various classifications. Like DORFMAN's classification, it included follicular lymphoma as an entity, a concept we had advocated since 1964.[23]

Subsequently, further Letters to the Editor have appeared in *Lancet*. Written

[20] GÉRARD-MARCHANT, HAMLIN, LENNERT, RILKE *et al.*, 1974.
[21] 1974a.
[22] BENNETT, FARRER-BROWN, HENRY and JELLIFFE, 1974.
[23] LENNERT, 1964a, 1969a, c, 1971, 1973a.

Table 7. Kiel Classification of non-Hodgkin's lymphomas, compared with RAPPAPORT's classification (roughly corresponding to GÉRARD-MARCHANT *et al.*, 1974)

| Kiel Classification | Rappaport equivalent |
|---|---|
| *Low-grade malignancy* | |
| M.L. lymphocytic (CLL and others) | M.L. well differentiated lymphocytic, diffuse |
| M.L. lymphoplasmacytoid (immunocytic) | {M.L. lymphocytic type with dysproteinemia<br>Lymphoproliferative diseases with dysproteinemia} |
| M.L. centrocytic | M.L. {well / poorly} differentiated lymphocytic {nodular / diffuse} |
| M.L. centroblastic/centrocytic[a]<br>follicular<br>follicular and diffuse<br>diffuse | M.L. {well and poorly differentiated lymphocytic; mixed-cell histiocytic-lymphocytic; histiocytic} {nodular / diffuse} |
| *High-grade malignancy* | |
| M.L. centroblastic | {M.L. histiocytic, nodular or diffuse<br>M.L. undifferentiated, nodular or diffuse} |
| M.L. lymphoblastic<br>Burkitt type<br>Convoluted-cell type<br>Others | {M.L. undifferentiated<br>M.L. poorly differentiated lymphocytic, diffuse} |
| M.L. immunoblastic | M.L. histiocytic, diffuse |

[a] With or without sclerosis

with or without humor, they have reflected all too well the degree of confusion and feeling of helplessness that now permeate the field of lymphoma research.[24]

At about the same time, DIEBOLD[25] in Paris recommended a nomenclature that differed again from all other suggestions (Table 10). It also clearly showed that a return to former concepts had become impossible. Further classifications were given by HAMILTON-FAIRLY and FREEMAN,[26] BEARD,[26a] and SCHNITZER.[27]

These presentations appeared at the time when KAPLAN's group at Stanford had published several comprehensive papers on non-Hodgkin's lymphoma, basing them on a very large amount of clinically well-studied material.[28] Other large clinicopathologic studies followed.[29] All of these investigations were still morphologically based on RAPPAPORT's classification. The Stanford group repeatedly stressed how clinically useful this classification proved to be. They emphasized especially that differentiating the nodular forms of malignant lymphoma from the diffuse forms revealed that the nodular forms had a significantly

[24] KAY, 1974; BRADFIELD, 1974; DORFMAN, 1974b; KATAYAMA and PECHET, 1974.
[25] 1974a, b.
[26] 1974.
[26a] 1975.
[27] 1975.
[28] JONES, FUKS, BULL, KADIN *et al.*, 1973; GLATSTEIN, KIM, DONALDSON, DORFMAN *et al.*, 1974; KIM and DORFMAN, 1974; SOUTHARD, BROOKS, NICKLAS and HOCH, 1974; ROSENBERG, DORFMAN and KAPLAN, 1975.
[29] BLOOMFIELD, GOLDMAN, DICK, BRUNNING *et al.*, 1974; PATCHEFSKY, BRODOVSKY, MENDUKE, SOUTHARD *et al.*, 1974.

Table 8. Working classification of non-Hodgkin's lymphomas of DORFMAN, 1974a

| Follicular lymphomas[a] (follicular or follicular and diffuse) | Diffuse lymphomas[a] |
|---|---|
| Small lymphoid | Small lymphocytic (S.L.) (C.L.L.)<br>S.L. with plasmacytoid differentiation |
| Mixed small and large lymphoid | Atypical small lymphocytic<br>Convoluted lymphocytic (thymic) |
| Large lymphoid | Large lymphoid (pyroninophilic)<br>Mixed small and large lymphoid<br>Histiocytic<br>Burkitt's lymphoma<br>Mycosis fungoides<br>Undefined |

[a] Composite lymphomas, comprising two well-defined and apparently different types of lymphoma within the same tissue and lymphomas associated with sclerosis, are suitably designated.

Table 9. Lymphoma classification of BENNETT *et al.*, 1974

| | |
|---|---|
| *Follicular lymphomas* | Grade 1 |
| Follicle cell predominantly small | Grade 1 |
| Follicle cell mixed small and large | Grade 1 |
| Follicle cell predominantly large | Grade 1 |
| *Diffuse lymphomas* | Grade 1 |
| Lymphocytic well differentiated (small round lymphocyte) | Grade 1 |
| Lymphocytic intermediate differentiation (small follicle cell) | Grade 1 |
| Lymphocytic poorly differentiated | Grade 2 |
| Mixed small lymphoid and undifferentiated large cell | Grade 2 |
| Undifferentiated large cell | Grade 2 |
| Plasma cell | Grade 2 |
| True histiocyte | Grade 2 |
| Unclassified | Grade 2 |

Plasmacytoid differentiation in lymphocytic tumors, and banded or fine sclerosis are recorded.

Table 10. Classification of lymphoid non-Hodgkin's hematosarcomas (translated from DIEBOLD, 1974a)

1. Lymphosarcoma with atypical nuclei (small lymphocytes with distorted nuclei)
2. Pleomorphic lymphocytosarcoma (association of lymphocytes and lymphoblasts)
3. Lymphoblastosarcoma
4. Pleomorphic lymphoblastosarcoma (lymphoblasts and immunoblasts)
5. Immunoblastosarcoma with atypical nuclei
6. Immunoblastosarcoma with plasmacytic differentiation
7. Plasmacytic sarcoma
8. Histiocytosarcoma (corresponding to some of the former reticulosarcomas)

better prognosis. That did not surprise us. On the contrary, from our studies we had expected the clinical behavior of follicular lymphoma, which we regarded as a definite entity, to be quite different from that of many diffuse lymphomas, although the latter would show great variability depending on the cell type.

Table 11. Somewhat modified Kiel Classification as used in this book. The subclassification of lymphocytic lymphoma and the adjuncts "B" and "T" are not sanctioned by the members of the European Lymphoma Club

*I. Low-grade malignancy*

*M.L. lymphocytic*
- B-CLL
- T-CLL
- Hairy-cell leukemia (?)
- Mycosis fungoides and Sézary's syndrome
- T-zone lymphoma

*M.L. lymphoplasmacytic/lymphoplasmacytoid* (LP immunocytoma)

*M.L. plasmacytic* (plasmacytoma[a])

*M.L. centrocytic*

*M.L. centroblastic/centrocytic*
- follicular
- follicular and diffuse
- diffuse
- with or without sclerosis

*II. High-grade malignancy*

*M.L. centroblastic*
- primary
- secondary

*M.L. lymphoblastic*
- B-lymphoblastic, Burkitt type and others
- T-lymphoblastic, convoluted-cell type and others
- Unclassified

*M.L. immunoblastic*
- with plasmablastic/plasmacytic differentiation (B)
- without plasmablastic/plasmacytic differentiation (B or T)

[a] Only extramedullary plasmacytoma

Accordingly, the results of the Stanford group and other clinicopathologic studies may be considered further evidence that follicular lymphoma is a distinct entity that must be differentiated from the diffuse forms of malignant lymphoma. We must admit now, however, that the types of tumors arising from germinal centers are more numerous than we had originally thought. Furthermore, we know that germinal center-cell neoplasms, especially the purely centrocytic and centroblastic lymphomas, can exhibit a diffuse pattern. The prognoses of the latter lymphomas may vary little or greatly from that of malignant lymphoma of the centroblastic/centrocytic type, which usually shows a follicular pattern. The studies of LUKES and COLLINS[30] and our own comparative electron-microscopic and immunologic studies[31] have made a major contribution to this realization.

It soon became evident that the cells in some immunoblastic lymphomas show signs of differentiation towards plasma cells or large plasmablast-like

[30] 1973, 1974a, b, 1975a, b.

[31] LENNERT, 1973b, c; LENNERT, MOHRI, STEIN and KAISERLING, 1975; LENNERT, STEIN and KAISERLING, 1975.

cells with rough endoplasmic reticulum in the cytoplasm on electron microscopy. At a meeting of the European Lymphoma Club in Paris in February, 1975, it was therefore decided to distinguish two subtypes of immunoblastic lymphoma:

1. That with plasmablastic and/or plasmacytic differentiation.
2. That without plasmablastic and/or plasmacytic differentiation.

Whereas the lymphomas of the first subtype (with plasmablastic and/or plasmacytic differentiation) may always be interpreted as B-immunoblastic lymphomas, the second subtype (without plasmablastic and/or plasmacytic differentiation) includes the probably very rare T-immunoblastic lymphomas as well.[32]

At the meeting in Paris, the European Lymphoma Club also generally agreed to add another group of low-grade malignant lymphomas, namely, the primary plasmacytomas of lymphatic tissue (M.L. plasmacytic).

In the present monograph we use the Kiel Classification with some slight modifications (see Table 11). In several respects it differs from the nomenclature we originally proposed. The reason is that we felt obliged to sacrifice some of our terms to clear the way for a generally acceptable approach to a new nomenclature, at least for some European lymphoma experts. At the same time, we have endeavored to simplify the overwhelming complexities without surrendering scientific accuracy. From previous data accumulated regarding the prognosis of non-Hodgkin's lymphoma, it seemed quite obvious to the European Lymphoma Club that the new classification would prove clinically relevant and useful.[33] Final proof, however, was needed.

# II. Some Ideas for a Modern Lymphoma Classification

As far as we know, Cooper *et al.*[34] were the first to call for a classification of lymphomas based on their *relationship to the B- and T-cell systems*. Since then, this demand has been accepted almost everywhere. Pioneers in its realiza-

---

[32] Since the writing of this monograph, Mathé, Rappaport, O'Conor and Torloni (1976) have published a WHO classification. It distinguishes tumors from chronic lymphocytic leukemia (CLL) and other lymphoproliferative diseases (macroglobulinemia of Waldenström, myeloma, plasma-cell leukemia, heavy-chain diseases, and Sézary's syndrome). The tumors include "lymphosarcomas," mycosis fungoides, plasmacytoma, reticulosarcoma, and Hodgkin's disease. The lymphosarcomas are subdivided as follows: 1. nodular; 2. diffuse: a) lymphocytic, b) lymphoplasmacytic, c) prolymphocytic, d) lymphoblastic, e) immunoblastic, f) Burkitt's tumor. We consider the publication of this classification to be not particularly appropriate. The mixing of old and new terms and the presented division into "lymphoproliferative diseases" and "tumors" will hardly lessen the current confusion. There is no reason to assume that this classification, which, as far as we know, is used only in the institution of Mathé, will find the worldwide acceptance that a WHO classification should have. We shall have to wait and see what the second edition of the "Blue Book" has to offer. The reader may also refer to the critical comments made by Chelloul, Diebold, Flandrin, Gérard-Marchant *et al.* (1976).

[33] Lennert, 1973c, Fig. 8.

[34] Cooper, Peterson, Gabrielsen and Good, 1966.

tion included the following groups. The research teams of SELIGMANN (in Paris) and AISENBERG (in Boston) engaged in studies of surface immunoglobulin. Various rosette techniques were applied by LUTZNER and BÉRARD and co-workers (in Bethesda). At the institute of ROBB-SMITH (in Oxford), TAYLOR succeeded in demonstrating intracytoplasmic immunoglobulin in routine paraffin sections.[34a] Many authors still have reservations, however, as to whether the time is ripe for a grouping into B- and T-cell lymphomas, such as the one we proposed together with LUKES in London in 1973 (Table 6). Nevertheless, we agree with LUKES that it is quite possible at the present time to ascribe many malignant non-Hodgkin's lymphomas to the B- and T-lymphocyte series by means of morphologic methods alone. When that is impossible, we must avail ourselves of all methods used in modern immunologic research and morphology in order to reach our goal. We are convinced that such complicated studies will soon make it possible, at least in most cases, to extrapolate to morphology and to clearly separate B- and T-cell lymphomas. This appears to be more feasible for lymphomas of the B-cell series than for those of the T-cell series, since the relationship of morphology and function in B-cell forms is better understood. In addition, the morphology, cytochemistry, and immunochemistry of the development of T-cells and T-cell variants must be studied more extensively in order to find the counterparts of the various kinds of neoplastic T-cells.

Such endeavors should not beguile us into complacency. We must remember that all cells of the B-cell and T-cell systems in "normal" lymphatic tissue are disposed to *cooperate* and that every reaction of lymphatic tissue involves several cell types, either simultaneously or one after the other. Accordingly, that must also be true to a certain degree for malignant lymphomas, since at least most of them represent more or less distorted reflections of normal reactions seen in lymphatic tissue.[35] The higher the degree of differentiation, the better a malignant lymphoma will reproduce the normal pattern of the lymphatic reaction (immune reaction). In anaplastic tumors the normal intercellular cooperation is often only fragmentary or vague. The following are examples.

Firstly, follicular lymphoma (M.L. centroblastic/centrocytic, follicular) is almost a complete mirror image of the normal germinal center. The neoplastic germinal centers contain centroblasts, centrocytes, dendritic reticulum cells, a few macrophages, sometimes a few plasma cells, and even occasionally immune precipitates (see p. 331). That was the reason why, until the fundamental studies of RAPPAPORT *et al.*,[36] follicular lymphoma and follicular hyperplasia could often not be told apart. If the tumor cells become more anaplastic, then a monotonous, chiefly centroblastic tumor (previously called germinoblastic sarcoma, but now referred to as M.L. centroblastic) may develop from the original mingling of different cells. Dendritic reticulum cells are then missing. Therefore, there is no longer cellular cooperation with these cells.

Somewhat less well "differentiated" in the sense of intercellular cooperation is M.L. centrocytic. The typical centroblast is absent, and dentritic reticulum cells are present in only a number of cases. Usually no follicles are formed.

[34a] For literature, see Part Six and the chapters on each lymphoma.

[35] LENNERT, 1973c.

[36] RAPPAPORT, WINTER and HICKS, 1956.

Consequently, the degree of differentiation and therefore the grade of malignancy can be ascertained from the extent to which the normal follicle is reproduced.

A second example of this kind is T-zone lymphoma. In this tumor, besides atypical T-lymphocytes, we find interdigitating reticulum cells, epithelioid venules, reticulin fibers, and sometimes T-associated plasma cells. In other words, the tumor completely imitates the T-cell regions of normal lymph nodes and, in particular, reactive T-cell regions, which can be found in many different types of nonspecific lymphadenitis. This is occasionally reflected in the abundance of T-associated plasma cells.

Follicular lymphoma and T-zone lymphoma therefore imitate their normal counterparts. Organoid structures belonging to the B-cell and T-cell regions develop, undoubtedly owing to an interaction between various cells. The dendritic or interdigitating reticulum cells may well exert a certain guiding influence.

We can go a step further with follicular and T-zone lymphomas. It seems plausible that highly differentiated organoid lymphomas of one cell system can induce the proliferation of another cell system.[37] For example, the neoplastic follicles of typical M.L. centroblastic/centrocytic are surrounded by highly developed T-cell tissue. That is to say, they are surrounded by numerous T-lymphocytes, some interdigitating reticulum cells, epithelioid venules, and fibers. In contrast, T-zone lymphoma is associated with follicles rich in B-lymphocytes; sometimes numerous germinal centers showing regressive changes and surrounded by thick collars of lymphocytes may even be found among the tumor cells of the T-lymphocytic type and the contiguous venules. The lymphocytes surrounding the germinal centers can definitely be interpreted as B-lymphocytes on the basis of their immunologic markers.

In both of the examples referred to, it seems that, at least in highly differentiated states, the organoid neoplasm of either the B-cell or T-cell system is associated with a nonneoplastic increase in cells of the other system (T-cell or B-cell, respectively).

Another example of the imitation of normal reactions is the appearance of *epithelioid cells* in malignant lymphomas. We can find epithelioid cells in lymphomas producing IgM, such as lymphoplasmacytoid or immunoblastic lymphoma. Epithelioid cells are most prominent in so-called epithelioid-cell lymphogranulomatosis,[38] in which we see proliferations of lymphocytes, larger transformed basophilic lymphocytic forms, and epithelioid cells (see p. 467). We assume that the lymphocytes play the leading role, and we believe it is possible that they might secrete a mediator substance, which attracts monocytes and induces them to transform into epithelioid cells. Initially, we thought of the migration inhibitory factor (MIF), but, so far, we have not been able to demonstrate it. Undoubtedly, we know very little about such interrelationships. Thus, we should make every attempt to learn more about them. By this means we may also obtain insight into normal reactions, as was the case with the investigation of plasmacytoma.

A last example, immunoblastic lymphoma, illustrates how easily the close association of nonneoplastic cells can obscure the true appearance of the tumor. For decades this tumor was misinterpreted in two ways: the large tumor cells

[37] Kaiserling, 1975.
[38] Lennert and Mestdagh, 1968.

were equated with the associated macrophages that showed evidence of phagocytosis and an intensely positive esterase reaction; thus, many investigators concluded that the tumor was histiocytic in nature. In contrast, from the increase in reticulin fibers in the tumor, others held the opinion that the tumor was reticular in nature. Both viewpoints were wrong, since they were based on the characteristics of *associated* cells and not on the tumor cells themselves. The tumor cells, however, cause the macrophages to accumulate and induce the formation of reticulin fibers, changes that often occur in many types of inflammation. Consequently, it is essential to determine which cell is really neoplastic in each tumor; the associated nonneoplastic cells should not lead us astray. We presume that the same axiom holds true for extralymphatic lymphomas, for example, for microgliomatosis of the central nervous system. Here, the intense proliferation of microglial cells results only because of the presence and function of the tumor cells, which in our opinion are lymphocytes and plasma cells (LP immunocytoma; see p. 224).

Lymphomas not only shed new light on immunologic reactions and cellular interactions, they also show direct relationships to pathologic immune conditions.[39] For example, it has been known for a long time that malignant lymphomas frequently occur in immune-deficiency disorders.[40] Hodgkin's disease and other malignant lymphomas also frequently develop in conditions of increased and pathologic immune activity, such as autoimmune diseases.[41] Reticulosarcoma, follicular lymphoma, and lymphosarcoma have been reported in systemic lupus erythematosus. The development of malignant lymphomas, chiefly chronic lymphocytic leukemia, but occasionally reticulosarcoma, has also been described in cases of rheumatoid arthritis. The lymphomas associated with Sjögren's syndrome were mostly reticulosarcomas, but they also included chronic lymphocytic leukemia and macroglobulinemia of Waldenström. A large number of so-called reticulosarcomas have been recorded following treatment with immunosuppressive drugs after organ transplantation,[42] and a number of Hodgkin's and non-Hodgkin's lymphomas have been reported after diphenylhydantoin treatment[43] (but not all cases were proved to be malignant lymphomas). Finally, the graft-versus-host reaction in animals is sometimes followed by the development of a malignant lymphoma, probably immunoblastic sarcoma.[44] Apparently, most of these lymphomas are of B-cell nature, except perhaps for the lymphomas in congenital immune-deficiency syndromes. In these disorders, we find a still-unestimated number of T-cell lymphomas. Study of the manifold immune-deficiency disorders will perhaps enrich the study of malignant lymphomas, and vice versa.[45] Consideration of the different classes of immune-response genes might play a key role in such studies.

---

[39] Schwartz and André-Schwartz, 1968; Hoerni and Laporte, 1970, Lit.; Aisenberg, 1973.

[40] Miller, 1967a; Krüger, 1972; Good, 1973; Kersey, Gajl-Peczalska and Nesbit, 1974.

[41] Talal and Bunim, 1964; Miller, 1967b; Jones, 1973.

[42] Penn, Halgrimson and Starzl, 1971; Krüger, 1972; Reis, 1972; Videbaek, 1973.

[43] Lit.: see Aisenberg, 1973; Leder and Lennert, 1972; experiments: see Krüger, Harris and Sussman, 1972.

[44] Gleichmann, Gleichmann, André-Schwartz and Schwartz, 1972; Gleichmann, Gleichmann and Schwartz, 1972; Grundmann and Hobik, 1973; Solnik, Gleichmann, Kavanah and Schwartz, 1973.

[45] See Oliver, 1975.

Another basic problem with malignant lymphomas is the definition of *leukemia.* We wish to avoid participating in the disputes among clinicians, who disagree on the number of neoplastic cells needed in the blood for a diagnosis of leukemia and on whether the bone marrow must be involved or not. We are more concerned with the nature of leukotic and nonleukotic neoplasms of similar cells. In other words, are there fundamental differences between nonleukotic lymphomas ("sarcomas") and leukoses (leukemias)? Our answer to this question is "yes" and is based on the following reasons.

From pathoanatomic, histologic, and cytologic standpoints, we define a leukemia (leukosis) as follows. It is seen grossly as a diffuse infiltration of bone marrow, liver, spleen, lymph nodes, and so forth, without any recognizable formation of nodules or localized tumor masses. Histologically, there is uniform infiltration, which often preferentially involves certain regions, for example, the portal areas of the liver; destructive growth is not seen. Destruction of the stroma is essential for the diagnosis of sarcoma, but not for the diagnosis of leukemia.[46] When infiltrates are unusually massive, they can cause "pressure atrophy" of preexistent structures. In lymph nodes the leukemic cells either appear to "skip" the capsule and crowd as massive infiltrates about it (as in chronic lymphocytic leukemia) or they extensively permeate the capsule, widening it but causing no destruction (as in acute lymphoblastic leukemia). Cytologically, the cells of chronic leukemias range in maturity from "-blasts" to "-cytes" (chronic myeloid leukemia, chronic lymphocytic leukemia) or are exclusively mature cells (for example, plasma-cell leukemia). In acute leukemias the cells are virtually always "blast cells."

In contrast to leukemia (leukosis), sarcomas of the blood-forming organs are defined as tumor nodules or masses that destroy the preexistent tissue. In addition, there are two varieties of combinations of "leukemia" and "sarcoma." (1) There are cases in which the disease appears primarily as a tumor and in which a leukemic blood picture is found at some time during the course of the disease. (2) There are cases in which typical leukemia exists over a longer period of time with diffuse infiltration of organs, etc., and in which autopsy reveals a tumorous picture, with nodules of neoplastic cells in organs, and tumor masses as well as still-existent diffuse infiltrates.

So-called thymic lymphosarcoma (M.L. lymphoblastic, convoluted-cell type) can serve as an example of the first group of cases, in which the eventual leukemia may be regarded as a "spilling over"[47] rather than evidence of increased cellular differentiation.

In the second group of cases, the ability of the leukemic cells to enter the blood might be interpreted as a sign of their differentiation. As the cells develop, they acquire surface properties enabling them to emigrate into the blood. If in such cases of leukemia we find masses or nodules of tumor at autopsy, then we may consider this to be a sign of dedifferentiation. The cells have lost the surface properties enabling them to emigrate into the blood and have therefore "stuck together" in the tissue in the form of cell masses, which no longer show purely infiltrative growth, but instead destructive growth.

---

[46] Robb-Smith, 1964. [47] Galton, 1964.

In 1908, STERNBERG[48] referred to the first variety as leukosarcomatosis, a term appropriate at the time. The second variety embraces tumor-forming leukemias.[49] Although the blood picture is "leukemic" in both types, the nature of the "leukemia" is basically different. We should try to express this difference when we formulate our concepts about leukemia. We should avoid regarding leukemia and hyperleukocytosis of the blood as synonyms, just as we should refrain from depriving leukopenic leukemia of its leukemic nature merely because at certain times in its course great numbers of proliferating cells fail to appear in the blood. We mention this problem now, since in the Kiel Classification use of the adjective leukemic for all lymphomas may introduce an equating factor that is practical, but obscures the nature of the various lymphomas. The same holds true for applying the term lymphoma to both leukemias and nonleukotic neoplasms of the lymphatic tissue.

# III. A Simplified Cellular Scheme as a Basis for a Modern Classification of Lymphomas

As described in Part One, two cell series, namely, the T- and the B-lymphocyte series develop from a still poorly defined stem cell of the bone marrow (see Fig. 33). The "virgin" T- and B-cells are called $T_1$- and $B_1$-lymphocytes, respectively. When these lymphocytes encounter antigenic stimulation for the first time, they transform into blast cells. $T_1$-lymphocytes develop into T-immunoblasts, i.e., large basophilic cells as we know them from studies of tissue cultures with phytohemagglutinin (PHA). These immunoblasts either fulfill their function and die, or they become $T_2$-lymphocytes. The latter react more intensely and more quickly when stimulated a second time by the same antigen. They represent the memory cells of the T-cell series. Inclusion of the so-called T-associated plasma cell[50] in our scheme is meant to be provocative. This type of cell has not yet been fully defined, although we presume that it is related to the T-cell system. We realize, however, that the term plasma cell is not compatible with that assumption. Furthermore, it has not been proved by any means that T-associated plasma cells produce immunoglobulin (see p. 31).

When B-lymphocytes encounter antigenic stimulation for the first time, they also transform into immunoblasts (B-immunoblasts), which so far cannot be morphologically distinguished from T-immunoblasts. B-immunoblasts give rise to plasma cells, which develop *via* plasmablasts and proplasmacytes. The plasma cells are relatively small at first and have a relatively small Golgi body. These

[48] Also 1916.
[49] LENNERT, 1964a.
[50] MÜLLER-HERMELINK, KAISERLING and LENNERT, 1973; LENNERT, KAISERLING and MÜLLER-HERMELINK, 1975.

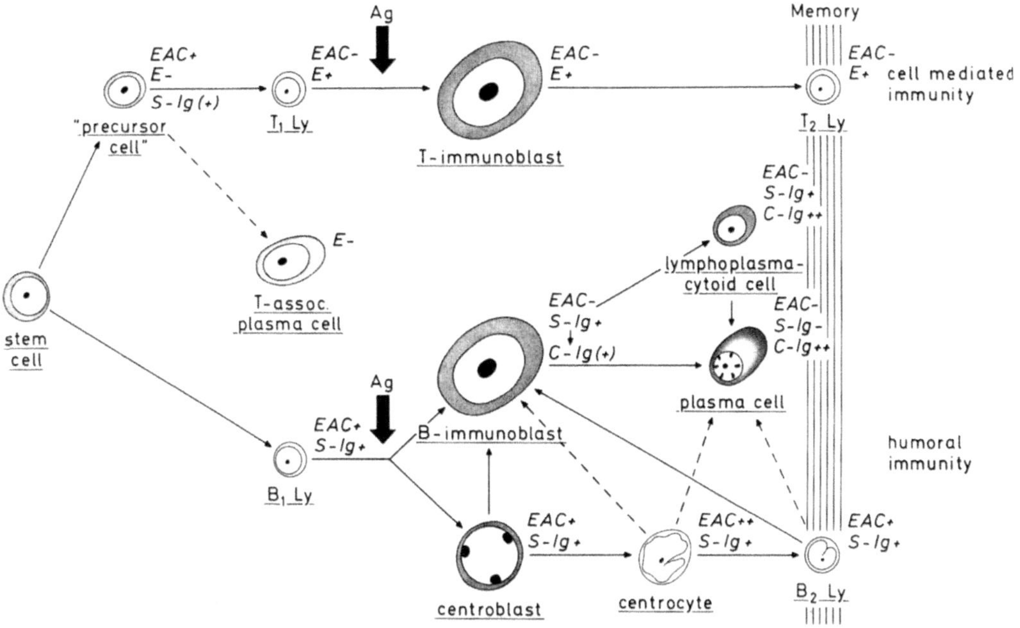


Fig. 33. Preliminary, simplified scheme of the T- and B-lymphocyte systems. The subtypes of T-lymphocytes are not shown. *EAC+* = complement receptor-positive (cell forms rosette with EAC). *EAC−* = complement receptor-negative (cell does not form rosette with EAC). *E+* = sheep-E receptor-positive (cell forms spontaneous rosette with sheep erythrocytes). *E−* = sheep-E receptor-negative (cell does not form spontaneous rosette with sheep erythrocytes). *S-Ig* = surface immunoglobulin. *C-Ig* = intracytoplasmic immunoglobulin. *Ag* = antigenic stimulation. *Ly* = lymphocyte

cells used to be called lymphatic plasma cells, plasmacytoid lymphocytes, or lymphoplasmacytoid cells, which correspond to the plasma cells circulating in the blood. They initially bear surface IgM and secrete chiefly IgM. The small plasmacytoid cells enlarge, becoming the plasma cells previously called the "reticular" or Marschalkó type. These are the cells that are chiefly responsible for producing IgG, IgA, IgD, and IgE. They may, however, also produce IgM. Only relatively few plasma cells, mainly of the lymphoplasmacytoid type, are produced in the primary immune response; consequently, the amount of immunoglobulin they produce is small.

A further response to the first antigenic stimulation is the development of germinal centers. In germinal centers, centroblasts originate from small lymphocytes. In turn, the centroblasts give rise to centrocytes and these ultimately to $B_2$-lymphocytes, which are the memory cells of the B-cell system. In addition, lymphocytes, probably of random antigen specificity, develop in germinal centers.[50a] Thus, germinal centers are first a site of B-lymphocyte multiplication. They also produce the precursors of the plasma-cell series. It seems likely that large centroblasts can transform directly into immunoblasts and thereby join the plasma-cell series. The formation of plasma cells can, however, proceed by way

[50a] Keuning, 1972.

of centrocytes and $B_2$-lymphocytes. An intermediate step between lymphocytes and plasma cells, considered to be the marginal-zone cell by NIEUWENHUIS and KEUNING,[51] is difficult to identify in human lymph nodes. According to our findings in malignant lymphomas, centrocytes can probably transform directly into immunoglobulin-secreting cells or plasma cells without going through a blastic or other intermediate stage. In any event, all agree that the germinal center is a site where plasma-cell precursors are produced. In human lymph nodes, mature plasma cells are also often produced *in* germinal centers.

Our scheme is an oversimplification and contains many flaws. Where should we include the various killer cells, for example? There is also no mention of T-helper cells or T-suppressor cells. Nonetheless, our scheme may help us to understand not only the main types of malignant lymphoma, but also the numerous possible borderline cases.

If we try to relate the various non-Hodgkin's lymphomas to the given cell scheme[52]—a similar attempt was made by SALMON and SELIGMANN[53]—a considerable number of the lymphomas can be more or less clearly linked. Most chronic lymphocytic leukemias (CLL) are derived from $B_1$- or $B_2$-lymphocytes; the blast cell of CLL represents an underdeveloped B-immunoblast that is not capable of further development into the plasma-cell series. When there is no block, however, plasmacytoid or plasmacytic cells develop. Together with lymphocytes, they characterize our lymphoplasmacytic/lymphoplasmacytoid type of lymphoma (immunocytoma). In contrast to the cells of chronic lymphocytic leukemia, these cells are able to produce immunoglobulin, mostly IgM. If, as rarely happens, pure populations of plasma cells proliferate in the lymph node (malignant lymphoma, plasmacytic), it is generally found, as expected, that the immunoglobulin produced is 7-S rather than 19-S type. Since plasma cells are often derived from germinal-center cells—corresponding to the secondary immune response—there is also a close relationship between the latter cells and immunocytoma. On the one hand, this relationship manifests itself in the polymorphic type of immunocytoma. On the other hand, immunoglobulin synthesis is occasionally found in germinal-center tumors, with or without retention of immunoglobulin. The tumors that arise from both main cell types of the germinal centers (centroblasts and centrocytes) usually show a follicular structure. These tumors correspond to the follicular lymphomas (Brill-Symmers disease) of the literature. Centrocytes, however, can also proliferate on their own. In this case we speak of M.L. centrocytic. Tumors composed of a pure population of centroblasts (M.L. centroblastic) are of high-grade malignancy. LUKES and COLLINS[54] also include Burkitt's tumor and other lymphomas in the group of "follicular-center cell" tumors. Most immunoblastic lymphomas (previously called reticulosarcoma) are derived from B-immunoblasts. Immunoblastic lymphomas seldom originate from T-immunoblasts. We are still uncertain where each of the T-lymphocytic lymphomas should be included in the scheme. There are probably several possibilities; to mention only two types of T-lymphocytes is no doubt to oversimplify. We still have more to learn in this area.

---

[51] 1974.
[52] LENNERT, 1975.
[53] 1974.
[54] 1974a, b.

# IV. The Kiel Classification and Its Clinical Relevance

The Kiel Classification is based primarily on cytology. Structural characteristics, such as formation of follicles or tendency to fibrosis, are used merely as adjuncts. Two main groups of tumors are distinguished: lymphomas of low-grade and those of high-grade malignancy. The terms used for the low-grade malignant lymphomas end with the suffix "-cytic" (or "-cytoid") and those for the high-grade with "-blastic." Generally, the cells of the low-grade tumors are small, with only occasional large blast forms intermingled among them. In contrast, the high-grade malignant types consist of a pure population of larger "blastic" cells. Nearly all malignant lymphomas may be associated with a leukemic blood picture.

The basic division into low- and high-grade malignancies corresponds well with results of kinetic studies recently presented by TREPEL and SCHICK.[55] Low-grade malignant lymphomas show a low to moderate rate of proliferation, a large percentage of cells in $G_0$-phase, and a low rate of cell death. The proliferation is restricted to basophilic cells ("blasts").[55] They are morphologically similar to the blast cells of high-grade malignant lymphomas, which show high mitotic activity and a high rate of cell death, whereas the percentage of $G_0$ cells is relatively low.

The kinetic data of SILVESTRINI *et al.*[56] correspond roughly with the concept of low- and high-grade malignancies. The question has been raised, however, as to whether a third, intermediate group should be introduced, in particular to include polymorphic immunocytoma and large-cell centrocytic lymphoma.

In fact, the group of low-grade malignant lymphomas is not homogeneous in comparison with the fundamentally uniform high-grade malignant lymphomas. Roughly speaking, one can say that the degree of malignancy is somewhat higher ("intermediate") when the lymphocytes or centrocytes are relatively large or when the number of "blasts" ("paraimmunoblasts," immunoblasts, centroblasts) is particularly large.

The author admits that the Kiel Classification represented a compromise in many respects. On the one hand, it was relatively easy to replace the names "germinocyte" and "germinoblast" with "centrocyte" and "centroblast," thus dispelling all misgivings of American colleagues who feared confusion with germ-cell tumors. On the other hand, other concessions were made with great reluctance. The present division into low-grade and high-grade malignant lymphomas does not fully correspond to the "irreversible progressive hyperplasia" and "sarcoma" that ROBB-SMITH[57] and the author[58] favored earlier. Malignant lymphoma of the centrocytic type is probably an intermediate form. Previously, it was regarded as a sarcoma. Now it is classed with the low-grade lymphomas. In addition, the author believes that equating leukemia with tumor poses a problem. This is discussed more thoroughly on pages 97f. and 407f.

[55] TREPEL and SCHICK, 1976.

[56] SILVESTRINI, PIAZZA, RICCARDI and RILKE, 1977.

[57] 1964.

[58] LENNERT, 1967.

Nevertheless, the Kiel Classification seems to us to provide the best compromise in terminology (but not in concept) that is possible at the present time. Its main advantage is that it allows tumors that are difficult to diagnose precisely at least to be classified in one of the main groups, either as a low-grade malignant lymphoma or as a high-grade type—low-grade malignant lymphomas consist of small or of small and large cells, whereas high-grade malignant lymphomas are relatively homogeneous proliferations of medium-sized or large basophilic cells. This possiblity is probably of the greatest clinical relevance. Even when working conditions are not optimal, a statement about the degree of malignancy of a lymphoma makes clinical predictions and appropriate treatment possible. Finally, the Kiel Classification leaves all avenues open for segregating lymphomas into B-cell and T-cell types by means of modern immunologic techniques. Actually, that should be the scientific aim of any classification of lymphomas. On this point we fully agree with LUKES and COLLINS and are encouraged by positive statements such as those made by HANSEN and GOOD.[59]

This leads us to a discussion of the clinical relevance of the Kiel Classification. No system of nomenclature should be pursued merely for its own sake. It must be clinically relevant and designed to help patients. Such aims, however, need not be immediately apparent. We would like to caution against prematurely rejecting a classification if it fails at first glance to show a clinical correlation. It is well known that some tumors of malignant appearance that progress rapidly are now more easily cured than more benign-appearing counterparts that progress more slowly. Here we need only recall to mind acute lymphoblastic leukemia (ALL), which is curable in some cases and shows longer remissions than "chronic" leukemias, all of which are still incurable. On the other hand, it is important to recognize subtle morphologic differences—correlating with definite immunologic or cytochemical markers—in the cells of malignant lymphomas, since therapy, both in kind and in dosage, as well as prognosis, depend to a considerable extent on a precise diagnosis. Accordingly, the value of a classification should not be measured *solely* by its *present* clinical relevance.

One should combine the approach that has produced such magnificent results under KAPLAN in Stanford,[60] and for which PETERS[61] was a crucial pioneer, with a subtle classification of lymphomas. That would mean an exact *staging* of non-Hodgkin's lymphomas, as has been practiced in Stanford and other places for years.[62] The combination of a lymphoma classification based on subtle morphology and immunology with precise staging procedures will benefit us in our understanding of non-Hodgkin's lymphoma and contribute to more cures than is possible at the present time. With non-Hodgkin's lymphoma, however, an additional parameter, the *blood picture,* must be taken into account. Whereas the changes in the peripheral blood in Hodgkin's disease are in most instances insignificant, in many non-Hodgkin's lymphomas they are of great importance. With adequate experience and good hematologic techniques, a large

[59] 1974.

[60] KAPLAN, 1972, Lit.

[61] 1963.

[62] FERGUSON, ALLEN, GRIEM, MORAN *et al.*, 1973; JONES, FUKS, BULL, KADIN *et al.*, 1973; DUMONT, DUFFILLOT, THIEBAUT, CHELLOUL *et al.*, 1974; KIM and DORFMAN, 1974; MUSSHOFF and SLANINA, 1974; TUBIANA and LE BOURGEOIS, 1974; VERONESI, MUSUMECI, PIZZETTI, GENNARI *et al.*, 1974.

number of non-Hodgkin's lymphomas can be diagnosed from the blood picture. Such studies of the peripheral blood make many investigations much easier, for example, those using cytochemistry, immune markers, and the electron microscope. They also spare the patient the distress of surgical procedures.

The histologic type and stage of a lymphoma are presumably the most important factors determining the prognosis. The data available for the Kiel Classification are not yet satisfactory. The results of three independent clinical studies show, however, that the Kiel Classification has at least some prognostic relevance. For a relatively small number of patients, MUSSHOFF *et al.*[63] demonstrated that there is a statistically significant difference between the prognoses of low- and high-grade malignant lymphomas (Fig. 34). The different types of lymphoma revealed different survival rates in the large series of VAN UNNIK *et al.*[64] M.L. centroblastic/centrocytic had the best prognosis, followed by M.L. centrocytic and M.L. lymphoplasmacytic/lymphoplasmacytoid. The shortest survivals were found with M.L. immunoblastic.

The series of the Kiel Lymphoma Study Group is the most homogeneous with respect to histologic diagnoses. It was studied by BRITTINGER *et al.*[65] and STACHER *et al.*[66] The results are given in Figure 35. The actuarial survival is by far the longest in M.L. centroblastic/centrocytic and chronic lymphocytic leukemia (CLL). The lowest survival rate is seen in M.L. lymphoblastic and M.L. immunoblastic. The curves for M.L. centrocytic, except towards the end, and M.L. lymphoplasmacytic/lymphoplasmacytoid lie between the extremes, but nearer those for the other low-grade malignant lymphomas.

The prognosis of non-Hodgkin's lymphomas is an important, but not the only, clinical criterion. The symptomatology shows significant differences in the various types of lymphoma. For example, the five subtypes of lymphocytic lymphoma have different clinical manifestations. CLL of the B-type always involves lymph nodes and the bone marrow, but rarely the skin. In contrast, tumor cells of CLL of the T-type have less of a tendency to infiltrate lymph nodes and the bone marrow, but frequently infiltrate the skin.[67] Hairy-cell leukemia is characterized by lymphoid myelofibrosis, splenomegaly, and pancytopenia, and it requires completely different treatment from other leukemias. Mycosis fungoides and Sézary's syndrome are clearly distinguished from the other lymphocytic lymphomas by their characteristic skin lesions. T-zone lymphoma hardly responds at all to conventional lymphoma therapy.

The other lymphomas of low-grade malignancy also have special clinical features. Hemolytic anemia is more often associated with LP immunocytoma than with B-CLL. LP immunocytoma has three clinical variants: (1) the lymph-node type, (2) the splenomegalic type, and (3) the oculocutaneous type, which may involve only the orbit and skin for many years. Only the first type has many features in common with B-CLL.

In contrast to patients with centroblastic/centrocytic lymphoma, those with

---

[63] MUSSHOFF, SCHMIDT-VOLLMER, LENNERT and SANDRITTER, 1976; MUSSHOFF, 1976.

[64] Preliminary data presented by the author at Airlie House Conference in 1975.

[65] BRITTINGER, BARTELS, BREMER, DÜHMKE *et al.*, 1976.

[66] STACHER, WALDNER and THEML, 1976.

[67] BROUET, FLANDRIN, SASPORTES, PREUD'HOMME *et al.*, 1975.

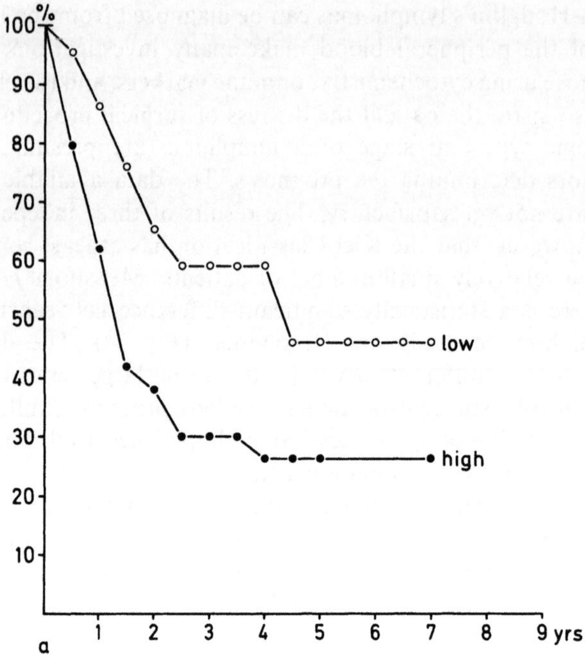


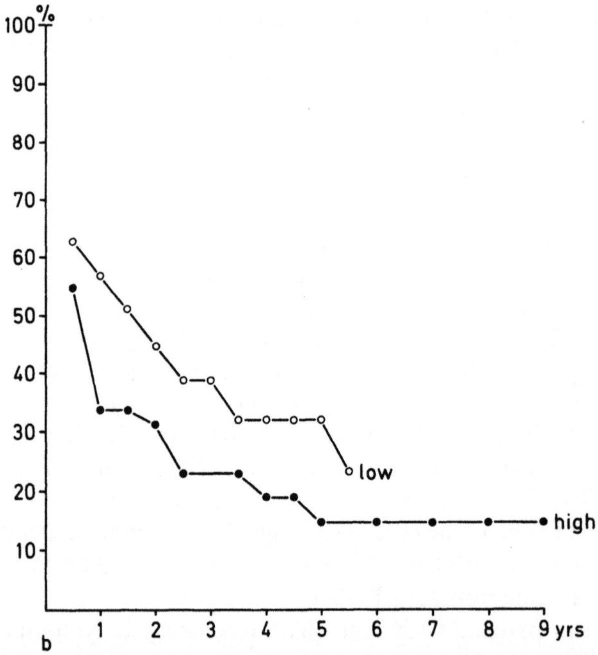


Fig. 34a and b. Actuarial survival (a) and disease-free survival rates (b) of patients with low- (n=22) and high-grade malignant lymphomas (n=53). The survival rates after 2 and 3 years for the patients with low-grade malignant lymphomas are significantly higher ($P<0.05$) than those for the patients with high-grade malignant lymphomas. (From MUSSHOFF, SCHMIDT-VOLLMER, LENNERT and SANDRITTER, 1976)

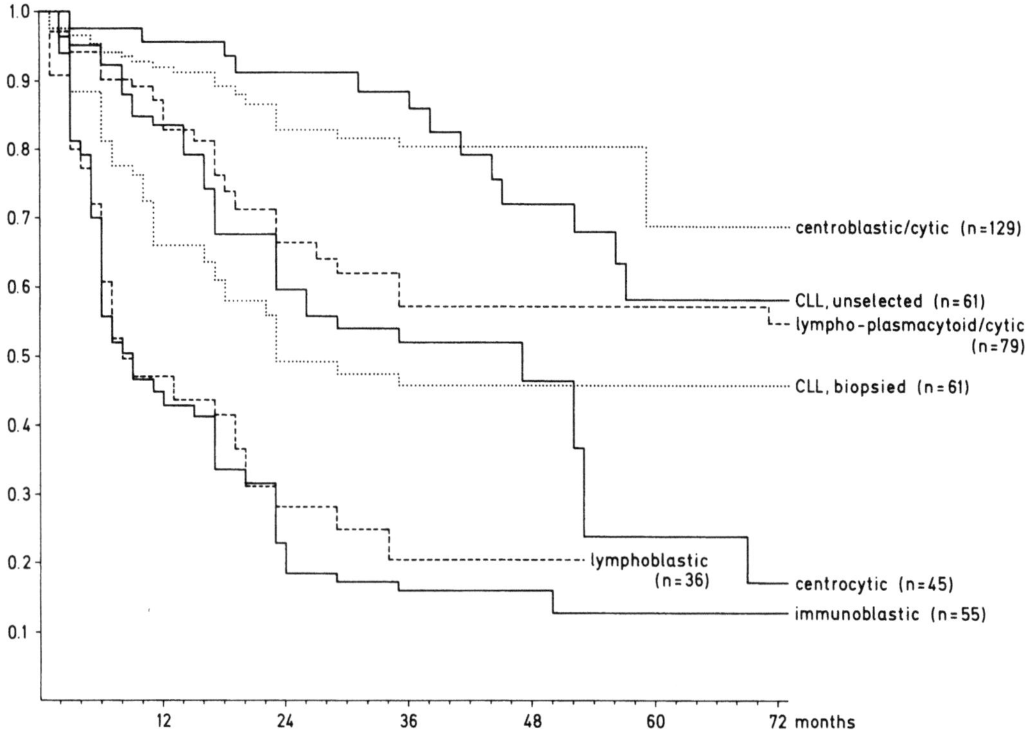


Fig. 35. Actuarial survival of patients with the main types of malignant lymphomas distinguished by the Kiel Classification. The group "CLL, unselected" consists of routine patients of the Department of Hematology, University of Essen. "CLL, biopsied" are contributed, as are all other types, by the Kiel Lymphoma Study Group. (From BRITTINGER, BARTELS, BREMER, DÜHMKE *et al.*, 1976)

centrocytic lymphoma usually present in stage IV at the time of biopsy. They almost always exhibit at least some centrocytes in the blood. Transformation into a lymphoma of higher-grade malignancy hardly ever occurs in cases of centrocytic lymphoma, whereas it is frequently observed in cases of centroblastic/centrocytic lymphoma. Nevertheless, centroblastic/centrocytic lymphoma often appears to be relatively benign for a long time, and it is sometimes confined to only one lymph-node region. It is now recognized everywhere that this type of lymphoma, which reveals a follicular pattern in 96% of the cases and is therefore by and large equivalent to "nodular lymphoma," is a special entity.

The clinical differences among high-grade malignant lymphomas are less well marked. The clinical manifestations of centroblastic lymphoma appear to largely coincide with those of immunoblastic lymphoma. Lymphoblastic lymphoma of the Burkitt type has been recognized for a long time as a distinct clinical entity because of the special manifestations of true African lymphoma. The non-African variety also appears to have particular clinical features—for example, the predominance of cervical and abdominal tumor masses. Patients with lymphoblastic lymphoma of the convoluted-cell type frequently present with a mediastinal tumor. This type of lymphoblastic lymphoma is more difficult to treat than lymphoblastic lymphomas of the Burkitt or unclassified type. According to MATHÉ *et al.*,[68] immunoblastic lymphoma is also a characteristic clinical entity. Paraproteinemia is occasionally found in the blood of patients with immunoblastic lymphoma.

An important difference between low- and high-grade malignant lymphomas lies in the age distributions (see p. 110). High-grade malignant lymphomas can occur in childhood and adolescence, whereas low-grade malignant lymphomas are observed only in adults.

All of these results are preliminary in some respects. They were obtained in retrospective studies without exact clinical staging and without standardized therapy. Nevertheless, they may give an idea of the usefulness and clinical applicability of the Kiel Classification. That encouraged us and our clinical lymphoma group to continue along the same path and to expand our studies to a prospective one with standardized staging procedures and therapy.

# V. Incidence of the Different Types of Lymphoma in Our Material

On the whole, malignant lymphomas are not very common neoplasms. During the three-year period 1964–1966, we diagnosed in Northern Germany (Schleswig-Holstein) 2.0 cases of Hodgkin's disease, 1.2 cases of non-Hodgkin's lymphoma excluding lymphocytic leukemia, and 1.7 cases of non-Hodgkin's lymphoma including lymphocytic leukemia per 100,000 population per year.[69] The total incidence of malignant lymphoma came to 3.2 and 3.7, respectively, per 100,000 per year. The number of lymphocytic leukemias was of course much higher than recorded here, since biopsies were made in only a small number of cases.

Statistical data on the incidence and age and sex distribution of malignant lymphomas are essential aids for diagnosis by the pathologist. Therefore, a summary of the most important data from each chapter will be given here.

The frequency of the various lymphomas in biopsy material is dependent on many factors. It does not reflect the true incidence of malignant lymphomas. For instance, in Germany, patients with chronic lymphocytic leukemia are often subjected to lymph-node biopsies, whereas that is not the case in Anglo-American countries. Nevertheless, a digest of the data on our material probably gives a rough idea of the relative frequency of the various lymphomas.

In our material (Table 12) Hodgkin's disease constitutes 43.6% and non-Hodgkin's lymphoma 56.4% of all malignant lymphomas. If we were to leave chronic lymphocytic leukemia (CLL) out of the non-Hodgkin's lymphomas, the

[68] MATHÉ, BELPOMME, DANTCHEV, POUILLART *et al.*, 1974.

[69] LENNERT, 1969b.

Table 12. Incidence of different types of malignant lymphoma in all material at the Lymph Node Registry in Kiel and in our routine material. First series, collected from July, 1965, through September, 1973

| Diagnosis | Total No. of biopsy cases | No. of routine lymph-node cases | Lymphomas (%) | Non-Hodgkin's lymphomas (%) |
|---|---|---|---|---|
| Hodgkin's disease | – | 651 | 43.6 | – |
| M.L. lymphocytic | 364 | 191 | 12.8 | 22.7 |
| CLL (B-type) | 261 | 176 | 11.8 | 20.9 |
| HCL | 33 | 3 | 0.2 | 0.4 |
| M.F. and Sézary's syndrome | 70 | 12 | 0.8 | 1.4 |
| M.L. lymphoplasmacytic/ -cytoid (LP immunocytoma) | 256 | 136 | 9.1 | 16.2 |
| M.L. plasmacytic (plasmacytoma) | 15 | 7 | 0.5 | 0.8 |
| M.L. centrocytic | 125 | 72 | 4.8 | 8.6 |
| M.L. centroblastic/ centrocytic | 606 | 184 | 12.3 | 21.9 |
| M.L. centroblastic | >23 | >10 | >0.7 | >1.2 |
| Primary | –[a] | >7 | >0.5 | >0.8 |
| Secondary | 23 | 3 | 0.2 | 0.4 |
| M.L. lymphoblastic | 211 | 107 | 7.2 | 12.7 |
| Burkitt type | 29 | 6 | 0.4 | 0.7 |
| Convoluted-cell type | 20 | 7 | 0.5 | 0.8 |
| Unclassified | 162 | 94 | 6.3 | 11.2 |
| M.L. immunoblastic | <187 | <134 | <9.0 | <15.9 |
| Unclassifiable | – | 150 | 9.9 | – |
| All non-Hodgkin's lymphomas | 1787 | 841 | 56.4 | – |
| All lymphomas | – | 1492 (+150) | – | – |

[a] Not estimated, included in M.L. lymphoblastic, unclassified and M.L. immunoblastic

frequency of Hodgkin's disease would be 49.5%, i.e., almost half of all malignant lymphomas. This percentage is, no doubt, relatively high when compared with the frequency in other countries.

M.L. centroblastic/centrocytic (follicular lymphoma of the old nomenclature) is the most common non-Hodgkin's lymphoma (21.9%). It is followed by chronic lymphocytic leukemia (20.9%), LP immunocytoma (16.2%), and immunoblastic lymphoma (< 15.9%). Immunoblastic lymphoma would probably come before LP immunocytoma if the uncertain cases were included. Next in frequency are lymphoblastic lymphomas (12.7%), most of which are unclassified, and then comes centrocytic lymphoma (8.6%). Centroblastic lymphoma is relatively rare (1.2%) in our material. This figure would

Table 13. Incidence of different types of malignant non-Hodgkin's lymphoma. Second series, collected from October, 1973, through December, 1976, at the Lymph Node Registry in Kiel

| Diagnosis | n | | % | |
|---|---|---|---|---|
| M.L. lymphocytic | 413 | | 20.7 | |
| B-CLL | | 345 | | 17.3 |
| T-CLL | | 5 | | 0.25 |
| Prolymphocytic leukemia | | 1 | | 0.05 |
| HCL | | 20 | | 1.0 |
| M.F. and Sézary's syndrome | | 16 | | 0.8 |
| T-zone lymphoma | | 26 | | 1.3 |
| M.L. lymphoplasmacytic/-cytoid | 355 | | 17.8 | |
| M.L. plasmacytic | 15 | | 0.8 | |
| M.L. centrocytic | 199 | | 10.0 | |
| M.L. centroblastic/centrocytic | 455 | | 22.8 | |
| M.L. centroblastic | 111 | | 5.5 | |
| M.L. lymphoblastic | 243 | | 12.1 | |
| Burkitt type (B) | | 42 | | 2.1 |
| Convoluted-cell type (T) | | 116[a] | | 3.8+2.0[b] |
| Unclassified | | 85 | | 4.2 |
| M.L. immunoblastic | 206 | | 10.3 | |
| Total | 1997 | | 100.0 | |
| Unclassifiable | 218 | | 9.8 | |
| Total | 2215 | | – | |

[a] Includes 40 cases where diagnosis was probable rather than certain
[b] Certain (3.8%) and probable cases (2.0%)

probably be much higher, however, if the cases earlier misdiagnosed as lymphoblastic and immunoblastic lymphomas were included. Mycosis fungoides (M.F.) and Sézary's syndrome make up 1.4% of our non-Hodgkin's lymphomas. Primary lymph-node plasmacytoma is very rare (0.8%). The Burkitt type and the convoluted-cell type of lymphoblastic lymphoma are recorded in Table 12 with about the same frequency. Undoubtedly, the figure for the convoluted-cell type is actually much higher (see Table 13), since a considerable number of lymphomas of this type cannot be diagnosed reliably when the techniques used are not optimal and when a cytochemical analysis is not performed. Such cases are included in the group of unclassified lymphoblastic lymphomas. Hairy-cell leukemia (HCL) is the rarest malignant lymphoma (0.4%).

Except for slight corrections, Table 12 is equivalent to the one we published in 1975.[70] The table presented here does not contain lymphoepithelioid-cell lymphoma, however, because the exact nature of the cases that cannot be classified as Hodgkin's disease has yet to be determined. The large number (150) of unclassifiable non-Hodgkin's lymphomas has not been altered, even though this has already been a reason for harsh criticism of our classification. The figure is an honest admission of fallibility and therefore we had no right

[70] Lennert, Mohri, Stein and Kaiserling, 1975.

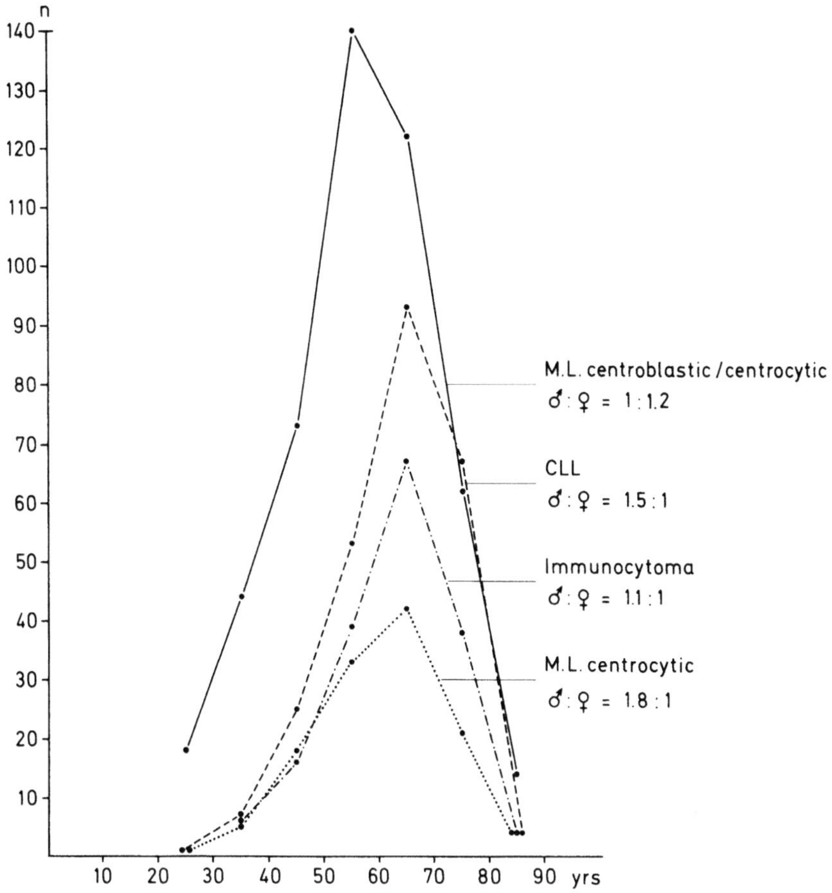


Fig. 36. Age distribution and sex ratio of low-grade malignant lymphomas. (From LENNERT, MOHRI, STEIN and KAISERLING, 1975)

to suppress it. The following factors were responsible for the large number of unclassifiable non-Hodgkin's lymphomas. Some cases could be diagnosed with only a certain degree of probability, either because the technical quality of the material was not good, or because there was not enough material. In other cases a definitive diagnosis could not be made because cytochemical or immunologic studies would have been necessary for specific classification of the lymphoma, and the relevant data were not available. Borderline cases between two defined entities made up another group of unclassifiable cases. Finally, our lack of experience and the present state of knowledge were not sufficient for a satisfactory diagnosis of a number of lymphomas.

The data given in Table 12 are based on the results of a joint study with MOHRI. After it was completed (September, 1973), we investigated another 2000 cases of non-Hodgkin's lymphoma (Table 13). We found that the incidence of the various low-grade malignant lymphomas was similar in the two series (Tables 12 and 13). The incidence of the different types of high-grade malignant

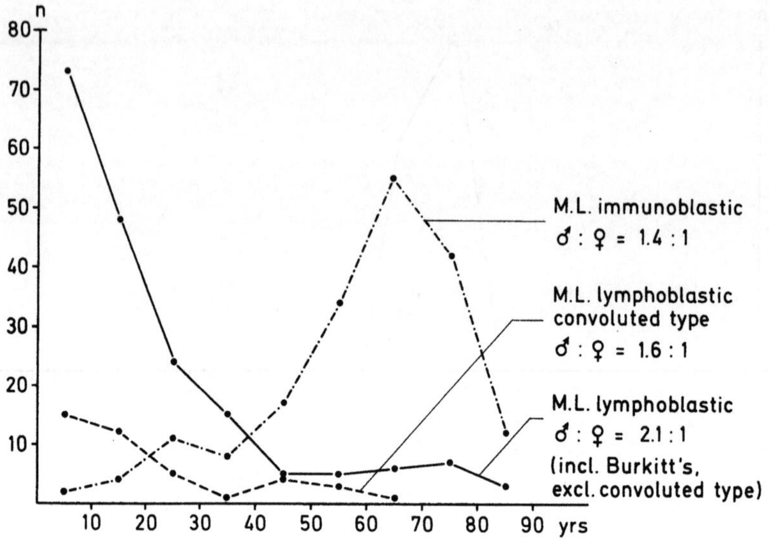


Fig. 37. Age distribution and sex ratio of high-grade malignant lymphomas. (Revised version of figure published by LENNERT, MOHRI, STEIN and KAISERLING, 1975)

lymphomas, however, revealed some differences that require comment here: centroblastic lymphoma made up 5.5% of the non-Hodgkin's lymphomas; lymphoblastic lymphoma of the Burkitt type, 2.1%; lymphoblastic lymphoma of the convoluted-cell type, 3.8% (certain cases) plus 2% (probable cases; i.e., in all about one third of the lymphoblastic lymphomas); and immunoblastic lymphoma, 10.3%. We add these data here, not merely in confirmation of the previously published incidence rates, but also because we would like to point out some trends that resulted from the use of better techniques (e.g., cytochemistry, electron microscopy, and immunologic analyses) and from a better understanding of the high-grade malignant lymphomas.

Looking at the age distribution of non-Hodgkin's lymphoma, the first thing we notice is an important principle: low-grade malignant lymphomas virtually do not occur before the age of 20 years (Fig. 36), whereas all high-grade malignant lymphomas can occur in youth, at times with marked predominance in the first decade (M.L. lymphoblastic; Fig. 37). In general, the peak frequency of low-grade malignant lymphomas and M.L. immunoblastic lies in the 7th decade, that of M.L. centroblastic/centrocytic (follicular lymphoma) in the 6th decade.

The sex ratio usually shows a slight to moderate predominance in males. The only lymphoma with a (slight) predominance of females is M.L. centroblastic/centrocytic.

Part Four

# Histopathology and Diagnosis of Non-Hodgkin's Lymphomas

K. LENNERT and N. MOHRI

## I. Malignant Lymphomas of Low-Grade Malignancy

### A. Malignant Lymphoma, Lymphocytic

Under this main heading we group all malignant lymphomas (M.L.) whose essential components are lymphocytes or variants of them. The lymphocytes may belong to either the B-cell or the T-cell series, or they may in exceptional instances have markers on their surfaces for both types of cells. Accordingly, in the following chapter, five subgroups of M.L. lymphocytic are discussed:

1. Chronic lymphocytic leukemia, B-cell type.
2. Chronic lymphocytic leukemia, T-cell type.
3. Hairy-cell leukemia.
4. Mycosis fungoides and Sézary's syndrome.
5. T-zone lymphoma.

#### *1. Chronic Lymphocytic Leukemia, B-Cell Type (B-CLL)*

*Synonyms:* Chronic lymphatic leukemia
M.L. lymphocytic, well differentiated, diffuse Lymphosarcoma, lymphocytic
M.L. small lymphocyte (LUKES and COLLINS)

**History, Terminology.** Chronic lymphocytic leukemia (CLL) has been a well-recognized entity since VIRCHOW,[1] although admittedly it has never been clearly delineated from "lymphocytic lymphosarcoma" and acute lymphoblastic leukemia. This failure is especially apparent in studies of autopsy material, for example, those of APITZ.[2] The reason is that in autopsy material the fine differences between CLL and lymphocytic lymphosarcoma (which we now call M.L. centrocytic) and between CLL and small-cell acute lymphoblastic leukemia are obliter-

[1] 1847.
[2] 1937a, 1940.

ated owing to autolysis (cf., POPKES,[3] Fig. 1). Nonetheless, the autopsy enables the pathologist to make macroscopic evaluations that allow him to distinguish neoplasms with and those without tumor nodules or masses. The types with tumor formation ("sarcomatous variants")[4] are characterized by nodular infiltrations or tumor masses as well as diffuse infiltrations. In contrast, typical CLL is distinguished by a purely diffuse infiltration of liver, spleen, and bone marrow. The lymph nodes are generally only moderately enlarged and well demarcated from one another. Histologically, the tumor nodules and masses show an infiltrative *and* destructive growth pattern, whereas the "pure" leukemia shows only infiltration of organs and tissues. Consequently, ROBB-SMITH[5] and one of the authors (K.L.)[6] included pure CLL without tumor formation among the irreversible progressive hyperplasias, and separated it from sarcoma and from CLL with tumor formation. Since, in agreement with the European Lymphoma Club, we disposed of the concept of sarcoma, the question that now confronts us is how to designate the cases of CLL with grossly visible formation of tumors and microscopic evidence of destructive growth.

In order to better understand tumor formation in CLL, we have studied our autopsy cases of CLL (a total of 107 in our collection). We found that 75.7% of these leukemias were devoid of any formation of tumor. In 15.9% tumor formation was obvious grossly, and in 8.4% it was questionable. Of the cases with definite formation of tumor, 3.8% showed development of what we previously called "lymphoblastic sarcoma" (see p. 131). In the remaining cases the tumor cells were characterized as so-called prolymphocytes, which are somewhat larger lymphocytes with relatively high mitotic activity, and there was destructive growth (destruction of walls of blood vessels, for example). In eight out of 88 cases of CLL, GALTON[7] found a locally aggressive behavior; they were probably equivalent to our cases of CLL with grossly evident tumor formation.

Whereas we did not find a transformation into "lymphoblastic" malignant lymphoma in any of our biopsy material (probably incidental), we saw sheets of prolymphocytes in several cases. They indicate a transition to a higher grade of malignancy, corresponding to grossly recognized CLL with tumor formation. We call this macroscopic and microscopic variant of CLL "tumor-forming CLL" (see p. 115).

Shortly after CLL was recognized as an entity, it became apparent that the disease develops in both leukemic and aleukemic forms. Therefore, a high lymphocyte count in the blood is not the decisive criterion for the disease. Accordingly, searches were made for other criteria. Lymphocytic infiltration of the bone marrow was then considered by many clinicians to be the essential criterion. Unfortunately, even that is unreliable, since every lymphoma can also metastasize to the bone marrow and be evident in sternal puncture material, without this meaning that a leukemia exists. Conversely, it is not yet clear whether there are variants of CLL that initially do not infiltrate the bone marrow.

[3] 1955.
[4] LENNERT, 1964a.
[5] 1964.
[6] LENNERT, 1967.
[7] 1964.

Consequently, the presence of neoplastic lymphocytes in the blood and infiltration of the bone marrow are not absolute criteria for CLL. In our opinion, the pathologist should base his diagnosis on the morphologic changes in the lymph nodes. Instead of speaking of CLL, we could be cautious and refer to malignant lymphoma of the CLL *type*. Thereby we would not presuppose that a chronic lymphocytic leukemia exists *clinically*. Nevertheless, we are convinced that the histologic picture of the CLL type cannot appear unless CLL is clinically manifest at some time or other. Future studies will have to prove whether there are *formes frustes* that can behave like sarcomas described in the earlier literature.

**Origin of the Neoplastic Cells.** We interpret the lymphocytes of the lymphoma of the CLL type described here as B-lymphocytes, since we, and many other investigators before us,[8] found B-cell markers on the surfaces of the neoplastic cells. In most cases a majority of lymphocytes in the blood have surface membrane-bound immunoglobulin (SIg). In addition, some have the complement receptor and/or the IgG-Fc receptor (they are EAC or EA rosette-positive). Conversely, T-cell markers (sheep-E rosettes, etc.) are not demonstrable on the neoplastic cells. The type of SIg is usually the same in all of the neoplastic lymphocytes; a monoclonal proliferation of cells is therefore present. In contrast to LP immunocytoma, the number of circulating lymphocytes containing intracytoplasmic Ig is very small[9] or nil. Other new data are presented in Part Six.

Whether the cells are $B_1$- or $B_2$-lymphocytes is a question that remains to be answered. Nevertheless, like SALMON and SELIGMANN,[10] we are inclined to assume that B-CLL as a rule is derived from $B_1$-lymphocytes. We cannot exclude the possibility, however, of a $B_2$-cell origin, which is highly probable for LP immunocytoma (see p. 213ff.). Irrespective of whether one regards them as $B_1$- or $B_2$-lymphocytes, they are incapable in the host of transforming into typical B-immunoblasts and joining the plasma-cell series. There is apparently a block in the switch from nonsecreting plasma-cell precursors to secreting plasma cells (Fig. 38).

Consequently, for us *the* criterion of CLL and *the* characteristic distinguishing it from LP immunocytoma is the inability of the cells to become actively secreting B-cells. The lymphocytes of CLL bear immunoglobulin only *on* the cell surface and not *in* the cytoplasm. Therefore, a monoclonal increase in immunoglobulin does not occur in typical CLL. The cases of CLL with paraproteinemia reported in the literature[11] are probably leukemic immunocytomas.

In compliance with common hematologic usage, we call the "blocked," underdeveloped immunoblasts of CLL "lymphoblasts." It would be better to call them "paraimmunoblasts." They differ from typical immunoblasts in the

---

[8] WILSON and NOSSAL, 1971; PREUD'HOMME and SELIGMANN, 1972; AISENBERG and BLOCH, 1972; AISENBERG, BLOCH and LONG, 1973; SILBERMAN and SCHREK, 1974; COHNEN, 1974, Lit.

[9] KNAPP, SCHUIT, BOLHUIS and HIJMANS, 1974; RUDDERS, 1976.

[10] 1974.

[11] E.g., HENNEMANN and RATHENOW, 1955; BRAUNSTEINER and SAILER, 1960; MICHAUX and HEREMANS, 1969, Lit.; WALDENSTRÖM, 1970, personal communication.

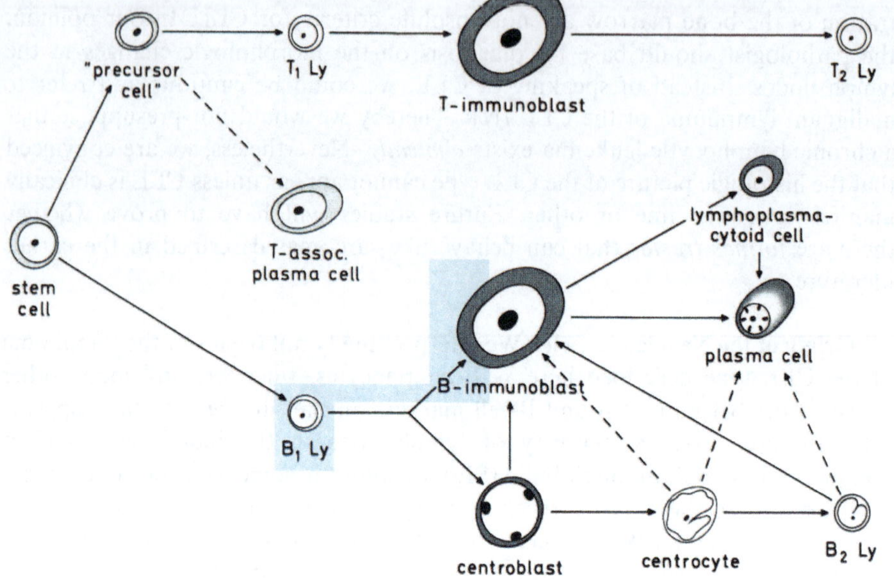


Fig. 38. Hypothetical origin of tumor cells of B-CLL is shown in the dark blue areas. A second possibility is shown in light blue. There is no evolution in the direction of plasma cells or lymphoplasmacytoid cells

weaker basophilia of the cytoplasm and nucleolus. Apparently, they can be produced from the lymphocytes of CLL in tissue culture.[12]

The lymphocytes of CLL have a number of special properties that distinguish them from normal lymphocytes.[13] Some of these properties express themselves in morphologic changes. First, the cell surface is profoundly altered.[14] That may explain why the lymphocytes of CLL fail either in large part or completely to recirculate.[15] Another explanation for the restricted recirculation might be the great decrease in the number of epithelioid venules in lymph nodes[16] involved by CLL. It seems unlikely, however, that such a decrease in venules is solely responsible for the restricted recirculation, since T-lymphocytes seem to recirculate freely through the veins of lymph nodes involved by CLL,[16] whereas leukemic B-lymphocytes do not. Secondly, greatly increased amounts of glycogen can be demonstrated in the leukemic cells,[17] representing that which is not utilized.[18]

---

[12] Cohnen, 1974, Lit.

[13] Gingold and Stoica, 1967; Rau, Mueller-Eckhardt, Huth and Löffler, 1968; Huber and Braunsteiner, 1972; Westerhausen, 1972; Perera and Pegrum, 1974, Lit.; Seeber and Schmidt, 1974, Lit.

[14] Gingold and Stoica, 1967; Rau, Mueller-Eckhardt, Huth and Löffler, 1968; Huber and Braunsteiner, 1972; Westerhausen, 1972; Perera and Pegrum, 1974, Lit.; Seeber and Schmidt, 1974, Lit.; Mintz and Sachs, 1975.

[15] Pfisterer, Nennhuber, Bolland and Stich, 1967; Harris and Bagai, 1972; Flad, Huber, Bremer, Menne *et al.*, 1973; Engeset, Frøland and Bremer, 1974.

[16] Söderström and Norberg, 1974; Bremer, Cohnen, Augener and Brittinger, 1975; Kaiserling, 1975.

[17] Astaldi, Bernardelli and Rondanelli, 1952; Storti, 1952; Mitus, Bergna, Mednicoff and Dameshek, 1958; Quaglino and Hayhoe, 1959; Bauer-Sic and Lambers, 1963; Heckner, 1963; Quaglino, Cowling and Hayhoe, 1964.

[18] Cf., Brody, Oski and Singer, 1969.

Thirdly, the number of acid phosphatase-positive lysosomes is greatly reduced and correlates with the low activities of acid phosphatase and β-glucuronidase in the leukemic lymphocytes.[19] The fragility of the lysosomal membranes is also increased.[20] Fourthly, there is a marked reduction in the number of protein-synthesizing ribosomes.[21] Fifthly, the activity of the surface enzyme ATPase is higher than that of normal lymphocytes.[22]

With respect to kinetics, TREPEL and SCHICK[23] emphasized that only blast cells larger than 9 μm proliferate and that the rate of proliferation is high in lymph nodes and low in bone marrow. BREMER[24] has presented a survey of the kinetic data.

**Definition.** CLL of the B-cell type (B-CLL) histologically shows proliferation of small lymphocytes, among which at least a few "lymphoblasts" (paraimmunoblasts) and prolymphocytes are *always* to be found. The pattern of the neoplasm is in principle diffuse; but in most cases it reveals small or large, light areas of proliferating cells (no follicles!). The blood lymphocyte count is usually higher than normal at the time of lymph-node biopsy. The bone marrow is always infiltrated. Paraproteinemia does not occur.

**Subclassification.** In analyzing our cases, we found that we could histologically distinguish three variants of CLL:

1. A diffuse type without focal proliferations (and with only occasional "lymphoblasts").
2. A pseudofollicular type with focal proliferations of "lymphoblasts" and prolymphocytes (Fig. 42).
3. A tumor-forming type with extensive areas of prolymphocytes and fewer "lymphoblasts" that occupy one third to three quarters of the lymph node, whereas the remaining part contains chiefly lymphocytes (Fig. 43).

These three subtypes reflect three grades of proliferative activity. The activity is low in the diffuse subtype, high in the tumor-forming subtype, and lies in between the extreme variants in the pseudofollicular type. The pseudofollicular and tumor-forming types probably correspond to so-called active CLL.[25]

**Occurrence.** B-CLL represents 11.8% of all malignant lymphomas, assuming second place among the non-Hodgkin's lymphomas in our first series, of which it makes up 20.9% (Table 14). The disease is actually considerably more common, since many cases are diagnosed clinically without biopsies of lymph nodes being made. In Schleswig-Holstein we diagnose 0.42 cases per 100,000 population from lymph nodes each year.[26]

Of the subtypes, the pseudofollicular type (2) predominates with 88.4%, followed by the diffuse type (1) with 4.1% and the tumor-forming type (3) with 2.3%. In 5.2% of our cases an exact subclassification was not possible.

---

[19] BRITTINGER, KÖNIG, ABERLE and ZIMMERSCHITT, 1970; BRITTINGER, KÖNIG, COHNEN and ABERLE, 1970; DOUGLAS, COHNEN, KÖNIG and BRITTINGER, 1973; COHNEN, 1974, Lit.
[20] KÖNIG, BRITTINGER and COHNEN, 1973.
[21] BILLINGTON and ITZHAKI, 1974.
[22] MÜLLER-HERMELINK and KAISERLING, 1975.
[23] 1976.
[24] 1975.
[25] KNOSPE, LOEB and HUGULEY, 1974.
[26] LENNERT, 1969b.

Table 14. CLL. Material and incidence

| | | |
|---|---|---|
| Total No. of cases | 368 | |
| Biopsy | | 261 |
| Autopsy | | 107 |
| Total No. of biopsies[a] | 273 | |
| Lymph nodes | | 261 |
| Extranodal | | 12 |
| Incidence in routine lymph-node biopsies[b] 176 | | |
| = 11.8% of malignant lymphomas | | |
| 20.9% of non-Hodgkin's lymphomas | | |

[a] In this and all other *material and incidence* tables, the number of biopsies means those collected at the Lymph Node Registry in Kiel. The material is, to some degree, selected.
[b] Unselected biopsy material routinely collected at our Department.

In 201 cases blood counts made at the time of biopsy and occasionally later were available to us for study. We rated lymphocyte counts of over 4000/μl with the leukemic forms. When the differential blood count was not available (infrequently), we regarded a total leukocyte count of over 11,000/μl as leukemic. Using these criteria, 75.5% of all cases were leukemic. Differences between the subgroups were not significant and must be investigated further.

The age distribution curve has a sharp peak in the seventh decade when both sexes are analyzed together (Fig. 39). The peak is the same as that when

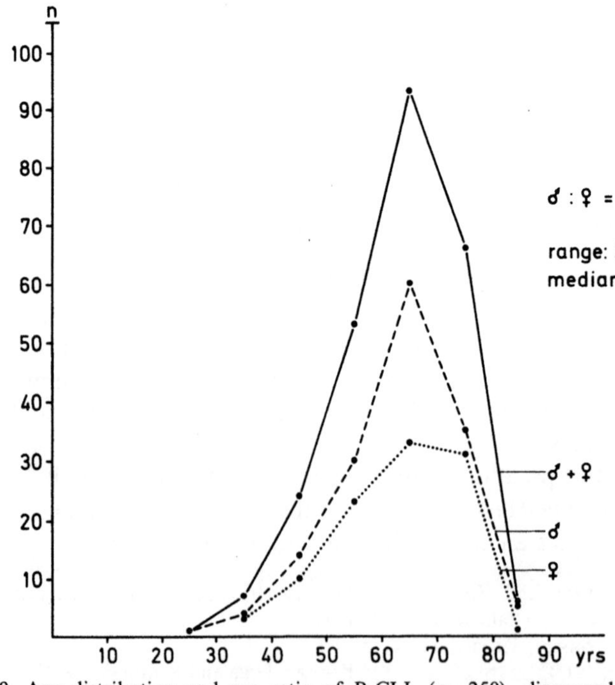


Fig. 39. Age distribution and sex ratio of B-CLL (n = 250), diagnosed in lymph-node biopsies at the Lymph Node Registry in Kiel

Table 15. Clinical symptoms of 66 CLL patients of the Kiel Lymphoma Study Group (STACHER, WALDNER and THEML, 1976)

| Symptom | n[a] | % positive |
|---|---|---|
| Fever >38° C | 52 | 19.2 |
| Weakness | 66 | 55.0 |
| Loss of appetite, weight loss | 38 | 26.3 |
| Night sweat | 23 | 39.1 |
| Symptoms of allergy | 15 | 20.0 |
| Arthralgia | 56 | 12.5 |
| Enlargement of lymph nodes | 50 | |
| Slow | | 78.0 |
| Rapid | | 22.0 |

[a] n = number of patients for whom data were available

men are analyzed alone, whereas for the women in our material there is a plateau between the seventh and eighth decades. The difference in frequency between the sexes may be due more to the makeup of the population than to the nature of the disease (the loss of men in World War I would affect the number living to the eighth decade). The youngest patient was only 24 years old, a most unusual exception. Even the number of patients in their thirties is very low. CLL actually never occurs before the third decade of life. On the other hand, it appears at all advanced ages. Our oldest patient subjected to biopsy was 84 years old. Some of those whom we autopsied were older than 90 years. The median age is 64.5 years. There seems to be a slight difference in age distribution of our patients with the pseudofollicular and diffuse types: the diffuse type shows an abrupt increase in the eighth decade.

That the male sex is more often afflicted is clearly evident from the male-to-female ratio of 1.47:1 (or 59.5%).

B-CLL is extremely rare in Japan. Among the Chinese and Japanese living in America the disease occurs much less often than among the Caucasians.[27]

**Clinical Manifestations.** The clinical picture of CLL is well known and will not be discussed here. Nevertheless, we shall present the clinical data on our material, which may differ from the clinical picture ordinarily seen in typical cases of CLL, since the lymph nodes in our collection were sometimes removed and investigated because of an unusual clinical presentation.

The following data of the Kiel Lymphoma Study Group were collected by THEML[28] and published by STACHER *et al.*[29] They were based on 66 patients. It should be mentioned that all values were not available in all cases. Table 15 shows the frequency of general symptoms, fever, and "allergic" phenomena. The lymph nodes enlarged slowly in 78% of the patients, rapidly in 22%. In 15% no increase in lymphocytes was evident in the blood (<4000 lymphocytes/µl; Table 16). Enlargement of lymph nodes both above and below

[27] SHIMKIN and LOVELAND, 1961.
[28] 1975, personal communication.
[29] STACHER, WALDNER and THEML, 1976.

Table 16. Lymphocyte counts in peripheral blood of 65 CLL patients of the Kiel Lymphoma Study Group (STACHER, WALDNER and THEML, 1976)

| Lymphocytes/μl | % |
|---|---|
| <2,000 | 7.7 |
| 2,000 – 4,000 | 7.7 |
| 4,000 – 5,000 | 7.7 |
| 5,000 – 10,000 | 18.5 |
| 10,000 – 20,000 | 12.3 |
| 20,000 – 50,000 | 15.4 |
| 50,000 – 100,000 | 12.3 |
| 100,000 – 200,000 | 7.7 |
| >200,000 | 10.7 |

Table 17. Hemoglobin, thrombocytes, RBC sedimentation rate, and immunoglobulin in blood of CLL patients of the Kiel Lymphoma Study Group (STACHER, WALDNER and THEML, 1976)

| Values | | n[a] | % |
|---|---|---|---|
| Hemoglobin | | 78 | |
| >13.1 g-% | | | 48.7 |
| 13.0 – 10.1 g-% | | | 35.9 |
| 10.0 – 8.1 g-% | | | 9.0 |
| <8.0 g-% | | | 6.4 |
| Thrombocytes <100,000/μl | | 65 | 23.1 |
| RBC sedimentation rate | | 74 | |
| Normal | | | 55.4 |
| Slightly accelerated (up to 20/33) | | | 27.0 |
| Moderately accelerated (up to 50/82) | | | 10.8 |
| Greatly accelerated | | | 6.8 |
| Immunoglobulin in serum | | 40 | |
| IgG | Normal | | 60.0 |
| | Increased | | 5.0[b] |
| | Decreased | | 35.0 |
| IgA | Normal | | 50.0 |
| | Increased | | 2.5[b] |
| | Decreased | | 47.5 |
| IgM | Normal | | 55.0 |
| | Increased | | 2.5 |
| | Decreased | | 42.5 |

[a] n = number of patients for whom values were available
[b] Increase in IgG and IgA in one case

the diaphragm was established in 80% of the cases. The bone marrow was infiltrated in all cases. Slight to severe anemia was found in only 51.3% of the cases (Table 17). Coombs-positive immune-hemolytic anemia was not demonstrated. In 23.1% the number of blood platelets was reduced. The RBC sedimentation rate was normal in 55.4%; otherwise it was slightly to highly elevated.

Table 18. Localization of biopsies in CLL

| Localization | n | | % | |
|---|---|---|---|---|
| Lymph nodes | 249 | | 95.4 | |
| Cervical | | 106 | | 49.3 |
| Axillary | | 60 | | 27.9 |
| Mediastinal | | 1 | | 0.5 |
| Abdominal | | 7 | | 3.2 |
| Inguinal | | 41 | | 19.1 |
| Cubital | | – | | – |
| Unknown | | 34 | | – |
| Extranodal | 12 | | 4.6 | |
| Bone marrow | | 2 | | – |
| Spleen | | 2 | | – |
| Tonsils | | 1 | | – |
| Others | | 7 | | – |
| Total | 261 | | 100 | |

The immunoglobulin level was normal or decreased. Only five cases, originally diagnosed as CLL, showed an increase in Ig, namely, monoclonal IgG in three cases, and IgE and monoclonal IgA in the other two cases. We therefore studied the slides again and realized that, in fact, three cases showed the features of LP immunocytoma. Two cases were still indistinguishable from typical CLL with a pseudofollicular pattern. In one of these two cases, however, a new biopsy was performed, and it clearly showed the morphology of LP immunocytoma. That permits the conclusion that a case of "CLL" with paraproteinemia is in all probability an "immunocytoma," even if we cannot identify it as such in a given lymph node. It might be identifiable in another localization of lymphoma proliferation. That demonstrates the close relationship between CLL and LP immunocytoma.

**Localization.** Table 18 lists the sources of the excised lymph nodes. It shows that 49.3% of the lymph nodes were removed from the cervical region, 27.9% from the axillary region, and 19.1% from the inguinal region. Lymph nodes from internal regions (mediastinal, abdominal) were submitted for study only rarely (0.5% and 3.2%, respectively). These numbers give us no information about the actual distribution of the disease in the various chains of lymph nodes.

**Gross Appearance.** In B-CLL the lymph nodes are usually only slightly to moderately enlarged and from soft to moderately firm. They are easily separated from one another. If large tumor masses or large lymph-node conglomerates have developed, then the histologic picture is in most cases that of the tumor-forming subtype. Sometimes there is also massive enlargement of lymph nodes in the pseudofollicular type.

**Histology.** In all subtypes of B-CLL the structure of the lymph nodes is completely effaced. Only rarely are remnants of noninfiltrated lymphatic tissue

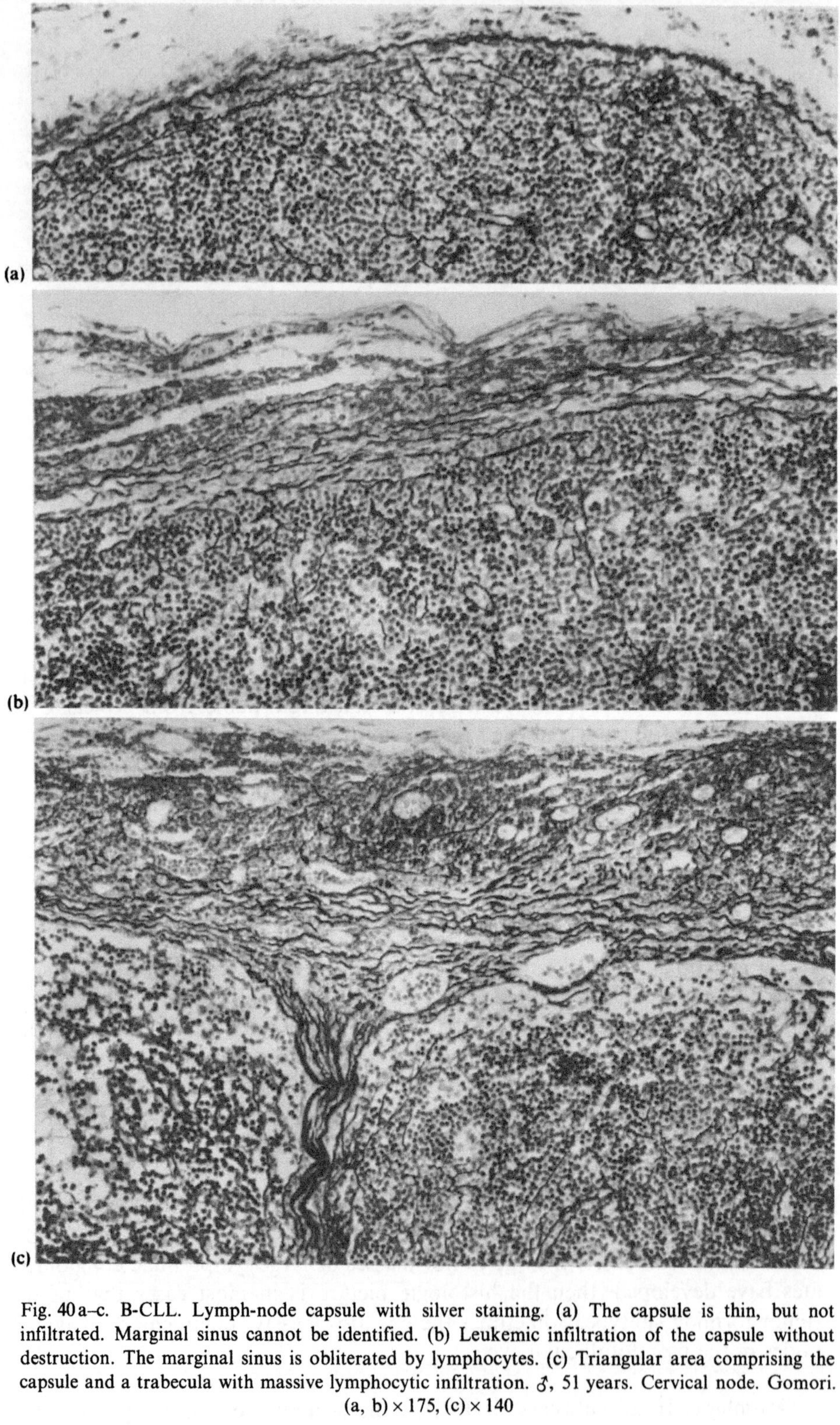


Fig. 40a–c. B-CLL. Lymph-node capsule with silver staining. (a) The capsule is thin, but not infiltrated. Marginal sinus cannot be identified. (b) Leukemic infiltration of the capsule without destruction. The marginal sinus is obliterated by lymphocytes. (c) Triangular area comprising the capsule and a trabecula with massive lymphocytic infiltration. ♂, 51 years. Cervical node. Gomori. (a, b) × 175, (c) × 140

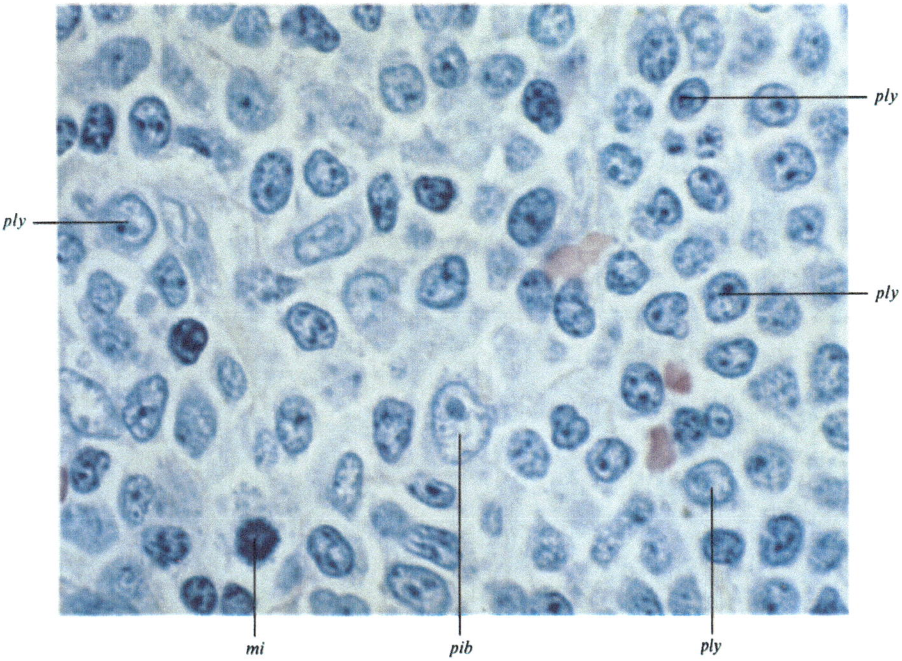


Fig. 41. B-CLL with Giemsa staining. Area of proliferation. Note one paraimmunoblast ("lymphoblast" *pib*), some prolymphocytes (*ply*), and one mitotic figure (*mi*). There are a moderate number of small lymphocytes. ♂, 70 years. Cervical node. × 1,550

left behind, for example, germinal centers with or without mantles of lymphocytes. It is difficult to decide where the infiltration begins. Sometimes one has the impression that it arose in the medullary region. In one case we found the infiltration exclusively in the outer cortex, in a somewhat nodular manner reminiscent of primary follicles. The sinuses are always narrow and hardly recognizable. That is especially true for the marginal sinus (Fig. 40). Here the lymphocytes accumulate up to the capsule, but do not destroy it. Infiltration of the capsule is only sometimes evident. On the other hand, lymphocytic infiltration is often found in triangular areas where the trabeculae branch off from the capsule. Rather massive infiltrates of lymphocytes are often demonstrable in the surrounding adipose tissue. The capsule of the lymph node usually remains intact and can be identified as such.

The reticulin fibers are few to moderate in number and mostly thin, at least thinner than in M.L. centrocytic. They form a relatively regular network throughout the lymphomatous tissue, in contrast to centrocytic lymphoma, in which they envelop large masses or groups of cells.

Cytologically, small lymphocytes predominate. They are, however, somewhat larger than the preexistent normal small lymphocytes they have replaced (Fig. 41). They are also larger than the leukemic lymphocytes circulating in the blood.[30] So-called lymphoblasts (paraimmunoblasts) are always found

[30] Popkes, 1955.

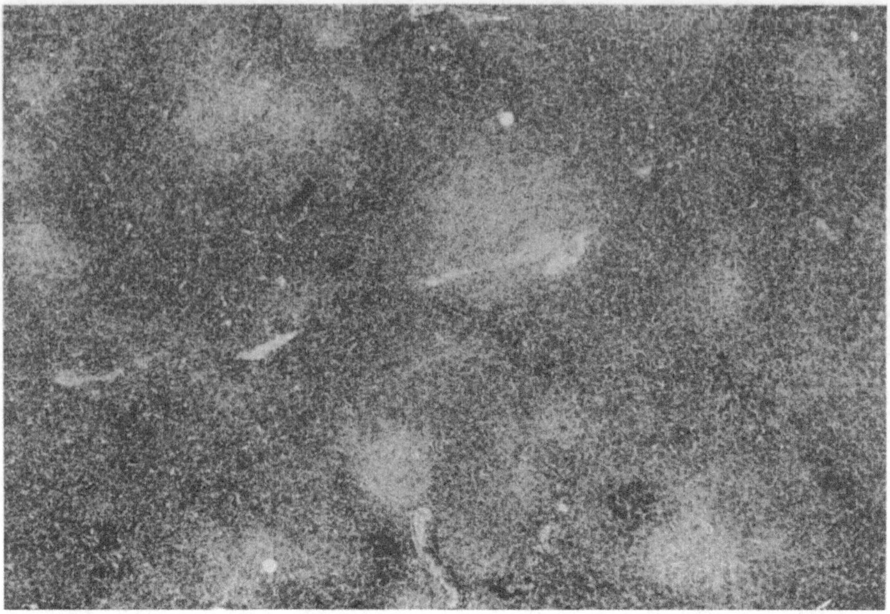

Fig. 42. B-CLL, pseudofollicular subtype. Note the light areas irregularly distributed throughout the lymph node. They should not be confused with neoplastic germinal centers. ♂, 41 years. Axillary node. Giemsa. ×56

among the lymphocytes. They have medium-sized to large, usually oval nuclei with fine chromatin and usually single, large, central nucleoli. These nucleoli are slightly basophilic, that is, they stain gray-blue to gray-violet with Giemsa. The cytoplasm is moderately abundant and, in contrast to that of lymphocytes, readily seen. With Giemsa it stains gray-blue, unlike the dark blue cytoplasm of immunoblasts or centroblasts.

Finally, so-called prolymphocytes are always present, particularly in the neighborhood of "lymphoblasts." They are a type of lymphocyte that is distinctly larger than the small lymphocytes, which predominate, and their chromatin is lighter. Their nuclei are generally round or oval, but are occasionally irregular, resembling somewhat those of centrocytes.

Mitotic figures are found chiefly among the "lymphoblasts" (paraimmunoblasts), at times also among the prolymphocytes, but not among the small lymphocytes.[31] The mitotic activity depends upon the number of these "immature" cells. The more numerous the "lymphoblasts" and prolymphocytes, the higher the mitotic activity, and vice versa.

The number of "lymphoblasts" and prolymphocytes also determines the *subtype* of CLL. When there are only very few "lymphoblasts" and prolymphocytes present, the picture is that of a diffuse type. When greater numbers

[31] Kinetics of CLL: see Rubin, Havemann and Dameshek, 1969; Cronkite and Schiffer, 1970; Trepel, Theml, Schick, Schneble *et al.*, 1972; Schick, 1973; Theml, Trepel, Schick, Kaboth *et al.*, 1973.

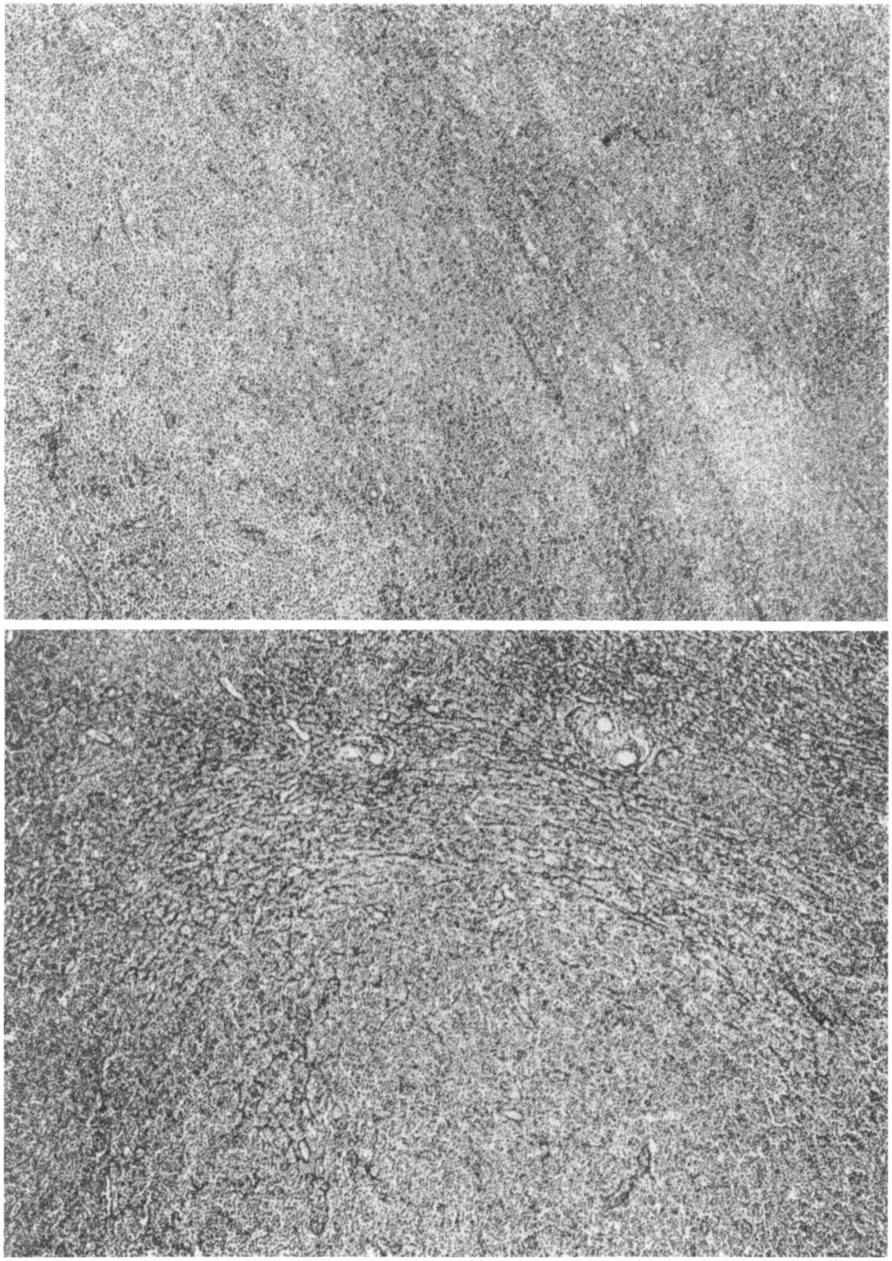

(a)

(b)

Fig. 43a and b. B-CLL, tumor-forming subtype. (a) The left half of the picture and a smaller focus at the lower right reveal cells that are lighter and larger than those in the rest of the field. (b) The same lymph node with silver staining. The lower half of the picture is equivalent to a lighter area of (a). Note the small number of reticulin fibers in this area, in contrast to the high fiber content of the surrounding lymphocytic infiltration. ♂, 51 years. Cervical node. (a) PAS, (b) Gomori. (a, b) ×56

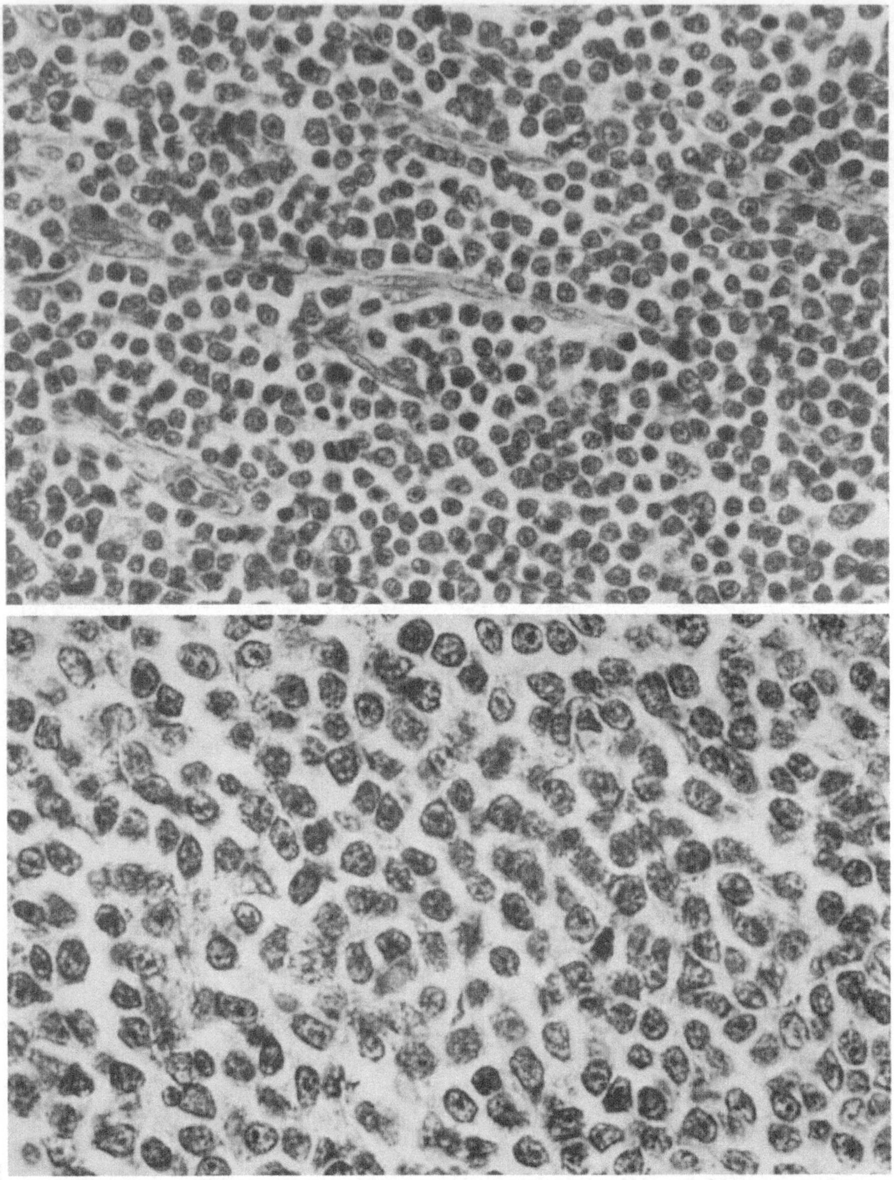

(a)

(b)

Fig. 44a and b. B-CLL, tumor-forming subtype. (a) Dark area containing chiefly lymphocytes and some prolymphocytes and paraimmunoblasts ("lymphoblasts"). ♂, 51 years. Cervical node. Giemsa. ×560. (b) Light area consisting only of polymorphic prolymphocytes. ♀, 52 years. Inguinal node. Giemsa. ×875

of these cells are evident, they are generally clustered as proliferating aggregates; this is the pseudofollicular type (Fig. 42). When prolymphocytes proliferate excessively, we speak of the tumor-forming type (Fig. 43). The "lymphoblasts" in this instance are relatively small and difficult to differentiate from the prolymphocytes (Fig. 44). When histologic sections from these cases are held up

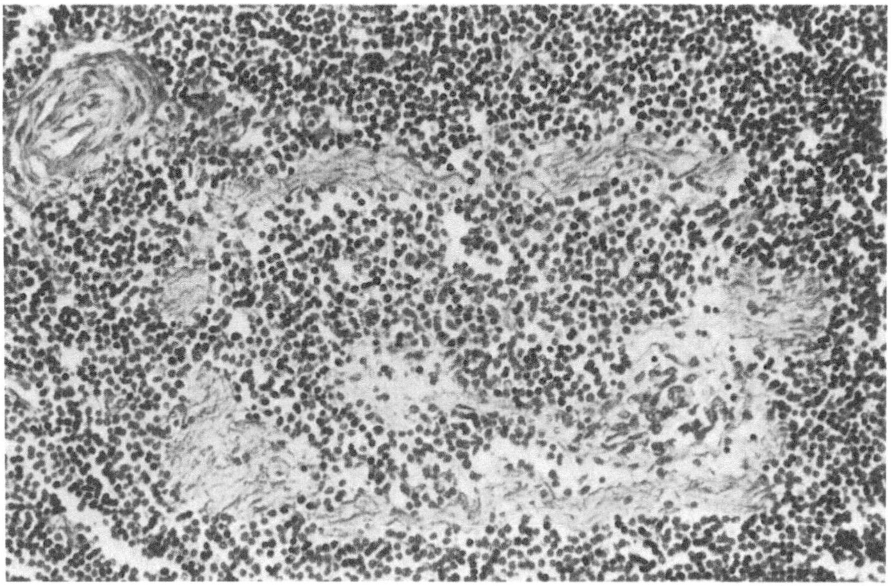

Fig. 45. B-CLL, tumor-forming subtype. Section of tumor mass in the pelvic region. A relatively large vein has been destroyed by the tumor. A small artery is intact. Autopsy case. ♂, 63 years. Van Gieson. ×70

against the light and examined with the naked eye, large lighter regions are conspicuous. TRUJILLO *et al.*[32] illustrated these regions well in Figure 4 of their paper.

Furthermore, the tumor-forming type is characterized by an especially prominent histologic feature that is probably not seen in the other types. The neoplastic cells grow destructively and destroy veins, especially the small and medium-sized vessels (Fig. 45). In addition, the adventitia of arteries and arterioles is often split open by tumor cells. In one case we encountered undifferentiated tumor cells of medium size, which we were unable to classify with the "lymphoblasts" or prolymphocytes. They had medium-sized polymorphic nuclei with medium-sized nucleoli. They were aggregated in and about small and medium-sized arteries and veins. Not only were the vascular lumina filled with tumor cells, but portions of their walls were also invaded and destroyed by them. Previously, one would have without doubt described this picture as sarcomatous transformation. The capsule and trabeculae of the lymph nodes from this case were notably still completely intact. The tumor cells directed their aggression apparently only at blood vessels.

The tumor-forming type also differs from the other types in its reticulin network. The sheets of prolymphocytes are virtually free of reticulin fibers and therefore contrast well with the relatively fiber-rich lymphocytic regions of the leukemically infiltrated lymph nodes (Fig. 43b).

Besides the lymphoid cells mentioned, other types of cells are rarely found. Mast cells are uncommon. There is no increase in reticulum cells. Occasionally, small clusters of interdigitating reticulum cells are found in remnants of T-re-

[32] TRUJILLO, BUTLER, AHEARN, SHULLENBERGER *et al.*, 1967.

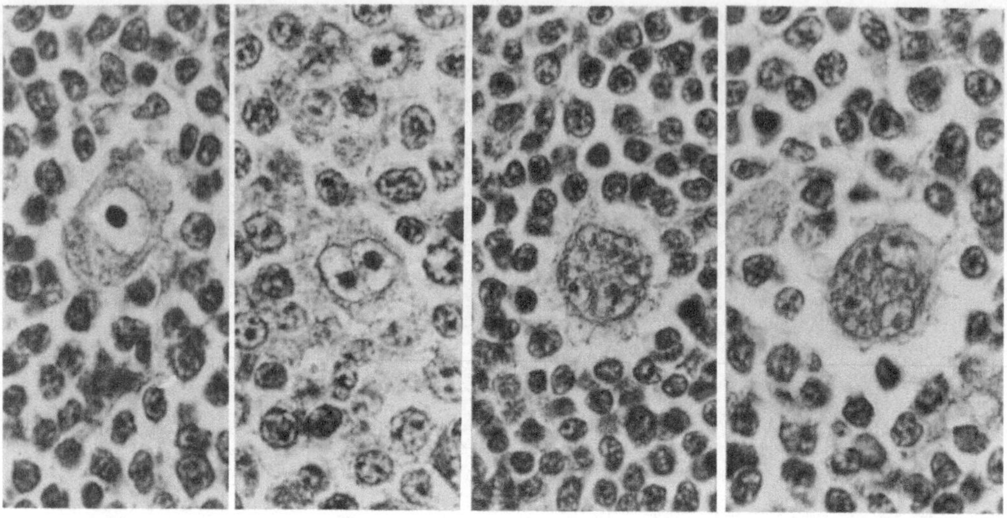

Fig. 46a–d. B-CLL. Giant cells that are very similar, if not identical, to Sternberg-Reed cells. A combination with Hodgkin's disease could be ruled out. (a, c, d) ♂, 56 years, treated with corticosteroids (Ultralan®). Axillary node. (b) ♀, 52 years. No previous treatment. (a) Giemsa, (b) methyl-green pyronine, (c) hematoxylin and eosin, (d) PAS. (a–d) ×875

gions. Neoplastic plasma cells or plasmacytoid cells are not present. Eosinophils are also not seen.

In three cases we found solitary or occasional multinucleate giant cells, which could not be distinguished from Sternberg-Reed cells (Fig. 46). The lymph-node pattern corresponded to the classic picture of B-CLL. Nothing indicated that there was a combination with Hodgkin's disease. One patient had been treated for at least a year with chlorambucil.

In two cases extramedullary hematopoiesis had developed and in one of them osteomyelosclerosis was suspected. In an autopsy case we also observed relatively marked hematopoiesis in myeloid metaplastic lymph nodes. Abundant megakaryocytes were most conspicuous. This was definitely a combination of CLL and osteomyelosclerosis (myelofibrosis; see p. 133).

**Smear/Imprint.**[32a] In smears B-CLL[33] reveals a large number of cells; thus, the staining of imprints macroscopically appears to be both dense and intense. That is also impressive at a low magnification. At the same time, the cells show marked uniformity at this microscopic level.

[32a] In this and all following chapters, *smear* means those taken from lymph-node puncture material, and *imprint* means those made by dabbing the fresh cut surface of biopsies onto glass slides.

[33] Guthrie, 1921; Forkner, 1927a, b; Pavlovsky, 1934; Tischendorf, 1938, 1939, 1951; Stahel, 1939; Schilling, 1943; Strunge, 1944, Lit.; Sundberg, 1947; Lorenz, 1949; Morrison, Samwick, Rubinstein, Stich *et al.*, 1952; Berman, 1953; Schoen, Heckner and Marsch, 1953; Bessis, 1954; André and Dreyfus, 1955; Heilmeyer and Begemann, 1955; Lucas, 1955; Lüdin, 1955; Klima and Herzog, 1956.

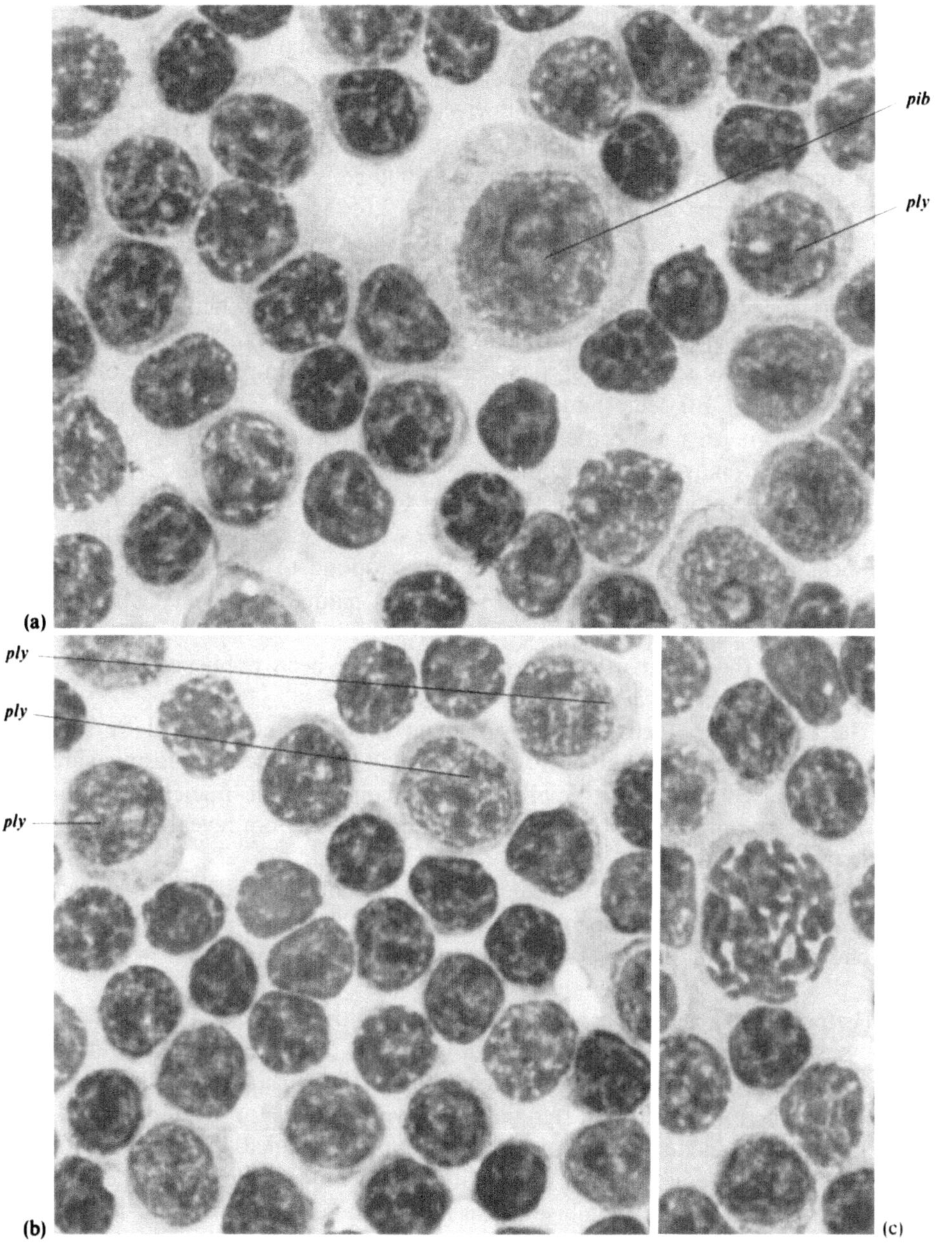


Fig. 47a–c. B-CLL in imprint. (a) One paraimmunoblast ("lymphoblast," *pib*), some prolymphocytes (*ply*), and many lymphocytes. (b) Some prolymphocytes (*ply*) and many lymphocytes. (c) Mitosis of a large cell (paraimmunoblast?). Note the plump chromosomes. ♂, 48 years. Pappenheim. × 1,460

The cytology of the lymph-node smear and imprint corresponds well to that of histologic sections (Fig. 47). The variations in cell size, however, are accentuated. The "lymphoblasts" (paraimmunoblasts) have a blue-gray to blue cytoplasm and "reticular" nuclei that usually contain a medium-sized or large light nucleolus. The lymphocytes and prolymphocytes differ from one another chiefly in size and in the density of the chromatin.

In imprints from 13 cases we counted 1000 cells per slide and found that the average number of "lymphoblasts" was 2.65%; the highest value lay at 10.4%.

STRUNGE[34] described a special variety of lymphocyte in CLL. He claimed that it is specific to leukemia and disappears after radiotherapy. He called the cells *cellules grumelées*, wanting to emphasize the clumped distribution of the chromatin. As a matter of fact, the chromatin clumps appear somewhat more clearly in CLL cells than in normal lymphocytes. The *cellules grumelées* are, however, neither a specific nor an obligatory feature of CLL.[35]

ANDRÉ and DREYFUS[36] mentioned another special feature of the lymphocytic nuclei that was supposed to be specific to CLL: the chromatin is *"pâteuse,"* i.e., thick and muddy, so that indistinct nuclei with a few dark spots are supposed to appear in imprints. These spots do not correspond to preexistent structures, but are artificially formed when the imprint is made. They are probably not specific to CLL.

Studies of the chromatin pattern of CLL have been published by SCHREK *et al.*[37] and by ZAJICEK *et al.*[38]

The fact that the cells are easily damaged has been mentioned by several authors.[39] This results in the occurrence of small, light blue cytoplasmic shreds. They are caused just as artificially as the changes in the nucleus mentioned previously. In contrast to blood smears, lymph nodes seldom reveal Gumprecht's shadows in large numbers.[40]

Mitotic figures are rarely found. When present, they are always seen in the larger cells. Typical azurophil granules have not been observed in leukemic lymphocytes of B-CLL.[41]

**Histochemistry and Cytochemistry.** In *sections* the PAS reaction of the lymphocytes, prolymphocytes, and "lymphoblasts" is negative. The reticulum cells lying among them sometimes contain globular PAS-positive inclusions, which could well be phagocytosed remnants of lymphocytes or accumulations of ingested Ig. The inclusions are of no diagnostic importance. With the reactions for nonspecific esterase or acid phosphatase it becomes evident that the sinuses are often destroyed and that histiocytic reticulum cells are sparse. The surface enzyme ATPase can be demonstrated in large amounts by both light and electron microscopy. In contrast, the enzyme 5-nucleotidase is found only in scanty amounts or not at all.[42]

---

[34] 1944.
[35] LUCAS, 1955.
[36] 1955.
[37] SCHREK, KNOSPE and TROBAUGH, 1970.
[38] ZAJICEK, BARTELS, BAHR, BIBBO *et al.*, 1972.
[39] TISCHENDORF, 1938, 1951; STAHEL, 1939.
[40] STAHEL, 1939.
[41] UNDRITZ, 1952; HEILMEYER and BEGEMANN, 1955.
[42] MÜLLER-HERMELINK and KAISERLING, 1975.

Table 19. Diagnostic criteria of B-CLL

1. Patients virtually not younger than 30 years, generally aged
2. In all cases lymphocytic infiltration of bone marrow
3. Blood picture generally reveals more than 4,000 lymphocytes/µl
4. Histologic picture
   a) diffuse (biopsy seldom made)
   b) pseudofollicular (biopsy often made)
5. Lymphocytes, prolymphocytes, and – always – "lymphoblasts" (paraimmunoblasts)
6. No plasma cells or plasmacytoid cells
7. PAS in lymphoid cells always negative in sections

Table 20. Cytologic criteria of B-CLL

| | Lymphocytes | Prolymphocytes | "Lymphoblasts" |
|---|---|---|---|
| Size | small | medium-sized | large |
| Nucleus | | | |
| Form | round | polymorphic | oval |
| Chromatin | coarse | fairly coarse | fine |
| Nucleolus | small | medium-sized | large, gray-blue, central |
| Cytoplasm | | | |
| Amount | small | small | moderate |
| Staining | light blue | light blue | deep gray-blue |

Although the cells of B-CLL in a *blood smear* generally exhibit an increased granular PAS reaction compared with that of normal lymphocytes,[43] the cells of lymph-node *imprints* or smears are usually negative or at most only weakly positive. The lysosomal enzymes acid phosphatase and β-glucuronidase reveal diminished activity in smears and imprints, in contrast to CLL of the T-cell type and to Sézary's syndrome.[44] The reaction for nonspecific esterase is negative.

**Diagnosis.** The diagnosis of B-CLL is based on clinical, histologic, and cytologic criteria (Tables 19 and 20). Clinically, the patients are mostly relatively old and always present leukemic infiltration of bone marrow and usually more than 4000 lymphocytes/µl in peripheral blood. Clinical information is not needed, however, for a histologic diagnosis. The latter is based on the following facts.

The structure of the lymph node is totally effaced, and particularly the sinuses are unrecognizable. The predominant cell is the small lymphocyte, but at least a few "lymphoblasts" and prolymphocytes are *always* detectable. The "lymphoblasts" and prolymphocytes usually proliferate focally (pseudofollicular picture). If the lymphocytic infiltration is diffuse throughout, immunocytoma should also be considered. Plasmacytoid cells or typical plasma cells do not appear

[43] WISLOCKI, RHEINGOLD and DEMPSEY, 1949; ASTALDI and VERGA, 1957; HAYHOE, 1960, Lit.; HECKNER, 1963; BAUER-SIC and LAMBERS, 1963.

[44] DOUGLAS, COHNEN, KÖNIG and BRITTINGER, 1973.

in CLL. PAS-positive inclusions in the nuclei and/or cytoplasm of the lymphoid cells rule out CLL. The occurrence of PAS-positive globular inclusions in the histiocytic reticulum cells is of no diagnostic importance.

The cytologic criteria of the different kinds of CLL cells are summarized in Table 20.

**Differential Diagnosis.** In the differential diagnosis, the following four lesions should be considered:

1. M.L. lymphoplasmacytic/lymphoplasmacytoid (LP immunocytoma; see p. 241 f).
2. M.L. centrocytic (see p. 298).
3. Hodgkin's disease with lymphocytic predominance.
4. Diffuse lymphatic hyperplasia.

As far as No. 3 is concerned, the picture presented by Hodgkin's disease with lymphocytic predominance is more polymorphic. Besides lymphocytes, which predominate, there are often a few or many epithelioid cells, always some Hodgkin's cells and Sternberg-Reed giant cells, and frequently small numbers of eosinophil leukocytes. In addition, one sometimes sees a nodular pattern, which greatly facilitates the diagnosis. Finally, in the lymphocyte-rich form of Hodgkin's disease one occasionally finds focal fibrosis, which does not occur in CLL.

Regarding No. 4, in diffuse lymphatic hyperplasia the sinuses are sharply demarcated and often markedly dilated. In addition, pseudofollicular proliferations are not apparent. A number of activated lymphocytes and cells of the plasma-cell series may be present, however, especially in the sinuses. The capsule and surrounding tissues may be infiltrated. This feature does not help to distinguish the two conditions.

**Borderline Cases.** Borderline cases between CLL and LP immunocytoma (see p. 244) and CLL and M.L. centrocytic exist. The former are more common than the latter. In our material (paraffin sections) 5.2% of the lymph nodes with a CLL-like appearance could not be definitely classified into either the group of CLL or that of LP immunocytoma.

Using methyl-green pyronine staining, SATODATE[45] studied 75 cases of B-CLL for pyroninophilic cells, namely, plasma cells and immunoblasts. Thirty-four of the 75 cases (45%) revealed a few pyroninophilic blast cells. In 47 cases (63%) he did not find any plasma cells at all. In 19 cases (25%) there were only a few plasma cells in the whole section (usually not more than 1–3). Nine cases, however, revealed more frequent plasma cells, often in small groups and usually near connective tissue or blood vessels. U. MÜLLER-HERMELINK[45a] showed that typical plasma cells at these locations were reactive, since they contained polyclonal intracytoplasmic Ig, demonstrated by means of the immunoperoxidase technique of TAYLOR. More about the differential diagnosis of borderline cases between B-CLL and LP immunocytoma is given on page 244.

**Development into a Lymphoma of Higher-Grade Malignancy.** As stated previously, in 15.9% of our autopsied cases we found a tumor-like gross appearance,

[45] Unpublished data.

[45a] Unpublished data.

which in past times would have been designated as sarcomatous transformation. Of these cases, 12.1% revealed the histologic picture that we described in biopsy material under *tumor-forming CLL*—they were characterized by a diffuse and destructive proliferation of prolymphocytes as well as by grossly evident nodules or masses of tumor. Therefore, we apply the *histologic* term "tumor-forming CLL" to cases of CLL with a tumor-like *gross* appearance when they also reveal a monotonous prolymphocytic proliferation. We cannot say to what extent our tumor form corresponds to the *formes ganglionnaires tumorales* of CLL described by RAIN *et al.*[46]

Of our autopsy cases, 3.8% had progressed into a monotonous proliferation of large basophilic cells, which one may characterize as "lymphoblastic." In conformity with the Kiel Classification, the picture that was presented would have to be specified as a high-grade malignant lymphoma. Accordingly, we might distinguish it as "M.L. lymphoblastic in CLL." We should not forget, however, that the "lymphoblasts" of CLL are by nature underdeveloped immunoblasts. So, strictly speaking, one should use the term *immunoblastic sarcoma* or *M.L. immunoblastic*.

The immunoblastic sarcoma developing terminally in CLL is identical to *Richter's syndrome*.[47] Under the name "generalized reticular cell sarcoma of lymph nodes associated with lymphatic leukemia," RICHTER[48] described a neoplasm of large cells that developed in conjunction with a preexisting CLL. Since his report, the combination is often referred to as Richter's syndrome, especially in Great Britain and France.

The cases published as Richter's syndrome appear to be heterogeneous, however, and do not always correspond to the description given by RICHTER. Especially combination cases with Hodgkin's disease have been mistakenly lumped together under the term Richter's syndrome. In our opinion, the term Richter's syndrome can be discarded. In any event, it represents the immunoblastic tumor variant of CLL and not a true histiocytic neoplasm (Fig. 48). This is evident from the membrane studies of CHELLOUL,[49] who found the same monoclonal light chain ($\lambda$) in lymphocytes and "sarcoma cells" from a case of CLL with Richter's syndrome. This may also be concluded from the observation of LONG and AISENBERG.[50] They found a monoclonal increase in IgM in the blood, together with the development of an immunoblastic lymphoma in a case of CLL.

The terminal transformation into a lymphoblastic phase[51] that is refractive to therapy is much less common in CLL than in chronic myeloid leukemia. In such cases the histologic picture reveals anaplasia of the lymphocytes; that is, they are relatively large and have light nuclei with larger nucleoli. In addition, the number of mitotic figures is large and the reticulin network scanty. The surface membrane-bound immunoglobulins (SIg) are of the same

[46] RAIN, FLANDRIN, BINET and BERNARD, 1971.

[47] RICHTER, 1928; LOESCH, 1933; AHLSTRÖM, 1938; LORTHOLARY, BOIRON, RIPAULT, LEVY *et al.*, 1964; GILVER, 1968; DUMONT, FLANDRIN, BASCH, RIPAULT *et al.*, 1971; LONG and AISENBERG, 1975.

[48] 1928.

[49] 1974.

[50] 1975.

[51] SCHOEN, HECKNER and MARSCH, 1953; CHIARI, 1964; LORTHOLARY, BOIRON, RIPAULT, LEVACHER *et al.*, 1966; KLAJMAN, YARETZKY, MANOR and STEINER, 1975.

(a)

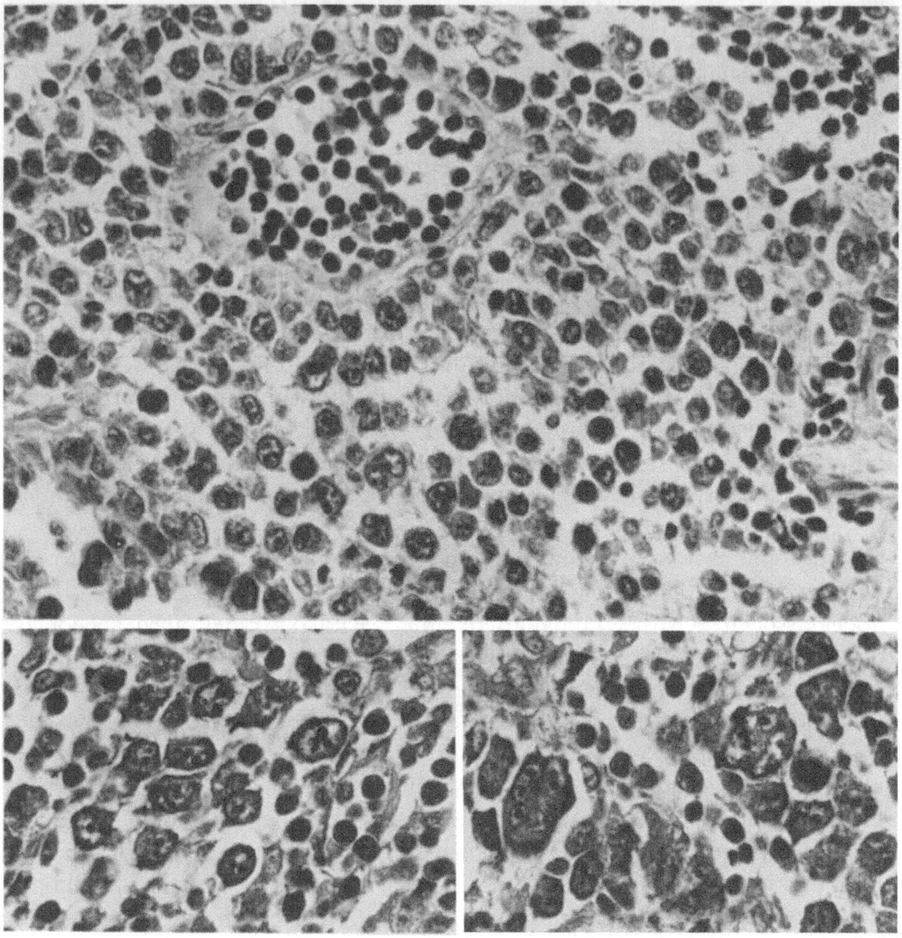

(b) (c)

Fig. 48a–c. Immunoblastic sarcoma (M.L. immunoblastic, Richter's syndrome) in CLL. Autopsy case. ♀, 47 years. (a) Large tumor cells. A vessel contains numerous lymphocytes, indicating persistence of CLL. Hematoxylin and eosin. ×440. (b) Note the intense basophilia and similarity to immunoblasts. Giemsa. ×560. (c) Immunoblastic giant cells simulating Hodgkin's disease. Giemsa. ×560

class as those detected before the blastic phase, indicating that further malignant transformation of the same clone has occurred.[52] The amount of SIg may be much reduced or even undetectable in the lymphoblastic phase.[53]

**Combination with Other Diseases.** In our lymph-node material obtained by biopsy, we found combinations with the following diseases:

1. Epithelioid-cell tuberculosis (twice).
2. Hodgkin's disease (3 times).
3. Adenocarcinoma (once).
4. Osteomyelosclerosis (questionable; once).

[52] BROUET, PREUD'HOMME, SELIGMANN and BERNARD, 1973.

[53] BRITTINGER, 1974, personal communication.

Regarding No. 2, the association with Hodgkin's disease is not so rare. It has been described a number of times in the literature.[54] In general, it is easy to recognize the combination. Besides the typical CLL lesion, such cases reveal a polymorphic neoplasm of reticulum cells, Sternberg-Reed cells, eosinophils, epithelioid cells, and lymphocytes. The reticulin pattern is also altered in focal areas, and there may be circumscribed sclerosis. Thus, it is clear that two independent processes are evident in combinations of CLL and Hodgkin's disease. Such cases are different from the rare CLL that reveal multinucleate giant cells resembling Sternberg-Reed cells. In the latter type of CLL, a uniform lymphocytic picture is found, and the fiber pattern is uniform throughout.

Regarding No. 3, the association of CLL with carcinoma has also been described many times, and a high rate of coincidence has been assumed, for instance, by KLIMA and HERZOG,[55] GUNZ and ANGUS,[56] and FRAUMENI.[57] GUNZ and ANGUS[56] found different kinds of cancer in 14.72% of their patients with CLL. This excess of cancer in CLL was statistically significant.

STACHER and BÖHNEL[58] have observed regression of the symptoms of CLL on appearance of carcinoma or of carcinoma metastases. Therefore, they interpreted the increase in lymphocytes as reactive, at least in part. Recently, however, STACHER[59] presumed that the "lymphocytosis" reflects an immunocytoma.

Regarding No. 4, the combination of CLL with osteomyelosclerosis was first described by VIDEBAEK and POULSEN.[60] It is certainly very rare and probably a chance occurrence (see p. 126).

**Prognosis.** Numerous clinical reviews concerned with the prognosis of CLL are available. According to them, a CLL with a relatively rapid course is distinguished from that which progresses slowly.[61] The 5-year survival rate reported for the large series (839 patients) of ZIPPIN *et al.*[62] was 44%. The survival rate fell with increasing age and was somewhat higher in women than in men.

Various authors have presented information on many different parameters for measuring prognosis.[63] A new attempt has been made to correlate the morphology of the circulating leukemic cells with survival.[64] PETERSON *et al.*[64] found that CLL presenting small lymphocytes has a poorer prognosis than CLL presenting large lymphocytes. Furthermore, a method of clinical staging was proposed and proved to be a reliable predictor of survival.[65] A correlation between histologic type and prognosis has yet to be made. The survival data of the Kiel Lymphoma Study Group, however, may give some information

[54] E.g., KEISER, UEHLINGER and VIRIEUX, 1961; TORNYOS, MACOSSAY and GYORKEY, 1967; LÖFFLER and KALTENBACH, 1969.

[55] 1956.

[56] 1965.

[57] 1969.

[58] 1966.

[59] 1975, personal communication.

[60] 1957; also LOUWAGIE, DESMET and VAN DEN BERGHE, 1973; cf., our autopsy case above (p. 126).

[61] GALTON, 1967; BOUTIS, OBRECHT, MUSSHOFF and JOCHMANN, 1968.

[62] ZIPPIN, CUTLER, REEVES and LUM, 1973.

[63] BOUTIS, OBRECHT, MUSSHOFF and JOCHMANN, 1968; FAYOLLE, CŒUR, BRYON, GENTILHOMME *et al.*, 1971; ZIPPIN, CUTLER, REEVES and LUM, 1973; GRAY, JACOBS and BLOCK, 1974.

[64] PETERSON, BLOOMFIELD, SUNDBERG, GAJL-PECZALSKA *et al.*, 1975.

[65] RAI, SAWITSKY, CRONKITE, CHANANA *et al.*, 1975.

about it. The prognosis of the cases of this group was poorer than that of the cases in the clinical lymphoma study by the Essen group (Fig. 35). We suppose that the cases of the Kiel group were chiefly lymphomas with an unusual and, in particular, shorter course than normal. The lymph nodes were often removed because of suspected sarcoma. Therefore, the survival data of our group are not representative of CLL as a whole. They might be representative of material that is composed mainly of the pseudofollicular variant of CLL, however, since most of the cases showed a pseudofollicular pattern. Thus, we venture to surmise that the diffuse, almost pure lymphocytic type has the best prognosis, the pseudofollicular type a poorer one, and the tumor-forming type the worst. In cytologic terms, on might say that the more lymphocytes there are, the better the prognosis is, and the more prolymphocytes and paraimmunoblasts there are, the poorer the prognosis is.

### *Addenda*

#### *a) The Prolymphocytic Variant of B-CLL*

The term prolymphocytic leukemia covers two entities: (1) the prolymphocytic leukemia of MATHÉ *et al.*,[66] which was claimed to be a variant of acute lymphoblastic leukemia and which is probably equivalent to the leukemic variant of M.L. centrocytic, and (2) the prolymphocytic leukemia of GALTON *et al.*[67] In our opinion, only the latter leukemia (2) should be called prolymphocytic leukemia, since it alone shows neoplasia of the type of cell that we are able to distinguish in CLL as the prolymphocyte.

After comparing material from our cases with blood smears kindly sent by Dr. GALTON, we are fully convinced of the existence of this entity. We agree with GALTON *et al.*[67] that prolymphocytic leukemia can be distinguished from classic CLL, from lymphosarcoma-cell leukemia (our M.L. centrocytic with leukemia), and from acute lymphoblastic leukemia. We regard most cases as relatively rare, *immature variants of CLL of the B-cell type*;[68] but there are also cases of prolymphocytic leukemia of the T-type (see p. 138).[69] In agreement with RAPPAPORT,[70] we would prefer to use the term *chronic* prolymphocytic leukemia, in contrast to the *acute* type of MATHÉ.

Instead of describing the features of the disease ourselves, we prefer to quote verbatim the summary given by GALTON *et al.*[67] in their paper:

> The disease predominantly affects males in the sixth and seventh decades of life and presenting symptoms include fatigue, weakness, weight loss, sweats, and fevers. Massive enlargement of the spleen (mean weight at autopsy 1383 g, range 227–3500 g) and to a lesser extent of the liver (mean weight 2445 g, range 2030–3079 g) are regular findings. In contrast, peripheral lymphadenopathy is inconspicuous or absent. The characteristic cell in the peripheral blood is a relatively

---

[66] MATHÉ, POUILLART, STERESCU, AMIEL *et al.*, 1971; MATHÉ, POUILLART, WEINER, HAYAT *et al.*, 1973.

[67] GALTON, GOLDMAN, WILTSHAW, CATOVSKY *et al.*, 1974.

[68] See also CATOVSKY, GALETTO, OKOS, GALTON *et al.*, 1973.

[69] BROUET, FLANDRIN, SASPORTES, PREUD'HOMME *et al.*, 1975.

[70] 1975, personal communication.

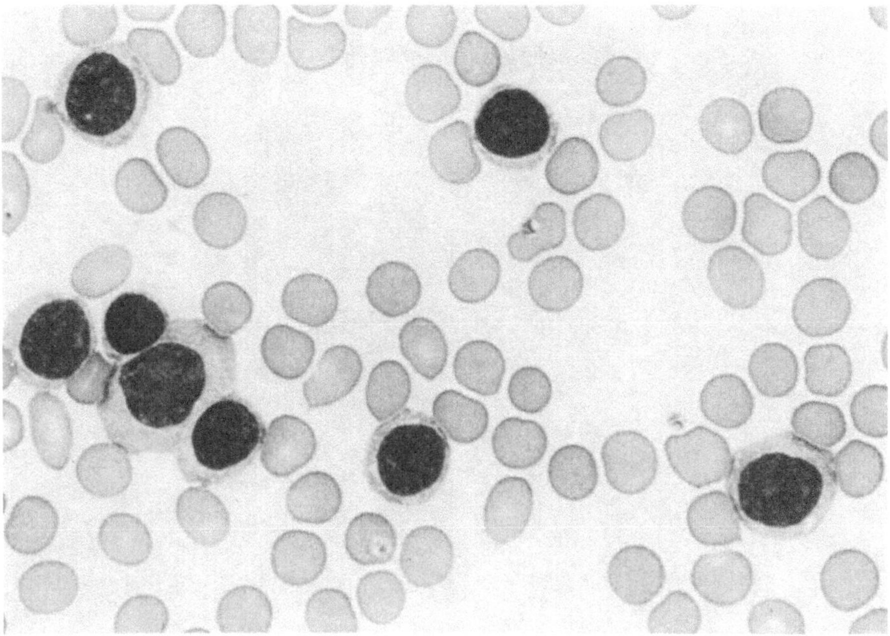

Fig. 49. Prolymphocytic leukemia. Blood smear. The leukemic cells are relatively large and have a distinct light nucleolus and a moderately broad rim of cytoplasm. On the left there is a "lymphoblast"-like cell with larger nucleoli. ♀, 72 years. Pappenheim. ×875

large lymphoid cell with a large vesicular nucleolus, relatively well-condensed nuclear chromatin and moderate amount of cytoplasm [see Fig. 49]. The counts of these cells in the peripheral blood at the time of diagnosis are very high (mean 355,000/μl, range 26,000 – 1,110,000/μl). The clinical response to methods of treatment that are usually effective in classical CLL (particularly alkylating agents and corticosteroid drugs) is uniformly poor and the patients' survival after diagnosis is in most cases quite short. On the basis of a single case we suggest that further trials of splenectomy are indicated.

In contrast to the massive splenomegaly, the involvement of the lymph nodes in such cases is minimal. Only during later stages of the disease may larger lymphomas develop.[71] Histologically, one then finds great numbers of prolymphocytes, perhaps mingled with a few lymphoblasts (Fig. 50). The lymphocytes in the blood of one of our patients were PAS-positive, as they are in B-CLL. CATOVSKY *et al.*[72] made in the same observation, and reported that in two cases 95% of the cells were strongly PAS-positive. Their illustrations showed the positive staining to vary from fine to coarse granularity. The reaction for acid phosphatase was positive in some or many cells, with or without resistance to tartaric acid. In contrast to the cells of typical B-CLL, the leukemic cells revealed more surface Ig and formed spontaneous rosettes with mouse erythrocytes.[73]

---

[71] GALTON, 1974, personal communication.

[72] CATOVSKY, GALETTO, OKOS, MILIANI *et al.*, 1974.

[73] BUSKARD, CATOVSKY, OKOS, GOLDMAN *et al.*, 1976.

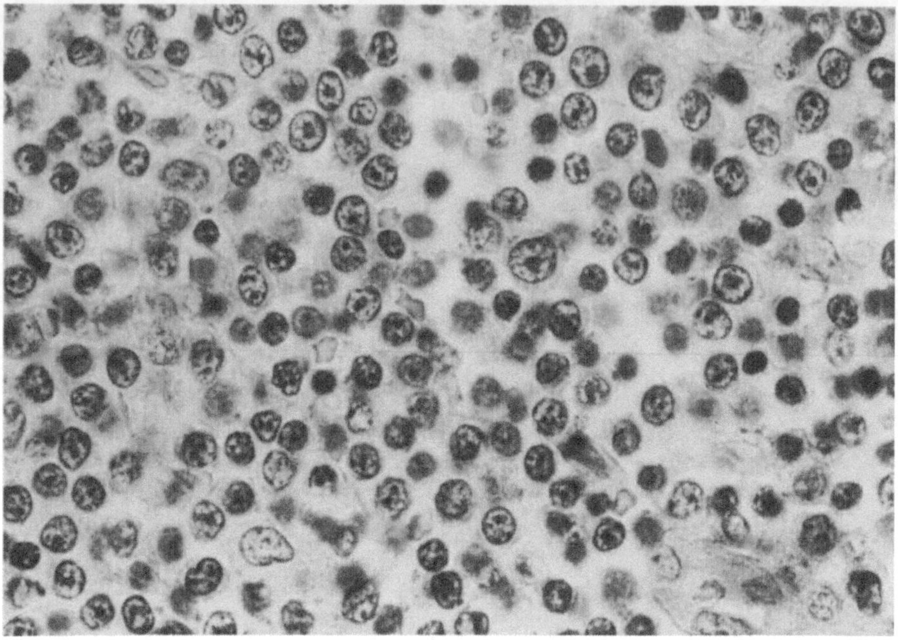

Fig. 50. Prolymphocytic leukemia? (anaplastic CLL?). Relatively large lymphocytoid cells and some "lymphoblast"-like cells. ♀, 53 years. Axillary node. Hematoxylin and eosin. ×875

It would be interesting to find out whether such cases of prolymphocytic leukemia are to be found among the forms of LP immunocytoma with splenomegaly, or vice versa. Likewise, one must keep the distinction between prolymphocytic leukemia and hairy-cell leukemia in mind, especially in cases of leukemia with a tartrate-resistant acid phosphatase reaction and a prolymphocyte-like picture. Such uncertainties imply that further studies are needed in this area.

### *b) Is There a Nonleukemic Lymphoma of the CLL Type?*

Although the clinical impression is at times only that of localized lymph-node tumors and although at first a marked increase in lymphocytes in the blood is occasionally absent, our observations leave no doubt that malignant lymphoma of the CLL type *always* sooner or later becomes generalized *like leukemia,* involves the bone marrow, and shows at least a slight increase in lymphocytes in the blood. Thus, we do not have any evidence for the existence of a nonleukemic lymphoma of the CLL type. The term lymphosarcoma is still used in some places for the relatively immature forms of CLL, but should be avoided in the future.

## *2. Chronic Lymphocytic Leukemia, T-Cell Type (T-CLL)*

**History.** Sézary's syndrome undoubtedly accounts for many chronic lymphocytic leukemias of the T-cell type (T-CLL). This syndrome is characterized not only by a special type of cell (the Lutzner cell), but also by erythroderma. Some cases, however, despite an associated erythroderma, cannot be accepted as belonging to Sézary's syndrome because of the morphology of the lymphocytes. A case in point is the observation of SHEVACH *et al.*,[74] who described lymphocytes that formed both sheep-E and EAC rosettes.

Clinically, the patient had suffered an eczematous dermatitis for 9 years prior to the development of leukemia with more than 300,000 WBC/µl. As the leukemia appeared, the dermatitis changed into exfoliative erythroderma. The lymphocytes did not resemble Lutzner cells of Sézary's syndrome on electron microscopy, but instead showed round nuclei. Nevertheless, this type of lymphocytic leukemia is undoubtedly closely related to Sézary's syndrome.

In another case, published by DEWAR *et al.*,[75] the lymphocytes also gave a mixed rosette reaction (EA + E rosettes).

Generalized purpura, splenomegaly, and enlargement of all lymph nodes developed in a 67-year-old man. The WBC count rose from 17,000 to 234,000/µl; the differential count revealed 55% lymphocytes and 44% prolymphocytes with no morphologic signs of Sézary cells. The PAS reaction was positive in the neoplastic lymphocytes. Ten percent of these lymphocytes showed mixed rosettes, namely, with IgG-coated human erythrocytes (EA rosettes) and sheep erythrocytes (sheep-E rosettes).

According to BROUET and PRIEUR,[76] the combined demonstration of surface Ig and sheep-E rosettes needs to be carefully studied for its validity. The surface Ig can adhere to the surface of T-lymphocytes secondarily; then the CLL is really of the T-cell type. The CLL may be of a B-cell type, however, when the surface Ig shows anti-sheep erythrocyte activity.

In the last few years, several reports have appeared describing CLL purely of the T-cell type.[77] Often, however, no mention was made of whether erythroderma existed or not. Moreover, the reports generally lacked careful and detailed cytologic descriptions of the lymphocytes and a precise histologic account. In addition, statements were often not made about the cytochemistry of the tumor cells, especially their content of acid phosphatase. Consequently, it is difficult to compare the published cases with one another.

It is commendable that BROUET *et al.*[78] observed 11 cases of T-CLL and have now published a study of these cases, including cytochemical findings on the lymphocytes. BROUET *et al.*[78] established that nine cases showed a characteristic clinicohematologic pattern, whereas two cases showed no special clini-

[74] SHEVACH, EDELSON, FRANK, LUTZNER *et al.*, 1974; EDELSON, LUTZNER, KIRKPATRICK, SHEVACH *et al.*, 1974.

[75] DEWAR, HABESHAW, YOUNG, STUART *et al.*, 1974.

[76] 1974.

[77] E.g., MOORE and MINOWADA, 1972; BENTWICH and KUNKEL, 1973; DICKLER, SIEGAL, BENTWICH and KUNKEL, 1973; FOULIS, COCHRAN and ANDERSON, 1973; LILLE, DESPLACES, MEEUS, SARACINO *et al.*, 1973; SELIGMANN, PREUD'HOMME and BROUET, 1973; SUMIYA, MIZOGUCHI, KOSAKA, MIURA *et al.*, 1973; YODOI, TAKATSUKI and MASUDA, 1974; INSEL, MELEWICZ, LA VIA and BALCH, 1975.

[78] BROUET, FLANDRIN, SASPORTES, PREUD'HOMME *et al.*, 1975.

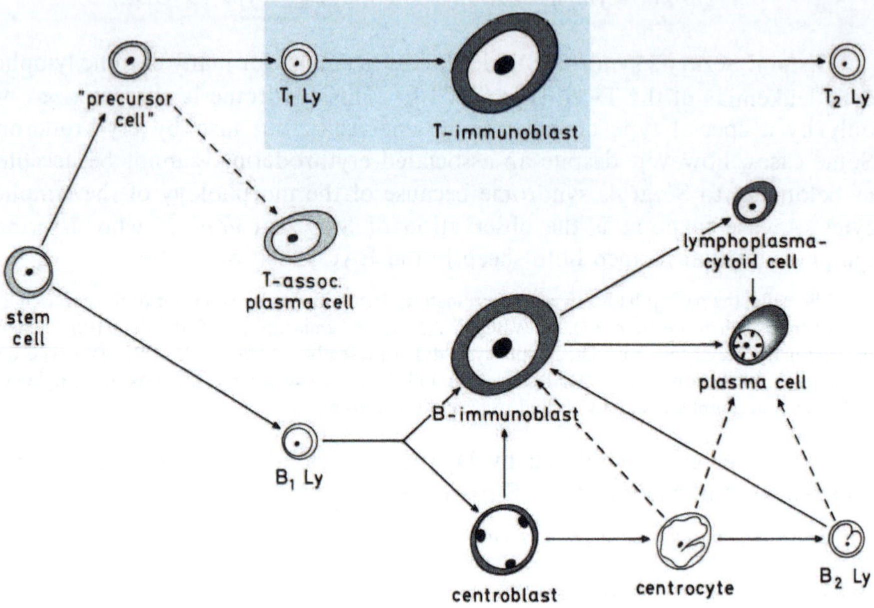


Fig. 51. Hypothetical origin of tumor cells of T-CLL. It is not definite whether the lymphocytes are actually $T_1$-lymphocytes; they might also be the $T_2$-lymphocytes of this scheme. Furthermore, it is not clear to which subtype or subtypes of T-lymphocytes the tumor cells of T-CLL belong

cal features, but instead gave the same impression as the prolymphocytic leukemia of GALTON (see p. 134). Therefore, one can distinguish a lymphocytic and a prolymphocytic variant of T-CLL.

We were able to study lymph nodes from three patients with T-CLL. The blood pictures showed that one case could be interpreted as lymphocytic, the other two cases as prolymphocytic. The three cases will be discussed together, however, since there were no significant differences in the histology, cytology, and cytochemistry of the lymph nodes between the lymphocytic and prolymphocytic types.

**Origin of the Neoplastic Cells.** Using numerous methods (see Part Six), it has been proved that the cells of both variants of T-CLL are definitely T-lymphocytes (Fig. 51). They are SIg-negative, form sheep-E rosettes and also H rosettes,[79] and bear surface T-antigen. The concentration of T-cell antigen on the lymphocyte surface is lower than it is on normal T-lymphocytes.[80] BROUET *et al.*[81] found it remarkable that the lymphocytes reacted very differently with various anti-T-sera. They therefore suggested that different subsets of T-lymphocytes might be affected and that there might also be counterparts of these subsets among normal T-lymphocytes. The findings of TAKATSUKI

[79] SHELDON and HOLBOROW, 1975.
[80] RODT, THIEL, THIERFELDER, HUHN *et al.*, 1976; THIEL, RODT, HUHN and THIERFELDER, 1976.
[81] BROUET, FLANDRIN, SASPORTES, PREUD'HOMME *et al.*, 1975.

*et al.*[82] indicate that, at least in some cases of T-CLL, the tumor cells are derived from T-suppressor cells.

**Occurrence.** T-CLL occurs much less frequently than B-CLL. SELIGMANN *et al.*[83] found only three cases of T-CLL in a collection of 150 cases of CLL. BROUET *et al.*[84] were of the opinion, however, that T-CLL is somewhat more common than was evident from the data obtained in 1973 from the same hospital. We estimate the ratio of T-CLL to B-CLL to be about 1:20. It is remarkable that several cases of T-CLL have been described in Japan,[84a] where B-CLL is extremely rare; the ratio of T-CLL to B-CLL appears to be about 1:1 in Japan.[82]

The patients observed so far were 25–78 years old.[84] A predominance of one age group has not been determined, and a predominance of one sex cannot yet be substantiated on the basis of the cases published so far.

The prolymphocytic variant is evidently considerably rarer than the lymphocytic variant (prolymphocytic:lymphocytic ~ 1:5?). Prolymphocytic leukemia of the T-type is considerably rarer than that of the B-type in the material of the Paris group [84] and of the London group (T:B ~ 1:5).[84b]

**Clinical Manifestations.** On the basis of their 11 cases, BROUET *et al.*[84] sketched the following clinical picture of T-CLL. In contrast to B-CLL, there is usually no enlargement of lymph nodes. BROUET *et al.* found a moderate enlargement of superficial lymph nodes only once, and abnormal lymphangiograms and therefore probable involvement of deep lymph nodes in three out of five patients. On the other hand, there is almost always splenomegaly. It may be very prominent. In exceptional cases, however, it may be completely absent. The liver was moderately enlarged in four patients. There were skin lesions in four cases. One patient had mild erythroderma. In two cases skin biopsies revealed lymphocytic infiltration; in one of these patients it was chiefly localized to the ears and face. The fourth patient had multiple lymphocytic skin nodules with itching.

In the *lymphocytic variant* (nine cases), BROUET *et al.*[84] found a slight to moderate increase in lymphocytes (4000–20,000/μl) in the peripheral blood of eight patients. In one case the lymphocyte count was only 3000/μl. There were plump azurophil granules in almost all leukemic cells from six patients. Four patients had extreme neutropenia (<400/μl). The bone marrow was only slightly to moderately infiltrated; the percentage of lymphocytes was >35% in six cases, and the highest value of 70% was reached in only one case. In the other three patients, the value was under 25%. Histologically, when the bone marrow was infiltrated, the infiltration was more often diffuse than nodular.

BROUET *et al.*[84] found the highest lymphocyte counts (400,000 and 500,000/

---

82 TAKATSUKI, UCHIYAMA, SAGAWA and YODOI, in press.

83 SELIGMANN, PREUD'HOMME and BROUET, 1973.

84 BROUET, FLANDRIN, SASPORTES, PREUD'HOMME *et al.*, 1975.

84a YODOI, TAKATSUKI and MASUDA, 1974.

84b GALTON, personal communication.

μl) in the *prolymphocytic variant*. The blood lymphocytes chiefly showed the morphology of prolymphocytes (large solitary nucleoli). Evidently, they did not contain azurophil granules. The bone marrow was infiltrated to a greater degree than it was in the lymphocytic variant. Otherwise, the clinical picture of the prolymphocytic variant of the T-type appears to be largely equivalent to that of the prolymphocytic variant of the B-type.

**Localization.** There are not enough data available. We studied one cervical, one axillary, and one inguinal lymph node.

**Gross Appearance.** The gross appearance is similar to that of lymph nodes from B-CLL.

**Histology.** Before discussing the histology of T-CLL, it may be pertinent to give a brief summary of the clinical findings in our three cases, which formed the basis of this study.

*Case 1* (R 1750/74):[85] The patient was a 34-year-old man. He had complained of weakness for one year. Cervical and axillary lymph nodes showed very protracted, slight to moderate enlargement. The liver and spleen were not enlarged. There was no involvement of the tonsils, skin, or mediastinum. Hemoglobin 16.1 g-%. Erythrocytes $5.1 \times 10^6$/μl. Platelets 106,000/μl. Leukocytes 11,300/μl; 70% lymphocytes. Ninety-eight percent of the lymphocytes formed sheep-E rosettes. Sternal bone marrow: 70% lymphocytes. ESR 3/6 mm. The patient responded well to COP therapy and later to CP alone. Twenty-four months after the diagnosis was made, he was back at work and required only CP therapy at 3-month intervals.

*Case 2* (R 3854/75):[85] The patient was a 69-year-old man. He showed generalized enlargement of lymph nodes 9 months before biopsy. There was moderate splenomegaly (3–4 cm) and no hepatomegaly. Leukocytes 280,000/μl; 99% lymphocytes and prolymphocytes. Eighty percent of the lymphocytes formed sheep-E rosettes and were killed by anti-T-serum. ESR 21/60 mm. There was no significant improvement in the patient's condition after extracorporeal irradiation of his blood, irradiation of the spleen, leukopheresis, and cytostatic therapy (Knospe regimen). The liver and spleen were greatly enlarged, and the blood lymphocyte count increased to 450,000/μl after treatment. Three months after lymph-node biopsy, the patient underwent surgery for a perforated stomach ulcer and then died.

*Case 3* (R 1580/76):[86] The patient was a 41-year-old man. He presented with generalized lymphadenopathy, splenomegaly (12 cm), and hepatomegaly (4 cm). Leukocytes 350,000/μl; 99% lymphocytes and prolymphocytes ("prolymphocytic leukemia"). ESR 55/86 mm. The patient showed resistance to treatment with chlorambucil and cyclophosphamide. The biopsy was performed after chemotherapy. Blood lymphocytes did not have B-cell markers and only 3% of them formed sheep-E rosettes. Additional data are provided by LÖFFLER *et al.*[87] The patient died a few weeks after biopsy.

The lymph-node structure was obliterated in all three cases. Some germinal centers were found in case 2 and remnants of dermatopathic lymphadenitis were seen in case 3. The lymph-node tissue was diffusely infiltrated by small lymphocytes. In the prolymphocytic type the lymphocytes were somewhat larger and more weakly stained, so that the first impression (under low magnification) was

[85] We wish to thank Dr. THEML, Department of Internal Medicine I (Head: Prof. Dr. H. BEGEMANN), City Hospital, München-Schwabing, for providing the clinical data.

[86] We are grateful to Prof. Dr. H. LÖFFLER, Department of Internal Medicine, University of Gießen, for providing the clinical data.

[87] LÖFFLER, GRAUBNER, DESAGA and JUNG, 1977.

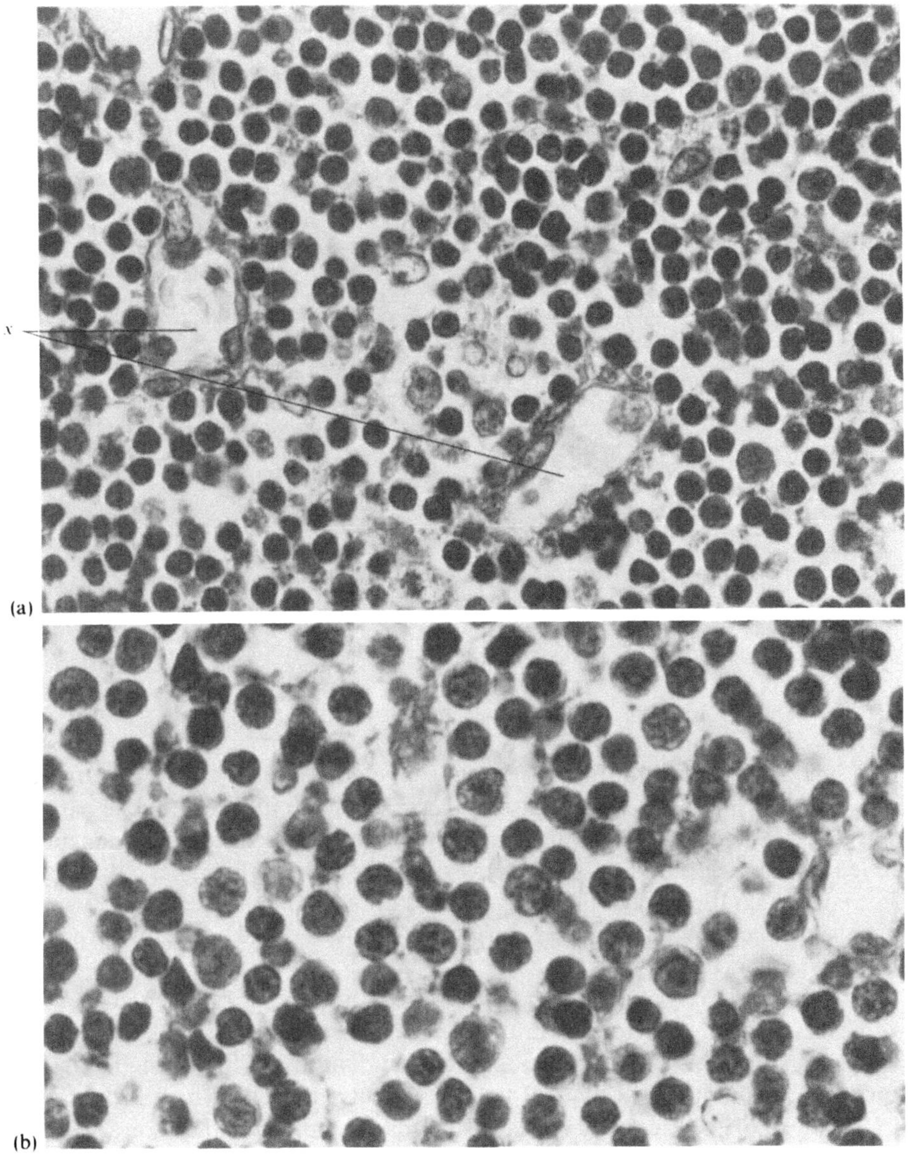


Fig. 52a and b. T-CLL. Case 1. Note the narrow atypical venules (*x*) in (a) and the polymorphism of the often convoluted nuclei in (b). ♂, 34 years. Retroauricular node. PAS. (a) ×560, (b) ×875

reminiscent of M.L. centrocytic. Pseudofollicular structures like the ones in B-CLL were not found. In case 1 almost no mitotic activity was present. In cases 2 and 3 there were large numbers of mitotic figures, which showed plump chromosomes. The lymphocytes had spread from the lymph-node parenchyma, through the obliterated marginal sinus, to the capsule. The capsule showed focal infiltration by lymphocytes without destruction. Outside the capsule there was also

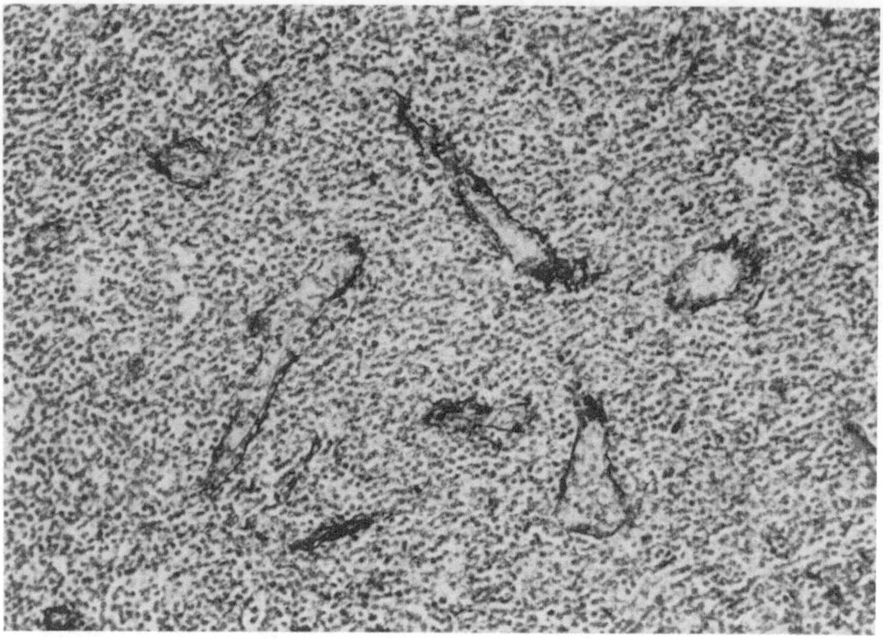

Fig. 53. T-CLL. Case 2. Numerous PAS-positive epithelioid venules. ♂, 69 years. Axillary node. PAS. ×175

focal lymphocytic infiltration of the connective and adipose tissue. The trabeculae of the lymph node from case 2 were heavily infiltrated and expanded.

In case 1 we saw abundant thin-walled blood vessels with prominent or flat endothelial cells and only a very weak PAS reaction (Fig. 52a). The vessels showed no migration of lymphocytes. Silver staining demonstrated that they were atypical venules and not wide capillaries. A few thin-walled vessels were packed full of lymphocytes.

In contrast, cases 2 and 3 showed a great increase in epithelioid venules with excessive lymphocyte migration (Figs. 53 and 54). It was most easily seen with silver and PAS stains. There were abundant thick fibers encircling the venules. The endothelial cells had typical vesicular nuclei. In case 3 there was a normal number of endothelial cells. In case 2, however, they were reduced in number in some venules (anaplastic venules?). There were often tightly packed lymphocytes in the lumina of the venules. The lymphocytes were evidently migrating in large numbers through the walls of the venules. Then, their nuclei often appeared in typical "hand-mirror" form or in elongate thin forms. Among the encircling fibers of the venular walls there were massive numbers of lymphocytes, which had pushed the fibers apart. Numerous venules were also seen in perinodal fat infiltrated by lymphocytes.

With silver staining cases 1 and 2 showed relatively abundant, fine to moderately coarse fibers. In case 1 some of them certainly belonged to preexistent vessels, which were overrun by tumor cells that often left the connective-tissue fibers intact. In case 2 the high fiber content corresponded to the large number

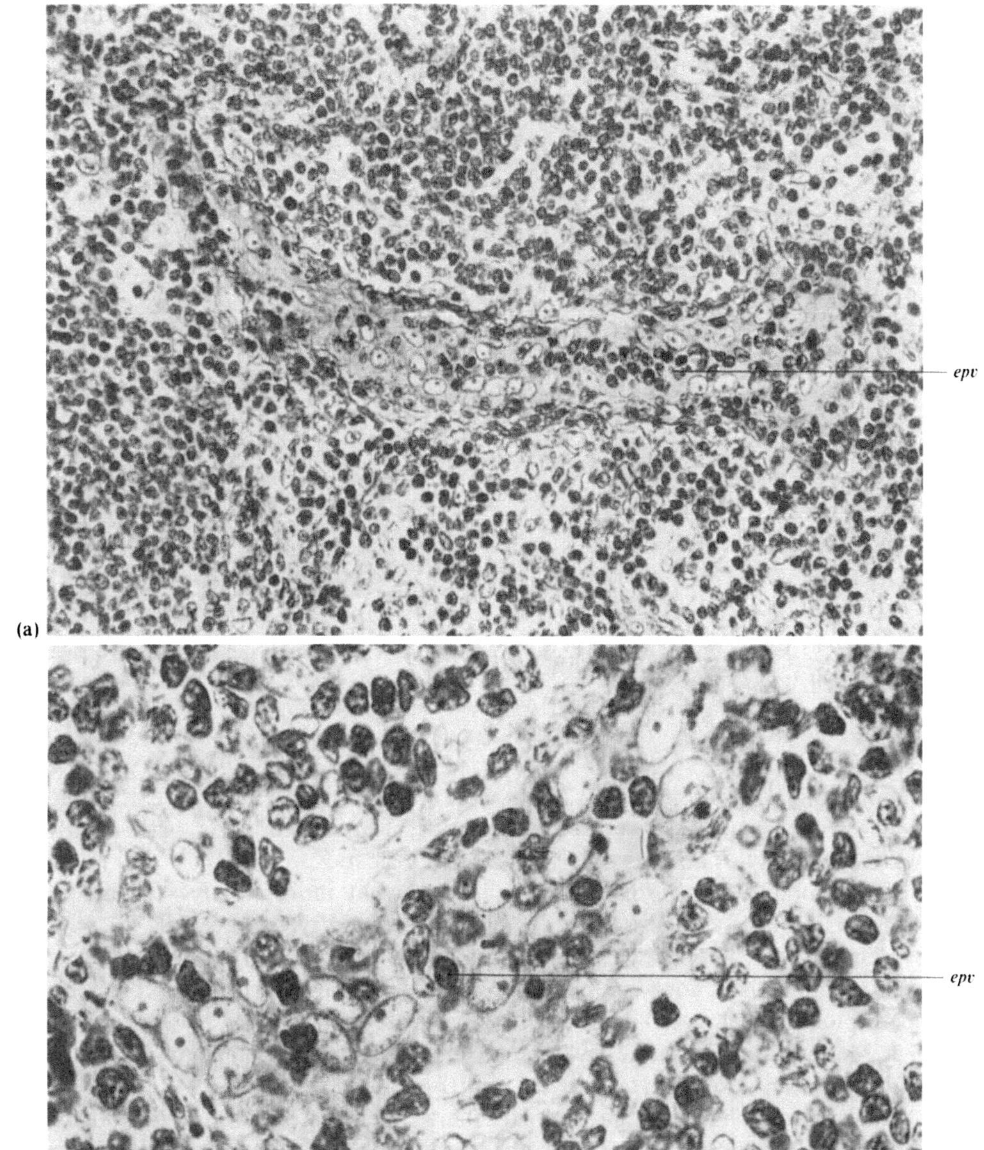


Fig. 54a and b. T-CLL. Case 3. Almost PAS-negative epithelioid venule (*epv*) with numerous recirculating lymphocytes in the wall. ♂, 41 years. Inguinal node. (a) PAS. ×350. (b) Giemsa. ×875

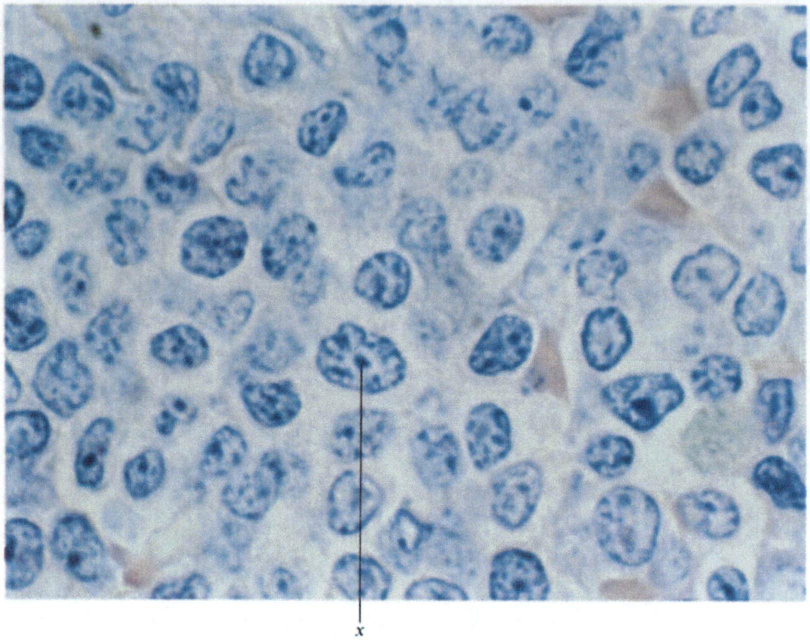


Fig. 55. T-CLL with Giemsa staining. Case 2. Note the polymorphism of the relatively large lymphoid cells (prolymphocytes). In the middle, the large convoluted nucleus of a lymphocyte (*x*; hyperdiploid?). ♂, 69 years. Axillary node. × 1,550

of epithelioid venules. In case 3 fibers were numerous only around epithelioid venules. Furthermore, there were fiber-poor, venule-free areas with tightly packed lymphocytes and extremely sparse thick fibers.

If one looks at the proliferating cells somewhat more closely—the use of oil immersion is advisable—one recognizes three main types of cells:

1. Small cells: lymphocytes—predominant.
2. Medium-sized nonbasophilic cells: cells with convoluted nuclei, probably hyperdiploid lymphocytes—only a few (see Fig. 55).
3. Medium-sized to large basophilic cells: blast cells—a small or moderate number; more in the prolymphocytic type (Fig. 56).

The small cells have the characteristic coarse nuclear structure and the narrow rim of cytoplasm of lymphocytes. In the "prolymphocytic" variant, the solitary nucleoli are somewhat larger and the rim of cytoplasm is somewhat broader. It is gray-blue with Giemsa staining. In case 1 the nuclei were often not round, but instead pleomorphic and irregularly angular or convoluted.

The medium-sized nonbasophilic cells have large nuclei with the dense chromatin structure of lymphocytes and a very narrow rim of cytoplasm. The nucleus usually does not contain a nucleolus. On the other hand, it shows manifold variations in contour, e.g., protuberances, and may be described as "convoluted." Since these variations can be recognized in more detail in imprints, they will be described and illustrated more fully below.

The medium-sized to large basophilic cells have round or oval nuclei, mostly

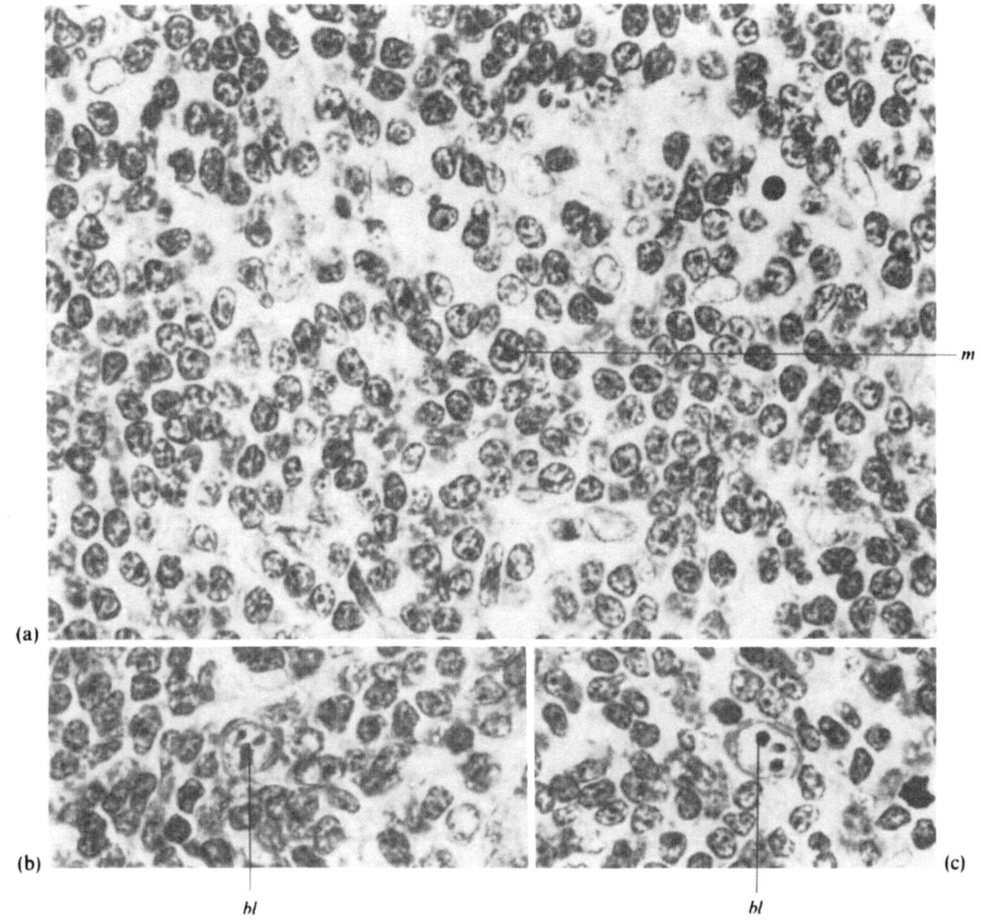


Fig. 56a–c. T-CLL. Case 3. Note the medium-sized cell (*m*) in the center of (a). It has a prominent nucleolus and a convoluted nucleus. (b, c) Two large blast cells (*bl*; T-immunoblasts?). ♂, 41 years. Inguinal node. (a) PAS, (b, c) Giemsa. (a–c) ×875.

with one moderately basophilic, medium-sized nucleolus. These cells are somewhat reminiscent of the paraimmunoblasts of B-CLL. The variable rim of cytoplasm is usually moderately wide and may be finely vacuolated. In case 1 we saw a few mononuclear giant forms of this cell.

Whereas the small cells are definitely lymphocytes, the medium-sized to large basophilic cells may be interpreted as T-immunoblasts (Fig. 56). The medium-sized nonbasophilic cells with convoluted nuclei are probably hyperdiploid lymphocytes.

**Smear/Imprint.** Lymphocytes are also predominant in imprints (Fig. 57). In the prolymphocytic variant, one sees a relatively wide rim of cytoplasm and, above all, solitary large light nucleoli. There is some variation in cell size, with transitional forms ranging up to the medium-sized cells with convo-

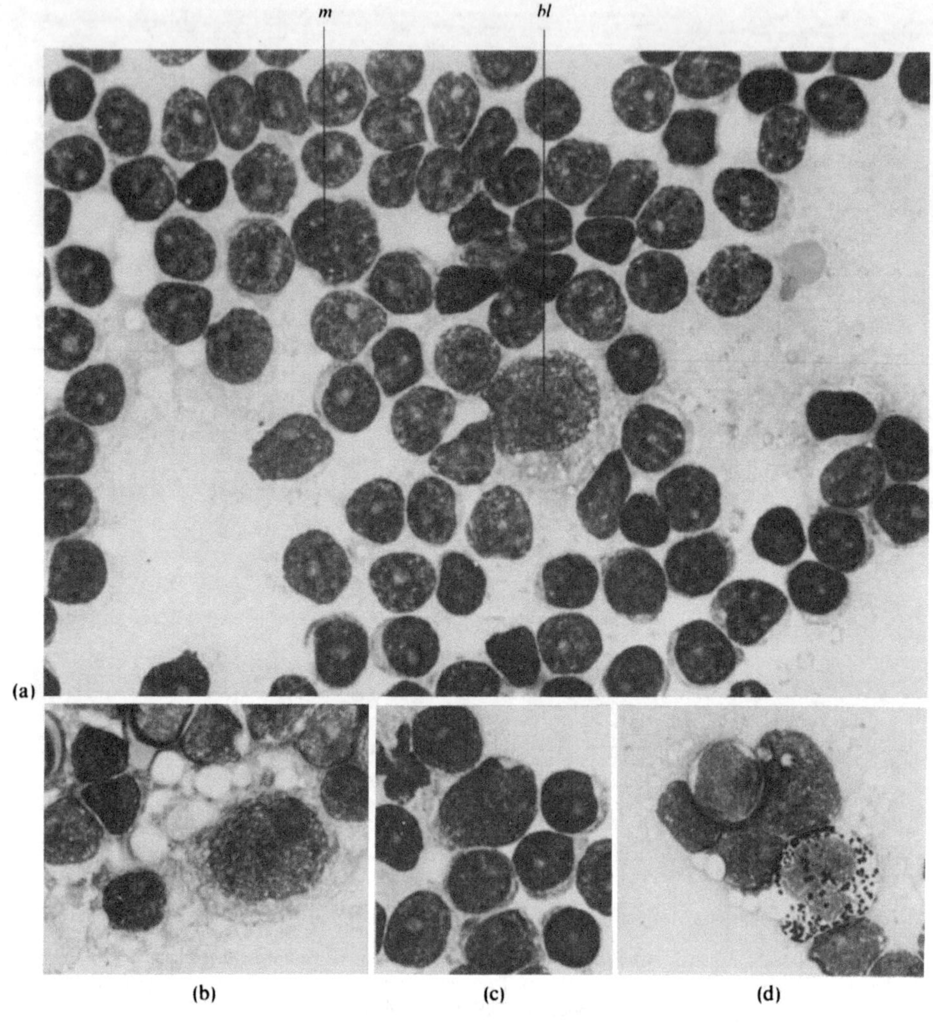


Fig. 57a–d. T-CLL in imprint. Cases 2 (a, c) and 3 (b, d). Lymphoid cells have large solitary nucleoli and thus fulfill one criterion of prolymphocytes. In both (a) and (c) there is a medium-sized lymphoid cell (*m*) with a convoluted nucleus (hyperdiploid lymphocyte). In (a) and (b) there is a large blast cell (*bl*) with several prominent nucleoli (T-immunoblast?). A basophil granulocyte is demonstrated in (d). Pappenheim. ×910

luted nuclei. These cells have an irregularly angular nuclear contour. On the whole, the nucleus appears ungainly. Occasionally, the nuclei also have rounded protuberances, which may overlap each other to some extent. The chromatin is dense like that of lymphocytes. There is usually no nucleolus, but occasionally a nucleolus of the same size as those of lymphocytes is seen. The rim of cytoplasm is very narrow and gray to gray-blue. The medium-sized to large basophilic blast cells occasionally have irregular nuclei. Most of the large forms, however, show oval nuclei with fine chromatin and several large blue nucleoli. These cells have a moderately wide rim of basophilic cytoplasm, which often contains numerous small vacuoles.

In the lymphocytes of case 1, one could occasionally detect a barely stained, roundish region in the cytoplasm that looked like a conglomerate of tiny soap bubbles (on electron microscopy there were clusters of mitochondria). In cases 2 and 3 there was a great increase in mitotic figures, which revealed markedly plump chromosomes.

Case 1 exhibited a few interdigitating reticulum cells, identified by their morphology and cytochemistry, and some medium-sized cells that might be interpreted as T-associated plasma cells.

A functionally significant finding was a definite increase in blood basophils, which were found in imprints in cases 1 and 3. No corresponding increase in eosinophils was present. In case 3 there was also some increase in mast cells.

**Histochemistry and Cytochemistry.** In sections the PAS reaction occasionally showed positive globules of moderate size in the cytoplasm of reticulum cells. All of the tumor cells were negative.

In imprints the PAS reaction of tumor cells was negative in case 1. Cases 2 and 3 showed granular PAS positivity in lymphocytes, although the number of positive lymphocytes was small (less than 1%). The PAS-positive material was in the form of fine, occasionally coarser, granules, densely packed in the cytoplasm.

Focal reactivity in lymphocytes for acid phosphatase,[88] acid nonspecific esterase, and β-glucuronidase[88] seems to be characteristic of T-CLL (Fig. 58). The pattern of activity is about the same in all three reactions, but it is most striking in the acid nonspecific esterase reaction. The activity is often seen as a paranuclear, small roundish spot, which appears to consist of a few coarse granules; but there is occasionally coarse granular enzyme positivity scattered over the cytoplasm, as SCHWARZE[89] found in 20%, 63%, and 69%, respectively, of the peripheral lymphocytes from our three cases. The granular pattern was found only in EFRATI's case[90] with many azurophil granules, mentioned on page 151. Not only the lymphocytes, but also the medium-sized cells with convoluted nuclei are focally positive, whereas the blast cells are enzyme-negative. The acid phosphatase reaction may be tartrate-sensitive or -resistant. LÖFFLER *et al.*[91] demonstrated tartrate resistance in our case 3. We found it in another case in our collection. The focal positivity of the lymphocytes approximately corresponds to that seen in lympho*blastic* lymphoma of the T-type, except that the diameter of the "focus" is smaller.

In contrast to the acid nonspecific esterase reaction, the neutral nonspecific esterase reaction is negative in the tumor cells, but shows a few strongly positive histiocytic reticulum cells, clearly positive venular endothelial cells, and sparse, slightly positive monocytes. In case 2 interdigitating reticulum cells could be

---

[88] BROUET, FLANDRIN, SASPORTES, PREUD'HOMME *et al.*, 1975.

[89] Unpublished data.

[90] 1976, personal communication.

[91] LÖFFLER, GRAUBNER, DESAGA and JUNG, 1977.

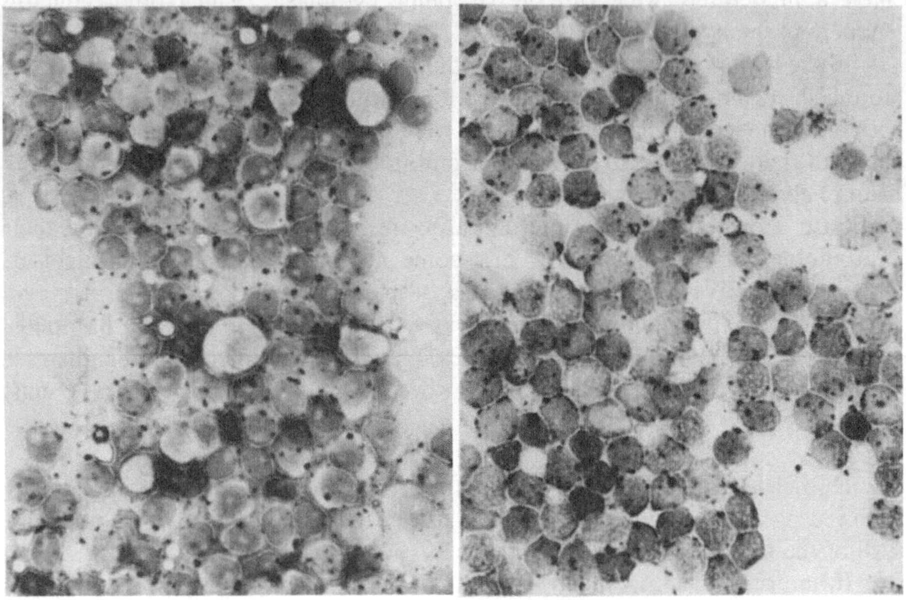

(a) (b)

Fig. 58a and b. T-CLL in imprint. Case 2. Acid nonspecific esterase (a) and acid phosphatase reactions (b). Note the focal coarse positivity in both reactions. ×525

clearly identified by their weakly positive neutral esterase and acid phosphatase reactions.

**Blood Picture.** The morphology of the leukemic cells is best studied in peripheral blood smears, since the cells are well spread out and not mechanically altered (Fig. 59).

We found mainly small lymphocytes or prolymphocytes and only a few medium-sized convoluted cells. The ratio of lymphocytes to convoluted cells was about 200–500:1. The small lymphocytes reveal two special features that were hardly noticeable in imprints: the nuclei often have small protuberances or clefts. The clefts do not penetrate more than halfway into the diameter of the nucleus, however, and the high degree of nuclear cleavage seen in the Lutzner cells of Sézary's syndrome is not observed in the lymphocytes. In particular, we did not find the lateral "sulci" on the upper side of the nuclei. Brouet *et al.*[92] and Insel *et al.*[93] also detected no features of Sézary cells in lymphocytes on light and electron microscopy.

The medium-sized cells with convoluted nuclei have a certain resemblance to large Lutzner cells. They are so characteristic that they alone—together with the nonconvoluted lymphocytes—allow a preliminary diagnosis of T-CLL.

The enzyme reactions (acid phosphatase, acid nonspecific esterase, β-glucuronidase) are more striking and more clearly recognizable in blood smears than

92 Brouet, Flandrin, Sasportes, Preud'Homme *et al.*, 1975.

93 Insel, Melewicz, La Via and Balch, 1975.

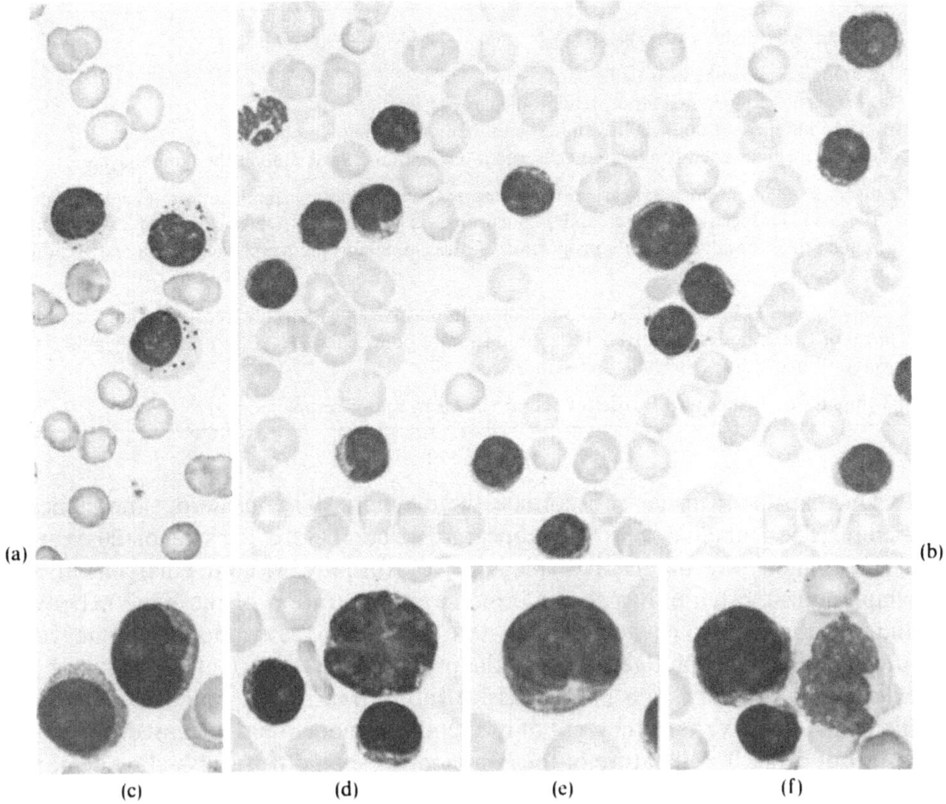


Fig. 59a–f. T-CLL. Blood smear. (a) Smear kindly provided by Dr. EFRATI, Rehovot. Large lymphocytes with coarse azurophil granules. (b–f) Case 2. Besides small lymphoid cells, note the medium-sized cells with convoluted nuclei. For comparison, a monocyte is shown in (f). Pappenheim. (a, b) ×805, (c–f) ×1,030

in imprints. The PAS reaction was negative in case 1; in case 2 it was positive in a small percentage of the cells, and in case 3 it was positive in most of the lymphocytes.

**Diagnosis.** Histologically (Table 21), the most prominent feature, when present, is an increase in epithelioid venules, which should immediately arouse the suspicion of T-CLL when seen with a monotonous lymphocytic infiltration. This suspicion is strengthened by the demonstration of medium-sized convoluted lymphocytes. Because these cells occur in small numbers, they must be looked for with oil immersion, but they are easier to demonstrate in blood smears or imprints. The decisive cytochemical reactions are also possible with the latter. Most of the leukemic lymphocytes and the convoluted cells contain small clumps of acid phosphatase, acid nonspecific esterase, and $\beta$-glucuronidase activity. Thus, a diagnosis can be made on the basis of these morphologic and cytochemical findings.

Table 21. Diagnostic criteria of T-CLL

1. Patients older than 20 years
2. Histologic picture: as in B-CLL, but
   a) no proliferation centers (no pseudofollicular pattern)
   b) large numbers of epithelioid venules with many migrating lymphocytes
   c) some medium-sized convoluted cells and a few immunoblasts among the lymphocytes
3. Imprints and blood smears: nearly all lymphocytes contain solitary small clumps of acid phosphatase, acid nonspecific esterase, and $\beta$-glucuronidase activity. In a proportion of cases, azure granulation is found. In another proportion of cases, polymorphic lymphocytes with convolutions are seen.
4. Clinical findings in favor of T-CLL: moderate to massive splenomegaly (mostly without enlargement of lymph nodes), relatively little infiltration of bone marrow (except in the prolymphocytic variant), marked neutropenia, and skin lesions
5. Lymphocytes form sheep-E rosettes and are killed by anti-T-serum

One can then further substantiate the diagnosis by considering the clinical picture. The leukemia does not appear to occur before the age of 20 years. There is moderate to massive splenomegaly (usually without enlargement of lymph nodes), often only a slight to moderate infiltration of the bone marrow, and sometimes marked neutropenia and skin lesions. Peripheral lymphocytes often contain azurophil granules. In the prolymphocytic variant blood lymphocyte counts are very high (with massive infiltration of the bone marrow). In the lymphocytic variant they are only slightly to moderately increased.

Proof of the T-cell nature of the lymphocytes should be furnished by demonstrating that they form sheep-E rosettes and are killed by anti-T-sera.

**Differential Diagnosis.** In the differential diagnosis one must distinguish T-CLL above all from B-CLL and Sézary's syndrome, but also from T-zone lymphoma, LP immunocytoma, centrocytic lymphoma, and lymphoblastic lymphoma of the T-type.

In B-CLL lymph-node involvement is clinically prominent. Histologically, there is usually a pseudofollicular picture. In contrast to T-CLL, a great increase in epithelioid venules is not evident. Medium-sized lymphocytes with convoluted nuclei do not occur. In imprints and blood smears the acid phosphatase, acid nonspecific esterase, and $\beta$-glucuronidase reactions of lymphocytes show only a few positive granules or are negative; one never sees solitary clumps of enzyme activity. The PAS reaction of blood lymphocytes is positive in B-CLL, whereas it may be positive or negative in T-CLL. So far, we have seen an increase in blood basophils only in imprints from T-lymphocytic neoplasms and not in those from B-CLL. With common methods, such an increase cannot be determined in sections.

Sézary's syndrome is always associated with erythroderma, which apparently does not, or only rarely occurs in T-CLL. Other skin lesions, however, which still need to be more clearly defined, are observed in T-CLL. Histologically, the skin lesions in T-CLL show lymphocytic infiltration of the deeper skin layers, whereas infiltration of the subepidermal cutis and the inner epidermis (pseudoabscesses) is typical of Sézary's syndrome. The morphologic distinction between

Sézary's syndrome and T-CLL can be made with blood lymphocytes. In Sézary's syndrome these cells show a high degree of nuclear convolution (with lateral and diagonal "sulci" on the nuclear surface), whereas the lymphocytes of T-CLL may reveal only small nuclear protuberances or shallow nuclear grooves. The lymphocytes of T-CLL usually cannot be distinguished from typical lymphocytes or prolymphocytes.

Medium-sized convoluted lymphocytes appear to occur in both Sézary's syndrome and T-CLL. In any event, they cannot be clearly told apart. Nevertheless, the lymphocytes can be differentiated in blood smears and imprints, especially with cytochemical methods. In T-CLL one usually finds solitary clumps of acid phosphatase, acid nonspecific esterase, and $\beta$-glucuronidase activity. In Sézary's syndrome one sees a few randomly distributed positive granules in the cytoplasm. Histologically, Sézary's syndrome shows a much more heterogeneous picture, in contrast to the monotonous picture of T-CLL. In most cases of Sézary's syndrome, the whole lymph node is not infiltrated by Sézary cells. The remaining noninfiltrated tissue may contain some remnants of dermatopathic lymphadenitis (increase in interdigitating reticulum cells, active germinal centers, sheets of plasma cells, etc.). A very varied cell picture with numerous interdigitating reticulum cells and diverse inflammatory cells is also noticeable in imprints. The increase in venules is not as prominent in Sézary's syndrome as it can be in T-CLL.

In T-zone lymphoma an increase in venules is also prominent, but the cytology is clearly different. The neoplastic lymphocytes are larger and are interspersed with numerous blast cells, possibly with formation of giant cells. Furthermore, T-zone lymphoma often reveals numerous remnants of follicles, which occur only very occasionally in T-CLL, if at all. In T-CLL we did not find the relatively marked eosinophilia often observed in T-zone lymphoma.

LP immunocytoma is more like B-CLL and is characterized by the presence of plasma cells or plasmacytoid cells. The tumor cells often contain intranuclear and/or intracytoplasmic PAS-positive globular inclusions. Epithelioid venules are occasionally increased in number.

M.L. centrocytic does not contain basophilic blast cells. The nuclei are cleaved and not convoluted. In practice, however, the distinction between cleavage and convolution is less clear than the different names imply.

M.L. lympho*blastic* of the convoluted-cell type has the focal positivity for acid phosphatase, acid nonspecific esterase, and $\beta$-glucuronidase in common with T-CLL. The area of activity is clearly larger, however, in the former lymphoma. In addition, the cells are of "blastic" nature: the chromatin is fine and the cytoplasm is basophilic. Typical lymphocyte nuclei with clumped chromatin do not occur. Furthermore, there is no increase in venules. Finally, the clinical picture is completely different. The course of M.L. lymphoblastic of the convoluted-cell type is rapid. There is often a mediastinal tumor, which has never been described in T-CLL. The lymphoblastic neoplasm occurs especially in the first two decades of life, whereas T-CLL does not develop in young patients.

**Prognosis.** Antileukemic therapy is essential in most cases. It led to a quick, complete remission in our case 1. EFRATI[94] observed a 50-year-old woman

[94] 1972, personal communication (later publication planned).

who had splenomegaly and blood lymphocytosis of about 90,000/μl but no other symptoms, and required no treatment for many years. A similar observation was made by BROUET *et al.*[95] in one case in which the disease did not progress for 5 years without therapy, although there was a great decrease in B-lymphocytes and neutrophil leukocytes.

In cases of the prolymphocytic variant, the prognosis is much worse than in cases of the lymphocytic variant. Our patients 2 and 3 responded only poorly to cytostatic treatment and died within a few months.

### 3. *Hairy-Cell Leukemia (HCL)*[96]

*Synonyms:* Leukemic reticuloendotheliosis (EWALD)
Lymphoid reticulosis (German literature, MITUS *et al.*)
*Myélofibrose lymphoïde* (DUHAMEL)
*Histiolymphocytose de l'adulte* (CHELLOUL *et al.*)
and many others

**History, Terminology.** In 1923, EWALD described a case of hemoblastosis as "leukemic reticuloendotheliosis." He claimed that it was derived from reticuloendothelial cells and regarded it as an acute hemoblastosis, since, like other leukemias, the disease terminated rapidly with sepsis. The spleen was the main organ involved, but infiltrates were also found in the liver and bone marrow. EWALD mentioned nothing about changes in the lymph nodes.

The term reticuloendotheliosis is still used to this day, despite the many modified names suggested to replace it, such as histiocytic leukemia, malignant reticulosis, etc. In German-speaking countries the term lymphoid reticulosis found special favor.

So-called reticuloendotheliosis has certainly been misinterpreted many times as monocytic leukemia. It has not even been proved that the case of EWALD was one of monocytic leukemia, as LÖFFLER *et al.*[97] believed. Only in the last few years has it become apparent that the lymphoid myelofibrosis of DUHAMEL[98] was the same entity. On the other hand, most investigators outside France failed to note that WAITZ *et al.* had already described the same entity under the names *myélophthise à réaction lymphoïde*[99] and *myélosclerose à forme lymphoïde.*[100] In similar fashion the "splenic lymphoma" of SÖDERSTRÖM[101] went ignored.

---

[95] BROUET, FLANDRIN, SASPORTES, PREUD'HOMME *et al.*, 1975.

[96] BOURONCLE, WISEMAN and DOAN, 1958; IIJIMA, 1966, 1973; PLENDERLEITH, 1970; CHELLOUL, DANIEL and FLANDRIN, 1973; EMBERGER, NAVARRO, RIZKALLA and IZARN, 1973; FLANDRIN, DANIEL, FOURCADE and CHELLOUL, 1973; TANAKA, 1973; BURKE, BYRNE and RAPPAPORT, 1974; CATOVSKY, PETTIT, GALTON, SPIERS *et al.*, 1974; DÜLLMANN, WULFHEKEL, DRESCHER and HAUSMANN, 1974; DUHAMEL, 1974; HAEGERT, CAWLEY, COLLINS, FLEMANS *et al.*, 1974; KATAYAMA and FINKEL, 1974; LÖFFLER, ROUX, FISCHER, DESAGA *et al.*, 1976.

[97] LÖFFLER, ROUX, FISCHER, DESAGA *et al.*, 1976.

[98] DUHAMEL and GUERRA, 1966; DUHAMEL, 1969, 1974.

[99] WAITZ, MAYER and MAYER, 1955.

[100] WAITZ, MAYER, BIGEL and FITZENKAM-SAITO, 1963.

[101] 1970.

In the meantime, the term hairy-cell leukemia (HCL) has been accepted by many authors. PLENDERLEITH[102] suggested the name after SCHREK and DONNELLY[103] had described the leukemic cells of reticuloendotheliosis as "hairy cells." On the other hand, KATAYAMA and NAGY[104] strongly opposed the term hairy-cell leukemia. Notwithstanding, we have endorsed the name, since "hairy cell" does not prejudge the origin of the cells involved, which, in our opinion, probably do not arise from reticuloendothelial cells. Consequently, the term hairy cell may be used as a descriptive name, even though in some cases the "hairy" surface of the cells is not prominent.

Of even greater diagnostic importance than the hairy surface of the leukemic cells is the demonstration of tartrate-resistant acid phosphatase in the cytoplasm.[105] We diagnose HCL with certainty only if we are able to demonstrate this enzyme.

**Origin of the Neoplastic Cells.** Until recently, EWALD's[106] assumption that the cells of this type of leukemia stem from reticuloendothelial, reticular, or histiomonocytic cells was accepted as highly probable, if not proved, most recently by TRUBOWITZ *et al.*,[107] CHELLOUL *et al.*,[108] KING *et al.*,[109] RAPPAPORT and BRAYLAN,[110] and SCHEINBERG *et al.*[111] A few investigators believe that the leukemia represents a combined proliferation of lymphocytes and reticular cells (e.g., DUHAMEL[112]). The ability to phagocytose[113] is assumed to support the interpretation of the proliferating cells as histiocytic elements. From our studies, however, the essential enzyme of histiocytic cells, nonspecific esterase, is absent, or present in small amounts only.

The studies of RUBIN *et al.*,[115] in our opinion, have shown that hairy cells are probably of lymphocytic origin. New investigative techniques (e.g., demonstration of immunoglobulin on the cell membrane, synthesis and secretion of IgM/$\lambda$,[116] rosette formation with mouse erythrocytes,[117] and other methods) have provided arguments indicating that the hairy cell may be a *special form of B-lymphocyte*[118] (see Part Six). Our histologic studies have contributed further evidence. The proliferation of hairy cells clearly begins in the outer cortex of lymph nodes, that is, in the B-cell region. It spares initially the T-cell regions. Scanning electron-microscopic pictures of the cells have been interpreted by some as showing their B-cell nature,[119] by others as indicating a cell type more compatible with a monocytic-histiocytic origin.[120] Because hairy cells have

[102] 1970.
[103] 1966.
[104] 1974.
[105] YAM, LI and LAM, 1971.
[106] 1923.
[107] TRUBOWITZ, MASEK and FRASCA, 1971.
[108] CHELLOUL, DANIEL and FLANDRIN, 1973.
[109] KING, HURTUBISE, SAGONE, LOBUGLIO *et al.*, 1975.
[110] 1975.
[111] SCHEINBERG, BRENNER, SULLIVAN, CATHCART *et al.*, 1976.
[112] 1974.
[113] DANIEL and FLANDRIN, 1974.
[115] RUBIN, DOUGLAS, CHESSIN, GLADE *et al.*, 1969.
[116] DEBUSSCHER, BERNHEIM, COLLARD-RONGÉ, GOVAERTS *et al.*, 1975.
[117] CATOVSKY, PAPAMICHAIL, OKOS, MILIANI *et al.*, 1975.
[118] CATOVSKY, PETTIT, GALETTO, OKOS *et al.*, 1974; HAAK, DE MAN, HIJMANS, KNAPP *et al.*, 1974; STEIN and KAISERLING, 1974; SCHMALZL, HUHN, ASAMER and BRAUNSTEINER, 1975.
[119] SCHNITZER and HAMMACK, 1974; CATOVSKY, FRISCH, OKOS and VAN NOORDEN, 1975.
[120] POLLIACK, BRAYLAN and GOLOMB, 1974; GOLOMB, BRAYLAN and POLLIACK, 1975.

Table 22. Hairy-cell leukemia. Material and incidence

| | | |
|---|---|---|
| Total No. of cases | 39 | |
| Biopsy | | 33 |
| Autopsy | | 6 |
| Total No. of biopsies | 52 | |
| Lymph nodes | | 7 |
| Extranodal | | 45 |
| Incidence in routine lymph-node biopsies | | 3 |
| =0.2% of malignant lymphomas | | |
| 0.4% of non-Hodgkin's lymphomas | | |

features of both B-lymphocytes and monocytes, it has also been postulated that they are derived from an unknown subpopulation of mononuclear cells.[121] Actually, the question still awaiting solution is: which cell of the hemopoietic tissue is the normal equivalent of the hairy cell?

If hairy cells are really lymphocytic variants, then where in our scheme should we best fit the proliferating hairy cells? We would place them near centrocytes, $B_2$-lymphocytes, and ("reticular") plasma cells, without yet being able to specify the exact spot. Indications for such a relationship are provided by the facts that cases with coincident proliferation of plasma cells have been described[122] and that there seem to be borderline cases between HCL and macroglobulinemia of Waldenström.

**Occurrence.** Hairy-cell leukemia accounts for about 2% of all leukemias.[123] We diagnose HCL more frequently on sections from bone marrow than on those from lymph nodes; we also often diagnose it on extirpated spleens and sometimes on liver biopsies.

In our material (Table 22) there were seven biopsies of lymph nodes and six autopsies in which sections of lymph nodes were also available for study. For every 58 lymph nodes showing a lymphoma of the CLL type, usually one is found with the picture of HCL. It made up about 0.2% of the malignant lymphomas and 0.4% of the non-Hodgkin's lymphomas among our routine biopsies. HCL occurs most frequently in the sixth decade, that is, about 10 years earlier than CLL (Fig. 60). Our youngest patient was 22 years old; our oldest, a woman, was 80. According to the literature, the male-to-female ratio is about 4:1. In our material, however, it was 1.36:1.

**Clinical Manifestations.** The disease begins insidiously and runs a slow chronic course. In most cases extreme splenomegaly and panhemocytopenia are the paramount signs. An aspiration biopsy of the bone marrow is usually dry

[121] RIEBER, V. HEYDEN, LINKE, SAAL *et al.*, 1976.
[122] CATOVSKY, PETTIT, GALTON, SPIERS *et al.*, 1974; own observation.
[123] BOURONCLE, WISEMAN and DOAN, 1958; CATOVSKY, PETTIT, GALTON, SPIERS *et al.*, 1974.

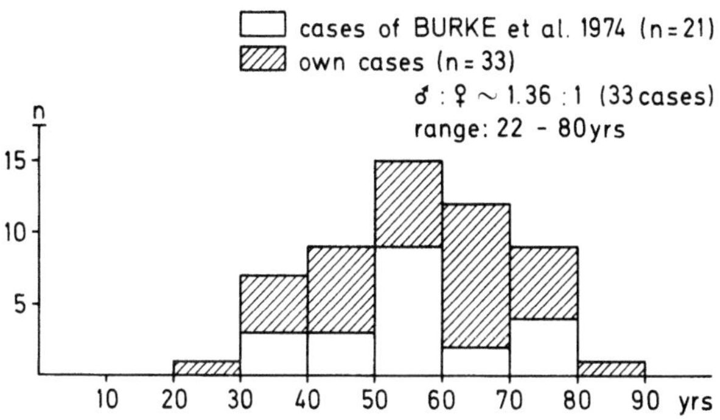


Fig. 60. Age distribution and sex ratio of hairy-cell leukemia. Data on 21 patients from BURKE, BYRNE and RAPPAPORT (1974) and on 33 patients in our series

and therefore unrewarding. In advanced stages, however, histologic study of the bone marrow reveals massive leukemic infiltration and a great increase in reticulin fibers. Because the disease apparently begins in the spleen, the bone marrow may show merely focal infiltration, even when the spleen is very large. In the spleen the white pulp and cords of the red pulp are both infiltrated. As a result, the volume of the red pulp is greatly increased and the passage of blood cells through the infiltrated red pulp is retarded.[124] Thus, more platelets and erythrocytes perish than normal. Peripheral lymph nodes are usually small, at times slightly enlarged. Although the total white blood cell count may be low, normal, or moderately increased, one can always find hairy cells in scanty or modest numbers. The cells contain at least some tartrate-resistant acid phosphatase. In contrast to B-CLL, there is no decrease in serum Ig for a long time, and, in fact, there is often a slight polyclonal increase.

**Localization.** It is generally agreed that peripheral lymph nodes are only slightly enlarged, if at all. Five of the lymph nodes we studied came from the axilla and two from the splenic hilum of extirpated spleens. In their large series of cases KATAYAMA and FINKEL[125] found that only splenic lymph nodes were involved, never peripheral lymph nodes.

Occasionally, at autopsy the para-aortic lymph nodes are found to be enlarged,[126] confirming results of lymphographic studies that indicate at times extensive involvement of retroperitoneal lymph nodes.[127] Involvement of the mediastinal lymph nodes apparently does not occur.[128]

**Gross Appearance.** The lymph nodes involved are seldom much enlarged. They exhibit a delicate smooth capsule and a homogeneous, fleshy, pale gray cut surface.[129]

[124] BURKE, MACKAY and RAPPAPORT, 1976.
[125] 1974.
[126] CATOVSKY, PETTIT, GALTON, SPIERS *et al.*, 1974.
[127] DÜLLMANN, WULFHEKEL, DRESCHER and HAUSMANN, 1974.
[128] FLANDRIN, DANIEL, FOURCADE and CHELLOUL, 1973; DUHAMEL, 1974.
[129] NAEIM and SMITH, 1974.

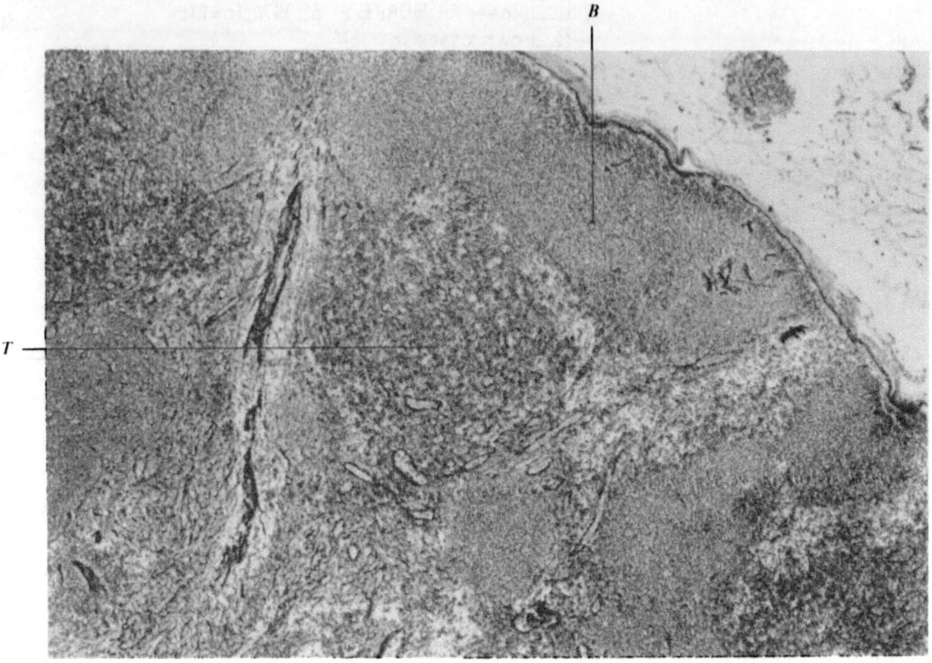


Fig. 61. Hairy-cell leukemia. Early lymph-node infiltration. The leukemic infiltration is localized in the B-areas (*B*), whereas the T-areas (*T*) are well preserved. ♀, 51 years. Axillary node. Gomori. ×70

**Histology.**[130] Since the lymph nodes become infiltrated relatively late, if at all, one often has the opportunity to study early changes. The hairy cells settle at first in the B-cell region, often leaving the T-cell region intact (Fig. 61). The most typical primary site of localization in the lymph node is the lymphatic tissue beneath the marginal sinus. Here the hairy cells establish themselves in small nodules (resembling the primary follicles) or in broad bands directly under the marginal sinuses. Remnants of germinal centers and extensive portions of intact T-nodules may lie among them. In the primary follicle-like areas one sometimes detects bizarre fiber networks that probably come from small vessels and perhaps originate from involuted germinal centers. In advanced stages the entire lymphatic parenchyma becomes infiltrated, but remains of nodules may often still be visible. Only in the late phases are the capsule and trabeculae infiltrated, and in these structures the infiltrates are sometimes markedly perivascular (Fig. 62). Important is the fact that, in general, the marginal sinus remains intact and does not become attenuated. With further infiltration, the proliferation spreads out into the surrounding adipose tissue.

[130] Bouroncle, Wiseman and Doan, 1958; Duhamel, 1969, 1974; Chelloul, Daniel and Flandrin, 1973; Emberger, Navarro, Rizkalla and Izarn, 1973; Burke, Byrne and Rappaport, 1974; Catovsky, Pettit, Galton, Spiers *et al.*, 1974; Naeim and Smith, 1974.

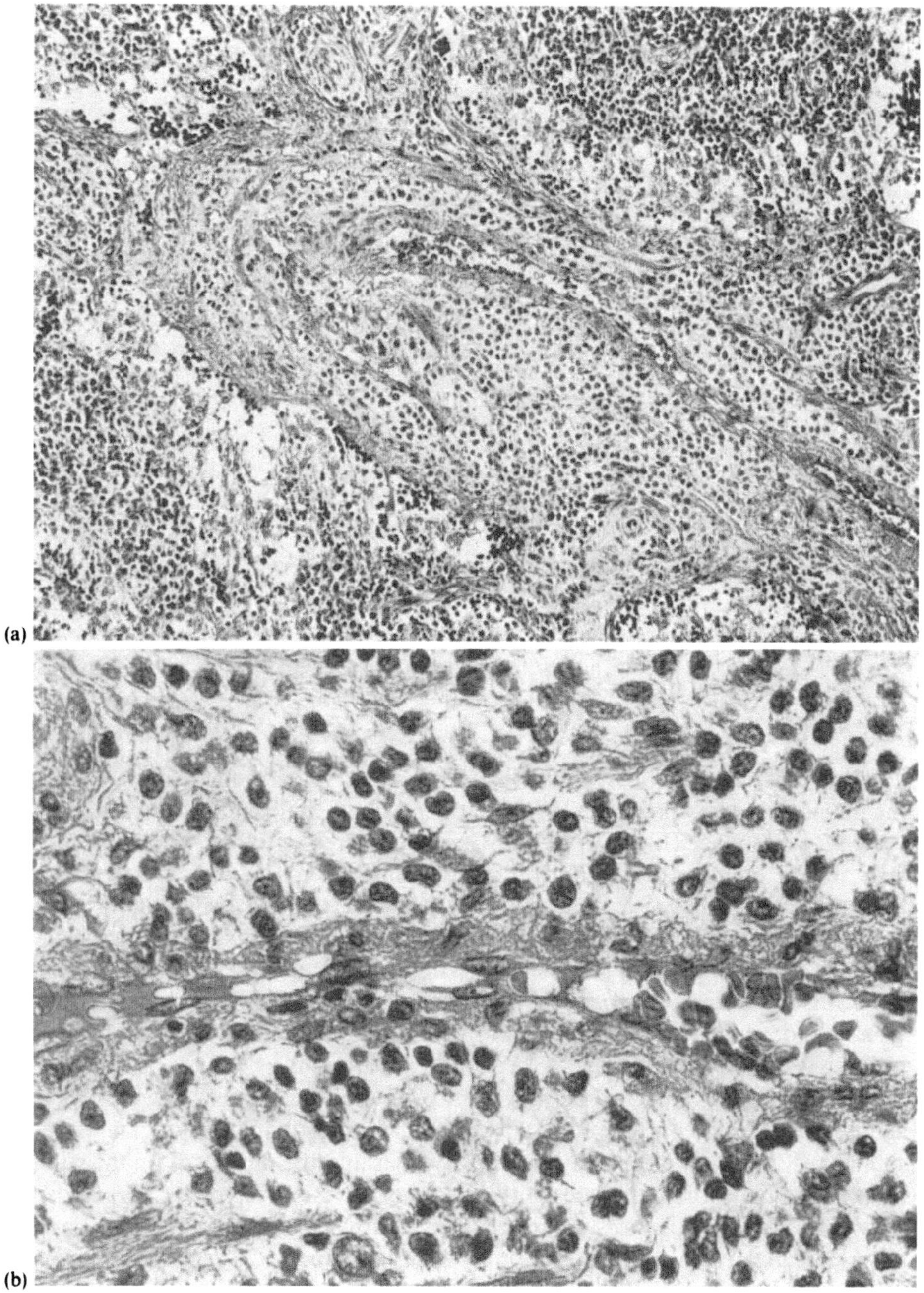

Fig. 62a and b. Hairy-cell leukemia. Perivascular leukemic infiltration of a trabecula. The nuclei of the hairy cells are fairly far apart in comparison with those in the surrounding lymphatic tissue at upper right and lower left in (a). Note the polymorphic, sometimes reniform nuclei in (b). ♂, 61 years. Axillary node. Hematoxylin and eosin. (a) ×140, (b) ×560

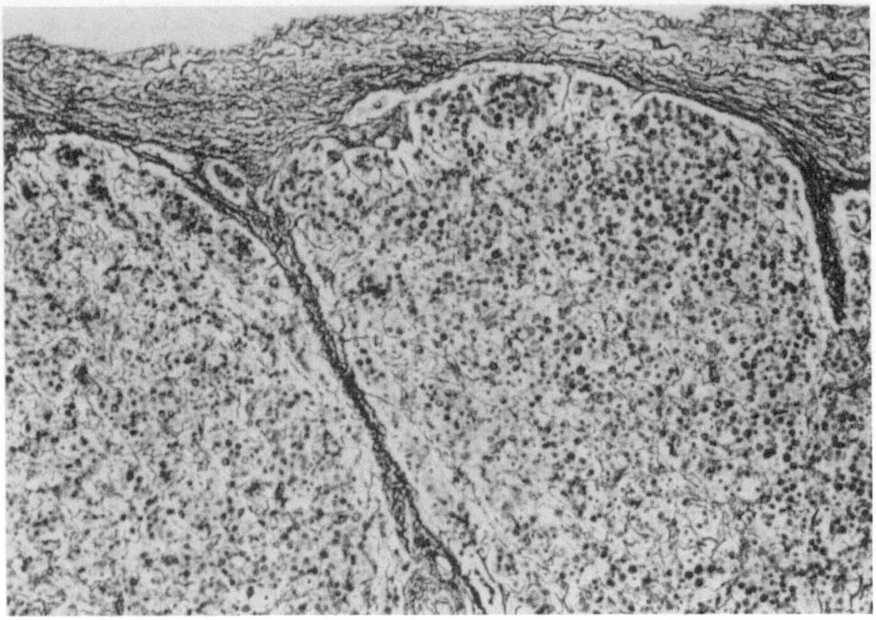

Fig. 63. Hairy-cell leukemia. Fiber pattern. Specimen kindly provided by Professor Dr. DUHAMEL, Paris. ♂, age unknown. Abdominal node. Gomori. ×140

Although the regions first infiltrated reveal very few reticulin fibers, when the disease becomes protracted a more or less intense formation of fibers (and vessels?) takes place (Fig. 63). Initially, such an increase in fibers is seen particularly in the regions about the infiltrates. Only when the disease lasts for a long time is the entire lymph node rich in fibers. The formation of fibers can then be seen particularly in perivascular regions and is often associated with distinct hyalinization (deposition of immunoglobulin?). DUHAMEL[131] compares this tendency to fibrosis with the changes that occur in the bone marrow. In a case described by ANDERSON and WALFORD[132] the fibrosis was especially pronounced in all regions where there were infiltrations.

The infiltrating cells are strikingly monotonous and somewhat larger than typical lymphocytes (Figs. 64 and 65). Their nuclei are often slightly bean-shaped, sometimes round. The chromatin is usually finer and the nucleus is on the whole lighter than that of lymphocytes in the neighboring T-cell regions. Characteristically, the hairy cells are distinguished by a relatively broad rim of cytoplasm, but unfortunately this feature cannot always be made out. Nevertheless, because of the broad rim of cytoplasm and the special qualities of the surface of hairy cells, one has the impression that their nuclei are fairly far apart. If at the same time the nuclei are bean-shaped, then it is understandable how the infiltrates could be misinterpreted as monocytic leukemia.

[131] 1974. [132] 1963.

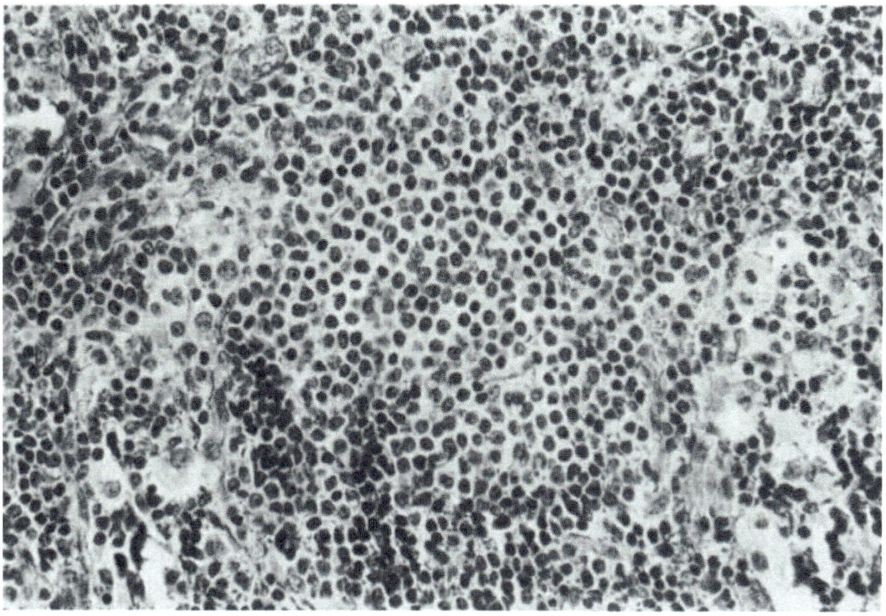

Fig. 64. Hairy-cell leukemia. Early lymph-node infiltration. There is an accumulation of hairy cells in the middle of the picture. Same node as Fig. 61. Hematoxylin and eosin. ×350

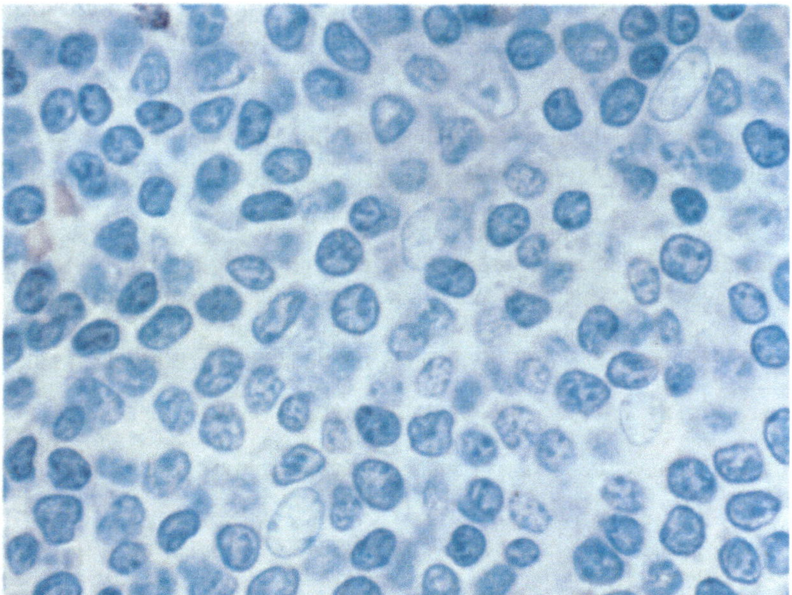

Fig. 65. Hairy-cell leukemia with Giemsa staining. Same node as Figs. 61 and 64. ×1,550

Hairy cells have only small, usually solitary nucleoli. Mitotic figures are virtually absent. CATOVSKY *et al.*,[133] however, illustrated a mitotic figure in the bone marrow. The rate of cellular proliferation is extremely low, as BERG and BRANDT[134] were able to demonstrate by *in-vitro* studies of splenic and liver biopsy material. Fewer than 1% of the hairy cells incorporated $^3$H-thymidine, that is, were synthesizing DNA. Apparently, hairy cells divide directly without "blast cells" appearing, much as plasma cells do in myeloma.

KATAYAMA *et al.*[135] were able to visualize by light microscopy, in three out of 11 cases of HCL, the cytoplasmic inclusions that they have described on electron microscopy as "ribosome-lamella complexes."[136] These are rod-shaped structures that vary somewhat in length and thickness. Thus, they may resemble either needles or cigars. Apparently, they are cylindrical and exhibit a central space, which can be recognized as a translucency only in imprints. That explains why the inclusions look like two pieces of cord lying next to one another. In histologic sections the cytoplasmic inclusions are amphophilic with the hematoxylin and eosin stain, presumably gray-blue with the Giemsa stain, and pyroninophilic as well.[137] They have been accorded a certain diagnostic importance, much like the Auer bodies in acute myeloid leukemia.[135] The inclusions have also been observed, however, in cases of each of the following: CLL,[138] LP immunocytoma,[139] and an undefined "lymphosarcoma."[140]

In three cases we found an increased number of plasma cells, which in one case were smaller than typical (reticular) plasma cells. In one lymph node mast cells were also increased in number. A large number of fibers and capillaries were seen in this case.

In a surgically removed lymph node and in a lymph node removed at autopsy we found considerable myelopoiesis. In the biopsy this led to a false diagnosis of myeloproliferative disease. We consider the myelopoiesis to be a compensatory reaction to the bone-marrow infiltration and myelofibrosis.

**Smear/Imprint.** In lymph-node smears and imprints one sees the same cells as in blood smears or in fine-needle biopsies of the liver, spleen, or bone marrow.[141]

The hairy cells in a blood smear[142] vary from 10–20 µm in size and are by no means uniform. In some cases the cells resemble plasma cells. In other cases, however, the cells look more like monocytes. Finally, there are cases in which some of the cells contain coarse azurophil granules.[143] As STEIN and KAISERLING[144] have observed, it is chiefly the cells with azurophil granules that

[133] CATOVSKY, PETTIT, GALTON, SPIERS *et al.*, 1974.
[134] 1970; also RUBIN, DOUGLAS, CHESSIN, GLADE *et al.*, 1969.
[135] KATAYAMA, NAGY and BALOGH, 1973.
[136] KATAYAMA, LI and YAM, 1972b; later e.g., DANIEL and FLANDRIN, 1974.
[137] CHELLOUL, DANIEL and FLANDRIN, 1973.
[138] ZUCKER-FRANKLIN, 1963; KAISERLING, 1975.
[139] KAISERLING, 1975.
[140] ANDAY, GOODMAN and TISHKOFF, 1973.
[141] BERG and BRANDT, 1970; SÖDERSTRÖM, 1970; BURKE, BYRNE and RAPPAPORT, 1974; and others.
[142] MITUS, MEDNICOFF, WITTELS and DAMESHEK, 1961; CATOVSKY, PETTIT, GALTON, SPIERS *et al.*, 1974.
[143] MITUS, MEDNICOFF, WITTELS and DAMESHEK, 1961.
[144] 1974.

have horseshoe-shaped nuclei, although the relatively small agranular cells may have them too. Furthermore, they noted a striking increase in lymphocytes with azurophil granules after passage through nylon fiber columns in three cases of HCL.

The cells that are somewhat reminiscent of plasma cells have a round nucleus lying eccentrically in the oval cell. The cytoplasm, however, stains gray-blue, in contrast to that of plasma cells, and is occasionally replete with innumerable vacuoles. The nucleus has finely granular chromatin with a moderately large, pale to gray-blue nucleolus.

The cells that look more like monocytes have bean-shaped or dumbbell-shaped[145] nuclei and a gray-blue cytoplasm, which at times has a reddish tinge and which is relatively plentiful. The surface of these cells is particularly "hairy."

The term hairy cell was coined after studies under the phase-contrast microscope[146] revealed that the cells possessed many irregular fine and coarser villus-like projections on the surface of the cytoplasm. This feature is not specific to the hairy cells of the leukemia now under discussion, nor can it be easily recognized in all cases when the slides are stained by Pappenheim's method. Above all, the cells containing azurophil granules show no projections. If one wants to visualize the hairy surface of the cells particularly well, as one can with a phase-contrast microscope, then slides stained for acid phosphatase prove particularly good for this purpose.

Since the hairy surface is not specific to HCL and not all the cells of HCL show this characteristic, we need other, more reliable criteria for identifying the leukemia with certainty. Cytochemical methods and electron microscopy offer such criteria.

**Histochemistry and Cytochemistry.** Performing histochemical reactions on paraffin sections is of little value. The PAS reaction is always negative. Occasionally, the chloroacetate esterase reaction confirms extramedullary myelopoiesis.

In contrast, the use of cryostat sections from unfixed tissue is most useful. They are ideal for carrying out the acid phosphatase reaction with or without pretreatment with tartaric acid. The neoplastic cells contain moderate amounts of tartrate-resistant acid phosphatase, as KATAYAMA *et al.*[147] convincingly described and illustrated. All other lymphomas have been found to be negative for tartrate-resistant acid phosphatase. Only Hodgkin's disease is said to exhibit a focal positive reaction. YAM *et al.*,[148] however, detected tartrate-resistant acid phosphatase in healthy persons and in patients with CLL, lymphosarcoma, chronic myeloid leukemia, and infectious mononucleosis. LÖFFLER *et al.*[149] also doubted that all other non-Hodgkin's lymphomas are negative. NANBA *et al.*[150] found tartrate-resistant acid phosphatase in "reticulum-cell sarcomas," and CATOVSKY *et al.*[151] described it in prolymphocytic leukemia (see p. 135).

[145] ANDERSON and WALFORD, 1963.
[146] SCHREK and DONNELLY, 1966.
[147] KATAYAMA, LI and YAM, 1972a.
[148] YAM, LI and FINKEL, 1972.
[149] LÖFFLER, ROUX, FISCHER, DESAGA *et al.*, 1976 (see References to Part Five).
[150] NANBA, ITAGAKI and IIJIMA, 1975.
[151] CATOVSKY, GALETTO, OKOS, MILIANI *et al.*, 1974.

From the studies by MITUS *et al.*,[152] we know that the hairy cells in a *blood smear* contain fairly large amounts of acid phosphatase. Only through the demonstration of its tartrate-resistance did this enzyme become a marker enzyme.[153] After pretreatment with L(+) tartaric acid, all other types of leukocytes (neutrophil granulocytes, monocytes), which otherwise give a positive reaction, become negative for acid phosphatase, whereas hairy cells retain the enzyme activity. The explanation why they do so was given by YAM *et al.*,[153] who were able to demonstrate that hairy cells contain the isoenzyme 5 of acid phosphatase.

According to the quantitative studies of CATOVSKY *et al.*,[154] not all of the hairy cells circulating in the blood were positive for acid phosphatase. Generally, 60% of the cells were moderately to strongly positive for acid phosphatase. In one case, only 20–25% of the cells were still positive after pretreatment with L(+) tartaric acid. In addition, the degree of activity is considerably diminished after pretreatment. Only the hairy cells with strong acid phosphatase activity are tartrate-resistant. Consequently, it is possible, when only a few leukemic cells are found in the blood, that only a rare cell will give a positive reaction, and then only a weak one. Perhaps these facts explain why in some cases a tartrate-resistant acid phosphatase reaction allegedly could not be demonstrated.[155]

All other cytochemical reactions are much less important for diagnostic purposes. Nevertheless, all favor a lymphocytic rather than a histiocytic derivation of the neoplastic cells. In about half of the cases the PAS reaction shows fine positive granules and, less often, a weakly positive, diffuse staining of the cytoplasm. At other times it is negative. Such variations probably depend on the technique of staining employed. The Sudan black stain either is negative or discloses a few granules.[152] The methyl-green pyronine stain shows even less pyroninophilia than it does in CLL.[152] The nonspecific esterase (α-naphthyl acetate esterase) reaction exhibits slight diffuse positivity that is not inhibited by sodium fluoride.[156] The acid variant of nonspecific esterase, however, was negative in one of our cases. β-Glucuronidase activity is extremely low or negative in hairy cells.[157] Abundant ATPase has been found on the surfaces of tumor cells.[157a] The phosphorylase, peroxidase, and chloroacetate esterase reactions are negative. Lysozyme activity (as in monocytes) and NBT reduction were not observed.[158]

**Diagnosis.** In typical cases the diagnosis of HCL is easily made (Table 23); at other times, however, it is extremely difficult. Consequently, one should not rely entirely on histologic studies of lymph nodes, but should instead resort to additional histologic studies, especially of the bone marrow, liver, and, when

[152] MITUS, MEDNICOFF, WITTELS and DAMESHEK, 1961.

[153] YAM, LI and LAM, 1971.

[154] CATOVSKY, PETTIT, GALTON, SPIERS *et al.*, 1974.

[155] E.g., BURKE, BYRNE and RAPPAPORT, 1974; DÜLLMANN, WULFHEKEL, DRESCHER and HAUSMANN, 1974.

[156] FLANDRIN, DANIEL, FOURCADE and CHELLOUL, 1973; SCHNITZER and KASS, 1974; VON HEYDEN, WALLER, PAPE, BENÖHR *et al.*, 1976.

[157] LÖFFLER, ROUX, FISCHER, DESAGA *et al.*, 1976 (see References to Part Five).

[157a] MÜLLER-HERMELINK and KAISERLING, unpublished data.

[158] CATOVSKY and GALTON, 1973.

Table 23. Diagnostic criteria of hairy-cell leukemia

1. Late and only partial infiltration of the lymph node
2. First infiltration in outer cortex (B-cell region), paracortical zone often not infiltrated
3. Monomorphic proliferation of lymphoid cells
4. Lymphoid cells somewhat larger than normal, nuclei sometimes reniform, chromatin finer than that of typical lymphocytes
5. No "lymphoblasts"
6. No mitotic activity
7. PAS reaction negative in paraffin sections
8. Tartrate-resistant acid phosphatase in cryostat sections and smears
9. Splenomegaly
10. Lymphoid myelofibrosis of the bone marrow

possible, of an extirpated spleen. Knowledge of the clinical manifestations of the disease and of the cytologic and cytochemical changes in the blood helps greatly in establishing the diagnosis. That is particularly true for the tartrate-resistant acid phosphatase reaction, for in doubtful cases it may be decisive.

Histologically, the architecture of the lymph nodes is usually preserved, with intact sinuses and an intact connective-tissue network. The infiltrates begin in the cortex (B-cell region) and usually leave remnants of the T-cell region intact. Fibrosis occurs in later phases of the disease. The infiltrating cells are somewhat larger than normal lymphocytes and sometimes have reniform nuclei.

The bone marrow discloses the changes described by DUHAMEL[158a] as "lymphoid myelofibrosis," a picture characterized by massive infiltration by hairy cells and a marked degree of fibrosis. The normal hematopoiesis is greatly reduced. In the liver the periportal spaces show a slight to moderate, often loose-looking infiltration, which also penetrates into the neighboring sinusoids. On the other hand, there may also be intrasinusoidal infiltration without the periportal spaces being affected to any significant degree. In typical cases one finds in the spleen massive infiltration of the pulp cords and white pulp; thus, at times no normal lymphocytes can be detected. The type of infiltration closely resembles that seen in ("reticular") plasma-cell leukemia.

Classic signs of the disease are gross splenomegaly, panhemocytopenia, and merely discrete enlargement of lymph nodes. The panhemocytopenia is adequately explained by the infiltration of the bone marrow (reduced hematopoiesis) and the splenic enlargement (increased destruction of blood cells).

The blood picture may be either aleukemic or leukemic. The characteristic hairy cells are usually easily recognized in slides stained by Pappenheim's method. The acid phosphatase reaction, however, is even better for this purpose. It is also a key diagnostic enzyme in that it is resistant to L(+) tartaric acid. Only when this criterion is fulfilled may we be sure that the disorder under investigation is hairy-cell leukemia. The presence of pyroninophilic, double-stranded inclusions sustains the diagnosis of HCL.

**Differential Diagnosis.** HCL must be differentiated from all neoplasms that consist chiefly of lymphocytes or lymphocyte-like cells, as well as from monocytic leukemia.

[158a] 1969, 1974.

*1. B-CLL:* The clinical picture of this leukemia is quite different from that of HCL. In B-CLL the peripheral lymph nodes are heavily involved. Hypogammaglobulinemia may develop in the course of CLL, but not in HCL. The peripheral lymphocytes in CLL show a weak granular acid phosphatase reaction, which, however, is not tartrate-resistant. Histologically, the architecture of the lymph nodes involved by CLL is totally altered. We have not yet seen an early involvement in this disease restricted only to the B-cell regions. The marginal sinuses in CLL are compressed and narrow and usually difficult to delineate. Remnants of the original normal lymphatic tissue cannot as a rule be distinguished. The tissues around the lymph nodes are infiltrated much earlier in CLL. Cytologically, at least a few "lymphoblasts" are always present and often small focal proliferations can be seen as well. In contrast, in HCL "lymphoblasts" are always absent. In CLL small to moderate numbers of mitotic figures can be found. In HCL, however, there are practically no mitotic figures. The hairy cells are somewhat lighter and usually contain a finer chromatin and sometimes a more bean-shaped nucleus. Nevertheless, the distinction between individual cells may be difficult, sometimes for technical reasons. The nuclei of the cells of HCL are less closely packed than those of the lymphocytes of CLL, mainly because of their abundant cytoplasm and villous surface. In advanced cases the fiber content in HCL is greater than that in CLL. In addition, the appearance of the fiber pattern differs somewhat in the two diseases. In CLL the reticulin fibers are not as regularly associated with small vessels as they are in HCL.

*2. Sézary's syndrome:* In this disease the infiltration begins in the T-nodules. The sinuses, especially the marginal sinuses, are obliterated by the tumor cells that have entered *via* the lymphatics and continued to proliferate. The infiltrating cells disclose irregular nuclei (Lutzner cells) and sometimes show mitosis. Among them one finds large cells, including so-called mycosis cells. The tumor cells do not contain tartrate-resistant acid phosphatase.

*3. M.L. centrocytic:* Although this condition resembles HCL somewhat, the two types of neoplasm can be distinguished by the cytologic features. The centrocytes have a narrower rim of cytoplasm and characteristic so-called cleaved nuclei. At least a few mitotic figures are always evident. The fibrous network is much coarser.

*4. LP immunocytoma:* Occasionally, the two conditions look somewhat alike. Plasma cells have also been found in HCL.[159] Immunocytoma always contains at least some immunoblasts and frequently shows PAS-positive inclusions, whereas HCL never does.

*5. Monocytic leukemia:* In a blood smear monocytic leukemia is easily distinguished from HCL. First, the monocytic cells give a relatively intense, diffuse esterase reaction, which is inhibited by sodium fluoride. In sections monocytes appear to be larger than hairy cells. The involved lymph nodes show a tendency to new formation of blood vessels and more marked fibrosis. The nuclei of the monocytic cells are more pleomorphic than those of hairy cells, and they exhibit deep indentations. There are practically always at least

---

[159] Catovsky, Pettit, Galton, Spiers *et al.*, 1974.

a few myelocytes or promyelocytes with a positive naphthol-AS-D-chloroacetate esterase reaction (see p. 297 and Table 50 for further criteria).

**Development into a High-Grade Malignant Lymphoma.** So far, there have been no reports on development of HCL into a high-grade malignant lymphoma.

**Prognosis.** Hairy-cell leukemia characteristically runs a chronic course. The patients, however, are often able to exert themselves physically to a surprising degree. Among our patients we had a deep-sea diver, who after each confinement to the hospital resumed his rigorous physical activity without trouble.[160]

The cases described in the literature with acute clinical courses[161] are, according to BURKE *et al.*,[162] probably best classified as malignant histiocytosis, or perhaps as prolymphocytic leukemia; they should not be included under the entity of HCL. CATOVSKY *et al.*[163] express similar skepticism about the possibility of HCL with a rapidly fatal course. Death usually follows from the consequences of the panhemocytopenia (sepsis, pneumonia, hemorrhages, and anemia) and not from reduced function of the immune system, as in B-CLL.

Older publications report the median survival time to be from 3–5 years. A good many patients, however, have survived longer than 10 years.[163] The treatment of choice at present is splenectomy. Cytostatic therapy is contraindicated. Corticosteroids may be useful.

### *Addendum*

### *Is There a Nonleukemic Lymphoma of the HCL Type?*

This question is still difficult to answer, since hairy-cell leukemia is as a rule defined according to morphologic and cytochemical criteria of blood smears. Reports on systematic studies of a nonleukemic tumor of the same type of cell are not available as yet. If the tumor occurs at all, it certainly must be rare.

## *4. Mycosis Fungoides (M.F.)*

**Definition.** Mycosis fungoides[164] is a type of lymphoma that primarily involves the skin and after an unpredictable period spreads to the lymph nodes and internal organs. Both clinically and histologically, the disease exhibits three phases: (1) a premycotic phase, with only nonspecific changes in the skin, (2) an infiltrative phase, in which a band-shaped infiltrate is found in the upper dermis with infiltrates in the adjoining epidermis, and (3) a tumor phase, charac-

---

[160] WALLER, personal communication.

[161] E.g., BOURONCLE, WISEMAN and DOAN, 1958.

[162] BURKE, BYRNE and RAPPAPORT, 1974.

[163] CATOVSKY, PETTIT, GALTON, SPIERS *et al.*, 1974.

[164] Review papers: GANS and STEIGLEDER, 1955, 1957; KNOTH, 1959; CYR, GEOKAS and WORSLEY, 1966; EICHENBERGER-DE BEER and STORCK, 1970; THOMAS and RAPPAPORT, 1975.

terized by multiple nodular infiltrates in the skin and frequent involvement of lymph nodes and internal organs. The primary tumor variant (*mycosis fungoides d'emblée*) is still a controversial subject. Leukemic blood pictures are rare in M.F.; some so-called Lutzner cells, however, are frequently found in the blood.[165]

**Origin of the Neoplastic Cells.** Electron-microscopic studies have revealed that a majority of the proliferating cells in M.F. are morphologically identical with Sézary cells. Since Sézary cells are more easily obtained for immunocytologic studies, they have been used to disclose information about the nature of the tumor cells of M.F., which are often referred to as Lutzner cells.[166]

Without a doubt, Sézary cells are derived from a subset of T-lymphocytes (T-helper cells? See p. 187). Accordingly, one may assume that M.F. is also a neoplasm of T-lymphocytes. Studies by ZUCKER-FRANKLIN *et al.*[167] support this assumption. In cases of M.F. that lacked the clinical manifestations of Sézary's syndrome, they encountered the same type of cells with similar immunologic and cytologic properties as are seen in typical cases of Sézary's syndrome. Using the rosette technique, EDELSON *et al.*[168] found only T-lymphocytes in the organs involved by M.F. VAN LEEUWEN *et al.*[169] demonstrated specific T-cell membrane characteristics on Lutzner cells in infiltrated lymph nodes.

**Occurrence.** Mycosis fungoides is a rare disease. In the USA an average of 71 patients die of M.F. each year.[170] Besides the cutaneous changes, enlargement of lymph nodes is the most frequent clinicopathologic sign.[171] RAPPAPORT *et al.*[172] found the lymph nodes involved in 24 out of 45 autopsy cases. Of the 30 lymph nodes we studied from cases of M.F., only one failed to show specific infiltration by tumor cells. Among the almost 250 cases of dermatopathic lymphadenitis in our collection we are unable to state how often M.F. involved the skin, but the number is probably not very high.

In our routine biopsy material (Table 24) the frequency of unequivocal cases of M.F. is 0.1% of all lymph-node biopsies; that is, 0.5% of the malignant lymphomas and 0.9% of non-Hodgkin's lymphomas.

According to the literature, M.F. occurs most commonly between the ages of 40 and 60 years[173] (Fig. 66). In our material the reason why the peak in incidence of M.F. (and Sézary's syndrome) falls about 10 years later may be that the lymph nodes become involved late in the course of the disease. The male-to-female ratio reported in the literature varies from 1.4:1[170]–2.1:1.[174]

[165] LANE and GREENWOOD, 1933; CLENDENNING, BRECHER and VAN SCOTT, 1964; FLANDRIN and BROUET, 1974; VARIAKOJIS, ROSAS-URIBE and RAPPAPORT, 1974.

[166] After they were described by LUTZNER and JORDAN, 1968 (see p. 172).

[167] ZUCKER-FRANKLIN, MELTON III, and QUAGLIATA, 1974.

[168] EDELSON, KIRKPATRICK, SHEVACH, SCHEIN *et al.*, 1974.

[169] VAN LEEUWEN, MEIJER and DE MAN, 1975.

[170] EPSTEIN, LEVIN, CROFT and LUTZNER, 1972.

[171] BLOCK, EDGCOMB, EISEN and VAN SCOTT, 1963.

[172] RAPPAPORT, EDGCOMB and THOMAS, 1968; THOMAS and RAPPAPORT, 1975.

[173] EPSTEIN, LEVIN, CROFT and LUTZNER, 1972; FUKS, BAGSHAW and FARBER, 1973.

[174] FUKS, BAGSHAW and FARBER, 1973.

Table 24. Mycosis fungoides (M.F.) and Sézary's syndrome. Material and incidence

| | M.F. | | Sézary's syndrome | |
|---|---|---|---|---|
| Total No. of cases | 79 | | 12 | |
| Biopsy | | 60 | | 10 |
| Autopsy | | 19 | | 2 |
| Total No. of biopsies | 60 | | 10 | |
| Lymph nodes | | 30 | | 8 |
| Extranodal | | 30 | | 2 |
| Incidence in routine lymph-node biopsies | 8 cases | | 4 cases | |
| = % of malignant lymphomas | 0.53 | | 0.26 | |
| % of non-Hodgkin's lymphomas | 0.9 | | 0.5 | |

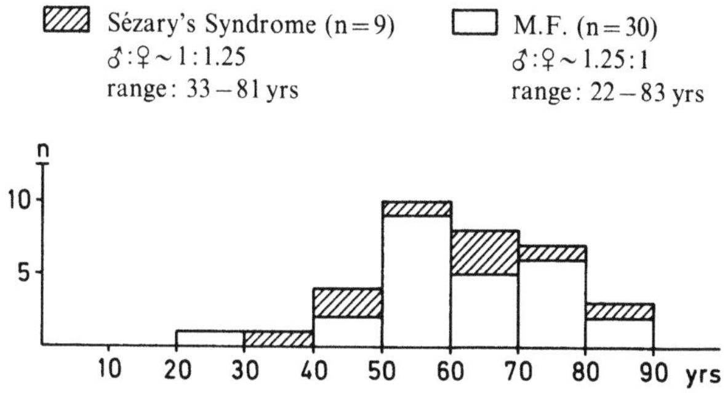


Fig. 66. Age distribution and sex ratio of 30 patients with mycosis fungoides (*M.F.*) and of nine patients with Sézary's syndrome

Table 25. Localization of excised lymph nodes in mycosis fungoides (M.F.) and Sézary's syndrome

| Localization | M.F. | Sézary's syndrome |
|---|---|---|
| Cervical | 6 | 1 |
| Axillary | 5 | 2 |
| Mediastinal | – | – |
| Abdominal | – | – |
| Inguinal | 10 | 3 |
| Cubital | – | 2 |
| Unknown | 9 | – |
| Total | 30 | 8 |

**Localization.** As shown in Table 25, we studied lymph nodes removed from the cervical, axillary, and inguinal regions. In the literature it is also reported that chiefly peripheral lymph nodes are involved in M.F. That is understandable, since the skin is affected first and since the histologic picture often indicates the lymphogenous influx of Lutzner cells into the lymph nodes. In staging laparotomies, however, VARIAKOJIS *et al.*[175] found that abdominal lymph

[175] VARIAKOJIS, ROSAS-URIBE and RAPPAPORT, 1974.

nodes—together with the spleen—were affected in three out of 13 cases of M.F. In two cases the involvement was only focal, and in one the lymph-node structure was partially effaced. In two of the patients lymphangiographic studies had already led to a diagnosis of lymph-node involvement.

Whether M.F. can also develop without the skin becoming involved is still questionable; it is more likely that it cannot, although repeated statements to the contrary have been made.[176]

Spread to the lymph nodes takes place not only *via* lymph channels, but also by the blood *via* epithelioid venules. That is especially true for the deeper lymph nodes, as well as for the spleen, liver, and other internal organs that can be infiltrated by the hematogenous route.

**Gross Appearance.** The involved lymph nodes seldom exceed 2—3 cm in diameter. They are moderately firm, and in the gray-white tissue of the freshly sectioned node one may occasionally recognize black stippling or flecks due to melanin deposits from a preceding or persisting dermatopathic lymphadenitis.

**Histology.**[177] When one studies the relatively few published reports on the histology of the lymph nodes in M.F., one becomes somewhat bewildered. Not only are the cells given different names—they are usually called histiocytes or reticulum cells—but the morphologic descriptions are also by no means congruent. Such variations are understandable to a certain degree, since in the lymph nodes (as in the skin) the changes appear at first nonspecific and resemble chiefly those of dermatopathic lymphadenitis.

The following description is essentially based on our own observations. We have made these from a study of 30 lymph nodes from patients who had clinically and/or histologically proven M.F. of the skin. To facilitate an understanding of the subject, we shall discuss the changes in the lymph nodes in four sections:

1. Dermatopathic lymphadenitis (lipomelanic reticulocytosis) as a nonspecific reaction of the regional lymph nodes.
2. The fully developed picture of M.F.
3. The early changes of M.F.
4. The anaplastic late stages of M.F.

*1. Dermatopathic Lymphadenitis (Lipomelanic Reticulocytosis).* Mycosis fungoides begins often, or perhaps always, with the regional lymph nodes presenting the histologic picture of dermatopathic lymphadenitis (Fig. 67). This lymphade-

[176] E.g., Faber, 1939.

[177] Paltauf and von Zumbusch, 1913; Pautrier and Woringer, 1939; Robb-Smith, 1964; de Graciansky, Timsit, Daniel, Revuz *et al.*, 1967; Duhamel, 1969; Gomez Orbaneja, Sanchez Yus, Diaz-Flores and Simon Huarte, 1972; Long and Mihm, 1974; Variakojis, Rosas-Uribe and Rappaport, 1974; Thomas and Rappaport, 1975.

Fig. 67a—c. Dermatopathic lymphadenitis with early M.F. infiltration (a, b) and without M.F. infiltration (c). Note the very large T-nodule in (a) and the large number of polymorphic lymphocytes with three mitotic figures (*m*) and with some interdigitating reticulum cells (*irc*) in (b). (c) Dermatopathic lymphadenitis in dermatitis herpetiformis Duhring. The number of interdigitating reticulum cells (*irc*) is larger, the number of lymphocytes is smaller. (a, b) ♀, 59 years. Inguinal node. (c) ♀, 17 years. Lymph node removed at autopsy. (a) Giemsa. × 70. (b) Hematoxylin and eosin. × 560. (c) Goldner. × 560 ▷

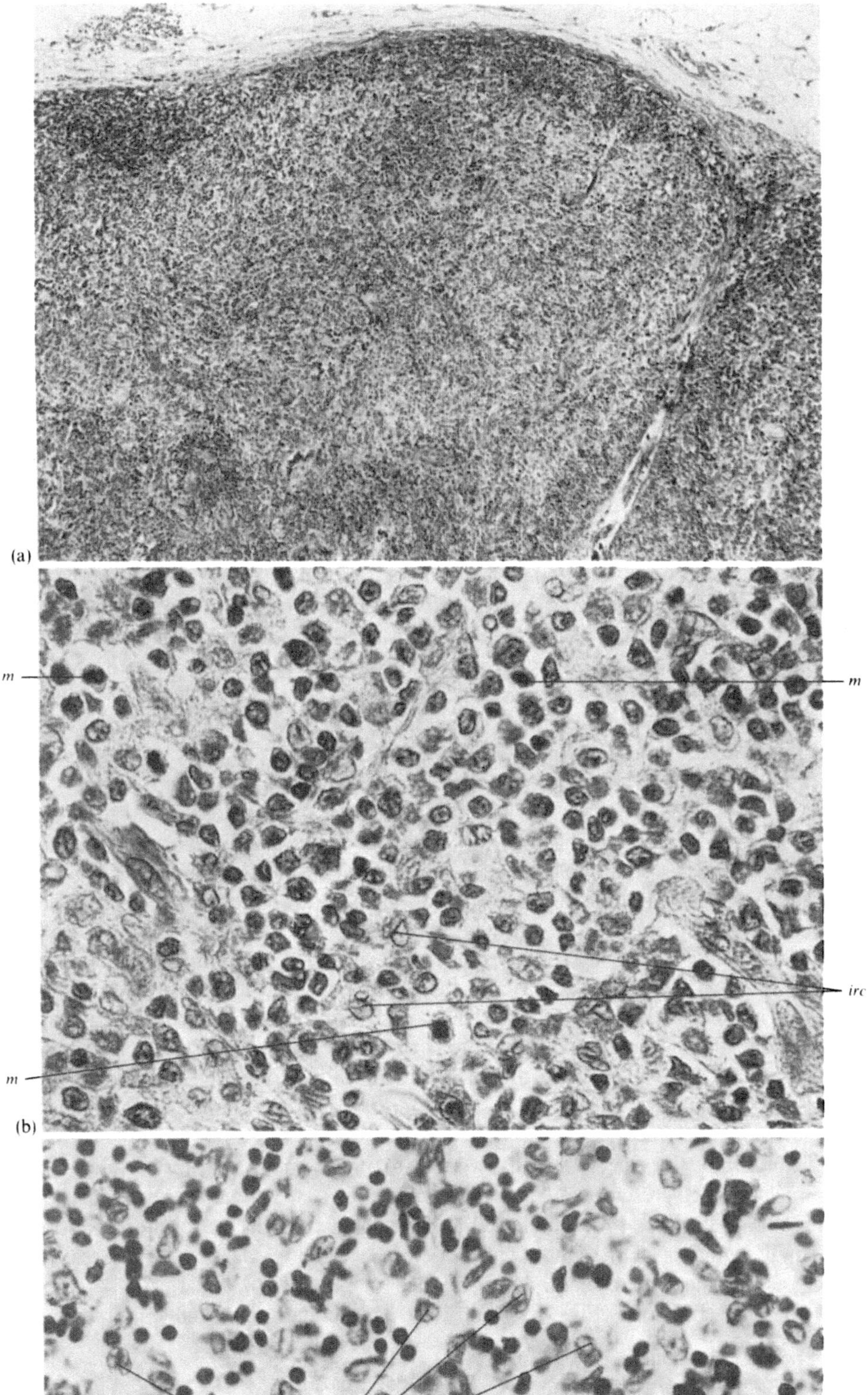
(a)
m
m
irc
m
(b)
(c)
irc

nitis associated with M.F. differs in no way from the dermatopathic lymphadenitis that develops with other pruritic skin diseases. In both conditions it has to be regarded as a special response of the T-cell areas (T-nodules, formerly called tertiary follicles)[178] of the lymph node, in which T-specific interdigitating reticulum cells increase in number until they ultimately dominate the histologic picture.

Since LUTZNER *et al.*[179] were able to demonstrate by electron microscopy the cells characteristic of M.F. (Lutzner cells) in a series of lymph nodes that had revealed only dermatopathic lymphadenitis on light microscopy, the question has arisen as to whether a neoplastic proliferation like M.F. can occur undetected in what appears to be a straightforward inflammatory lymph node. The results of studies by ERKMAN-BALIS and RAPPAPORT[180] emphasize the importance of this question, for they were able to find by cytogenetic studies distinctly atypical lymphocytes in a lymph node that seemed to present only the picture of dermatopathic lymphadenitis. This shows that dermatopathic lymphadenitis may, at times, represent involvement by M.F. and not merely a response to the disease localized in the skin. Accordingly, we must search for histologic criteria that enable us to recognize the earlier stages of M.F. involvement. In the third section (p. 173) we report on our attempts to define such criteria. We should be cautious about interpreting the electron-microscopic findings of LUTZNER *et al.*[179] as evidence of lymph-node involvement by M.F., since LUTZNER *et al.*[179] themselves, FLAXMAN *et al.*,[181] and ROSAS-URIBE *et al.*[182] showed that so-called Lutzner cells can be found in inflammatory reactions both in and outside the lymph node and also in histologically "normal" spleens.[182] Thus, they are not specific to M.F.

*2. The Fully Developed Picture of Mycosis Fungoides.* The architecture of the lymph node is completely effaced. The M.F. infiltration involves primarily paracortical areas, but may spill over into the cortex, the medulla, and occasionally even into the tissues surrounding the lymph node. The capsule is generally infiltrated only slightly or not at all, but it may show a fibrous thickening. There is often a marked increase in the number of epithelioid venules, which contain numerous lymphocytes, especially in the walls. There is a variable increase in reticulin fibers. Occasionally, portions of the sinuses are obstructed by infiltrates of Lutzner cells. That often results in dilatation and sclerosis of the parts of the sinuses behind the obstruction. The dilated lumina of the sinuses contain chiefly reticulum cells, but some Lutzner cells as well. In one case, in the region of the marginal sinus, we found an extreme formation of vessel-like channels, which resembled those we described as vascular transformation (Fig. 68).[183] Perhaps they developed as a result of the obstruction and sclerosis of small segments of the sinus wall. On rare occasions, we saw large areas of necrosis involving most of the lymph node.

The M.F. infiltrate (Figs. 69 and 70) usually consists of small polymorphic

---

178 LENNERT and ELSCHNER, 1954.
179 LUTZNER, HOBBS and HORVATH, 1971.
180 1970, 1974.
181 FLAXMAN, ZELAZNY and VAN SCOTT, 1971.
182 ROSAS-URIBE, VARIAKOJIS, MOLNAR and RAPPAPORT, 1974.
183 HAFERKAMP, ROSENAU and LENNERT, 1971.

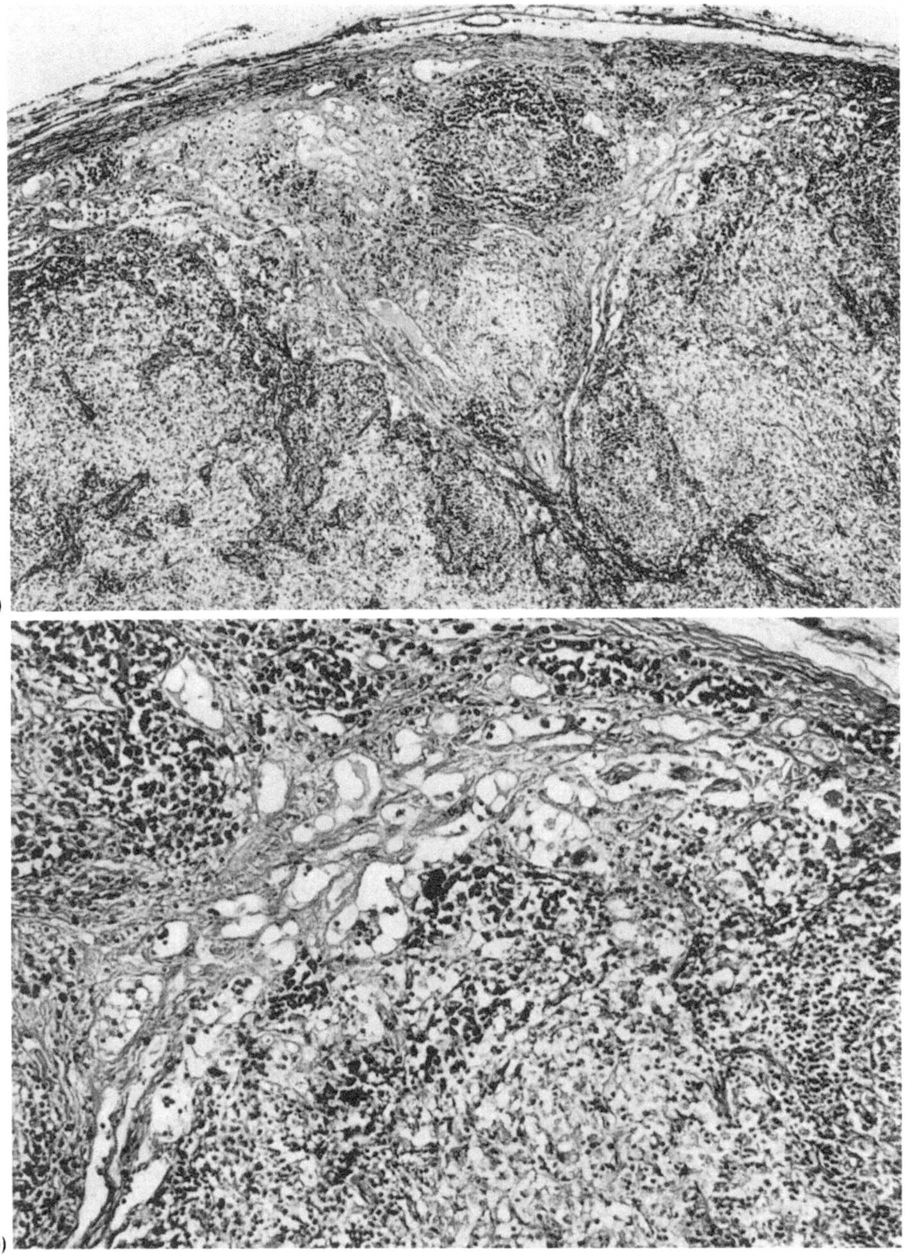

(a)

(b)

Fig. 68a and b. Mycosis fungoides. Sclerosis and many vessel-like channels in marginal sinuses like vascular transformation. In (a) there is M.F. infiltration in a "triangle" of the capsule. ♀, 53 years. Axillary node. Giemsa. (a) ×56, (b) ×140

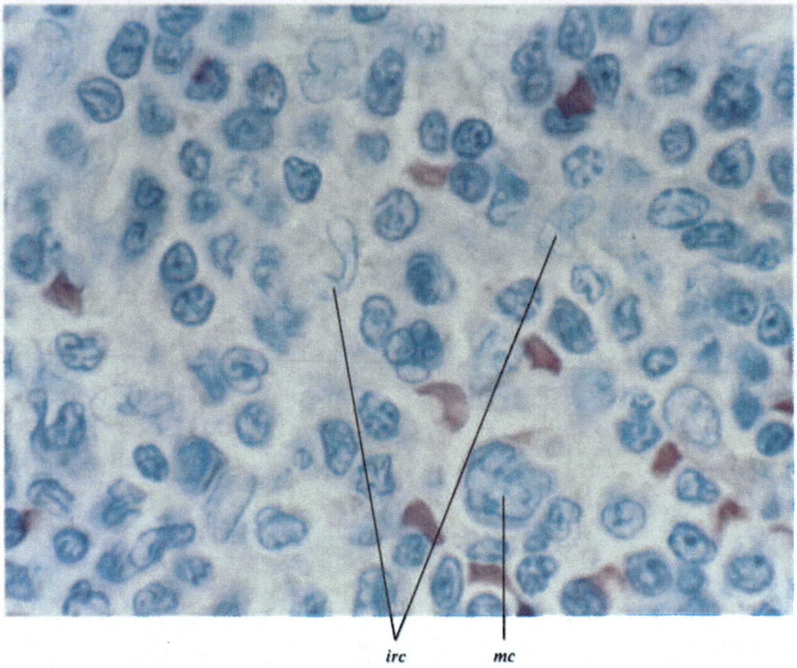


Fig. 69. Mycosis fungoides with Giemsa staining. Numerous polymorphic lymphocytes (Lutzner cells). Many, at least eight, interdigitating reticulum cells (*irc*). One so-called mycosis cell (*mc*). ♀, 79 years. Clinically, the patient had leukemia, but did not have Sézary's syndrome. Inguinal node. × 1,550

lymphoid cells (Lutzner cells).[184] In addition, larger polymorphic cells are present, and these are customarily called mycosis cells. Mitotic figures are generally numerous, occurring in both the small and the large cells. Among the special lymphoid cells (Lutzner cells), we always find some interdigitating reticulum cells, which may be part of the neoplasm and not merely remnants of dermatopathic lymphadenitis. That is also suggested by the occurrence of interdigitating reticulum cells together with Lutzner cells in the skin infiltrations of M.F.[185]

On electron microscopy, Lutzner cells have a nucleus "which appears serpentine with lobulations and indentations, often interconnected by narrow bridges composed of rows of dense nuclear particles and nuclear membranes."[186] With the light microscope the nucleus seems "cerebriform with overlapping folds and clefts."[186]

On light microscopy, *Lutzner cells* (T-lymphocytes) are usually small, being only slightly larger than B-lymphocytes still present in the follicles; but they may also be distinctly larger. LUTZNER *et al.*[187] now distinguish two sizes of cells and, consequently, a small- and a large-cell type of M.F.

[184] LUTZNER and JORDAN, 1968; LUTZNER, HOBBS and HORVATH, 1971; LUTZNER, EMERIT, DUREPAIRE, FLANDRIN *et al.*, 1973.
[185] GOOS, KAISERLING and LENNERT, 1976.
[186] LUTZNER and JORDAN, 1968.
[187] LUTZNER, EMERIT, DUREPAIRE, FLANDRIN *et al.*, 1973.

The nuclei of the larger cells appear to be considerably paler than those of normal lymphocytes. In contrast, the nuclei of the small cells are only slightly lighter, and in Giemsa-stained slides their chromatin is more gray in comparison with the blue chromatin seen in the nonneoplastic lymphocytes. In addition, as our studies revealed, the nuclei are frequently indented and notched, occasionally incompletely segmented. The nucleoli are small. The cytoplasm is so faintly basophilic that in the usual Giemsa-stained slides it can scarcely be perceived as such.

In contrast, the *mycosis cells* are much less clearly defined, and one feels compelled to ask what type of cell they represent. It is difficult to reach any definite conclusions from the published accounts, especially since only hematoxylin and eosin staining was mentioned.

In our studies of the large cells found in M.F. we were able to differentiate four types, although these were not always easily distinguished from one another (Fig. 70). The four types are:

a) Large cells with polymorphic giant nuclei that are crumpled or folded ("convoluted"), small nucleoli, and a narrow, barely visible, pale rim of cytoplasm. These cells differ from the lymphoid Lutzner cells only in their abnormal size; consequently, we interpret them as polyploid Lutzner cells.

b) Large cells that are strongly basophilic, usually with only one round or oval nucleus containing one or more large nucleoli (Fig. 70a). Their moderately broad rim of cytoplasm is easily made out. They are most probably some type of blast cell (T-immunoblasts?).

c) Large, slightly to moderately basophilic cells, in which the nuclei are very variable. The nuclei may be round, oval, or irregular with numerous indentations (Fig. 70b, c). There are one or more medium-sized or large nucleoli. The cytoplasm of these cells is moderately abundant and often displaced more to one side. It is impossible to state the origin of these cells. They are probably equivalent, however, to the "mycosis cells" described in the literature.

d) Large, moderately basophilic cells with elongate cytoplasmic processes and large, round or oval, clear nuclei containing medium-sized or large nucleoli, which stain gray with Giemsa. Occasionally, some of these cells are multinucleate. They are perhaps atypical reticulum cells.

In addition, we found in a few cases very occasional cells that fulfilled the criteria of Hodgkin or Sternberg-Reed cells: they had one or more large nuclei containing a clear karyoplasm and voluminous, slightly basophilic nucleoli. Their cytoplasm stained gray-blue with Giemsa. In imprints we also occasionally found similar cells with very prominent nucleoli in the giant "reticular" nuclei with fine chromatin. These cells, however, no more indicate that Hodgkin's disease is associated with M.F. than do similar cells in infectious mononucleosis.[188]

*3. The Early Changes of Mycosis Fungoides* (Fig. 67a, b). As a source of material we restudied eight lymph nodes that had been removed from patients diagnosed clinically as having M.F., but in whom we had made the histologic diagnosis of dermatopathic lymphadenitis. By restudying the lymph nodes we intended to find out whether or not subtle changes were in reality present

[188] TINDLE, PARKER and LUKES, 1972.

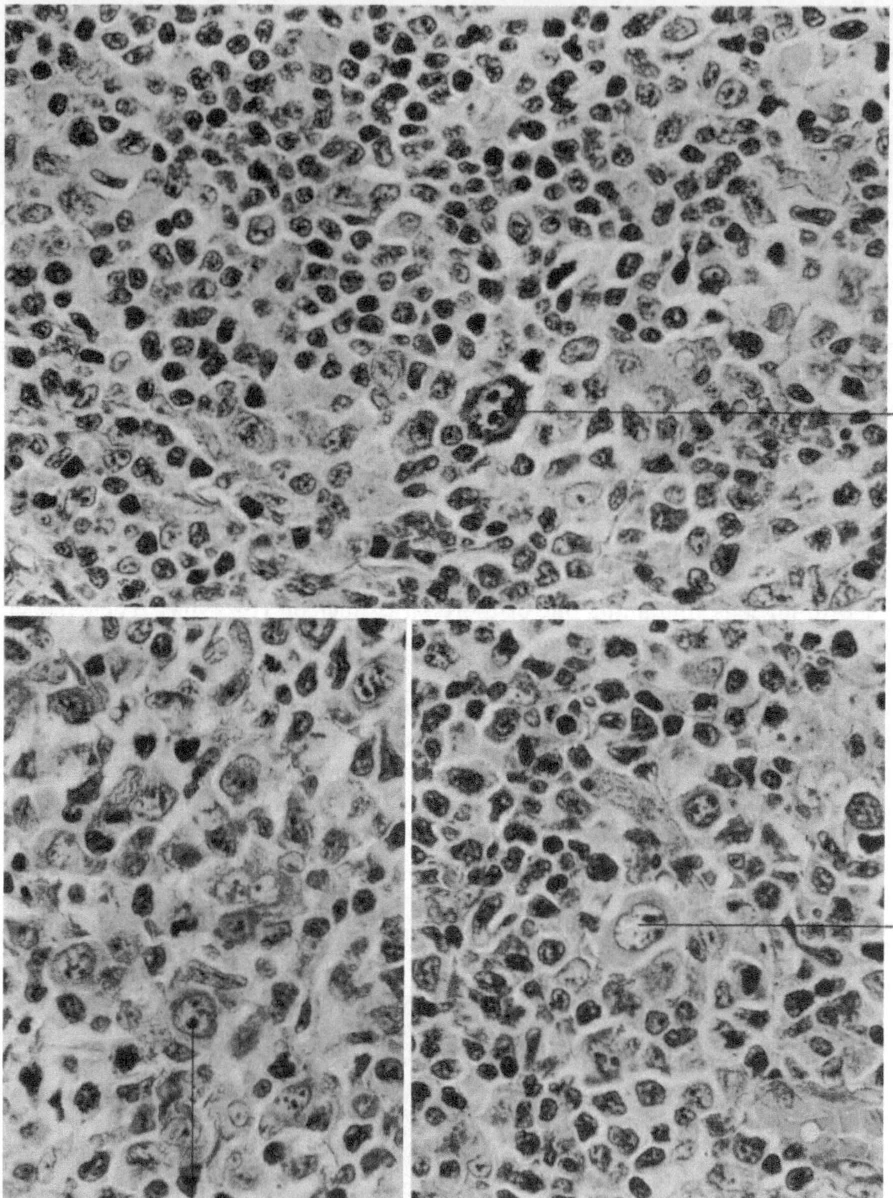

Fig. 70a–c. Mycosis fungoides. Various kinds of large cells ($x$; "giant cells," "mycosis cells") among polymorphic lymphocytes. (a) A very basophilic variant (T-immunoblast?). (b, c) Slightly basophilic cells. A relatively anaplastic pattern is seen in (b); other fields revealed a definitely anaplastic stage of M.F. (cf., Fig. 71). ♂, 54 years. Lymph node. Giemsa. ×560

that would have warranted our diagnosing M.F. From our review we concluded that in four lymph nodes we could have diagnosed M.F. with certainty, in three lymph nodes with likelihood, whereas in one, M.F. could not have been suspected.

What criteria enable us to distinguish the dermatopathic lymphadenitis associated with M.F. from that associated with other, nonneoplastic diseases of the skin? The following criteria seem to us to be especially helpful in diagnosing M.F. at an early stage:

a) In M.F., Lutzner cells – sometimes hardly distinguishable from lymphocytes – can be found in large numbers in the outer cortex and particularly in the marginal sinus. They lead to obliteration of the sinus with frequent focal fibrosis. They destroy the marginal sinus and sometimes form a narrow band above the T-nodules opposite the capsule. At times they appear to "nibble away" at the adjacent capsule. These changes are best seen with reticulin stains.

b) Large numbers of Lutzner cells can also be identified in the T-nodules. In the dermatopathic lymphadenitis of M.F., Lutzner cells are more numerous in the reticulum cell-rich T-nodules than they are in dermatopathic lymphadenitis of other causes. The Lutzner cells stand out because of their polymorphism. Polyploid Lutzner cells are of particular diagnostic value, whereas the other large basophilic cells are of little help in the differential diagnosis, since we know too little about the origin or significance of similar cells in reactive dermatopathic lymphadenitis. Strongly basophilic blast cells sometimes appear in particularly large numbers in dermatopathic lymphadenitis not associated with M.F.

c) Numerous mitotic figures (in Lutzner cells) within the T-nodules are suggestive of M.F.[189]

d) Occasionally, there is cellular infiltration of the lymph-node capsule, especially in the triangular areas formed by the junction of capsule and trabecula; or there may be infiltration outside the node, often perivascular. Such infiltrates are particularly suggestive of M.F. when they contain atypical cells (Fig. 68a). The atypical cells include not only Lutzner cells, but also larger cells with convoluted, crumpled-looking, or folded nuclei and relatively abundant gray cytoplasm. The larger cells are interdigitating reticulum cells.

e) In M.F. other inflammatory changes in the lymph node are generally less marked or entirely absent. Consequently, the germinal centers are often small or have completely vanished. Plasmacytosis of the medulla is usually slight, if present at all. Eosinophils are also few in number.

The most important sign is the presence of some or many Lutzner cells in marginal sinuses, in subsinusoidal regions of the cortex, and in T-nodules. In M.F. the latter appear to contain fewer reticulum cells and a greater number of mitotic figures than they do in nonneoplastic dermatopathic lymphadenitis.

*4. The Anaplastic Late Stages of Mycosis Fungoides.* The small-celled histologic picture may persist until death. We saw this picture in 22 out of 30 lymph-node biopsies and in five out of 14 lymph nodes removed at autopsy (see Table 26).

[189] Variakojis, Rosas-Uribe and Rappaport, 1974.

Table 26. Histologic types of M.F. infiltration in lymph nodes

| Histologic type | Biopsies | Autopsies |
|---|---|---|
| Small-celled | 22 | 5 |
| Intermediate or partially anaplastic | 3 | 4 |
| Anaplastic | 5 | 5 |
| Total | 30 | 14 |

On the other hand, in many patients the cells are larger from the very start, or become so as the disease progresses. Consequently, a variety of morphologic pictures can develop. We found anaplastic features in eight out of 30 lymph-node biopsies and in nine out of 14 lymph nodes at autopsy (Table 26). The great majority of the cells may be of medium size and moderately basophilic (Figs. 71 and 72). The round nuclei then contain three or four nucleoli (anaplastic Lutzner cells?). In such cases, the cytologic picture may be very heterogeneous, since there may be many eosinophils as well as some epithelioid cells. In addition, especially with this polymorphic picture, one can sometimes detect mononuclear and multinucleate giant cells that closely resemble Hodgkin and Sternberg-Reed cells. In some cases we found areas composed of relatively uniform-appearing, medium-sized cells between areas of small cells. The cytoplasm of the larger cells was moderately basophilic and their oval nuclei contained medium-sized nucleoli (T-associated plasma cells?). Finally, a picture like that of T-zone lymphoma (with large atypical lymphocytes) may be found.

Whereas the histologic features of M.F. with small-cell infiltrates are quite well characterized, the very varied morphology of the anaplastic late stages may mislead one into assuming that a transformation into another malignant lymphoma has occurred. This assumption is certainly unjustified. The situation here is like that of follicular lymphoma, in which the "sarcomatous" end stages can also present rather different pictures from those seen earlier in the disease.

In this context, we should mention the so-called *mycosis fungoides d'emblée*. We have had the opportunity to examine three lymph nodes from patients diagnosed clinically as having *M.F. d'emblée*. We shall not discuss this subject here, however, because it is necessary that modern cytologic techniques should be employed before we can be sure that the changes seen in this supposedly special form of M.F. actually belong in the spectrum of M.F. Such cytologic studies should be performed for the anaplastic late stages of M.F. to enable easier recognition of the various cell types in relation to their normal counterparts.

**Smear/Imprint**[190] **and Cytochemistry.** So far, we have had the opportunity of studying imprints of only four lymph nodes from patients with M.F. We found that the cytology of M.F. is more difficult to evaluate in imprints than it is in sections. In no instance were we able to classify all of the cells—and that is perhaps one of the most valuable criteria for the diagnosis of M.F.

[190] DEGOS, OSSIPOVSKI, CIVATTE and TOURAINE, 1957.

(a)

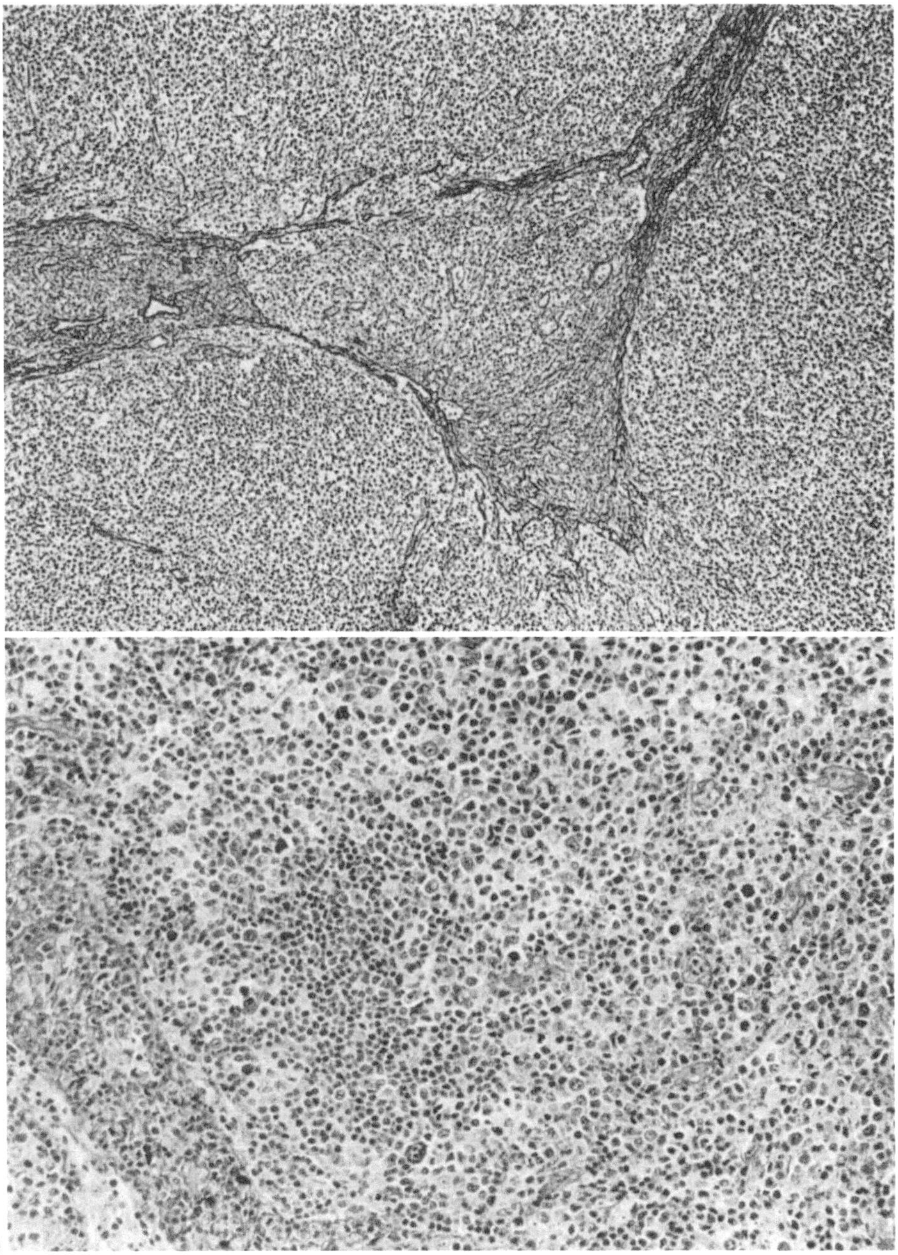

(b)

Fig. 71a and b. Mycosis fungoides, anaplastic stage. (a) A trabecula is infiltrated and destroyed. (b) Numerous anaplastic Lutzner cells of medium size, only some remnants of small lymphoid cells (small Lutzner cells?), and some large cells ("mycosis cells"). Same node as Fig. 70. (a) Gomori. ×70. (b) Giemsa. ×175

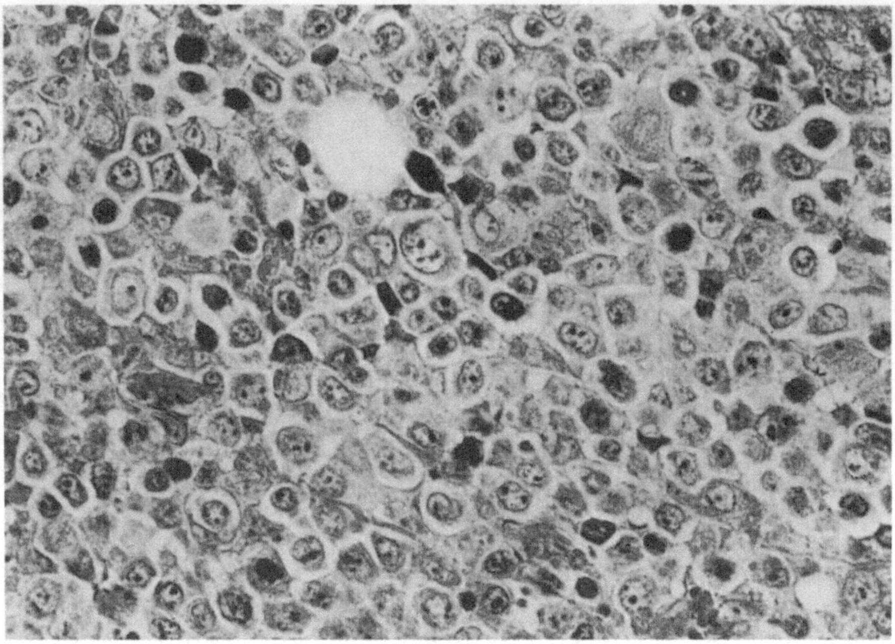

Fig. 72. Mycosis fungoides, sarcoma-like anaplastic end stage. Pure population of medium-sized or large cells (anaplastic Lutzner cells?). No small lymphoid cells. Many mitotic figures. ♂, 56 years. Skin biopsy. Giemsa. ×560

In the cases studied we found a population of cells that was chiefly lymphocytoid and pleomorphic, interspersed with large numbers of cells of moderate size. These cells had a grayish, rather wide rim of cytoplasm. The lymphocytoid cells often appeared quite large and resembled the larger Sézary cells, as will be described in the blood (p. 193). They were polymorphic and revealed three to five small to medium-sized acid phosphatase-positive granules that were irregularly distributed in the cytoplasm. The neutral nonspecific esterase and PAS reactions were negative.

Among the lymphocytoid cells there were large round cells with single nuclei and a very narrow rim of cytoplasm. Other large mononuclear cells had irregular convoluted nuclei. In addition, we saw a few basophilic cells of medium or large size that contained several, usually pale, medium-sized or large nucleoli in their round or oval nuclei. Very occasionally, we detected binucleate giant cells with large, sharply outlined, basophilic nucleoli. We could not distinguish these cells from Sternberg-Reed giant cells.

Besides these lymphoid cells we also found many large reticulum cells with abundant gray-blue-staining cytoplasm. The nuclei were conspicuously polymorphic, sometimes cleaved. The cells tended to form giant nuclei, which then contained particularly large nucleoli. Now and then we could visualize numerous small vacuoles in their cytoplasm, also occasionally small, dark blue, spherical structures. That these cells were interdigitating reticulum cells was shown by cytochemistry. The cytoplasm of the reticulum cells showed a *faint*, diffusely

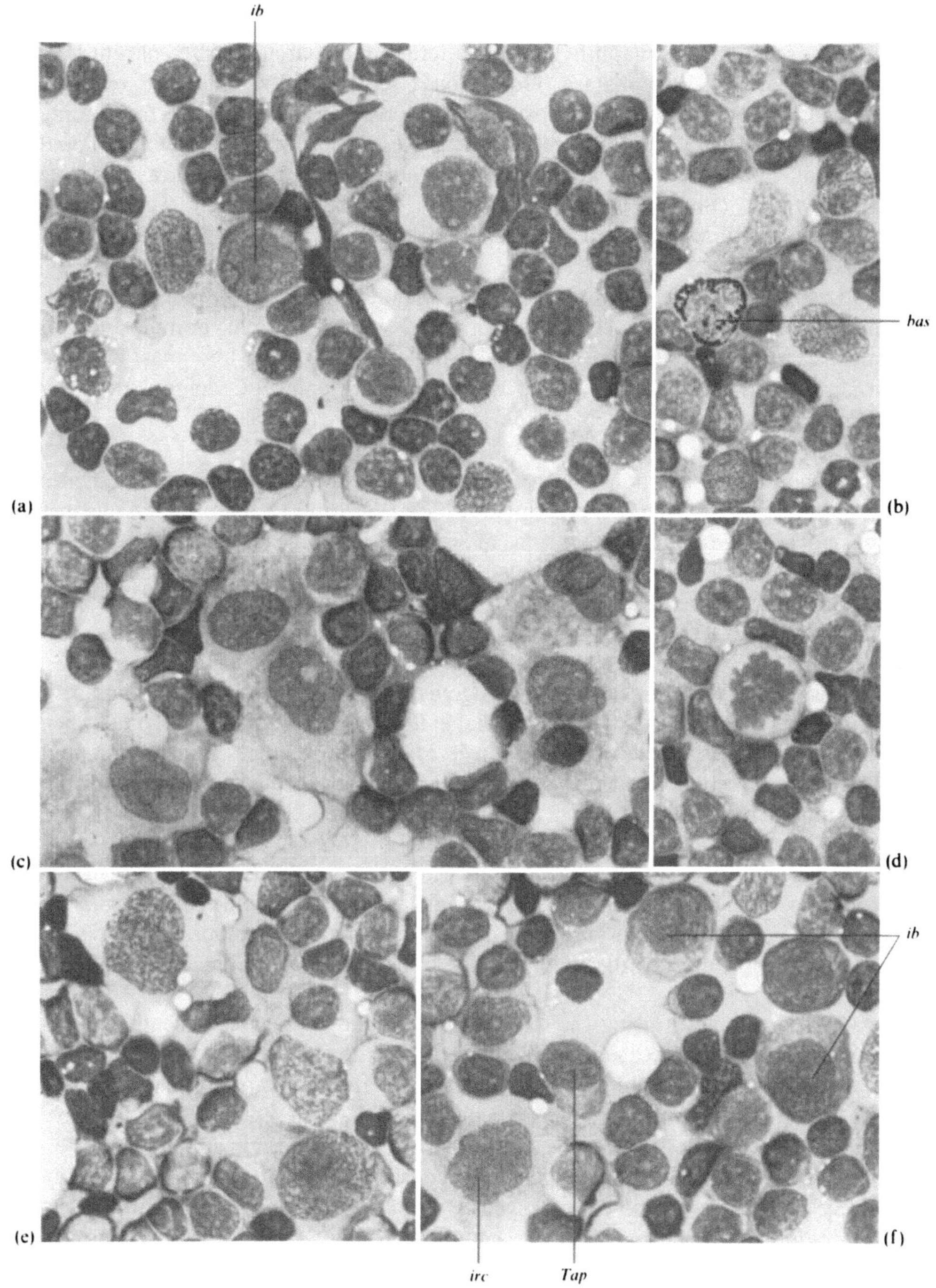


Fig. 73a–f. Mycosis fungoides in imprint. (a) Small lymphocytes, some medium-sized cells (partly vacuolated), one strongly basophilic cell (T-immunoblast? *ib*). To the left of this cell there is probably an interdigitating reticulum cell. (b) Basophil granulocyte (*bas*; blood basophil). At the upper right, an eosinophil granulocyte. (c) Five interdigitating reticulum cells. (d) Mitotic figure with plump chromosomes. (e) Two small giant cells, probably of type c described on p. 173 and illustrated in Fig. 70b and c. (f) Large blast cells (T-immunoblasts? *ib*). A medium-sized cell, probably T-associated plasma cell (*Tap*). A large interdigitating reticulum cell (*irc*). ♂, 59 years. Axillary node. Pappenheim. ×745

positive reaction for α-naphthyl acetate esterase and a circumscribed paranuclear reaction for acid phosphatase (Golgi body; see Fig. 23b). The PAS reaction, although weak, was diffusely positive; PAS-positive granules were found only occasionally. The vacuoles were PAS-negative and probably represented lipoid material. In addition, we encountered time and again strongly esterase-positive histiocytic reticulum cells with oval nuclei. Furthermore, there were macrophages, sometimes clustered together, that contained pigment and vacuoles of fat.

Lastly, we always saw more or less plentiful typical lymphocytes, a few plasma cells and plasma-cell precursors, and some neutrophil granulocytes. In most cases we found some eosinophils, blood basophils, and mast cells—a finding that perhaps corresponds with the increase in IgE demonstrated by STEIN in the tissue homogenate from such a case.

**Blood Picture.** In about 20% of the cases[191] of M.F. one finds that Lutzner cells have emigrated into the peripheral blood, leading to more or less distinct leukemic changes, but no other signs of Sézary's syndrome (see p. 193). In each of the cases described by VARIAKOJIS *et al.*[192] a leukemic blood picture was associated with involvement of the spleen. Lymphopenia often develops in advanced cases.

**Diagnosis.** The clinical picture, together with the histologic findings in a *skin* biopsy, may be sufficient to make the diagnosis of M.F. Thus, when the disease is suspected, one will inquire about skin changes and itching, and encourage thereby biopsy of the skin. An ample literature is available supplying a comprehensive discussion of the histology of the skin in M.F. The criteria offered by RAPPAPORT[193] have served us well:

1. The epidermis is often profoundly altered by acanthosis, keratosis, hyperkeratosis, elongation of rete pegs, spongiosis, and intraepidermal clusters of Lutzner cells. These clusters are often called Pautrier's abscesses, or better pseudoabscesses. In contrast, the epidermis in other types of malignant lymphoma is atrophic.

2. The cells infiltrating the cutis form bandlike aggregates beneath the epidermis and wander occasionally from there into the epidermis. In the infiltrative stages they are limited to the upper dermis, but in the tumor stage they invade the subcutis. In contrast, other types of malignant lymphoma usually leave a more or less wide space between upper cutis and epidermis uninvolved.

3. The infiltrates of M.F. generally consist chiefly of Lutzner cells. They always contain some so-called mycosis cells as well, and occasionally a few cells of moderate size that are at present unclassifiable. At times there is considerable infiltration by eosinophils and/or plasma cells.

4. M.F. of the skin tends to ulcerate, especially in the tumor stage. Other types of lymphoma rarely manifest this tendency.

The most important histologic characteristic of cutaneous M.F. is the so-

[191] CLENDENNING, BRECHER and VAN SCOTT, 1964; see also LANE and GREENWOOD, 1933.

[192] VARIAKOJIS, ROSAS-URIBE and RAPPAPORT, 1974.

[193] 1966.

called Pautrier's pseudoabscess. If we fail to find this lesion, we hesitate in diagnosing M.F. or Sézary's syndrome.

In lymph nodes, the typical (nonanaplastic) form of M.F. can be recognized primarily by means of the following characteristic features:

1. The infiltration begins from the marginal sinus on the one hand and in the paracortical area (T-nodules) on the other hand, and spreads from these sites to involve the whole lymph node. In many cases, however, there are remnants of preexistent lymphatic tissue, often showing signs of dermatopathic lymphadenitis and germinal centers. That is an important diagnostic criterion.[194]

2. The Lutzner cell is by far the most prevalent type of cell. It looks much like a lymphocyte. Its nucleus, however, is generally larger and paler than that of typical lymphocytes, which at times still persist in the remnants of uninvolved lymphatic tissue.

3. Among this relatively monotonous proliferation of Lutzner cells, there are *always* occasional cells with a large nucleus, or rarely with several nuclei. Some of these are so-called mycosis cells.

4. There is usually an increase in epithelioid venules and reticulin fibers.

Without clinical information and skin biopsy material, the anaplastic variants of M.F. are difficult to diagnose in a lymph node. The most important characteristic is the fact that the cytology cannot be accommodated in any of the usual pigeonholes of lymphoma classification.

If one is in doubt whether a lymph node is involved by M.F., cytogenetic study of the lymph-node cells may prove useful. In lymph nodes involved by M.F., ERKMAN-BALIS and RAPPAPORT[195] found five cases with 47 chromosomes and one case with 50 chromosomes per cell. In addition, in one lymph node out of three involved by dermatopathic lymphadenitis numerous cells revealed abnormal karyotypes. This means that the proliferating cells were probably malignant. Thus, only by chromosome analysis can such lymph nodes, which do not appear to be suspicious in histologic sections, be recognized as containing abnormal cells that establish the diagnosis of M.F.

In contrast, an electron-microscopic analysis proves helpful only when clusters or sheets of Lutzner cells are present. Occasionally, Lutzner cells can also be found in reactive hyperplasia of lymph nodes.[196]

**Differential Diagnosis.** The lymphomas that particularly need to be considered in the differential diagnosis of M.F. are CLL, hairy-cell leukemia, M.L. centrocytic, and LP immunocytoma. Differentiating these from M.F. will, in general, pose no problems, particularly if one takes advantage of histopathologic studies of the skin. Two diseases, however, may cause great difficulty in the differential diagnosis, since both are accompanied by itching of the skin and often by cutaneous lesions. These are Hodgkin's disease and what we refer to as lymphogranulomatosis X.

*Hodgkin's disease* of the mixed type may prove difficult to distinguish from an anaplastic type of M.F., if this consists primarily of large cells, some of which may resemble Sternberg-Reed cells. Since abundant infiltrates of eosinophils

[194] RAPPAPORT and THOMAS, 1974.
[195] 1970, 1974.
[196] ROSAS-URIBE, VARIAKOJIS, MOLNAR and RAPPAPORT, 1974.

can also occur in such cases, the diagnosis may become exceptionally difficult. What is important is to focus one's attention on the main type of cell; that is, on the Lutzner cells already described as lymphocyte-like cells that are difficult to identify histologically. They apparently differ in their morphology from the lymphoid cells of Hodgkin's disease. In any event, histologic study of the skin is indicated and usually helps in arriving at a definitive diagnosis.

Hodgkin's disease with lymphocytic predominance may also be somewhat similar to M.F., especially in early stages of development. The essential distinguishing feature of M.F. in this differential diagnosis is the existence of itching skin lesions, which do not occur in Hodgkin's disease with lymphocytic predominance.

*Lymphogranulomatosis X*[197] is equivalent, at least in many cases, to *immunoblastic lymphadenopathy*[198] or *angioimmunoblastic lymphadenopathy.*[199] It is in general clinically characterized by fever, pruritus, exanthematous lesions of the skin, blood eosinophilia, generalized lymphadenopathy, and hepatosplenomegaly. Hypersensitivity to drugs is sometimes found. Histologically, the basic structure of the lymph node appears to be destroyed. The most prominent feature is a conspicuous increase in epithelioid venules throughout the lymph node and also in the lymph-node capsule and in other organs (e.g., bone marrow or skin). The endothelial cells of the venules are surrounded by PAS-positive, basement membrane-like deposits. Between the vessels we always find immunoblasts, plasmablasts, and plasma cells, and in most cases a variable number of eosinophils and mast cells. About half of our cases showed clusters of epithelioid cells and diffuse infiltration by "activated lymphocytes." PAS-positive deposits have been described among the cells.[198] Germinal centers are absent or show regressive transformation. Necrosis occurs occasionally. Based on this histologic description, M.F. can be ruled out in most cases. The essential feature of lymphogranulomatosis X, i.e., the striking increase in PAS-positive epithelioid venules in the lymph-node parenchyma and capsule, is not found to such a degree in M.F.

**Development into a High-Grade Malignant Lymphoma.** Whereas the cytologic picture of M.F. usually tends to become more heterogeneous and its cells larger (clinically "tumor-forming") the longer the disease lasts, it can also develop into a high-grade malignant lymphoma of more uniform, medium-sized or large cells. First, there is a tumor consisting of *medium-sized* moderately basophilic cells, which may best be interpreted as anaplastic Lutzner cells (see Fig. 72). In addition to this, there were, in our material, three distinct types of *large-celled* high-grade malignant tumors that developed in patients with M.F.: (1) a tumor consisting of strongly basophilic cells resembling immunoblasts – M.L. immunoblastic, T-type (Fig. 74), (2) a tumor of moderately basophilic cells with abundant cytoplasm, often spindle-shaped, together with multinucleate giant cells (reticulum cells? fibroblasts? see Fig. 75), and (3) a tumor containing slightly basophilic

---

[197] Lennert, 1973c; Lennert and Mohri, 1974; Radaszkiewicz and Lennert, 1975.

[198] Lukes and Tindle, 1973, 1975.

[199] Frizzera, Moran and Rappaport, 1974; Rappaport and Moran, 1975.

(a)

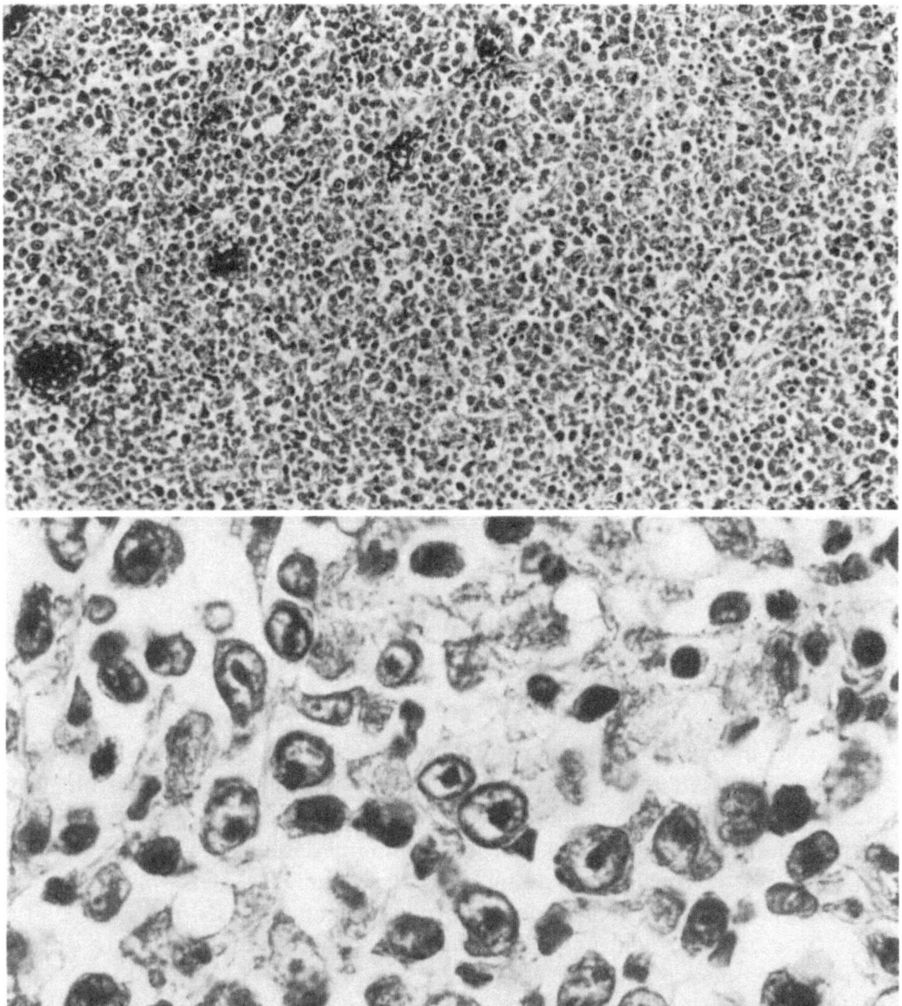

(b)

Fig. 74a and b. Immunoblastic lymphoma (immunoblastic sarcoma) following typical M.F. There is a uniform proliferation of large, strongly basophilic cells that are morphologically identical with immunoblasts. ♂, 75 years. Clinically, the patient had leukemia. Node removed at autopsy. Giemsa. (a) × 140, (b) × 875

cells with extremely polymorphic, contorted nuclei that were identical with interdigitating reticulum cells (see p. 485; Figs. 232 and 233).

We had the opportunity to study the case of immunoblastic lymphoma published by SCHWARZE and UDE[200] (Fig. 74). In brief, the tumor arose in a 75-year-old man afflicted for years with M.F., which ran a typical clinical course. The tumor consisted of large cells, and there were large numbers of

[200] 1975.

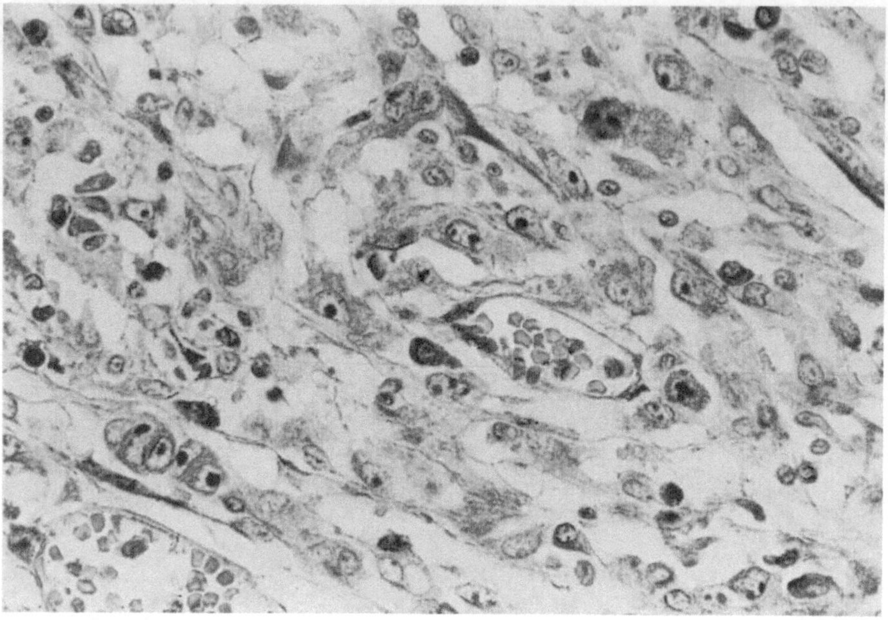

Fig. 75. Large-cell sarcoma supervening on M.F. Elongate polymorphic cells with multinucleate giant cells. Age and sex unknown. Inguinal node removed at autopsy. Giemsa. ×560

these cells in the blood. Terminally, the white blood cell count was 57,000/μl, 36% of which were atypical, large, strongly basophilic cells. Histologically, the tumor in the lymph nodes and other organs was composed entirely of large, intensely basophilic blast forms with moderately abundant cytoplasm and mostly oval nuclei containing very large nucleoli. These blast cells gave the same cytochemical reactions as normal T-immunoblasts in a PHA culture, namely, a granular acid phosphatase reaction and a weak, diffuse or granular nonspecific esterase reaction. The tumor is probably a T-immunoblastic malignant lymphoma with leukemic outpouring of immunoblasts into the blood.

**Combination with Other Diseases.** In one of our cases we found a noncaseating tubercle in a lymph node that otherwise showed the typical picture of M.F. The alleged transitions and combinations of M.F. with lymphosarcoma, reticulum-cell sarcoma, and Hodgkin's disease have not been proved.[201] The morphologic spectrum of M.F. is so broad, particularly in the late stages, that it sometimes gives the false impression that the M.F. has transformed into another type of malignant lymphoma.

**Prognosis.**[202] EPSTEIN *et al.*[203] and FUKS *et al.*[204] have recently published comprehensive reports reviewing the statistics on the prognosis of M.F. The

[201] E.g., BLOCK, EDGCOMB, EISEN and VAN SCOTT, 1963; CYR, GEOKAS and WORSLEY, 1966.
[202] BLOCK, EDGCOMB, EISEN and VAN SCOTT, 1963; EPSTEIN, LEVIN, CROFT and LUTZNER, 1972; FUKS, BAGSHAW and FARBER, 1973.
[203] EPSTEIN, LEVIN, CROFT and LUTZNER, 1972.
[204] FUKS, BAGSHAW and FARBER, 1973.

survival times fluctuate greatly from patient to patient. Death may result within the first year after the diagnosis is made, but it can also occur 20 to 30 years later. Finally, the successful cure of M.F., as occasionally reported, is certainly possible.

Patients under 50 years of age have the best prognosis, as do those without palpable lymph nodes and without tumorous skin lesions (with or without ulceration).[205] When ulcerated cutaneous tumors and enlargement of lymph nodes are present, 50% of the patients die within a year.[205] An extreme lymphopenia is also a bad omen.[206] Furthermore, the prognosis depends on the type of involvement of the skin. FUKS *et al.*[206] reported an 8-year survival (after the first therapy) for 85% of the patients with eczematous and limited plaques. The 8-year survival was 51% for those patients with generalized plaques, 39% for those with the erythematous form, and only 5% for those with the tumorous form of the disease. If death occurred, it was within the first 4 years after therapy had been discontinued.

FUKS *et al.*[206] found in their series of cases that the average time from the histologic diagnosis of M.F. of the skin to the development of generalized lymphoma was 31 months. When the cutaneous lesions were generalized plaques, the interval was somewhat longer (4 years). With cutaneous lesions of the erythematous type the interval was shorter (1 year). All patients showing involvement of lymph nodes and internal organs died, except for one. On average, the patients lived only 7.5 months after the diagnosis of extracutaneous involvement was made.

FUKS *et al.*[206] distinguished two groups of patients: those with and those without lymphadenopathy before therapy was started. Of a total of 54 patients 28 had lymphadenopathy. An actuarial analysis of this group showed only 39% with complete regression of skin lesions and relapse in all cases within 30 months. In contrast, patients without lymphadenopathy showed 80% initial complete regression. There was also a statistically significant difference in survival between those with and those without lymphadenopathy. The actuarial survival of patients with enlarged nodes at presentation was only 43%, in contrast with a figure of 67.6% for patients without lymphadenopathy at presentation, both figures relating to patients at risk 5–10 years after treatment. In the first group 36% developed extracutaneous dissemination, compared with only one patient (4%) in the second group.

About half of the deaths in M.F. are due to pneumonia and/or sepsis (especially from staphylococci).[205] In about a third of the patients death is a direct result of the malignant lymphoma (e.g., generalized lymphoma with cachexia, etc., lymphoma in the brain, heart, or lungs, etc.).

Unfortunately, the data presented here are not wholly satisfactory. Lymphadenopathy can have many meanings. The histologic type of M.F. has not yet been related to the clinical course. A systematic classification of M.F. into stages, as proposed by FUKS *et al.*, [206] and histologic types, in combination with lymphangiography,[207] should be made.

---

[205] EPSTEIN, LEVIN, CROFT and LUTZNER, 1972.
[206] FUKS, BAGSHAW and FARBER, 1973.
[207] FUKS, CASTELLINO, CARMEL, FARBER *et al.*, 1974.

## *Addendum*

### *Sézary's Syndrome, a Leukemic Variant of Mycosis Fungoides*

**Definition.** Sézary's syndrome[208] was described in 1938 by SÉZARY *et al.*,[209] in 1949 by SÉZARY, and in 1939 by BACCAREDDA as a distinct disease entity. It is characterized by generalized erythroderma with intense itching and a tendency to extreme pigmentation, by lymphadenopathy, and by a leukemic blood picture. Moderate splenomegaly often develops. In contrast to B-CLL, the leukemic cells of Sézary's syndrome do not infiltrate the bone marrow for a long time, and the marrow may remain free up until death. A so-called tumor stage, such as often appears in M.F., never develops in Sézary's syndrome. SÉZARY and many others interpreted the blood cells as reticular cells. Today we know that they are the lymphocytes with cerebriform nuclei previously described in M.F.[210] For this reason, and because the histology of the cutaneous changes of Sézary's syndrome is like that of M.F. (including Pautrier's pseudoabscesses), it seems probable that Sézary's syndrome is closely related to, if not fundamentally the same as mycosis fungoides.[211] Like LÖFFLER *et al.*,[212] we regard Sézary's syndrome as a leukemic variant of M.F. Classifying Sézary's syndrome with the reticuloses, as has been done in European literature[213] for decades, is now unjustifiable.

**Nature of Sézary's Syndrome.** If we regard Sézary's syndrome as a leukemic variant of M.F., we imply that it is *a priori* malignant. Some authors are of the opinion, however, that Sézary's syndrome is not in itself malignant. CLAUDY,[214] for example, felt he could not decide whether the Sézary cell is a tumor cell or the result of chronic immunologic stimulation. WINKELMANN[215] reported that among his 28 patients with Sézary's syndrome, a "lymphoma" developed in only four. He advised that low-intensity therapy should therefore be applied before a lymphoma appears. WINKELMANN's patients, however, failed to fulfill all three criteria of Sézary's syndrome. For example, he found lymphadenopathy in only 16 of his 28 patients, and in all 16 cases the lymph nodes merely showed dermatopathic lymphadenitis.

Large reviews [216] do touch on the question of the origin and nature of Sézary's syndrome, but discuss the subject cautiously. The question has not

[208] Review papers: TASWELL and WINKELMANN, 1961; FLEISCHMAJER and EISENBERG, 1964; HUHN, DOBBELSTEIN and ENGELHARDT, 1972; LÖFFLER, MEYHÖFER, LANGE, EHLERS *et al.*, 1974; see also Symposium on the Sézary Cell, Mayo Clinic Proceedings **49**, 499–592 (1974).

[209] SÉZARY and BOUVRAIN, 1938; SÉZARY, HOROWITZ and MASCHAS, 1938.

[210] LUTZNER and JORDAN, 1968; LUTZNER, HOBBS and HORVATH, 1971; GOMEZ ORBANEJA, SANCHEZ YUS, DIAZ-FLORES and SIMON HUARTE, 1972; HUHN, DOBBELSTEIN and ENGELHARDT, 1972; LUTZNER, EMERIT, DUREPAIRE, FLANDRIN *et al.*, 1973.

[211] LUTZNER, EMERIT, DUREPAIRE, FLANDRIN *et al.*, 1973; ZUCKER-FRANKLIN, MELTON III, and QUAGLIATA, 1974.

[212] LÖFFLER, MEYHÖFER, LANGE, EHLERS *et al.*, 1974.

[213] SÉZARY, 1949; MUSGER, 1954, 1956, 1966; DEGOS, OSSIPOVSKI, CIVATTE and TOURAINE, 1957; NEUHOLD and WOLFRAM, 1952; KNOTH, 1959; and others.

[214] 1974.

[215] 1974.

[216] EDELSON, LUTZNER, KIRKPATRICK, SHEVACH *et al.*, 1974; WINKELMANN, PERRY, MULLER, SCHROETER *et al.*, 1974.

yet been answered definitively. Cytogenetic studies should provide the final answer.

**Origin of the Sézary Cells.** Sézary cells[217] are nonphagocytic and do not transform into macrophages or adhere to glass.[218] Cytochemically, they resemble lymphocytes.[219] They can be stimulated with PHA in various amounts,[220] and a large[221] or small[222] number form spontaneous rosettes with sheep erythrocytes (sheep-E rosettes). That has also been observed on electron microscopy.[223] Occasionally, Sézary cells fail to form sheep-E rosettes and also lack the surface-marker characteristics of B-cells (such cells are called "null cells").[224] It has also been reported that Sézary cells form H rosettes (rosettes with homologous group-0 Rh-negative erythrocytes), which is a characteristic of a subgroup of T-lymphocytes.[225] In one case, BERARD[226] found that 90% of the lymphocytes formed sheep-E and EAC rosettes. Sézary cells cannot be stimulated with pokeweed mitogen.[227] The cells do not bear immunoglobulin[228] or complement[229] or IgG-Fc receptors.[223] Most cells are destroyed by specific anti-T-cell sera.[230] Sézary cells produce migration-inhibitory factors (MIF).[231]

The results of all these studies indicate that Sézary cells are T-derived lymphocytes.[233] This notion receives further support from our histologic observation that infiltration of the lymph node by Sézary cells occurs first in the T-cell region (Fig. 78a).[234]

In their review of 13 patients presenting the triad of exfoliative erythroderma, atypical circulating lymphocytes, and generalized lymphadenopathy, EDELSON *et al.*[235] reported on the electron-microscopic characteristics and immunologic markers of the lymphocytes circulating in the blood. In eight patients the cells were relatively large and had highly convoluted nuclei, like the cells described by SÉZARY. In four patients the lymphocytes were smaller and their nuclear irregularities less conspicuous. Such lymphocytes are regarded as the small cell variant of the Sézary cell. In one patient the cells had polar cytoplasmic

---

[217] Review: CLAUDY, 1974.

[218] LÖFFLER, 1972a.

[219] LÖFFLER, 1972a, b; ZUCKER-FRANKLIN, MELTON III and QUAGLIATA, 1974.

[220] LÖFFLER, 1972a, b; LUTZNER, EMERIT, DUREPAIRE, FLANDRIN *et al.*, 1973; ZUCKER-FRANKLIN, MELTON III and QUAGLIATA, 1974; BRAYLAN, VARIAKOJIS and YACHNIN, 1975.

[221] BROOME, ZUCKER-FRANKLIN, WEINER, BIANCO *et al.*, 1973; BROUET, FLANDRIN and SELIGMANN, 1973; MICHLMAYR, PATHOULI, FALKENSAMMER, HUBER *et al.*, 1976.

[222] BRAYLAN, VARIAKOJIS and YACHNIN, 1975.

[223] ZUCKER-FRANKLIN, MELTON III and QUAGLIATA, 1974.

[224] GOLDSTONE, CAWLEY, ROBERTS, LEVENTINE *et al.*, 1976.

[225] SHELDON and HOLBOROW, 1975.

[226] 1973, personal communication.

[227] CROSSEN, MELLOR, FINLEY, RAVICH *et al.*, 1971.

[228] PREUD'HOMME and SELIGMANN, 1972; BROOME, ZUCKER-FRANKLIN, WEINER, BIANCO *et al.*, 1973; BROUET, FLANDRIN and SELIGMANN, 1973.

[229] BROOME, ZUCKER-FRANKLIN, WEINER, BIANCO *et al.*, 1973.

[230] BROUET, FLANDRIN and SELIGMANN, 1973.

[231] YOSHIDA, EDELSON, COHEN and GREEN, 1975.

[233] BROOME, ZUCKER-FRANKLIN, WEINER, BIANCO *et al.*, 1973; LUTZNER, EMERIT, DUREPAIRE, FLANDRIN *et al.*, 1973; BROUET, PREUD'HOMME and SELIGMANN, 1975. Recently, BRODER, EDELSON, LUTZNER, NELSON *et al.* (1976) found evidence that the Sézary cells from a majority of patients originate from a subset of T-cells programmed exclusively for helper-like interactions with B-cells ("helper cells").

[234] LENNERT, 1974a.

[235] EDELSON, LUTZNER, KIRKPATRICK, SHEVACH *et al.*, 1974.

projections and nonindented nuclei (see p. 193). In addition to the customary involvement of the skin, the bone marrow of all patients revealed a remarkably modest infiltration. In contrast, the lymph nodes from 11 patients were heavily infiltrated, and in six patients other viscera were involved. In one of the six patients autopsied was there involvement of the thymus. The neoplastic cells in the blood and tissues exhibited properties typical of T-cells: they formed sheep-E rosettes and were killed by anti-T-serum. In the one case manifesting a somewhat different morphology, 40–68% of the counted cells formed mixed rosettes (E+EAC).

Cytogenetic and DNA studies of Sézary cells have been performed by CROSSEN *et al.*,[236] LUTZNER *et al.*,[237] BROUET *et al.*,[238] PRUNIERAS,[239] and BOSMAN and VAN VLOTEN.[240] In their investigations, LUTZNER *et al.*[237] distinguished two types of cells: (1) a larger cell with a serpentine and cerebriform nucleus, near-tetraploid DNA values, and near-tetraploid chromosome counts; (2) a smaller cell with an indented nucleus, diploid DNA values, and pseudodiploid or hyperdiploid chromosome counts. They also found that the neoplastic cells possessed A and B as well as Gq markers. A recent publication reports on measurements of the nuclear contour index of Sézary cells and compares the results with those made on cells of CLL.[241]

**Occurrence.** In our collection of lymphoma cases we examined eight lymph nodes from patients with Sézary's syndrome. All of the lymph nodes were totally overrun by the infiltrating Sézary cells.

In our material from routine biopsies the incidence is 0.26% of malignant lymphomas and 0.5% of non-Hodgkin's lymphomas, i.e., half the frequency in our series of M.F. lymph nodes (see Table 24).

According to the literature, the disease shows a peak frequency in the sixth decade.[242] In our material the peak incidence falls 10 years later (see Fig. 66), but the number of cases was too small to determine whether the difference was significant. The ratio of men to women is reported to be 1.8 to 1.[243]

**Localization.** As Table 25 indicates, cervical, axillary, inguinal, and cubital lymph nodes were submitted for examination. According to SÉZARY, the inguinal lymph nodes are the first to enlarge. From these the tumor cells apparently infiltrate the deeper iliac chain of nodes. Spread to the axillary and epitrochlear (cubital) lymph nodes soon follows. With the primary manifestations FLEISCHMAJER and EISENBERG[244] include not only the involvement of the axillary and inguinal lymph nodes, but that of the cervical lymph nodes as well.

[236] CROSSEN, MELLOR, FINLEY, RAVICH *et al.*, 1971.
[237] LUTZNER, EMERIT, DUREPAIRE, FLANDRIN *et al.*, 1973; see also FLANDRIN and BROUET, 1974.
[238] BROUET, FLANDRIN and SELIGMANN, 1973.
[239] 1974.
[240] 1975.
[241] LITOVITZ and LUTZNER, 1974.
[242] FLEISCHMAJER and EISENBERG, 1964.
[243] FLEISCHMAJER and EISENBERG, 1964; HUHN, DOBBELSTEIN and ENGELHARDT, 1972.
[244] 1964.

**Gross Appearance.** SÉZARY[245] described the lymph nodes of the inguinal region and axilla as enlarged and not adherent. According to WINKELMANN,[246] the lymph nodes are generally 1 – 3 cm in diameter, but exceptionally the nodes may be very large (6 – 10 cm). Nonetheless, he emphasized that the enlarged lymph nodes showed signs only of dermatopathic lymphadenitis.

**Histology.** In the literature concerned with Sézary's syndrome, histologic changes in lymph nodes are mostly confined to descriptions of nonspecific inflammatory changes and dermatopathic lymphadenitis.[247] We, however, have found dermatopathic lymphadenitis in many cases of erythroderma without detectable abnormalities in the blood picture, i.e., in cases that did not show the complete triad of Sézary's syndrome. Instead, in our cases clinically diagnosed as leukemia we always found in the lymph nodes a specific infiltration characterized primarily by its monomorphism and small-cell composition. In contrast, the diagnostic features pointing to a dermatopathic lymphadenitis were either rudimentary or lacking completely in our slides. This differs from typical M.F., in which we often found conspicuous remnants of a preceding dermatopathic lymphadenitis. In brief, the degree of lymph-node infiltration in Sézary's syndrome was considerable, and there was relative monomorphism with a lymphoid aspect (Figs. 76 and 77). There were relatively few large mononuclear and multinucleate cells exhibiting slight to strong basophilia (mycosis cells). Large numbers of epithelioid venules were always evident (Figs. 77 and 78b), filled with lymphocytes (predominantly Lutzner cells) in the process of emigration.

The obstruction of the sinuses, with dilatation and sclerosis, as described previously in M.F., was prominent in some cases of Sézary's syndrome (Fig. 79). In addition, the leukemic cells appeared to encroach upon the thickened capsule in a few cases, but only once infiltrated it. The afferent lymphatics and sinuses were often unusually conspicuous, since they were greatly dilated and stuffed with innumerable lymphocytes (Lutzner cells). Eosinophils were occasionally seen. The amount of fiber was generally large.

If we ask ourselves how the Lutzner cells get to the lymph nodes in Sézary's syndrome and in M.F., our histologic slides suggest that two routes are possible, namely, the lymphogenous and the hematogenous routes. The lymphocytic cells infiltrating the skin might reach the marginal sinus by way of the afferent lymphatics. On the other hand, they certainly invade the parenchyma of the lymph node in great numbers through the increased epithelioid venules, especially in the T-cell regions. In fact, the T-cell regions are at first the only site of infiltration (Fig. 78a), whereas the B-cell regions (follicles) initially remain intact. As the disease progresses, however, the B-cell regions are gradually destroyed by the T-cell proliferation.

**Smear/Imprint.** The cell pictures resemble in many respects those of M.F. They can be even more monotonously uniform, however, when the lymph nodes are more heavily infiltrated. The Lutzner cells are the predominant cell type.

[245] 1949.

[246] 1974.

[247] MARSHALL, 1956; TASWELL and WINKELMANN, 1961; FLEISCHMAJER and EISENBERG, 1964; RAPPAPORT, 1966.

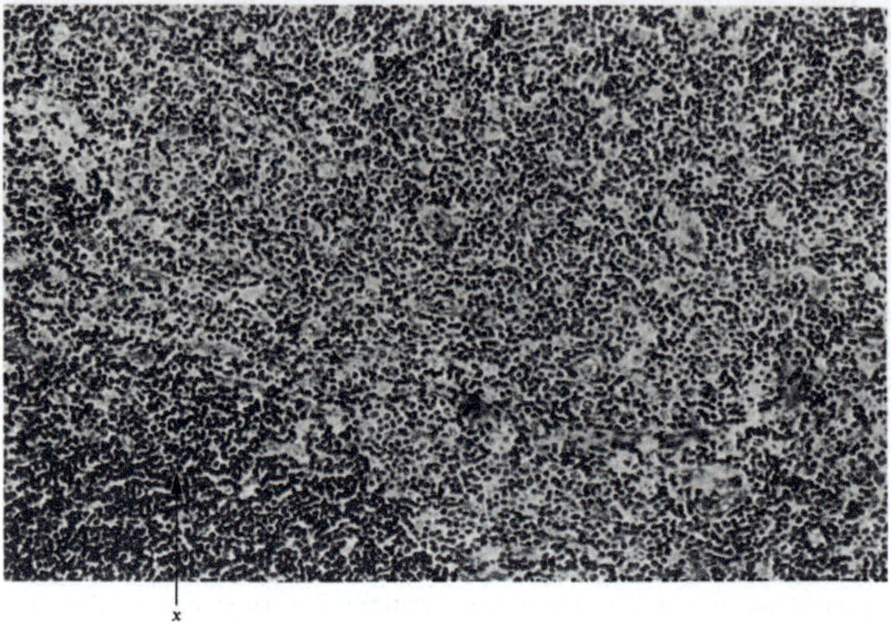


Fig. 76. Sézary's syndrome, first diagnosed 10 years earlier. At the lower left, remnant of noninfiltrated lymphatic tissue (*x*). Here the lymphocytes are smaller and they lie closer together than in the infiltrated area. ♀, 64 years. Supraclavicular node. Giemsa. ×140

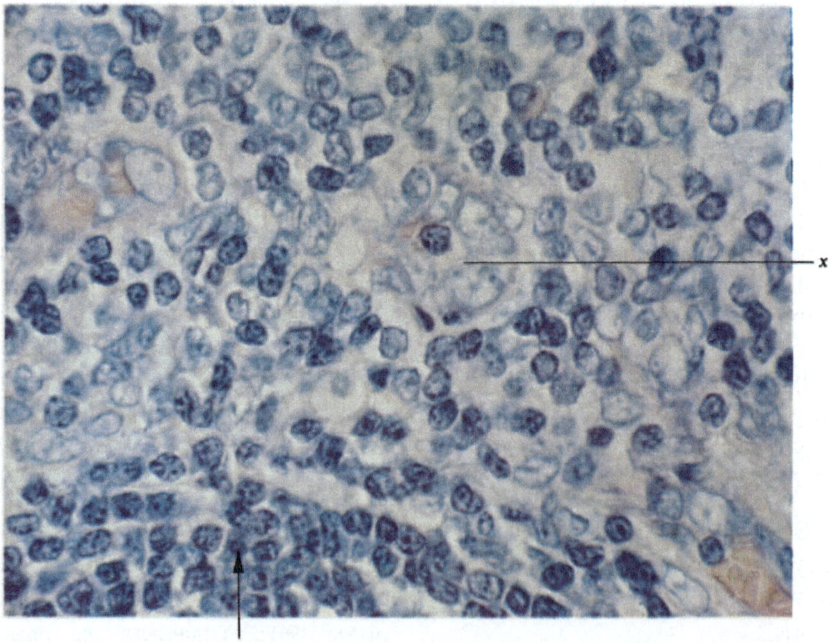


Fig. 77. Sézary's syndrome with Giemsa staining. The arrow points to residual lymphocytes. The lymphoid infiltration reveals marked pleomorphism of the nuclei. Epithelioid venule (*x*). Same node as Fig. 76. ×1,000

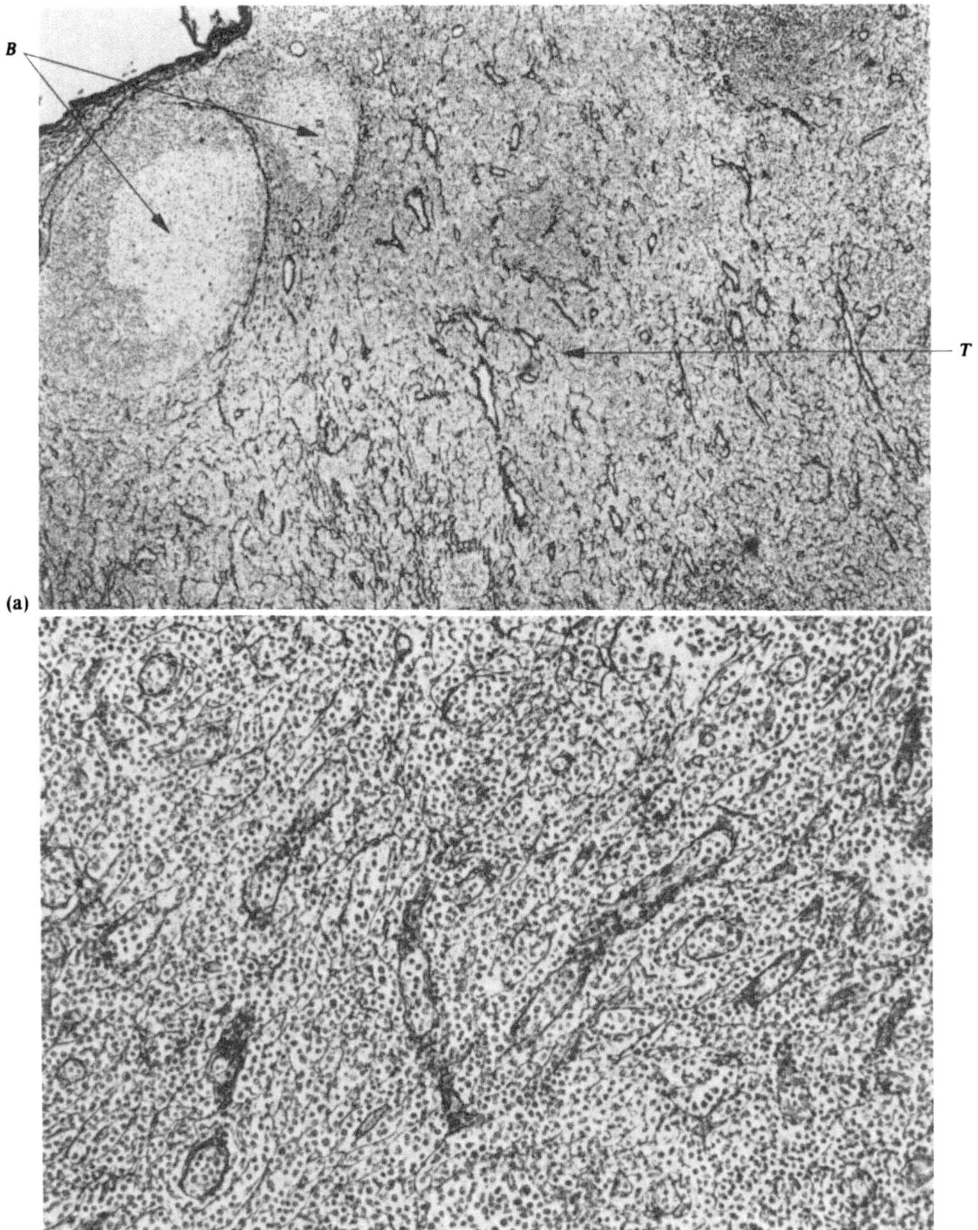


Fig. 78a and b. Sézary's syndrome. Infiltration of the expanded T-cell region (*T*) with many epithelioid venules and fibers. In the cortex there are remnants of lymph follicles with germinal centers (*B*). (a) ♀, 55 years. Inguinal node. Gomori, ×56. (b) ♀, 46 years. Axillary node. Gomori. ×140

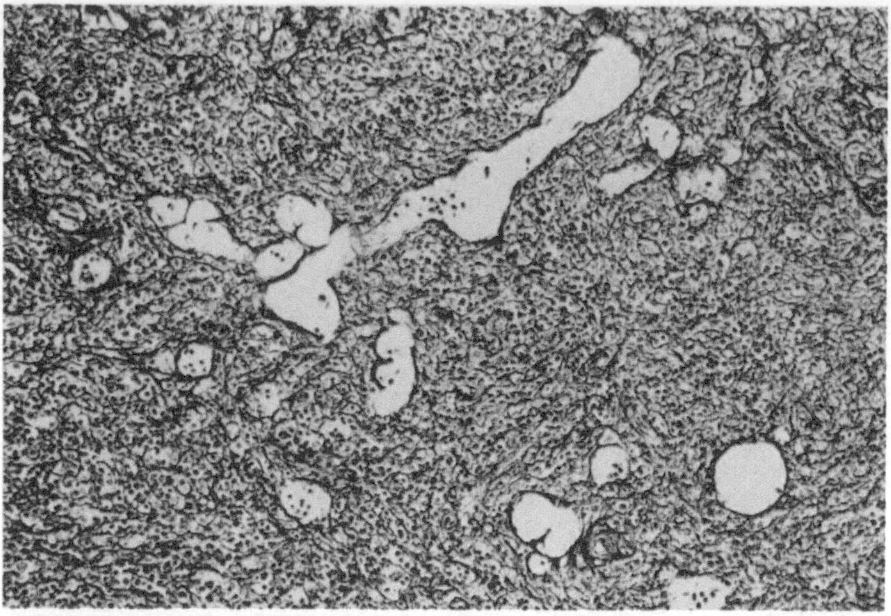

(a)

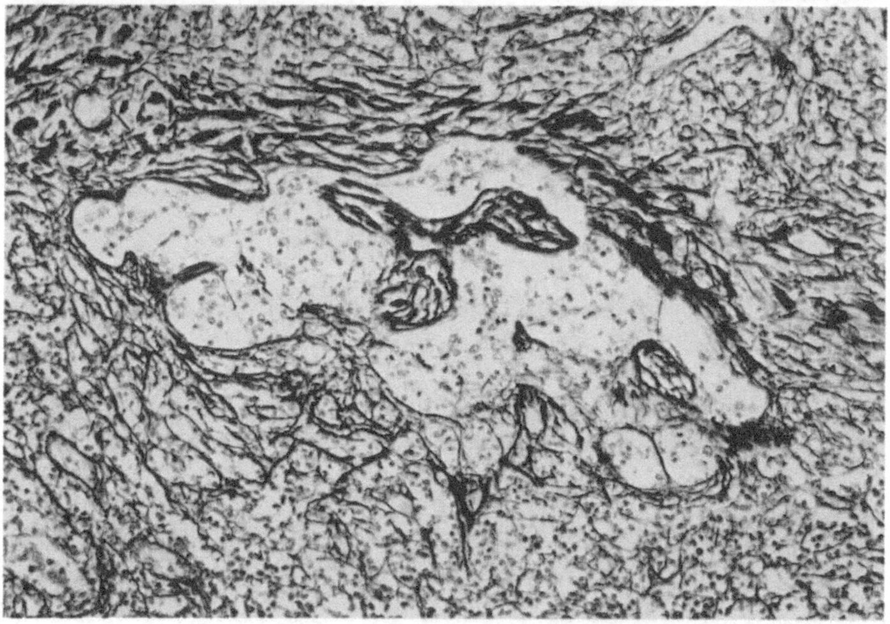

(b)

Fig. 79a and b. Sézary's syndrome. Sinus dilatation and sclerosis. (a) Same node as Fig. 78b. (b) ♂, 62 years. Axillary node. (a, b) Gomori. ×140

**Blood Picture.**[248] The increase in lymphocyte-like cells is one of the three cardinal signs of Sézary's syndrome. The white blood cell count can range from 8400–142,000/μl, but it usually remains within moderate limits.

[248] Hoagland, 1974; Flandrin and Brouet, 1974; Löffler, 1972a, b.

(a) (b) (c)

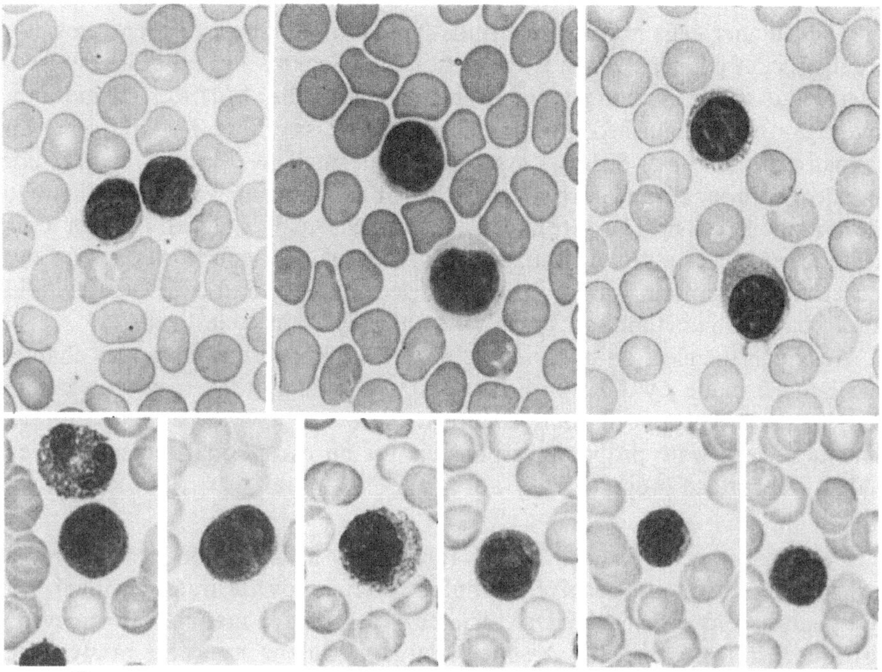

(d) (e) (f) (g) (h) (i)

Fig. 80a–i. Sézary cells in blood smear. Note the convoluted nuclei in (a), (f), (g), (h), and (i). Other nuclei are slightly indented, round, or oval. In (e) the nucleus is subdivided into two parts. In (c) the Sézary cells are vacuolated. (a, b) ♀, 69 years. (c) ♀, 55 years. (d–i) ♀, 64 years. (a–i) Pappenheim. ×825

In smears the Lutzner cells are generally somewhat larger than small lymphocytes (Fig. 80). In proportion to the width of their rim of cytoplasm, their nuclei seem too large. The nuclei mostly appear round (for technical and other reasons). In some cells, however, the nuclei have "a swirled chromatin pattern that has a notched, folded, or cleft-like appearance, being at times compared to the convolutions seen on the surface of the human brain."[249] The nuclei are therefore also described as cerebriform. This special nuclear configuration is sometimes easily recognizable, sometimes hardly visible in Pappenheim smears. It is then advisable to apply the acid phosphatase reaction, which reveals the nuclear contours better. The most characteristic finding is that the "sulci" on the surface of the cerebriform nuclei appear as diagonal lines across the nucleus, either centrally or peripherally. The chromatin may appear to be either fine or coarse like that of lymphocytes. The nucleoli are small to medium-sized and clear. In Pappenheim staining they generally cannot be recognized. They are much better visualized in PAS-stained slides. The cytoplasm is gray-blue and may be vacuolated. The vacuoles apparently contain glycogen, as revealed

[249] HOAGLAND, 1974.

in PAS-stained slides. Then, the cytoplasm has "a beading appearance that surrounds the nucleus."[250]

The Lutzner cells may be small like lymphocytes. Some of them, however, are significantly larger, which is the reason why SÉZARY and other investigators referred to them as monocytoid or histiocytoid cells. EDELSON[251] and other investigators distinguished a large-cell variant (classic Sézary's syndrome) and a small-cell variant of Sézary's syndrome. The small-cell variants in our series revealed both small and larger cells (the latter made up about one tenth of the lymphoid cells). The larger cells resembled small Lutzner cells in every detail except size (tetraploid Lutzner cells?). Some of them, however, had oval nuclei, fine chromatin, solitary medium-sized nucleoli, and a moderately wide rim of basophilic cytoplasm. These we would regard as "blast cells."

Although the electron-microscopic results are not discussed in this chapter, one remark made by ZUCKER-FRANKLIN[252] should not be overlooked here: lymphocytoid plasma cells were found in the blood of two patients. She said that these cells were probably responsible for an exceptional increase in cells with B-cell surface properties.

**Cytochemistry.**[253] The small and large Sézary cells in blood smears reveal a slight, but distinctly positive, granular reaction for (tartrate-sensitive) acid phosphatase and $\beta$-glucuronidase. The enzyme-positive granules are unevenly distributed in the cytoplasm. A solitary large granule is seen only rarely. Electron-microscopic studies[254] have confirmed the positive reaction for acid phosphatase. The reaction for neutral nonspecific esterase is negative or weakly positive and granular, not diffusely positive as it is in monocytes. The PAS reaction, positive in a variable proportion of the cells, appears as a granular deposit, which may probably be looked upon as glycogen according to the electron-microscopic findings of LUTZNER and JORDAN.[255] This view receives support from CLENDENNING *et al.*,[256] who reported that the PAS-positive granules are sensitive to diastase. Both the chloroacetate esterase and peroxidase reactions are negative.

**Diagnosis.** The diagnosis of Sézary's syndrome (Table 27) is based on the clinical triad of erythroderma, lymphocytosis of the blood, and enlargement of lymph nodes. Histologically, most of the neoplastic cells resemble normal lymphocytes and display marked uniformity. Under high magnification they can usually be differentiated from normal lymphocytes, particularly by their irregular nuclei. Epithelioid venules and reticulin fibers are always increased in number.

In every case one should ask for a skin biopsy,[257] in which bandlike infiltrates

[250] HOAGLAND, 1974.
[251] 1976.
[252] 1974.
[253] TASWELL and WINKELMANN, 1961; HUHN, DOBBELSTEIN and ENGELHARDT, 1972; LÖFFLER, 1972a, b; FLANDRIN and BROUET, 1974.
[254] HUHN and STICH, 1969.
[255] 1968.
[256] CLENDENNING, BRECHER and VAN SCOTT, 1964.
[257] HOLDAWAY and WINKELMANN, 1974.

Table 27. Diagnostic criteria of Sézary's syndrome

1. Patients middle-aged and older
2. In all cases pruritic skin lesions (erythroderma)
3. In all cases increase in small or large lymphocytoid cells in the blood
4. Bone marrow usually free of infiltration
5. Lymph nodes reveal
   a) increase in polymorphic lymphocytes (Lutzner cells), first in T-region
   b) a few large mono- and multinuclear, slightly to strongly basophilic cells (mycosis cells)
   c) in occasional cases eosinophils
   d) increase in fibers and venules
   e) in some cases increase in interdigitating reticulum cells (remnants of dermatopathic lymphadenitis)

of Lutzner cells in the upper dermis and frequent Pautrier's pseudoabscesses are found.

Finally, study of a blood smear enables the experienced investigator to make a quick diagnosis, particularly when he takes advantage of cytochemical reactions (PAS and acid phosphatase with and without tartrate inhibition).

**Differential Diagnosis.** Diseases that may resemble Sézary's syndrome and from which it must be differentiated are CLL, hairy-cell leukemia, centrocytic lymphoma, LP immunocytoma, and small-cell lymphoblastic lymphoma including ALL. Since the histology of the cutaneous involvement and the blood smear make a precise diagnosis of Sézary's syndrome possible, we may dispense with a lengthy discourse about the differential diagnosis.

**Development into a High-Grade Malignant Lymphoma.** We have not observed such a development in our cases. Of the patients studied by WINKELMANN,[258] however, four developed a malignant "lymphoma" during the course of the Sézary syndrome. The tumors were classified as "reticulum-cell sarcoma," Hodgkin's disease, myelomonocytic leukemia, and lymphosarcoma. We do not know whether they should be interpreted as further development of Sézary's syndrome or as independent neoplasms.

**Combination with Other Diseases.** WINKELMANN[258] reported on a patient who had a nodular lymphocytic gastric "mass" 3 years before developing Sézary's syndrome. A second patient had a mass in the temporal region 11 years before Sézary's syndrome appeared. A "benign lymphocytosis" of the skin associated with a parapsoriasis of many years' standing finally changed into mycosis fungoides. Two patients presented with sarcoid-like granulomata, which in one case involved the lymph nodes as well. According to WINKELMANN,[258] these granulomata appear more commonly after therapy of Sézary's syndrome. Among our collection of cases we have no instances of Sézary's syndrome combined with other diseases.

---

[258] 1974.

**Prognosis.** FLEISCHMAJER and EISENBERG[259] report patients surviving from 6 months to 16 years. HUHN *et al.*[260] regard thc prognosis as somewhat more favorable than with M.F.

### *5. Malignant Lymphoma, Lymphocytic, T-Zone Type (T-Zone Lymphoma)**

**History, Definition.** Follicular lymphoma has been known for a long time as an organoid lymph-node tumor that reveals follicles as the chief proliferating element. Between the follicles, however, there are more or less developed T-zones that seem to be essential parts of the tumor. The T-zone counterpart of follicular lymphoma is the tumor that we call M.L. lymphocytic, T-zone type or, for short, T-zone lymphoma. In this tumor, the T-zones show neoplastic proliferation, while nonneoplastic lymph follicles or follicle remnants can often be found in between. Like follicular lymphoma, which is composed of all of the elements of the follicles (centroblasts, centrocytes, dendritic and histiocytic reticulum cells), T-zone lymphoma shows the essential components of the T-region, i.e., T-lymphocytes, at times with T-associated plasma cells,interdigitating reticulum cells, epithelioid venules, and fairly abundant reticulin fibers. Thus whereas the essential neoplastic element in follicular lymphoma is the B-cell region, in T-zone lymphoma it is the T-area. Both tumors may be considered to be relatively well-differentiated lymphomas, since they each contain the two essential basic structures of the lymph node, namely, the B- and T-regions, side by side.

We first presented T-zone lymphoma for discussion during a lymph-node seminar at the 10th International Congress of the International Academy of Pathology in Hamburg in September, 1974. We then demonstrated it in London in August, 1975, at the 3rd Meeting of the European and African Division of the International Society of Haematology, and in Bad Nauheim in September, 1975,[261] at the Congress of the German and Austrian Society of Hematology.[262]

**Origin of the Neoplastic Cells.** The development of the tumor in the T-cell region leads one to expect that it is derived from T-lymphocytes. In fact, in three of our cases it could be shown that practically all of the tumor cells formed sheep-E rosettes (Fig. 81), but no EAC or mixed rosettes. The IgM content of the tumor homogenate also ranged from normal to extremely reduced. Thus, this is no doubt a malignant lymphoma of T-lymphocytes (Fig. 82).

* In collaboration with R. SATODATE and D. HELBRON.

259 1964.

260 HUHN, DOBBELSTEIN and ENGELHARDT, 1972.

261 LENNERT, 1976.

262 Recently, after we had finished writing this monograph, COLLINS told us about a malignant lymphoma that appeared to be related to the T-zone lymphoma of our classification. It was described by WALDRON, LEECH, GLICK, FLEXNER *et al.* (in press) as a malignant lymphoma of peripheral T-lymphocyte origin.

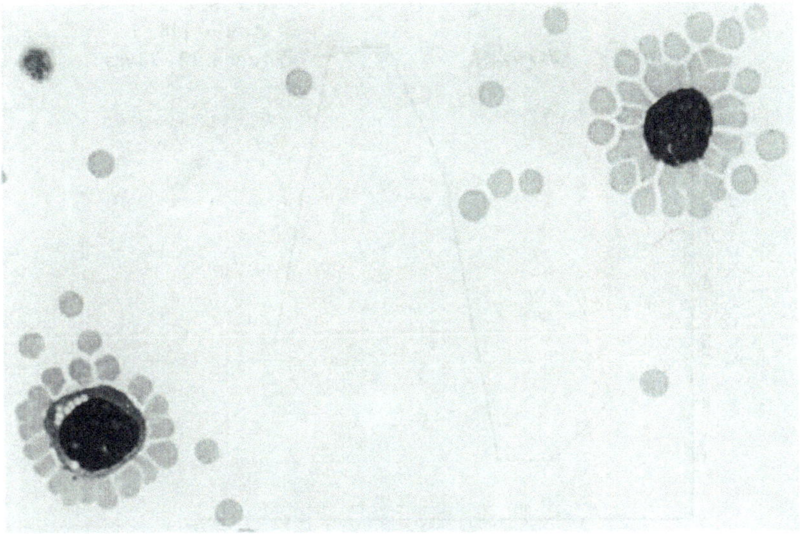

Fig. 81. T-zone lymphoma. Lymphoid cells forming sheep-E rosettes. Note the vacuoles in the cytoplasm of the cell at lower left. ♂, 56 years. Cell suspension. Pappenheim. ×875

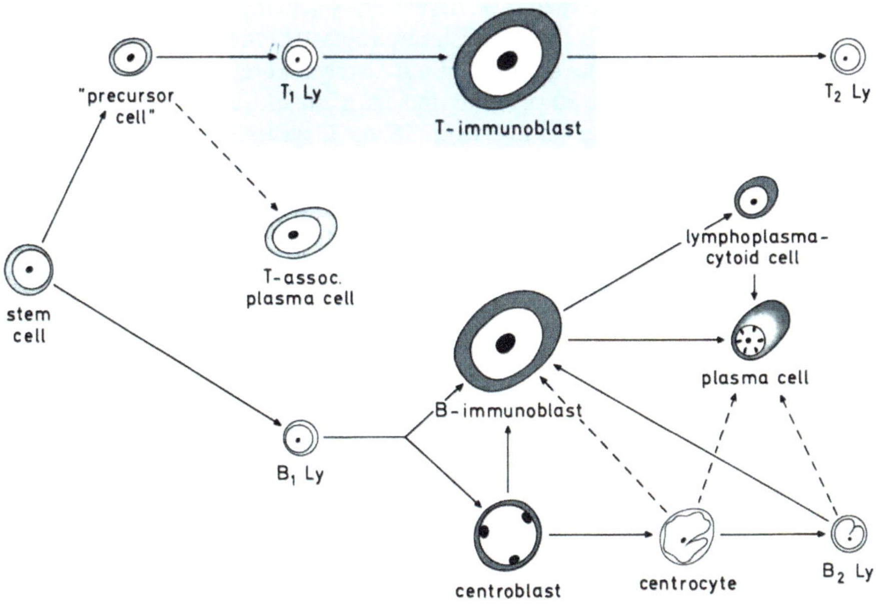


Fig. 82. Hypothetical origin of tumor cells of T-zone lymphoma. This scheme provides only a rough orientation. It merely indicates that the tumor cells are T-lymphocytes and related blast cells ("T-immunoblasts"), and occasionally T-associated plasma cells

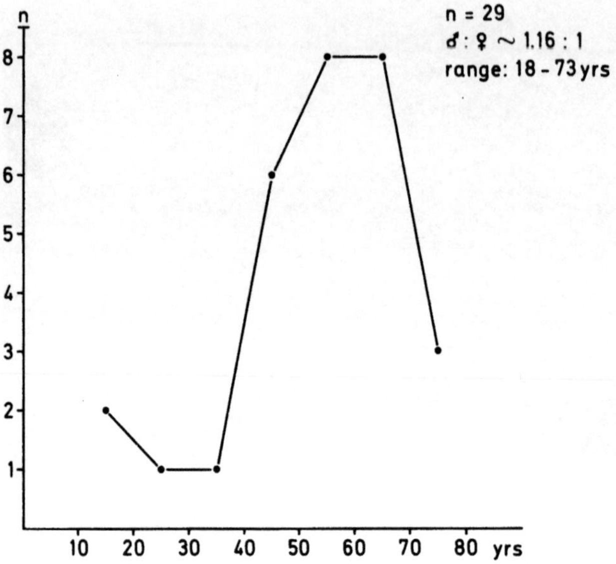


Fig. 83. Age distribution and sex ratio of T-zone lymphoma (29 patients)

**Occurrence.** Between January 1, 1974, and July 1, 1976, we observed 25 cases of T-zone lymphoma, i.e., 1.1% of a total of 2273 non-Hodgkin's lymphomas. In addition, we found four cases in a series of 400 non-Hodgkin's lymphomas from VAN UNNIK, giving an incidence of 1%. The true incidence must be somewhat higher than 1%, however, since there are probably cases misdiagnosed as Hodgkin's disease or immunoblastic lymphadenopathy.[263]

Fourteen of the patients were male and twelve were female (Fig. 83). The sex was not given in three cases. This means a male-to-female ratio of about 1.16:1. The patients ranged in age from 18 to 73 years. Most of the patients were between the ages of 40 and 70 years.

**Clinical Manifestations.** The available data are still meager. The following findings are worth mentioning. Sixteen out of 28 patients had general symptoms (unexplained fever, weakness, weight loss). Lymphadenopathy often developed quickly (within 0.5—3 months). It usually progressed rapidly, in some cases with symptoms of lymphatic obstruction. At the time of lymph-node biopsy, six patients were in stage I, six in stage II, 15 in stage III, and five in stage IV. Enlargement of mediastinal lymph nodes was reported in 11 out of 32 patients. Only 15 out of 30 patients were said to have splenomegaly or hepatomegaly. One patient, however, later had a greatly enlarged spleen and severe Coombs-positive hemolytic anemia. In the spleen removed from this patient, we found both lymphoma infiltrates in the T-region and remnants of follicles (B-cells), as well as extremely active erythropoiesis and massive infiltration of the red pulp by eosinophils. Of 32 patients, eight presented with tumor infiltrates in the tonsils;

[263] We have examined another eight cases of T-zone lymphoma since the writing of this monograph. The only data that could be included here were those on clinical manifestations, localization, and survival.

four, with infiltrates in the lungs and pleura; and two, with enlargement of the parotid gland. The bone marrow was free of lymphatic infiltration in 18 out of 24 cases studied. In seven cases, however, it showed marked eosinophilia. Atypical lymphocytes were seen in the blood of nine patients. Excessive eosinophilia of 44% was found in one patient with a leukocyte count of 17,000/μl; 4–8% eosinophils were demonstrated in four, and more than 8% eosinophils in five out of 25 patients. Marked lymphopenia was seen in seven out of 24 patients. There was a polyclonal increase in immunoglobulin in the blood of six out of 15 patients (IgA once, IgM twice, IgG twice, and IgG and IgA once). Three patients showed a decrease in serum Ig. The $\alpha_2$-globulin level was increased in 14 out of 24 patients. The erythrocyte sedimentation rate of 25 patients was normal (six patients), moderately elevated (11 patients), or highly elevated (eight patients).

**Localization.** All of the lymph nodes we studied were peripheral (22 cervical, seven axillary, and five inguinal). We also examined one biopsy from the nasopharynx and one from the tonsil.

**Gross Appearance.** The lymph nodes are moderately to greatly enlarged. They are variable in consistency. The cut surface is uniformly gray-white.

**Histology.** Even at a low magnification, two essential changes can often be perceived. (1) One sees sparse or abundant follicles or follicle remnants, which stand out as dark blue in Giemsa-stained slides and which are also particularly

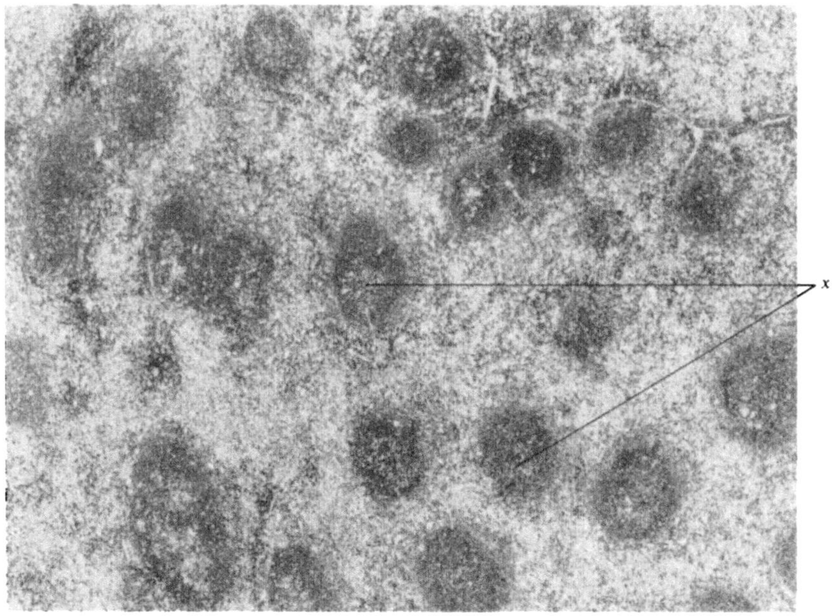


Fig. 84. T-zone lymphoma at a low magnification. The follicles (*x*) are not neoplastic, but simulate a follicular lymphoma. Actually, the interfollicular areas (T-zones) are neoplastic (light). ♂, 68 years. Submandibular node. Giemsa. ×14

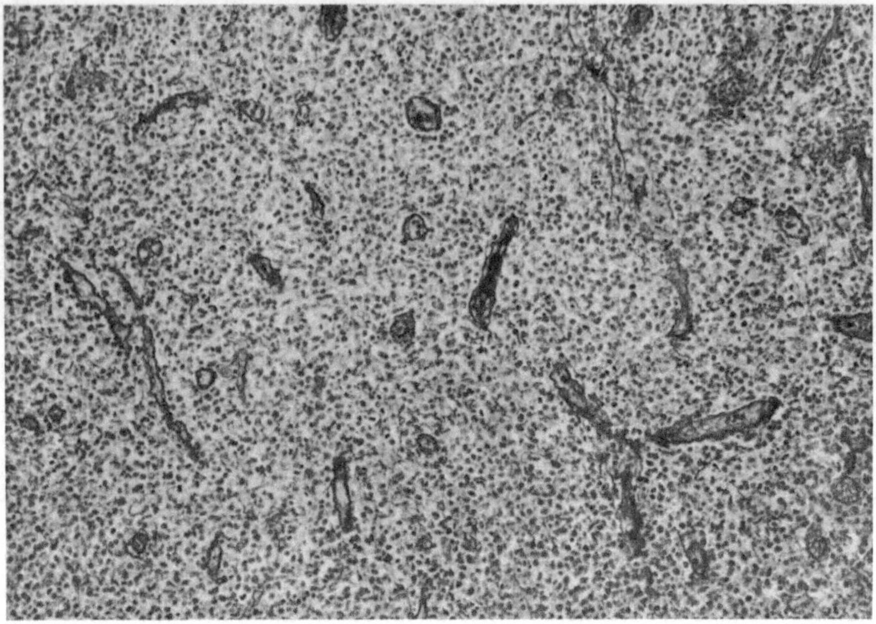

Fig. 85. T-zone lymphoma. Numerous epithelioid venules. ♂, 48 years. Cervical node. PAS. ×56

well shown by silver staining (Fig. 84, see also Fig. 91). Sometimes this pattern is evident even when the Giemsa-stained slide is held against the light and viewed with the naked eye: the follicles look like blue islands in a sea of gray. (2) There is a great increase in venules in the interfollicular tissue (Fig. 85). This can be observed equally well in Giemsa-stained slides, in the PAS reaction, and with silver stains.

The lymph-node architecture is destroyed. There is a somewhat polymorphic, but on the whole relatively monotonous-seeming cell proliferation. The cells show frequent to very frequent mitotic figures.

The proliferating cells include three types:

1. T-lymphocytes.
2. Large blast cells, occasionally with giant cells.
3. T-associated plasma cells.

1. Neoplastic lymphocytes—T-lymphocytes according to results of marker studies—usually predominate (Figs. 86 and 87). They are always larger than normal lymphocytes; they can be twice as large as lymphocytes or even larger. The nuclei appear somewhat convoluted. As a rule, the cytoplasm cannot be clearly defined in Giemsa-stained slides. The chromatin is coarse and consists of several medium-thick to thick clumps. Among these clumps there are also one or two medium-sized nucleoli, which can be hardly recognized in sections but may be clearly identified in smears. The pleomorphism of the T-lymphocytes is considerable. Giant nuclei with the same nuclear structure and with a markedly irregular (convoluted) contour are occasionally seen.

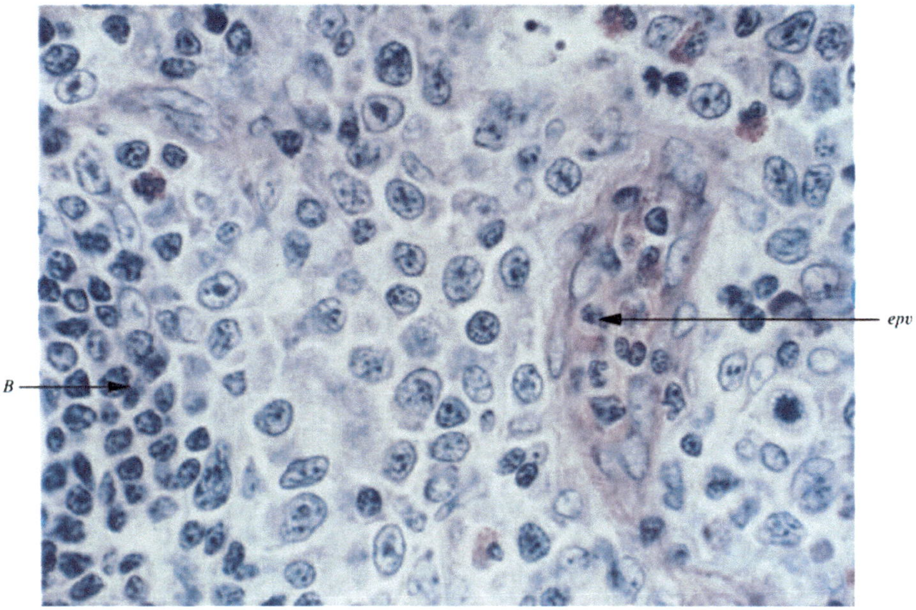


Fig. 86. T-zone lymphoma with Giemsa staining. Polymorphic medium-sized lymphocytes and a few blast cells and eosinophils around an epithelioid venule (*epv*). On the left, the remnant of a lymph follicle (*B*). Same node as Fig. 85. ×1,000

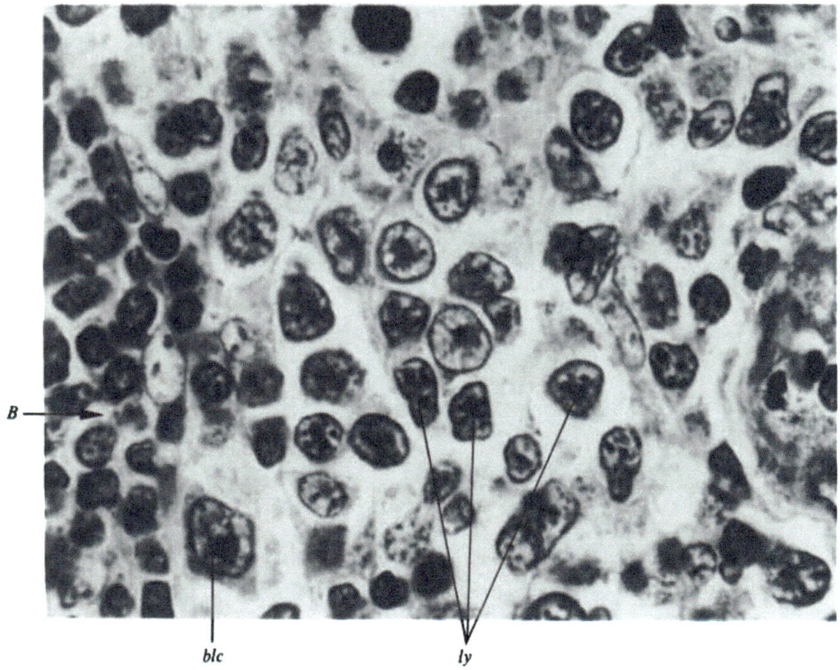


Fig. 87. T-zone lymphoma. Same area of the lymph node illustrated in Fig. 86. Blast cell (*blc*) and polymorphic lymphocytes (*ly*). On the left, the remnant of a follicle (*B*) with small, typical (B-) lymphocytes. Giemsa. ×1,550

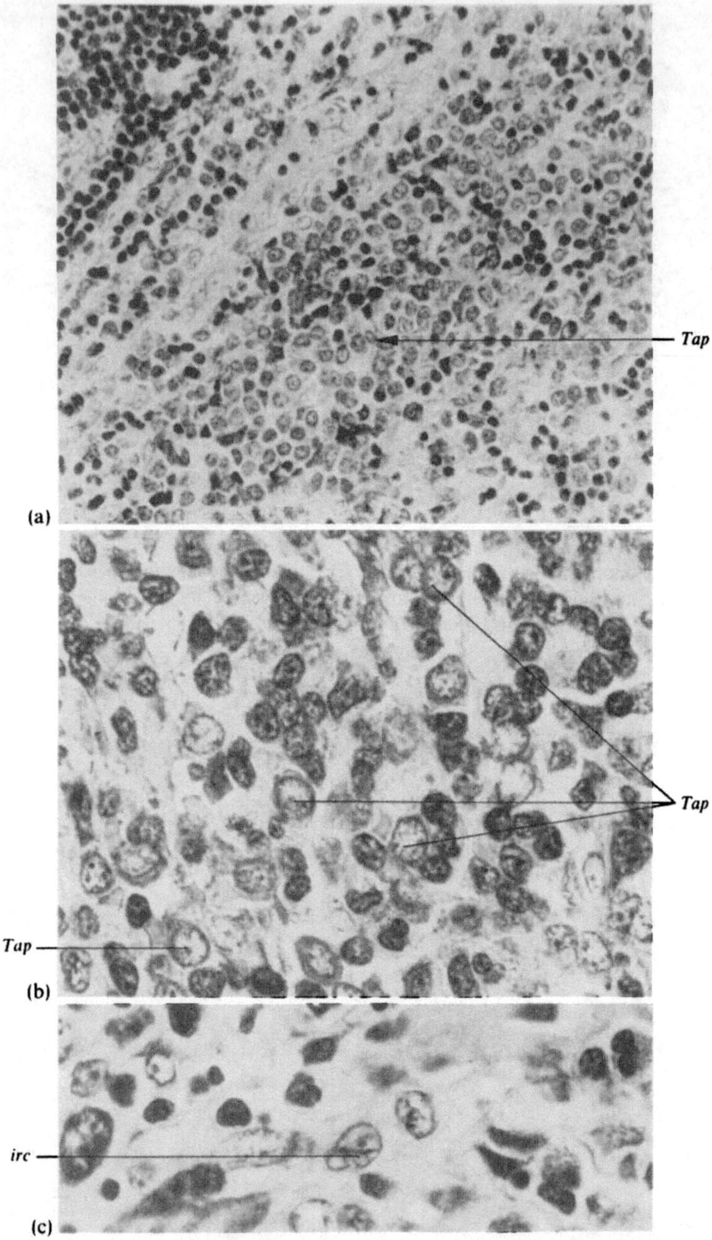


Fig. 88a–c. T-zone lymphoma. (a, b) A sheet of T-associated plasma cells (*Tap*). (c) Interdigitating reticulum cell (*irc*). ♂, 55 years. Cervical node. Giemsa. (a) ×350, (b, c) ×875

2. Compared with the T-lymphocytes, the large blast cells are in the minority. They make up 5–10% of the lymphocytes. They have large oval nuclei with large central gray-stained nucleoli and marginal chromatin condensation. The chromatin is finer than that of the T-lymphocytes. There is a moderate amount of cytoplasm, which is often poorly defined, frequently accumulated on one

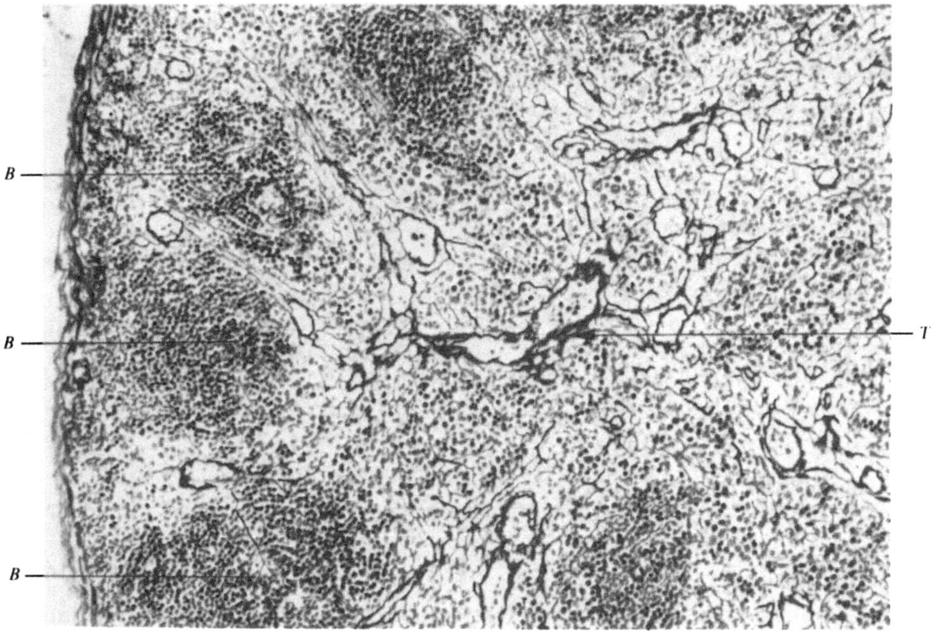


Fig. 89. T-zone lymphoma. Tumor area (*T*) with numerous epithelioid venules. Some nonneoplastic follicles (*B*). ♂, 55 years. Cervical node. Gomori. ×140

side, and clearly gray-blue with Giemsa staining, i.e., moderately basophilic. The blast cells occasionally form binucleate and multinucleate giant cells, which reveal a certain similarity to Sternberg-Reed giant cells. We found such giant cells in about one fourth of our cases. Their nucleoli are also gray, but usually not as large as those of the mononuclear blast cells. The chromatin is also not as fine, so the nucleus is not as light as in Hodgkin's disease.

3. T-associated plasma cells are occasionally present in small numbers. In one of our cases, however, they formed fairly large clusters (Fig. 88a, b). These cells are medium-sized and have oval nuclei with medium-sized, usually solitary nucleoli, and a moderately broad, well-defined rim of gray-blue cytoplasm. The chromatin is fairly fine.

Among the proliferating cells there are at least some interdigitating reticulum cells (Fig. 88c). It is easier to recognize them on electron microscopy or in imprints (cytochemically). They have characteristic polymorphic nuclei with deep indentations.

The sinuses are destroyed and cannot be recognized as such. In the venules one often sees active cell migration, in particular of small lymphocytes and eosinophils.

With silver stains fairly abundant, fine reticulin fibers are found among the tumor cells (Fig. 89). These fibers sometimes surround broad groups of cells. There can be a great increase in fibers, especially after therapy. Occasionally, there is fibrosis in part of the capsule and the adjacent lymphatic tissue.

Satodate studied the tissue and cell components of T-zone lymphoma in 25 cases from our series. The results are given in Table 28. Remnants of follicles

Table 28. Histologic features in lymph nodes with T-zone lymphoma. 25 cases studied by SATODATE

| Component | No. of cases |
|---|---|
| Follicles or follicle remnants | |
| abundant | 15 |
| sparse | 8 |
| none | 2 |
| Germinal centers present in follicle remnants | 13 |
| abundant | 6 |
| Eosinophils | |
| abundant | 11 |
| sparse | 4 |
| none | 10 |
| Increase in neutrophil granulocytes | 6 |
| Epithelioid cells | 2 (+2?) |
| Multinuclate giant cells | 7 |

were found in moderate or large numbers in 15 cases and in small numbers in eight cases. Only two cases revealed no remnants of follicles. The follicles contained germinal centers in 13 cases, in six relatively numerous. Generally, however, these germinal centers showed regressive transformation. Here KAISERLING found numerous dendritic reticulum cells by means of electron microscopy.

Among the proliferating cells there were often a few (four cases) or numerous (11 cases) eosinophils. The eosinophilia was not consistent in subsequent multiple biopsies from the same patients. An increase in mast cells was sometimes found together with the eosinophils. The mast cells could be immature (small, paucity of granules). Small numbers of neutrophils were seen in six cases. In two cases we recognized a few typical plasma cells among the tumor cells.

A small focal proliferation of epithelioid cells, particularly in the B-cell regions, was observed in two cases. It was also slightly developed between the T-lymphocytes. In one case the initial picture was that of plasma cell-poor lymphogranulomatosis X (immunoblastic lymphadenopathy) with numerous epithelioid cells, but without any sign of an obvious T-cell proliferation. A lymph node examined later revealed that a relatively monotonous T-zone lymphoma had developed. In another case we could observe the gradual change from "lymphogranulomatosis X" to T-zone lymphoma in three biopsies taken at 2-week intervals. The T-cell proliferation was hardly recognizable in the first biopsy, but fully developed and easily seen in the third biopsy.

**Smear/Imprint.** Most of the tumor cells are polymorphic lymphocytes (Figs. 81, 90, 91). They have coarse chromatin and round to oval, occasionally deformed and twisted nuclei. Very clearly contrasted, solitary, medium-sized nucleoli can be seen in the nuclei, particularly in enzyme cytochemical slides. These nucleoli are light in Pappenheim staining. The cytoplasm is not always definable since it is very fragile. When it is seen, the rim of cytoplasm is narrow

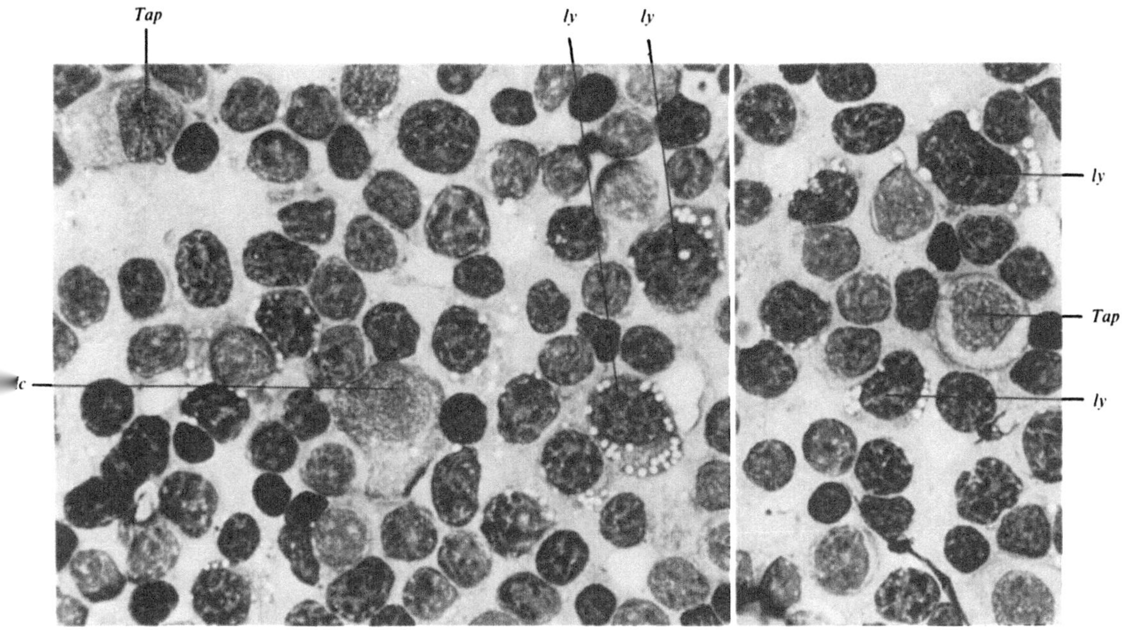


Fig. 90. T-zone lymphoma. Imprint of a lymph node from the same patient as Figs. 81, 88, 89, and 91. Neoplastic lymphocytes (*ly*) with marked anisocytosis and often with cytoplasmic vacuoles. Large blast cell (*blc*). T-associated plasma cells (*Tap*)? Pappenheim. ×760

and stains bright gray-blue or even blue. It contains no granules. In a few cases the cytoplasm showed large numbers of vacuoles of equal size (fat droplets). The large blast cells are basophilic and have a few large light or blue nucleoli. Their rim of cytoplasm is relatively narrow to moderately broad, often accumulated on one side. The T-lymphocytes and blast cells can—without changes in their principal morphology—occasionally form mononuclear, or more rarely multinucleate giant cells. The T-associated plasma cells have a fairly broad rim of deep gray cytoplasm with an eccentric nucleus. The nuclei are round and contain one or two small to medium-sized, light nucleoli.

Among the tumor cells there are more or less numerous eosinophils, as well as a few basophil leukocytes, mast cells, and typical plasma cells. Furthermore, B-lymphocytes from the follicle remnants can be demonstrated. Interdigitating reticulum cells are seen in most cases.

**Histochemistry and Cytochemistry.** When the alkaline phosphatase and 5-nucleotidase reactions are performed simultaneously (Fig. 91), the T- and B-areas can be identified quite clearly. The alkaline phosphatase reaction is positive (red) in and around large vessels in the neoplastic T-zones, whereas the lymphocytes in the nonneoplastic follicles show a brown 5-nucleotidase reaction.

With the acid phosphatase reaction in imprints most of the T-lymphocytes contain several to fairly abundant, positive, coarse granules. The granules are occasionally found in a nuclear indentation. This type of reaction clearly differs,

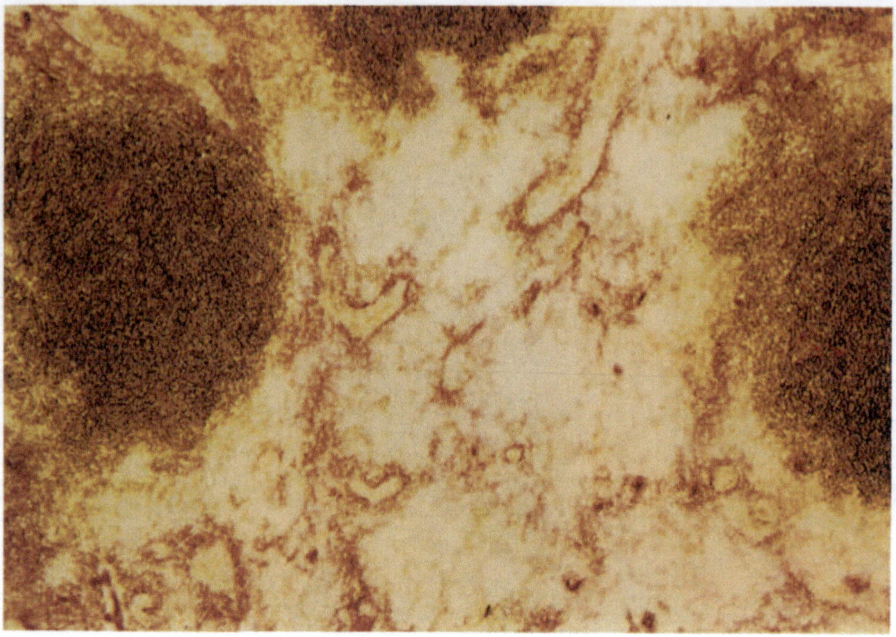

Fig. 91. T-zone lymphoma. Alkaline phosphatase (*red*) and 5-nucleotidase (*brown*) reactions. The light area represents the tumor with an increase in vessels and fibroblastic reticulum cells (*red*). The dark brown nodules are nonneoplastic follicles. Photograph made by Dr. H.-K. MÜLLER-HERMELINK. Same patient as Figs. 81, 88, 89, and 90. ×56

however, from that seen in lymphoblastic lymphoma of the convoluted-cell type. In the latter, the focal accumulation of acid phosphatase activity is much more pronounced. Neutral nonspecific esterase (α-naphthyl acetate esterase) is completely negative in the tumor cells. In one case numerous tumor cells showed a strongly positive, granular PAS reaction (Fig. 92b). In another case the tumor cells were PAS-negative.

The interdigitating reticulum cells can be identified by their weak α-naphthyl acetate esterase and acid phosphatase reactions and their uniformly weak PAS reaction.

**Diagnosis.** Remnants of lymph follicles, an increase in venules, and eosinophilia lead one to suspect T-zone lymphoma. This suspicion is confirmed by the demonstration of characteristic medium-sized T-lymphocytes with polymorphic nuclei. Further criteria are listed in Table 29.

**Differential Diagnosis.** Essentially, T-zone lymphoma must be distinguished from two other lymph-node diseases, namely, from plasma cell-poor lymphogranulomatosis X (immunoblastic lymphadenopathy) and from Hodgkin's disease.

A great increase in venules is characteristic of both T-zone lymphoma and lymphogranulomatosis X (immunoblastic lymphadenopathy). Eosinophilia also

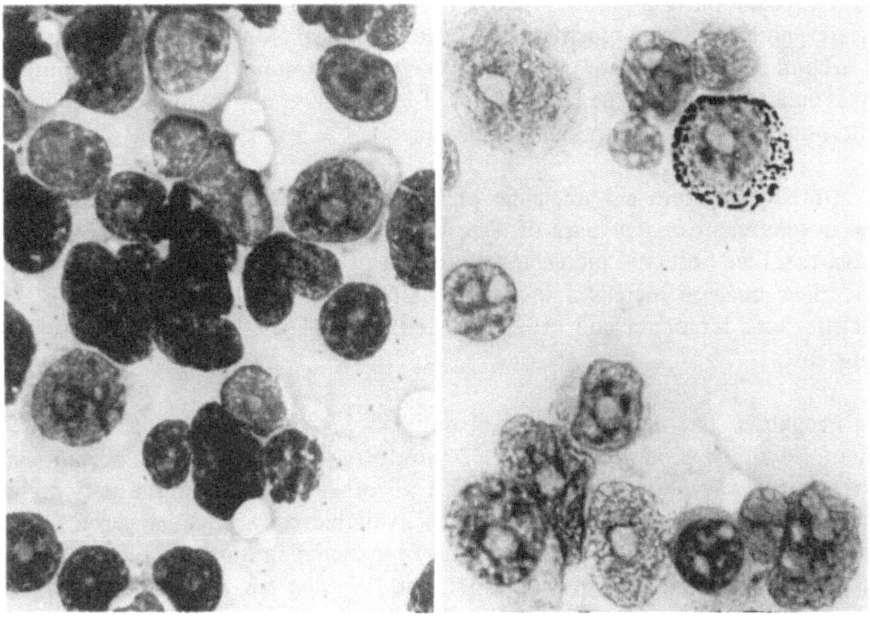

(a) (b)

Fig. 92a and b. T-zone lymphoma. Imprint of a lymph node removed a year later from the same patient as Fig. 90. (a) The lymphocytes are larger and more anaplastic. They have large solitary nucleoli. Pappenheim. ×875. (b) Same imprint with PAS reaction. One cell reveals coarse granular PAS positivity. ×875

Table 29. Diagnostic criteria of T-zone lymphoma

1. Bone marrow not infiltrated until late stages
2. Blood picture not leukemic
3. Histology:
   Selective infiltration of T-regions; follicles or follicle remnants are seen in most cases
   Great increase in venules (PAS+)
   Despite polymorphism, a relatively monotonous picture (in contrast to immunoblastic lymphadenopathy)
4. Cytology:
   Polymorphic lymphocytes (larger than normal)
   Blast cells
   Interdigitating reticulum cells
   In most cases: eosinophils
   In some cases: T-associated plasma cells
   In some cases: multinucleate giant cells
5. Neoplastic lymphocytes form sheep-E rosettes

fits into the picture of both diseases. On the other hand, a relatively monotonous proliferation of T-lymphocytes can be demonstrated only in T-zone lymphoma. That is the decisive criterion for the differential diagnosis. The picture of lymphogranulomatosis X is much more polymorphic, comprising typical hyperbasophilic immunoblasts and often numerous plasma cells.

The eosinophilia and the existence of mononuclear and occasionally multinucleate giant cells lead much too easily to the suspicion of Hodgkin's disease. It is contradicted, however, by the *relatively* monotonous increase in T-lymphocytes and, above all, the demonstration of a certain regularity in the proliferation intermingled with remnants of follicles.

**Development into a Lymphoma of Higher-Grade Malignancy.** We followed the development of ten cases of T-zone lymphoma in subsequent biopsies. In most cases we observed increasing anaplasia of the lymphocytes. Both the cells and their nucleoli increased in size. Finally, there was a monotonous blastic picture with large nucleoli; such markedly anaplastic variants were seen in four cases.

**Prognosis.** The actuarial survival data on 27 patients are given in Fig. 93. The follow-up period was at most 32 months. At the end of that period, only one patient was definitely still alive. In all other cases either the patient had died earlier (16/27) or information was available only up to a certain point after biopsy. The median survival time of patients in stages I and II was 16 months, that of patients in stages III and IV was 5.8 months, and that of all patients was 9.4 months. None of the patients in stages III and IV survived more than 20 months.

There have not been enough systematic studies to say which is the best therapy. It appears, however, that large doses of corticosteroids and the COP regime provide the best results. Radiotherapy did not induce complete remission. In some cases, the clinicians informed us that their patients survived for many months or a few years although they did not show complete remission. It was pointed out that the response to therapy was very poor in most patients.

Because of the evidently poor prognosis, classifying T-zone lymphoma as a low-grade malignant lymphoma is problematical. Our reason for doing so

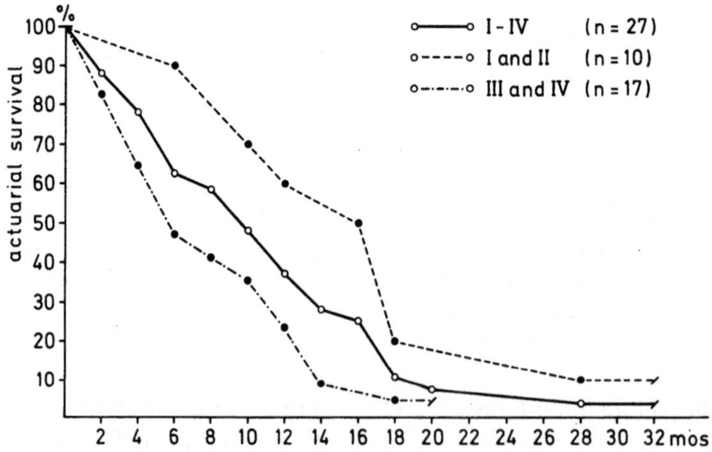


Fig. 93. Actuarial survival of 27 patients with T-zone lymphoma

was that there is not a pure population of blast cells as in other high-grade malignant lymphomas. Instead, T-zone lymphoma reveals lymphocytes, although atypical ones, in addition to blast cells and characteristic structural elements of the T-zone (interdigitating reticulum cells, epithelioid venules).

## B. Lymphomas of Immunoglobulin-Secreting Cells

Tumors whose cells are capable of secreting immunoglobulin were called immunocytoma by HEREMANS.[264] HOBBS[265] adopted the term and distinguished between malignant and benign immunocytomas. We use the term only for a malignant neoplasm, namely, for lymphoplasmacytic/lymphoplasmacytoid immunocytoma (LP immunocytoma). We designate other Ig-producing tumors either as plasmacytoma or as M.L. immunoblastic on the basis of their cytology. This is probably contrary to the practice of HEREMANS, who called an apparently immunoblastic or plasmablastic lymphoma of the ileocecal region of the rat an immunocytoma.

All tumors of Ig-secreting cells contain plasma cells or their direct precursors up to B-immunoblasts. The term immunocytoma does not imply merely an assumed functional property of the tumor cells, as DORFMAN[266] erroneously interpreted; instead, it stands for a morphologically recognizable property of the tumor cells, which, to be sure, necessarily includes the function of Ig production: plasma cells are *qua definitione* Ig-secreting cells.

Whereas LP immunocytoma always contains abundant lymphocytes as well as plasma cells or plasmacytoid cells, lymph-node plasmacytoma consists of a pure population of ("reticular") plasma cells. Both tumors, in our opinion, belong to the low-grade malignant lymphomas. They are discussed in the following two sections. On page 421ff. we present the high-grade malignant lymphomas of Ig-secreting cells (M.L. immunoblastic).

### *1. Malignant Lymphoma, Lymphoplasmacytic/Lymphoplasmacytoid (LP Immunocytoma)*

*Synonyms:* M.L. lymphocytic, well differentiated (RAPPAPORT)
M.L. plasmacytoid-lymphocytic (LUKES and COLLINS)
Lymphoplasmacytoid immunocytoma (LENNERT, STEIN and KAISERLING, 1973)
Macroglobulinemia of Waldenström (some cases)

**History, Terminology.** In 1944, WALDENSTRÖM[267] reported a new entity that he distinguished from plasmacytic myeloma. He described the disease as characterized by elevated levels of IgM in the blood and by a proliferation of cells,

[264] Cited by HOBBS, 1971.
[265] 1971.
[266] 1974b.
[267] Later reviews: WALDENSTRÖM, 1958, 1968.

principally lymphocytic, in the bone marrow, lymph nodes, spleen, and liver, as well as in other organs. Eventually, the entity became known as macroglobulinemia of Waldenström or Waldenström's disease. Pathoanatomic studies were relatively rare. Not until 1959 was a study published in the USA.[268] Several reports and reviews on the pathology of macroglobulinemia had already been published in Europe.[269]

According to the descriptions presented, macroglobulinemia of Waldenström was a neoplasm mainly of lymphocytes and was therefore to be differentiated from plasmacytoma. On the other hand, since plasma cells were also present along with the lymphocytes, it could be differentiated from chronic lymphocytic leukemia. SCHAMAUN,[270] and later LELBACH,[271] DUTCHER and FAHEY,[268] and others, detected as a characteristic of macroglobulinemia of Waldenström the intracytoplasmic and particularly intranuclear inclusions of protein in many of the cells. These inclusions proved to be PAS-positive and were subsequently described many times in malignant lymphomas of other types as well.[272]

In the years 1956–1958, one of us (K.L.) and H. MARTIN had the opportunity to study lymph nodes from three patients with leukemia. The lymph nodes were particularly remarkable because sections revealed a proliferation of lymphoplasmacytoid cells, many of which were heavily laden with intracellular inclusions of protein. Clinically, the leukemias ran relatively benign courses lasting 6–20 years. The occurrence of hemolytic anemia in two of the three patients was remarkable. The disease had arisen in the lymph nodes, and in one of the patients the spleen and bone marrow were still free of involvement when the patient died. The blood picture manifested a slight to massive increase in lymphocytes, with numerous plasmacytoid forms and their precursors. The serum-IgM level was not elevated, and the techniques used at that time provided no hint of a monoclonal increase in other immunoglobulins. Because we were unable to present a rational interpretation of these leukemias at the time, we left our manuscript unfinished and unpublished. We now know that the three cases were excellent examples of the lymphoma we shall discuss in this section.

RAPPAPORT, first with JOHNSON[273] and later with BUFFA,[274] has already published two accounts of such malignant lymphomas with associated acquired hemolytic anemia and with protein inclusions resembling Russell bodies in the cells. With BUFFA's assistance, RAPPAPORT has also chemically analyzed the proteins in homogenates of lymph nodes and found the same "dysproteinemia" as in the blood. With KIM and HELLER,[275] RAPPAPORT reported on globular PAS-positive inclusions in the nuclei in a series of lymphomas. Unfortunately, RAPPAPORT did not continue the immunochemical analysis of lymphomas by means of modern techniques. The systematic immunochemical study of homogenates of malignant lymphomas then surprisingly opened a new door.[276] Using

[268] DUTCHER and FAHEY, 1959.

[269] BICHEL, BING and HARBOE, 1950; SCHAUB, 1952, 1953; SCHAMAUN, 1954; LENNERT, 1955; OETTGEN and QUITMANN, 1956; LELBACH, 1957; WUKETICH and SIEGMUND, 1957; ŠVEJDA, KOSTELNÍK and CHURÝ, 1958; ZOLLINGER, 1958.

[270] 1954.

[271] 1957.

[272] KIM, HELLER and RAPPAPORT, 1973; and others.

[273] 1955.

[274] BUFFA and RAPPAPORT, 1957.

[275] KIM, HELLER and RAPPAPORT, 1973.

[276] STEIN, LENNERT and PARWARESCH, 1972; STEIN, KAISERLING and LENNERT, 1973; LENNERT, STEIN and KAISERLING, 1974, 1975.

these methods, it was also possible to clarify many monoclonal gammopathies of the blood, which have been reported to be associated with various lymphomas,[277] and to look at them from the same point of view. Perhaps DE OLIVEIRA[278] described the same entity as "retothelsarcoma with hemopoietic differentiation." Finally, the figures given by HOBBS[279] must be considered. He reported finding among his nonplasmacytic immunocytomas only 32 cases of macrogloublinemia of Waldenström, but 26 cases of lymphosarcoma and five cases of CLL.

Our studies with STEIN and KAISERLING[276] disclosed that there is a type of lymphoma that is characterized in light- and electron-microscopic studies by an intermingling of lymphocytes with plasmacytoid cells or typical plasma cells and that produces immunoglobulin. This Ig proved to be monoclonal. What was new from these investigations was that the tumor cells may synthesize large amounts of IgM, but may be unable to release it into the blood because of disturbances in polymerization and/or secretion. Consequently, there may even be an absence of the corresponding Ig classes in the blood.[280] DIEBOLD *et al.*[281] had already proved such a case of IgM-storing lymphoma without an increase in IgM in the blood by means of immunofluorescence microscopy in 1971.

The second new result of our studies was that, besides IgM, the lymphoma cells can also produce IgG, IgA, or IgE and can release them into the blood.

Furthermore, it has become evident that a monoclonal increase in IgM in the blood may be associated with malignant lymphomas that are not composed of lymphocytes and plasma cells or plasmacytoid cells, such as immunoblastic sarcoma.

From these facts we may conclude the following:

1. There is a type of malignant lymphoma that morphologically corresponds to the description of macroglobulinemia of Waldenström, but which only produces IgM in order to store it and is therefore not associated with macroglobulinemia. It represents, so to speak, a "macroglobulinemia without macroglobulinemia." Such cases are, in essence, identical with Waldenström's disease. Nevertheless, we do not consider the term macroglobulinemia compatible with the definition.[282] Therefore, we recommended calling the lymphoma "lymphoplasmacytoid immunocytoma," since the definition of a neoplasm should be based on its morphology.

2. If the cells of the lymphoma are able to produce not only IgM but also IgG, IgA, or IgE, then the term macroglobulinemia is meaningless, whereas the term LP immunocytoma fully covers these Ig-producing variants.

---

[277] AZAR, HILL and OSSERMAN, 1957; OLMER, MONGIN, MURATORE and DENIZET, 1961, review of older cases; KRAUSS and SOKAL, 1966; GINGOLD and STOICA, 1967; RAU, MUELLER-ECKHARDT, HUTH and LÖFFLER, 1968; MICHAUX and HEREMANS, 1969, Lit.; MALDONADO, WILLIAMS, SILVERSTEIN and HARRISON, 1970; MOORE, MIGLIORE, SHULLENBERGER and ALEXANIAN, 1970; HOBBS, 1971; FITZGERALD, RASTRICK and HAMER, 1973; BRAUN, BRUCHHAUS and ALY, 1973; PALUTKE and MCDONALD, 1973; and many others, review: FATEH-MOGHADAM, 1974.

[278] 1936.

[279] 1971.

[280] STEIN, KAISERLING, LENNERT and PARWARESCH, 1973.

[281] DIEBOLD, ZITTOUN, FINE, TRICOT *et al.*, 1971.

[282] DAMESHEK, 1964; and others.

3. Since a monoclonal increase in IgM can also occur in other types of malignant lymphoma, as WALDENSTRÖM himself reported several times,[283] the clinical finding of an increase in macroglobulin in the blood is not suitable for the definition of these neoplasms. At most, the term macroglobulinemia of Waldenström may be used for a *clinical syndrome* when both a lymphoplasmacytic proliferation and a monoclonal increase in IgM can be demonstrated.

In rejecting the concept of a Waldenström's *disease*, as KRAUSS and SOKAL[284] have already recommended, we do not want in any way to detract from the valuable contributions made by WALDENSTRÖM, who greatly stimulated the research in this field with his clinical and immunochemical studies.

Among the LP immunocytomas we also include those cases of chronic lymphocytic leukemia in which we find in paraffin sections cells containing globular PAS-positive inclusions. Our reasons for doing so are:

1. Frequently, in light-microscopic studies, unmistakable plasmacytoid or plasmacytic cells can be identified among the typical lymphocytes (also evident in cases published in the literature, for example, in Figure 2 of BUFFA and RAPPAPORT[284a]).

2. When we found no plasmacytoid or typical plasma cells on light microscopy, we were able to detect at least some plasmacytoid forms by means of electron microscopy. We had failed to recognize these cells on light microscopy because the histologic sections were not of high quality and because the cells were too small.

3. After eliminating the cases with globular PAS-positive inclusions from our collection of chronic lymphocytic leukemias, it no longer contained any cases with a monoclonal increase in IgM in the blood.

We interpret the accumulations of Ig in the cells as a result of a disturbance in secretion. Accordingly, we include the lymphoplasmacytoid cells of immunocytoma with the secreting derivatives of B-lymphocytes. The lymphocytes of CLL are unable to secrete, but do bear Ig on the cell surface. We regard this difference as being not only important but also essential. It allows us to make a distinction between malignant lymphomas with the fundamental capability to secrete Ig from those that lack this capability. The fact that the switch from the non-secreting to the secreting cell is "blocked" in typical CLL[285] should not prevent us from distinguishing the "blocked" cells from "unblocked" cells. Otherwise we would not be justified in differentiating plasma-cell leukemias from lymphocytic leukemias.

In accordance with these thoughts, we classify all "chronic lymphocytic leukemias" of the literature in which globular PAS-positive protein inclusions were found in the cells of blood smears, bone-marrow smears, or histologic sections as LP immunocytoma.[286] We are not sure, however, whether one may classify all those "CLL" in which PAS-negative, crystalline inclusions are seen in lymphocytes of blood smears or on electron microscopy, as immunocytoma.[287]

[283] 1968, 1970.
[284] 1966.
[284a] 1957.
[285] SALMON and SELIGMANN, 1974.
[286] LASZLO, GERBER and SOMMER, 1967; HUREZ, FLANDRIN, PREUD'HOMME and SELIGMANN, 1972.
[287] BESSIS, 1951; DE MAN and MEINERS, 1962; HUREZ, FLANDRIN, PREUD'HOMME and SELIGMANN, 1972; COHNEN, 1975.

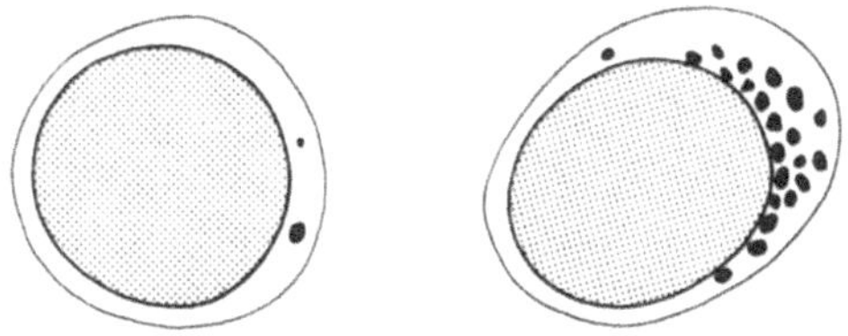

Fig. 94. Acid phosphatase reaction in B-CLL (left) and immunocytoma (right). Schematic drawing of lymphoid cells in lymph-node imprint

We have such reservations, even though these inclusions also represent immunoglobulin, which, in the two cases of KNAPP *et al.*,[288] contained the same heavy and light chains as did the Ig on the surface of the lymphocytes.

In our opinion, the cases that were defined by SELIGMANN *et al.*[289] as intermediate lymphomas between CLL and macroglobulinemia should be classified as LP immunocytoma, because of the monoclonal increase in immunoglobulin in the blood. This increase is probably caused by proliferation of a large number of Ig-producing plasmacytoid cells or plasma cells. Such cases do not exclude the existence of borderline cases between CLL and LP immunocytoma (see p. 243ff.) with a minimal number of plasmacytoid cells.

There are other arguments for an essential difference between B-CLL and LP immunocytoma. For example, it was recently shown in our laboratory that the lymphocytes of LP immunocytoma contained larger amounts of acid phosphatase than did the lymphocytes of CLL. This was demonstrated by light microscopy in lymph-node imprints[290] (Fig. 94) as well as by means of biochemical techniques in tissue homogenates (Fig. 95).[291] A similar significant difference was found between the amounts of acid nonspecific esterase in the two tumors.[292] With the acid phosphatase and esterase reactions we found many positive granules (lysosomes) that were often accumulated at one side of the cytoplasm of lymphocytoid cells. Such reactions are not seen in B-CLL lymphocytes. There were significant differences ($p < 0.05$) between the amounts of acid phosphatase exhaustively extracted from B-CLL, M.L. centroblastic/centrocytic, and LP immunocytoma, with the highest values in LP immunocytoma (Fig. 95).

Finally, a clinical argument was provided by GUNZER *et al.*,[293] who investigated in lymphoma patients the antibody titers against Epstein-Barr virus (VCA and EA). They found that the values for LP immunocytoma were significantly lower than those for all other malignant lymphomas, including B-CLL.

**Origin of the Neoplastic Cells.** LP immunocytoma is, without doubt, a lymphoma that originates from B-lymphocytes, in particular from $B_2$-lymphocytes.

[288] KNAPP, SCHUIT, BOLHUIS and HIJMANS, 1974.

[289] SELIGMANN, PREUD'HOMME and BROUET, 1976.

[290] SCHWARZE, unpublished data.

[291] PARWARESCH, STEIN, SCHWARZE and LENNERT, to be published; PARWARESCH, STEIN and SCHMIDT, to be published.

[292] SUGIYAMA, MÜLLER-HERMELINK and SCHWARZE, to be published.

[293] GUNZER, NÜRNBERGER and THIEMANN, 1975.

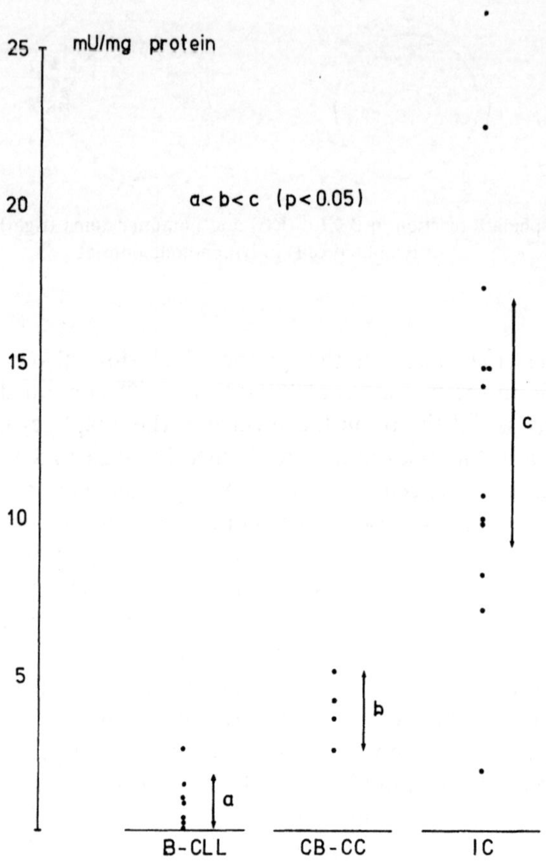


Fig. 95. Distribution of specific activity of acid phosphatase in terms of mU per mg protein, extracted from tissue samples of B-CLL (n = 7), centroblastic/centrocytic lymphoma (*CB-CC*; n = 4), and immunocytoma (*IC*; n = 12). Statistical computation considering 95% confidence limits pertains to $p < 0.05$

The strong granular positivity for acid phosphatase and esterase is perhaps a characteristic feature of $B_2$-lymphocytes. According to our subclassification (see the following section), LP immunocytoma can have various components: (1) lymphocytes, (some) immunoblasts, and Marschalkó plasma cells (Fig. 96), (2) lymphocytes, (some) immunoblasts and lymphoplasmacytoid cells (Fig. 97), or (3) lymphocytes, many immunoblasts, lymphoplasmacytoid cells or plasma cells, often with centroblasts and centrocytes (Fig. 98). This polymorphic tumor demonstrates the close relationship between germinal centers and plasmacytopoiesis. The focal EAC rosetting by cells of such tumors indicates that they are derived from germinal-center cells. Other immunologic data on LP immunocytoma are presented in Part Six.

**Definition.** We define LP immunocytoma, which the members of the Kiel Conference of 1974 renamed malignant lymphoma, lymphoplasmacytoid (immunocytic), as follows:

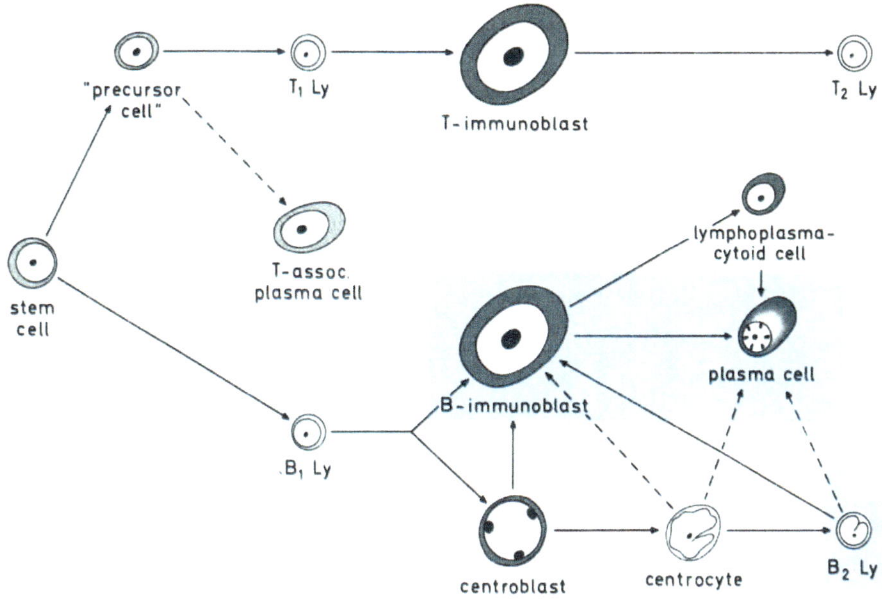


Fig. 96. Hypothetical origin of tumor cells of lymphoplasmacytic immunocytoma

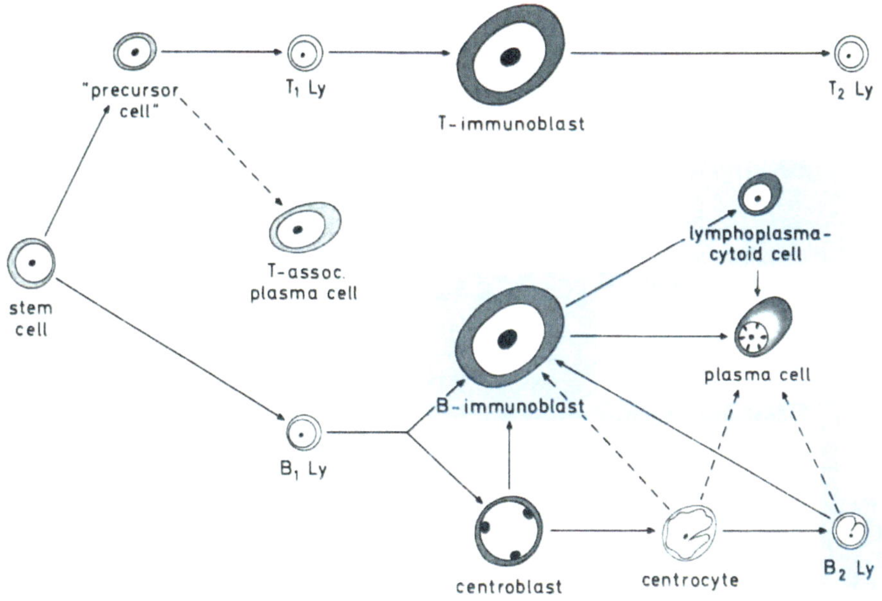


Fig. 97. Hypothetical origin of tumor cells of lymphoplasmacytoid immunocytoma

1. It is a malignant lymphoma composed predominantly of lymphocytes, but containing *also* plasmacytoid or typical plasma cells as essential components. It shows a diffuse growth pattern.

2. It *may* be associated with an increase in monoclonal Ig in the blood

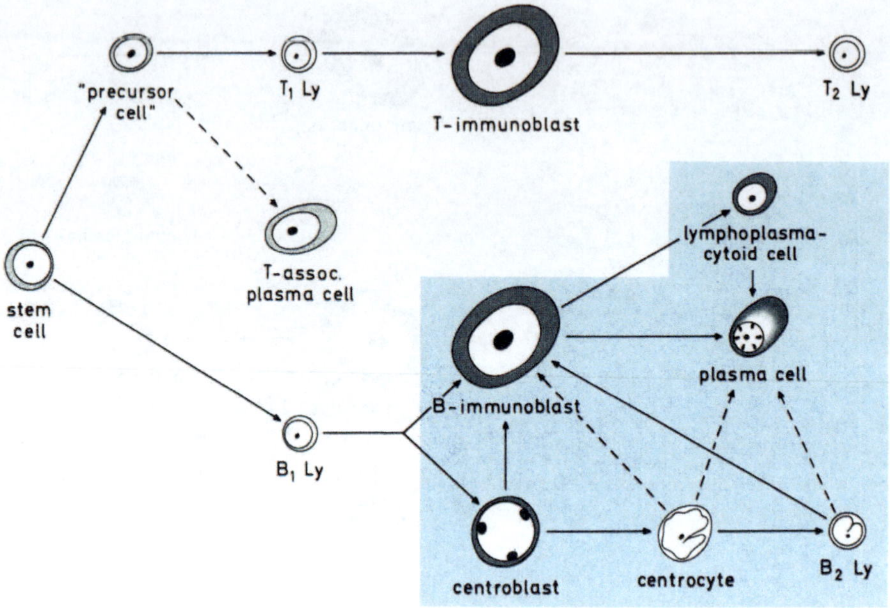


Fig. 98. Hypothetical origin of tumor cells of polymorphic immunocytoma

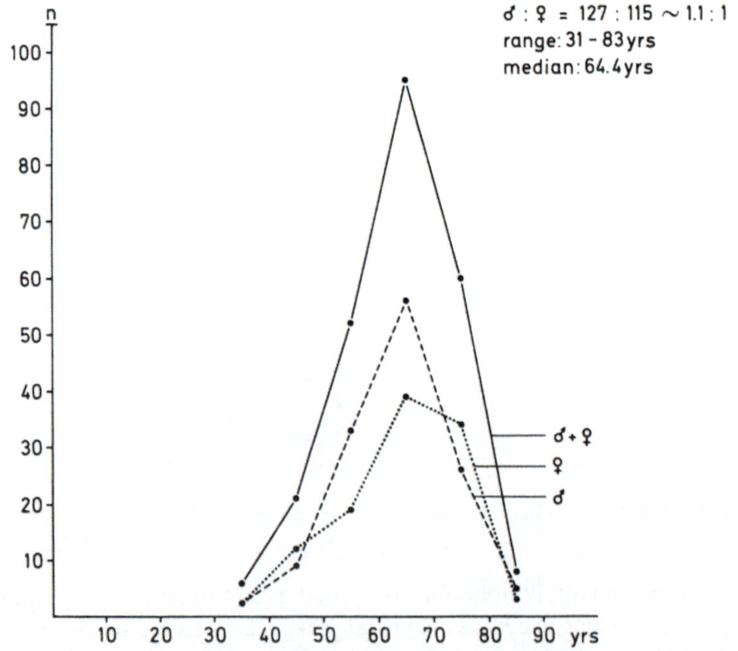


Fig. 99. Age distribution and sex ratio of all types of LP immunocytoma (n=242)

and/or tissue. This increase occurs more frequently in the tissue than in the blood.

3. The blood *may* exhibit a leukemic picture.

4. The disease chiefly affects the elderly and usually runs a very chronic course.

By comparing the results of our electron-microscopic studies of these tumors with those of our immunochemical analyses, we learned in time what an immunocytoma looks like. We then carefully searched our entire Lymph Node Registry for all lymphomas of this type. We discovered that immunocytoma occurs in three morphologic variants, which we shall discuss separately:

1. A lymphoplasmacytic lymphoma, containing in addition to lymphocytes typical ("reticular," Marschalkó) plasma cells and some immunoblasts. The morphology corresponds to earlier descriptions of macroglobulinemia of Waldenström.

2. A lymphoplasmacytoid lymphoma, containing along with lymphocytes small lymphocyte-like plasma cells with scanty cytoplasm and some immunoblasts.

3. A polymorphic variant, containing in addition to lymphocytes and plasmacytoid cells numerous cells of moderate or large sizes. Some of them resemble centroblasts and centrocytes, whereas others have a morphology like that of immunoblasts and of more mature plasma-cell precursors.

Thus, we distinguish three subgroups of LP immunocytoma. As we shall see, these subgroups are also of clinical and epidemiologic relevance.

**Occurrence.** LP immunocytoma is by no means a rare tumor (Table 30). When the non-Hodgkin's lymphomas were ranked according to frequency, it occupied fourth place in our first series after M.L. centroblastic/centrocytic, CLL, and M.L. immunoblastic. It constituted 9.1% of all malignant lymphomas and 16.2% of non-Hodgkin's lymphomas.

The incidence of each of the three subgroups is as follows. Lymphoplasma*cytoid* immunocytoma is by far the most common (63%). The polymorphic variant is the next most common (25.6%). The variant exhibiting the lymphoplasma*cytic* picture, which is regarded as typical of Waldenström's

Table 30. M.L. lymphoplasmacytic/lymphoplasmacytoid (LP immunocytoma). Material and incidence

| | | |
|---|---|---|
| Total No. of cases | 268 | |
| Biopsy | | 256 |
| Autopsy | | 12 |
| Total No. of biopsies | 401 | |
| Lymph nodes | | 324 |
| Extranodal | | 77 |
| Incidence in routine lymph-node biopsies | | 136 |
| =9.1% of malignant lymphomas | | |
| 16.2% of non-Hodgkin's lymphomas | | |

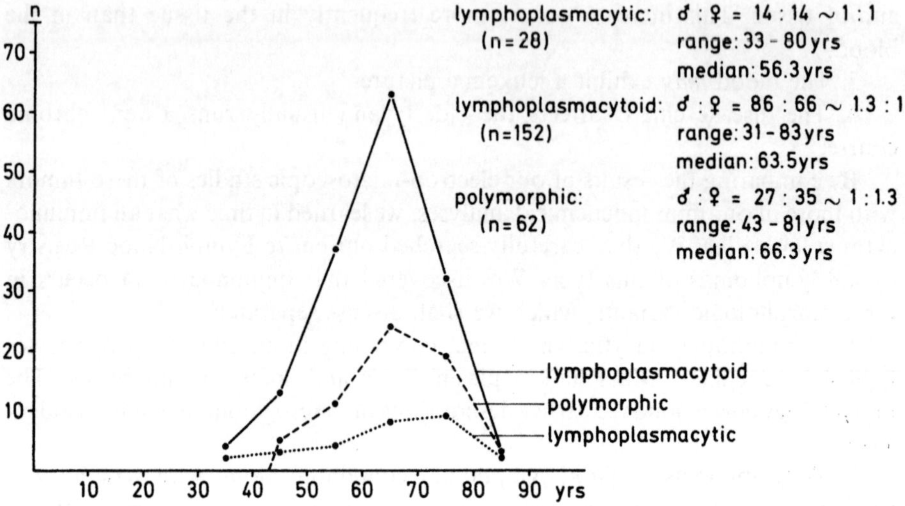


Fig. 100. Age distribution and sex ratio of the three subtypes of LP immunocytoma (n=242)

disease, is the rarest (11.4%). In addition to these variants, we have found some cases that we interpreted as transitional stages between LP immunocytoma and "blastic" sarcoma (see p. 243).

When we group all immunocytomas of both sexes together, the age curve peaks quite sharply in the seventh decade (Fig. 99). The patients ranged in age from 31 to 83 years. The incidence in women in the eighth decade seems to be greater than in men of the same age, a difference we also detected in B-CLL. The male-to-female ratio is 1.1:1.

When we plot the curves of the age distribution in the three subgroups (Fig. 100), we find that the curve for the lymphoplasmacytoid type is like the one for all the immunocytomas together. In contrast, the lymphoplasmacytic curve forms a plateau between the ages of 60 and 80. The polymorphic type does not occur before the age of 40 and its curve is flatter than the lymphoplasmacytoid curve. In addition, its sex ratio differs from those of the other types, for it occurs in women somewhat more commonly than in men (male-to-female ratio 1:1.3). The sex ratio of the lymphoplasmacytoid type shows a slight predominance of men (1.3:1). The lymphoplasmacytic type does not seem to show a preference for either sex.

**Clinical Manifestations.** Stacher[294] and Stacher *et al.*[295] evaluated 80 cases of the Kiel Lymphoma Study Group and obtained the following data. In 86% of the cases the disease had begun insidiously, in 14% abruptly. In about half of the patients objective symptoms (enlarged spleen or lymph nodes, development of cutaneous tumors) appeared only a short time before diagnosis; in the other half of the patients, one or more years earlier (in one patient more than 10 years before diagnosis).

[294] 1974, personal communication.

[295] Stacher, Waldner and Theml, 1976.

Table 31. Symptoms of 80 LP-immunocytoma patients of the Kiel Lymphoma Study Group (STACHER, WALDNER and THEML, 1976)

| Symptom | % |
|---|---|
| Unexplained fever >38° C | 42 |
| Fatigue, weakness | 71 |
| Loss of appetite, weight loss | 48 |
| Night sweats | 31 |
| Allergic phenomena | 17 |
| Arthralgia | 35 |
| Itching | 16 |

Table 32. Rate of enlargement of lymph nodes in LP-immunocytoma patients of the Kiel Lymphoma Study Group (STACHER, WALDNER and THEML, 1976)

| | All subtypes (n=77) | Subtype | | |
|---|---|---|---|---|
| | | Lymphoplasmacytic (n=7) | Lymphoplasmacytoid (n=50) | Polymorphic (n=20) |
| | % | % | % | % |
| Slow | 66 | 85 | 72 | 45 |
| Rapid | 34 | 15 | 28 | 55 |

The subjective complaints of the patients are listed in Table 31. Fever was reported by 42% of the patients; thus, it was more frequent than in CLL. Other constitutional symptoms (weakness, loss of weight, etc.) were also somewhat more frequent. The same was true for arthralgia. Sixteen percent of the patients complained of itching. Ten percent of the patients had received vaccinations. The lymph nodes enlarged slowly in 66% and rapidly in 34% of the patients. Enlargement of lymph nodes occurred more rapidly in the polymorphic subtype than in the others (Table 32). There was splenomegaly in 41.3% and hepatomegaly in 43.5% of the patients. These figures are surely too low, however, since they were based only on palpation findings. The bone marrow was infiltrated in 71.6%. This is in remarkable contrast to the infiltration of the marrow in 100% of the patients with B-CLL.

The hemoglobin concentration roughly corresponded to that of CLL, but there were some patients with more severe anemia (Table 33). Most of the anemia patients were Coombs-positive. Seven out of 28 cases showed a positive Coombs test. Furthermore, there was cryoglobulinemia in three patients and a large amount of cold agglutinins in two. Occasionally, analyses were made for antibodies against leukocytes, thrombocytes, vessels, or thyroid gland, and the results were sometimes positive.

The thrombocyte counts were—as in B-CLL—somewhat reduced in 22.4% of the patients (Table 33). The RBC sedimentation rate was more often accelerated and less frequently normal than in CLL. The lymphoplasmacytic type never showed normal or merely slightly elevated values. The amount of total

Table 33. Blood values of LP-immunocytoma patients of the Kiel Lymphoma Study Group (STACHER, WALDNER and THEML, 1976)

| | All subtypes | Subtype | | |
|---|---|---|---|---|
| | | Lympho-plasma-cytic | Lympho-plasma-cytoid | Poly-morphic |
| | (%) | (%) | (%) | (%) |
| Hemoglobin g-% | (n=78) | (n=9) | (n=50) | (n=19) |
| >13.1 | 42.3 | 11 | 50 | 36 |
| 13.0–10.1 | 34.2 | 44 | 28 | 47 |
| 10.0–8.1 | 9.0 | 22 | 10 | — |
| <8.0 | 14.5 | 22 | 12 | 15 |
| Thrombocytes/μl | (n=67) | (n=8) | (n=43) | (n=16) |
| <100,000 | 22.4 | 19 | 21 | 32 |
| RBC sedimentation rate | (n=78) | (n=9) | (n=50) | (n=19) |
| Normal | 16 | — | 24 | 4 |
| Slightly accelerated (at least 10/15) | 17 | — | 20 | 21 |
| Moderately accelerated (at least 32/58) | 29 | 11 | 28 | 42 |
| Greatly accelerated (at least 90/—) | 35 | 89 | 28 | 35 |
| Total protein g-% | (n=70) | (n=8) | (n=38) | (n=17) |
| <6 | 12 | 25 | 13 | 6 |
| 6–8 | 65 | 12.5 | 68 | 82 |
| >8 | 21 | 62.5 | 17 | 12 |
| Increase in serum Ig | (n=58) | | | |
| IgM | 28.0 | | | |
| IgG | 7.5 | | | |
| IgA | 3.0 | | | |
| IgM+IgG | 1.5 | | | |
| IgM+IgA | 1.5 | | | |
| IgE | 1.5 | | | |
| not detected | 56.0 | | | |

protein in the serum was decreased in 12%, about normal in 65%, and increased in 21% of the patients. Of the patients of the Kiel Lymphoma Study Group, 44% presented an increase in serum Ig (Table 33). Of the cases in our whole series, only 20% showed a *monoclonal* increase in serum Ig. Bence-Jones proteinuria had often developed, even when paraproteinemia was not demonstrated. In this context, it is interesting that WESTERHAUSEN[296] found paraproteinemia in 16 out of 90 (17.7%) patients with CLL; IgG was detected in four patients, IgA in one, IgM in 10, and Bence-Jones protein in one patient.

---

[296] 1973.

According to the clinically predominant site of lymphoma manifestation, we can distinguish three main types:

1. Lymph-node type (68 cases in the series of STACHER *et al.*[297]).
2. Splenomegalic type (7 cases in the series of STACHER *et al.*[297]).
3. Oculocutaneous type (5 cases in the series of STACHER *et al.*[297]).

Most patients with the *lymph-node type* manifested generalized enlargement of the lymph nodes, although the nodes were relatively small, indolent, and not mutually adherent. Only some patients presented rather large lymph nodes, which were seen in only two or three lymph-node regions, rather than generalized enlargement. These cases were generally of the polymorphic subtype, and the prognosis was relatively poor. The skin was involved secondarily in five patients.

The distinctive characteristic of the *splenomegalic type* is an excessively enlarged spleen. In four patients the bone marrow was normal (proved by biopsy) and peripheral lymphadenopathy was not evident. This splenomegalic type is apparently equivalent to the special type of CLL described by HITTMAIR[298] and LEIBETSEDER and TUBA,[299] which was said to involve only the spleen. If the spleen is not removed, infiltration of the bone marrow and lymph nodes will develop. Cases with splenomegaly *and* lymphadenopathy from the beginning are not included in this group.

Patients with the *oculocutaneous type* have primary tumors in the orbit and/or skin, including the subcutis or skeletal muscles. The orbit may reveal development of retrobulbar tumors. We have also seen tumor infiltration of the whole bulb. Furthermore, the conjunctiva and eyelids may be involved.[300] The tumor sometimes proceeded from the orbit to the skin, e.g., of the face or elsewhere. In addition, there were patients who had tumors only in the skin and skeletal muscles, especially in the extremities. The tumors appeared as nodules, either singly or widely spread over the body. The disease often ran a course of many years, sometimes 10–20 years. Definite recovery seems to be possible. Sometimes (regional or deep) lymph nodes and other organs are involved secondarily.

**Blood Picture.** The data of the Kiel Lymphoma Study Group are listed in Table 34. In contrast to B-CLL, the absolute number of lymphocytes in the peripheral blood was lower than 4000/μl in 71.0% of the patients. That is nearly the same as the percentage we found by analyzing the blood values of all the cases recorded at our Lymph Node Registry (68.8%). Of these cases, 31.2% were accompanied by a leukemic blood picture. It was found most commonly in the lymphoplasmacytoid subtype (37.1%), least commonly in the lymphoplasmacytic subtype (9.5%). The polymorphic subtype showed an intermediate proportion of 19%. The highest white blood cell count observed was 241,000/ μl with 88% lymphocytes and 4% "blast cells." All other counts were below 100,000/μl.

[297] STACHER, WALDNER and THEML, 1976.
[298] 1952.
[299] 1956.
[300] SCHWARZE, RADASZKIEWICZ, PÜLHORN, GOOS *et al.*, 1976.

Table 34. Number of lymphocytes in peripheral blood of LP-immunocytoma patients of the Kiel Lymphoma Study Group (STACHER, WALDNER and THEML, 1976)

| Lymphocytes/μl | All Subtypes (n=76) | Subtype | | |
|---|---|---|---|---|
| | | Lymphoplasma-cytic (n=7) | Lymphoplasma-cytoid (n=50) | Polymorphic (n=19) |
| | (%) | (%) | (%) | (%) |
| <2,000 | 43.4 | 71 | 44 | 31 |
| 2,000– 4,000 | 27.6 | 14 | 24 | 42 |
| 4,000– 5,000 | 1.3 | – | – | 5 |
| 5,000– 10,000 | 6.5 | – | 6 | 10 |
| 10,000– 20,000 | 13.1 | – | 18 | 5 |
| 20,000– 50,000 | 5.2 | – | 6 | – |
| 50,000–100,000 | 2.6 | 14 | 2 | 5 |

The morphology of the lymphoid cells in peripheral blood smears is sometimes not distinguishable from that of CLL lymphocytes. At times there are somewhat larger lymphoid cells similar to plasma cells ("plasmacytoid cells"). In cases of the polymorphic subtype we can also find large numbers of centrocytes, sometimes with plasmacytoid cells and plasmablasts. These cells of the plasma-cell series are, in certain cases, more numerous in bone-marrow smears than in the blood. In many cases the diagnosis of LP immunocytoma is not possible by investigation of blood smears alone, even when a leukemic blood picture is found. In the future some help will definitely be provided by systematic cytochemical [301] and immunocytologic studies.

**Localization.** If we consider immunocytoma as a whole (Table 35), then almost half of the lymph nodes removed for study originated from the cervical region (45.5%). Axillary and inguinal lymph nodes together made up about half of our collection (25.4% and 21.3%, respectively). Noteworthy is the infrequency with which abdominal (4.5%) and mediastinal (1.6%) lymph nodes were represented in our material, whereas cubital lymph nodes constituted 1.6%, a remarkable percentage.

When we consider the subtypes, it is notable that we never diagnosed a lymphoplasma*cytic* immunocytoma in a supraclavicular, mediastinal, or abdominal lymph node, whereas we diagnosed it most frequently in axillary lymph nodes. The large number of cervical lymph nodes involved by the polymorphic type (55.9%) is remarkable.

Concerning *extranodal involvement*—biopsies of tissues other than lymph nodes made up a relatively large proportion (19.1%) of the material we have received for study. Worthy of mentioning are specimens from the skin and subcutis (23), orbit (4), gastrointestinal tract (4), and nasopharynx (3).

At this juncture, we would like to make special reference to the immunocy-

[301] HELLER, 1972.

Table 35. Localization of biopsies in LP immunocytoma

| Localization | Lymphoplasma-cytic | | Lymphoplasma-cytoid | | Polymorphic | | Total | |
|---|---|---|---|---|---|---|---|---|
| | n | % | n | % | n | % | n | % |
| Lymph nodes | 24 | 61.5 | 189 | 81.1 | 83 | 88.3 | 296 | 80.9 |
| Cervical | 7 | 36.8 | 66 | 42.0 | 38 | 55.9 | 111 | 45.5 |
| Axillary | 8 | 42.1 | 45 | 28.7 | 9 | 13.3 | 62 | 25.4 |
| Mediastinal | – | – | 3 | 1.9 | 1 | 1.5 | 4 | 1.6 |
| Abdominal | – | – | 10 | 6.4 | 1 | 1.5 | 11 | 4.5 |
| Inguinal | 4 | 21.1 | 30 | 19.1 | 18 | 26.5 | 52 | 21.3 |
| Cubital | – | – | 3 | 1.9 | 1 | 1.5 | 4 | 1.6 |
| Unknown | 5 | | 32 | | 15 | | 52 | |
| Extranodal | 15 | 38.5 | 44 | 18.9 | 11 | 11.7 | 70 | 19.1 |
| Skin and subcutis | 9 | | 11 | | 3 | | 23 | |
| Spleen | – | | 9 | | 1 | | 10 | |
| Tonsils | 2 | | 1 | | 4 | | 7 | |
| Bone marrow | 2 | | 4 | | – | | 6 | |
| Orbit | – | | 4 | | – | | 4 | |
| Gastrointestinal tract | 2 | | 1 | | 1 | | 4 | |
| Liver | – | | 3 | | 1 | | 4 | |
| Nasopharynx | – | | 3 | | – | | 3 | |
| Lung | – | | 2 | | – | | 2 | |
| Others | – | | 6 | | 1 | | 7 | |

tomas of the *orbit*. They have usually been misinterpreted as benign lymphomas or pseudolymphomas.[303] We have had the opportunity to follow up patients with such orbital lymphomas and have found that similar infiltrates may appear years later at other sites, such as the skin or abdominal lymph nodes, often with an associated IgM paraproteinemia. Comparable reports on single case studies are accumulating in the literature.[304]

Two further important localizations do not appear in our list of extranodal immunocytomas: the lungs and the central nervous system. The group of primary lymphocytic lymphomas of the *lung* includes a subgroup that in fact represents typical lymphoplasmacytoid or lymphoplasmacytic lymphoma. Examples of this entity have been published by a number of authors, for instance, by HEINE[305] and THIERBACH and HUTH.[306] The so-called primary pulmonary variant of macroglobulinemia of Waldenström[307] is the corresponding variant with IgM paraproteinemia, although, as in other immunocytomas, this is not obligatory.

[303] Lit.: SCHWARZE, RADASZKIEWICZ, PÜLHORN, GOOS *et al.*, 1976.

[304] PAUFIQUE, GIRARD, SCHOTT, CREYSSEL *et al.*, 1969; GODEAU, SICARD, HERREMAN and SLAMA, 1972; BLATRIX, FINE, YEME and LAMBIN, 1973; GARNER, 1973; VAN HEERDE, HIJMANS, WAGENAAR, SCHUIT *et al.*, 1974.

[305] 1957.

[306] 1963.

[307] FATEH-MOGHADAM, PRECHTEL, WOLF-HORNUNG, LAMERZ *et al.*, 1974, Lit.

A distinction between this subgroup and pseudolymphoma may be difficult to make and is not yet sufficiently understood. The mixture of lymphocytes and plasma cells, which sometimes contain Russell bodies, is typical of immunocytoma, but may lead to the misinterpretation of the picture as that of an inflammatory infiltration.

The demonstration of numerous so-called primary lymphomas of the *CNS* at the International Symposium on Malignant Lymphomas of the Nervous System in Vienna, 1974, made it very likely that a large number of these lymphomas can be interpreted as immunocytomas. That is probably particularly true for microgliomatosis, which can practically always be classified as a lymphoplasmacytic neoplasm (immunocytoma). The increase in glial cells observed in this disease is probably reactive. According to JELLINGER *et al.*,[308] the primary lymphomas of the CNS besides lymphoplasmacytic immunocytoma are either immunoblastic or lymphoblastic lymphomas.

HEENAN *et al.*[309] added to three previous publications on "macroglobulinemias associated with *small-bowel* malignancy" a further case with an isolated tumor in the jejunum. This case revealed a monoclonal increase in IgM in the blood and IgM/$\kappa$ in the plasma cells of the tumor. Histologically, there were *lymphocytes,* plasma cells, and intermediate forms (features characteristic of immunocytoma).

**Gross Appearance.** The lymph nodes are usually only slightly to moderately enlarged. They are of the same consistency as the nodes in CLL, and, when sectioned, their fresh surface is gray-white.

**Histology.** Several publications have already dealt comprehensively with the histologic changes in the lymph nodes in macroglobulinemia of Waldenström.[310] These reports described mainly our first subtype, lymphoplasmacytic immunocytoma. For a description of the other subtypes we must depend on our own studies of the last few years.

In the lymphoplasmacytic and lymphoplasmacytoid subtypes the proliferation apparently begins in the pulp. In any event, we have examined cases in which the pulp was infiltrated, while the follicles and T-areas were nearly intact. There is usually a monotonous small-cell picture. It is somewhat less uniform only in the polymorphic subtype. In this subtype we cannot yet decide whether the proliferation actually begins in the pulp. In principle, the follicles could also be the site of origin. Several cases in our series revealed a great increase in epithelioid venules. That should not lead to the false conclusion that they are T-lymphocytic neoplasms. Sometimes there are epithelioid cells, either solitary or in small groups, but there are no epithelioid-cell granulomas (Fig. 101). An increase in mast cells is often observed (see p. 233). Occasionally, we found amyloid deposits, especially in the lymphoplasmacytic subtype (Fig. 102; see p. 247).

[308] JELLINGER, RADASZKIEWICZ and SLOWIK, 1975.

[309] HEENAN, MASON, SKINNER and TAYLOR, 1976.

[310] LENNERT, 1955, 1964a; LELBACH, 1957; RAPPAPORT, 1966; HARRISON, 1972.

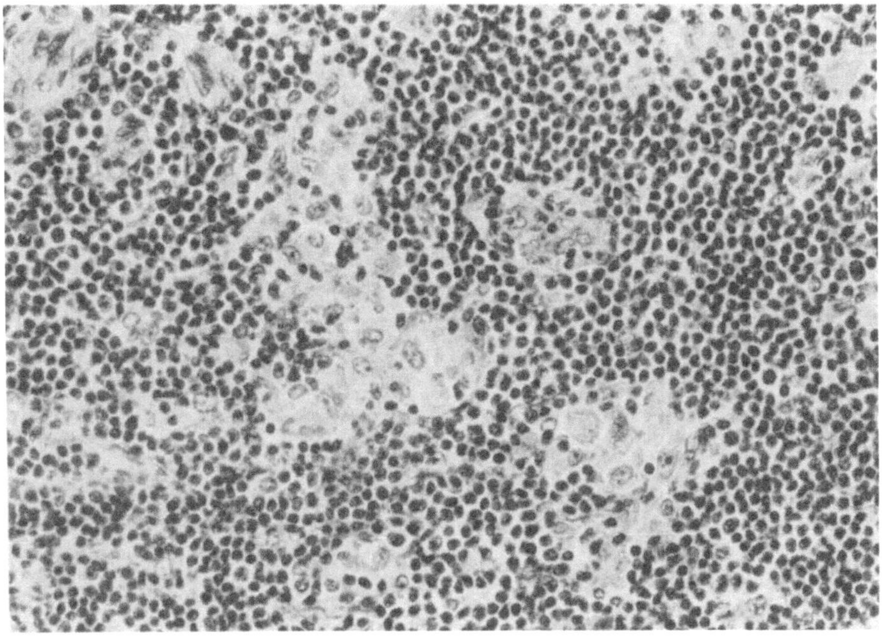

Fig. 101. Epithelioid-cell clusters in LP immunocytoma (lymphoplasmacytoid subtype). ♂, 46 years. Cervical node. Hematoxylin and eosin. ×350

### *a) Lymphoplasmacytic Subtype (Figs. 103 and 104)*

In this subtype of immunocytoma the lymph-node architecture and especially the pattern of reticulin fibers are often relatively well preserved. That holds true particularly for the sinuses, which are often well defined and sometimes markedly or extremely dilated (Fig. 105).[311] Occasionally, they contain inspissated lymph, which stains intensely PAS-positive ("protein lakes"[312]). Follicles are barely evident, if at all. The lymphatic parenchyma, as well as the capsule and adjacent regions around the lymph nodes, are infiltrated by neoplastic lymphocytes, among which a few to many typical Marschalkó plasma cells are found. Often these plasma cells form distinct aggregates. Immunoblasts or plasmablasts are less plentiful. Occasionally, one finds small foci of epithelioid cells with or without Langhans' giant cells. An increase in reticulum cells is not apparent. A pseudofollicular picture like that seen in B-CLL is found only very rarely; when it is evident, it is not pronounced. The number of mitotic figures is very low, as Harrison[313] proved in quantitative studies comparing these tumors with other types of malignant lymphoma. A proportion of the plasma cells often[314] or always[313] contain intranuclear PAS-positive inclusions

[311] Lennert, 1955; Haas and Knorre, 1956; Lelbach, 1957; Harrison, 1972.
[312] Lennert, 1955; Lelbach, 1957.
[313] Harrison, 1972.
[314] Krämer, 1971.

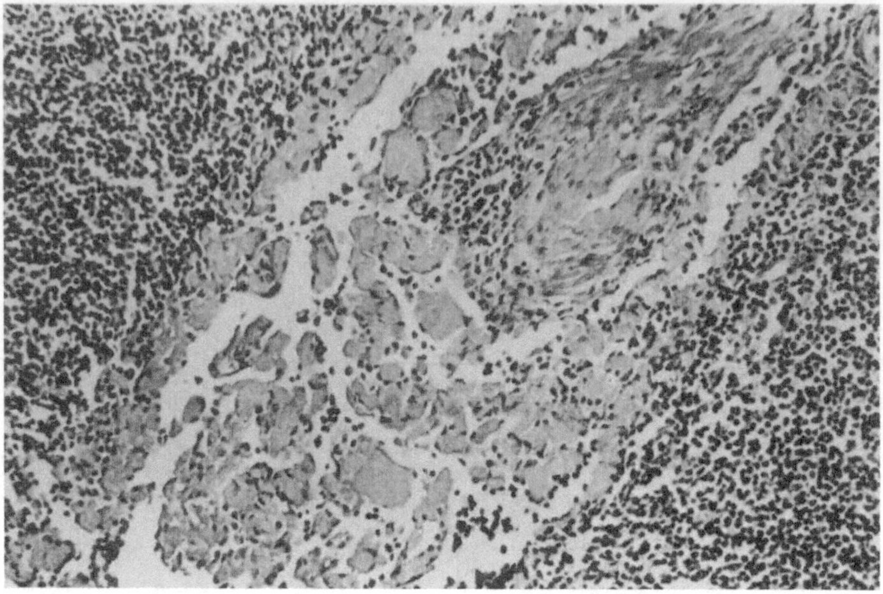

Fig. 102. Amyloid deposits in a dilated sinus in LP immunocytoma (lymphoplasmacytic subtype). ♂, 61 years. Axillary node. Congo red. ×350

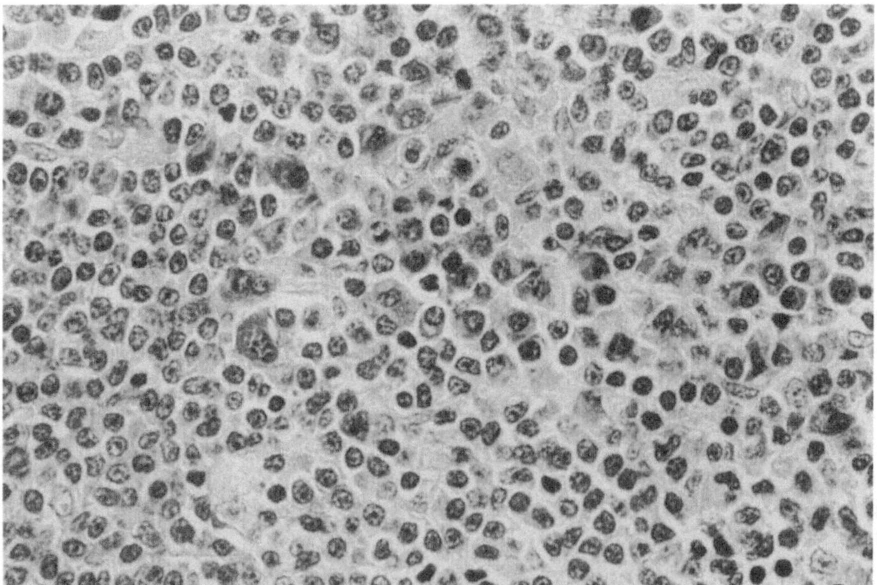

Fig. 103. LP immunocytoma, lymphoplasmacytic subtype. Typical, but pleomorphic Marschalkó plasma cells among lymphocytes. ♂, 66 years. Cervical node. Giemsa. ×560

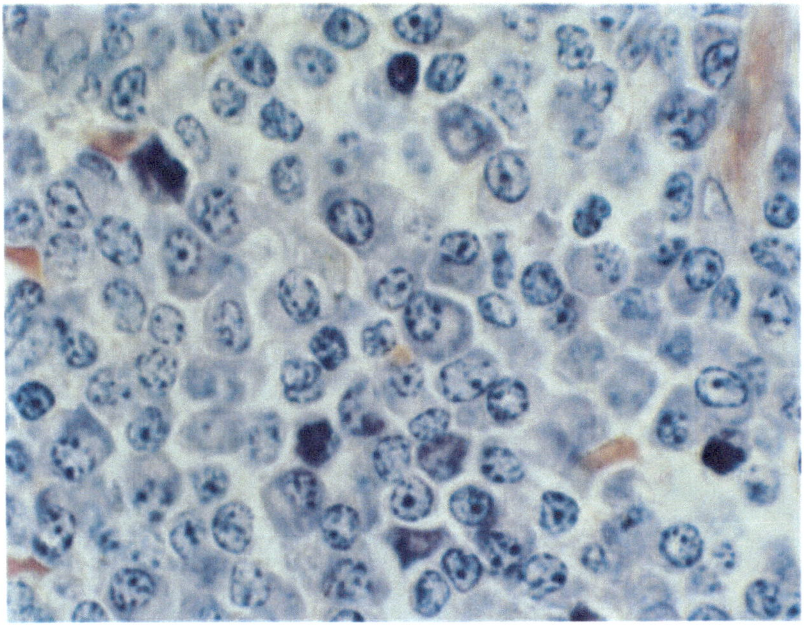

Fig. 104. LP immunocytoma, lymphoplasmacytic subtype, with Giemsa staining. Note typical Marschalkó plasma cells among lymphocytes. Same case as Fig. 103. ×1,550.

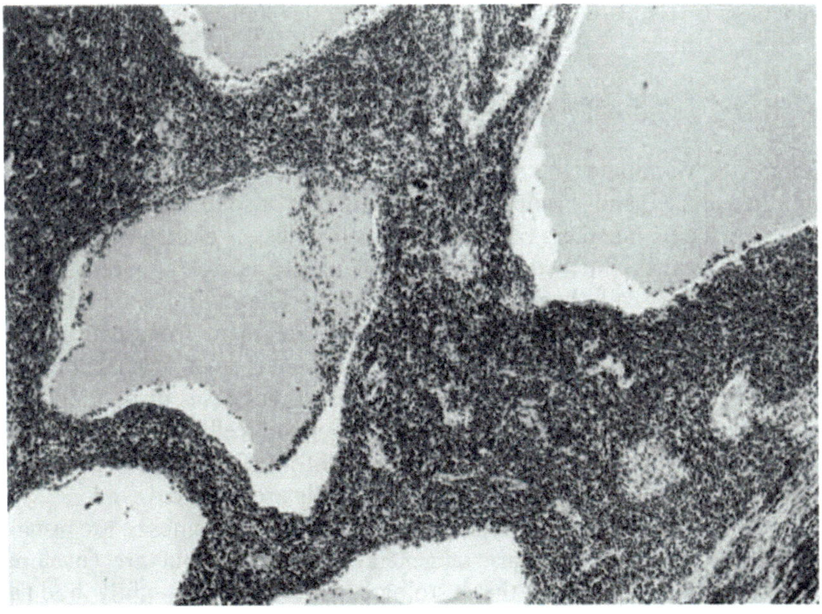

Fig. 105. LP immunocytoma, lymphoplasmacytic subtype. Cavernous dilatation of the sinuses. ♂, 65 years. Inguinal node. Clinically, the patient had macroglobulinemia of Waldenström. Hematoxylin and eosin. ×56

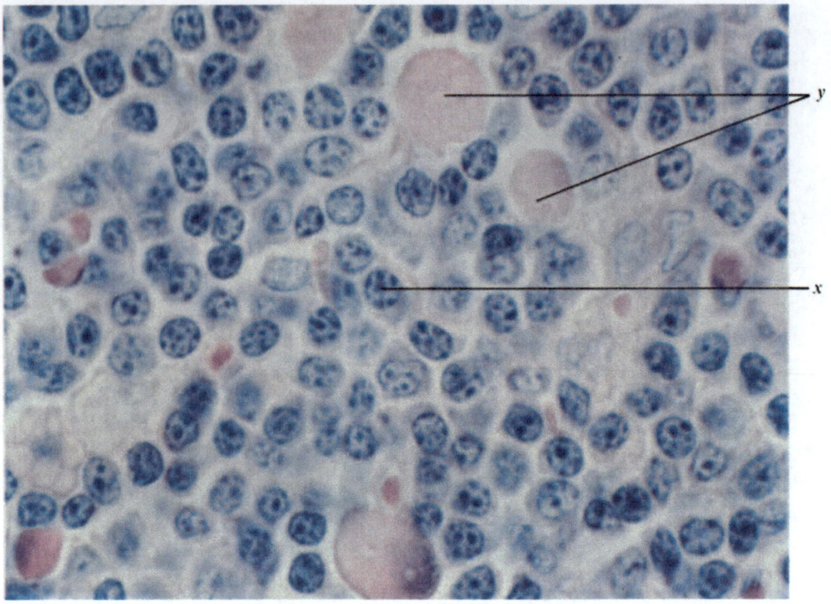


Fig. 106. LP immunocytoma, lymphoplasmacytoid subtype, with Giemsa staining. A few plasmacytoid cells ($x$) and some large Russell bodies ($y$) among lymphocytes. ♂, 69 years. Axillary node. ×1,550

or show a diffuse positive PAS reaction in the cytoplasm (see p. 235ff.). Hemosiderosis is frequently evident, especially in the sinuses.

### *b) Lymphoplasmacytoid Subtype (Fig. 106)*

Lymphocytes dominate the histologic picture, but *somewhat* larger cells with rounded nuclei and basophilic cytoplasm are also present. These cells can be interpreted as members of the plasma-cell series, as electron-microscopic studies have revealed. Since their plasma-cell nature is not apparent at first glance, we prefer to call them plasmacyt*oid* cells. The cytoplasm may be so scanty that it is virtually impossible to differentiate them from lymphocytes by means of light microscopy. When we use the Giemsa or, even better, the methyl-green pyronine stain, however, it is easier to make this distinction.

In addition to the lymphocytes and plasmacytoid cells one always finds at least some immunoblasts or plasmablasts. Mitotic figures are seen rarely or in moderate numbers. At times a few eosinophils are observed.

Certain differences from subtype (a) are evident. The sinuses are usually not preserved, or at least they are in general not dilated, but are enveloped by the infiltration. Sometimes the histologic pattern looks slightly nodular, and the nodular regions seem to contain few reticulin fibers, whereas the remaining lymphatic tissues appear to be replete with them.

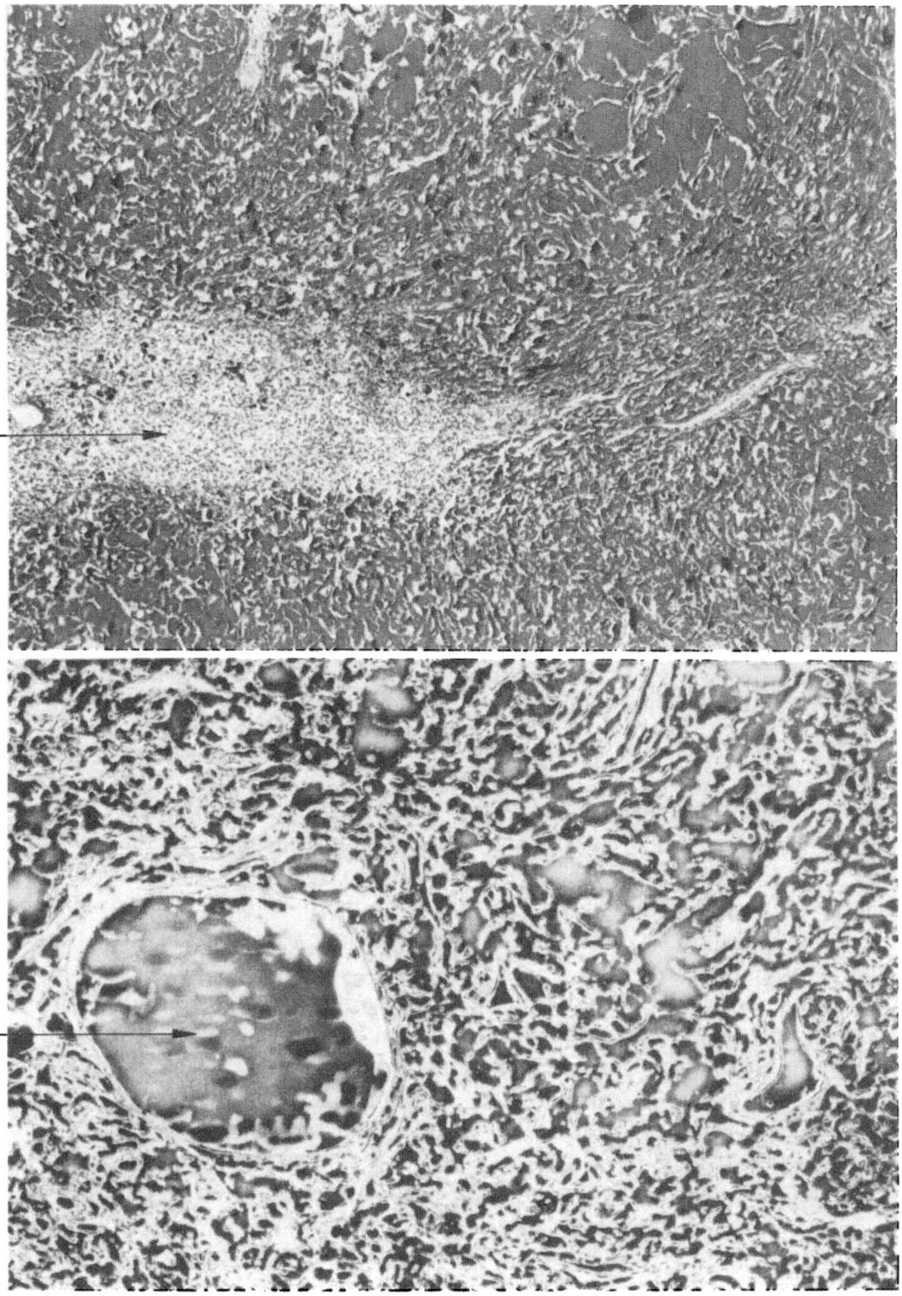

(a)

(b)

Fig. 107a and b. LP immunocytoma, lymphoplasmacytoid subtype. Protein masses, probably immunoglobulin, in the tumor. ♂, 64 years. Axillary node. (a) Only a small part of the section still shows remnants of tumor cells (arrow) with large PAS-positive Russell bodies. PAS. ×56. (b) The same node with Ladewig staining. The red-stained protein masses are situated among fibers and cells as well as in a dilated lymph vessel (arrow). ×140

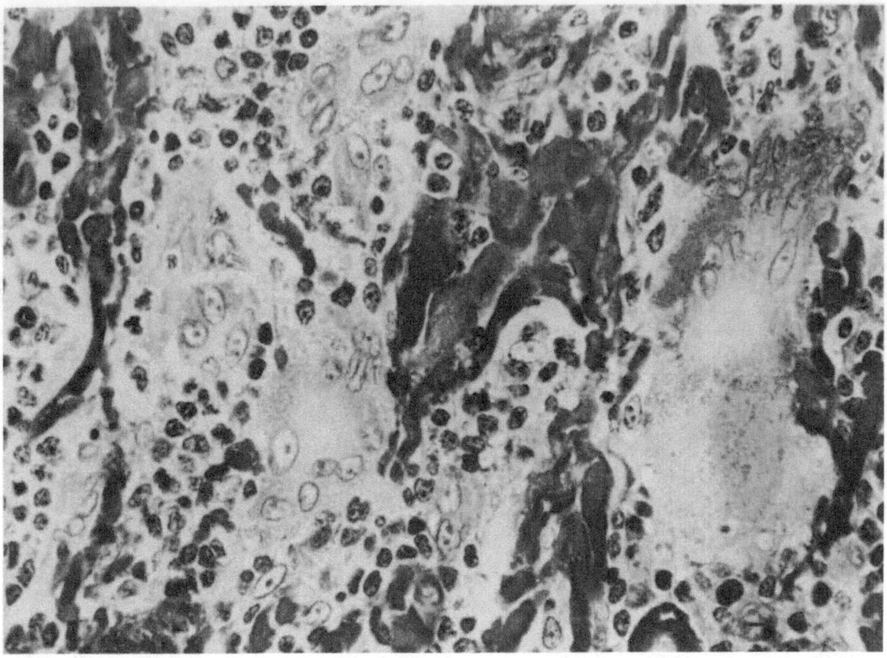

Fig. 108. LP immunocytoma, lymphoplasmacytoid subtype. Among the lymphocytes there are protein masses, probably immunoglobulin, apparently attacked by histiocytes and foreign-body giant cells. ♀, 70 years. Supraclavicular node. PAS. ×560

A pseudofollicular picture like that seen in CLL of the B-type is not uncommon. In such cases the clusters of proliferating cells include cells that are similar to those of CLL (prolymphocytes, "paraimmunoblasts"), sometimes intermingled with typical (strongly basophilic) immunoblasts and centroblasts. The borderline between these cases and the third, the polymorphic, subtype is therefore not very sharp.

In one case we found total necrosis of the infiltrated lymph node, an occasional, but characteristic finding in M.L. centroblastic/centrocytic.

A proportion of the lymphocytoid or plasmacytoid cells usually contain at least a few PAS-positive globular inclusions in the nuclei and/or cytoplasm. In several examples of this subtype of immunocytoma we found large numbers of cells with Russell body-like inclusions (Fig. 114). Sometimes these cells were so plentiful that they formed broad sheets. In a few of these tumors there were extensive extracellular deposits of protein that stained just like the intracellular deposits of immunoglobulin. In contrast, amyloid stains were negative. The protein deposits were found both in grossly dilated lymph channels and in the meshes of reticulin fibers (Fig. 107). Le Beux and Ganter[316] described a similar massive deposit of protein in a lymph node in macroglobulinemia. In one of our cases the immunoglobulin was definitely not IgM, however, since the protein masses stained red with Ladewig staining. In another case

[316] 1963.

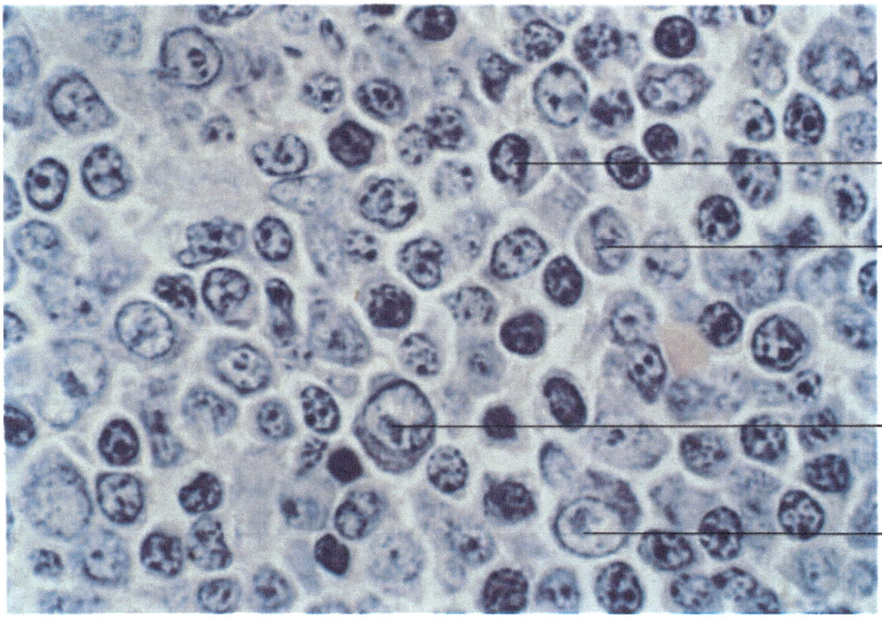


Fig. 109. LP immunocytoma, polymorphic subtype, with Giemsa staining. Large cells (immunoblasts; *ib*), medium-sized cells (proplasmacytes; *ppc*), plasma cells (*plc*), and lymphocytes. Note the polymorphism. ♀, 80 years. Supraclavicular node. ×1,750

we found abundant extracellular protein deposits as well as large histiocytes and foreign-body giant cells, which attacked the "paraprotein" (Fig. 108). In addition, there were some groups of epithelioid cells and occasional Langhans' giant cells.

### *c) Polymorphic Subtype (Figs. 109 and 110)*

Associated with the lymphocytes and plasmacytoid cells or plasma cells, there are still other cells that create a more variegated picture. In addition to immunoblasts and plasmablasts, there are often cells that fulfill all the morphologic criteria of centroblasts (multiple, medium-sized, membrane-associated nucleoli; narrow rim of basophilic cytoplasm) and centrocytes (cleaved nuclei). These centroblasts and centrocytes are often congregated in sheets and show EAC-rosette formation. There are also cells (centrocytes?) that resemble the cells of the marginal zone of splenic follicles ("marginal-zone cells" of KEUNING[317]). Finally, there are a number of lymphoid cells that are somewhat larger than typical small lymphocytes. Mitotic figures are more numerous than in subtypes (a) or (b).

PAS-positive protein inclusions in the neoplastic cells are generally demonstrable, but are not as conspicuous as in subtype (b). Diffuse PAS-positive staining of the cytoplasm is sometimes found in plasmacytoid cells.

[317] KEUNING and BOS, 1967.

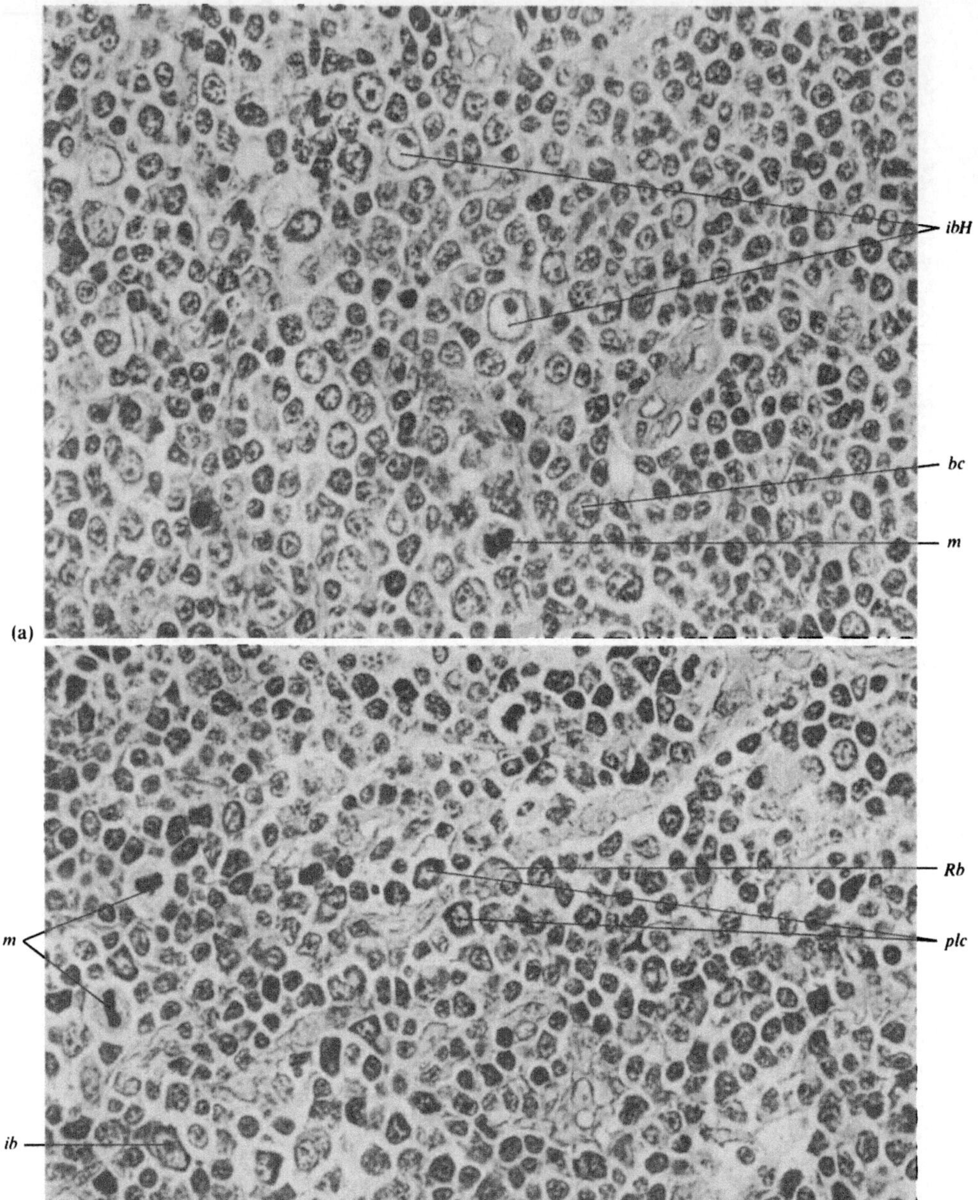


Fig. 110a and b. LP immunocytoma, polymorphic subtype. Polymorphic impression at first glance. Immunoblasts (*ib*), some giant immunoblasts resembling Hodgkin cells (*ibH*), medium-sized blast cell (*bc*), plasmacytoid cells (*plc*), plasma cell with globular cytoplasmic inclusions (Russell bodies; *Rb*), and numerous mitotic figures (*m*). ♀, 72 years. Axillary node. Giemsa. ×560

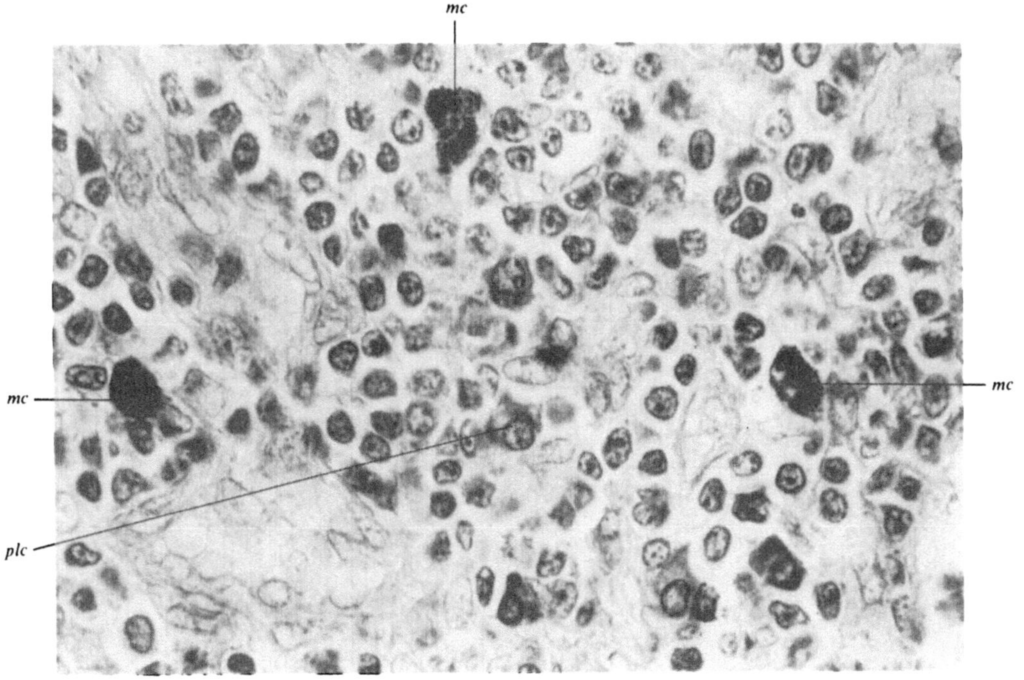


Fig. 111. Increase in mast cells (*mc*) in LP immunocytoma, lymphoplasmacytic subtype. Numerous lymphocytes and some Marschalkó plasma cells (*plc*). ♂, 73 years. Inguinal node. Giemsa. ×880

The reticulin-fiber pattern is usually diffuse; but sometimes it appears somewhat nodular, and thus, under low magnification, the histologic picture may be mistaken for a follicular lymphoma. Fully developed follicles, however, are not found. The nodular regions are either poor in fibers or devoid of them entirely, whereas the surrounding tissues and diffusely infiltrated parts are rich in fibers.

## *Mast Cells in LP Immunocytoma*

Many years ago, we showed that mast cells are unusually numerous in the lymph nodes in macroglobulinemia of Waldenström[318] (see Fig. 111), as had already been reported by TISCHENDORF and HARTMANN[319] in smears of bone marrow. More mast cells were found in this disease than in any other malignant lymphoma. That was confirmed by HARRISON.[320] We must now examine whether it is also true for all immunocytomas, irrespective of the morphologic subtype. SATODATE *et al.*[321] estimated the number of mast cells in Giemsa-stained sections from 58 cases of immunocytoma and compared them with 34 cases of CLL. The results are given in Fig. 112. They found more than four mast cells per

[318] LENNERT and ILLERT, 1959.
[319] 1950.
[320] 1972.
[321] SATODATE, SCHWARZE and LENNERT, 1977.

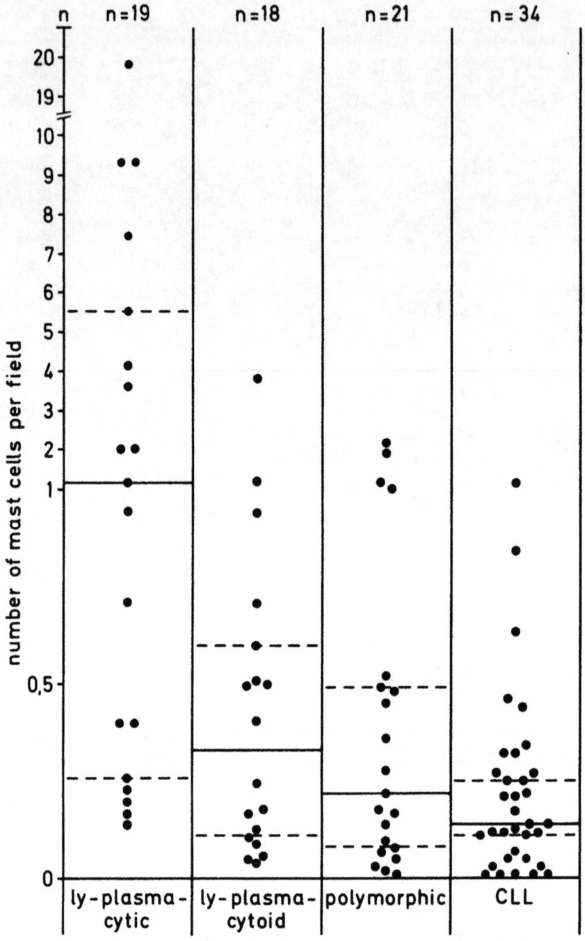


Fig. 112. Number of mast cells in LP immunocytoma (lymphoplasmacytic, lymphoplasmacytoid, and polymorphic subtypes) and B-CLL, determined with ×25 objective and ×10 ocular. The horizontal solid lines indicate the median values; the dashed lines, the 3$\sigma$ deviation. The U-test of WILCOXON[322] and MANN and WHITNEY[323] (two-sided, $\alpha = 0.05$) showed that the difference between the median values for the lymphoplasmacytic and lymphoplasmacytoid subtypes of immunocytoma and that for CLL was significant, whereas the difference between the values for the polymorphic subtype and CLL was not significant. (Cf., SATODATE *et al.*[324])

field (determined at a magnification of ×312) only in the lymphoplasmacytic subtype. The median value was 1.14 mast cells per field. This value was significantly higher than those for the other subtypes of immunocytoma and for CLL. There was not such a great difference between the values for the lymphoplasmacytoid and polymorphic subtypes and those for CLL. Another finding was that the number of mast cells appeared to be roughly correlated with the amount of IgM, which STEIN demonstrated in tissue homogenates of the lymphomas he studied.

[322] 1945.

[323] 1947.

[324] SATODATE, SCHWARZE and LENNERT, 1977.

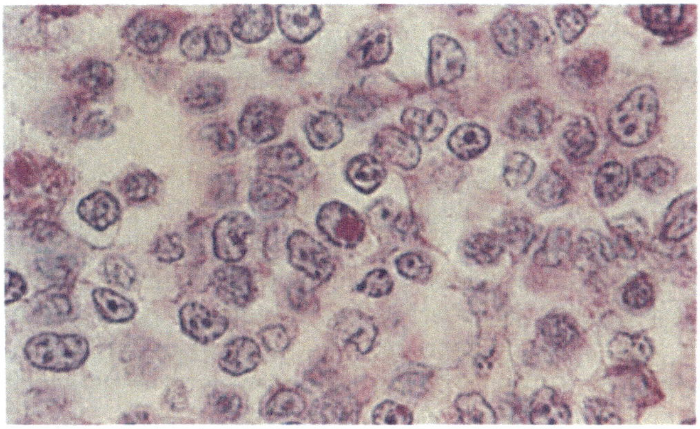

Fig. 113. Intranuclear PAS-positive inclusion in LP immunocytoma with μ-chain disease. ♂, 43 years. Cervical node. PAS. × 1,000

Therefore, a great increase in mast cells is a good indicator of lymphoplasmacytic immunocytoma, especially if large amounts of IgM are produced. Apparently, that does not hold true for the other subtypes, in which the number of mast cells is not significantly greater than in CLL.

The mast cells are usually large and highly metachromatic with Giemsa staining (and also with toluidine blue staining). Sometimes there are immature, smaller forms with sparse, light reddish-violet granules. These cells are more easily recognized in the chloroacetate esterase reaction, but should not be confused with precursors of neutrophils.

### *Globular PAS-Positive Inclusions in the Nucleus and Cytoplasm*

One of the most important morphologic characteristics of immunocytoma is the presence of globular PAS-positive inclusions in the lymphoid, plasmacytic, or plasmacytoid cells, a property previously described as protein inclusions in plasmacytomas of the bone marrow[325] and also frequently in macroglobulinemia.[326] Evidence of these inclusions in the nuclei of the cells mentioned has great diagnostic importance (Fig. 113). On the other hand, the presence of PAS-positive globules in the reticulum cells and histiocytes scattered here and there is of no diagnostic significance. Great care is needed always to insure that the PAS-positive inclusions are located within cells of the lymphoplasmacytic series.

One of us (N.M.) studied 184 cases of immunocytoma for globular PAS-positive inclusions and found them in 56% of the tumors. This figure is perhaps somewhat too low, however, for not only must one search long and hard for them, but the protein inclusions are sometimes very small. Consequently, when looking for them, we like to use the high-power oil-immersion lens in order to make

[325] APITZ, 1937b; BRASS, 1943a, b, 1947/48.

[326] SCHAMAUN, 1954; LELBACH, 1957; BRITTIN, TANAKA and BRECHER, 1963; HARRISON, 1972; DIEBOLD, REYNES, KALIFAT and TRICOT, 1974.

certain of PAS-positivity in doubtful cases. Since even a few cells showing a positive PAS reaction represent the strictest histologic criterion for distinguishing an immunocytoma from CLL, the time spent in searching for PAS-positive inclusions is well worth it.

When we examine the subtypes for the frequency of PAS positivity, we find that the lymphoplasmacytic subtype has the highest rate, with 73.7% positive cases. The polymorphic subtype is second with 57.4%, and the lymphoplasmacytoid subtype has the lowest rate of 52.5%, although the reaction is strongest in this type. We have in our present collection three lymphoplasmacytoid tumors and four others from an earlier series that contained extraordinary numbers of PAS-positive cells. In these tumors the PAS-positive cells were so numerous that they dominated the histologic picture in large parts of the slide. Since the nucleus and cytoplasm were often barely visible or had already disintegrated, certain cases revealed only masses of red globular structures in hematoxylin and eosin- or Giemsa-stained slides. Such structures puzzle the uninitiated. Usually, however, the globular PAS-positive inclusions were sparse (in 47.8% of the cases) or moderately plentiful (in 6.5% of the cases) in the lymphoplasmacytoid subtype.

The globular inclusions were found in the nucleus and/or cytoplasm. The intranuclear inclusions are of particular diagnostic significance. They may lie in the center or more at the periphery of the nucleus. They frequently reveal a light corona, which sets off the PAS-positive substance against the chromatin. According to electron-microscopic findings, the nuclear inclusions are formed because of synthesis and accumulation of immunoglobulin in the perinuclear space, which then expands and makes a dent in the nucleus. As far as we know, no one has proved the second possibility, namely, that the nucleus is invaginated by cytoplasm that contains rough endoplasmic reticulum showing secretory activity. When large globules form in the nucleus, they may ultimately cause it to burst, destroying it.

The intracytoplasmic inclusions can be solitary or multiple. They range in size from very small ("granular") to very large, filling almost the entire cell.

The cells with globular PAS-positive inclusions are congregated remarkably often in the sinuses, especially the marginal sinus, and in the connective tissue of the adjacent capsule.

That the globular PAS-positive inclusions represent retained immunoglobulin is supported by the results of many studies. The inclusions are diastase-resistant and do not diminish during processing for paraffin embedding. On electron microscopy they correspond to protein precipitates.[327] By means of immunofluorescent techniques they can also be identified as immunoglobulin.[328]

In addition, the cells of immunocytoma may contain intracytoplasmic, finely globular or dust-like deposits of PAS-positive material that are also resistant to paraffin embedding, but actually represent glycogen. KAISERLING was able to prove this repeatedly in electron-microscopic studies of our tumors.

The PAS-positive globules mostly represent IgM. In some tumors we were able to show that the globules consisted of 8 S IgM monomer. In several

[327] MORI and LENNERT, 1969; STEIN, KAISERLING, LENNERT and PARWARESCH, 1973.

[328] DIEBOLD, REYNES, KALIFAT and TRICOT, 1974.

Table 36. Staining properties of PAS-positive and PAS-negative immunoglobulin deposits

| Substance | PAS | Goldner (Masson) | Ladewig (Mallory) |
|---|---|---|---|
| IgG | + | Red | Red |
| IgA | + | Red | Red |
| IgM (19 S and 8 S) | + | Green | Blue |
| Light chains and other Ig fragments | – | Red | Red |

of these tumors the deposits were extremely abundant. We could demonstrate IgG/κ in one of the PAS-positive tumors, which was associated with a leukemic blood picture. Retained IgA also gives a positive PAS reaction, as we know from studies of IgA plasmacytoma.[329] Furthermore, retained proteins in μ-chain disease show a positive PAS reaction (see p. 259ff.).

When the PAS-positive globules are abundant, it is certainly worth the effort to try to determine with staining methods what type of immunoglobulin is present. For such studies Ladewig's modification of Mallory's connective-tissue stain and the modified Masson trichrome stain according to Goldner are of some value (Table 36; Fig. 114). With the Ladewig and Goldner methods IgM stains gray-blue or green, respectively. Only occasional cells take on a reddish hue (light chains?). In addition, 8 S IgM (IgM monomer) and μ-chains stain like the 19 S pentamer of macroglobulin. In contrast, deposits of IgG and IgA usually stain orange-red to bright crimson with both methods. Retained light chains and other incomplete components of immunoglobulin may take on the same colors. In such cases, however, the PAS reaction of the globular deposits may be negative. PAS-negative protein deposits may be found in the nucleus and/or cytoplasm, for example, in so-called Bence-Jones myeloma. They also occur in various immunocytomas because of disturbances in Ig secretion that are not yet fully understood.

PAS-positive, intranuclear inclusions are by no means specific to immunocytoma and plasmacytoma. They can be found as well in other types of malignant lymphoma,[330] for example, in M.L. centroblastic/centrocytic,[331] and in plasma cells of nonmalignant diseases.[332]

The biologic significance of the intranuclear inclusions is generally thought to lie in a disturbance of secretion. Diebold *et al.*[333] believe that it is possible that an initial, abnormally rapid secretion might cause the disturbance.

In rare instances the PAS-positive substances are detected as crystalline deposits. We saw this type of reaction in an immunocytoma that had produced IgG/κ. In addition to the crystalline deposits, however, there were some large PAS-positive globules resembling Russell bodies. With the immunoperoxidase

[329] Brittin, Tanaka and Brecher, 1963; Krämer, 1971; Diebold, Reynes, Kalifat and Tricot, 1975.

[330] Lennert, Stein and Kaiserling, 1975.

[331] Rappaport and Johnson, 1955.

[332] Harrison, 1972; Kim, Heller and Rappaport, 1973; Diebold, Reynes, Kalifat and Tricot, 1974.

[333] Diebold, Reynes, Kalifat and Tricot, 1974.

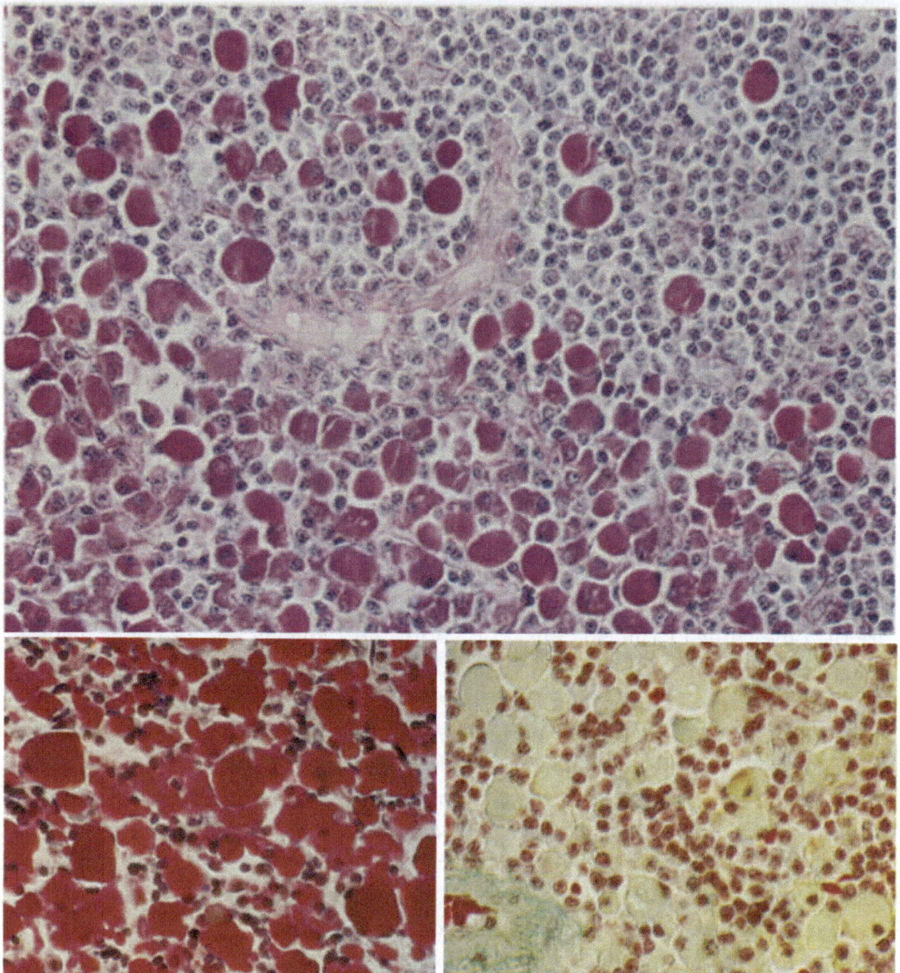

(a) (b) (c)

Fig. 114a–c. PAS-positive globules (Russell bodies) in LP immunocytoma, lymphoplasmacytoid subtype. (a) ♀, 74 years. Inguinal node. Increase in IgM in tissue. PAS. ×350. (b) With Goldner staining, (PAS-positive) globules are red. ♀, 40 years. Abdominal node. Monoclonal increase in IgG/κ in blood serum. ×350. (c) With Goldner staining, (PAS-positive) globules are green and thus represent IgM inclusions. Same node as (a). ×350

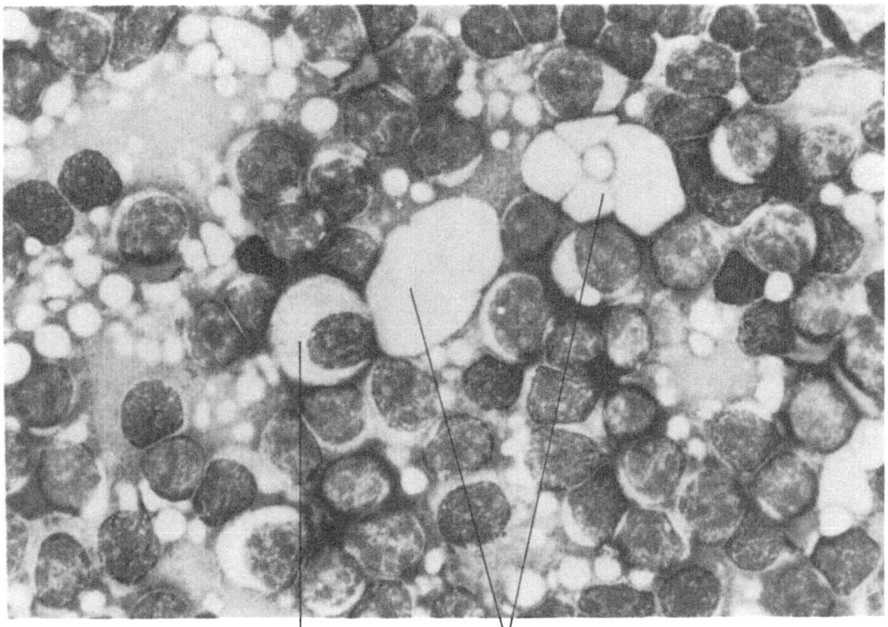


Fig. 115. LP immunocytoma, lymphoplasmacytoid subtype, in imprint. Numerous lymphocytes. Two immunoglobulin deposits, corresponding to the large globules (Russell bodies; *x*) in the section. Plasmacytoid cell with foamy cytoplasm (*plc*). Same node as Fig. 107. Pappenheim. ×875

technique the crystalline deposits were positive for $\gamma$- and $\kappa$-chains, whereas the globular inclusions were negative.[333a]

At times, plasma cells stain *diffusely* to a slight or moderate degree. Only rarely are they strongly positive. Such diffuse staining suggests, however, marked synthesis of immunoglobulin and serves as another aid in the diagnosis of immunocytoma.

**Smear/Imprint.** The cytologic picture seen in the *lymphoplasmacytic* subtype is like that described for the lymph nodes in Waldenström's disease.[334] The predominant cells are small lymphocytes and somewhat larger, round lymphoid cells, which were erroneously referred to in years past as lymphoid reticulum cells. Scattered here and there among them are a few typical "reticular" plasma cells and some plasmablasts and immunoblasts. Occasionally, some of the plasma cells contain Russell bodies; these globular deposits of protein stain light gray-blue and often deform the nucleus. There is also an increase in mast cells and blood basophils in many cases.

In the *lymphoplasmacytoid* subtype (Fig. 115), by virtue of their relatively scanty, although distinctly basophilic cytoplasm, the plasmacytoid cells can be distinguished from the typical lymphocytes in imprints easier than in sections. In addition, there are lymphocytic cells that are somewhat larger or medium-

[333a] Fuchs, unpublished data. [334] Lelbach, 1957.

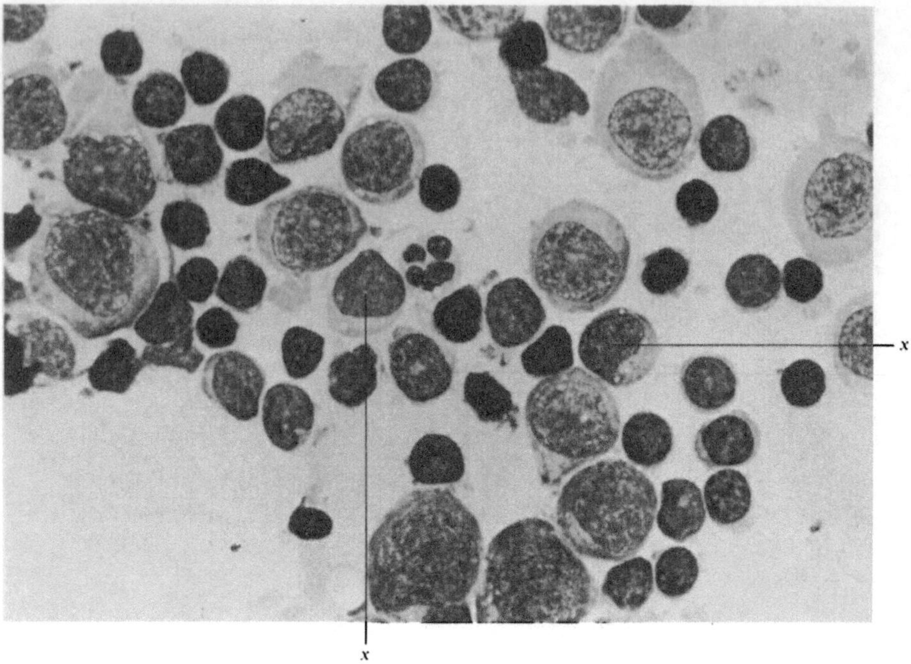


Fig. 116. LP immunocytoma, polymorphic subtype, in imprint. Medium-sized and large basophilic cells of the plasma-cell series. Some plasmacytoid cells (*x*). Numerous lymphocytes. ♀, 48 years. Supraclavicular node. Increase in IgM in tissue homogenate and blood. Pappenheim. ×875

sized and contain a fairly broad rim of gray-blue cytoplasm. The reduced basophilia of the cytoplasm readily sets them apart from the dark blue plasmablasts and immunoblasts. In some cases one finds abundant plasmacytoid cells with a broad basophilic rim of cytoplasm containing large vacuoles or droplets.

Imprints of the *polymorphic* subtype present a remarkably variegated picture (Fig. 116). In addition to the lymphocytes and plasmacytoid forms, there are polymorphic cells of medium size. Some of these cells fulfill the criteria for centroblasts; some, the criteria for plasmablasts or immunoblasts. It is usually impossible to classify them precisely. Among these cells there are great numbers of lymphoid cells, which are distinctly larger than lymphocytes. They reveal a very narrow rim of gray cytoplasm and sometimes an indented nucleus (centrocytes).

**Histochemistry and Cytochemistry.** The PAS reaction in sections is discussed on page 235 ff. Detailed cytochemical studies of imprints have yet to be made. An important finding is that small, medium-sized, and large cells can reveal slight to moderately strong, diffuse PAS positivity or an intranuclear or intracytoplasmic globular reaction. That is helpful in establishing the diagnosis. Furthermore, in imprints the lymphoid cells reveal a granular acid phosphatase reaction, as in some cases of M.L. centroblastic/centrocytic. The acid and neutral nonspecific esterase reactions are weakly positive and diffuse in plasma cells.

Table 37. Diagnostic criteria of LP immunocytoma

1. Age ≈ B-CLL
2. Three clinical types:
   a) lymph-node type
   b) splenomegalic type
   c) oculocutaneous type
3. Leukemia ≧ 1/3 of cases
4. Sometimes autoimmune hemolytic anemia
5. Paraproteinemia in about 20% of cases, most frequently IgM
6. Sometimes Bence-Jones proteinuria, even when decrease in corresponding Ig in blood
7. Predominant cells always lymphocytes
8. Always some or a moderate number of plasmacytoid cells or plasma cells
9. Always some immunoblasts
10. In polymorphic type: many immunoblasts, often centroblasts and centrocytes in addition to (7) and (8)
11. Mast cells increased in number
12. Diffuse diastase-resistant PAS positivity or globular inclusions in nuclei or cytoplasm of plasmacytoid or plasma cells
13. Occasionally paramyloidosis

**Diagnosis.** For the diagnosis of lymphoplasma*cytoid* and polymorphic immunocytoma, a Giemsa stain or methyl-green pyronine stain is indispensable. The lymphoplasma*cytic* subtype can usually be recognized in a hematoxylin and eosin-stained slide. The PAS reaction has great diagnostic importance.

The diagnosis is based on both the clinical data and the following histologic features (Table 37):

1. The predominant type of cell is a small (or slightly enlarged) lymphocyte.

2. Besides lymphocytes, one can always find typical Marschalkó plasma cells or plasmacytoid cells. A few plasma-cell precursors (immunoblasts, plasmablasts) are always present as well.

3. In addition to the cells already mentioned, the polymorphic subtype abounds with germinal-center cells (some centroblasts, numerous centrocytes), plasmablasts, and immunoblasts.

4. Mast cells can be more plentiful in LP immunocytoma than in any other type of malignant lymphoma.

5. In many cases the PAS reaction reveals at least a few globular diastase-resistant inclusions. The intranuclear inclusions are of particular diagnostic importance, although they are not specific.

6. In the lymphoplasmacytic subtype the pattern of the reticulin fibers is hardly changed, but the sinuses are often dilated. In the lymphoplasmacytoid and polymorphic subtypes the fiber pattern is destroyed; occasionally, nodular fiber-poor and diffuse fiber-rich regions appear side by side. In most cases, however, the growth pattern is completely diffuse without any nodularity.

7. Localized (or generalized) amyloid deposits favor the diagnosis of LP immunocytoma.

**Differential Diagnosis.** The most important disease to be considered in the differential diagnosis of LP immunocytoma (all histologic subtypes) is B-CLL

Table 38. Differential diagnosis of LP immunocytoma/B-CLL

| Morphology | LP immuncytoma | B-CLL |
|---|---|---|
| Pseudofollicular pattern | Often − | Mostly + |
| Plasma cells or plasmacytoid cells | ± to ++ | − |
| Plasmablasts/immunoblasts | + | − (paraimmunoblasts) |
| Centroblasts, centrocytes | Mostly −, in polymorphic type sometimes + | − |
| Mast cells | Often increased | Normal or subnormal number |
| Globular PAS+protein in nucleus and/or cytoplasm | Mostly ± to +++ | − |
| Cavernous sinus dilatation | Occasionally + | − |
| Amyloid deposits | Occasionally + | − |

(see Table 38). Although many of the criteria listed in the table possess only a certain degree of probability, a few data are essential. The lymph node in CLL contains neither neoplastic plasma cells or plasmacytoid cells, nor definite immunoblasts (plasmablasts) or germinal-center cells. The neoplastic cells never reveal globular, PAS-positive, intranuclear inclusions. CLL usually presents a pseudofollicular picture, which develops less frequently in immunocytoma. Therefore, a monotonously diffuse type of growth is, from the first, suggestive of immunocytoma. When there is a pseudofollicular pattern of CLL and when there are typical plasma cells, the plasma cells usually have to be interpreted as reactive. An increase in mast cells definitely suggests immunocytoma, especially the lymphoplasmacytic subtype. Extreme sinus dilatation and amyloid deposits occur only in LP immunocytoma.

Borderline cases between CLL and immunocytoma that are difficult to classify will be discussed below. In addition, there are borderline cases to germinal-center tumors. That is particularly true for the *polymorphic subtype* of immunocytoma. The latter should not be confused with lymph-node reactions that contain numerous plasma cells and plasma-cell precursors, in particular with lymph-node lesions of infectious mononucleosis. The number of strongly basophilic cells and of mitotic figures is, as a rule, much larger, and the histologic picture is usually much more polymorphic in infectious mononucleosis. Typical lymphocytes may show maximal reduction in infectious mononucleosis, whereas they always constitute the majority of cells in immunocytoma. Moreover, in infectious mononucleosis, the sinuses often contain accumulations of basophilic cells. In contrast, the sinuses are narrow or unrecognizable in polymorphic immunocytoma. We have not seen intranuclear PAS-positive inclusions in infectious mononucleosis.

The polymorphic subtype is often misinterpreted as Hodgkin's disease. The large basophilic cells (immunoblasts) can be distinguished from typical Hodgkin and Sternberg-Reed cells in Giemsa-stained slides, however, by the more intense basophilia of the cytoplasm and nucleoli, by the strongly stained nuclear membrane, and by the strongly stained and thus clearly identifiable chromatin.

Furthermore, in polymorphic immunocytoma there is neither marked sclerosis nor infiltration by eosinophils.

A false diagnosis of acute myeloid leukemia may result from the use of the chloroacetate esterase reaction. That happened to us in a case of LP immunocytoma with numerous immature mast cells, which were not recognizable in Giemsa-stained slides, but revealed a positive chloroacetate esterase reaction.

**Development into a High-Grade Malignant Lymphoma ("Sarcomatous" Transformation).** In addition to the 268 cases listed in Table 30, we have studied 11 cases that were regarded as transitional forms into blastic "sarcoma." Two of these tumors were associated with increased levels of immunoglobulin (IgM or IgG) in the blood. Five cases were leukemic. Histologically, there was a particularly large number of large basophilic cells (immunoblasts, plasmablasts, centroblasts), so that the general impression went beyond the picture of the polymorphic subtype, with a larger number of large cells and greater basophilia. Intermingled with them, however, were relatively abundant lymphocytes and plasma cells or plasmacytoid cells. Twice we were able to follow the development of an immunocytoma into such a transitional form. In one patient the transitional form evolved further into a pure immunoblastic "sarcoma" (M.L. immunoblastic).

Thus, we see that an immunocytoma may evolve into a *fully developed blastic "sarcoma."* In four cases we saw this picture in the initial lymph-node biopsy, and in five cases in a later biopsy from patients previously diagnosed as having typical LP immunocytoma. The sarcomatous components or the final sarcoma consisted entirely of medium-sized to large, intensely basophilic cells. These cells usually resembled immunoblasts or plasmablasts. In one of our leukemic cases the clinical picture changed into a fulminant one 6 weeks before death. The patient had gigantic lymph-node masses, there was a monotonous plasmablastic morphology of the infiltrates, and hyperbasophilic blast cells were seen in the blood ("plasmablastic leukemia," "immunoblastic leukemia"). Once we also found centroblast-like sarcoma cells. In an autopsied case the cells were quite small and looked more like anaplastic centrocytes. In another autopsied case the classic picture of LP immunocytoma with macroglobulinemia and abundant Russell bodies in sections was followed by blastic sarcoma without Russell bodies and without continuation of the macroglobulinemia. Similar cases were observed by WALDENSTRÖM himself[335] and by other authors.[336] About 3.6% of our immunocytomas underwent change into a fully developed blastic malignant lymphoma ("sarcoma"). Transitional forms between immunocytoma and blastic sarcoma constituted 3.9% of the immunocytomas in our material.

**Borderline Cases and Extreme Variants.** Immunocytoma always consists of at least three types of cells: lymphocytes, plasma cells or plasmacytoid cells, and some immunoblasts. In the polymorphic subtype there are numerous immunoblasts and there may also be relatively abundant centroblasts and centrocytes. When one of the cell components just mentioned appears to be exceptionally

[335] 1968; 1970, personal communication. [336] BÖSKEN and NOLTENIUS, 1968.

numerous or even to dominate the picture, this may be regarded as a borderline case between immunocytoma and another low-grade malignant lymphoma.

In the first type of extreme case lymphocytes occur practically alone, and the question arises as to whether the tumor might really be *B-CLL*. Plasma cells in small numbers are easily overlooked in hematoxylin and eosin-stained sections, and even with Giemsa staining. We can identify them only at a high magnification. The methyl-green pyronine stain, however, makes it possible to quickly identify even minimal numbers of plasma cells by their bright red cytoplasm. With the immunoperoxidase technique of TAYLOR, plasma cells can also be identified more easily than in routinely stained sections. Only when the intracytoplasmic Ig has one light chain and one heavy chain (or two heavy chains), i.e., when it is monoclonal, may the plasma cells be interpreted as part of the neoplasm and not as reactive. This interpretation can be substantiated by comparing the intracytoplasmic Ig in the plasma cells with the surface Ig on lymphocytes in the tumor. If the heavy and light chains are the same in both types of cell, then one may assume that the plasma cells belong to the same tumor-cell clone as the lymphocytes, and a diagnosis of LP immunocytoma is therefore justified.

In contrast to typical plasma cells, plasma*cytoid* cells should always be interpreted as components of LP immunocytoma. In some cases it is extremely difficult to identify them. Here, we find the PAS reaction and electron microscopy of diagnostic help. If PAS-positive globules are found in the cytoplasm and particularly in the nuclei of the "lymphocytes," we feel justified in diagnosing immunocytoma, even when no definite plasmacytoid cells can be demonstrated by light microscopy. In such cases electron-microscopic study usually reveals that some of the "lymphocytes" contain relatively abundant rough endoplasmic reticulum, so that the plasmacytoid nature of the cells can be confirmed.

In the second type of extreme case, plasma cells prevail in such great numbers that one tends to assume a *plasma-cell neoplasm* ("lymphatic" plasma-cell leukemia, see pp. 250 and 279). We observed two such cases with a monoclonal increase in IgM in the blood and a leukemic blood picture (see p. 250f.). These cases showed an increase in small, strongly basophilic plasma cells and their precursors in the blood and tissue. Typical lymphocytes did not belong to the neoplasm. These tumors must be differentiated from the plasma-cell leukemias of the bone marrow, i.e., the leukemic equivalents of multiple myeloma, which we call "reticular" plasma-cell leukemias. In the latter type of leukemia, the plasma cells have a somewhat broader rim of cytoplasm and are also larger; plasmablasts do not occur.

In rare cases the distinction between immunocytoma and plasmacytoma is not clear. There are lymphoplasmacytic immunocytomas in which typical plasma cells containing many Russell bodies are so numerous that, at first glance, the tumors may be mistaken for plasmacytomas. Plasmacytoma, however, does not contain lymphocytes. Even a small number of lymphocytes, together with some immunoblasts, lead us to classify the lymphoma in the group of immunocytomas.

In the third type of extreme case there can be a *follicular centroblastic/centro-*

*cytic lymphoma* that reveals marked proliferation of plasma cells in the follicles and/or in the lymphatic tissue between them. At the same time, the tumor cells may contain more or less abundant PAS-positive globules.

We have seen the following variants of this type:

Cases I and II presented the picture of a follicular centroblastic/centrocytic lymphoma, in which the follicles themselves contained sheets of "Russell bodies." In one of the tumors the PAS-positive globules were red with the Goldner stain and therefore probably represented IgG or IgA. A paraprotein was found in the patient's blood, but it could not be clearly defined.

Cases III and IV were partly follicular, partly diffuse centroblastic/centrocytic lymphomas with sclerosis and also revealed extreme plasmacytosis of the interfollicular lymphatic tissue with many PAS-positive inclusions, as well as a monoclonal increase in IgM in the blood.

Case V was a nodular lymphoma, which—similar to nodular paragranuloma—consisted of large, closely packed nodules (Figs. 117 and 118). They were bounded by fibers, but contained few fibers themselves. Morphologically, the nodules were somewhat reminiscent of the progressively transformed germinal centers seen in reactive hyperplasia of lymph nodes, but they did not contain as many lymphocytes.

The predominant cells in case IV were centrocytes with a relatively wide rim of cytoplasm and often round or merely indented nuclei. There were also some typical centroblasts and a small number of very plump histiocytic reticulum cells (electron microscopy also revealed dendritic reticulum cells; see p. 509). Small to medium-sized centrocyte-like cells were gathered in the inner parts of the nodules. The cytoplasm of these cells exhibited moderately strong, diffuse PAS positivity. The PAS-positive material appeared to make some dents in the nuclei (Fig. 118a). When the nucleus was indented on only one side, it had a reniform contour; when the nucleus was indented on many sides, it had a bizarre contour. The nuclei showed small nucleoli and relatively fine chromatin. They were hardly reminiscent of nuclei of plasma cells. Now and then, the centrocyte-like cells contained strongly PAS-positive globules. We occasionally found ghost cells of such diffusely PAS-positive cells. Among the cells there were often abundant oval or round extracellular bodies that were somewhat smaller than erythrocytes and that revealed strong PAS positivity. With Goldner and Ladewig stains the PAS-positive material, both inside and outside the cells, was not stained red, indicating that it was IgM. In fact, Stein demonstrated 350 times the normal amount of IgM in tissue homogenates, but found no monoclonal increase in serum IgM. In imprints (Fig. 118b), besides typical centroblasts and less typical centrocytes, we found some small to medium-sized centrocyte-like cells with a deep gray-blue rim of cytoplasm that was wider on one side. Occasionally, a poorly outlined reddish-violet streak or fleck was observed at the periphery of the cytoplasm. The tint and the appearance of the red-violet deposits was reminiscent of the so-called flaming plasma cells described in the hematologic literature. The nuclei of the cells with and without cytoplasmic inclusions were round, oval, or indented, and had fine chromatin and apparently no nucleoli. We consider these cells to be centrocytes with certain plasmacytoid

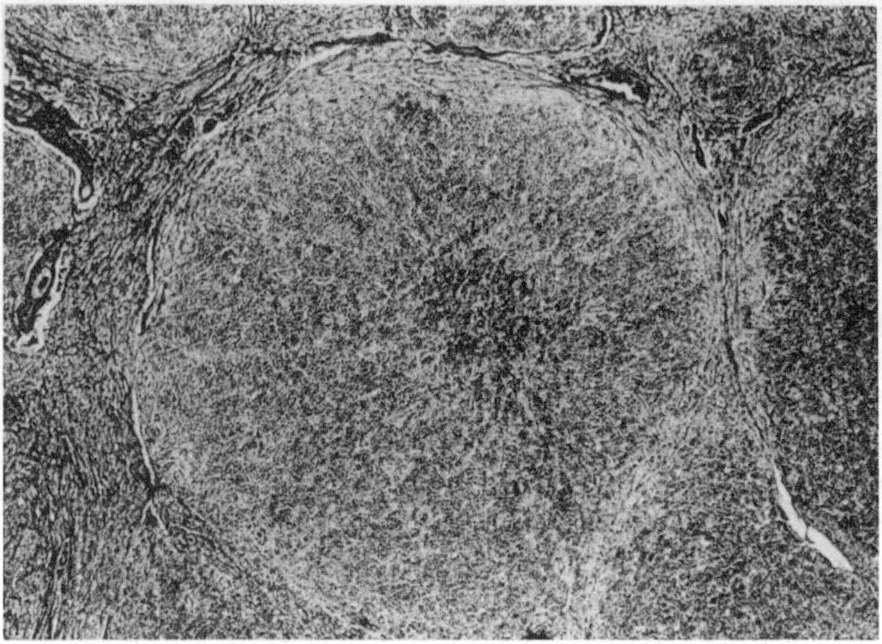

Fig. 117. Borderline case between M.L. centroblastic/centrocytic and LP immunocytoma. Case V. Nodular appearance. Amount of IgM in tissue homogenate was 350 times greater than normal; there was no increase in serum IgM. ♀, 48 years. Axillary node. Gomori. ×56.

features. They definitely synthesize large amounts of immunoglobulin (see p. 509). Among them we found only one cell that resembled a reticular plasma cell. There was strong, chiefly coarse, granular acid phosphatase activity in the centrocyte-like cells. The neutral nonspecific esterase reaction was negative. Sections and imprints revealed an increase in mast cells. In imprints we also found an increase in basophils.

We classified all of these cases as M.L. centroblastic/centrocytic because they contained either obvious or progressively transformed germinal centers. We must admit, however, that the borderline to immunocytoma was somewhat arbitrarily drawn.

It is understandable that the boundary between immunocytoma and centroblastic/centrocytic lymphoma is not stable, since germinal centers produce the precursors of the plasma-cell series. Therefore, it is not surprising that in several cases of centroblastic/centrocytic lymphoma a few plasma cells were found in the neoplastic germinal centers on electron microscopy (see p. 509). The findings of Taylor[336a] should also be mentioned here. Using the immunoperoxidase technique, he found intracytoplasmic Ig in cells from 12 out of 17 follicular lymphomas. In a few cases monoclonal Ig was detected in numerous interfollicular plasma cells.

The blastic (sarcomatous) variants of immunocytoma disclose another rela-

[336a] 1974.

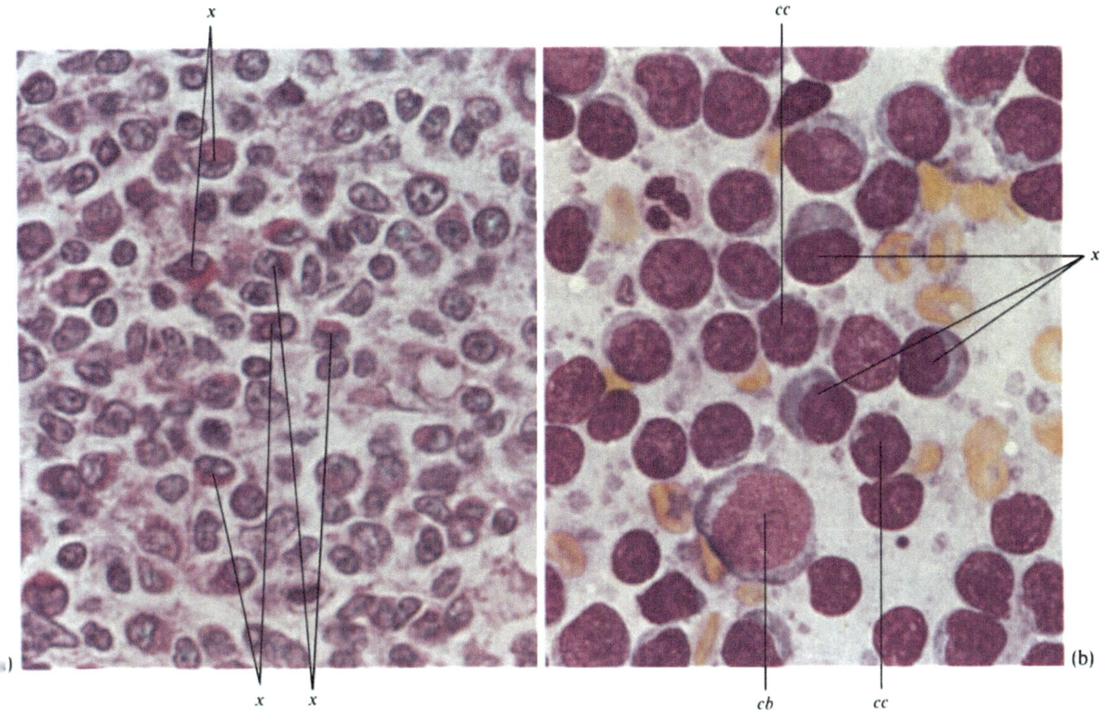


Fig. 118a and b. Same case as Fig. 117. (a) PAS reaction in section. Some centrocyte-like cells (*x*) with diffusely positive cytoplasm, often on one side of nucleus. ×875. (b) Imprint. One large centroblast (*cb*). Some typical centrocytes (*cc*). Three centrocyte-like cells (*x*) with gray-blue, wider rim of cytoplasm; they correspond to the PAS-positive cells in the section. Pappenheim. ×875.

tionship to centroblastic/centrocytic lymphoma. We found one case in which the "sarcoma" was composed chiefly of anaplastic centrocytes, and a second case in which the large "sarcoma cells" could be interpreted morphologically as large centroblasts.

The fact that there are *centrocytic lymphomas* with abundant plasma cells is another indication of a relationship between LP immunocytoma and germinal-center tumors. We encountered the relationship between M.L. centrocytic and LP immunocytoma in one patient. This 42-year-old man showed merely unilateral enlargement of axillary lymph nodes. Part of the tumor represented an LP immunocytoma with foci of epithelioid cells, while the other part was a classic large-cell M.L. centrocytic.

**Combination with Other Diseases.** In three out of 401 biopsies (0.75%) studied, we found along with the tumor the development of epithelioid-cell *granulomas*, whose etiology we could not interpret (tuberculosis? sarcoidosis? sarcoid-like lesions?).

*Amyloid* deposits were present in the lymph nodes five times (1.25%). These call to mind the frequency of secondary paramyloidosis (the pericollagenous and mixed types of amyloidosis according to MISSMAHL[337]) in macroglobulinemia of Waldenström.[338] In 13 monoclonal gammopathies[339] the amyloid deposits were of the pericollagenous type in 10 and of the pericollagenous/perireticular mixed type in three cases. In our autopsy material we found amyloidosis in 12.5% of all cases of macroglobulinemia, but in only 3% of our cases of multiple myeloma. BRAUN *et al.*[340] reported detecting paramyloidosis in 1/7 of their macroglobulinemias running a protracted course and in 4/8 with a rapid course. These generalized amyloidoses must be distinguished from localized amyloid deposits, as observed in plasmacytoma, and from localized immunoglobulin deposits, as we have described in immunocytoma. In addition, they are probably different from the tumor-like lymph-node amyloidosis with a monoclonal increase in IgM in the blood, as described by SCHEURLEN *et al.*[341] Here we should mention the findings of ISOBE and OSSERMAN,[342] who found M components (IgM seven times, once with Bence-Jones/κ) in the blood and urine in secondary amyloidosis and in the mixed type paramyloidosis/secondary amyloidosis.

Combinations of immunocytoma with *plasmacytoma* (multiple myeloma) have been reported many times.[343] On the other hand, combinations with so-called reticulosarcoma[344] are to be interpreted as malignant transformations of immunocytoma into immunoblastic sarcoma.

According to the statistics given by KAPPELER *et al.*,[345] 8% of the patients with macroglobulinemia of Waldenström develop *carcinomas*. In his review of the literature, FATEH-MOGHADAM[346] estimated the coincidence of macroglobulinemia and other malignant tumors to be 10%. MOESCHLIN[347] described two carcinomas (one in the upper lip, one in the cecum).

**Prognosis.** It is not yet possible to make definite statements about the prognosis of immunocytoma, since the period of follow-up is still not long enough. The curves of the Kiel Lymphoma Study Group[348] are based only on some previously available information (Fig. 34). On the whole, however, it seems that immunocytoma has a somewhat poorer prognosis in comparison with CLL and M.L. centroblastic/centrocytic. It is probably not wrong to assume that the polymorphic type, which reveals relatively high mitotic activity corresponding to the large number of blast cells, has the worst prognosis of the three subtypes of immunocytoma.

From some findings on macroglobulinemia of Waldenström presented in the literature, we may assume that the course of immunocytoma varies. For the immunocytomas that are equivalent to macroglobulinemia of Waldenström

337 MISSMAHL and GAFNI, 1964; MISSMAHL, 1967.
338 E.g., LELBACH, 1957; BRAUN, BRUCHHAUS and ALY, 1973.
339 ALY, BRAUN and MISSMAHL, 1969; see FATEH-MOGHADAM, 1974, for further literature.
340 BRAUN, BRUCHHAUS and ALY, 1973; BRAUN, 1976.
341 SCHEURLEN, HAUN, MÄUSLE and WOLFF, 1973.
342 1974.
343 SCHUBERT and MONDORF, 1969, Lit.; MCNUTT and FUDENBERG, 1973.
344 WALDENSTRÖM, 1968.
345 KAPPELER, KREBS and RIVA, 1958.
346 1974.
347 1966.
348 STACHER, WALDNER and THEML, 1976.

the available data show that there are two clinical types. The first runs a protracted course and responds well to therapy or requires hardly any or only minimal doses of chlorambucil[349] or procarbazine[350] for its control. The second progresses rapidly and requires active therapy.

The first type with a relatively benign course is probably far more common than the other. At the conclusion of their study of patients with macroglobulinemia, BRAUN *et al.*[351] calculated that the geometric mean of life expectancy was 32.2 months. For their patients who responded well to treatment, MACKENZIE and FUDENBERG[352] reported an average life expectancy of 49.2 months.

For the second type of macroglobulinemia with the less favorable prognosis, BRAUN *et al.*[351] estimated at the end of their study that the geometric mean of life expectancy was 8.6 months. MACKENZIE and FUDENBERG[352] found that their patients who responded poorly to therapy lived an average of 24.1 months.

## *Addenda*

### *a) The Leukemic Variants of LP Immunocytoma*

As explained above, about one third of all cases of LP immunocytoma are accompanied by a leukemic blood picture or at least by some neoplastic lymphoplasmacytoid cells in the blood. The nonleukemic form does not seem to differ in its clinical or pathoanatomic manifestations from the leukemic form.

The leukemic variants often exhibit the picture of *CLL*; at least it is difficult to make a morphologic distinction. An important indication of the correct diagnosis is, however, the presence of plasma-cell precursors or a *plasmacytoid appearance of the lymphocytes*. Such cases show somewhat larger lymphocytes with relatively abundant cytoplasm that stains gray-blue. One is not sure whether to classify these cells as lymphocytes or plasma cells.[353] Some large basophilic cells are often intermingled (Figs. 119 and 120). This pleomorphic picture was recently described by RUDDERS[354] as "atypical" CLL. It is apparent from RUDDERS' own findings that the cases of this type of "CLL" were actually leukemic immunocytomas. The leukemic cells always revealed intracytoplasmic Ig and usually IgG/κ on the surface. There were M components in the blood of four out of six cases (IgG/κ in three cases, free light chains in one case). In "typical" CLL, RUDDERS found chiefly IgM/κ on the cell surface and intracytoplasmic Ig in only one third of the cases. Capping was less pronounced than in "atypical" CLL. The other symptoms of both types of "CLL" were also different. In "atypical" CLL, general symptoms were more severe and there was more often generalized lymphadenopathy, clinically palpable hepatosplenomegaly, and myelophthisis requiring frequent transfusions of red blood cells and platelets. Infections were also more frequent in "atypical" CLL. These

---

349 MACKENZIE and FUDENBERG, 1972; BRAUN, BRUCHHAUS and ALY, 1973.

350 MITROU, SCHUBERT and MARTIN, 1972.

351 BRAUN, BRUCHHAUS and ALY, 1973.

352 1972.

353 STEIN, KAISERLING, LENNERT and PARWARESCH, 1973.

354 1976.

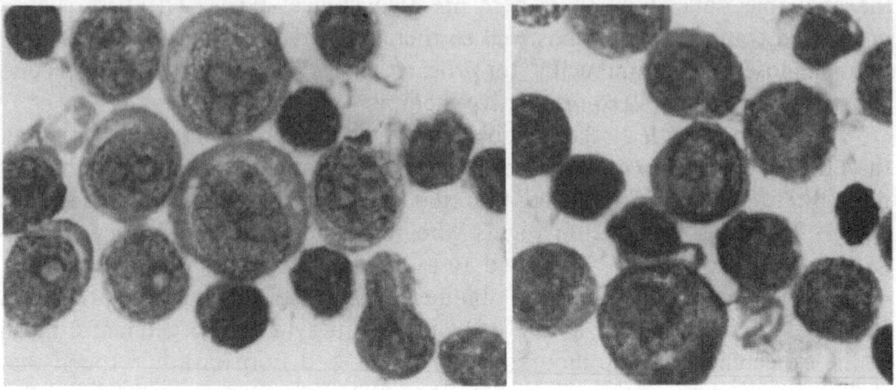

Fig. 119. Leukemic variant of LP immunocytoma, polymorphic subtype, in imprint. Hyperbasophilic, large and medium-sized cells of the plasma-cell series and lymphocytes. ♀, 58 years. Cervical node. Pappenheim. ×1,250

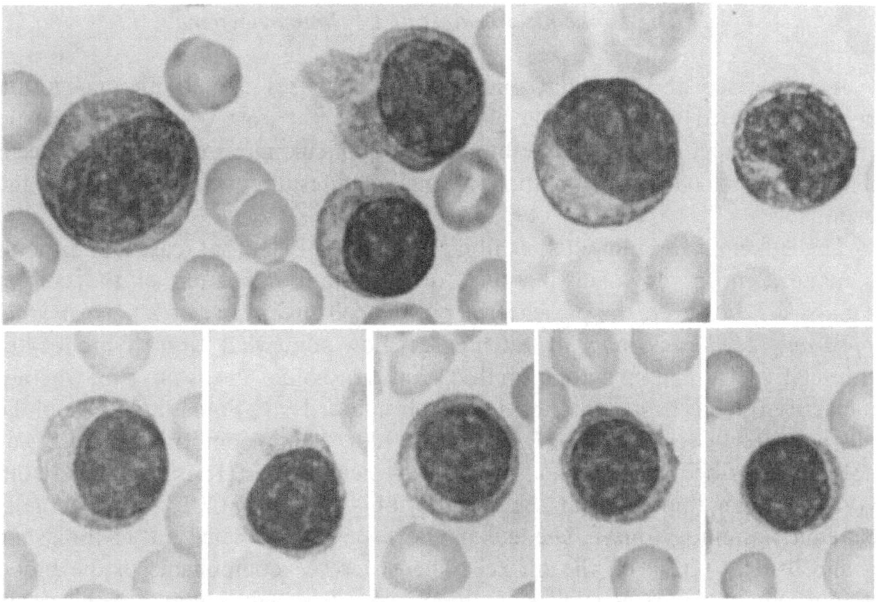

Fig. 120. Leukemic LP immunocytoma. Blood smear. Note the different sizes and grades of basophilia of the plasmablastic, plasmacytoid, and lymphoid cells. Same case as Fig. 119. Pappenheim. ×1,400

findings unintentionally emphasize how important (and clinically relevant) it is to distinguish LP immunocytoma from CLL.

The most extreme of the leukemic variants of immunocytoma is (true) *lymphatic plasma-cell leukemia.*[355] The blood (and the tissue) contains chiefly small

[355] Wanner and Siebenmann, 1957; Marchal, Fine and Bilski-Pasquier, 1962; Fritze and van de Loo, 1965; Moeschlin, 1966.

plasma cells with some proplasmacytes and plasmablasts, and therefore does not reveal the monotonous "pure-cell" picture of "reticular" plasma-cell leukemia, the leukemic equivalent of multiple myeloma. "Lymphatic" plasma-cell leukemias have in general been described with an associated macroglobulinemia of Waldenström.[355] We have personally observed two patients with so-called lymphatic plasma-cell leukemia accompanied by macroglobulinemia. SCHLEICHER[356] reported on an extraordinary case of this type. In the blood and tissue he found an enormous number of cells with globular PAS-positive inclusions like those we have already described in immunocytoma. A similar case with globular IgG deposits in blood lymphocytes was recently described by NIES *et al.*[357] In a corresponding case in our series the peripheral blood contained numerous lymphoid cells with solitary or multiple, medium-sized vacuoles that were weakly PAS-positive. Lymph nodes, however, revealed only a small number of such cells, but many strongly basophilic plasmacytoid cells and precursors.

Finally, leukemias have been found in association with macroglobulinemia of Waldenström that have been called stem-cell leukemia[358] or paraleukoblastic leukemia.[359] The "blast cells" in these cases were most probably plasmablasts. Perhaps such leukemias approximately correspond to the observation of FITZGERALD *et al.*,[360] who described a case of CLL without paraproteinemia that eventually showed a leukemic picture with plasmablasts and a monoclonal increase in IgM in the blood.

### *b) The Heavy-Chain Diseases*

Monoclonal gammopathy with an increase in complete immunoglobulins is found in multiple myeloma (plasmacytoma) and in various malignant lymphomas. So far, light chains alone have been demonstrated mostly in patients with myeloma and in rare cases of immunocytoma. Conditions with heavy chains alone have been described as $\gamma$-, $\alpha$-, and $\mu$-chain diseases. A brief description of these diseases follows.

*1. $\gamma$-Chain disease (Franklin's disease).*[361] In 1964, FRANKLIN *et al.*[362] and, a short time later, OSSERMAN and TAKATSUKI[363] described the occurrence of monoclonal free heavy chains of the $\gamma$ type in the blood. Since then about 30 cases have been reported in the literature. The patients were from 18 to 80 years old. The male-to-female ratio was 13:9. In most cases there was hepatosplenomegaly and enlargement of superficial and sometimes of deep lymph nodes. In almost half of the cases there was edema of the soft palate and uvula. Intercurrent infections were reported in many cases. The blood frequently revealed anemia and leukopenia. The bone marrow was often infiltrated by lymphocytes and plasma cells as well as by lymphoplasmacytoid cells (as in macro-

[356] 1965.
[357] NIES, MARSHALL, OBERLIN, HALPERN *et al.*, 1976.
[358] VIDEBAEK, 1971.
[359] MÄRKI and SIEGENTHALER, 1964.
[360] FITZGERALD, RASTRICK and HAMER, 1973.
[361] Reviews: SELIGMANN, 1972b; FRANGIONE and FRANKLIN, 1973; WARNER, POTTER and METCALF, 1974; LOYAU, BARRÉ, L'HIRONDEL, LANIÈCE *et al.*, 1975.
[362] FRANKLIN, LOWENSTEIN, BIGELOW and MELTZER, 1964.
[363] 1964.

globulinemia of Waldenström). The γ-chain occurs as a dimer in which the Fc fragment is present but the Fab fragment and a large part of the Fd fragment are missing. The hexose component is variable in quantity.

Neither the nature nor the morphology of this condition, now known as Franklin's disease, are very well defined. On the one hand, the disease appears like a malignant tumor of the lymphoreticular tissue. On the other hand, there are cases in which the disease develops slowly and occasionally recedes spontaneously, and which are perhaps to be interpreted as benign.[364] Considering this clinical heterogeneity, it is not surprising that there is also no uniform morphologic picture among the cases reported in the literature. Whereas in a few cases a malignant neoplasm could not be histologically demonstrated, in the majority of cases there were lymphoproliferative disorders of the following types:

a) In numerous cases typical plasma cells and plasma-cell precursors (plasmablasts or immunoblasts) and eosinophil leukocytes were demonstrated in addition to lymphocytes. The lymph-node structure was not always destroyed. Thus, the alterations were cautiously interpreted as not definitely malignant. FRANKLIN *et al.*[365] and DELMAS-MARSALET *et al.*[366] reported coarse PAS-positive granules within lymphoid and plasmacytic cells in blood and bone-marrow smears as well as in needle biopsies of lymph nodes. Some of these lymph-node lesions can probably be interpreted as signs of a lymphoplasmacytic immunocytoma, especially since alterations in the bone marrow like those seen in macroglobulinemia of Waldenström have also been described. Recently, SHIRAKURA *et al.*[367] described lymph-node infiltrates that on electron microscopy consisted of small lymphocytes and large "lymphoplasmablastic" cells.

b) "Reticulosarcoma" was described in several cases. Accordingly, the lesion is probably to be interpreted as immunoblastic sarcoma.

c) There were a few reports of plasma-cell leukemia. In the case of KELLER *et al.*[368] IgM/κ paraproteinemia was associated with the γ-chain disease.

We have had the opportunity of studying two cases of γ-chain disease, although both cases were atypical. The first case[369] (Fig. 121) presented the clinical picture of a malignant lymphoma. No paraprotein was found in fresh serum. Under refrigeration (+4° C), however, a paraprotein (cryoglobulin) precipitated that showed all of the properties of γ-chains, although the Fc fragment of IgG was not detected in the blood—an atypical finding. The urine contained only the Fc fragment and no light chains. Histologically, the lymph-node structure was effaced. There were enormous numbers of epithelioid venules among abundant round cells. Cytologically, small lymphocytes predominated. There were also abundant typical Marschalkó plasma cells with a widened, vacuolated Golgi body. Now and then, vacuoles were found elsewhere in the cytoplasm. The plasma cells were occasionally multinucleate. Sometimes they

[364] SELIGMANN, 1972a.

[365] FRANKLIN, LOWENSTEIN, BIGELOW and MELTZER, 1964.

[366] DELMAS-MARSALET, VOISIN, HENNACHE, BAUTERS *et al.*, 1971.

[367] SHIRAKURA, KOBAYASHI, MURAI, INOUE *et al.*, 1976

[368] KELLER, SPENGLER, SKVAŘIL, FLURY *et al.*, 1970.

[369] The slides and clinical data were kindly provided by Dr. J. BOHINJEK, Lubljana.

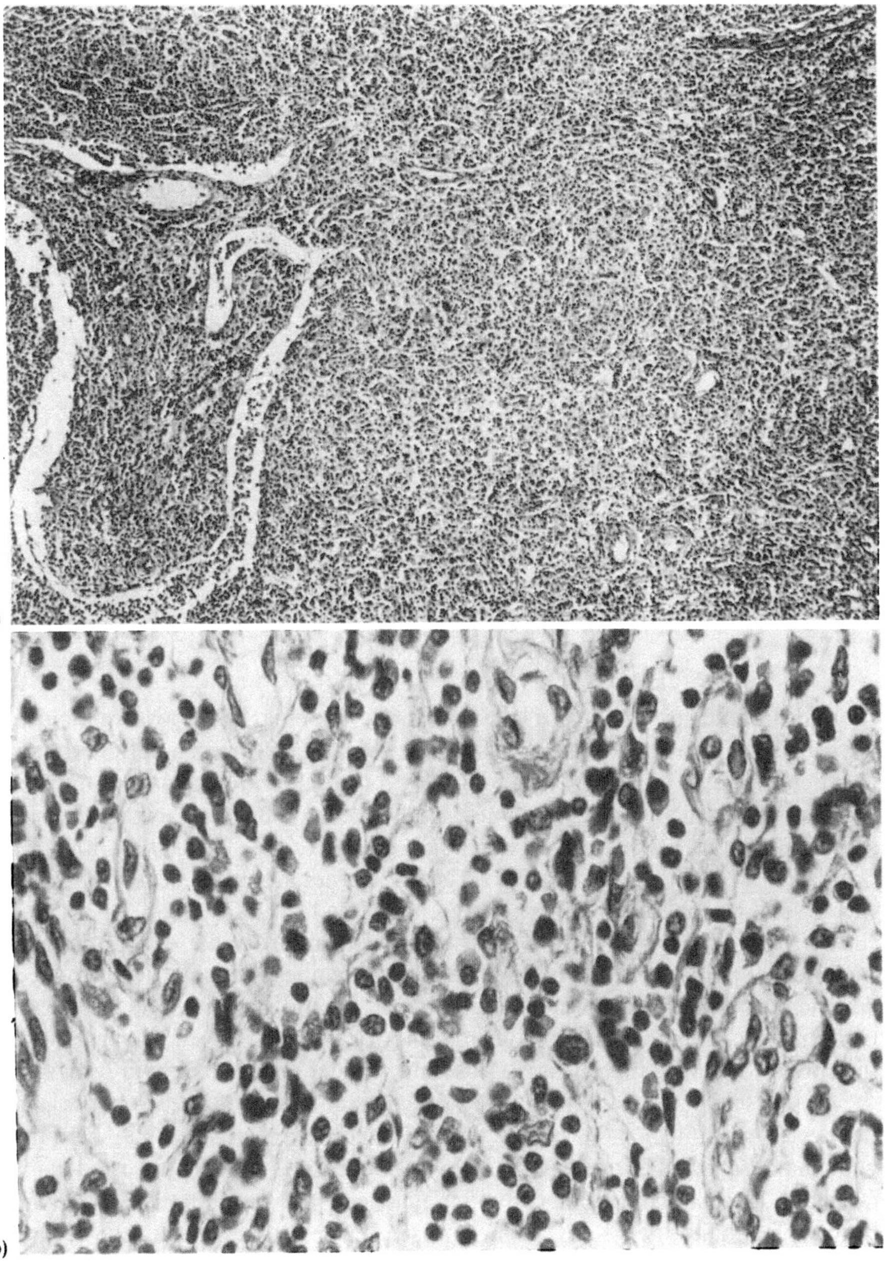

(a)

(b)

Fig. 121a and b. γ-Chain disease (?). The lymph-node structure is effaced (a). Chiefly lymphocytes, one immunoblast, and some typical plasma cells (b). Section kindly provided by Dr. BOHINJEK, Lubljana. ♂, 72 years. Axillary node. Hematoxylin and eosin. (a) ×70, (b) ×560

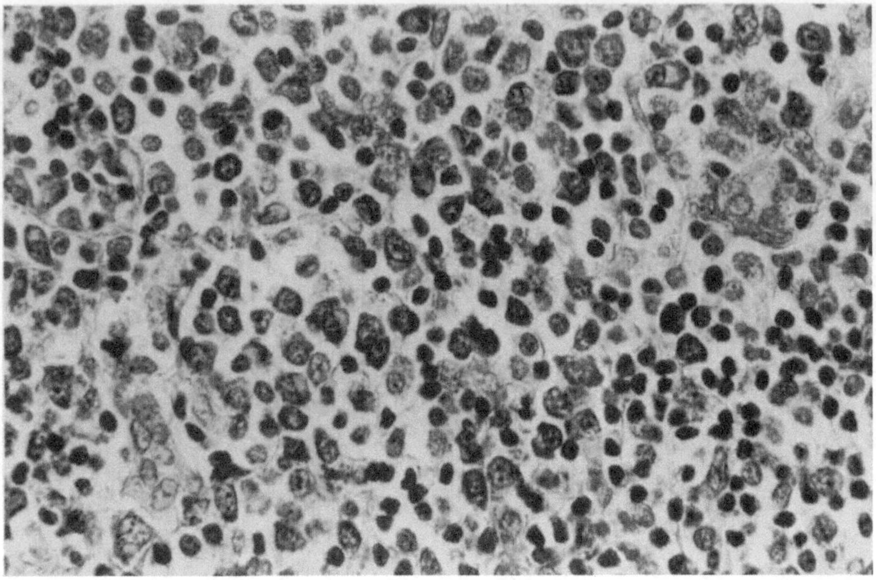

Fig. 122. $\gamma$-Chain disease. Numerous plasma cells and lymphocytes, and some plasmablasts. Section of Dr. Röttger, Frankfurt. Turkish ♀, 12 years. Mesenteric node. Giemsa. ×560

showed slight to strong, diffuse PAS positivity. Globular PAS-positive inclusions were absent. Occasional plasmablasts were found. There was a definite increase in reticulum cells. In imprints we found both typical lymphocytes and numerous plasma cells, which were sometimes small like lymphoplasmacytoid cells and sometimes large like classic Marschalkó plasma cells. There were also some proplasmacytes as well as a few large indeterminate blast cells. Finally, we saw several lymphoid cells that we were not able to classify.

*Epicrisis:* The histologic picture was largely similar to that of immunoblastic lymphadenopathy because of the numerous venules. It is difficult to decide whether the lymphoplasmacytic proliferation should be interpreted as reactive or neoplastic (lymphoplasmacytic immunocytoma?). We lean toward the first interpretation, since there was no absolute clinical proof of $\gamma$-chain disease.

In the second case[370] (Fig. 122) the patient was a 12-year-old girl from Turkey. The clinical picture was that of Mediterranean intestinal lymphoma with malabsorption syndrome, but immunochemical analysis revealed $\gamma$- (not $\alpha$-) chain disease.[371] Histologically, the picture in the lymph node corresponded to that of $\alpha$-chain disease, i.e., numerous plasma cells and plasma-cell precursors were found, whereas the lymph-node structure was relatively well preserved. This case still needs further clarification.

In summary, a complete picture of the morphology and nature of $\gamma$-chain disease cannot be formulated at present. Therefore, it would be helpful to collect all known cases at a central place and to evaluate them uniformly.

[370] The slides and clinical data were kindly provided by Dr. Röttger, Frankfurt/Main.

[371] Analyzed by Prof. Dr. M. Seligmann, Paris.

*2. α-Chain disease.*[372] In 1968, SELIGMANN *et al.*[373] described α-chain disease. Since then more than 70 additional cases have been published.[374] α-Chain disease is definitely the most frequent of the heavy-chain diseases. In contrast to all other paraproteinemias, it occurs in young people, especially in the second and third decades. In the cases reported, males were affected 1.65 times more frequently than females.[375] The disease affects primarily the secretory IgA system of the digestive tract. The respiratory tract was involved in only two reported cases;[376] both patients were children who came from areas where intestinal lymphoma is infrequent, namely, from Holland and the USA. Clinically, there is chronic diarrhea when the intestinal tract is involved, often with severe malabsorption syndrome and sometimes with abdominal tumors. The small-intestinal mucosa shows massive infiltration by mature plasma cells (Marschalkó type) as well as secondary villous atrophy and crypt sparsity. Later, the picture of immunoblastic sarcoma may also appear in the intestine. A description of the changes in mesenteric lymph nodes is given below. Peripheral lymph nodes are not infiltrated, or perhaps rarely in late stages. There is a striking predilection for certain geographic areas (North Africa, Middle East, Far East, South America, Southern Europe). This strongly suggests that environmental factors (frequent intestinal infections?) in these areas play an etiologic role. Several reports of the reversibility of the disease in response to antibiotic therapy also support the assumption of some such initially reactive process.

α-Chain disease occurs with similar symptoms in countries where so-called Mediterranean (intestinal) lymphoma with malabsorption[377] has been reported. This suggests that the two diseases are identical and that α-chains had merely not been looked for in most cases of Mediterranean intestinal lymphoma.[375] It does not appear to be true in such a broad sense, however; only some of the Mediterranean lymphomas are probably to be interpreted as α-chain disease. DUTZ[378] estimated the percentage of α-chain disease to be about 10–15% and RAMOT,[379] about 25% of all cases of Mediterranean lymphoma. Therefore, α-chain disease is a variant of primary intestinal lymphoma,[380] which may also be associated with the formation of complete IgA molecules.[381]

*Lymph-node lesions:*[382] At first, the lymph nodes appear to reveal only an increase in plasma cells of the Marschalkó type and in plasma-cell precursors. Evidently, such plasmacytosis may look at first like reactive hyperplasia. We had the opportunity of examining a case from the series of RAMOT, however,

---

372 Reviews: WARNER, POTTER and METCALF 1974; SELIGMANN, 1975.

373 SELIGMANN, DANON, HUREZ, MIHAESCO *et al.*, 1968.

374 SELIGMANN, 1972a, b, 1975.

375 SELIGMANN, 1975.

376 STOOP, BALLIEUX, HIJMANS and ZEGERS, 1971; FAUX, CRAIN, ROSEN and MERLER, 1973.

377 RAMOT, SHAHIN and BUBIS, 1965; EIDELMANN, PARKINS and RUBIN, 1966; DUTZ, ASVADI, SADRI and KOHOUT, 1971; RAMOT, 1971; RAMOT and MANY, 1972; RAPPAPORT, RAMOT, HULU and PARK, 1972; DOE, 1975; RAMOT and HULU, 1975; KHARAZMI, HAGHIGHI, HAGHSHENAS, NASR *et al.*, 1976.

378 1974, personal communication.

379 1976, personal communication.

380 SHAHID, ALAMI, NASSAR, BALIKIAN *et al.*, 1975.

381 CHANTAR, ESCARTÍN, PLAZA, CORUGEDO *et al.*, 1974.

382 BOGNEL, RAMBAUD, MODIGLIANI, MATUCHANSKY *et al.*, 1972; DOE, HENRY, HOBBS, AVERY JONES *et al.*, 1972; RAPPAPORT, RAMOT, HULU and PARK, 1972; RAPPAPORT, 1974, 1976.

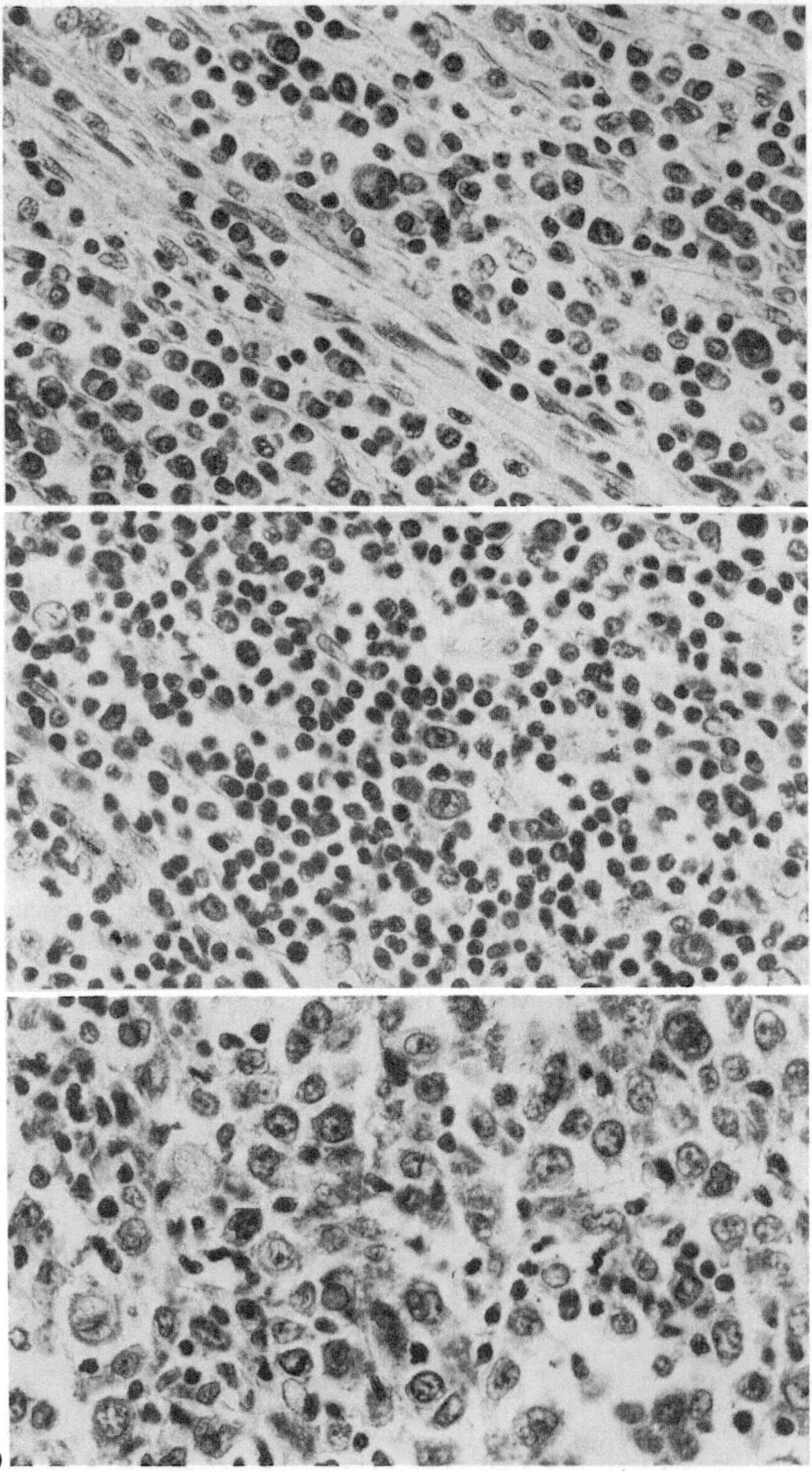

(a)

(b)

(c)

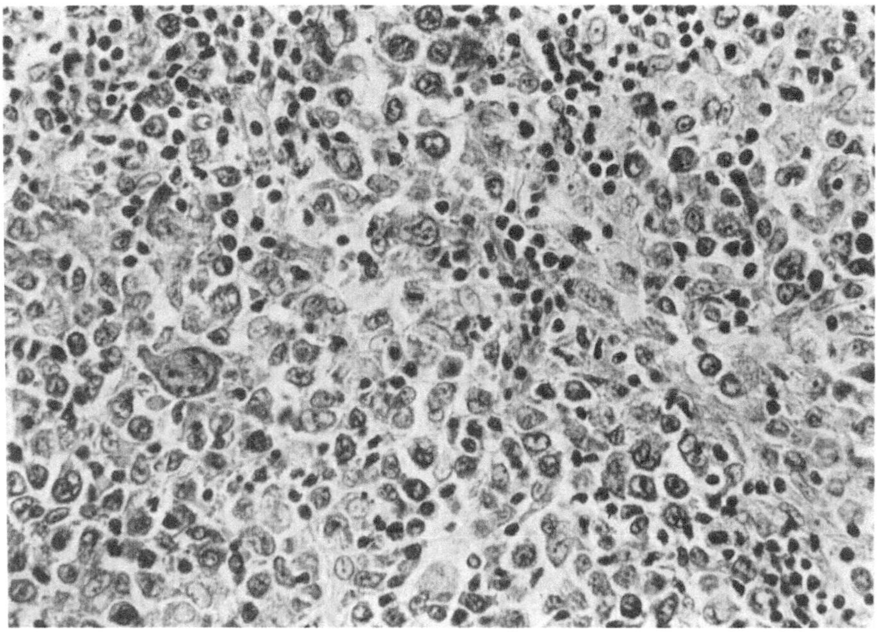

Fig. 124. α-Chain disease. Sarcomatous appearance is reminiscent of immunoblastic lymphoma. Note the giant cell. Same case as Fig. 123. Mesenteric node. Giemsa. ×350

that showed lymphomatous infiltration with a completely destroyed lymph-node structure in addition to reactive changes and follicular lymphatic hyperplasia. Cytologically, the lymphoma consisted chiefly of lymphocytes, but it also contained relatively large numbers of plasma cells, plasmablasts, and immunoblasts and could therefore be considered to be a lymphoplasmacytoid immunocytoma. We also suspect that the intestinal tumor described by SKINNER *et al.*[383] was an immunocytoma with abundant plasma cells. In another case, which was kindly shown to us by Dr. PRATSIKA-OUGOURLOGLOU from Athens, the number of more or less typical plasma cells was larger, but they were seen in all areas with lymphocytic infiltration (Fig. 123).

Finally, there is the development of a large-celled "blastic" proliferation, which was at first interpreted as reticulosarcoma or as Hodgkin's disease (Fig. 124). This interpretation is understandable, since the cytology is sometimes relatively polymorphic and since there are occasionally multinucleate giant cells that are reminiscent of Sternberg-Reed giant cells. Most of the cells, however, resemble plasmablasts, i.e., immunoblasts that already show some plasmacytic

[383] SKINNER, MANOUSOS, ECONOMIDOU, NICOLAOU *et al.*, 1976.

◁ Fig. 123a–c. α-Chain disease. (a) Lymphoplasmacytic infiltration of the muscularis intestini. Predominance of plasma cells. (b) Predominance of lymphocytes and some immunoblasts in a mesenteric lymph node. (c) Sarcomatous appearance in another part of the same mesenteric lymph node. Note the polymorphism as in so-called Hodgkin's sarcoma. Case of Dr. PRATSIKA-OUGOURLOGLOU, Athens. ♂, 32 years. Giemsa. ×560 differentiation. According to RAPPAPORT,[384] one should probably interpret the lesions as those of immunoblastic sarcoma. The cases we observed were remarkable for the intense basophilia of the cells and certain plasma cell-like features in the small and medium-sized cells, features that are seen only very rarely in immunoblastic lymphomas in other sites. According to our classification, the tumor has to be called immunoblastic lymphoma with plasmablastic or plasmacytic differentiation.

Between the initial plasmacytosis of the lymph node (and the mucosa of the small intestine) and the final immunoblastic sarcoma there are probably intermediate stages in which both pictures are mixed.

Our material includes two cases that are of interest in this context. In one case there was γ-chain disease; otherwise, the clinical picture was typical of Mediterranean lymphoma (see p. 254). In another patient, a 66-year-old man of German descent, we diagnosed malabsorption syndrome showing massive plasmacytosis, villous atrophy, and crypt sparsity in a biopsy from the small intestine 6 months before death. At autopsy there was malignant lymphoma in the small intestine and regional lymph nodes and in other lymph nodes and organs. The histologic picture was that of a highly pleomorphic immunoblastic sarcoma with plasmablastic features and with some similarity to "Hodgkin's sarcoma." Therefore, it may be assumed that intestinal lymphoma with malabsorption occurs not only in Mediterranean countries, but also in Central Europe, as shown years ago in England by HARRIS *et al.*[385]

*3. μ-Chain disease.*[386] This disease was independently discovered in 1969 in the laboratories of FRANKLIN, KUNKEL, and KOCHWA[387] and at the New York Veterans Administration Hospital.[388] Since then more than 10 cases have been published.[389] Usually, there was "chronic lymphocytic leukemia." In the case of BONHOMME *et al.*[390] the blood picture was normal and there was merely splenomegaly, which, however, was not examined histologically. In contrast to γ- and α-chain disease, Bence-Jones protein was found in the urine in seven out of ten published cases. This means that light chains are also formed, but they are not joined with the μ-chains. Amyloidosis (paramyloidosis), which was even described in the first case of FORTE *et al.*,[387] is perhaps related to the presence of light chains in the blood. We studied three cases of μ-chain disease that will be described in detail here, since morphologic changes in the lymph nodes have received little consideration in the literature. A case of nonneoplastic μ-chain disease will also be presented (case 4).

*Case 1:*[391] Male, 41 years old; left supraclavicular lymph node. Clinically, there was subleukemic "CLL" (see GERMANN *et al.*[392] for further clinical data). Histologically, we found a destroyed

[384] 1974.

[385] HARRIS, COOKE, THOMPSON and WATERHOUSE, 1967.

[386] Reviews: GERMANN, WESTERHAUSEN and KICKHÖFEN, 1972; DAMMACCO, BONOMO and FRANKLIN, 1974; WARNER, POTTER and METCALF, 1974.

[387] FORTE, PRELLI, YOUNT, JERRY *et al.*, 1970.

[388] BALLARD, HAMILTON, MARCUS and ILLES, 1970.

[389] E.g., LEE, ROSNER, RUBERMAN and GLASBERG, 1971; GERMANN, WESTERHAUSEN and KICKHÖFEN, 1972; JØNSSON, VIDEBAEK, AXELSEN and HARBOE, 1976, Lit.

[390] BONHOMME, SELIGMANN, MIHAESCO, CLAUVEL *et al.*, 1974.

[391] The histologic slide was kindly provided by Prof. Dr. W. SANDRITTER, Freiburg. The case was published by GERMANN *et al.*, 1972.

[392] GERMANN, WESTERHAUSEN and KICKHÖFEN, 1972.

lymph-node structure. The sinuses were still well defined, however, and contained a greatly increased number of mast cells. The capsule was massively infiltrated by small tumor cells, occasionally in a somewhat nodule-like arrangement. A majority of the cells were lymphocytoid, perhaps also plasmacytoid. There were also definite Marschalkó plasma cells, including several mononuclear giant forms. There was pronounced hemosiderosis. The lymph in the sinuses was strongly PAS-positive. Poorly defined, amorphous PAS-positive deposits were found in greatly enlarged macrophages. Silver staining revealed abundant fine fibers (of no diagnostic value since the infiltration of the lymph node was only slight and most of the fibers were certainly preexistent).

**Epicrisis:** We interpreted this as a case of immunocytoma, probably of the lymphoplasmacytic type.

*Case 2*[393] (Figs. 125–127): Male, 43 years old. Clinically, there were no general symptoms, but moderately rapid enlargement of lymph nodes in both groins (1st biospy) and in the left supraclavicular region. The liver and spleen were not enlarged. Scintigraphic analysis also revealed no enlargement of the spleen and, in addition, no skeletal infiltration. Histologically, the bone-marrow trephine biopsy showed no infiltration. RBC sedimentation rate was 10/28; leukocytes 6350/ml, 23% lymphocytes, no atypical forms. Rheumatic complaints in some joints. The Waaler-Rose test was positive. Lymphography revealed widespread retroperitoneal infiltration. Stage III had therefore been reached. After three courses of combined chemotherapy (vincristine, methotrexate, cyclophosphamide, and prednisone), there was full remission for 6 months, but then recurrence in the left cervical region (2nd biopsy). Demonstration of free μ-chains in the blood; no Bence-Jones proteinuria.

Histologically, the lymph nodes from both groins (R 2367/73) showed the same picture. The normal architecture was effaced. The sinuses could not be identified. The degree of basophilia of the cytoplasm could not be determined for technical reasons. Cytologically, part of the lymph node consisted of lymphocytes, while the appearance of other parts was similar to that of polymorphic immunocytoma. With fiber staining, large foci that were somewhat reminiscent of germinal centers could be recognized among a monotonous proliferation of small cells. Argyrophil fibers were scanty. Venules could be demonstrated only in foci as remnants of T-cell areas. The infiltration appeared to begin in the outer cortex. The PAS reaction was negative, except in a few large typical plasma cells that contained intracytoplasmic globular inclusions. These cells were probably to be interpreted as preexistent plasma cells.

In the second biopsy (supraclavicular, R 1560/74) the lymph-node structure was also destroyed. Roundish areas containing cells with larger nuclei were often found (Fig. 125). They were slightly reminiscent of germinal centers, but the cells were not clearly distinguishable from the surrounding small lymphoid cells. Unexpectedly, such apparently lighter foci were also found in the capsule and spread from there into the adipose tissue and the marginal sinus. Mast cells were found only occasionally. On the other hand, we saw a few eosinophils.

Cytologically, the cells consisted of lymphoid cells that were clearly larger than typical lymphocytes and sometimes had cleaved nuclei. There were also smaller cells with round nuclei, a somewhat broader band of basophilic cytoplasm, and one or two small but distinct nucleoli. The nuclear "sap" was light, the chromatin fine. In addition, there were a few typical proplasmacytes and plasmablasts. Especially in the areas containing large cells we also saw some typical centroblasts and a few polymorphic, larger or giant cell (mononuclear) forms with strong or moderate basophilia, many oval nuclei, and very large nucleoli (atypical centroblasts?). There were a few definite dendritic reticulum cells. Mitotic activity was quite high. Mitotic figures were found chiefly in larger cells. Finally, the blastic foci and the sinuses contained very large macrophages that had abundant cytoplasm and were closely packed together.

Very abundant PAS-positive material was seen in the macrophages. It often formed crystals (Fig. 126). In profile these crystals were often shaped like the needle of a compass; in cross-section they were rhomboid or square. Frequently, they also formed very narrow needle-like structures, up to 30 μm long. They were found in an amorphous or granular-appearing mass. Like the crystals, this mass was PAS-positive. Most of the crystals and the granular-appearing aggregates of macrophages were gray-blue with Ladewig staining and green with Goldner staining. Only some of the crystals showed a patchy or even total orange-red staining with these methods.

The lymphoid cells contained moderately abundant intranuclear PAS-positive globules, which

---

[393] The clinical data were kindly provided by Prof. Dr. C.G. SCHMIDT, Essen. We also thank Prof. Dr. C.J. LÜDERS, Berlin, for the first lymph-node biopsy.

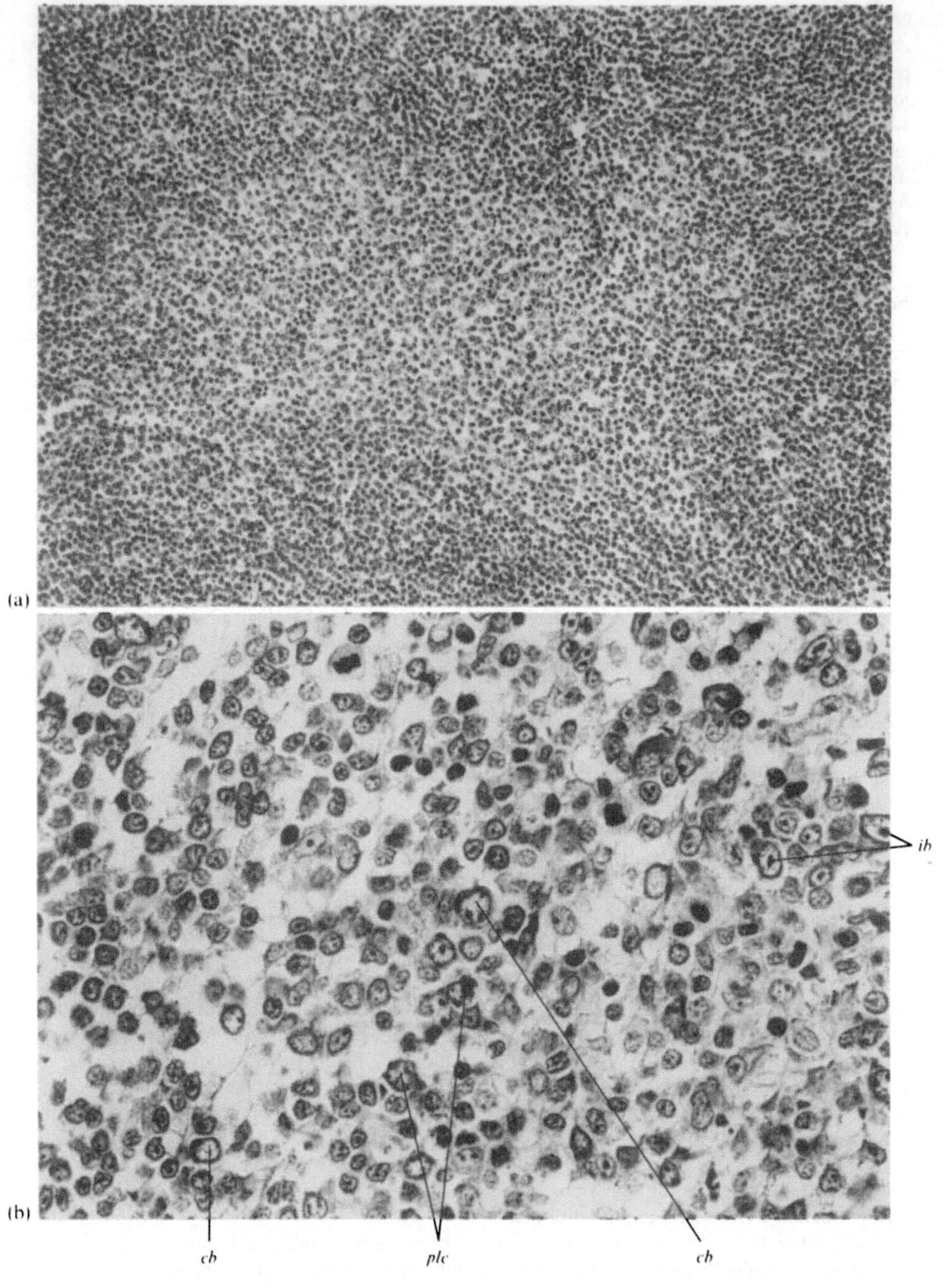


Fig. 125a and b. μ-Chain disease. Case 2. (a) Lymph-node architecture effaced. Large proliferation center. (b) Centroblasts (*cb*) and immunoblasts (*ib*). Plasmablast and plasma cell (*plc*). ♂, 43 years. Cervical node. (a) Ladewig. ×140. (b) Giemsa. ×560

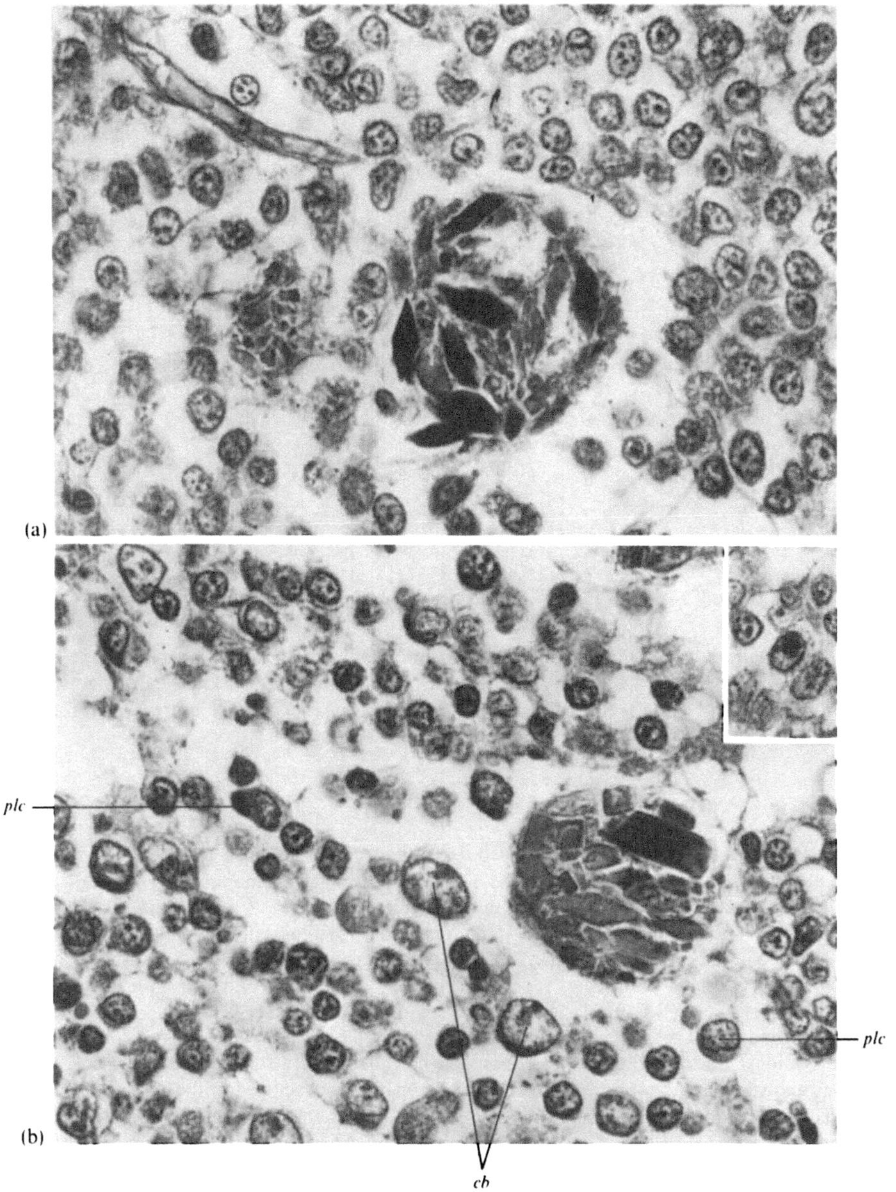


Fig. 126a and b. μ-Chain disease. Large macrophages filled with PAS-positive immunoglobulin crystals. Note two centroblasts (*cb*) and plasma cells (*plc*) in (b). Inset: PAS-positive intranuclear inclusion. Same node as Fig. 125. PAS. ×875

were gray-blue with Ladewig staining. The cytoplasm of some medium-sized lymphoid or plasmacytoid cells showed a strong, diffuse PAS-positive reaction. In the sinuses probably extracellular conglomerates of crystals with strong PAS positivity were occasionally found. The lymph and the blood serum were strongly PAS-positive.

The fiber picture was largely similar to that of Burkitt's tumor, i.e., there were hardly any fibers in the neoplastic proliferation (Fig. 127). The tumor grew in the form of large cohesive

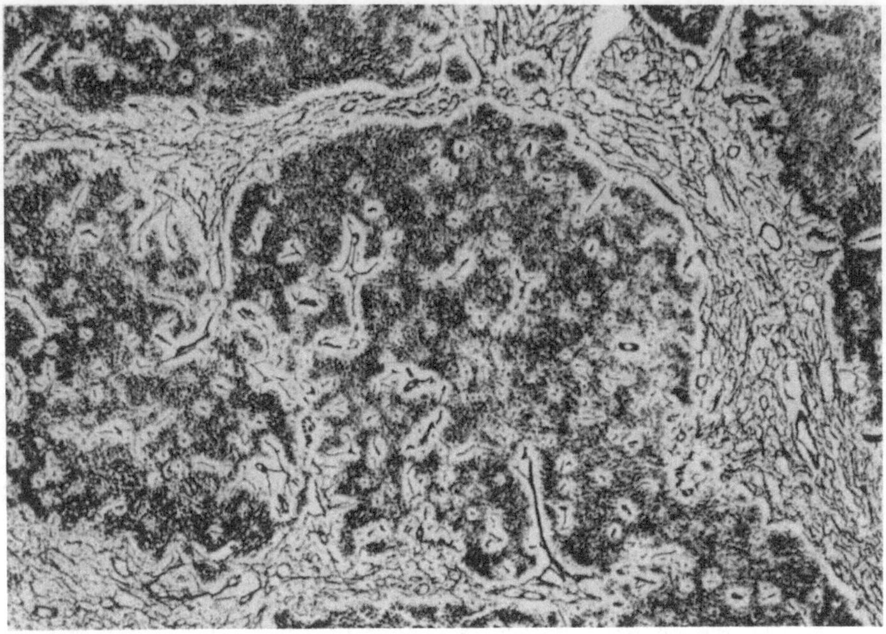

Fig. 127. μ-Chain disease. Silver staining of the tumor infiltration closely resembles that of other B-cell lymphomas (e.g., M.L. centrocytic or M.L. lymphoblastic, Burkitt type). T-zones (with numerous fibers and vessels) are seen as remnants between the neoplastic areas. Same node as Fig. 125. Gomori. ×70

masses that were traversed and subdivided by a few capillaries and scanty fibers. Remnants of lymphatic tissue with abundant venules and fibers were seen among the tumor cells. Active lymphocyte emigration could be observed in the venules.

**Epicrisis:** This was a polymorphic immunocytoma. Cytologically, it contained the following cells, listed in the order of frequency: lymphocyte-like cells, often basophilic ++++, lymphoplasmacytoid cells++, centrocytes++, centroblasts (with atypia and transitions into plasmablasts)+, plasmablasts (+), proplasmacytes (+), dendritic reticulum cells (+). Germinal center-like accumulations of blast cells suggested a relationship to lymph follicles, which was not fully supported by the cytology. Furthermore, the fiber structure did not reveal a follicular arrangement. Instead, this was an extremely fiber-poor neoplasm, which apparently developed in the B-region and whose fiber picture showed a certain similarity to that of Burkitt's tumor. Clinically, the absence, both of a leukemic blood picture and of infiltration of the bone marrow, as well as the mild rheumatoid symptoms speak for our interpretation of immunocytoma and against CLL.

*Case 3:*[394] Female, 54 years old; cervical lymph node (R 2393/74). Clinically, there were lymphomas in the cervical and mediastinal regions without leukemic changes. Free μ-chains were found in the blood. Partial remission was achieved through combined chemotherapy.

Histologically, the lymph-node structure was destroyed. Small lymphoid round cells dominated the picture. Among them, however, there were some large blast cells with large central nucleoli (immunoblasts). Further, we recognized some typical plasma cells and plasmacytoid cells. There was a small amount of fiber. Mitotic figures were abundant. The PAS reaction revealed several PAS-positive plasmacytoid cells, sometimes with a diffuse red staining of the cytoplasm and some-

[394] The clinical data were kindly provided by Prof. Dr. O. WETTER, Essen. We thank Prof. Dr. Dr. H.A. HIENZ, Krefeld, for the histologic slides.

times with red globular deposits in the cytoplasm. Intranuclear PAS-positive inclusions and protein crystals were not found. The serum was strongly PAS-positive.

**Epicrisis:** This was also an immunocytoma, specifically of the lymphoplasmacytoid type, but there was not the picture of CLL.

*Case 4:* A 16-year-old girl with "μ-chain disease" was described by WETTER in 1973. Clinically and histologically, it does not fit into the picture of other μ-chain diseases. Histologically, the lymph-node structure was well preserved. The germinal centers were hyperplastic and, like the pulp, contained an enormous number of plasma cells. There was also a small focal increase in epithelioid cells.

**Epicrisis:** The histologic features were not those of a malignant neoplasm and we would regard this case as a vigorous immunologic reaction. According to this interpretation, it is probable that free μ-chains can also appear under nonneoplastic conditions.

**Summary and Conclusions.** In our view, when μ-chain disease is neoplastic, as it is in most cases, the basic lesion is an immunocytoma, which may be lymphoplasmacytoid, lymphoplasmacytic, or polymorphic. We presume that the alleged cases of CLL reported in the literature are actually leukemic immunocytomas, especially since an abundance of plasma cells was often mentioned. For instance, in the bone marrow of their first case, FORTE *et al.*[395] found not only 45% lymphoid cells, but also 33% plasma cells, which frequently contained vacuoles and Russell bodies. Histologically, our case 1, which was clinically interpreted and published as CLL, did not in fact show the picture of CLL, but instead that of macroglobulinemia of Waldenström with an increase in typical plasma cells and mast cells and with well-preserved sinuses. The patient of BONHOMME *et al.*,[396] who showed splenomegaly but a normal blood picture, probably had the splenomegalic variant of immunocytoma. The mild rheumatic symptoms (case 2) also agree with the interpretation of μ-chain disease as an immunocytoma. Furthermore, the finding of paramyloidosis in μ-chain disease[395] would fit this interpretation.

The presence of crystalline protein deposits in macrophages of our case 2 deserves particular attention. The reactions of these crystals for different stains indicated that they were precipitates of μ-chains containing carbohydrates. They might have been derived from cells that had perished (after chemotherapy?) or from the extracellular space, and were deposited in macrophages because heavy chains are practically insoluble when they are not bound to light chains.

## 2. *Malignant Lymphoma, Plasmacytic (Plasmacytoma)*

**Definition.** Ultimately, every plasmacytoma is derived from B-lymphocytes and is thus, strictly speaking, a "lymphoma." Most authors, however, use the term plasmacytoma and do not include this neoplasm among the lymphomas. In addition, one finds that a clinically important distinction is made between plasmacytomas of the bone marrow (myeloma) and extraskeletal (extramedullary) plasmacytomas. The plasmacytomas arising primarily in the lymph nodes belong to this extraskeletal type.

---

[395] FORTE, PRELLI, YOUNT, JERRY *et al.*, 1970.

[396] BONHOMME, SELIGMANN, MIHAESCO, CLAUVEL *et al.*, 1974.

In addition, a large proportion of the remaining *extraskeletal (extramedullary) plasmacytomas*[397] also arise from lymphatic tissue, for example, from the tonsils or from the gastrointestinal tract. WILTSHAW[398] showed that 75% originate in the submucosa of the upper respiratory tract, evidently multifocally in many cases. Other localizations are the salivary glands, stomach, small and large intestine, breast, lung, thyroid, genital organs, and orbit. Some of the plasmacytomas of the orbit and other sites are probably LP immunocytomas. Extraskeletal plasmocytomas occur most frequently between the ages of 40 and 70 years.[399] Men are affected four times more frequently than women.[399] Evidently, the sex ratio of extramedullary plasmacytoma differs from that of medullary plasmacytoma, which shows only a slight to moderate predominance in men.[400]

Extraskeletal plasmacytoma metastasizes to the regional lymph nodes in about 80% of cases and may later spread to other lymph nodes. Hematogenous metastasis to the bones, bone marrow, subcutis, and other organs occurs occasionally.[401]

Studies of the immunoglobulins in the blood of patients with gut plasmacytoma have revealed IgG, Bence-Jones protein, or 7S IgA.[402] In the blood and urine of an alleged case of lymph-node plasmacytoma, HOBBS and JACOBS[403] found a special IgG/κ, in which the γ-chain represented only half of a molecule. The published photograph actually revealed a polymorphic immunocytoma, however, and not a plasmacytoma.

The so-called plasmacytomas of the gastrointestinal tract distinguished by HENRY *et al.*[404] have to be separated from the extramedullary plasmacytoma we are discussing here. These tumors do not consist of pure populations of plasma cells, for they also contain plasmablasts and probably always lymphocytes. Thus, they are more closely related to LP immunocytoma than to extramedullary plasmacytoma. We should point out here that all malignant lymphomas of the gastrointestinal tract have a special morphology and clinical behavior. Therefore, they cannot be identified with the seemingly equivalent malignant lymphomas of the lymph nodes.

In this section we discuss only the primary plasmacytomas of lymph nodes and shall consider the metastases of extramedullary or intramedullary plasmacytomas in the section on differential diagnosis. There will also be a section on multiple myeloma and one on the leukemic variant of plasmacytoma, namely, plasma-cell leukemia.

The plasmacytomas of lymph nodes,[405] like the other extraskeletal plasmacytomas, consist of pure populations of plasma cells of the Marschalkó type ("reticular" plasma cells; Fig. 128). Precursors of plasma cells (plasmablasts, etc.) are never found. From this definition we can disregard the numerous cases referred to in the literature as lymphatic plasmacytoma,[406] lymphatic plasma-cell leukemia,[407] *sarcomatose ganglionnaire diffuse à différenciation plasmocytaire,*[408] *plasmocytome ganglionnaire,*[409] and the like,[410] since their diag-

[397] Reviews: JAEGER, 1942; HELLWIG, 1943; JACKSON and PARKER, 1947; STOUT and KENNEY, 1949; EWING and FOOTE, 1952; WILTSHAW, 1969.
[398] 1971.
[399] STOUT and KENNEY, 1949.
[400] SNAPPER and KAHN, 1971, Lit.
[401] WILTSHAW, 1969.
[402] DOE, HENRY, HOBBS, AVERY JONES *et al.*, 1972.
[403] 1969.
[404] HENRY, HOWARTH and FARRER-BROWN, 1976.
[405] MARESCH, 1909; KAUFMANN, 1928/29; JACKSON, PARKER and BETHEA, 1931 (same case: JACKSON and PARKER, 1947); BASSET and SCAPIER, 1937; WEISZER, 1942; JÉQUIER-DOGE, NICOD and CHAPUIS, 1947; ANDERSEN, 1949; SIMON and EIDLOW, 1950; HIRSCHER, 1953/54; ROWLANDS and SHAW, 1954; NELSON and LYONS, 1957; FRUHLING and CHADLI, 1963 (questionable!); SUISSA, LAROSA and LINN, 1966; POOLE and MARCHETTA, 1968; GASTON, DOLLINGER, STRONG and HAJDU, 1969; SNAPPER and KAHN, 1971; WILTSHAW, 1969, 1971.
[406] FORSTER and MOESCHLIN, 1954; MOESCHLIN, 1961.
[407] LENNERT, 1964a, b.
[408] FLANDRIN, DANIEL, EL YAFI and CHELLOUL, 1972.
[409] LEJEUNE, TURPIN, LECOUTURIER, BOUVIER *et al.*, 1972.
[410] E.g., WIDMANN, 1957.

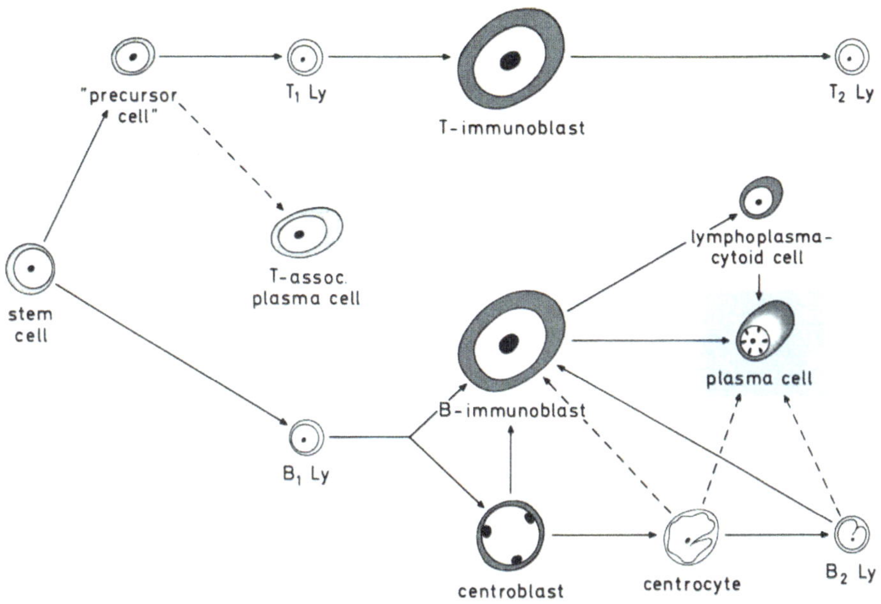


Fig. 128. Hypothetical origin of tumor cells of primary lymph-node plasmacytoma.

noses depended upon the demonstration of plasma cells *and* their precursors in needle biopsies or imprints of lymph nodes. We shall discuss these conditions in a later chapter under the term lymphogranulomatosis X with excessive plasmacytosis. It is too early yet, however, to state whether indeed a malignant lymphoma does occur that is composed of plasma cells and plasma-cell precursors. The case described by HECKNER[411] might possibly fulfill the criteria.

**Occurrence.** Compared with plasmacytomas of the bone marrow, primary lymph-node plasmacytomas are extraordinarily rare. Of the extraskeletal plasmacytomas, those of the lymph nodes make up only a small percentage. Among 192 plasmacytomas of the head and neck, only four involved the cervical lymph nodes,[412] whereas 72 arose in the paranasal sinuses and nasal cavity, 41 in the nasopharynx, and 26 in the pharyngeal tonsil. Other localizations were the palate and maxillary gingiva (11), larynx (8), oropharynx (6), combined (6), fauces (4), tongue (1), and trachea (1). Primary lymph-node plasmacytoma is thus extremely rare. Plasmacytoma of the lymphatic tissue in the pharynx and nasopharynx, namely, that of the tonsils, is much more frequent.

Our first series contained eight cases of primary lymph-node plasmacytoma (Table 39). In our routine material we had seven primary lymph-node plasmacytomas, i.e., 0.5% of all malignant lymphomas and 0.8% of non-Hodgkin's lymphomas. In the same period we received two lymph-node metastases of bone-marrow plasmacytomas as routine material. Metastases of extraskeletal

[411] 1951.

[412] EL CASTRO, LEWIS and STRONG, 1973.

Table 39. M.L. plasmacytic (plasmacytoma). Material and incidence

| | | |
|---|---|---|
| Total No. of biopsies | 15 | |
| Lymph nodes | | 8 |
| Extranodal | | 7 |
| Incidence in routine lymph-node material | 7 | |
| = 0.5% of malignant lymphomas | | |
| 0.8% of non-Hodgkin's lymphomas | | |

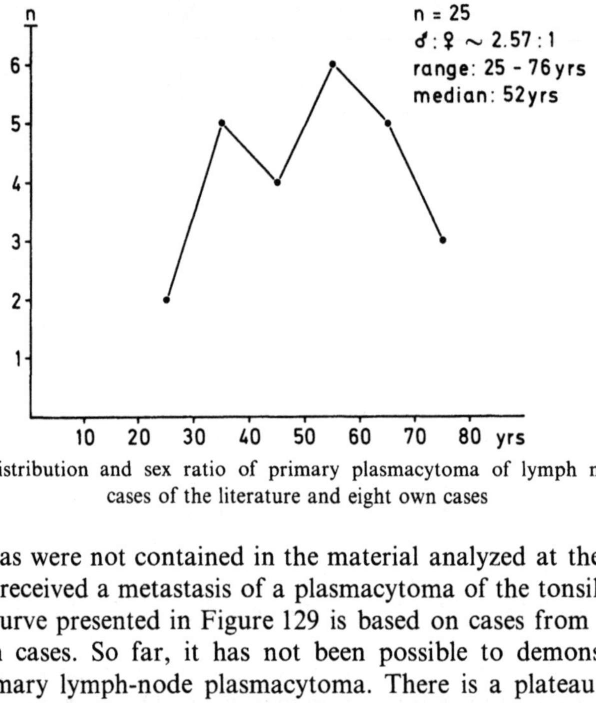


Fig. 129. Age distribution and sex ratio of primary plasmacytoma of lymph nodes. Seventeen cases of the literature and eight own cases

plasmacytomas were not contained in the material analyzed at the time. Later, however, we received a metastasis of a plasmacytoma of the tonsil.

The age curve presented in Figure 129 is based on cases from the literature and our own cases. So far, it has not been possible to demonstrate a clear peak for primary lymph-node plasmacytoma. There is a plateau between the ages of 30 and 70 years. The youngest patient was 25 years old (see p. 605, however), the oldest was 76; the median lay at 52 years. The male-to-female ratio was 2.6:1.

**Clinical Manifestations.** In general, at the time of biopsy of the lymph node the patient has no general symptoms. The tumors usually develop slowly. The RBC sedimentation rate may be slightly or greatly increased. Often the blood shows no paraproteinemia, although occasionally a monoclonal increase in Ig, for instance, IgG, exists and then disappears after the tumor is excised.[413] The detection of an M-component in the blood probably depends on the size of the tumor mass.[414] Bence-Jones proteinuria develops only occasionally. At the time of lymph-node involvement there is no evidence of plasmacytoma of the bone marrow. If the marrow is involved at all, it is only in the late

[413] Nelson and Lyons, 1957; Gaston, Dollinger, Strong and Hajdu, 1969.

[414] See Hobbs, 1969.

Table 40. Localization of excised lymph nodes in primary lymph-node plasmacytoma (17 reported in the literature and eight from the present series)

| Localization | n |
|---|---|
| Cervical | 15 |
| Axillary | 7 |
| Mediastinal | 1 |
| Inguinal | 1 |
| Unknown | 1 |
| Total | 25 |

stages of the disease, when metastases may develop. The liver and spleen are—at least at first—not enlarged. The blood picture shows no increase in plasma cells.

**Localization.** The situations of the extirpated lymph nodes are presented in Table 40. It shows that the cervical region is the most frequent site of involvement (15 lymph nodes), followed by the axilla (7 lymph nodes). Mediastinal and inguinal plasmacytomas were excised in only one case each. In three cases it was reported that two lymph-node regions were involved at the time of lymph-node biopsy, and in two cases multiple lymph-node regions were said to be affected.

**Gross Appearance.** The involved lymph nodes may become exceptionally large (up to the size of an orange). When freshly sectioned, the exposed surface is gray-white to gray-red as in multiple myeloma. Occasionally, the surface is described as irregularly lobulated.[415] The consistency of the lymph nodes is soft.

**Histology.** The architecture of primary lymph-node plasmacytoma is characteristic, so that even at low magnification one can suspect this type of tumor. The tumor cells form compact clusters, which are enclosed in the meshes of a rather regular network of fibers and small blood vessels (Fig. 130). The resulting picture is consequently relatively repetitious. Often remnants of lymphatic tissue are demonstrated in the form of germinal centers with a mantle of lymphocytes. At times, the thick hyalinized capsule is enveloped by tumor tissue, which penetrates adjacent areas. There is occasionally band-forming sclerosis extending from the sclerotic capsule into the lymph node.

The tumor cells themselves appear quite monotonous. This can also be recognized at low magnification (Fig. 131). The tumor cells are exclusively relatively typical plasma cells of the Marschalkó type ("reticular plasma cells"). Only rarely can one make out among them a few small histiocytic reticulum cells. Mast cells are either absent or extremely rare. Only in a plasmacytoma

[415] Nelson and Lyons, 1957.

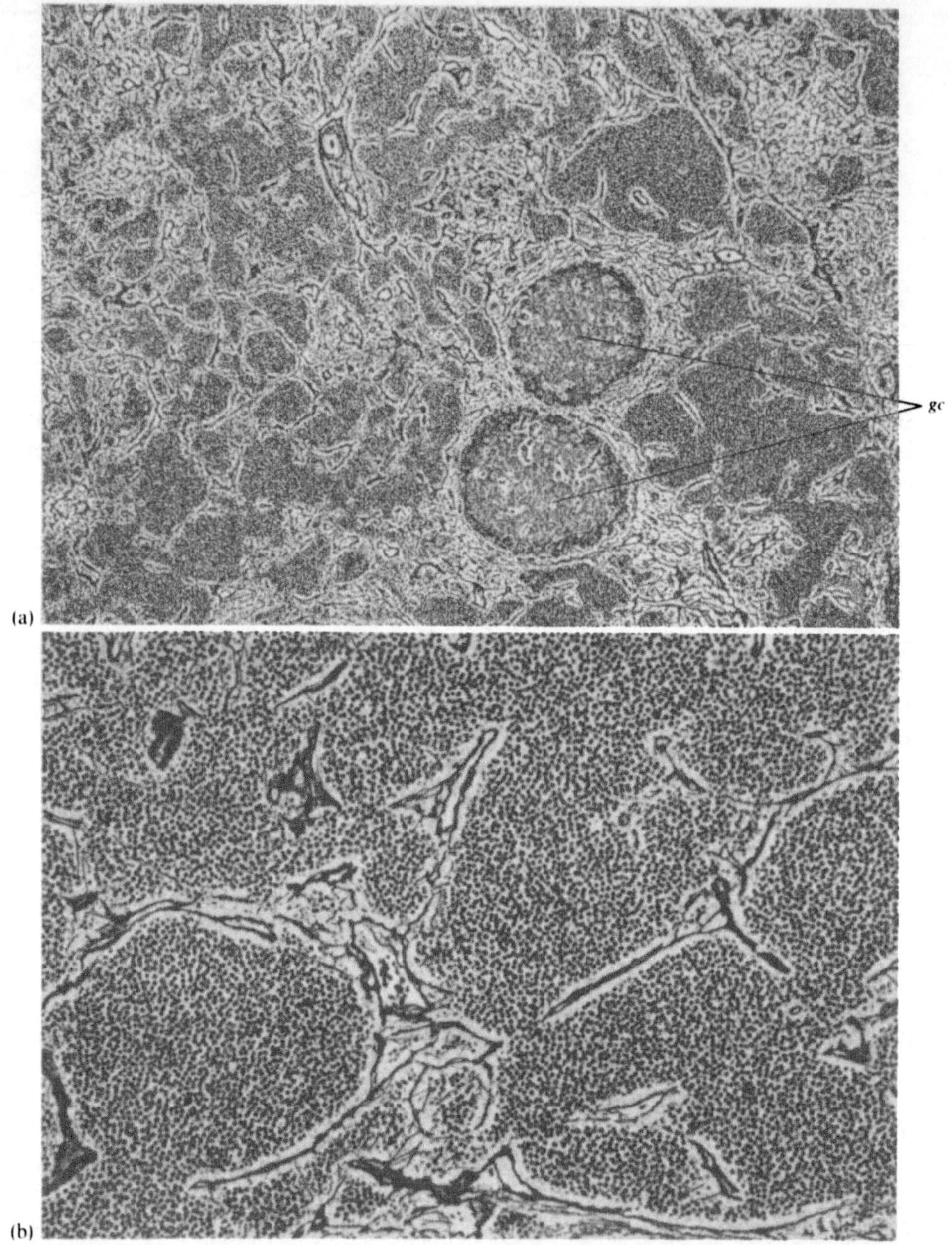


Fig. 130a and b. Primary lymph-node plasmacytoma. Note some residual germinal centers (*gc*). The uniform, closely packed tumor cells form large clusters and masses surrounded by thick fibers and vessels producing a coarse alveolar pattern. ♂, 70 years. Cervical node. Gomori. (a) ×56, (b) ×140

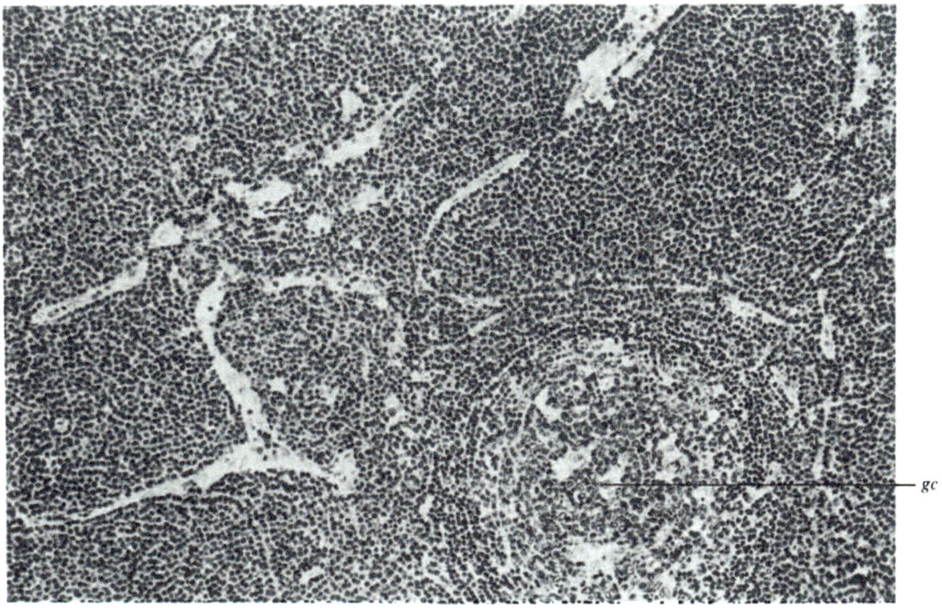


Fig. 131. Primary lymph-node plasmacytoma. At the lower right, a residual germinal center (*gc*). The picture corresponds to the fiber pattern shown in Fig. 130b. Same node as Fig. 130. Giemsa. × 140

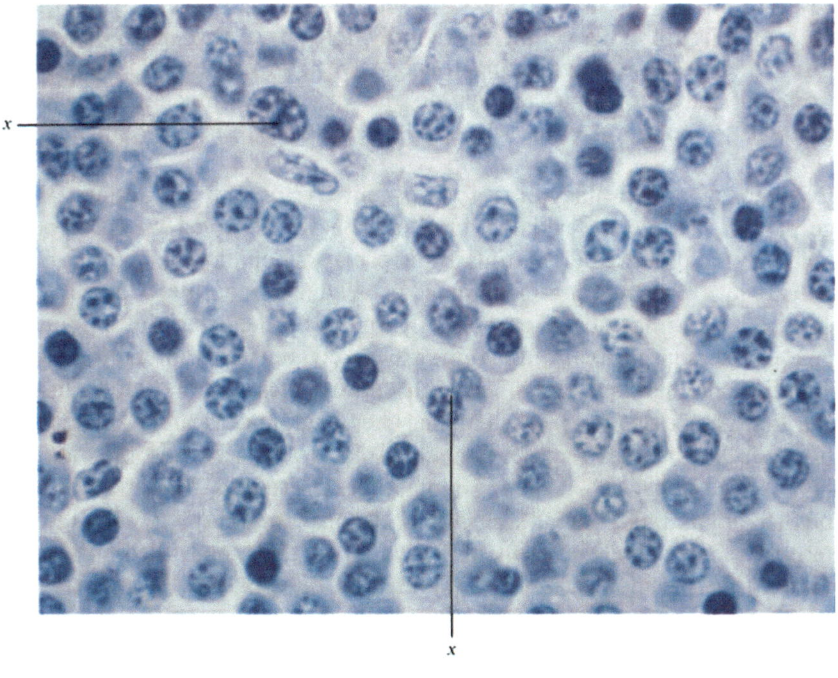


Fig. 132. Primary lymph-node plasmacytoma with Giemsa staining. Somewhat polymorphic plasma cells. Two plasma cells with two nuclei (*x*). Same node as Figs. 130 and 131. × 1,550

of the tonsil with large deposits of protein in dilated lymph vessels did we find a definite increase in mast cells.

The neoplastic plasma cells differ from normal plasma cells by their narrower rim of cytoplasm, by the not always clearly visible perinuclear halo, and by an increase in the nuclear/cytoplasmic ratio (Fig. 132). All the nuclei are round and have the typical chromatin structure of plasma cells ("spoked" structure); that is, the nuclear chromatin is dispersed in coarse, uniformly sized clumps with a regular arrangement, and there are one or two nucleoli of about equal size. This classic picture of the plasma cells is often best seen in central parts of the section, namely, where a certain degree of autolysis has occurred due to insufficient fixation. Occasionally, the number of chromatin clumps appears to be greater than normal (increased DNA content?). The nuclei lie towards one side of the rather intensely basophilic cytoplasm. At times one finds larger, polyploid nuclei that have the same chromatin pattern as the small nuclei, which shows that they are not nuclei of plasmablasts. In addition to the polyploid mononuclear plasma cells, there are also always a few or some multinucleate plasma cells whose nuclei are usually of equal size. GASTON *et al.*[416] illustrated multinucleate plasma cells in their paper. A small to moderate number of mitotic figures may be evident. Russell bodies were never found in large numbers, but sometimes in small or moderate numbers in our cases.

With silver stains the plasma-cell clusters prove to be free of fibers, but are enmeshed in a loose or tight network of fibers with small blood vessels. The tumor cells are deep gray and therefore show a certain argyrophilia. Silver staining also discloses another important feature of plasmacytoma, namely, a tendency of the cells to invade the walls of veins without destroying them. That is apparent not only within the lymph node, but also in the veins of the capsule and those in neighboring tissue. Silver staining reveals, moreover, that groups of plasmacytoma cells within the vascular lumina are enveloped by their own "stroma," in other words by reticulin fibers in alveolar arrangement.

The tendency of plasmacytoma to grow into veins and to occlude them in large part or completely explains an alteration we observed on three occasions—namely, a pseudoangiomatous transformation of the tumor (Fig. 133). This we saw in a tonsillar plasmacytoma, in a lymph-node metastasis from a nasopharyngeal plasmacytoma, and in a lymph-node metastasis of a multiple myeloma. One sees large areas of the tumor relatively uniformly interspersed with anastomosing channels that are filled with erythrocytes and/or blood plasma, so that at first glance one suspects a capillary hemangioma. At higher magnification, however, it becomes apparent that plasmacytoma cells line the vascular spaces, not endothelial cells. Silver staining further reveals that the channels have neither a basement membrane nor a fibrous boundary. In two tumors innumerable vacuoles were evident at the edges of the blood-filled spaces. In our opinion, this pseudoangiomatous picture can be explained by two factors. First, the flow of blood is hindered due to the obstruction of the veins. The second factor is the very regular fiber network of the tumor.

---

[416] GASTON, DOLLINGER, STRONG and HAJDU, 1969.

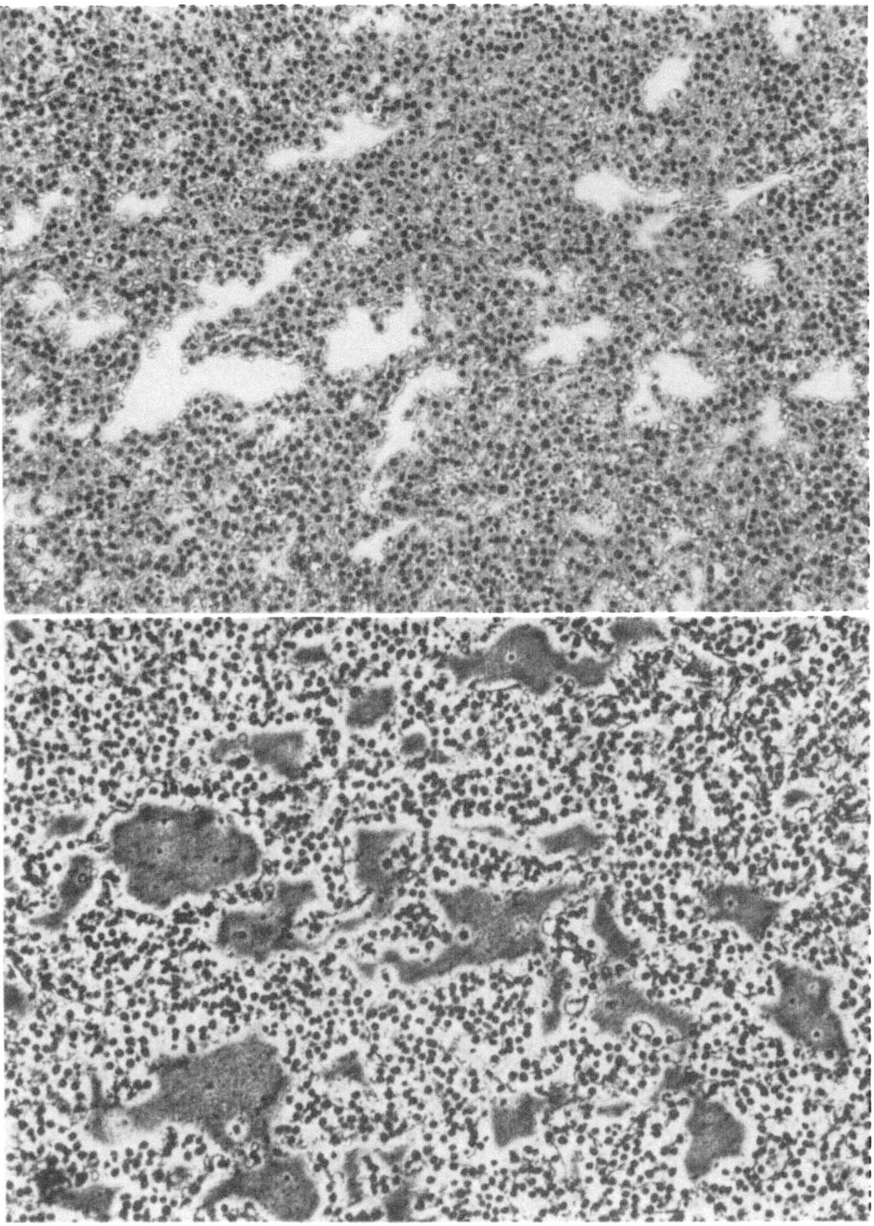

(a)

(b)

Fig. 133a and b. Metastasis of a plasmacytoma of the nasopharynx 15 years after removal of the primary tumor. Pseudoangiomatous pattern. ♂, 66 years. Cervical node. (a) Van Gieson. ×140. (b) Gomori. ×140

Another feature of plasmacytoma of the lymph nodes—like plasmacytoma of the bone marrow—is the accumulation of amyloid. This substance may be deposited in greatly thickened venous walls and occasionally in arterial walls, as well as in the broadened fibrous capsule and in surrounding fat and connective

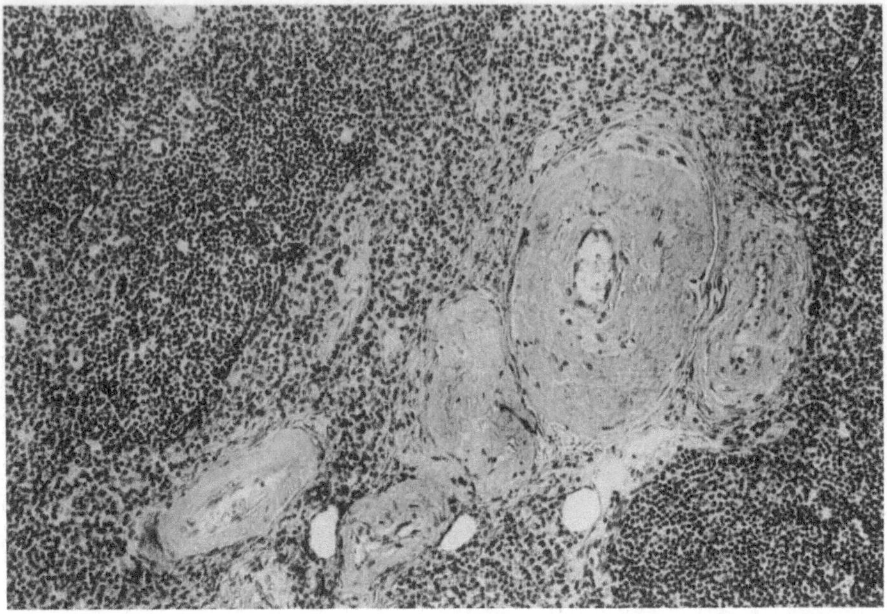

Fig. 134. Pericollagenous amyloidosis in primary lymph-node plasmacytoma. Note the amyloidosis in the vessel walls. ♂, 75 years. Cervical node. Congo red. ×140

tissue (Fig. 134). As with paramyloidosis, this distribution corresponds to the pericollagenous amyloid of MISSMAHL.[417] In addition, however, there may be deposits of amyloid generally regarded as the tumor amyloid of plasmacytoma (Fig. 135). One sees all grades from accumulated masses of protein to Congo red-positive amyloid. This is exemplified by two cases:

In a plasmacytoma of the tonsil the lymph vessels were filled with inspissated protein and were very dilated. With Ladewig staining they were deep red; with Giemsa staining, blue. The material was Congo red-negative. It was surrounded by histiocytes and foreign-body giant cells.

In a primary lymph-node plasmacytoma we found similar inspissated masses of protein in the dilated lymph vessels. There were also large deposits of similar protein throughout the whole lymph node, but they usually showed no relation to lymph channels. With Ladewig staining some of the central protein masses were pale red, whereas the peripheral masses were gray-blue. With Giemsa staining the protein masses were gray-blue to deep blue. The peripheral areas and sometimes all of the masses showed a positive reaction for Congo red with green dichroism on polarization. The peripheral protein masses were more PAS-positive than the faintly stained central areas. Numerous histiocytes and foreign-body giant cells were found near these protein masses. Silver staining disclosed abundant argyrophil fibers. The histiocytes in neighboring areas contained in their cytoplasm numerous coarsely granular PAS-positive deposits that gave a negative reaction with Congo red. The foreign-body giant cells contained

[417] 1968 and earlier.

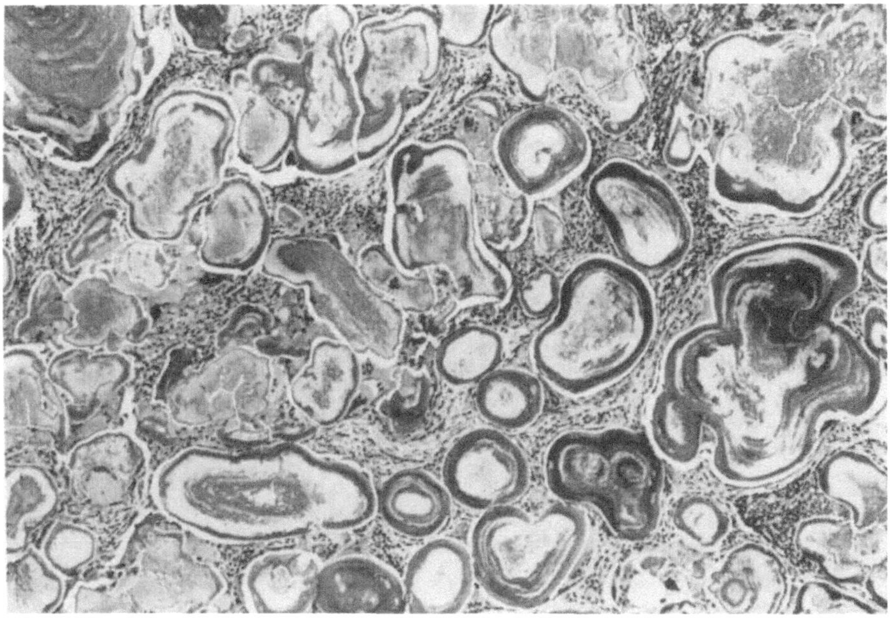

Fig. 135. Primary lymph-node plasmacytoma. Many sharply demarcated deposits of amyloid in a variety of shapes. Some deposits show a laminated structure. Note foreign body-type giant cells eroding some of the amyloid masses. Between the amyloid deposits there are only a few strands of residual tumor cells. ♂, 52 years. Axillary node. Congo red. × 56

chiefly finely granular PAS-positive deposits. Some of the giant cells were monstrous in size. It appeared as if the histiocytes and foreign-body giant cells were nibbling away at the protein masses and "dissecting" them. That resulted in bizarre, indented or grooved structures, similar to those observed in dilated tubules of myeloma kidneys. The amount of protein or amyloid deposited in the lymph node was so great that only remnants of tumor tissue could be recognized. This tissue showed typical plasma cells, but notably did not contain Russell bodies. Furthermore, there was still relatively abundant lymphatic tissue present that was not involved by the plasmacytoma. Besides the variable-sized protein or amyloid deposits, the walls of veins and some arteries also revealed amyloidosis. The large efferent lymphatics contained masses of amyloid, which were also attacked by foreign-body giant cells and histiocytes.

We interpret the protein or amyloid deposits in the following way. The tumor cells produce immunoglobulin with abundant light chains or exclusively light chains. These accumulate first in lymph vessels, causing congestion and stasis of the light chains that the tumor cells continue to secrete. The light chains, or their N-terminal fragments, then accumulate within the tumor itself and are transformed into amyloid.[418] The preamyloid and amyloid masses are perceived as foreign substances and, as far as possible, are destroyed by histiocytes and foreign-body giant cells.

[418] GLENNER, EIN and TERRY, 1972; GLENNER, TERRY and ISERSKY, 1973.

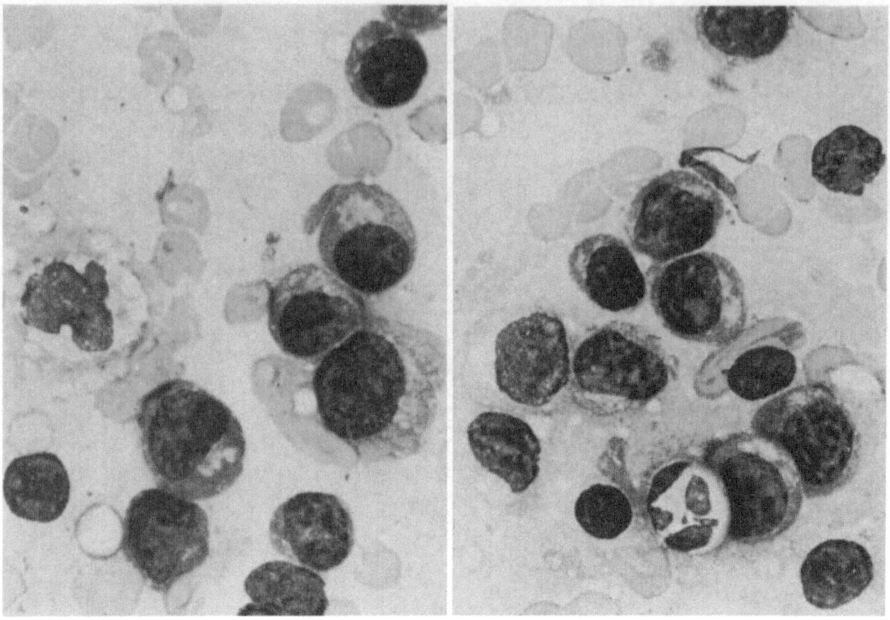

Fig. 136. Imprint of primary lymph-node plasmacytoma. Polymorphic plasma cells. No plasmablasts. ♂, 60 years. Pappenheim. ×875

**Smear/Imprint.**[419] The picture seen is relatively monotonous with ("reticular") plasma cells containing an eccentric nucleus and intensely basophilic cytoplasm (Fig. 136). Polymorphism and anisocytosis are occasionally quite pronounced. Typical plasmablasts are never found. At times there are remnants of uninvolved lymphatic tissue with lymphocytes, centroblasts, etc.

**Histochemistry and Cytochemistry.** The PAS reaction sometimes reveals Russell bodies in plasmacytoma. With Ladewig or Goldner staining they are as a rule reddish. In addition, the PAS reaction often shows a fine reddish to reddish-violet blush in the cytoplasm of plasmacytoma cells. In imprints the neoplastic plasma cells show numerous acid phosphatase-positive granules. The nonspecific esterase (α-naphthyl acetate esterase) reaction can be weakly to moderately positive and is diffuse.

**Diagnosis.** Primary plasmacytoma of lymph nodes is characterized by the following histologic features (see Table 41):

It presents a relatively organized, monotonous picture, produced by the uniform, relatively typical plasma cells and the coarsely to finely alveolar fiber network. Plasmablasts are absent, but polyploid plasma cells with one or more nuclei are almost always evident. Sometimes there is paramyloidosis or an accumulation of immunoglobulin with secondary transformation into amyloid. Occasionally, angioma-like structures are seen.

[419] Jackson and Parker, 1947.

Table 41. Diagnostic criteria of M.L. plasmacytic

1. All ages
2. Paraproteinemia or Bence-Jones proteinuria only when large tumor masses have developed
3. Bone marrow not infiltrated
4. Most common presenting site: cervical lymph nodes
5. Monotonous proliferation of small plasma cells
6. No plasmablasts
7. In many cases plasma cells with multiple or giant nuclei
8. Regular alveolar fiber pattern
9. PAS-positive cells (diffuse or globular reaction)
10. Occasionally amyloid deposits

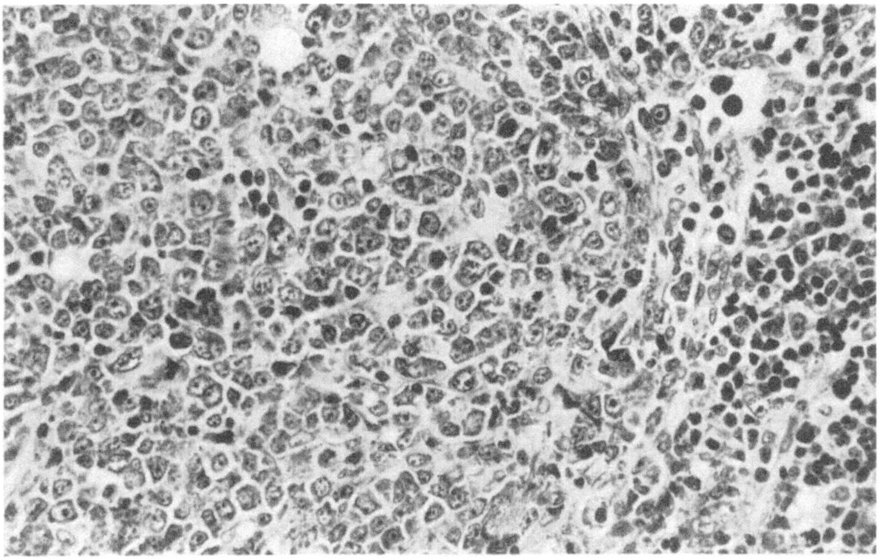

Fig. 137. Reactive plasmacytosis with many plasmablasts. ♂, 42 years. Supraclavicular node. Giemsa. ×350

The diagnosis of plasmacytoma is supported further by the finding of paraproteinemia or Bence-Jones proteinuria. Both disappear after the plasmacytoma is removed. By definition, the bone marrow, at least at the onset of the disease, must be free of infiltration by plasmacytoma cells.

**Differential Diagnosis.**

*1. Reactive Plasmacytosis.* A more or less preserved structure of the lymph node, which usually contains larger and more numerous germinal centers than in primary lymph-node plasmacytoma, suggests a reactive increase in plasma cells. More important is the presence of plasma-cell precursors (Fig. 137). These can often be recognized in sections only with an oil-immersion objective, but they are best seen in imprints. The plasma cells have a somewhat broader rim of cytoplasm than those of plasmacytoma, and their perinuclear halo (Golgi

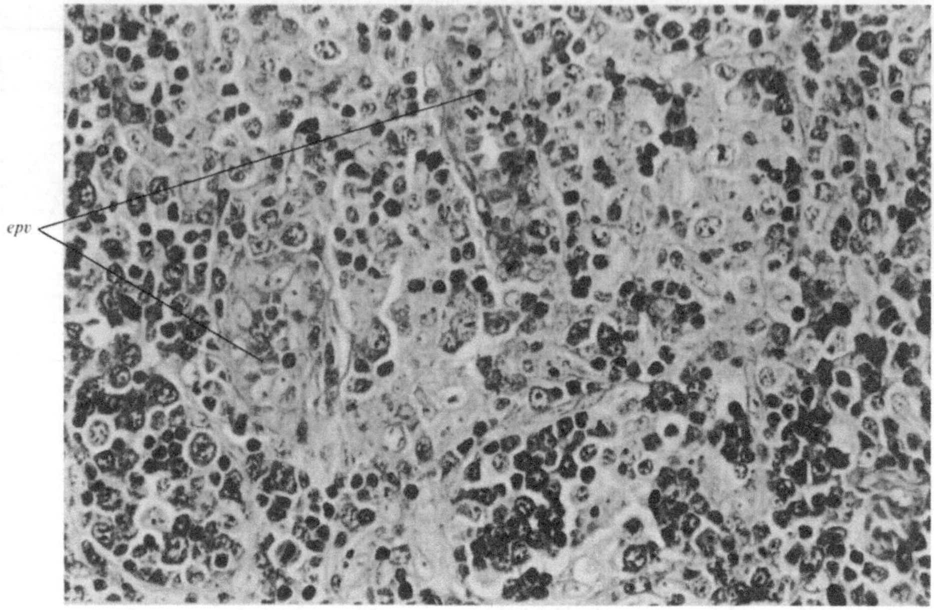


Fig. 138. Lymphogranulomatosis X (angioimmunoblastic lymphadenopathy) with excessive plasmacytosis. Note the epithelioid venules (*epv*). Many plasma cells and some plasmablasts. ♀, 57 years. Cervical node. Giemsa. ×560

apparatus) is more distinct. Sometimes eosinophils and mast cells are intermingled with the plasma cells. The blood often reveals a polyclonal increase in Ig. Bence-Jones protein cannot be demonstrated, even in concentrated urine. Like the lymph node, the bone marrow can also manifest slight to marked plasmacytosis.

2. *Lymphogranulomatosis X (immunoblastic lymphadenopathy) with excessive plasmacytosis.* In contrast to primary lymph-node plasmacytoma, in this condition there is a great increase in epithelioid venules (Fig. 138). The pulp reveals striking polymorphic hyperplasia with all types of stimulated lymphocytes and abundant plasma cells and plasma-cell precursors (proplasmacytes, plasmablasts, proplasmablasts = immunoblasts). These mature and immature forms of the plasma-cell series migrate in large numbers through the sinuses, which are often full of these cells and thereby dilated. The migration of plasma cells and their precursors is evident in the efferent lymphatics as well. Rubella infections can show a similar finding. Follicles and germinal centers are often not seen, or are, at most, only vaguely evident. There may be scattered eosinophils.

3. *Immunocytoma, lymphoplasmacytic subtype.* In general, it is easy to differentiate this disease from primary lymph-node plasmacytoma. Not only are plasma cells present, but also lymphocytes, as a rule in much larger numbers. In addition, one finds large basophilic cells (immunoblasts, plasmablasts). The decisive criterion, however, is the coexistence of lymphocytes, which are completely absent in the tumor masses in primary lymph-node plasmacytoma.

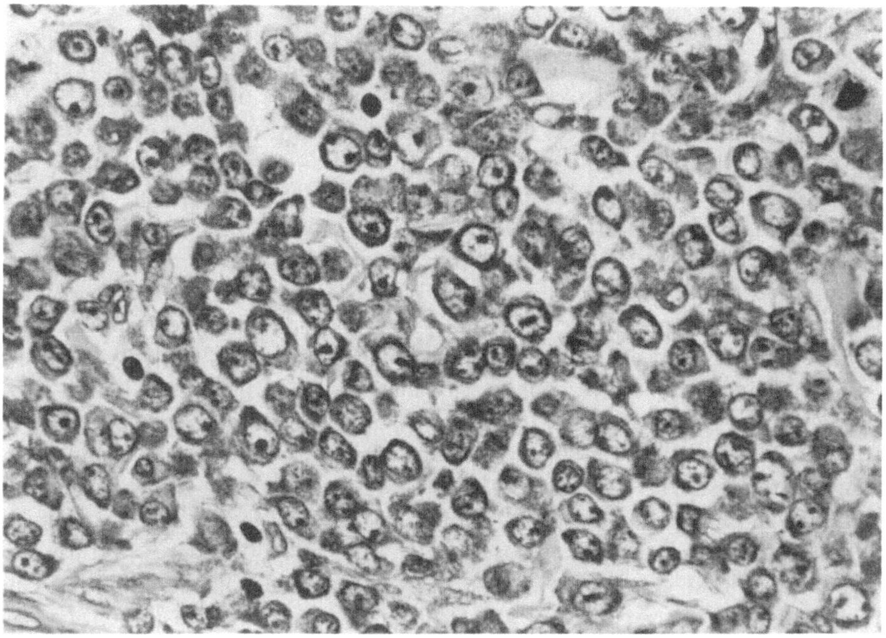

Fig. 139. Metastasis of an anaplastic myeloma ("plasmablastic" type of multiple myeloma). Chiefly large immunoblast-like cells with marked anisocytosis. Some small plasmacytoid cells. ♂, 74 years. Giemsa. ×560

In the earlier literature lymphoplasmacytic immunocytoma was occasionally described erroneously as extraskeletal plasmacytoma (e.g., case 15 of FRUHLING and CHADLI[420]).

4. *Metastasis of an extraskeletal plasmacytoma.* From our experience, metastases of extraskeletal plasmacytomas cannot be distinguished from primary lymph-node plasmacytomas. That is especially true for metastases of tonsillar plasmacytomas.

5. *Metastasis of a multiple myeloma.* Such metastases can be identical with those of extraskeletal plasmacytomas and therefore with primary lymph-node plasmacytomas. The cells of multiple myeloma are often more anaplastic, however; i.e., they are *larger,* assuming the form of large basophilic cells, which, in essence, do not represent true plasma-cell precursors (plasmablasts), but are instead extremely undifferentiated plasma cells (Fig. 139). Regardless of whether the tumor cells are small or large, the picture is monotonous, since it is always composed of a pure population of only *one* type of cell, never of cells at different stages of maturity simultaneously. Sometimes multinucleate giant cells are observed, which should not be mistaken for megakaryocytes or Sternberg-Reed giant cells. This error can be easily avoided if one compares the giant cells with the neighboring mononuclear tumor cells: their cytoplasmic and nuclear structures are identical. The diagnosis is easily substantiated by

[420] 1963.

demonstrating infiltration of the bone marrow by plasma cells and the generally associated paraproteinemia.

6. *Plasma-cell leukemia.* The infiltration in "reticular" plasma-cell leukemia is very similar to that of nonleukemic primary lymph-node plasmacytoma. That is to say, the infiltration consists of small plasma cells. In general, however, the infiltration of trabeculae and the capsule as well as of tissue surrounding the lymph node is greater in plasma-cell leukemia—a finding similar to that in acute leukemias. The infiltration in "lymphatic" plasma-cell leukemia consists of a mixture of plasma cells and plasma-cell precursors.

**Prognosis.** The prognosis of primary lymph-node plasmacytoma appears to be better than that of multiple myeloma. Reports exist of patients surviving $2^1/_2$–26 years. One of the reasons for this may be that patients with lymph-node plasmacytoma generally enter treatment in stage I, namely, when only one group of lymph nodes is involved. In contrast, multiple myeloma usually first becomes manifest after it is already widespread in the bone marrow. According to the calculations of HOBBS,[421] however, it takes a long time (one or more decades) for this to happen. Consequently, multiple myeloma is not treated until it is at least generalized in the bone marrow. Another reason for the better prognosis of primary lymph-node plasmacytoma is the feasibility of surgically removing the tumor completely, since most arise in readily accessible sites (neck, axilla).

## *Addenda*

### *a) Metastases of Myeloma in Lymph Nodes*

Metastases of a multiple myeloma in lymph nodes are seldom diagnosed while the patient is still alive, because multiple myeloma rarely causes large tumor masses in lymph nodes and because the diagnosis of multiple myeloma is made by other means before a lymph-node biopsy is performed. It is noteworthy that several such myeloma metastases in our material were from the axilla.

Even at autopsy one rarely finds greatly enlarged lymph nodes with myeloma infiltration—in our material we were able grossly to detect myeloma metastases in 6%. A scrupulous histologic analysis, however, often discloses slight or moderate myeloma infiltration of lymph nodes that are only slightly enlarged or not enlarged at all. HAYES *et al.*[422] reported infiltration in 46% of autopsy cases in the literature and their own series. The percentage is probably even greater if one includes only the cases one has studied oneself. CHURG and GORDON[423] found myeloma infiltration in 18 out of 28 cases, particularly of retroperitoneal and rarely of peripheral lymph nodes. We have, in addition, frequently detected extramedullary hemopoiesis in retroperitoneal lymph nodes, especially megakaryocytes and granulocyte precursors, less frequently erythropoiesis. The lymph nodes also often disclose marked hemosiderosis.[424]

The finding that the lymph nodes are frequently only slightly enlarged or

[421] 1969.
[422] HAYES, BENNETT and HECK, 1952, Lit.
[423] 1950.
[424] OLMER, MONGIN, MURATORE and DENIZET, 1961.

are even atrophic[425] in myeloma is in remarkable contrast to the widespread enlargement of lymph nodes regularly demonstrated in plasma-cell leukemia.[426]

The morphology of myeloma metastases in lymph nodes has already been discussed (see p. 277).

### *b) The Leukemic Variant of Plasmacytoma: Plasma-Cell Leukemia*[427]

Plasma-cell leukemia is characterized by a moderate or large number of neoplastic plasma cells in the blood and by systemic extraskeletal plasmacytic proliferation with generally diffuse infiltration by plasma cells, but without any formation of tumor nodules. The extraskeletal infiltration affects the liver and spleen and usually lymph nodes. The bone marrow also shows only a diffuse proliferation of plasma cells. The plasma cells are of the Marschalkó type ("reticular").

The weakest link in the chain of definition is the plasma-cell count in the blood. Since in practically every multiple myeloma—as often in malignant tumors of nonhemopoietic tissue—some tumor cells may be found in the blood, the question arises at what level of cell count one should begin to refer to "leukemia." The answer has to be just as arbitrary as for other leukemias or lymphomas. In any event, subleukemic plasma-cell counts (less than 10,000/μl) seem to be much more common than high leukemic values.[425] Consequently, the systemic character of the neoplasm is probably more important than the plasma-cell count in the blood.

This "reticular" plasma-cell leukemia must be distinguished from two other entities that have also been called plasma-cell leukemia, and specifically *lymphatic* plasma-cell leukemia. Both entities are characterized by an increase not only in small plasma cells ("lymphatic" or "lymphoid" plasma cells) but also in their precursors (proplasmacytes and plasmablasts) in the blood and lymph nodes.

The first of these two entities has already been discussed in the chapter on LP immunocytoma. It has been seen as "lymphatic" plasma-cell leukemia in several cases of macroglobulinemia of Waldenström (see p. 250f.). It definitely represents a malignant neoplasm and may thus properly be called lymphatic plasma-cell leukemia.

The second entity with a leukemia-like blood picture has been described in company with autoimmune phenomena as lymphatic plasmacytoma,[428] *akute subleukämische Plasmocytose,*[429] lymphatic plasma-cell leukemia,[430] *sarcomatose ganglionaire diffuse à différenciation plasmocytaire,*[431] lymph-node plasmacytoma,[432] and hyperbasophilic malignant lymphoma.[433] AZAR[425] reported on

[425] AZAR, 1973.

[426] OLMER, MONGIN, MURATORE and DENIZET, 1961.

[427] Reviews: MOSS and ACKERMAN, 1946; BICHEL, EFFERSØE, GORMSEN and HARBOE, 1952; PRUZANSKI, PLATTS and OGRYZLO, 1969; AZAR, 1973; FÜLLE and PRIBILLA, 1973.

[428] HECKNER, 1951; FORSTER and MOESCHLIN, 1954.

[429] WIDMANN, 1957.

[430] LENNERT, 1964a, b.

[431] FLANDRIN, DANIEL, EL YAFI and CHELLOUL, 1972.

[432] LEJEUNE, TURPIN, LECOUTURIER, BOUVIER *et al.*, 1972.

[433] BROUET, LABAUME and SELIGMANN, 1975; DUMONT, DUFFILLOT, FLANDRIN, CHELLOUL *et al.*, 1975.

similar cases in a chapter on "Immune disorders simulating a plasmacytic neoplasm." The histologic picture is described on page 276.

Clinically, a greatly accelerated erythrocyte sedimentation rate is caused by a polyclonal increase in Ig. In one case, however, we saw the transition from a polyclonal increase in Ig in the blood into monoclonal IgG/$\kappa$ paraproteinemia, which was then correlated with a changed histologic picture. Instead of the plasma cells *and* precursors that were seen in the biopsy, pure populations of plasma cells were found in lymph nodes, spleen, and bone marrow at autopsy. Frequently, cold agglutinins may be detected in the blood. A positive Coombs' test and anti-smooth muscle antibodies are often found. In addition, the patient usually has fever and often a skin rash. The enlargement of lymph nodes is usually generalized and associated with hepatosplenomegaly. Small to moderate numbers of "lymphatic" plasma cells and their precursors circulate in the blood. They are also evident in the bone marrow in smaller numbers. BROUET *et al.*[434] demonstrated polyclonal membrane-bound Ig on these cells.

The disease may run an extremely rapid (fulminating), acute, or subchronic course. It may end in death in a few weeks or within a year. Remissions may occur with or without therapy. Corticosteroids have proved to be the most effective treatment.

It has not been proved that this second entity is a malignant neoplasm. The spontaneous recovery we have observed in two cases suggests a nonneoplastic nature of the disease. Furthermore, using a hybridization technique, ZUR HAUSEN demonstrated a relatively small amount of Epstein-Barr virus (EBV) in lymph-node cells in two representative cases from our series.[435] That allows the assumption that in these cases the EBV had caused a B-cell overreaction (with insufficient T-cell reaction?) and that these cases therefore represent an unusual form of infectious mononucleosis. The future will have to show what proportion of cases of this second variant of "lymphatic plasma-cell leukemia" reveal EBV in the lymph nodes and whether or not other infections or immune reactions can also cause the same picture. Since there is a great increase in epithelioid venules in all cases of this variant—we observed the greatest increase in a case of MOESCHLIN[436]—one might consider the disease to be a special variant of immunoblastic lymphadenopathy. Therefore, we used the term immunoblastic lymphadenopathy with excessive plasmacytosis[435] (see p. 276). We no longer employ this term, however, because it hinders thinking more about the still unknown nature of the lesion. In London in 1973, RAPPAPORT and LUKES said that they could not yet determine whether immunoblastic lymphadenopathy is a malignant or a reactive process. This uncertainty and other reasons (cf., T-zone lymphoma) have caused us to continue to use the term we proposed in 1971, namely, lymphogranulomatosis X.[437]

**Occurrence.** "Reticular" plasma-cell leukemia is extremely rare. For every 100 multiple myelomas reported, there are about two plasma-cell leukemias.[438]

[434] BROUET, LABAUME and SELIGMANN, 1975.
[435] BORNKAMM, STEIN, LENNERT, RÜGGEBERG *et al.*, 1976.
[436] 1961.
[437] RADASZKIEWICZ and LENNERT, 1975.
[438] BICHEL, EFFERSØE, GORMSEN and HARBOE, 1952.

The age and sex distribution of plasma-cell leukemia appears to be the same as that of multiple myeloma.[439] Its peak incidence is in the 7th decade. The youngest patient of BICHEL *et al.*[440] was 25 years old, their oldest was 80. In one patient plasma-cell leukemia developed 3 years after treatment with thorium X.[441] Immunochemically, light chains were found most frequently in the blood, occasionally IgG and IgD. Most of the IgE-plasmacytic neoplasms described so far have been leukemic.[442]

**Involvement of Lymph Nodes.** PRUZANSKI *et al.*[443] reported that the lymph nodes were involved in 28 out of the 32 autopsied patients described in the literature. Such involvement is characterized by diffuse infiltration of all lymph-node regions with destruction of the lymph-node architecture. There may also be marked infiltration of trabeculae and surrounding fatty tissue. In the lymph node from one of our patients, we found foci of erythropoiesis and megakaryocytes in the sinuses. The plasma cells are small. Some or numerous mononuclear or multinucleate polyploid forms are seen.

The site of infiltration in the spleen is the same as that seen in hairy-cell leukemia, i.e., the neoplastic cells are found in Billroth's cords in the red pulp. Occasionally, one finds an associated paramyloidosis.

**Prognosis.** The disease usually progresses rapidly. Almost all patients die within the first 6 months of clinical observation. Only the patient of FÜLLE and ALBRECHT[444] survived longer than 2 years.

## C. Lymphomas of Germinal-Center Cells

The cells we call centroblasts and centrocytes are the cells that proliferate or develop in germinal centers. These two types of cells can produce malignant lymphomas. There are three possibilities. In the first there is the formation of both centroblasts *and* centrocytes, as in normal germinal centers; this results in a germinal-center tumor in the true sense, namely, M.L. centroblastic/centrocytic (previously known as germino*blastoma,* follicular lymphoma, or Brill-Symmers disease). The second possibility is a proliferation only of centrocytes; the formation of germinal centers is not realized, and we speak of M.L. centrocytic (germino*cytoma*). Finally, the proliferation can consist either exclusively or chiefly of centroblasts: M.L. centroblastic.

Whereas we distinguish between M.L. centroblastic/centrocytic and M.L. centrocytic, LUKES and COLLINS[445] are of the opinion that all germinal center-cell tumors consist of cleaved *and* noncleaved follicular-center cells (FCC). They speak of the cleaved-cell (centrocytic) type when less than 25% of the cells are noncleaved (centroblastic) and when no large areas with noncleaved FCC (centroblasts) can be demonstrated. Furthermore, LUKES and COLLINS have

[439] MOSS and ACKERMAN, 1946.
[440] BICHEL, EFFERSØE, GORMSEN and HARBOE, 1952.
[441] RIEGEL, 1956.
[442] SALMON, MCINTYRE and OGAWA, 1971.
[443] PRUZANSKI, PLATTS and OGRYZLO, 1969.
[444] 1972.
[445] 1974a, b, 1975a, b.

so far included centrocytic lymphoma together with centroblastic/centrocytic lymphoma, claiming that both can show a follicular, follicular and diffuse, or diffuse growth pattern. The reason for our distinction of two tumors is that they are to be interpreted as biologically different neoplasms, despite all of the morphologic similarities and despite the existence of borderline cases that are difficult to classify as one or the other type of tumor. The differences are:

1. The lymphomas have different age and sex distributions.
2. In *histologic slides* M.L. centrocytic does not show any centroblasts (with basophilic cytoplasm), whereas M.L. centroblastic/centrocytic always shows at least a few. In M.L. centrocytic the cells undergoing mitosis are therefore centrocytes; in M.L. centroblastic/centrocytic the dividing cells are centroblasts.
3. M.L. centrocytic has a fundamentally diffuse growth pattern, but it may occasionally exhibit slight nodularity. In 96% of the cases of M.L. centroblastic/centrocytic at least part of the tumor shows follicular growth. The diffuse variant of M.L. centroblastic/centrocytic is very rare. When it is found, it is often localized at one site, while a follicular pattern has developed at another.
4. "Sarcomatous" transformation occurs frequently in M.L. centroblastic/centrocytic, but very rarely in M.L. centrocytic.
5. M.L. centroblastic/centrocytic occurs more frequently in a sclerotic variant.
6. Involvement of the bone marrow is clinically demonstrated more frequently in M.L. centrocytic than in M.L. centroblastic/centrocytic.
7. In M.L. centrocytic extramedullary hemopoiesis occasionally appears in the lymph node and other sites, with corresponding changes in the blood picture. That was not observed in any of our (more than 800) cases of M.L. centroblastic/centrocytic.
8. Cytologic findings, especially those provided by electron microscopy, show that M.L. centrocytic is often definitely more anaplastic than M.L. centroblastic/centrocytic (see Part Five).
9. The clinical data (B symptoms, stage of disease at time of first examination) and the survival data demonstrate the different, more malignant behavior of M.L. centrocytic.

These differences do not exclude an intimate relationship between the two tumors. This relationship is also evident from the morphology of the tumor cells often found in the blood, which have notched or cleaved nuclei ("cleaved cells"). In some cases there is a great increase in these cells in the blood, so one may speak of a leukemia (see p. 301 ff.).

### *The Morphology of Centroblasts and Centrocytes*

Both types of cells have many features in common with their normal counterparts. As they become malignant, however, deviations appear that do not affect the principle of their origin.

The *centroblasts* of our definition are largely equivalent to the noncleaved follicular-center cells (FCC) of LUKES and COLLINS.[446] The latter term is also used by LUKES and COLLINS, however, for the germinal-center cells with round nuclei that we shall describe and illustrate in the chapter on lymphoblastic lymphoma of the Burkitt type (see p. 365 and Fig. 180). According to our definition, centroblasts are generally medium-sized, but occasionally large, and seldom multinucleate (centroblastic giant cells). Their rim of cytoplasm is narrow, or at most moderately broad, and *intensely* basophilic. With Giemsa staining it is deep blue and with methyl-green pyronine staining it is red. The nuclei are round to oval and are not indented. In typical centroblasts the nuclei contain several medium-sized, strongly basophilic nucleoli, which lie at the nuclear membrane. In some of the cells the nucleoli are located in the center of the nucleus and are then larger, but also strongly basophilic; the question arises as to whether we should interpret these cells as immunoblasts.

All of these criteria can also be reproduced in imprints. Of diagnostic importance are the deep blue, quite narrow rim of cytoplasm and the medium-sized nucleoli. Cytochemically, centroblasts are almost inert. Only the acid phosphatase reaction reveals a few fine to coarse granular structures in the cytoplasm.

*Centrocytes* (cleaved follicular-center cells according to LUKES and COLLINS[446]) are small to medium-sized. Their cytoplasm is so faintly stained that it can hardly be seen in Giemsa sections. It is never as basophilic as the cytoplasm of centroblasts. The nuclei are very polymorphic, often showing deep clefts ("cleaved"). They contain up to three small central nucleoli. The nuclei always stain much less intensely with the Giemsa stain than do those of lymphocytes; that is, they appear more gray-blue in contrast to the deep blue nuclei of lymphocytes.

Centrocytes are more difficult to recognize in imprints, since the irregular nuclei become rounded when the imprints are made or when the cells are spread, and therefore only some of the nuclei retain their original form. Nevertheless, the nuclei often reveal irregular indentations. Occasionally, one finds deep fissures and clefts in the nuclei. Nucleoli are not visible in most cells; but sometimes we find up to three small or medium-sized, light nucleoli. The cytoplasm is sparse and appears clear and gray-blue. Cytochemically, there is no marked difference between centrocytes and centroblasts.

The significance of cleaved nuclei must not be overestimated. The phenomenon of cleavage is by no means a specific cytologic criterion. We have to look at the cytologic picture as a whole, and not only for nuclear clefts, which occur in a number of lymphomas. Otherwise, we would include centrocytes and Lutzner cells of Sézary's syndrome in one group, as HAMBURG *et al.*[447] recently did. The frequency of cleaved nuclei depends, furthermore, on the quality of the histologic technique. In reviewing a large collection of poorly fixed and embedded lymphomas, we found many more cleaved cells

---

[446] 1974a, b, 1975a, b.

[447] HAMBURG, BRYNES, REESE and GOLOMB, 1976.

than in our own material. Moreover, we have occasionally found some nuclear cleavage and nuclear irregularities in lymphocytes in peripheral blood smears of patients with histologically typical B-CLL.

### *1. Malignant Lymphoma, Centrocytic (Centrocytoma)*

*Synonyms and related terms:*

Lymphocytic lymphosarcoma
Malignant lymphoma, lymphocytic, well and poorly differentiated
Malignant lymphoma, lymphocytic, intermediate
Malignant lymphoma, FCC, cleaved, diffuse
Malignant lymphoma, atypical small lymphocytic
Lymphosarcoma-cell leukemia
Germinocytoma

**Origin of the Neoplastic Cells and Terminology.** For a long time this tumor was called lymphocytic lymphosarcoma. Even now, in accordance with RAPPAPORT's concept, it is regarded as a well or poorly differentiated or, according to DORFMAN,[448] an atypical small lymphocytic malignant lymphoma. We agree with LUKES and COLLINS,[449] however, that it is a tumor formed of germinal-center cells, specifically of centrocytes (germinocytes, cleaved follicular-center cells).

We consider the tumor to be a neoplasm of centrocytes (Fig. 140) for the following reasons:

1. The proliferating cells are essentially centrocytes. That is not definitely apparent at first glance in all cases. In sections from well-fixed and -embedded tissue, however, the proliferating cells can be clearly identified as centrocytes in most cases. They are the dividing cells. Furthermore, on electron microscopy, the tumor cells of M.L. centrocytic most closely resemble centrocytes of germinal centers. They frequently contain nuclear pockets as do normal centrocytes.[450]

2. As KAISERLING[450] was able to show in electron-microscopic studies in 12 out of 20 cases, dendritic reticulum cells with desmosomes can be demonstrated among the centrocytes. Since these reticulum cells occur only in or near the follicles in normal lymph nodes, they are an important indication of the follicular origin of the proliferating cells.

3. Occasionally, in lymph-node imprints it is possible to identify a few "blast cells" that resemble centroblasts in their narrow rim of basophilic cytoplasm and medium-sized multiple nucleoli. They also look like centroblasts in electron micrographs. In routine histologic sections, however, these cells cannot be recognized. We may interpret these "blast cells" as rudimentary centroblasts or as centrocytes in a "blastic," i.e., premitotic phase.

4. Silver staining occasionally reveals some nodularity (but no true follicles) in the growth pattern.

---

[448] 1974a.

[449] 1974a, b; see also GLICK, LEECH, WALDRON, FLEXNER *et al.*, 1975; LEECH, GLICK, WALDRON, FLEXNER *et al.*, 1975.

[450] KAISERLING, 1975.

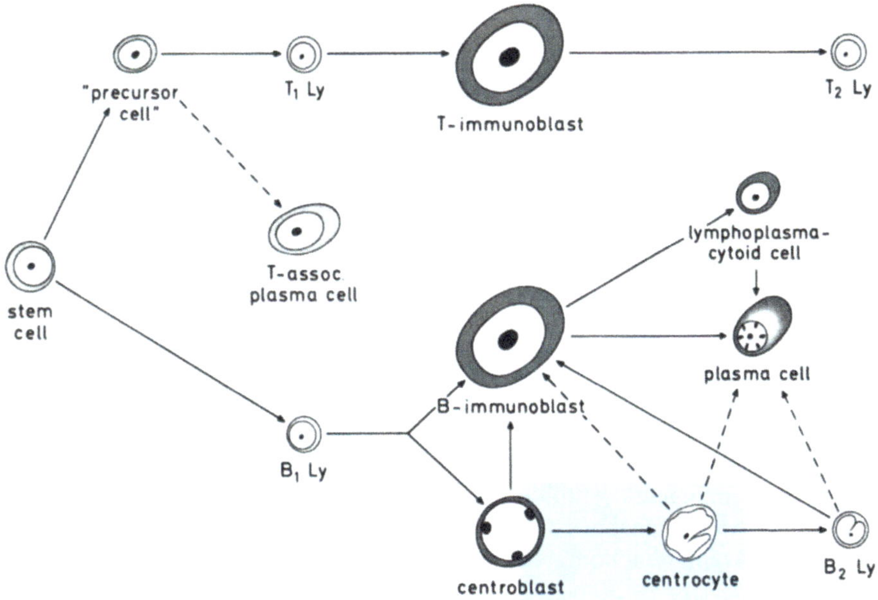


Fig. 140. Hypothetical origin of tumor cells of M.L. centrocytic

5. There are borderline cases between centroblastic/centrocytic and centrocytic lymphoma in which the tumor in one region shows a follicular centroblastic-centrocytic picture, whereas in another region a diffuse, purely centrocytic picture may be evident. We have also seen a few cases in which a centroblastic/centrocytic lymphoma was later followed by the appearance of a centrocytic lymphoma.

6. The results provided by our immunologic studies not only proved the B-cell nature of the tumor cells, but also supported their germinal-center origin. The tumor homogenates revealed a usually slight, rarely marked, increase in IgM, but hardly ever a marked decrease. For the most part, this IgM must be interpreted as surface Ig, since we always found an increase in IgM in the second extract (see Part Six for further details). In addition, in all the tumors we studied with the immunoperoxidase technique, we detected a remarkably large amount of surface IgM. Furthermore, we were able to demonstrate complement receptors in all tumors analyzed. A number of authors have reported similar findings. LEECH *et al.*[451] and HOPPER[452] found chiefly IgM and IgD, occasionally IgG on the surfaces of cleaved follicular-center cells; in contrast to the nodular type, their cases showed mainly λ-chains. AISENBERG and LONG[453] reported larger amounts of surface Ig (IgM) in 10 out of 11 cases than in B-CLL; the 11th case was Ig-negative.

[451] LEECH, GLICK, WALDRON, FLEXNER *et al.*, 1975.
[452] 1974.
[453] 1975; earlier: AISENBERG and BLOCH, 1972; AISENBERG, BLOCH and LONG, 1973.

The former term lymphosarcoma emphasized that the tumor is quite malignant. In the Kiel Classification centrocytic lymphoma is classified in the "low-grade malignancy" group. Nevertheless, we regard the tumor as somewhat more malignant than the other low-grade malignant lymphomas, e.g., centroblastic/centrocytic lymphoma, CLL, and LP immunocytoma, for the following reasons:

1. The tumor does not grow in an organoid manner forming germinal centers. Instead, the tumor cells are "emancipated" and show a disorganized growth pattern.

2. The centrocytes are often somewhat more anaplastic than those of centroblastic/centrocytic lymphoma. They reveal greater anisocytosis and, as electron-microscopic studies disclosed, they generally lack rough endoplasmic reticulum.

3. Dendritic reticulum cells are not always present. *Typical* centroblasts also cannot be seen in sections.

4. The sinuses are completely destroyed by tumor cells.

5. On average, the prognosis is poorer than that of the other four types of low-grade malignant lymphomas. It lies at the lower limit of all low-grade malignant lymphomas, but is significantly poorer than the prognosis of centroblastic/centrocytic lymphoma and B-CLL.

**Occurrence.** Among every 1000 lymph nodes studied, we find eight centrocytic lymphomas. They represent 4.8% of all our malignant lymphomas and 8.6% of our non-Hodgkin's lymphomas (Table 42). In the larger series we analyzed later (see Table 13), 10% of the non-Hodgkin's lymphomas were centrocytic. We estimate that in Northern Germany each year one M.L. centrocytic develops for every one million inhabitants.

The age curve shows a pronounced peak in the 7th decade (Fig. 141). Our youngest patient was 22, our oldest 86 years old. Males predominate (1.8:1), in contrast to centroblastic/centrocytic lymphoma, which shows a slight predominance in females.

Table 42. M.L. centrocytic. Material and incidence

| | | |
|---|---|---|
| Total No. of cases | 128 | |
| Biopsy | | 125 |
| Autopsy | | 3 |
| Total No. of biopsies | 175 | |
| Lymph nodes | | 139 |
| Extranodal | | 36 |
| Incidence in routine lymph-node biopsies | | 72 |
| = 4.8% of malignant lymphomas | | |
| 8.6% of non-Hodgkin's lymphomas | | |

**Clinical Manifestations.** Brittinger *et al.*[454] reviewed the clinical data accumulated by the Kiel Lymphoma Study Group on centrocytic lymphoma and reported the following (see Table 43). Lymph-node enlargement occurred slowly in 40% and rapidly in 33% of the cases. Lymph nodes above and below the

[454] Brittinger, Bartels, Bremer, Dühmke *et al.*, 1976.

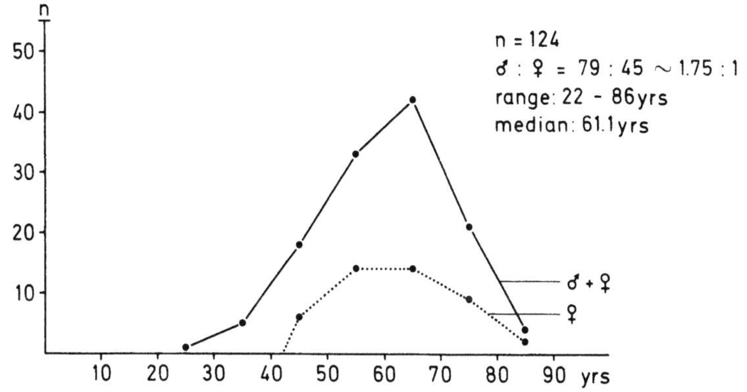


Fig. 141. Age distribution and sex ratio of M.L. centrocytic (124 patients)

Table 43. Clinical data on M.L. centrocytic (28 – 36 usable cases) of the Kiel Lymphoma Study Group (BRITTINGER *et al.*, 1976)

| | | % |
|---|---|---|
| Enlargement of lymph nodes (n = 30) | | |
| | Rapid (1 – 3 months) | 33 |
| | Average (3 – 5 months) | 27 |
| | Slow (> 6 months) | 40 |
| Splenomegaly (n = 36) | | 47 |
| B-symptoms (n = 28) | | 54 |
| Bone-marrow involvement (n = 31) | | 68 |
| Immunoglobulin in blood (n = 23) | | |
| IgG | Normal | 83 |
| | Increased | – |
| | Decreased | 17 |
| IgA | Normal | 61 |
| | Increased | 13 |
| | Decreased | 26 |
| IgM | Normal | 67 |
| | Increased | 4 |
| | Decreased | 29 |
| Hemoglobin g-% (n = 36) | | |
| | > 13 | 44 |
| | 10–13 | 42 |
| | < 10 | 14 |
| Thrombocytes/μl (n = 30) | | |
| | < 100,000 | 17 |

Table 44. Blood lymphocyte counts of 34 patients with M.L. centrocytic. Estimated by Dr. KÖNIG, Kiel Lymphoma Study Group (BRITTINGER *et al.*, 1976)

| | No. of cases Total | % |
|---|---|---|
| Total lymphocytes/µl | | |
| < 1000 | 3/34 | 9 |
| 1000 – 4000 | 22/34 | 65 |
| > 4000 | 9/34 | 26 |
| Small and large lymphocytes/µl | | |
| < 1000 | 7/19 | 37 |
| 1000 – 4000 | 10/19 | 53 |
| > 4000 | 2/19 | 10 |
| Centrocytes/µl | | |
| 0 | 3/19 | 16 |
| < 1000 | 7/19 | 37 |
| 1000 – 4000 | 5/19 | 26 |
| > 4000 | 4/19 | 21 |

diaphragm were generally involved. Splenomegaly was diagnosed by palpation in 47% of the patients. The bone marrow was infiltrated in at least 68%. Most of the cases were stage IV, but a few were stage III at the time of initial diagnosis. B symptoms (according to the Ann Arbor definition[455]) were found in 54% of the patients. About half of the patients were slightly to moderately anemic, but only 17% had thrombocytopenia. The erythrocyte sedimentation rate could be slightly to greatly increased. The level of Ig in the serum was lower than in all other non-Hodgkin's lymphomas. In particular, the IgM level was usually slightly subnormal or even further reduced.

**Blood Picture.** Generally, the number of lymphocytes in the blood is normal. Careful study, however, reveals almost always that some or many lymphoid cells are typical centrocytes with cleaved or notched nuclei and one to three light nucleoli of small or medium size. They are probably identical with the lymphosarcoma cells of SCHREK and DONNELLY,[456] SCHNITZER *et al.*,[457] and AISENBERG and LONG.[458]

The centrocytes are of different sizes in different cases, but in each case all cells will be relatively monotonous and of nearly the same size. Centroblasts do not occur.

KÖNIG[459] analyzed blood smears of the cases of the Kiel Lymphoma Study Group and found the values given in Table 44. Nine percent of the patients showed severe lymphopenia, and 26%, lymphocytosis with counts higher than 4000/µl. In 16 out of 19 cases the "lymphocytes" included small or relatively large numbers of centrocytes: < 1000/µl in seven cases, 1000 – 4000/µl in five

[455] CARBONE, KAPLAN, MUSSHOFF, SMITHERS *et al.*, 1971.
[456] 1966.
[457] SCHNITZER, LOESEL and REED, 1970.
[458] 1975.
[459] Unpublished data.

Table 45. Localization of biopsies in M.L. centrocytic

| Localization | n | | % |
|---|---|---|---|
| Lymph nodes | 139 | | |
| Cervical | | 51 | 45.1 |
| Axillary | | 24 | 21.2 |
| Mediastinal | | — | — |
| Abdominal | | 3 | 2.7 |
| Inguinal | | 34 | 30.1 |
| Cubital | | 1 | 0.9 |
| Unknown | | 26 | — |
| Extranodal | 30 | | |
| Skin | | 7 | — |
| Intestine, including rectum | | 7 | — |
| Stomach | | 3 | — |
| Tonsils | | 4 | — |
| Others | | 9 | — |

cases, and more than 4000/μl in four cases. In most cases the proportion of centrocytes lay between 35 and 55%.

In a double-blind study KÖNIG, and later SCHWARZE,[460] could not distinguish the leukemic centrocytes of M.L. centroblastic/centrocytic from the centrocytes occurring in the blood in M.L. centrocytic. That is further evidence of the identity of the circulating cells in both lymphomas. We should add, however, that we observed a number of cleaved lymphocytes in the peripheral blood in some cases of B-CLL with a pseudofollicular histologic pattern. Cleaved lymphocytes are also found in some cases of LP immunocytoma, especially that of the polymorphic subtype.

We found leukocyte counts between 22,800 and 182,000/μl in six out of 93 cases at the Lymph Node Registry. The number of lymphocytes was estimated to be between 6310 and 71,600/μl. According to the available data, 23.7% of the patients had lymphocyte counts of more than 4000/μl.

Myeloid precursors (promyelocytes, myelocytes) and normoblasts may be found occasionally in addition to the centrocytes. We found them in three cases.

**Localization.** The lymph nodes sent to us for study came most frequently from the cervical region, but almost as frequently from the inguinal or axillary regions (Table 45). In contrast, only rarely did we receive mediastinal or abdominal lymph nodes. Our material also includes specimens other than lymph nodes removed from many organs and tissues, particularly the skin, tonsils, rectum, and stomach.

**Gross Appearance.** The lymph nodes are slightly or moderately enlarged and rather soft. When sectioned, the fresh surface is mostly gray-white.

[460] Unpublished data.

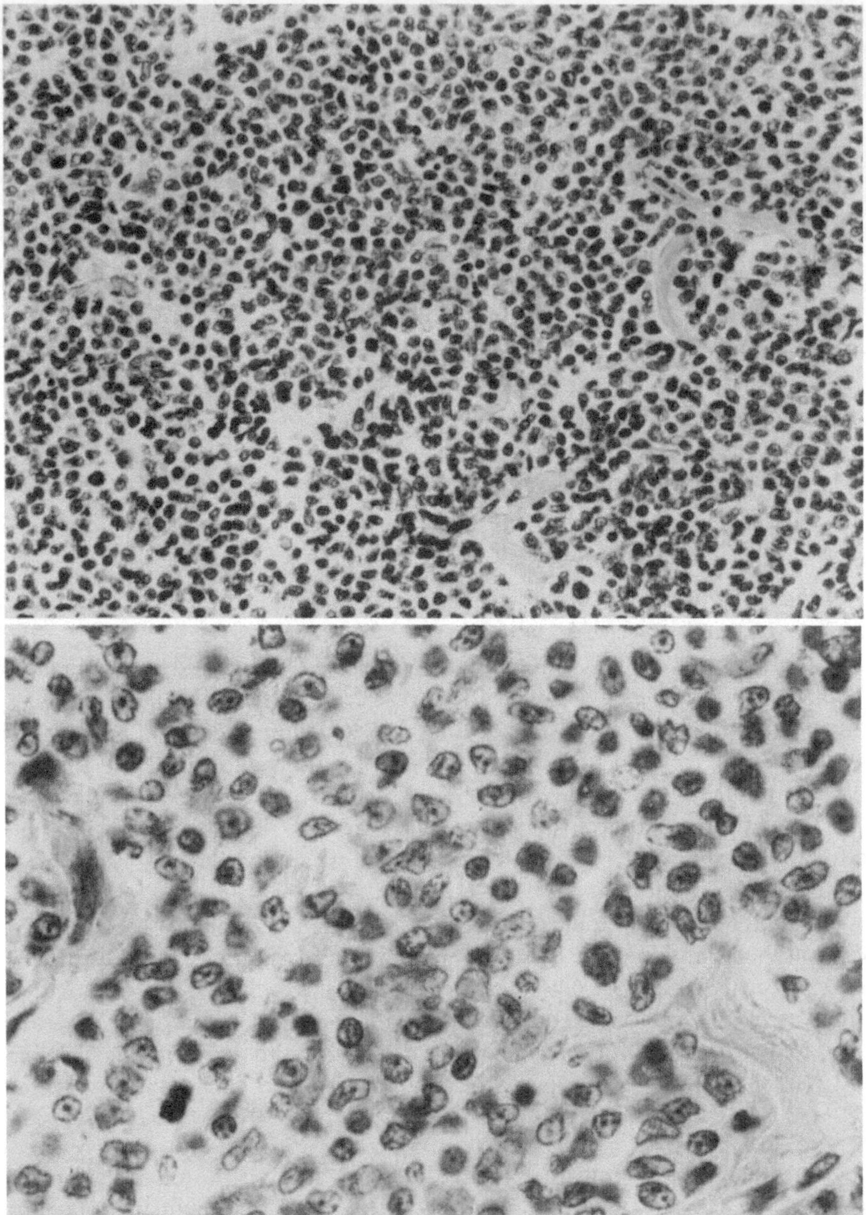

(a)

(b)

Fig. 142a and b. M.L. centrocytic, small cell. Monotonous picture. Some hyalin strands (around small vessels). At higher magnification one sees some pleomorphism with some cleaved nuclei. Note the uniformity of cell size. ♂, 44 years. Axillary node. Giemsa. (a) ×350, (b) ×875

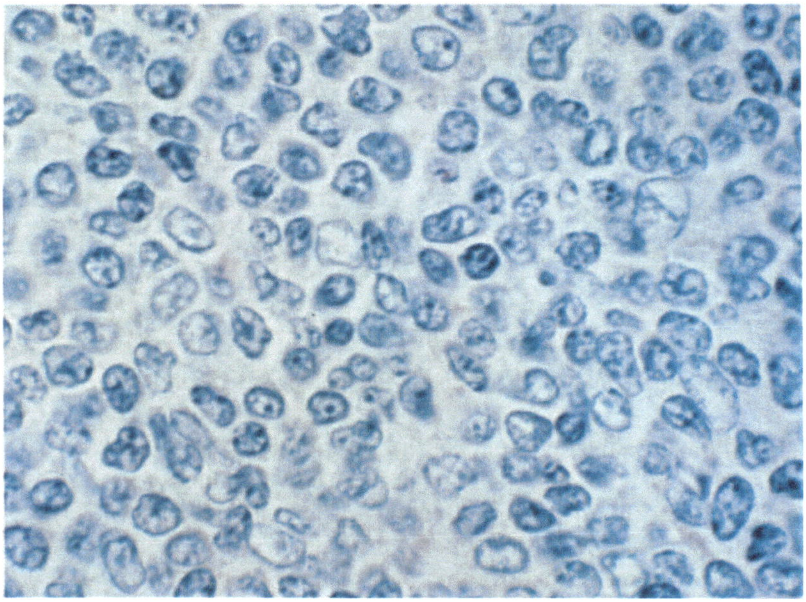

Fig. 143. M.L. centrocytic, small cell, with Giemsa staining. The overall impression suggests uniformity, but the individual nuclei vary considerably. Some cells contain cleaved nuclei. The chromatin pattern is fine, the nucleoli are small. Cytoplasm cannot be identified. ♂, 53 years. Axillary node. × 1,550

**Histology.** Even at a low magnification, it is possible to make a tentative diagnosis of M.L. centrocytic. This requires a Giemsa section—on the whole, the centrocytes appear more gray-blue and not as deep blue as, for example, the cells of CLL or immunocytoma. That produces a relatively uniform ("boring") first impression, which must then be substantiated by cytologic analysis.

There is another histologic feature that may support the first cytologic impression: the tumor cells are more or less regularly interspersed with small blood vessels (capillaries, arterioles) that are often surrounded by a distinct sheath of hyalin. Epithelioid venules are almost completely absent. The sinuses are destroyed by the proliferation and cannot be recognized as such.

Cytologically, the centrocytes are small to medium-sized (Figs. 142 and 143). Although in one tumor the nuclei may be fairly uniform in size, in another they may vary greatly. As already described above, the nuclei are polymorphic with irregularly angular or cleaved shapes. With Giemsa staining the cytoplasm can hardly be recognized, in other words, it is not basophilic; there is also little of it. Generally, there are small or moderate numbers of mitotic figures, although at times they may be abundant. Typical centroblasts are absent. A few typical plasma cells are sometimes found, especially around small vessels with thick hyalinized walls. The T-associated plasma cells that KAISERLING detected by electron microscopy in one third of his cases are generally overlooked in light-microscopic studies. Finally, among the neoplastic centrocytes there are reticulum cells with light oval nuclei and an ill-defined, but generally narrow

Table 46. Nodularity in large- and small-cell variants of centrocytic lymphoma. 98 cases of the Lymph Node Registry, Kiel, investigated by Dr. SATODATE

| Nodularity | Large-cell variant | Small-cell variant | Total |
|---|---|---|---|
| Negative | 14 | 61 | 75 |
| Questionable | 1 | 10 | 11 |
| Definite, but slight | 2 | 4 | 6 |
| Definite, found in more than half of the section | – | 6 | 6 |
| Total | 17 | 81 | 98 |

rim of cytoplasm. Some of these cells may be regarded as dendritic reticulum cells.

Infiltration undoubtedly begins in the outer cortex. Occasionally, the infiltration is seen as wide bands encircling preexistent germinal centers containing few cells or remnants of germinal centers. That may give a coarsely nodular impression. Besides this phenomenon, in about 12% of cases[461] silver staining brought out some nodularity in a part of the lymph node (Table 46). What was seen, however, was not the picture of germinal centers, but instead that of solid tumor nodules, deficient or lacking in fibers, but surrounded by tumor tissue abounding in fibers. The nodules and the surrounding tissue were composed of the same cells. The nodules themselves were slightly reminiscent of primary follicles. In most cases (75%), however, the proliferation was undoubtedly diffuse. Silver staining then revealed only sparse but thick fibers that either were widely dispersed or formed a coarse alveolar pattern (Fig. 144). With silver staining the destructive growth of the tumor, especially where it reached the capsule, could also be recognized. Defined areas of the capsule were destroyed.

Band-forming sclerosis similar to that seen in sclerosing centroblastic/centrocytic lymphoma sometimes develops (Table 47). That was also the experience of BENNETT,[462] who found sclerosis in eight out of 20 cases of centrocytic lymphoma—an incidence of 40%. He reported that sclerosis is more frequent in the large-cell type (75%) than in the small-cell type (17%). SATODATE[461] investigated 98 biopsies of centrocytic lymphoma and found pronounced band-forming sclerosis in 6% of the cases. In addition, he could demonstrate marked diffuse fibrosis in 3% of the cases. This fibrosis was characterized by a diffuse increase in thick bundles of argyrophil fibers circumscribing small groups of cells or even single tumor cells. It is equivalent only in part to the "fine sclerosis" of BENNETT,[463] since apparently this also includes the commonly observed alveolar pattern of a few coarse fibers, which we have so far not recorded as sclerosis or fibrosis. Moreover, SATODATE demonstrated slight band-forming sclerosis in 10% of the cases and slight diffuse fibrosis in 32%.

In two centrocytic lymphomas we studied, we found a rather pronounced extramedullary hematopoiesis, with abundant chloroacetate esterase-positive

[461] SATODATE, unpublished data.
[462] 1975a, b.
[463] 1975b.

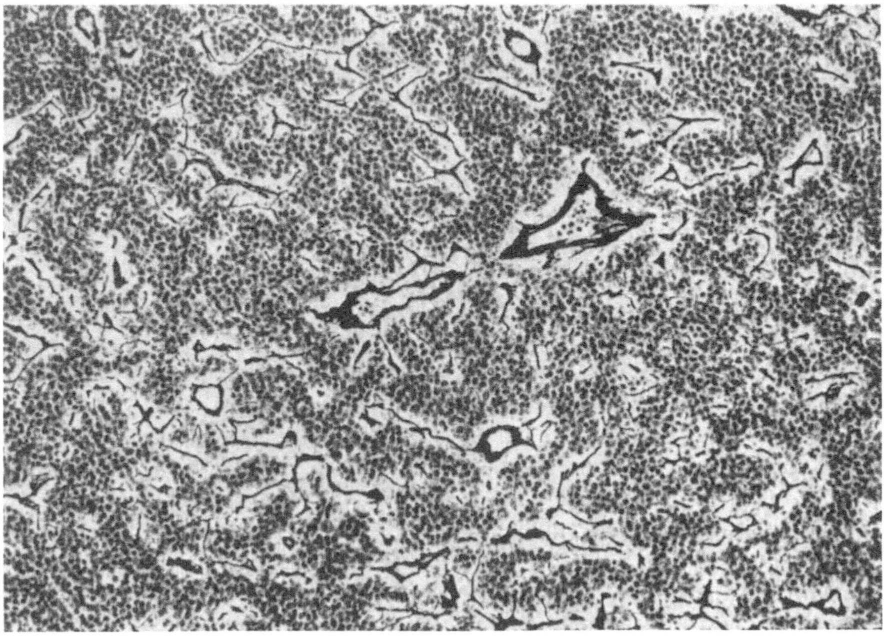

Fig. 144. M.L. centrocytic with silver staining. The tumor cells form closely packed masses without any follicular arrangement. The fibers are thick and very sparse, mostly around small vessels. Same node as Fig. 142. Gomori. × 140

Table 47. Sclerosis and fibrosis in large- and small-cell variants of centrocytic lymphoma. 98 cases of the Lymph Node Registry, Kiel, investigated by Dr. SATODATE

| Sclerosis/Fibrosis | Large-cell variant | Small-cell variant | Total |
|---|---|---|---|
| Negative | 10 | 30 | 40 |
| Negative, with some scars | – | 7 | 7 |
| Slight band-forming sclerosis | – | 10 | 10 |
| Slight diffuse fibrosis | 5 | 27 | 32 |
| Marked band-forming sclerosis | – | 6 | 6 |
| Marked diffuse fibrosis | 2 | 1 | 3 |
| Total | 17 | 81 | 98 |

myelocytes and in one case also with some normoblasts. In the latter case these findings corresponded to the clinical finding of normoblasts in the peripheral blood.

Because we had the subjective impression that there are two subtypes of centrocytic lymphoma, namely, a small- and a large-cell subtype, SATODATE was asked to review our material and to clarify the following questions in quantitative studies:

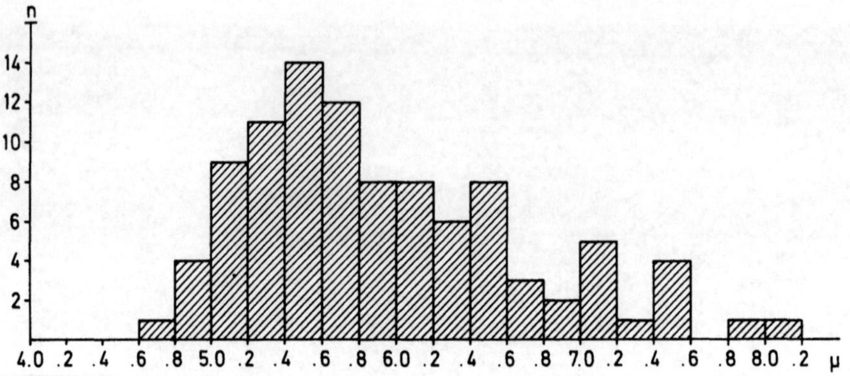


Fig. 145. Nuclear diameters in M.L. centrocytic. $n$ = number of cases. μ = mean value for 30–70 nuclear diameters in microns, measured in photomicrographs at a magnification of ×800 by Dr. SATODATE

1. Do we have to distinguish a small- and a large-cell variant of centrocytic lymphoma? If so—
2. How many mitotic figures are found in each variant?
3. How often is fibrosis or sclerosis found in each variant?
4. How often is some nodularity found in each variant?

1. The maximal nuclear diameter was estimated in 98 specimens. The results are shown in Figure 145. The largest nuclear diameters ranged from 4.6 to 8.2 μm. Although there is no clear bimodal distribution, the graph might suggest grouping together large-cell variants with a diameter of >6.5 μm and small-cell variants with a diameter of <6.5 μm. The large-cell tumors can have a maximum diameter of 8.2 μm, the small-cell variants a minimum diameter of 4.6 μm.

2. The number of mitotic figures varied greatly (Table 48). SATODATE[464] found 0–2 mitotic figures per field (at a magnification of ×500) in 59 cases and more than two mitotic figures (up to five per field) in 39 cases. The small-cell type revealed more than two mitotic figures per field in about one third of the cases (34.6%), and the large-cell type, in about two thirds of the cases (64.7%). No mitotic figures were seen in 20 cases. Nineteen of these were of the small-cell type. Therefore, the average rate of proliferation, as measured by the number of mitotic figures, is clearly higher in the large-cell type than in the small-cell type. That is in agreement with the kinetic studies presented by SILVESTRINI *et al.*[465] In large-cell centrocytic lymphoma, they observed a spread of cells through the cell cycle and a faster rate of proliferation than in small-cell centrocytic lymphoma, which showed a very low labeling index. Therefore, they suggested that the degree of proliferation of large-cell centrocytic lymphoma (together with polymorphic immunocytoma) lies between that of the other low-grade malignant lymphomas and that of the high-grade lymphomas.

[464] Unpublished data.

[465] SILVESTRINI, PIAZZA, RICCARDI and RILKE, 1977.

Table 48. Number of mitotic figures in 98 nodal biopsies of M.L. centrocytic

| No. of mitotic figures[a] | Large cells $>6.5\ \mu m$ | Small cells $<6.5\ \mu m$ | Total |
|---|---|---|---|
| $<2$ | 6 | 53 | 59 |
| $>2$ | 11 | 28 | 39 |

[a] Number of mitotic figures per field at a magnification of $\times 400$; mean value for 10 fields.

3. Among 17 large-cell centrocytic lymphomas SATODATE found only two cases with marked diffuse fibrosis and five cases with slight diffuse fibrosis, but no case with band-forming sclerosis (Table 47). In contrast, small-cell centrocytic lymphoma showed striking band-forming sclerosis in six cases and slight band-forming sclerosis in 10 cases, whereas only one case revealed marked diffuse fibrosis and 27 cases, slight diffuse fibrosis.

4. The tendency to form small nodules was seen in about 12% of the small- and large-cell variants, but it was found to a greater extent in the small-cell variant (Table 46).

Thus, we may conclude that there are some differences between the small- and the large-cell variants of M.L. centrocytic (see also Fig. 147). The validity of this subdivision needs to be substantiated by clinical studies.

**Smear/Imprint.** The centrocytes form a relatively monotonous picture (Fig. 146). They are somewhat larger than lymphocytes and, above all, have lighter nuclei. These usually contain a clear, small or medium-sized nucleolus, sometimes two or three. The nuclei often appear round, but are sometimes indented or irregular in shape. The cytoplasmic rim is very narrow and often not even visible. Scattered among these centrocytes are rare centroblast-like cells with narrow haloes of clearly basophilic cytoplasm and several nucleoli. These are of medium size and lie at the nuclear membrane. The centroblast-like cells are somewhat larger than the centrocytes and their cytoplasm can be clearly seen. Finally, a few histiocytic reticulum cells may be encountered.

**Histochemistry and Cytochemistry.** In sections and imprints the tumor cells as a rule are PAS-negative. In particular, there is no fine or coarse granular PAS reaction as in lymphoblastic neoplasms. The centrocytes give a weakly to moderately positive, granular reaction for acid phosphatase in imprints. The reaction for ATPase in sections is generally positive, that for 5-nucleotidase is negative or at most extremely weak.

**Diagnosis.** Initital clues pointing to the diagnosis are the uniformity of small to medium-sized cells and the relatively weak staining in Giemsa slides. The main cytologic criteria are the polymorphism of the gray-blue, relatively light nuclei and the lack of blast cells with basophilic cytoplasm in sections. The cleavage of nuclei is often not clearly visible or is absent, especially after poor fixation. After poor embedding, all nuclei may be cleaved or rounded. Silver

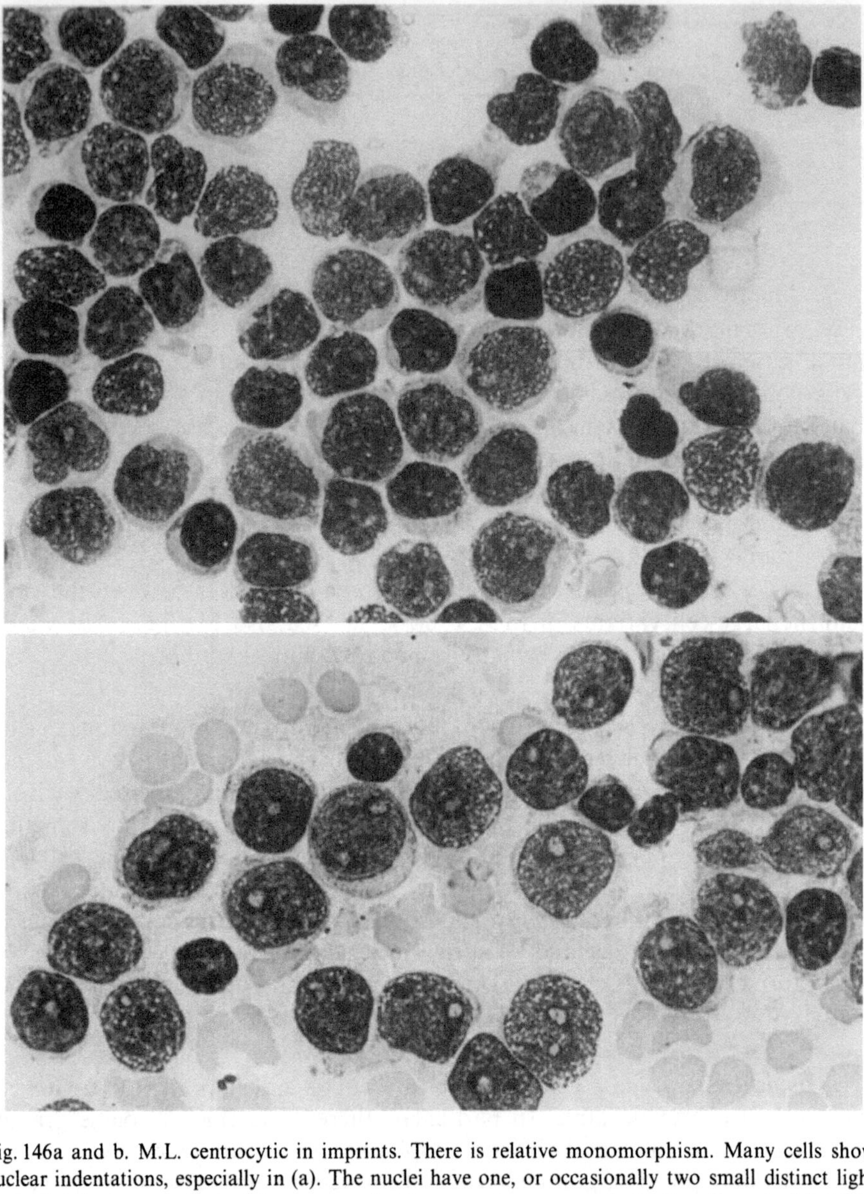

(a)

(b)

Fig. 146a and b. M.L. centrocytic in imprints. There is relative monomorphism. Many cells show nuclear indentations, especially in (a). The nuclei have one, or occasionally two small distinct light nucleoli. The tumor cells in (b) are somewhat larger and more anaplastic than those in (a). (a) ♀, 72 years. Cervical node. (b) ♀, 78 years. Tonsil. Pappenheim. ×875

staining reveals in most cases only a few thick fibers that are in coarse alveolar patterns. Further criteria are listed in Table 49.

**Differential Diagnosis.** The *unclassified type of lymphoblastic lymphoma (including ALL)* causes the greatest problem in the differential diagnosis, especially the small-cell type. In this disease one also finds relatively light, polymorphic

Table 49. Diagnostic criteria of M.L. centrocytic

| |
|---|
| 1. No patients younger than 20 years |
| 2. Only one kind of tumor cell: centrocytes (cleaved nuclei, small nucleoli, cytoplasm not visible) |
| 3. Prominent polymorphism and anisocytosis of the centrocytes |
| 4. No blast cells |
| 5. Low to high mitotic activity |
| 6. Few but very thick fibers in most cases; sometimes diffuse fibrosis or band-forming sclerosis |
| 7. Diffuse growth pattern, but at times somewhat nodular |

nuclei. The cells are very similar to those of centrocytic lymphoma, which tempted us to infer a kinship between the two tumors. At present, however, this relationship cannot be proved.

The best criterion for differentiating the two lymphomas is the stainability of the cytoplasm. That of the centrocytes scarcely becomes colored with Giemsa staining, whereas the cytoplasm of the cells of lymphoblastic lymphoma is clearly basophilic. Although the cytoplasm of lymphoblastic lymphoma cells is a bright blue, it is so narrow that an oil-immersion objective is necessary for its recognition; but even then it is sometimes hardly visible in sections. The use of imprints makes the differentiation considerably easier. In these the cytoplasm of the centrocytes is bright gray-blue. In contrast, that of lymphoblasts is definitely blue.

Three other criteria help to differentiate these two tumors. Centrocytic lymphoma often displays relatively few mitotic figures, whereas lymphoblastic lymphoma always shows high mitotic activity. Centrocytic lymphoma reveals relatively sparse, thick fibers and occasionally shows some nodularity. In lymphoblastic lymphoma we find only small to moderate numbers of very fine fibers; nodularity is not seen. Centrocytic lymphoma does not appear before the third decade, whereas lymphoblastic lymphoma occurs most frequently before the age of 20.

In contrast to nonleukemic lymphoblastic lymphoma ("sarcoma"), the leukemic variant of lymphoblastic lymphoma (unclassified type) often shows a uniform infiltration and widening of the connective tissue of the capsule and trabeculae, which are not observed in centrocytic lymphoma. On the other hand, centrocytic lymphoma shows definitely destructive growth when the capsule is invaded. When this is seen, it is an important point of distinction from ALL. The same holds true for distinguishing *acute myeloid leukemia* (AML), which can be very similar to ALL. Some similarity to centrocytic lymphoma can be seen when the myeloid cells include a large number of monocytes (myelomonocytic leukemia), since monocytes look somewhat like centrocytes owing to the sometimes deeply cleaved nuclei. The most important reaction for distinguishing AML, including myelomonocytic variants, from centrocytic lymphoma is the chloroacetate esterase reaction. It is positive in myeloid precursor cells, although not invariably so.

The similarity between centrocytic lymphoma and AML is particularly striking when there are no, or almost no, other cells present besides monocytes *(monocytic leukemia)*. In such cases the differential diagnostic criteria listed

Table 50. Diagnostic criteria of monocytic leukemia

1. All ages
2. In peripheral blood increased numbers of monocytes and some or many myeloid precursors
3. First infiltration in the pulp, especially of the medulla
4. Monotonous, but polymorphic neoplasm of atypical monocytes:
   Nucleus: relatively large, sometimes cleaved or bilobated, anisocytotic and polymorphic; contains one large nucleolus
   Cytoplasm: less abundant than normal, not basophilic (gray with Giemsa staining)
5. Some or many chloroacetate esterase-positive cells:
   (+) some precursors of monocytes
   ++ promyelocytes, myelocytes, mast cells
6. Great increase in fibers and capillaries
7. Monocytes are positive for nonspecific esterase in blood smears, imprints, or cryostat sections

in Table 50 are of help. In contrast to centrocytic lymphoma, which involves the cortex first, monocytic leukemia first infiltrates the medullary pulp. With silver staining the infiltrated areas are immediately conspicuous owing to the large number of reticulin fibers and blood vessels (especially capillaries). Neoplastic monocytes are somewhat larger than centrocytes. The chromatin pattern of monocytes is finer and their polymorphic nuclei are sometimes cleaved or even bilobed. In contrast to the nuclei of centrocytes, those of monocytes contain relatively large, solitary nucleoli. The cytoplasm of monocytes is more abundant, but its reddish violet color with Giemsa staining is clearly recognizable. The chloroacetate esterase reaction usually reveals at least a few strongly positive promyelocytes and myelocytes. In immature monocytes there is sometimes a weakly positive chloroacetate esterase reaction. In blood smears or imprints the monocytic nature of the leukemia is easily confirmed by means of the nonspecific esterase reaction.

In contrast, the differentiation of centrocytic lymphoma from *chronic lymphocytic leukemia, immunocytoma,* and *centroblastic/centrocytic lymphoma* is relatively easy. None of these tumors consists of a "pure population" of tumor cells like centrocytic lymphoma. Instead, they always contain blast cells as well ("lymphoblasts," immunoblasts, centroblasts), which are readily recognized by their prominent basophilic cytoplasm. In addition, the blast cells are larger than the majority of the proliferating centrocytes. For recognizing the blast cells, however, one needs thin sections (3–4 μm) and good Giemsa staining.

**Development into a Lymphoma of Higher-Grade Malignancy.** In occasional cases we have seen a change in the cytology of the tumor a few years after diagnosis. In a later biopsy the tumor cells were more polymorphic and there was a very large number of mitotic figures (Fig. 147). Even giant cells could be found. Such anaplastic variants probably signify a poorer prognosis.

Once we observed an immunoblastic lymphoma in a patient with centrocytic lymphoma. The immunoblastic lymphoma revealed a large number of globular PAS-positive inclusions and was therefore confirmed as being a B-immunoblastic lymphoma.

**Borderline Cases.** The boundary separating centrocytic lymphoma from *centroblastic/centrocytic lymphoma* is not sharp. Sometimes the distinction can be made only with great difficulty. We found such borderline cases in about 10% of our centrocytic lymphomas. In such instances one finds primary follicle-like structures with a few centroblasts, in addition to diffuse regions consisting only of centrocytes. These patterns may be realized in two different lymph-node regions. We observed one case, for instance, in which the tonsils revealed a chiefly follicular picture with a few centroblasts, while an associated nuchal lymph node showed a diffuse centrocytic picture.

A second type of borderline case, namely, centrocytic lymphoma with some immunoblasts, plasmablasts, and plasma cells, was occasionally found in our material. One of these cases showed a great increase in IgM in the tissue homogenate. A few other cases showed a relatively large number of typical Marschalkó plasma cells. Because of the lack of typical lymphocytes, none of these cases has so far been listed as *LP immunocytoma*. Nevertheless, these cases show the close relationship between centrocytes and the plasma-cell series, as is also indicated by the polymorphic type of immunocytoma.

Such borderline cases prove once again that centrocytic lymphoma is one of the types of tumors that arise from germinal centers and that it is not an anaplastic lymphocytic tumor as terms like lymphocytic sarcoma suggest.

**Combination with Other Diseases.** Except for one case with coincidental development of a squamous-cell carcinoma, our material contains no other diseases, in particular no cases of tuberculosis or Hodgkin's disease.

**Prognosis.** So far, we have only preliminary survival data on M.L. centrocytic. The probability of survival was calculated by BRITTINGER *et al.*[466] on the basis of 45 patients of the Kiel Lymphoma Study Group (Figs. 35 and 148). The median survival was 48 months. The difference between the probability of survival of centroblastic/centrocytic lymphoma and that of centrocytic lymphoma is statistically significant ($p<0.001$). There is no significant difference between centrocytic lymphoma and LP immunocytoma.

The second source of preliminary data is a series worked out by VAN UNNIK and his group.[467] We reviewed 77 cases and distinguished small centrocytic and large centrocytic types. In stages I and II the probability of survival was somewhat greater for the small centrocytic type. In all stages no difference was found between the small and large centrocytic types.

---

[466] BRITTINGER, BARTELS, BREMER, DÜHMKE *et al.*, 1976.

[467] Not yet published.

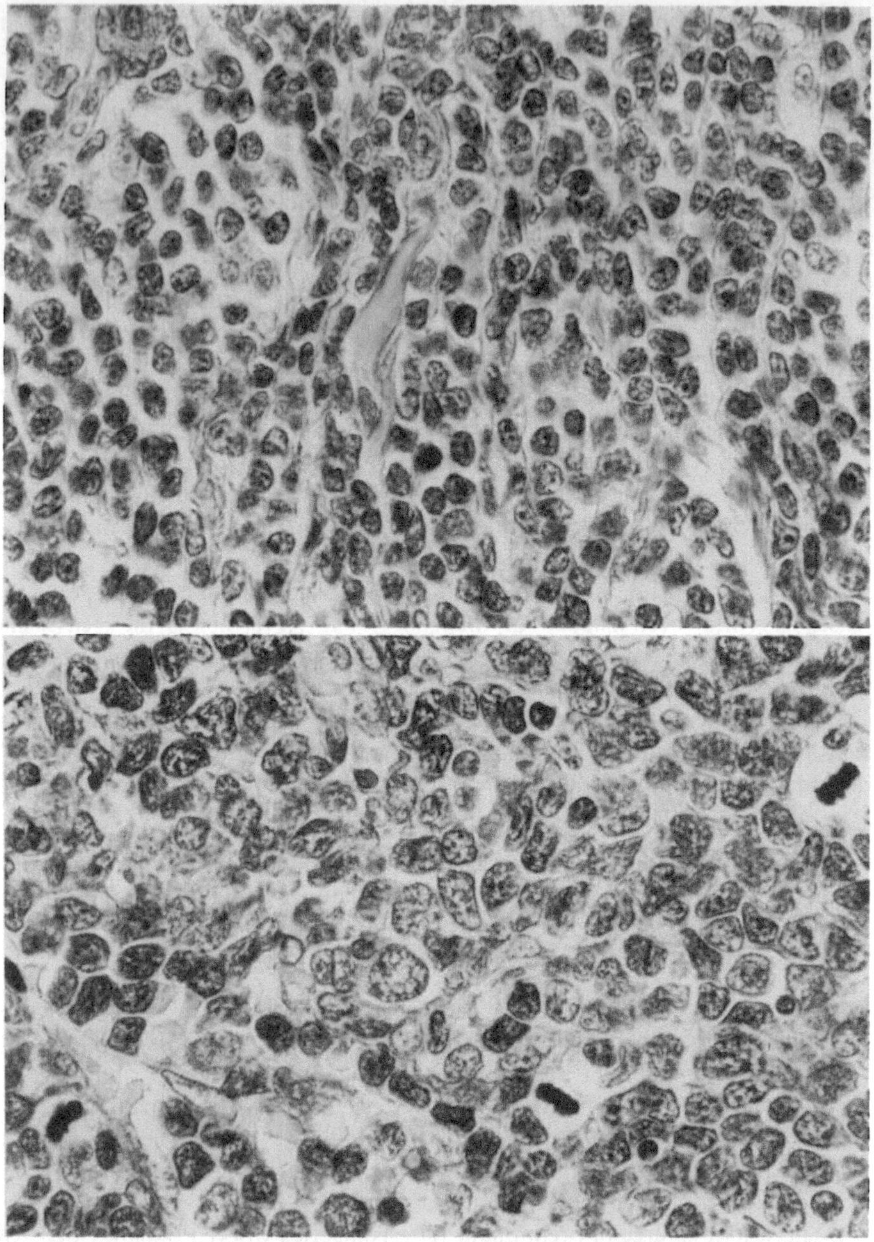

(a)

(b)

Fig. 147a and b. M.L. centrocytic. (a) Typical small-cell tumor. There are small centrocytes, sometimes with cleaved nuclei. In the center, a hyalin strand (around a small vessel). No mitosis. ♂, 42 years. Inguinal node. (b) Anaplastic large-cell variant, 2 years after the first diagnosis of M.L. centrocytic, small-cell type, was made. There is more pleomorphism, and three mitotic figures are seen. The average diameter of nuclei is greater than in the small-cell type. This picture does not differ from that found in cases in which the large-cell variant is seen from the beginning. ♂, 63 years. Inguinal node. (a, b) PAS. ×875

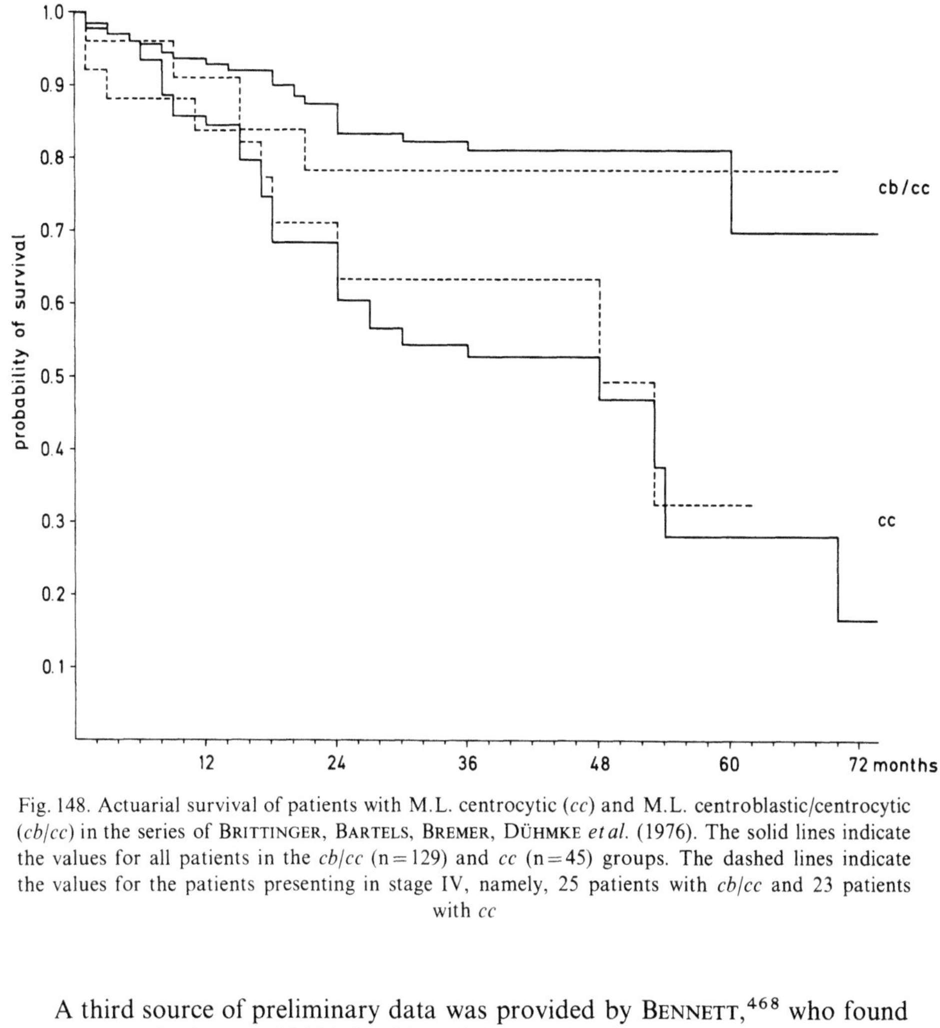


Fig. 148. Actuarial survival of patients with M.L. centrocytic (*cc*) and M.L. centroblastic/centrocytic (*cb/cc*) in the series of BRITTINGER, BARTELS, BREMER, DÜHMKE *et al.* (1976). The solid lines indicate the values for all patients in the *cb/cc* (n = 129) and *cc* (n = 45) groups. The dashed lines indicate the values for the patients presenting in stage IV, namely, 25 patients with *cb/cc* and 23 patients with *cc*

A third source of preliminary data was provided by BENNETT,[468] who found a 5-year survival rate of 31% for 20 nodal cases (against 43% for centroblastic/centrocytic lymphoma). The prognosis was somewhat better in cases with sclerosis than in those without.

## *Addendum*
## *The Leukemic Variant of M.L. Centrocytic*

As mentioned previously, M.L. centrocytic can have a leukemic blood picture. It then corresponds to the so-called lymphosarcoma-cell leukemia of some authors.[469] The term lympho*sarcoma*-cell is reasonable, since clinically and pathoanatomically one finds nodular infiltrates in the bone marrow, liver, spleen,

[468] 1975b.
[469] TISCHENDORF, 1946; SCHNITZER, LOESEL and REED, 1970; SCHREK and DONNELLY, 1971; AISENBERG and LONG, 1975.

and elsewhere, instead of generalized diffuse infiltration of these organs by tumor cells.

Another term for this leukemic variant was given by MATHÉ *et al.*[470] MATHÉ distinguished a prolymphocytic type of acute lymphoid leukemia (Type IV), which is probably identical with our centrocytic lymphoma.

The gross appearance and the histologic picture of both the leukemic and nonleukemic forms of M.L. centrocytic are identical. Even sclerosing variants of centrocytic lymphoma can be leukemic.

The data of SCHREK and DONNELLY[471] may be cited to give an idea of the prognosis of the leukemic variant of centrocytic lymphoma. They found that the cells of lymphosarcoma-cell leukemia usually showed less sensitivity to prednisolone and X-irradiation than the cells of CLL. Furthermore, the 5-year survival rates were lower (11%) than for CLL (51%).

### 2. *Malignant Lymphoma, Centroblastic/Centrocytic*[472]

*Synonyms:* Brill-Symmers disease
Follicular lymphoma
Nodular lymphoma
Germinoblastoma
Nodular variants of all malignant lymphomas (RAPPAPORT)
Malignant lymphoma, FCC, cleaved (LUKES and COLLINS)
Lymphoid follicular reticulosis (ROBB-SMITH)
Follicular reticulosis (ROULET)
Large follicular lymphoblastoma
Giant follicular lymphoma
In part: nodular sclerotic lymphosarcoma (BENNETT and MILLETT)

**History.** According to OBERLING and HAGUENAU,[473] M.L. centroblastic/centrocytic was probably first described by SABRAZÈS in 1899. The publication of BECKER, which appeared in 1901, was cited by BRILL *et al.*[474] It was probably the first case of follicular lymphoma observed in Germany, although the histology was described merely with the words "simple hyperplasia." In 1916, GHON and ROMAN described and illustrated a case of follicular lymphoma. Only after the publications of BRILL *et al.*[474] and D. SYMMERS,[475] however, did the morpho-

---

[470] MATHÉ, POUILLART, STERESCU, AMIEL *et al.*, 1971.

[471] 1971.

[472] Reviews and important papers: D. SYMMERS, 1938, 1948; MAYER and THOMAS, 1939; GALL, MORRISON and SCOTT, 1941; GALL and MALLORY, 1942; JACKSON and PARKER, 1947; ROBB-SMITH, 1947, 1964; RÜTTNER and VON ALBERTINI, 1947; VON ALBERTINI and RÜTTNER, 1950; VETTE, 1950; WETHERLEY-MEIN, SMITH, GEAKE and ANDERSON, 1952; BILGER, 1954; LUMB, 1954; OBERLING and HAGUENAU, 1954; FRESEN, 1956; RAPPAPORT, WINTER and HICKS, 1956; SLUITER, 1956; WRIGHT, 1956; LUMB and NEWTON, 1957; W.STC. SYMMERS, 1958; HURST and MEYER, 1961; BLUMENBERG, OLSON, STEIN and HAWKINS, 1963; DORFMAN, 1964b, 1973; LENNERT, 1964a, 1967, 1969a, 1971, 1973a; RAPPAPORT, 1964a, b, 1966; MORI and LENNERT, 1969; KOJIMA, IMAI and MORI, 1973; JONES, FUKS, BULL, KADIN *et al.*, 1973; LUKES and COLLINS, 1973, 1974a, b; SPIRO, GALTON, WILTSHAW and LOHMANN, 1975.

[473] 1954.

[474] BRILL, BAEHR and ROSENTHAL, 1925.

[475] 1927.

logic-clinical syndrome attract the attention of pathologists and clinicians. Even then, considerable time went by before the nature of the disease was correctly interpreted and diagnosed. The reason in part was that D. SYMMERS, one of the first to describe the disease, fell into the same trap as did HODGKIN 100 years earlier: SYMMERS recognized the special character of the follicular neoplasm, but was not yet able to distinguish it from apparently similar, but basically different lymph-node lesions, such as lipomelanic reticulocytosis. Therefore, SYMMERS' case studies include reactive lymph-node lesions along with neoplastic ones. The failure to make this distinction still continues in many places at the present time.

In this situation, the fundamental studies of RAPPAPORT *et al.*[476] could have brought a change. They laid down criteria for distinguishing reactive follicular lymphatic hyperplasia – the most important differential diagnosis – from centroblastic/centrocytic lymphoma. In their paper, which appeared at about the same time as the equally noteworthy review by WRIGHT,[477] RAPPAPORT *et al.* divided "nodular" lymphoma into five types: (1) lymphocytic, well differentiated; (2) lymphocytic, poorly differentiated; (3) mixed (lymphocytic and reticulum cell); (4) reticulum-cell type; (5) Hodgkin's type. The last variant is not discussed in this book. According to RAPPAPORT *et al.*, the other four types occur not only in a nodular (follicular) form, but also in a diffuse form. They therefore rejected the separate identity of follicular lymphoma. In our opinion, that was an unfortunate conclusion. Much as we admire the publication of RAPPAPORT *et al.* as a masterpiece of modern lymphoma research, we object to the cytologic equation of follicular and diffuse lymphomas. In our opinion, *every* follicular or nodular lymphoma of non-Hodgkin's type is a tumor of germinal-center cells. The existence of diffusely growing lymphomas of germinal-center cells does not allow the conclusion that all malignant lymphomas are to be regarded as nodular or diffuse variants of the same cell types. On the contrary, most diffusely growing lymphomas can be clearly distinguished from follicular lymphomas by their cytology alone.

The concept of RAPPAPORT[478] was accepted in the USA and many other countries. As a result, a diagnosis of follicular lymphoma was no longer made in these countries. We have repeatedly expressed our opposition to this concept with the following arguments:[479]

1. Cytologic analyses of follicular lymphomas in Giemsa-stained sections, in imprints, and in electron-microscopic studies all reveal the same – that follicular lymphoma is composed of cells that are characteristic of germinal centers, namely, centrocytes, centroblasts, dendritic reticulum cells, and macrophages. Whereas macrophages are not specific to germinal centers, dendritic reticulum cells appear to occur only in lymph follicles and surrounding B-cell areas. Consequently, they serve as useful markers, especially since, as far as we know, dendritic reticulum cells have not been found anywhere else except in tumors of germinal centers.

2. With Giemsa staining the centroblasts of follicular lymphoma can be readily distinguished from the "lymphoblasts" of CLL and from other "blast

[476] RAPPAPORT, WINTER and HICKS, 1956.
[477] 1956.
[478] Also 1966.
[479] LENNERT, 1964a, 1967, 1969a, d, 1971, 1973a, 1974b; MORI and LENNERT, 1969.

cells." The reactions for nonspecific esterase and acid phosphatase show that the cells that RAPPAPORT first called reticulum cells and later histiocytes are present in follicular lymphoma only in very small numbers. A follicular lymphoma composed of histiocytes that can be detected with enzyme-cytochemical methods does not exist.

3. A logarithmic plot of the age distribution of follicular lymphoma gives a straight line.[479a] That supports the assumption of one tumor entity and contradicts that of different tumor types.

We considered these arguments convincing enough for follicular lymphoma to be defined as a separate tumor of germinal-center cells. In principle, this concept also found agreement in Japan.[480] The same view is shared by GALTON, who with SPIRO, WILTSHAW, and LOHMANN,[481] produced powerful arguments in favor of the separate identity of follicular lymphoma in a convincing clinical study of 75 cases.

The view that follicular lymphoma is a tumor of germinal centers is beginning to take hold again in the USA. One fact that has helped to convince people was mentioned by RAPPAPORT *et al.* in their paper in 1956,[482] and also by other authors[483] in numerous recent papers, namely, that nodular lymphomas show a significantly better prognosis than diffuse lymphomas.

As late as 1971, in Nagoya, DORFMAN[484] still firmly adhered to the cytologic identity of nodular and diffuse lymphomas, and he referred to the idea that nodular lymphomas are derived from germinal-center cells, as KOJIMA, LUKES, and the author (K.L.) maintained, as "intriguing" but not yet proved. In 1973, at the CRC Symposium in London, however, DORFMAN admitted that follicular lymphoma is not only a structural, i.e., "nodular" variant of lymphoma, but also a cytologically distinct type of tumor.

LUKES and COLLINS[485] subscribed to our viewpoint, but even went beyond our interpretation. With the aid of a camera lucida they had sketched the cells of germinal centers and of malignant non-Hodgkin's lymphomas. They found that in germinal centers there are small to medium-sized cells with cleaved nuclei (cleaved FCC; the same as our centrocytes) and medium-sized to large basophilic cells with rounded nuclei (noncleaved FCC; the same as our centroblasts). LUKES and COLLINS were able to identify similar cells in follicular lymphomas and thus accepted our interpretation of this lymphoma. In addition, however, they postulated that most diffuse non-Hodgkin's lymphomas are also derived from germinal centers. Thus, Burkitt's tumor was said to consist of small noncleaved FCC, and a group of lymphoblastic sarcomas, of large noncleaved FCC.

The final proof that M.L. centroblastic/centrocytic is an entity in its own right came from studies of the lymphoma cells for complement receptors. The cells of follicular lymphomas reacted just like the cells of reactive germinal centers, as was first shown by JAFFE *et al.*[486] RAPPAPORT[487] now also considers

[479a] LENNERT, 1971.
[480] KOJIMA, IMAI and MORI, 1973.
[481] SPIRO, GALTON, WILTSHAW and LOHMANN, 1975.
[482] RAPPAPORT, WINTER and HICKS, 1956.
[483] E.g., JONES, FUKS, BULL, KADIN *et al.*, 1973.
[484] 1973.
[485] 1973.
[486] JAFFE, SHEVACH, FRANK, BERARD *et al.*, 1974; GREEN, JAFFE, SHEVACH, EDELSON *et al.*, 1975; JAFFE, SHEVACH, SUSSMAN, FRANK *et al.*, 1975.
[487] RAPPAPORT, 1974; RAPPAPORT and BRAYLAN, 1975.

it probable that the large cells in follicular lymphoma are not histiocytes, but transformed lymphocytes.

In 1969, BENNETT and MILLETT (later MILLETT *et al.*[488] and BENNETT[489]) presented an apparently new entity of malignant lymphoma, which they called *nodular sclerotic lymphosarcoma*. Although BENNETT and MILLETT had not declared the tumor as follicular lymphoma, one can read in their histologic description that diffuse and follicular patterns of growth could usually be demonstrated in the tumor. According to BENNETT and MILLETT, the distinctive feature of this variant of lymphoma is a band-like fibrosis, which divides a part of or the whole lymph node into irregular nodules and regions. Associated with the tumor are certain special characteristics regarding its occurrence and clinical manifestations. The tumor develops most commonly between the 5th and 7th decades, never before the 4th decade. Women are affected more often than they are with diffuse lymphosarcoma. The tumor is generally localized in the inguinal or retroperitoneal regions. The prognosis corresponds approximately to that of follicular lymphoma. In a second publication[488] the authors report, however, that the prognosis is even better than that of follicular lymphoma.

Through their distinction of "nodular sclerotic lymphosarcoma" BENNETT and MILLETT have undoubtedly performed a valuable service in calling attention to sclerosis in malignant lymphomas. This service should not be disparaged. Nevertheless, the tumor they describe is not a unique type of tumor, either in its cytology or in its nature. Our cytologic, electron-microscopic, and immunologic studies have revealed that almost all cases of "nodular sclerotic lymphosarcoma" are really centroblastic/centrocytic lymphomas. The few sclerosing lymphomas that are not centroblastic/centrocytic are usually centrocytic.

In 1972, on the basis of nine cases, ROSAS-URIBE and RAPPAPORT described a malignant lymphoma, histiocytic type with sclerosis. They compared this tumor, as a relatively slow-growing and less aggressive lymphoma, with the "lymphosarcoma" described by BENNETT and co-workers, without regarding the tumors as identical. From the illustrations published by ROSAS-URIBE and RAPPAPORT, however, their "histiocytes" are probably equivalent to our large centrocytes. Accordingly, this group of apparently histiocytic tumors should be classified with the neoplasms arising from germinal centers.

Recently, BENNETT[490] added a second type of fibrosis to band-forming nodular sclerosis (he also considered the cases of ROSAS-URIBE and RAPPAPORT to be of this second type) and called it "fine compartmentalizing fibrosis." In seven out of 13 cases, however, it was combined with the first type, i.e., fibrous band formation. BENNETT found this second type only in his "diffuse mixed" and "diffuse undifferentiated large cell" groups. His first, band-forming type was seen only in centroblastic/centrocytic and centrocytic lymphoma, which agrees with our findings.

**Definition.** By the term M.L. centroblastic/centrocytic (germinoblastoma) we understand a malignant tumor of germinal centers that is composed of the same mixed population of cells as is found in normal germinal centers,

[488] MILLETT, BENNETT, JELLIFFE and FARRER-BROWN, 1969.

[489] 1975a.

[490] 1975a, b.

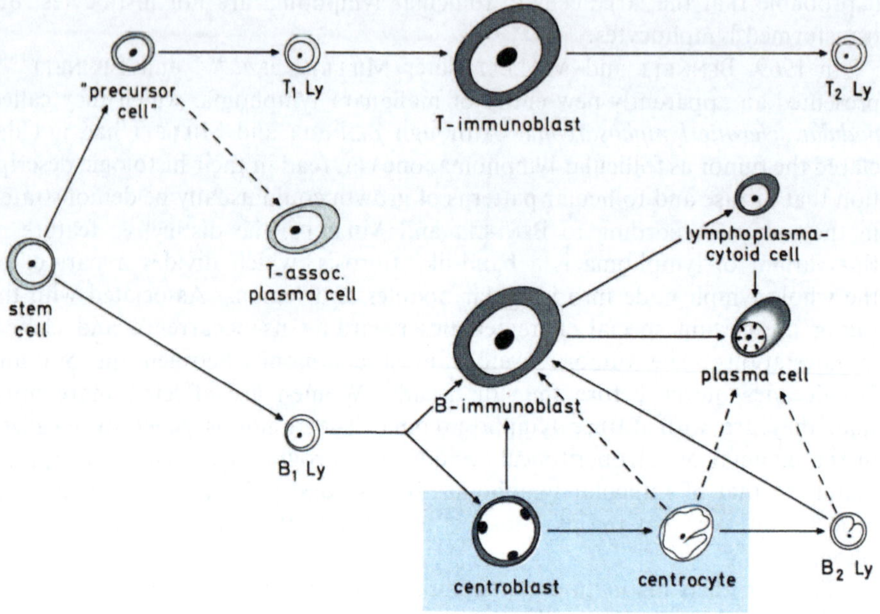


Fig. 149. Hypothetical origin of M.L. centroblastic/centrocytic. The main cellular constituents are shown in the dark blue area. Sometimes other cells, shown in the light blue area, can be found. That indicates the borderline between this tumor and LP immunocytoma

namely, of centroblasts, centrocytes, and dendritic and histiocytic reticulum cells. The proliferation can be follicular, follicular and diffuse, or diffuse. The diffuse type of growth, however, is very rare.

**Origin of the Neoplastic Cells.** M.L. centroblastic/centrocytic is the neoplastic equivalent of germinal centers and, consequently, it is definitely a B-cell lymphoma (Fig. 149). The tumor cells (centroblasts and centrocytes), like their normal counterparts, bear surface Ig and most of them have complement receptors on the cell surface. When the tumor cells differentiate further into $B_2$-lymphocytes—with or without release of cells into the blood—a number of centrocytes might lose their complement receptors.

Cell suspensions of centroblastic/centrocytic lymphoma always also contain 20–40% T-lymphocytes that form sheep-E rosettes.[491] This finding agrees well with the histologic picture, in which the neoplastic follicles are separated by more or less well-developed T-cell regions (with interdigitating reticulum cells and venules). In contrast to the neoplastic $B_2$-lymphocytes of M.L. centroblastic/centrocytic, the T-lymphocytes apparently recirculate back to the T-cell regions.[492]

**Subclassification of M.L. Centroblastic/Centrocytic.** Since, according to our definition, we refer only to those lymphomas composed of centroblasts and

[491] Jaffe, Shevach, Frank, Berard *et al.*, 1974.

[492] Kaiserling, 1975.

centrocytes as M.L. centroblastic/centrocytic, the distinction of follicular lymphomas of various cell types, as practiced, for instance, by RAPPAPORT *et al.*,[493] is eliminated at the outset. At most, one can subdivide according to the size of the centro*cytes* (centroblasts are always medium-sized or large) and distinguish a small-cell and a large-cell type of M.L. centroblastic/centrocytic. LUKES and COLLINS make such a distinction. They speak of small and large cleaved FCC types. The two types might well correspond to the nodular, well and poorly differentiated lymphocytic (small-cell) type and the nodular histiocytic (large-cell) type of RAPPAPORT *et al.*[493] and JONES *et al.*[494] The concept of a simply lymphocytic type of follicular lymphoma has been rejected[495] and may now be dropped.

In our opinion, the large-cell type is more anaplastic than the small-cell type. In the large-cell type it is often difficult to distinguish all of the large centrocytes from centroblasts, and the centroblasts are often atypical; whereas in the small-cell type the centroblasts are clearly distinguishable as large basophilic cells in contrast to the small nonbasophilic centrocytes. We do not need a mixed type, since *all* centroblastic/centrocytic lymphomas contain at least a few centroblasts; thus, all tumors are "mixed." Accordingly, most of the mixed-celled nodular lymphomas of JONES *et al.*[494] are to be included among our small-cell type, since the presence of both centroblasts and centrocytes is more readily apparent in the small-cell type than in the large-cell type.

In addition to these cytologic criteria, there are two histologic criteria that are suitable for characterizing M.L. centroblastic/centrocytic: the pattern of growth and the tendency to sclerosis. Depending on the way the tumor cells grow, we distinguish a follicular, a follicular and diffuse, and a diffuse type of M.L. centroblastic/centrocytic. As regards the tendency to sclerosis, the distinction of a sclerotic from a nonsclerotic type (M.L. centroblastic/centrocytic with or without sclerosis) is justified.

The histologically defined subtypes of centroblastic/centrocytic lymphoma are evidently not of great significance in the biologic behavior of the tumor. Thus, for example, "diffuse" does not imply a high grade of malignancy, as DORFMAN erroneously assumes.[496] Rather, it merely represents one of the variant patterns of the same tumor, which either before, at the same time, or later may display in other regions a different pattern of growth, although the cytology remains the same. Hence, we have seen follicular lymphomas that had proliferated in other tissues in a purely diffuse manner and could hardly be recognized as M.L. centroblastic/centrocytic. With respect to sclerosis, the variation may be even greater from lymph node to lymph node: in 28 cases of M.L. centroblastic/centrocytic in which more than one biopsy was examined, we found a nonsclerotic lymphoma on one occasion and a sclerotic lymphoma on another (Table 51). In 10 cases the discrepancy occurred in biopsies submitted at the same time, and in 15 cases, in biopsies submitted at different times from the same patient. In the latter group it was more usual for the second biopsy to show sclerosis (12 cases), but the reverse was true in three cases.

[493] RAPPAPORT, WINTER and HICKS, 1956.
[494] JONES, FUKS, BULL, KADIN *et al.*, 1973.
[495] E.g., BENNETT, 1973; FARRER-BROWN, 1973; LUKES, 1973; KOJIMA, IMAI and MORI, 1973.
[496] 1974b.

Table 51. Twenty-eight cases of M.L. centroblastic/centrocytic that were studied twice for tendency to sclerosis with different results. In 13 cases the two biopsies were examined at the same time, in 15 cases at different times. Of the latter cases, sclerosis was found in the first biopsy in three and in the second biopsy in 12 cases

| Biopsy with sclerosis | | | Biopsy without sclerosis | |
|---|---|---|---|---|
| Localization | n | | Localization | n |
| Cervical LN | 9 | | Cervical LN | 4 |
| | | | Axillary LN | 2 |
| | | | Mesenteric LN | 1 |
| | | | LN of unknown origin | 2 |
| Axillary LN | 2 | | Axillary LN | 1 |
| | | | LN of unknown origin | 1 |
| Pectoral LN | 2 | | Cubital LN | 1 |
| | | | Inguinal LN | 1 |
| Inguinal LN | 6 | | Axillary LN | 1 |
| | | | Inguinal LN | 5 |
| LN of unknown origin | 5 | | Cervical LN | 1 |
| | | | Axillary LN | 1 |
| | | | LN of unknown origin | 2 |
| | | | Tonsil | 1 |
| Extranodal | 4 | | | |
| Salivary gland | | 2 | Salivary gland | 1 |
| | | | Cervical LN | 1 |
| Spleen | | 1 | Axillary LN | 1 |
| Tonsil | | 1 | Cervical LN | 1 |

LN = lymph node

**Occurrence.** M.L. centroblastic/centrocytic is the most common non-Hodgkin's lymphoma. In our first series (Table 52) it constituted 21.9% of the non-Hodgkin's lymphomas and 12.3% of all malignant lymphomas. In Northern Germany about three persons in every 1,000,000 inhabitants develop this tumor each year.[497]

In larger series from countries of the Western World nodular or follicular lymphoma made up from 13–44% of all non-Hodgkin's lymphomas (13.3%,[498] 14.6%,[499] 19%,[500] 25%,[501] 27%,[502] 44%[503]). Follicular lymphoma is rare in Japan. According to AKAZAKI,[504] it accounts for 4.2% of the non-Hodgkin's lymphomas and about 3.4% of all lymphomas. Up to 1963, only a little over 10 cases of follicular lymphoma had been reported in Japan.[505] In India, DESAI *et al.*[506] reported that only 1% of 800 malignant lymphomas were follicular

[497] LENNERT, 1969b.
[498] GALL and MALLORY, 1942; ROSENBERG, DIAMOND, JASLOWITZ and CRAVER, 1961.
[499] W.STC. SYMMERS, 1958.
[500] VAN UNNIK, BREUR, BURGERS, CLETON *et al.*, 1975.
[501] BROWN, PETERS, BERGSAGEL and REID, 1975.
[502] BUTLER, STRYKER and SHULLENBERGER, 1975.
[503] JONES, FUKS, BULL, KADIN *et al.*, 1973; ROSENBERG, DORFMAN and KAPLAN, 1975.
[504] 1973.
[505] AKAZAKI and WAKASA, 1964, see also 1974.
[506] DESAI, MEHER-HOMJI and PAYMASTER, 1965.

Table 52. M.L. centroblastic/centrocytic. Material and incidence

| | | |
|---|---|---|
| Total No. of cases | 635 | |
| Biopsy | | 606 |
| Autopsy | | 29 |
| Total No. of biopsies | 722 | |
| Lymph nodes | | 634 |
| Extranodal | | 88 |
| Incidence in routine lymph-node biopsies | | 184 |
| = 12.3% of malignant lymphomas | | |
| 21.9% of non-Hodgkin's lymphomas | | |

Table 53. Growth pattern and sclerosis in M.L. centroblastic/centrocytic (585 lymph nodes)

| Growth pattern | n | % | With sclerosis | |
|---|---|---|---|---|
| | | | n | % |
| Follicular | 427 | 73.0 | 98 | 23.0 |
| Follicular and diffuse | 134 | 22.9 | 47 | 35.1 |
| Diffuse | 24 | 4.1 | 9 | 37.5 |
| Total | 585 | | 154 | 26.3 |

lymphomas. Among Negroes follicular lymphoma is also rare.[507] In Brazil, MACHADO *et al.*[508] found only 5.5% follicular lymphomas among 524 cases.

The frequency of the various cytologic subtypes is as follows. The large-cell variant is considerably less common than the small- (and mixed-) cell variant. If one draws the borderline at a cell diameter of 8 μm, then only 7% of the cases in our material belong to the large-cell variant. If the histiocytic type in the material of JONES *et al.*[509] is regarded as the same as the large-cell variant, then one would expect 16% of the lymphomas to be of the large-cell type.

As to the pattern of growth, 73% of the centroblastic/centrocytic lymphomas were purely follicular, 22.9% follicular and diffuse, and 4.1% diffuse (Table 53). Of the 585 cases evaluated, 431 or 73.7% were nonsclerotic at the first examination and 154 or 26.3% were sclerotic. BENNETT reported that the incidence of the sclerotic variant of follicular lymphoma was 40.2%[510] or 54%.[511] On coding the frequency of sclerosis in our material according to the pattern of growth, we found that the tendency to sclerosis is greater in the follicular

[507] RAPPAPORT, WINTER and HICKS, 1956; DORFMAN, 1964b, 1973; TALERMAN, 1970.
[508] MACHADO, JAMRA, OKUYAMA and MARIGO, 1973.
[509] JONES, FUKS, BULL, KADIN *et al.*, 1973.
[510] 1975a.
[511] 1975b.

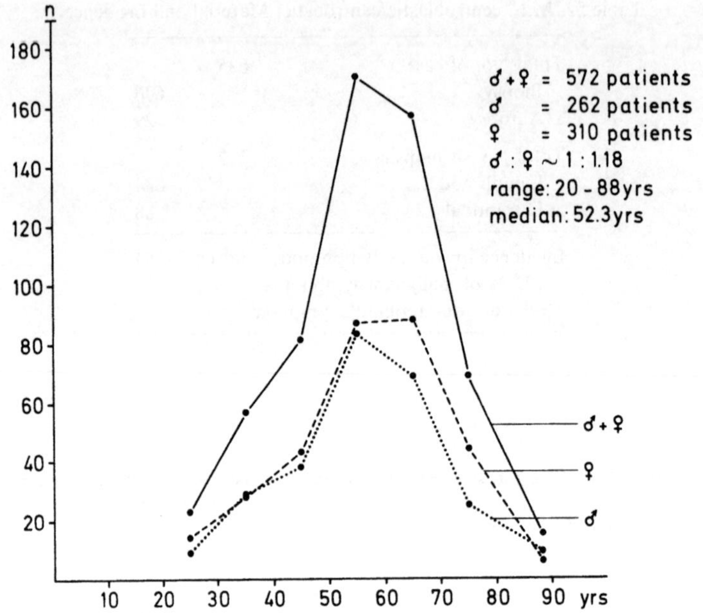


Fig. 150. Age distribution and sex ratio of M.L. centroblastic/centrocytic (572 patients of the Lymph Node Registry in Kiel)

and diffuse type (35%) and in the diffuse type (37.5%) of proliferation than in the purely follicular type (23%). In Italy the sclerosing diffuse type appears to be relatively common.[512]

In our material the *age* and sex distribution differs in some respects from that reported previously in collective statistics[513] (see Fig. 150). The age curve of M.L. centroblastic/centrocytic peaks in the 6th decade. The youngest patient in our series was 20 years old, the oldest was 88. We have never seen centroblastic/centrocytic lymphoma in patients younger than 20. The diseases occasionally described in the literature occurring in children and juveniles[514] are at least doubtful. In any event, one should be extremely cautious about diagnosing M.L. centroblastic/centrocytic in patients younger than 20 years of age.

Of the different subtypes based on the pattern of growth, Figure 151 shows the follicular and the follicular and diffuse types of M.L. centroblastic/centrocytic in relation to the age of the patients. There are no fundamental differences in the age distribution.

If we compare the sclerotic and the nonsclerotic variants (Fig. 152), we find that the sclerotic form peaks a decade later than the nonsclerotic form. That reflects the greater tendency to sclerosis in older patients, especially those in the 7th decade. As Table 54 indicates, 34.4% of the centroblastic/centrocytic lymphomas of patients in the 7th decade showed sclerosis, whereas only 17.4% were sclerotic in patients in the third decade.

[512] RILKE, personal communication.
[513] E.g., W.STC. SYMMERS, 1958.
[514] RAPPAPORT, WINTER and HICKS, 1956; MARSDEN and STEWARD, 1968; MILLETT, BENNETT, JELLIFFE and FARRER-BROWN, 1969; ROSENBERG, DORFMAN and KAPLAN, 1975.

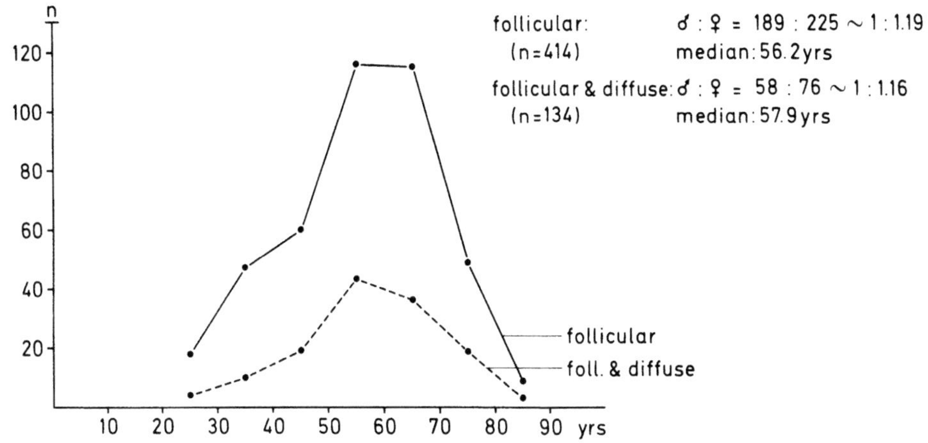


Fig. 151. Age distribution and sex ratio of 548 patients with follicular or follicular and diffuse growth pattern of M.L. centroblastic/centrocytic

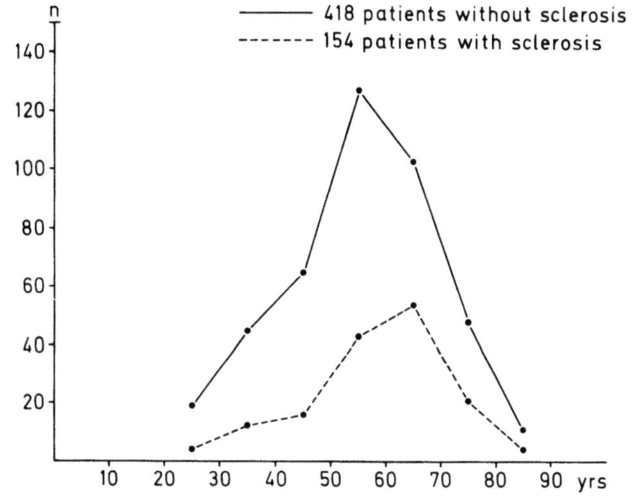


Fig. 152. Age distribution of 572 patients with M.L. centroblastic/centrocytic without or with sclerosis

With respect to the *sex* distribution, our findings agreed with those of SPIRO *et al.*[515] All forms show a slight predominance in women with an average of about 55% (♂:♀=1:1.18). This predominance in women holds true especially for those between the ages of 50 and 80 years. There are no substantial differences between the various histologic subtypes. Perhaps sclerosis develops somewhat more frequently in women than in men. We calculated a male-to-female ratio of 1:1.17 for the nonsclerotic type and a ratio of 1:1.23 for the sclerotic type.

[515] SPIRO, GALTON, WILTSHAW and LOHMANN, 1975.

Table 54. Frequency of tendency to sclerosis in M.L. centroblastic/centrocytic in the various age groups (572 cases)

| Age (years) | Without sclerosis | With sclerosis | |
|---|---|---|---|
| | n | n | % |
| 20–29 | 19 | 4 | 17.4 |
| 30–39 | 45 | 12 | 21.1 |
| 40–49 | 65 | 16 | 19.8 |
| 50–59 | 127 | 43 | 25.3 |
| 60–69 | 103 | 54 | 34.4 |
| 70–79 | 48 | 21 | 30.4 |
| 80–89 | 11 | 4 | 26.7 |
| | 418 | 154 | 26.9 |

**Clinical Manifestations.** There are numerous older,[516] sometimes quite detailed studies as well as a recent one[517] available on the clinical features of M.L. centroblastic/centrocytic. The last study stands out from the previous ones in that one of the authors, GALTON, held fast to the belief that follicular lymphoma is an entity, contrary to widespread practice. In many years of observation he discovered certain features in the clinical history, symptomatology, and physical signs that are characteristic of follicular lymphoma as distinct from the diffuse malignant lymphomas. This study had the added advantage for us that, owing to the kindness of the pathologists (HAMLIN, HARRISON) who first studied the cases, we had an opportunity to examine the histologic sections of all 75 cases ourselves. We recount almost verbatim the description given by SPIRO *et al.*[517]

They observed four phenomena in the *medical history* of the patients that they seldom found in cases of diffuse lymphoma:

1. Enlargement of a lymph node over many years, which did not lead the patient to consult a doctor until enlargement of additional lymph nodes appeared.

2. Generalized recurrent enlargement of lymph nodes since childhood, which caused the patient to seek medical care when the enlarged nodes persisted and grew larger (only one case).

3. Recurrent enlargement of lymph nodes at *one* site, usually in the groin, with repeated biopsies over several years. At the time of the first biopsy the diagnosis was merely follicular lymphatic hyperplasia; sometimes the possibility of follicular lymphoma was stressed. Later, when follicular lymphoma was recognized in a further biopsy, the first biopsy was retrospectively interpreted either as follicular lymphoma or still as follicular lymphatic hyperplasia.

4. In a few cases laparotomy was clinically indicated because of numerous large discrete lymph nodes in the mesentery and/or omentum.

---

[516] UHLMANN, 1948; BILGER, 1954; RAPPAPORT, WINTER and HICKS, 1956; ROSENBERG, DIAMOND, JASLOWITZ and CRAVER, 1961; DORFMAN, 1964b.

[517] SPIRO, GALTON, WILTSHAW and LOHMANN, 1975.

The most characteristic *finding,* particularly in patients younger than 40 years, was the demonstration of extensive, often massive enlargement of discrete, nonadherent lymph nodes in patients otherwise *free of symptoms.* In such cases there was also involvement of lymph-node sites that are rarely affected in diffuse lymphomas, namely, preauricular, mastoid, occipital, epitrochlear (cubital), infraclavicular, supra- and infrascapular lymph nodes as well as those along the medial margin of the scapula. Lymphography disclosed massive symmetrical involvement of the iliac and para-aortic lymph nodes. In older patients without symptoms the numerous large discrete lymph nodes in the mesentery and omentum felt like a sack of potatoes when the abdomen was palpated.

In addition to the widespread involvement of lymph nodes, a few patients revealed extranodal involvement. In diffuse lymphoma that would be a bad omen. In follicular lymphoma, however, it is easy to control. The following findings were also mentioned: infiltrates in the skin and subcutis, tumor masses formed of adherent lymph nodes resulting from spread of the growth, fixity of the lymph nodes, thickening of the overlying connective tissue, edema and sometimes reddening of the overlying skin, compression of veins, limb edema, and serous effusions.

In contrast to B-CLL, analysis of blood proteins often discloses no evidence of an immune defect for a long period of time. "Paraproteinemia" has been described occasionally. ROSSIER and SPÜHLER[518] probably described the first case, and a second case was reported by HEUCHEL and EITNER.[519] In those days, however, it was impossible to determine exactly what type of gammaglobulin was increased. Further cases were presented by KYLE *et al.*[520] and DANON *et al.*[521] HOBBS,[522] KIM *et al.*,[523] and PALUTKE and MCDONALD[524] each reported a case with a monoclonal increase in IgM/$\kappa$ in the blood. We also found in one of our cases a monoclonal increase in serum IgM.[525] In another case there was a great monoclonal increase in IgM and a slight increase in IgG.[526]

**Blood Picture.** The neoplastic cells of the follicles may migrate into the blood, which may result in a pronounced leukemic blood picture (see leukemic variant, p. 343ff.). Often, however, only a few centrocytes and sometimes also a few more or less characteristic centroblasts are found in the blood.[527] In such cases there is greater polymorphism and anisocytosis of the cells in the blood than there is in M.L. centrocytic. Nevertheless, the centrocytes cannot be clearly distinguished from the cells of centrocytic lymphoma. One third of the 15 cases analyzed did not show any atypical cells in the blood. See Table 55 for further details.

**Stage and Spread of the Disease.** JONES *et al.*[528] were the first to provide comprehensive statistics on the clinical stage of centroblastic/centrocytic lym-

[518] 1948; see also BARANDUN, SORDAT and SPENGLER, 1967.
[519] 1954.
[520] KYLE, BAYRD, MCKENZIE and HECK, 1960.
[521] DANON, CLAUVEL and SELIGMANN, 1967.
[522] 1971.
[523] KIM, HELLER and RAPPAPORT, 1973.
[524] 1973.
[525] LENNERT, STEIN and KAISERLING, 1975.
[526] LÖFFLER kindly provided this clinical information.
[527] BRITTINGER, BARTELS, BREMER, DÜHMKE *et al.*, 1976.
[528] JONES, FUKS, BULL, KADIN *et al.*, 1973.

Table 55. Blood lymphocytes and their variants in patients with M.L. centroblastic/centrocytic at the time of biopsy. Estimated by Dr. KÖNIG, Kiel Lymphoma Study Group (BRITTINGER *et al.*, 1976)

| Lymphocytes and variants | < 1000/µl | | 1000 – 4000/µl | | > 4000/µl | | 0 | |
|---|---|---|---|---|---|---|---|---|
| | n | % | n | % | n | % | n | % |
| All lymphoid cells | 12/78 | 15 | 56/78 | 72 | 10/78 | 13 | – | – |
| Lymphocytes (small and large) | 4/15 | – | 8/15 | – | 3/15 | – | – | – |
| Centrocytes | 6/15 | (40) | 1/15 | (7) | 3/15 | (20) | 5/15 | (33) |
| Centroblasts | 3/15 | (20) | – | – | – | – | 12/15 | (80) |
| Lymphocytoid plasma cells | 2/15 | – | – | – | – | – | 13/15 | – |

Table 56. Stage of disease at start of treatment in 178 cases of nodular lymphoma according to JONES *et al.* (1973)

| Stage | Lymphocytic, well differentiated | | Lymphocytic, poorly differentiated | | Mixed | | Histiocytic | | Total | | % |
|---|---|---|---|---|---|---|---|---|---|---|---|
| | A | B | A | B | A | B | A | B | A | B | A+B |
| I | 1 | – | 9 | – | 5 | – | 3 | – | 18 | – | 10.7 |
| $I_E$ | – | – | – | – | 1 | – | – | – | 1 | – | |
| II | 1 | – | 9 | – | 15 | – | 6 | 2 | 31 | 2 | 21.9 |
| $II_E$ | – | – | 2 | 1 | 2 | – | 1 | – | 5 | 1 | |
| III | 2 | – | 18 | 2 | 24 | 5 | 5 | 1 | 49 | 8 | 33.7 |
| $III_E$ | – | – | – | 1 | 1 | – | 1 | – | 2 | 1 | |
| IV | 2 | – | 16 | 11 | 18 | 3 | 6 | 4 | 42 | 18 | 33.7 |
| | 6 | 0 | 54 | 15 | 66 | 8 | 22 | 7 | 148 | 30 | |

A = without constitutional symptoms
B = with constitutional symptoms

phoma at the time of first treatment. That was the first attempt at classification into stages performed according to the Ann Arbor scheme on a retro- or prospective basis. They studied 178 "nodular lymphomas." The results are presented in Table 56. As we see, 10.7% of the patients were in stage I, 21.9% were in stage II, and stages III and IV had 33.7% in each. This means that two thirds of the patients were already in an advanced stage of the disease when they first visited a doctor. That is a much higher quota than that for Hodgkin's disease. The percentage agrees almost exactly with the data of WRIGHT[529] and SPIRO *et al.*[530] WRIGHT reported that 68% of 117 patients already had generalized disease at the time of biopsy. SPIRO *et al.* found that 72% of their 75 patients were already in stage III or IV.

[529] 1956.

[530] SPIRO, GALTON, WILTSHAW and LOHMANN, 1975.

Table 56 also indicates how frequently constitutional symptoms are present (unexplained fever and/or night sweats). A total of 17% of the patients experienced such general symptoms, usually in stages III and IV, but never in stage I. This percentage is exactly the same as that for M.L. centroblastic/centrocytic found by the Kiel Lymphoma Study Group.[531]

JONES *et al.*[532] did not provide any details as to the site of presentation of nodular lymphomas. From the figures provided we are only able to gather or calculate the following data: 75% of the nodular lymphomas were demonstrated in the lower cervical lymph nodes, including the supraclavicular region; of these 17.9% were on the right, 23.9% on the left, and 58.2% on both sides; 54% of the nodular lymphomas were identified in the upper para-aortic lymph nodes, 18% in the mediastinal (including hilar) lymph nodes.

JONES *et al.*[532] concerned themselves especially with the question of whether nodular lymphoma, like Hodgkin's disease, might spread progressively by the lymphogenous route, in particular from the upper para-aortic region into the inferior cervical lymph nodes, including the supraclavicular group; and whether the disease thereby skips, i.e., does not involve, the mediastinal lymph nodes, as the Stanford group under KAPLAN had shown for Hodgkin's disease. Indeed, JONES *et al.*[532] found that in 40% of the patients the mediastinal lymph nodes were bypassed; thus, nodular lymphoma probably spreads from the upper para-aortic region by way of the lymphogenous route directly into the inferior cervical lymph nodes. There was no statistically significant difference in the involvement of the lymph nodes on the left and right sides of the neck.

On the whole, JONES *et al.*[532] calculated that 81% of the nodular lymphomas spread progressively from lymph node to lymph node by way of lymphatic channels. The authors were unable to detect differences in spread between their various histologic subtypes of nodular lymphoma. "Random" spread appeared more frequently with the nodular lymphomas (19% of cases) than with either Hodgkin's disease ($<10\%$) or diffuse non-Hodgkin's lymphomas (10%). In particular, when nodular lymphoma was first diagnosed, there was sometimes infiltration of the bone marrow (22%) and of the gastrointestinal tract (12%). The frequency of involvement of the bone marrow varied somewhat according to the histologic type: 36% in M.L. lymphocytic, poorly differentiated, 13% in the mixed type, and 11% in M.L. histiocytic. The involvement of the gastrointestinal tract was usually a manifestation of stage IV disease; the small bowel was involved in six cases, the stomach in four cases, and the large bowel in two cases. In one patient there were multiple sites of involvement. The diagnosis of gastrointestinal involvement was usually made by laparotomy, less often by roentgenographic examination.

In a recent study by the Stanford group, KIM and DORFMAN[533] reported on the results of staging procedures with laparotomy and examination of bone marrow. They found that at the time of diagnosis of nodular lymphoma there is usually already widespread dissemination: 72% of the patients revealed abdominal involvement, and 28%, infiltration of the bone marrow. In the analysis

---

[531] BRITTINGER, BARTELS, BREMER, DÜHMKE *et al.*, 1976.

[532] JONES, FUKS, BULL, KADIN *et al.*, 1973.

[533] 1974.

of the Kiel Lymphoma Study Group only 34% of 113 patients showed bone-marrow involvement at the time of the first lymph-node biopsy.[534] This proportion is definitely smaller than the actual one, however, since trephine biopsies of the iliac crest were not performed in all cases.

**Localization.** The most important finding given in Table 57 is that the lymph nodes submitted for study came as often from the inguinal region as from the neck, each site contributing about 36% in our series. Axillary lymph nodes were next with 19.8% and abdominal lymph nodes (essentially retroperitoneal) with 6.8%.

In contrast, centroblastic/centrocytic lymphomas of the mediastinum were exceptionally rare in our material. Cubital lymph nodes were removed occasionally (0.8%). We received tissue from extranodal sites remarkably often, most frequently from spleens, tonsils, and skin including the subcutis. Specimens from the small bowel and stomach were next in frequency, and then numerous other organs with only a small number of cases.

We found that the tendency to sclerosis is most common in abdominal lymph nodes (39.4%). Those of the groin and axilla were next with 32.0% and 30.2%, respectively, whereas only 27.7% of the centroblastic/centrocytic lymphomas in the neck were sclerotic.

If we consider only the centroblastic/centrocytic lymphomas with marked sclerosis (last column of Table 57), abdominal lymph nodes were by far the most frequent site (27.3%). The cervical, axillary, and inguinal lymph nodes all showed a frequency of around 13–14% and therefore differed little from one another. It is remarkable that among the extranodal organs sclerosis was never observed in the spleen, whereas it occurred with variable frequency in other organs.

**Gross Appearance.** The lymph nodes are moderately to greatly enlarged and fairly well demarcated from one another. The consistency varies from pulpy to moderately firm. On sectioning, the fresh surface appears light gray and stippled. It looks as though it were studded with numerous tiny miliary nodules and thus has a certain resemblance to fresh sarcoidosis. Consequently, the diagnosis of centroblastic/centrocytic lymphoma can often be suspected from the gross appearance. This is especially evident in the spleen, which is dotted with numerous light gray, fairly prominent nodules. In the sclerotic type there may be some resemblance to the lymph nodes in nodular sclerosing Hodgkin's disease. The consistency is firm, and the cut surface may show bulging nodules between the sclerotic strands.

**Histology.** Typical follicular M.L. centroblastic/centrocytic reveals a destroyed lymph-node structure. The neoplastic follicles are rather uniformly distributed over the cortex and medulla. They can be small, and then there is usually abundant interfollicular lymphatic tissue. The follicles can also be very large, however, so only narrow bands of interfollicular tissue are recognized. The cells found in the interfollicular tissue vary from case to case. In the

[534] Brittinger, Bartels, Bremer, Dühmke *et al.*, 1976.

Table 57. Localization of 722 biopsies of M.L. centroblastic/centrocytic ±sclerosis

| Localization | Total No. of biopsies | | | | Biopsies with sclerosis, total | | | | Biopsies with marked sclerosis | | | |
|---|---|---|---|---|---|---|---|---|---|---|---|---|
| | n | | % | | n | | % | | n | | % | |
| Lymph nodes | 634 | | 87.8 | | 165 | | 26.0 | | 78 | | 12.3 | |
| Cervical | | 177 | | 36.5 | | 49 | | 27.7 | | 23 | | 13.0 |
| Axillary | | 96 | | 19.8 | | 29 | | 30.2 | | 13 | | 13.5 |
| Mediastinal | | 3 | | 0.6 | | 1 | | (33.3) | | 1 | | (33.3) |
| Abdominal | | 33 | | 6.8 | | 13 | | 39.4 | | 9[a] | | 27.3 |
| Inguinal | | 172 | | 35.5 | | 55 | | 32.0 | | 24 | | 14.0 |
| Cubital | | 4 | | 0.8 | | 2 | | (50) | | 2 | | (50) |
| Unknown | | 149 | | – | | 16 | | 10.7 | | 6 | | 4.0 |
| Extranodal | 88 | | 12.2 | | 24 | | 27.3 | | 6 | | 6.8 | |
| Spleen | | 29 | | 33.0 | | – | | – | | – | | – |
| Tonsils | | 25 | | 28.4 | | 11 | | 44 | | – | | – |
| Skin and subcutis | | 11 | | 12.5 | | 6 | | (55) | | – | | – |
| Intestine | | 5 | | 5.7 | | 2 | | – | | – | | – |
| Stomach | | 4 | | 4.5 | | 1 | | – | | – | | – |
| Others | | 14 | | 15.9 | | 4 | | – | | – | | – |
| Total | 722 | | | – | 189 | | | – | 84 | | | – |

[a] 6 mesenteric and 2 retroperitoneal

large centrocytic variant the interfollicular tissue contains chiefly lymphocytes, whereas in the variant with relatively small centrocytes the interfollicular tissue sometimes contains many of the same cells as are found in the follicles, i.e., small centrocytes. Usually the neoplastic follicles lie "naked" in the interfollicular tissue. Some, however, possess lymphocyte caps or rims. These can surround the newly formed germinal centers even in perinodal fat tissue. In analyses using the rosette technique, the lymphocyte "caps" can be either EAC-positive or EAC-negative.[535] The EAC-positive "lymphocytes" might be centrocytes, that is, still-immature cells, whereas the EAC-negative cells might already have differentiated into $B_2$-lymphocytes.

Our attention was drawn to the morphology of the interfollicular tissue by the electron-microscopic studies of KAISERLING. He found in this tissue not only lymphocytes, which he regarded as being most probably T-lymphocytes, but also numerous interdigitating reticulum cells, venules, and sometimes T-associated plasma cells. Abundant reticulin fibers were always demonstrated. Occasionally, a few eosinophils, mast cells, and typical lymphatic or reticular plasma cells were present. KAISERLING assumed that there is an association between the T-lymphocytic tissue and the proliferation of the B-region.

As silver staining reveals, the neoplastic follicles contain either very few or no argyrophil fibers. Sometimes the venules of the interfollicular tissue are increased in number focally, especially in the sclerotic form. Silver staining not only helps one identify the follicular structures; it also enables one to

[535] BERARD, 1973, personal communication.

recognize the nature of the process, even when the lymph node is totally necrotic, for even in a necrotic tumor the neoplastic follicles are as a rule easily distinguished. Such total necrosis is very characteristic of follicular lymphoma, since, although it is not very frequent, it is extremely rare in other lymphomas. Consequently, total necrosis is in itself of diagnostic importance. In addition to total necrosis, one occasionally finds partial coagulation necrosis.

The follicles consist of centrocytes, centroblasts, dendritic reticulum cells, and macrophages (Figs. 153 and 154). In contrast to many reactive germinal centers, there is no "zoning" with a light upper and a dark lower part. The morphology of the centrocytes and centroblasts has already been described. Usually the centrocytes greatly predominate. The centroblasts generally make up only a small percentage; they rarely reach a maximum of about one quarter of the germinal-center cells. There are a few to moderate numbers of mitotic figures in the neoplastic follicles. On electron microscopy it is evident that mitosis usually occurs in the centroblasts (rich in polyribosomes). Mitotic figures may also be seen in the follicular spaces when these are infiltrated by centrocytes.

The cells identified as dendritic reticulum cells with the electron microscope can only be suspected, but not definitely diagnosed as such with the light microscope. Their rim of cytoplasm is narrow, with very long, slender projections that can be seen best with enzyme reactions (nonspecific esterase). The nuclei are elongate and conspicuously light, with a sharply demarcated nuclear membrane and a solitary, medium-sized, slightly basophilic nucleolus in the middle. In addition, a few macrophages with a moderately wide to wide, pale band of cytoplasm can be found in the neoplastic germinal centers. These macrophages only rarely show pronounced phagocytosis of nuclear debris and are numerous only in extremely rare instances. Giant cells can be observed occasionally in the neoplastic follicles. They have nuclei like those of centroblasts and a strongly basophilic cytoplasm. At times they resemble the giant cells of the centroblast type seen in measles (Warthin-Finkeldey giant cells). They differ from Sternberg-Reed giant cells in their uniformly large nuclei and the basophilia of their cytoplasm and nucleoli. Finally, we have occasionally seen multinucleate reticulum cells whose cytoplasm was an intense gray-blue. KAISERLING[536] was able to identify these cells by electron microscopy as so-called dark reticulum cells.

Some lymphocytes are nearly always found in the neoplastic germinal centers. In several cases we also identified some plasma cells in them. These cells and centrocyte-like cells occasionally contained PAS-positive inclusions in their cytoplasm and nuclei.

Now and then, eosinophilic amorphous deposits of protein are found among the follicle cells.[537] These deposits are strongly PAS-positive and, according to ROSAS-URIBE *et al.*,[538] contain no fibrin; with the Masson trichrome stain they appear blue.[539] In electron-microscopic studies of one of their cases, ROSAS-URIBE *et al.*[538] reported that the fibrils of the deposits had a periodicity of

---

[536] 1975.

[537] DORFMAN, 1973; KOJIMA, IMAI and MORI, 1973; ROSAS-URIBE, VARIAKOJIS and RAPPAPORT, 1973; TALERMAN and PLATENBURG, 1974.

[538] ROSAS-URIBE, VARIAKOJIS and RAPPAPORT, 1973.

[539] ROSAS-URIBE, VARIAKOJIS and RAPPAPORT, 1973; DORFMAN, 1973.

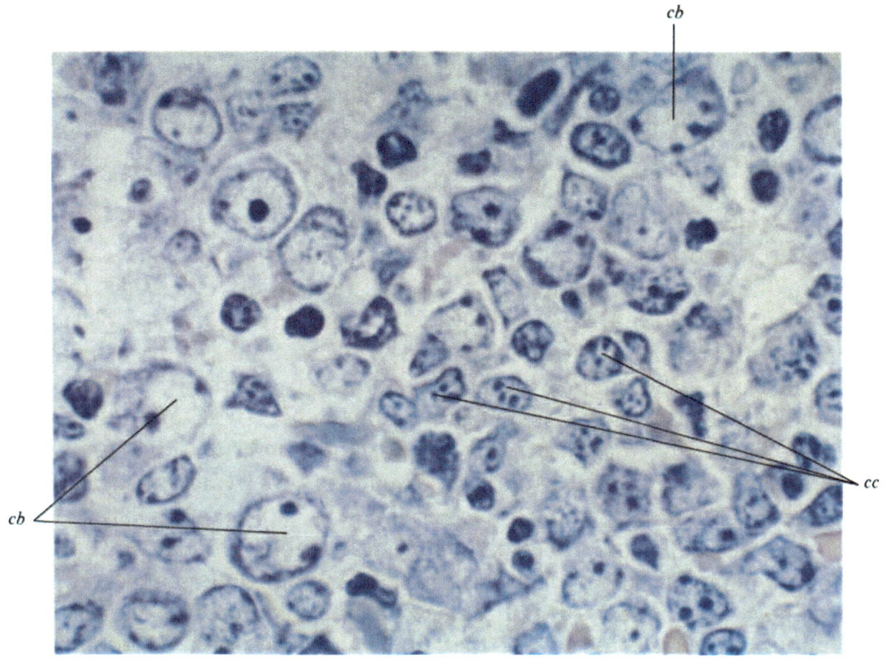


Fig. 153. M.L. centroblastic/centrocytic with Giemsa staining. Centrocytes (*cc*) and relatively numerous centroblasts (*cb*), ♀, 71 years. Cervical node: × 1,550

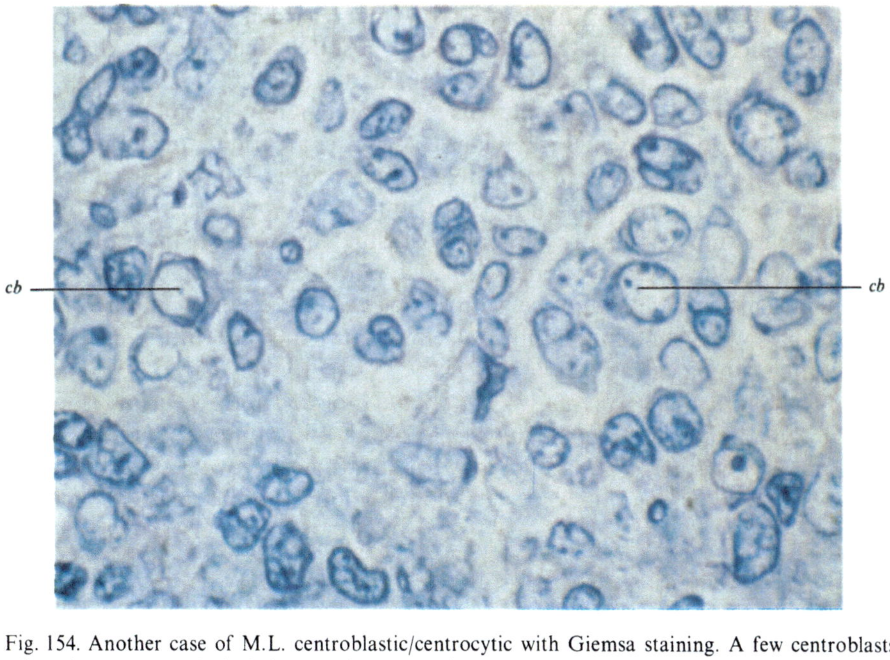


Fig. 154. Another case of M.L. centroblastic/centrocytic with Giemsa staining. A few centroblasts (*cb*) and numerous, relatively large and pleomorphic centrocytes. ♀, 26 years. Lymph node. × 1,550

150 Å and a thickness of 70 Å. In our opinion, they probably represent immunoglobulin or antigen-antibody precipitates with (partly degraded?) fibrin. The protein deposits are probably identical or related to deposits that one of us (K.L.) frequently demonstrated in the germinal centers of rabbits in previous immunization experiments[540] and which STUTTE and SCHLÜTER[541] recently analyzed in more detail in human spleens. These deposits contained fibrin that in part colored red, in part blue with the Ladewig modification of the Mallory stain for connective tissue. Electron microscopy showed that they contained fibrin as well as other substances.[542]

From the cytologic standpoint, a special variant of follicular lymphoma deserves our attention: M.L. centroblastic/centrocytic with marked plasma-cell differentiation or PAS-positive centrocyte-like cells. This is discussed under borderline cases in the chapter on immunocytoma (p. 245ff.).

Although we have not systematically studied the *effects of cytostatics* on follicular lymphoma, one case seems worth citing in brief (Fig. 155). A 70-year-old man with generalized follicular lymphoma was treated intensively with triaziquone (Trenimon®) and corticosteroids, and during treatment a lymph node was excised. It still revealed some typical lesions of relatively large-cell follicular lymphoma. Many of the neoplastic germinal centers appeared, however, to have been destroyed and replaced by shrunken nodules consisting of amorphous proteinaceous masses that stained weakly with eosin and were weakly Sudan-positive. These nodules contained a few reticulin fibers and vessels. Parts of neighboring germinal centers were often depopulated of cells, at times in a striplike fashion, and replaced by the weakly eosinophilic substance.

**Histologic Subclassification.**

*1. Subclassification According to Cell Size.* We regard as *small-cell* centroblastic/centrocytic lymphomas all those tumors whose cells measure less than 8 µm in diameter. Such tumors consist chiefly of small centrocytes and medium-sized to large centroblasts, whereas they usually contain only a small number of centroblasts. On electron microscopy the centrocytes are found to contain mainly monoribosomes.[543] *Large-cell* centroblastic/centrocytic lymphoma consists of numerous large bizarre centrocytes. In some cases these cells have a more oval nucleus, thus it is more difficult to distinguish them from centroblasts. Consequently, it is easy to understand why RAPPAPORT[544] and DORFMAN[545] believed them to be reticulum cells or histiocytes. On electron microscopy the large centrocytes contain mainly polyribosomes and are often hardly distinguishable from centroblasts.[543]

*2. Subclassification According to Pattern of Growth.* Typical centroblastic/centrocytic lymphoma grows in a *follicular* pattern (Fig. 156). A second variant reveals both follicular *and* diffuse patterns of tumor growth (Fig. 157). The diffuse growth demonstrated in such tumors should not be mistaken for the

---

[540] LENNERT, 1949, unpublished data.
[541] 1972.
[542] See also COOPER, HAQ and BAGNELL, 1969; HARMS, 1970.
[543] KAISERLING, 1975.
[544] RAPPAPORT, WINTER and HICKS, 1956; RAPPAPORT, 1966.
[545] 1964b.

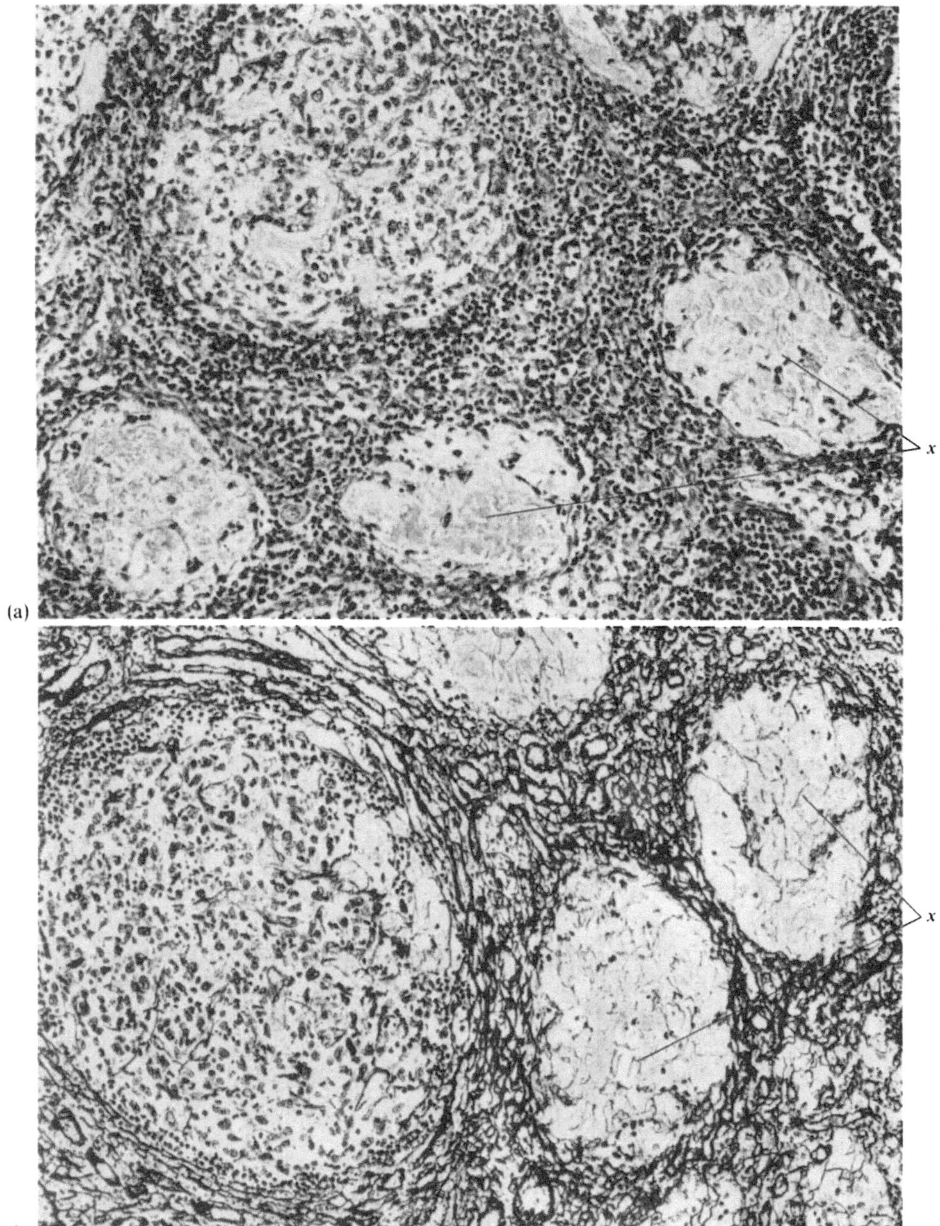


Fig. 155a and b. M.L. centroblastic/centrocytic, follicular, after treatment with triaziquone and corticosteroids. A number of neoplastic follicles are nearly free of cells and are replaced by structureless homogeneous masses containing proteins and lipoids ($x$). In the remaining follicles the number of cells is focally slightly reduced. Interfollicular lymphocytes are still present together with numerous fibers and venules. The patient was treated and biopsied by Prof. Dr. A. LINKE, Ludwigshafen. ♂, 70 years. Axillary node. (a) Hematoxylin and eosin, (b) Gomori. ×40

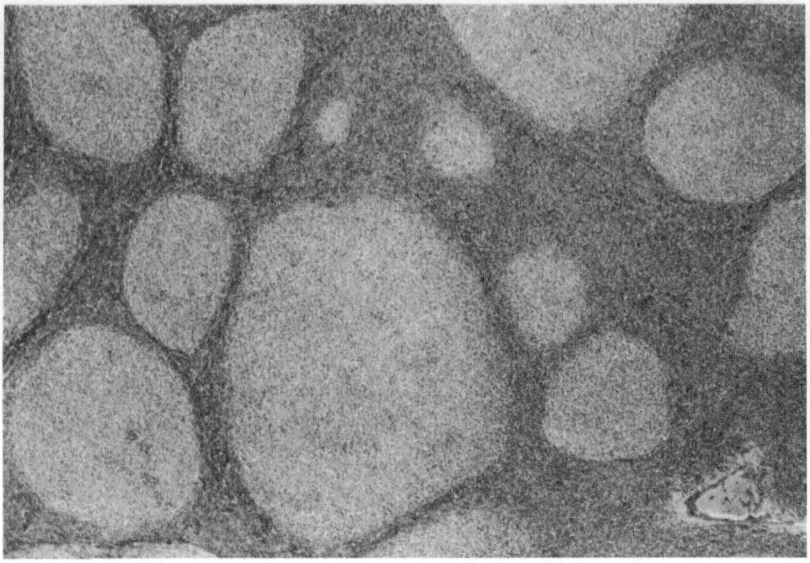

Fig. 156. M.L. centroblastic/centrocytic, follicular. ♀, 51 years. Axillary node. Giemsa. ×31

development of a "germinoblastic sarcoma," since the follicular and diffuse regions are made up of the same proliferating cells, namely, centrocytes, centroblasts, and some lymphocytes. In some cases an increase in reticulin and collagenous fibers is associated with the diffuse type of growth. One then often has the impression that the neoplastic follicles are dissected and disintegrated by the newly formed fibers; thus, the follicle cells finally seem to merge into the diffuse fibrous tissue.

A third variant is characterized from the beginning by an exclusively *diffuse* proliferation of centrocytes *and* centroblasts. This rare type of lymphoma poses diagnostic difficulties. We make the diagnosis only when we are sure that the great majority of cells are really centrocytes and centroblasts. Although the reticulin and collagenous fibers are more often sparse or moderately abundant than numerous, sclerosis is somewhat more frequent than in the first and second variants.

*3. Subclassification According to Tendency to Sclerosis.* By tendency to sclerosis we mean the occurrence of collagenous *fiber bundles,* as described by BENNETT and MILLETT.[546] Quite characteristic pictures develop that one should learn to recognize, especially in order to distinguish them from the nodular sclerosing type of Hodgkin's disease (Figs. 158 and 159). It seems best to quote

[546] 1969.

Fig. 157a–c. M.L. centroblastic/centrocytic, follicular and diffuse. (a) On the left diffuse, on the right follicular growth pattern. (b) Follicular area. (c) Diffuse area. There is no cytologic difference between (b) and (c). ♀, 57 years. Inguinal node. Giemsa. (a) ×31, (b, c) ×1,000 ▷

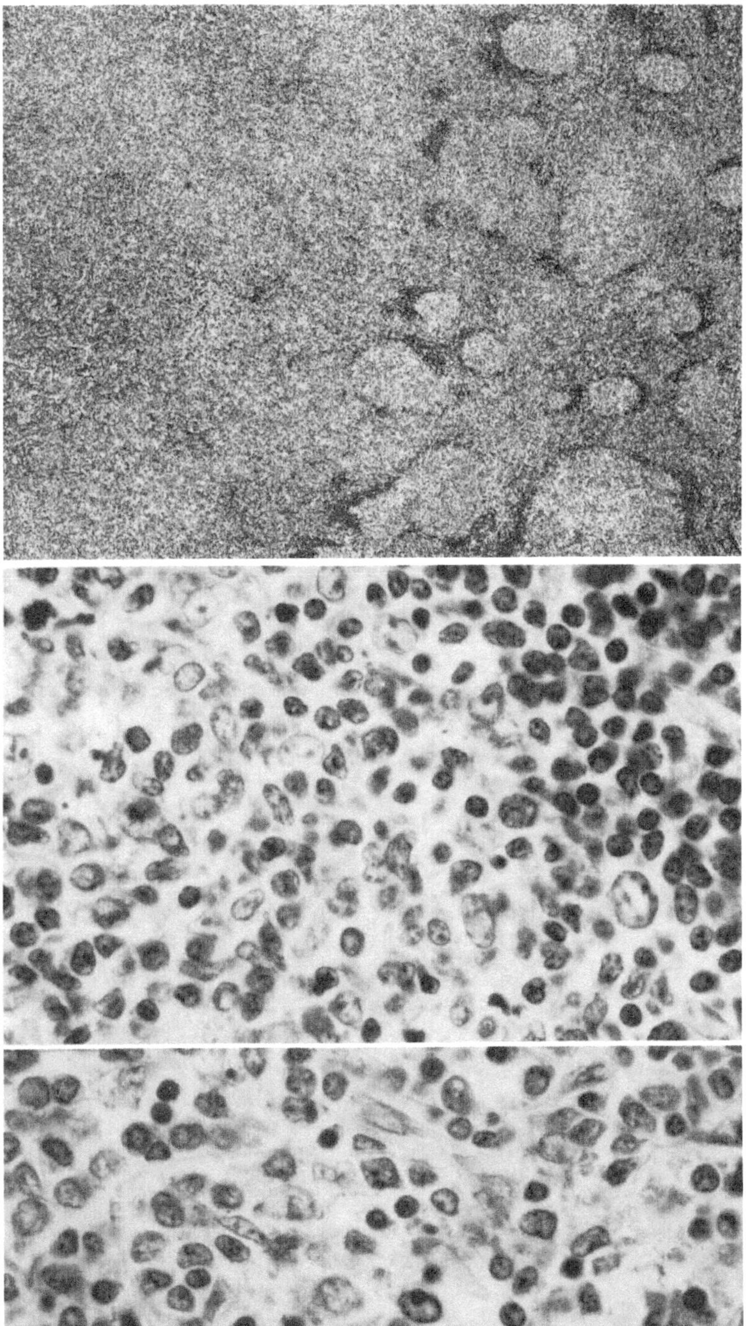

(a)
(b)
(c)

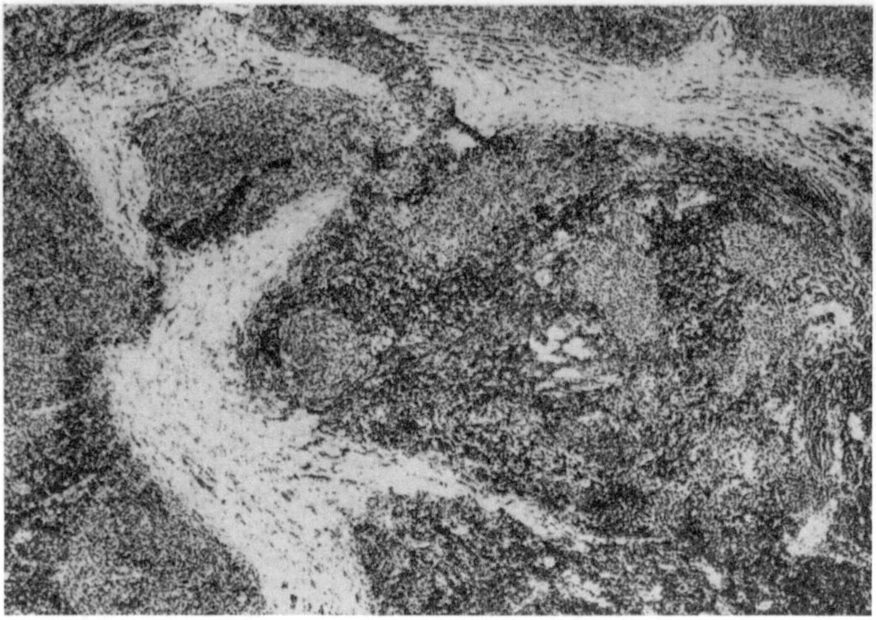

Fig. 158. M.L. centroblastic/centrocytic, follicular, with sclerosis. Sclerosis is band-forming. ♂, 69 years. Cervical node. Hematoxylin and eosin. ×56

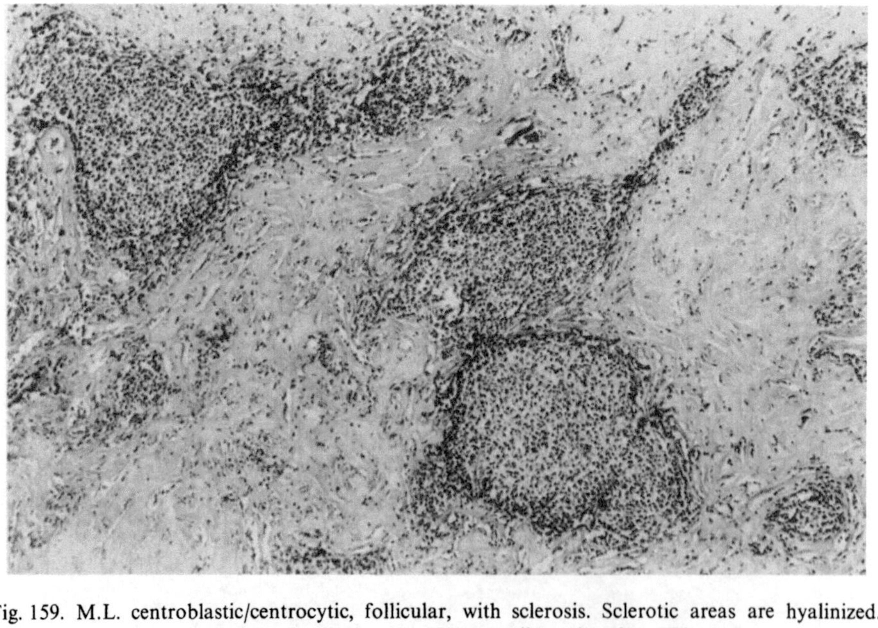

Fig. 159. M.L. centroblastic/centrocytic, follicular, with sclerosis. Sclerotic areas are hyalinized. ♀, 69 years. Inguinal node. Hematoxylin and eosin. ×96

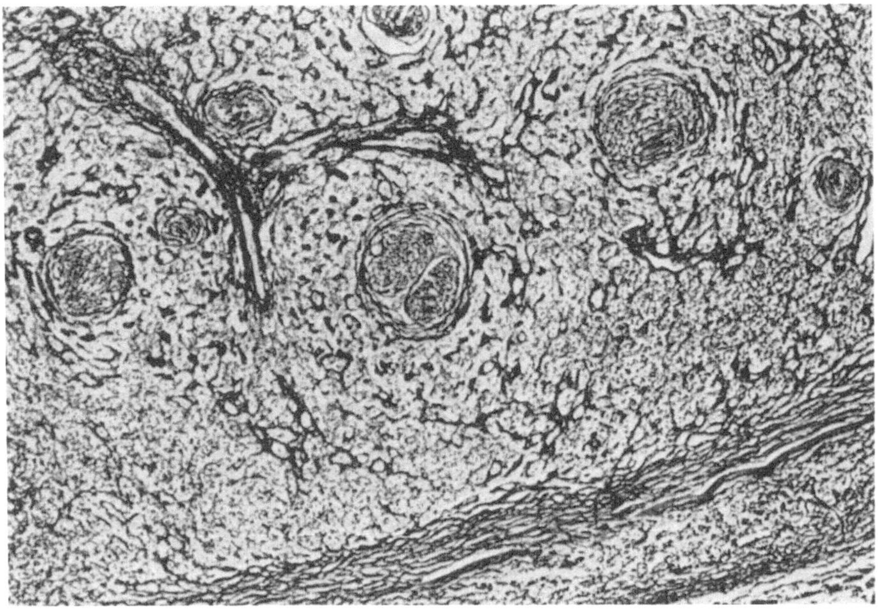

Fig. 160. M.L. centroblastic/centrocytic, follicular and diffuse, with sclerosis. Diffuse growth pattern around nerves in perinodal tissue. Band-forming sclerosis at the bottom. ♀, 63 years. Inguinal node. Gomori. ×56

the original description of "nodular sclerotic lymphosarcoma" given by BENNETT and MILLETT:[547]

All lymph nodes showing prominent fibrous bands dividing part or all of the gland into irregular nodules and areas were allocated to this group. The fibrous bands varied from 10 to several hundred μ, were doubly refractile and contained many reticulin fibres. The nodal pattern otherwise was either that of diffuse lymphosarcoma ... or follicular lymphoma but usually both patterns were present in different parts of the same node ... Frequently there was extensive invasion of tissues beyond the gland capsule and in these areas the fibrous bands were often more prominent. Usually the amount of gland showing the diffuse pattern was such that on previously accepted criteria they had been classified as diffuse lymphosarcoma before this present investigation.

We were able to confirm all of these details. From their histologic description, it is evident that BENNETT and MILLETT observed follicular as well as diffuse proliferations of neoplastic cells. We have also found all three types of growth patterns (follicular, follicular and diffuse, and diffuse) in the sclerotic variant. The combined follicular and diffuse centroblastic/centrocytic lymphoma shows sclerosis fairly often. The fiber production appears to be the "pacemaker" for the transformation of the follicles into diffuse structures.

The increase in fibers is often especially prominent beneath the capsule, and doubt sometimes arises whether the fibrous bands are newly formed or whether they are remnants of preexistent capsule. On the one hand, sclerotic bands extend into the lymph-node tissue; on the other hand, adjacent adipose tissue also contains numerous sclerotic bands as well as tumor tissue (Fig. 160). The sclerosis is often limited to one side of the lymph node. The sclerotic

[547] 1969.

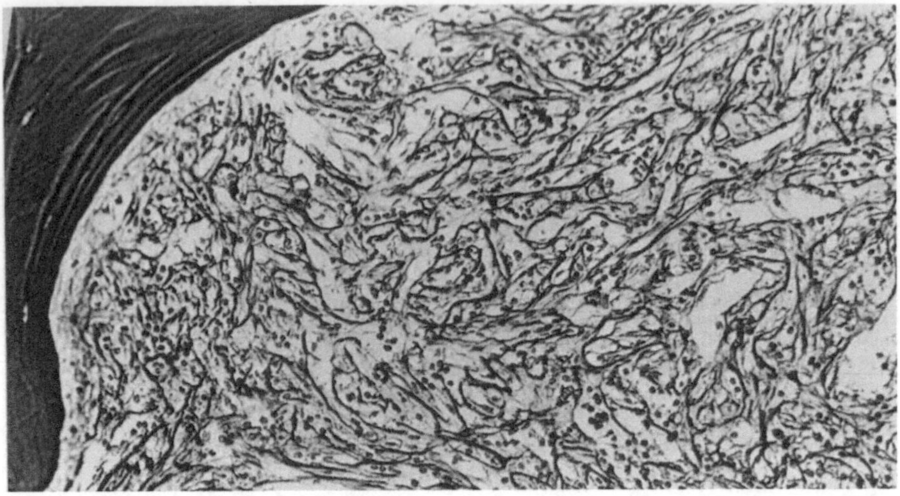

Fig. 161. M.L. centroblastic/centrocytic. Diffuse growth pattern in the bone marrow. Note the marked sclerosis, which was also found in a lymph node from this patient. ♀, 64 years. Trephine biopsy of iliac crest. Gomori. ×190

regions contain few cells and are somewhat hyalinized. With van Gieson staining and the PAS reaction they are colored deep red. Where cells are plentiful these are predominantly centrocytes. Nonetheless a few more or less typical centroblasts can always be identified. So far we have not found PAS-positive globules in the tumor cells.

The tendency to sclerosis appears to be a quality inherent in the tumor or in the patient with the tumor. In any event, we found sclerosis not only in lymph nodes but also in the bone marrow (Fig. 161) and in other extralymphatic sites. BENNETT[548] interprets the sclerosis as a product of "host resistance."

**Smear/Imprint.** Many authors[549] have reported on studies of the morphology of M.L. centroblastic/centrocytic in needle aspirates and imprints of excised lymph nodes. These reports suffer, however, from the fact that almost every author used his own nomenclature for the cells described; consequently, it is difficult to integrate the various descriptions. Therefore, we shall rely on our own studies of a large number of imprints.

One sees a relatively monotonous picture, dominated by centrocytes (Fig. 162), which have relatively light nuclei and fine, not very clearly granular ("reticular") chromatin. Often the nuclei are round, but sometimes they are irregular and show indentations, deep constrictions, or clefts. Sometimes one even gets the impression that the cells are binucleate or lobated.[550]

---

548 1975a.

549 STAHEL, 1948; LEIBETSEDER, 1949; MARTINI and WENDEROTH, 1950; MOESCHLIN (cited by COCCHI and MEIER, 1950); TISCHENDORF and HECKNER, 1950; HORSTER, 1951; ROSENTHAL, 1954; WÖCKEL and SCHREIBER, 1957; WILMS, 1970; SPIRO, GALTON, WILTSHAW and LOHMANN, 1975.

550 ISAACS, 1939.

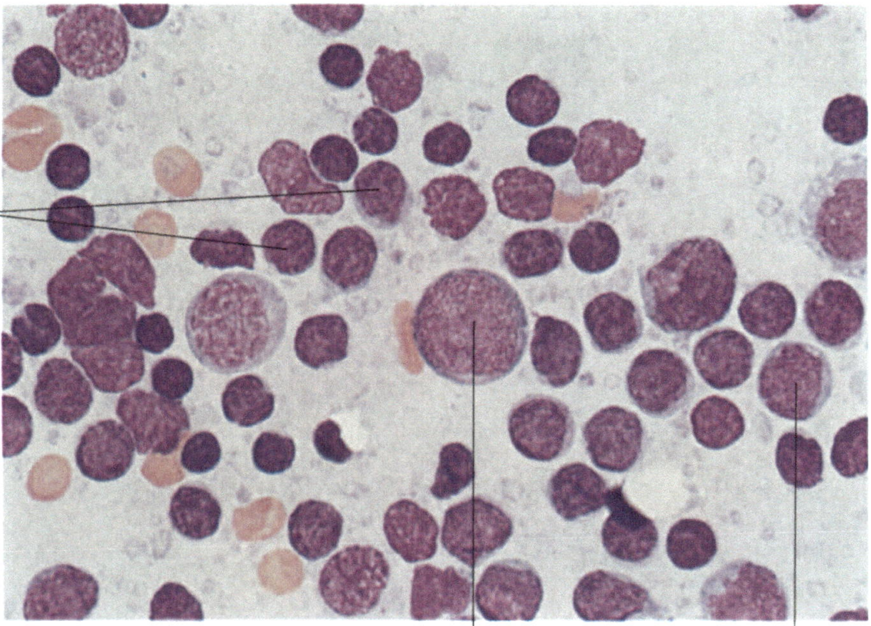


Fig. 162. M.L. centroblastic/centrocytic, follicular, in imprint. Numerous centrocytes (*cc*), one small centroblast or large centrocyte (*cb/cc*), and one typical large centroblast (*lcb*). The large centroblast contains four well-delineated light nucleoli. Note the narrow rim of strongly basophilic cytoplasm of centroblast. To the left of center, the prophase of a centroblastic mitosis. ♀, 34 years. Inguinal node. Pappenheim. ×920

Nucleoli are often lacking. At times, however, a small or medium-sized, light nucleolus may be visible. The rim of cytoplasm is narrow and stains only very faintly blue. It often cannot be recognized.

A few to moderately abundant centroblasts can always be found among the centrocytes. The centroblasts are medium to large in size and have round or oval nuclei. Their chromatin stains more brightly than that of the centrocytes and shows a distinctly reticular pattern. The nuclei contain one to several light, medium-sized or large nucleoli, which are sometimes found at the nuclear membrane. The rim of cytoplasm is narrow to moderately wide and stains deep blue. It frequently contains vacuoles.

In addition, one can always find a few macrophages and lymphocytes. Sometimes the nuclei of these lymphocytes are also indented or cleaved (cleaved lymphocytes). So far we have not been able to identify with certainty dendritic reticulum cells in imprints.

Occasionally, one finds giant cells,[551] which we believe to be derived from centroblasts.[552] Their nuclei are distinctly reticular, with large basophilic nucleoli, and their rim of cytoplasm is fairly broad and intensely basophilic.

---

[551] Stahel, 1948; Martini and Wenderoth, 1950; Lennert, 1960.

[552] Lennert, 1960.

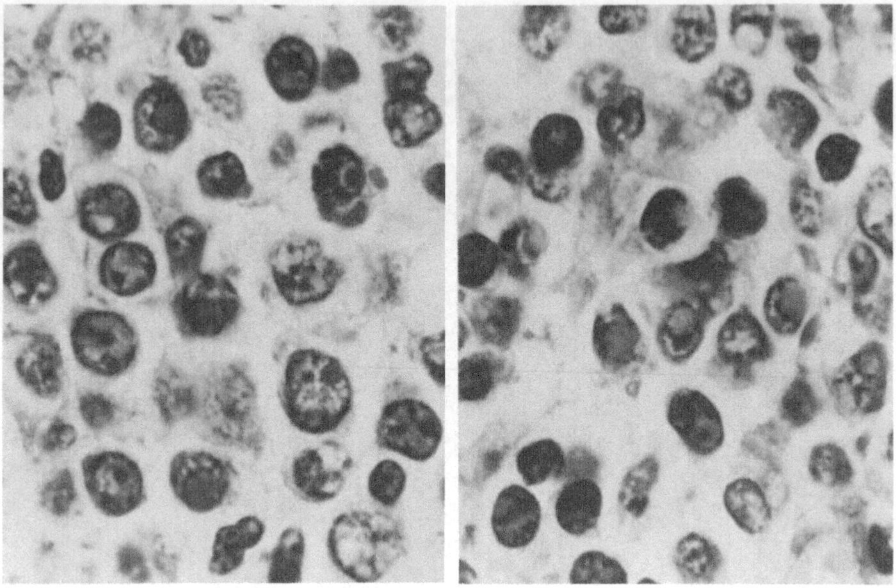

(a) (b)

Fig. 163a and b. M.L. centroblastic/centrocytic, follicular, without sclerosis. PAS-positive intranuclear inclusions in the follicular (a) and interfollicular (b) areas. ♀, 45 years. Inguinal node. PAS. × 1,400

LEIBETSEDER[553] measured the nuclear volumes in smears and found three distinct orders of size in the ratio 1:2:4. The greatest was at $K_1$ (diameter of 9.5 μm, volume of 449 $\mu m^3$).

**Histochemistry and Cytochemistry.** In paraffin sections from about 1% of the cases of centroblastic/centrocytic lymphoma, the centrocytes contain PAS-positive globular inclusions in their nuclei and/or cytoplasm (Fig. 163). RAPPAPORT and JOHNSON[554] had reported seeing similar PAS-positive inclusions. In one case with a follicular and diffuse pattern we saw innumerable centrocytes with diffuse or globular PAS positivity. There were more of these cells in the diffuse than in the follicular regions. This PAS positivity indicates that centrocytes may already start to synthesize immunoglobulin. The question therefore arises of whether the step from centrocyte to plasma cell must always be taken *via* large basophilic forms (plasmablasts) or whether a direct transition from centrocyte to plasma cell is possible (see p. 245ff.).

In cryostat sections, centrocytes and centroblasts were negative for all the enzyme reactions we have applied. In contrast, the macrophages (histiocytic reticulum cells) of the germinal centers gave a strongly positive reaction for acid phosphatase and nonspecific esterase.[555] Around the newly formed follicles – on the outer side of the mantle of lymphocytes – the reaction for alkaline

553 1949.

554 1955.

555 BRAUNSTEIN, FREIMAN, THOMAS and GALL, 1962a; LENNERT, LÖFFLER and GRABNER, 1962; LENNERT, LEDER and LÖFFLER, 1965.

Table 58. Cytologic criteria of M.L. centroblastic/centrocytic

1. Always centrocytes (highly predominant) *and* centroblasts
   Starry-sky cells absent (in 99% of cases)
   Dendritic and histiocytic reticulum cells present
2. Centrocytes:
   small to medium-sized;
   polymorphic, sometimes cleaved nuclei with fine chromatin and small nucleoli;
   cytoplasm not visible

   Centroblasts:
   medium-sized to large;
   round or oval nuclei with membrane-associated, medium-sized nucleoli or occasionally large central nucleoli;
   cytoplasm intensely basophilic, small to moderate amount
3. Sometimes small plasma cells or plasmacytoid cells in or among neoplastic germinal centers

phosphatase was strongly positive, resulting in a picture similar to that seen in reactive hyperplastic lymph nodes. There was a strongly positive ATPase reaction[556] in the neoplastic follicles; the activity was found on the surface of tumor cells. The results of ATPase studies to date are, however, not very uniform and need to be substantiated. The reaction for 5-nucleotidase[556] was only weakly positive.

In *smears* and imprints the PAS reaction is generally negative, but occasionally there is a fine granular reaction in centrocytes and centroblasts. There is a need for more precise studies on the PAS reaction. With the acid phosphatase reaction the centrocytes reveal moderately abundant fine granules, whereas the centroblasts show only sparse granules. In two cases we observed a strongly positive, granular acid phosphatase reaction in centroblasts and centrocytes. In contrast, macrophages give strongly positive reactions for both acid phosphatase and nonspecific esterase.

In quantitative determinations of DNA in imprints of lymph nodes, WILMS[557] was able to measure tetraploid values in only one out of four cases. In the other cases only a few DNA values barely reached the tetraploid mark. Consequently, WILMS presumed amitotic cell divisions, particularly since he found very few mitotic figures.

**Diagnosis.** The diagnosis of M.L. centroblastic/centrocytic depends in every case on the demonstration of centrocytes *and* centroblasts. The Giemsa stain is most suitable for revealing these cells. With it the nuclei of the centrocytes appear lighter and more polymorphic than those of lymphocytes. The centroblasts are strongly basophilic. In contrast to normal centroblasts, the nucleolus of neoplastic centroblasts is often centrally located. The cytologic criteria are summarized in Table 58. Silver impregnation aids considerably in recognizing the follicular structures that are usually present; thus fiber staining considerably facilitates the diagnosis. Further diagnostic criteria are listed in Table 59.

[556] MÜLLER-HERMELINK and KAISERLING, 1975. [557] 1970.

Table 59. Diagnostic criteria of M.L. centroblastic/centrocytic

1. Patients not younger than 20 years; peak in 6th decade
2. Growth pattern:
   73% follicular
   23% follicular and diffuse
   4% diffuse (often follicular in other lymph nodes)
3. Twenty-six percent with band-forming sclerosis
4. Small or large neoplastic germinal centers in all areas of lymph node, also often in surrounding fat

Table 60. Differential diagnosis of M.L. centroblastic/centrocytic and follicular lymphatic hyperplasia (chiefly based on data of RAPPAPORT, WINTER and HICKS, 1956)

| Histologic features | Follicular M.L. centroblastic/centrocytic | Follicular lymphatic hyperplasia |
|---|---|---|
| Lymph-node architecture | Destroyed | Largely preserved |
| Sinus histiocytosis | – | Often + |
| Follicles | | |
| Localization | In cortex and medulla | Chiefly in cortex |
| Boundaries | Usually unclear | Usually clear |
| In adjacent tissue | Often | Very rarely |
| Zonal architecture | Never seen | Often seen |
| Mitotic figures | Often only a few | Often very many |
| Protein precipitates | Rare | Frequent |
| Cytology of follicles: | | |
| Centrocytes | Large number | Relatively small number |
| Centroblasts | Often small number | Often very large number |
| Morphology of centroblasts | Often small and atypical | Often large, typical |
| Morphology of centrocytes | Sometimes larger than normal | Normal |
| Starry-sky cells | Absent or sparse | Often abundant |
| Interfollicular tissue | Monotonous, small cells | Sometimes polymorphic |
| Cytology of the interfollicular tissue (besides lymphocytes): | | |
| Plasma cells | – or (+) | Often + |
| Immunoblasts | – | Sometimes + |
| Neutrophil granulocytes | – | Occasionally + |
| Eosinophils | Occasionally (+) | Occasionally + |
| Mast cells | Occasionally (+) | Occasionally + |

**Differential Diagnosis.** First of all, *follicular* centroblastic/centrocytic lymphoma *without sclerosis* must be differentiated from reactive follicular hyperplasias. The distinction is often difficult and in a few cases impossible. In making this differential diagnosis we apply the criteria worked out by RAPPAPORT *et al.*,[558] which we have supplemented through our own observations (Table 60).

In every doubtful case we recommend going through the list of criteria shown in Table 60 step by step. One of the most important criteria is the

[558] RAPPAPORT, WINTER and HICKS, 1956.

number of starry-sky cells, which is equivalent to the number of tingible bodies. As a rule, starry-sky cells do not occur in follicular lymphoma;[559] usually macrophages are barely seen. In any event, they lack the abundant cytoplasm of the starry-sky cells as found in reactive germinal centers. Only in exceptional cases did we observe small or moderate numbers of true starry sky-cells. These appear more abundantly in tumors undergoing transition into "sarcoma," especially lymphoblastic lymphoma of the Burkitt type. Undoubtedly, they also represent the morphologic equivalent of a high rate of turnover of centroblasts. Neoplastic germinal centers do not show the zonal architecture of reactive germinal centers in the third phase (see p. 38).

Although we previously agreed with RAPPAPORT *et al.*[560] that the presence of plasma cells in the interfollicular tissue was incompatible with a follicular lymphoma, our experiences with the electron microscope have shown that, in addition to a few so-called T-associated plasma cells, a *few* lymphatic or reticular plasma cells can occur in the interfollicular tissue. There are even a few cases with a very large number of plasma cells (see also the sections on borderline cases, pp. 245ff. and 332).

Furthermore, the patient's *age* should always be taken into consideration. The greatest follicular hyperplasia develops during childhood or adolescence, at a time, in our experience, when follicular M.L. centroblastic/centrocytic never occurs.

In practice the most important differential diagnosis of centroblastic/centrocytic lymphoma is the enlargement of lymph nodes in *rheumatoid arthritis*. Here, the lymph nodes may enlarge to the size of a plum. These show marked follicular hyperplasia, but there is always at least a moderate increase in plasma cells. The prominent sinuses usually contain some neutrophil granulocytes. In accumulations of histiocytic reticulum cells[561] or macrophages one can often find large amounts of PAS-positive material.[562] It should not be difficult to identify such changes in lymph nodes as reactive and distinguish them from those of M.L. centroblastic/centrocytic. Experience teaches us, however, that the true nature of the disease is often not recognized and that a diagnosis of malignant lymphoma is often erroneously made, partly on account of the enormous size of the lymph nodes.

In doubtful cases, modern immunologic techniques may help at times to establish the diagnosis of follicular lymphoma or follicular hyperplasia. Whereas cryostat sections of reactive lymphatic hyperplasia reveal a positive reaction for Ig with a characteristic network pattern, the assay for Ig in M.L. centroblastic/centrocytic, follicular is (as a rule) negative.[563] The analysis of surface Ig should also be of help in this differential diagnosis: neoplastic germinal-center cells should bear monoclonal surface Ig.

The presence of *sclerosis* favors M.L. centroplastic/centrocytic. In rare instances, however, we have observed the same type of sclerosis in follicular hyperplasias.

---

[559] Also VETTE, 1950; WRIGHT, 1956.

[560] RAPPAPORT, WINTER and HICKS, 1956.

[561] LENNERT, LÖFFLER and GRABNER, 1962; see Fig. 3a.

[562] LENNERT, 1961.

[563] BRAYLAN and RAPPAPORT, 1973.

Very sclerotic centroblastic/centrocytic lymphoma should be simple to diagnose. It needs only to be differentiated from the nodular sclerosing type of Hodgkin's disease, which, however, is easily recognized because of its polymorphic cytology.

One may have great difficulties in differentiating *nonsclerotic diffuse* centroblastic/centrocytic lymphoma from other non-Hodgkin's lymphomas. It must be distinguished from CLL and from immunocytoma. In CLL there are no centroblasts, but instead "lymphoblasts," which have abundant cytoplasm and oval nuclei with large central nucleoli. The staining with Giemsa is important: "lymphoblasts" have gray-blue to gray-red nucleoli and a deep gray to gray-blue cytoplasm. In contrast, centroblasts usually reveal more basophilic, dark blue to blue-violet nucleoli and a strongly basophilic, dark blue cytoplasm. In typical centroblasts the nucleoli are multiple and are then usually found at the nuclear membrane. The rim of cytoplasm is narrow. The "prolymphocytes" of CLL may on occasions closely resemble centrocytes; consequently, they cannot be used for distinguishing these two neoplasms.

We need to learn more about how to differentiate diffuse M.L. centroblastic/centrocytic from immunocytoma, particularly since there are immunocytomas that contain abundant centrocytes.

**Histologic Evolution—Development into a High-Grade Malignant Lymphoma.** There have been several studies on repeated biopsies in M.L. centroblastic/centrocytic. The results are difficult to evaluate now, however, since the old cytologic criteria and old schemes of classification were used.[564] DORFMAN[565] reported that changes in the histologic picture could be observed during the course of the disease in 16% of the cases. In our opinion, the only sure evolution that takes place is that into a high-grade malignant lymphoma of germinal-center cells or of B-immunoblasts that are derived from them (see p. 354ff.).[566] The resultant tumor was previously often referred to as lymphoblastic sarcoma or reticulosarcoma, or the equivalent. Evolution into another type of tumor, such as true CLL, has, in our opinion, never been proved. That also applies to sclerosis, which evidently is not merely a function of time, but a quality characterizing the tumor or host from the very onset.

**Borderline Cases.** Three boundaries are not sharp: there are borderline cases between M.L. centroblastic/centrocytic and M.L. centrocytic (see p. 299), between M.L. centroblastic/centrocytic and immunocytoma, especially the polymorphic subtype (see p. 245ff.), and between M.L. centroblastic/centrocytic and the high-grade malignant variant of germinal-center tumors, i.e., M.L. centroblastic (see pp. 353 and 359). The third type of borderline case is a consequence of development of M.L. centroblastic/centrocytic into a lymphoma of higher-grade malignancy. Such development is particularly inherent in follicular lymphoma (see the preceding section on this page and p. 354ff.).

**Combination with Other Diseases.**[567] Among our 572 biopsied cases, M.L.

---

[564] E.g., WRIGHT, 1956; RAPPAPORT, WINTER and HICKS, 1956.
[565] 1973.
[566] In addition, COLLINS recently told us that one of his cases of follicular lymphoma developed into a true histiocytic reticulosarcoma (or a sarcoma of dendritic reticulum cells?), as proved by the nonspecific esterase reaction and immunocytologic investigations.
[567] See also FIRAT, STUTZMAN, STUDENSKI and PICKREN, 1965.

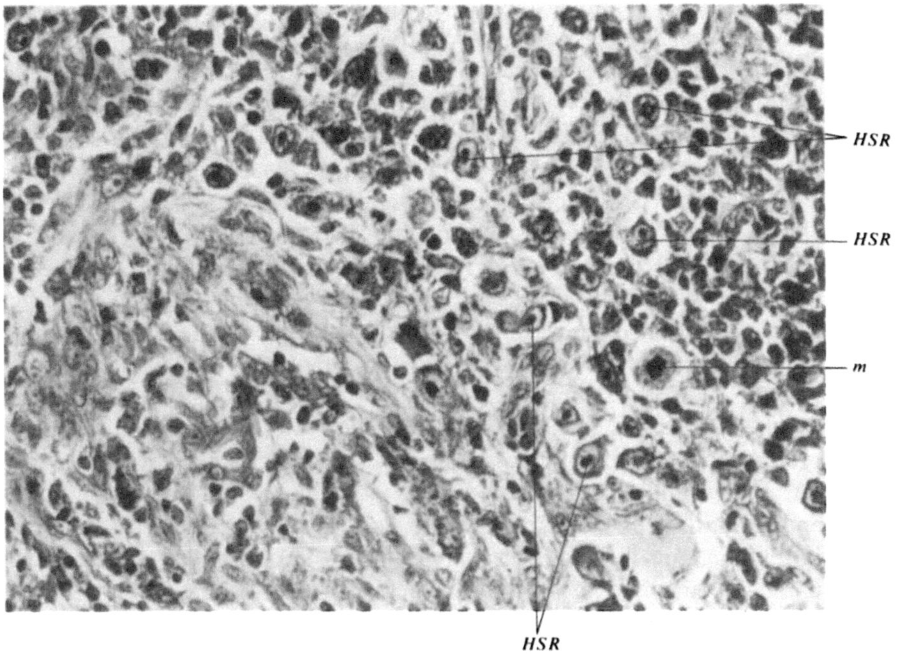


Fig. 164. M.L. centroblastic/centrocytic, follicular, with sclerosis (not seen in this figure), combined with Hodgkin's disease. Granulomatous appearance. Some Hodgkin and Sternberg-Reed cells (*HSR*), one in mitosis (*m*). ♀, 52 years. Cervical node. Giemsa. ×350

centroblastic/centrocytic occurred together with two other diseases: three times each with Hodgkin's disease and with a large focal (granulomatous) epithelioid-cell reaction.

The combination with *Hodgkin's disease* was described more often in the old literature, and sometimes a development into Hodgkin's sarcoma was assumed.[568] Most of these cases, however, fail to withstand critical analysis, and SLUITER[568] has already rejected them as true combinations. In particular, the cases reported as combinations with Hodgkin's sarcoma were rightly reinterpreted by SLUITER as sarcomatous transformations of follicular lymphoma. We are convinced, however, that centroblastic/centrocytic lymphoma and Hodgkin's disease do occur together. In our biopsy material three lymph nodes showed both the picture of follicular centroblastic/centrocytic lymphoma and that of Hodgkin's disease at the same time (Fig. 164). In one case we were able to confirm this finding in several subsequent biopsies. Definitely in one case and probably in two cases there was a mixed type of Hodgkin's disease. The case reported by WOLTER *et al.*[569] may also be regarded as a probable combination of M.L. centroblastic/centrocytic and Hodgkin's disease.

The combination of centroblastic/centrocytic lymphoma and Hodgkin's disease may be considered certain only when the latter has developed in interfollicular tissue. When giant cells are found only within the follicles, in case of doubt, these should be interpreted rather as centroblastic giant cells, since

[568] Lit. in SLUITER, 1956.

[569] WOLTER, HAMANN and OSTENDORF, 1970.

occasionally they cannot be clearly distinguished from Sternberg-Reed giant cells. In any event, one should be cautious about interpreting intrafollicular multinucleate giant cells as evidence for a combination with Hodgkin's disease.

The infiltrates of Hodgkin's disease can be recognized at a low magnification. There may be a discrete area in which the pattern of the interfollicular tissue is disturbed, for, in addition to the monotonous small round cells, there are larger reticulum cells, often epithelioid cells, and always Hodgkin and Sternberg-Reed cells. Usually a few eosinophils are also present. Finally, this region reveals a certain irregularity in the fiber pattern.

In Europe a *large focal (granulomatous) epithelioid-cell reaction* means formation of typical tubercles without marked caseation necrosis as found in *tuberculosis, sarcoidosis* (Boeck's sarcoid), or *sarcoid-like lesions.* In one of our three cases we may assume that there was tuberculosis: we found distinct small foci of caseation necrosis that exceeded the necrosis sometimes seen in sarcoidosis. In the other two cases there was no caseation necrosis. Therefore, we must leave undecided whether the epithelioid-cell granulomas indicated tuberculosis, sarcoidosis, or sarcoid-like lesions. KIM and DORFMAN[570] described such granulomas in five nodular lymphomas in lymph nodes, spleen, or liver and compared them to the epithelioid-cell granulomas of Hodgkin's disease. These authors regarded the granulomas as nonspecific in the sense of a "host response to the presence of a neoplastic process."

Epithelioid-cell tubercles are easy to recognize because of their oxyphilia. They also develop their own fiber network, which can be clearly distinguished from that of M.L. centroblastic/centrocytic.

In addition to these combinations in our biopsy material, we found in autopsy material a *carcinoma* combined with M.L. centroblastic/centrocytic more often than expected by chance. At times both diseases involved the same lymph node. In 40 autopsied cases of centroblastic/centrocytic lymphoma we found in addition to the lymphoma a carcinoma on five occasions, once in each of the following organs: stomach, colon, bile ducts, lung, and thyroid. Reports of combinations of M.L. centroblastic/centrocytic and carcinoma have also appeared in the literature. For example, WU[571] described follicular lymphoma associated with carcinoma of the uterus. The incidence of this combination therefore probably exceeds that expected by chance.

Other alleged combinations described in the literature have already been mentioned in the section on histologic evolution (p. 332).

**Prognosis.** From data reported in the literature and from our own studies we have compiled the figures given in Tables 61 and 62 regarding the prognosis of M.L. centroblastic/centrocytic. They indicate that the prognosis is better than that for all other non-Hodgkin's lymphomas, but that it is by no means as favorable as was believed in the days when one spoke of preblastomatosis. The survival rate previously thought to be so favorable and quoted in all textbooks certainly depended in part on the inclusion of a considerable number of false diagnoses (follicular hyperplasias). The median survival time of our patients with centroblastic/centrocytic lymphoma of the lymph nodes proved

[570] 1974. [571] 1942.

Table 61. Survival of patients with M.L. centroblastic/centrocytic according to the literature and our own data

| Authors | n | Survival | |
|---|---|---|---|
| | | Mean | Median |
| GALL and MALLORY (1942) | 42 | 5.6 years | 5.0 years |
| JACKSON and PARKER (1974) | | ~6.0 years | – |
| WRIGHT (1956) | 130 | – | 2.0 years |
| ROSENBERG *et al.* (1961) | 162 | – | 72.0 months |
| FIRAT *et al.* (1965) | 62 | 77.0 months | 53.0 months |
| SPIRO *et al.* (1975) | 54 | – | 5.5 years |
| Our series | | | |
| Deceased patients (nodal and extranodal biopsies) | 61 | 31.4 months | 18.0 months |
| Deceased and surviving patients: | | | |
| a) nodal biopsies | 82 | 48.1 months | 46.8 months |
| b) extranodal biopsies and splenectomies | 12 | 69.3 months | 61.5 months |

Table 62. Survival rate of patients with M.L. centroblastic/centrocytic according to the literature and our own data

| Authors | Survival rate (%) | | |
|---|---|---|---|
| | > 3 years | > 5 years | > 10 years |
| LUMB (1954) | 72.2 | 62.5 | – |
| RAPPAPORT *et al.* (1956) | | | |
| Type I (lymphocytic, well differentiated) | 77 | 55 | |
| Type II (lymphocytic, poorly differentiated) | 71 | 50 | |
| Type III (mixed) | 57 | 16 | |
| Type IV (reticulum cell) | 50 | 20 | |
| WRIGHT (1956) | 49 | 36.1 | 5.4 |
| LUMB and NEWTON (1957) | | 73 | |
| ROSENBERG *et al.* (1961) | | 54.4 | |
| FIRAT *et al.* (1965) | | 72[a] | 60[a] |
| SPIRO *et al.* (1975) | | 54 | 29 |
| QAZI *et al.* (1976) | | 54 | |
| Our series | 50.6 | 41.2 | |

[a] Percentage certainly too high, since 10 out of 64 patients were too young (< 20 years) to have centroblastic/centrocytic lymphoma

to be 46.8 months, whereas GALTON[572] reported $5^1/_2$ years. This difference is certainly the result of uniform and on average better therapy than that administered to the patients of our heterogeneous series. When M.L. centroblastic/centrocytic arose in extranodal sites (for example, in the spleen) the median survival in our series was longer, namely, 61.5 months.

[572] SPIRO, GALTON, WILTSHAW and LOHMANN, 1975.

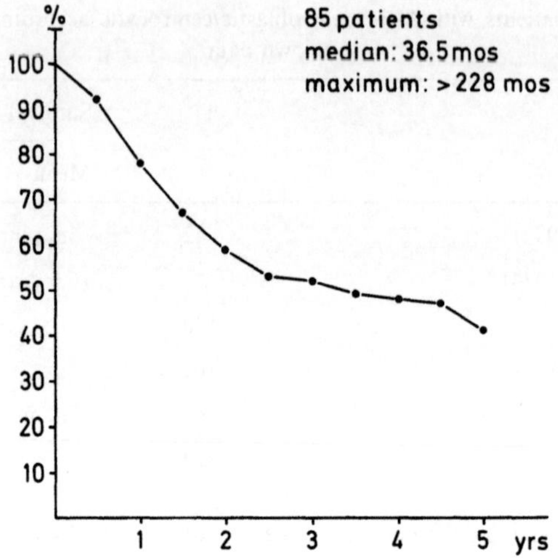


Fig. 165. Survival rate of 85 patients with M.L. centroblastic/centrocytic. Follow-up more than 5 years

In three published series, where the patients had received good treatment, the 5-year survival rate was 54% in each.[573] This concurrence is remarkable and does not seem to be merely by chance. The fact that a patient is still alive, however, does not mean that he is free of disease. QAZI *et al.*[574] reported that about 54% of their patients survived 5 years, but that only 18% were free of disease.

As shown in Figure 165, more patients die in the first two years after the histologic diagnosis is made than one would expect from the favorable prognosis generally assumed for M.L. centroblastic/centrocytic. After two years, however, the slope of the curve becomes gentler, that is, the death rate in subsequent years falls off. In our series the longest period a patient has been followed is 228 months. This patient is still alive and has probably been cured. Figure 35 shows the actuarial survival determined by the Kiel Lymphoma Study Group. It also demonstrates the relatively favorable prognosis of M.L. centroblastic/centrocytic, that is, of the lymphoma that is generally follicular.

According to our own findings on 94 cases and to those reported in the literature, the prognosis of M.L. centroblastic/centrocytic should be studied for correlations with histologic type, stage of the disease at the time of first examination, localization of the tumor (extranodal or nodal), and age and sex of the patient.

### *Histologic and Cytologic Parameters*

*a) Growth Pattern and Size of Follicles.* In the cases evaluated, we found that the average life expectancy of patients with purely follicular centroblastic/

[573] ROSENBERG, DIAMOND, JASLOWITZ and CRAVER, 1961; SPIRO, GALTON, WILTSHAW and LOHMANN, 1975; QAZI, AISENBERG and LONG, 1976.

[574] QAZI, AISENBERG and LONG, 1976.

Table 63. Survival rate of 89 patients with M.L. centroblastic/centrocytic. At the time of follow-up, 55 patients had died and 34 were still alive

| Type of growth | No. of patients | Survival rate (%) | | |
|---|---|---|---|---|
| | | > 3 years | > 5 years | > 10 years |
| Follicular | 81 | 59.3 | 40.0 | 12.5 |
| Follicular and diffuse | 8 | 50.0 | 42.9 | 0 |

Table 64. Mean survival of 55 patients who died from M.L. centroblastic/centrocytic of different histologic types of growth

| Type of growth | No. of patients | Mean survival (months) | Range (months) |
|---|---|---|---|
| Follicular | 50 | 33.3 | 1–143 |
| Follicular and diffuse | 5 | 29.2 | 5–68 |

centrocytic lymphoma differed slightly from that of patients with the follicular and diffuse types (Tables 63 and 64). Follicular and diffuse M.L. centroblastic/centrocytic revealed a somewhat shorter mean survival (29.2 months, compared with 33.3 months for the purely follicular type; the difference was not statistically significant). That can probably be attributed to the longest survivors' being among those with a purely follicular type; none of the cases of follicular and diffuse centroblastic/centrocytic lymphoma reached the 10-year mark. The longest period of observation was 68 months.

In contrast, as Figure 166 shows, the size of the neoplastic follicles correlates approximately with survival. None of the patients with very large follicles lived longer than 6 years, whereas there was a period of observation of up to 12 years for patients with the smallest follicles. We should point out, however, that even when the follicles of M.L. centroblastic/centrocytic are very small, death can occur within a few months. Therefore, the size of the follicles has only a limited prognostic value.

Van Unnik[575] found that the prognosis was better in cases that showed well-formed germinal centers than in those showing ill-defined germinal centers.

Butler *et al.*[576] distinguished three grades of follicular lymphoma. In grade I there was a distinct follicular pattern; the interfollicular areas were free of tumor cells. In grade II identical tumor cells were found both in and between the distinct follicles. In grade III the follicular growth pattern was confined to small areas. This grading was assumed to be of prognostic significance and of even more significance when it was related to the cytologic type of lymphoma.

*b) Tendency to Sclerosis.* According to Bennett[577] and his associates, as well as to Rosas-Uribe and Rappaport,[578] sclerotic follicular lymphoma or "histio-

[575] Personal communication, 1975.
[576] Butler, Stryker and Shullenberger, 1975.
[577] 1975a, b.
[578] 1972.

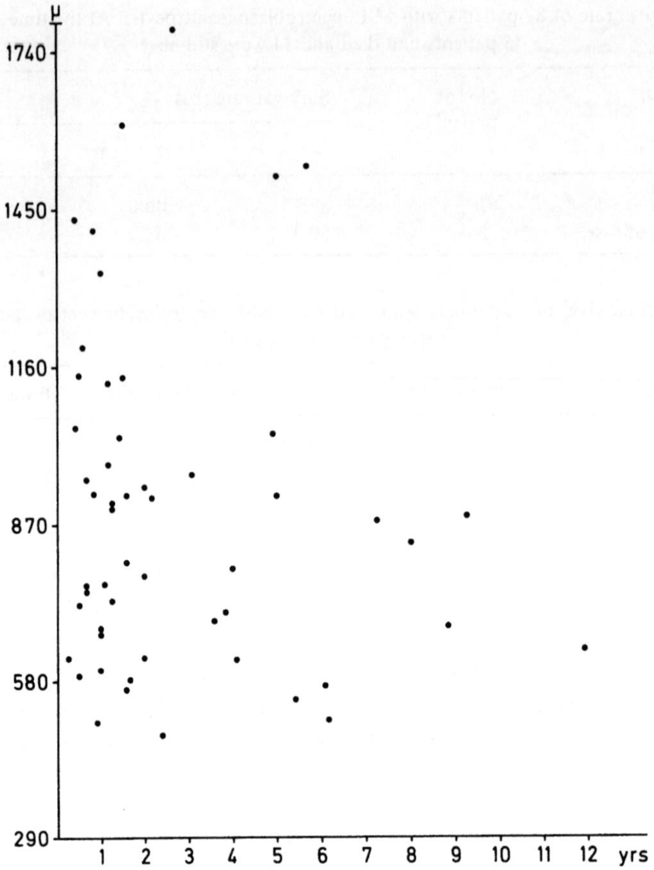


Fig. 166. Mean diameters of neoplastic follicles (ordinate) and survival times (abscissa) of 53 patients with M.L. centroblastic/centrocytic. Range: 471 – 1781 μm

cytic lymphoma" has a definitely better prognosis than nonsclerotic follicular lymphoma. As the most recent statistics of BENNETT[579] reveal, among 84 patients with follicular lymphoma, 58% of those with sclerotic tumors survived 5 years as compared with only 27% of those with nonsclerotic tumors. In our own series of cases (Table 65) sclerotic M.L. centroblastic/centrocytic that was diagnosed in lymph nodes showed a considerably better prognosis than the nonsclerotic variant. The median survivals were 46 and 36 months, respectively. The difference is statistically significant ($p < 0.05$). The number of extranodal lymphomas is too small for a statistical evaluation.

*c) Cell Size.* According to the average size of the proliferating cells, we have distinguished two groups. In the first group the cells measure 6 – 8 μm ("small cells"), those of the second group 8 – 10 μm ("large cells"). The results of our studies (Table 66) seem to indicate that the large-cell variant has a poorer prognosis than the small-cell variant. The number of cases is not sufficient

[579] 1975b.

Table 65. Survival of 94 patients with M.L. centroblastic/centrocytic with or without sclerosis. The patients either were deceased or had survived more than 3 years

| Histologic type | Lymph-node tumors | | | Extranodal tumors | | |
|---|---|---|---|---|---|---|
| | n | Survival | | n | Survival | |
| | | Mean (months) | Median (months) | | Mean (months) | Median (months) |
| With sclerosis | 23 | 52.5 | 46.0 | 3 | (45.0) | (61.0) |
| Without sclerosis | 59 | 46.3 | 36.0 | 9 | (77.4) | (62.0) |

Table 66. Survival rate of 89 patients with M.L. centroblastic/centrocytic, classified according to cell size. At the time of investigation, 55 of the patients had died and 34 were still living

| Cell size | No. of patients | Survival rate (%) | | |
|---|---|---|---|---|
| | | > 3 years | > 5 years | > 10 years |
| Small to medium-sized (6 – 8 μm) | 83 | 60.2 | 42.3 | 12.5 |
| Large (8 – 10 μm) | 6 | 33.3 | 16.7 | 0 |

for a significant conclusion; but our findings are supported by the studies of RAPPAPORT *et al.*,[580] JONES *et al.*,[581] and VAN UNNIK *et al.*[582] in larger groups of patients. The poorly differentiated lymphocytic type of RAPPAPORT certainly includes our small-cell type. RAPPAPORT *et al.* calculated for this type a 5-year survival rate of 50%. In contrast, only 20% of the patients with their reticulum-cell type, which probably includes our large-cell variant, survived for 5 years.

JONES *et al.*[581] found that patients with tumors of their poorly differentiated lymphocytic type lived as long as those with the mixed lymphohistiocytic type; both groups lived significantly longer than those with the histiocytic type of tumor. Their first two types probably correspond to our small-cell type, whereas their histiocytic type would be comparable to our large-cell variant.

From these facts we consider it safe to conclude that the small-cell type has a better prognosis than the large-cell type.

*d) Number of Centroblasts.* The number of centroblasts within the neoplastic follicles is a sure gauge of the prognosis (see Table 67, Fig. 167). The more numerous the centroblasts, the worse the prognosis. The difference is statistically significant ($p < 0.05$).

The idea that the number of centroblasts might correlate with the size of the follicles, in the sense that large follicles might be associated with a large number of centroblasts, could not be substantiated. Small follicles may contain

580 RAPPAPORT, WINTER and HICKS, 1956.
581 JONES, FUKS, BULL, KADIN *et al.*, 1973.
582 VAN UNNIK, BREUR, BURGERS, CLETON *et al.*, 1975.

Table 67. Survival rate of patients with M.L. centroblastic/centrocytic, classified according to the number of centroblasts in the neoplastic follicles

| Centroblasts | No. of patients | Survival rate (%) | | |
|---|---|---|---|---|
| | | >3 years | >5 years | >10 years |
| <10% | 69 | 61.0 | 39.7 | 12.5 |
| >10% | 17 | 35.3 | 31.2 | 7.7 |

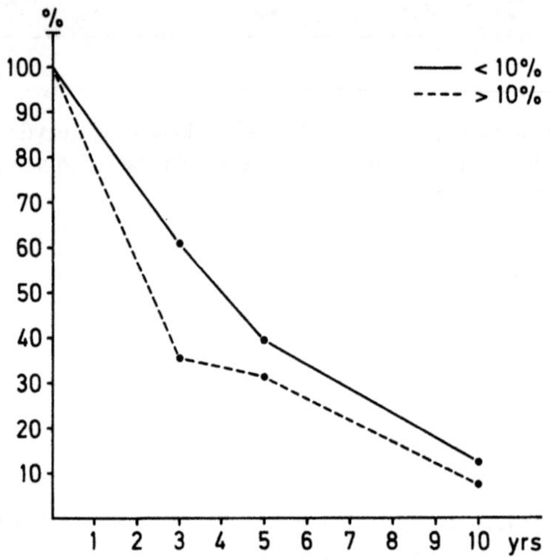


Fig. 167. Actuarial survival correlated with the percentage of centroblasts in M.L. centroblastic/centrocytic (n = 89 patients)

great numbers of centroblasts, just as very large follicles may contain only few centroblasts (see Fig. 168).

If at the time of biopsy "germinoblastic sarcoma" (M.L. centroblastic) is found along with follicular centroblastic/centrocytic lymphoma, then the prognosis is very poor. The average life expectancy was only 4.1 months in our cases.

## *Clinical Stage at the Time of Diagnosis*

The clinical stage at the time of first examination certainly plays as large a role in M.L. centroblastic/centrocytic as it does in many other types of malignant lymphoma.[583] WRIGHT[584] found many years ago that none of his 114 patients with generalized lymphoma at the time of biopsy were cured, whereas 16 patients with localized involvement of lymph nodes remained free of recurrence. Accordingly, WRIGHT calculated a recovery rate of 8.3%. JONES *et al.*[585] also reported that the localized centroblastic/centrocytic lymphomas (of the poorly differentiated lymphocytic and lymphocytic-histiocytic mixed types) had a relatively

[583] BLUMENBERG, OLSON, STEIN and HAWKINS, 1963.
[584] 1956.
[585] JONES, KAPLAN and ROSENBERG, 1972.

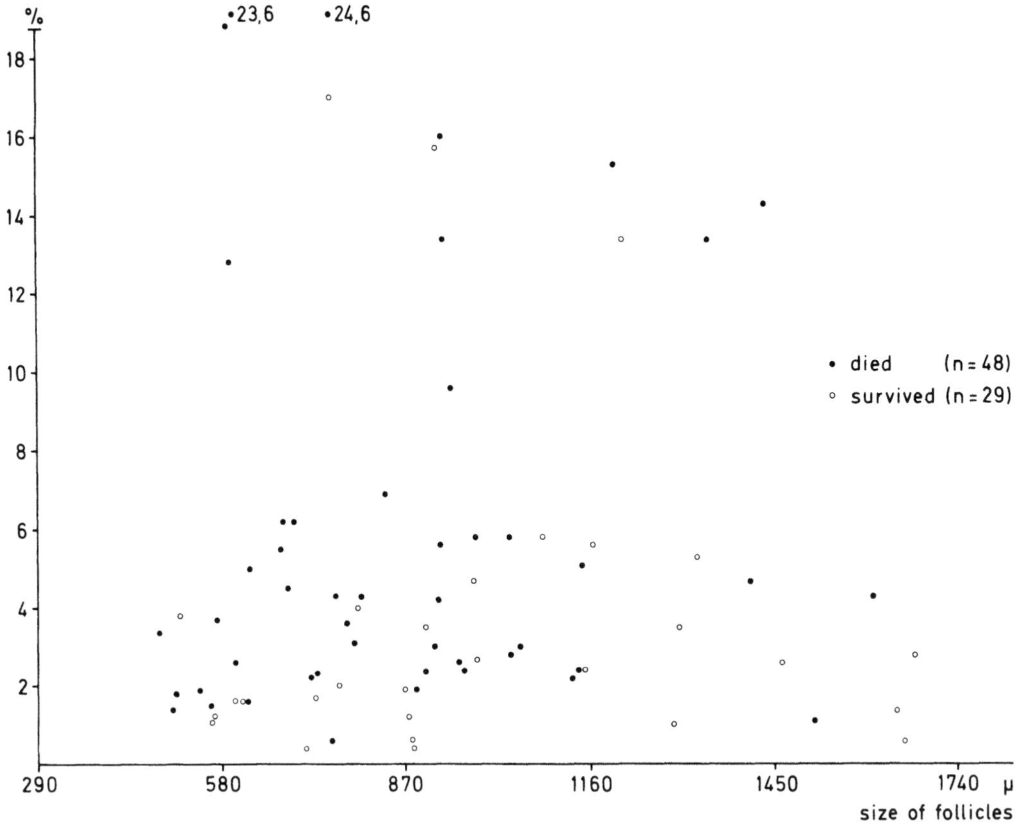


Fig. 168. Relation of percentage of centroblasts and size of follicles (77 patients)

favorable prognosis with a median survival of 80 months and a long relapse-free interval.

In the material of BENNETT,[586] 33 patients had a localized tumor and 31 showed generalization. Of the 33 localized tumors, 21 were sclerotic. Of the 31 generalized tumors, only 10 were sclerotic. The 5-year survival rate for the localized sclerotic follicular lymphomas was 86%. For the nonsclerotic follicular lymphomas it was 67%. In contrast, the 5-year survival rate for the generalized sclerotic follicular lymphomas was only 20% and for the nonsclerotic lymphomas it was as low as 14%. This means the prognosis is very much poorer when there is already generalization at the time of biopsy, but, nevertheless, as many as 14–20% of the patients survived 5 years. Since sclerotic centroblastic/centrocytic lymphoma is more commonly encountered in stages I and II than the nonsclerotic type, it is easy to understand why the prognosis is better for the former than for the latter. In general, the sclerotic form apparently grows and spreads more slowly.

It seems questionable whether generalization, for example, with involvement of the bone marrow or gastrointestinal tract, has the same serious consequences

[586] 1975b.

Table 68. Survival rate of 94 patients with follicular M.L. centroblastic/centrocytic, classified according to localization. The extranodal localizations were: tonsil (5 cases), spleen (3), salivary gland (2), lung (1), and intestine (1)

| Localization | No. of patients | Survival rate (%) | | |
|---|---|---|---|---|
| | | > 3 years | > 5 years | > 10 years |
| Nodal | 82 | 52.4 | 34.7 | 10.0 |
| Extranodal | 12 | 83.3 | 65.3 | 20.0 |

for the patient in cases of M.L. centroblastic/centrocytic as it does in cases of Hodgkin's disease or diffuse lymphoma.[587] The presence or absence of general symptoms (fever, etc.) seems to make little difference in the prognosis.[587]

### *Localization of the Presenting Tumor*

The prognosis is significantly ($p < 0.05$) better when the initial tumor is found at an extranodal site than when lymph nodes are involved (see Table 68). That holds especially true for follicular M.L. centroblastic/centrocytic of the spleen and probably also for that of the tonsils. According to JONES *et al.*,[588] however, there is no difference in the prognosis between primary extranodal localization and nodal involvement in stages I and II. Our experience is that splenectomy was often curative when only the spleen was involved. We have observed two such patients for 10 and 15 years, both without recurrence. Recently, BOUSSER *et al.*[589] drew attention to the favorable clinical course of isolated M.L. centroblastic/centrocytic of the spleen. JONES *et al.*[587] reported that with involvement of the mediastinal lymph nodes the prognosis is significantly ($p = 0.03$) worse than when they are not involved.

### *Age and Sex*

JONES *et al.*[587] compared the survival rate of patients under 40 years of age with that of those over 60 and found that the prognosis for the older patients with nodular lymphoma of the poorly differentiated lymphocytic and mixed types was significantly worse. This disparity could not be explained by a difference in stage at the onset of therapy.

Like SPIRO *et al.*,[590] we could not detect a definite correlation between age and prognosis. What did strike us as noteworthy, however, was that sometimes in very young patients the disease ran an extremely malignant course. For example, the initial biopsy of a tumor in a 21-year-old man revealed transition into a "germinoblastic sarcoma" (M.L. centroblastic). Although no such "sarco-

[587] JONES, FUKS, BULL, KADIN *et al.*, 1973.
[588] JONES, KAPLAN and ROSENBERG, 1972.
[589] BOUSSER, DELARUE, BILSKI-PASQUIER, DIEBOLD *et al.*, 1970.
[590] SPIRO, GALTON, WILTSHAW and LOHMANN, 1975.

Table 69. Survival rate of 94 patients with M.L. centroblastic/centrocytic, classified according to sex

| Sex | No. of patients | Survival rate (%) | | |
|---|---|---|---|---|
| | | > 3 years | > 5 years | > 10 years |
| Male | 49 | 42.9 | 31.8 | 7.9 |
| Female | 45 | 71.1 | 47.4 | 14.8 |

matous" transformation was evident in the tumor of another 22-year-old man, he died within 4 months.

In our series the disease has a significantly better prognosis in females ($p<0.1$) than in males (see Table 69). In contrast, JONES *et al.*[591] apparently were unable to detect any significant difference between the sexes.

*In conclusion*, the results of our studies and of those reported in the literature indicate that the prognosis is better for cases with a small-cell picture, with a small number of centroblasts, with sclerosis, in stages I and II, with an extranodal localization, and for women. Conversely, the prognosis is correspondingly poorer for cases with a large-cell picture, with a large number of centroblasts, without sclerosis, in stages III and IV, with primary involvement of lymph nodes, and for men.

### *Addendum*
### *The Leukemic Variant of M.L. Centroblastic/Centrocytic*

FLASHMAN and LEOPOLD[592] were perhaps the first to observe the leukemic variant of M.L. centroblastic/centrocytic. HORSTER,[593] however, definitely described and illustrated this disease. A short time later, ANDAY and SCHMITZ[594] described a patient with follicular lymphoma, whose blood at the onset of the illness contained large numbers of tumor cells with "notched nuclei," but who then remained aleukemic for 10 years. In the same year, ROSENTHAL *et al.*[595] published a report on the release of cells into the blood in follicular lymphoma. They called the cells hematogones. Later, numerous other investigators[596] described and illustrated leukemic cells in cases of malignant lymphoma of this type, but interpreted them differently, for example, as lymphosarcoma cells.[597]

The leukemic cells of M.L. centroblastic/centrocytic usually differ from the lymphocytes of CLL in blood smears by their *very* narrow rim of cytoplasm and by their irregularly angular, seldom round, nuclei that often reveal deep

[591] JONES, FUKS, BULL, KADIN *et al.*, 1973.
[592] 1929.
[593] 1951.
[594] 1952.
[595] ROSENTHAL, DRESKIN, VURAL and ZAK, 1952; see also ROSENTHAL, 1954.
[596] RAPPAPORT, WINTER and HICKS, 1956; WRIGHT, 1956; BLUMENBERG, OLSON, STEIN and HAWKINS, 1963; DORFMAN, 1964b, 1973; GALTON, 1964; RAPPAPORT, 1966; GAJL-PECZALSKA, BLOOMFIELD, COCCIA, SOSIN *et al.*, 1975; MCKENNA, BLOOMFIELD and BRUNNING, 1975.
[597] SCHNITZER, LOESEL and REED, 1970.

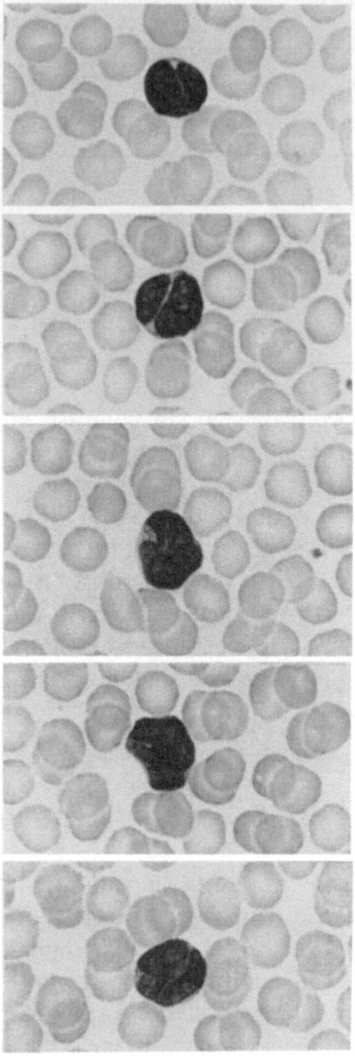

Fig. 169. Leukemic M.L. centroblastic/centrocytic, follicular. Blood smear. Note the polymorphic, mostly cleaved nuclei and the very scanty, nonbasophilic cytoplasm. ♂, 32 years. Pappenheim. ×875

indentations (Fig. 169). Consequently, various investigators have referred to the cells as notched-nucleus cells[598] and later as cleaved cells.[599] In a few of our cases, however, we could not clearly distinguish them from the cells of CLL. We then discovered that they gave a somewhat stronger reaction for acid phosphatase than the cells of CLL. The PAS reaction also helps some-

[598] GALTON, 1964; SPIRO, GALTON, WILTSHAW and LOHMANN, 1975.

[599] LUKES and COLLINS, 1973.

what in differentiating the two diseases. In the cases we have studied, the PAS reaction was almost always negative, whereas in CLL it was described as positive (see p. 128f.).

In addition to the small lymphoid cells, which we interpret as centrocytes and $B_2$-lymphocytes, one practically always finds a few basophilic cells of moderate to large size. These we interpret as centroblasts.

It is impossible to say from the histology of M.L. centroblastic/centrocytic whether or not the tumor releases large numbers of cells into the blood. Of 22 leukemic cases in our series, the growth was follicular in 19, and two of these also showed clerosis. In three cases the growth was follicular and diffuse.

The frequency of leukemic changes has been variously assessed. According to WRIGHT,[600] it is more than 5%. As calculated from the figures supplied by RAPPAPORT *et al.*,[601] it is about 15% (at the time of first hospitalization). ROSENBERG *et al.*[602] gave a rate of 8.6%. In our own material (507 cases) it proved to be 4.5%, a figure certainly too low, since blood counts were not available from all patients. The number of cases in which a few or moderately abundant "atypical lymphocytes" can be detected in the circulating blood is surely much higher. RAPPAPORT *et al.*[601] found 3–84% "abnormal lymphocytes" in the blood, with and without elevated leukocyte counts in 23 out of 35 patients.

It was only through careful studies pursued over several decades that GALTON and co-workers[603] were able to clarify questions about the frequency and time of appearance of a leukemic blood picture in M.L. centroblastic/centrocytic. They found among 75 cases an increase in "lymphocytes," with a variable proportion of "notched-nucleus cells," to 5000/μl or more in 36%. In other cases they detected "notched-nucleus cells" in blood smears, even without an increase in the total lymphocyte count. The highest lymphocyte count was 30,000/μl. On reexamining 11 cases, they discovered that the cells that were increased in number were not the typical "notched-nucleus cells," but instead lymphocytes with the usual morphology, as we have also experienced.

The increase in lymphocytes in the blood may be present at the very onset and then may disappear for good, either spontaneously or after therapy. It may also reappear after therapy, however, or may appear for the first time later in the course of the disease.[604]

The prognosis of the leukemic variant is not significantly different from that of M.L. centroblastic/centrocytic without leukemia.[604]

We must clearly distinguish this leukemic form of M.L. centroblastic/centrocytic from terminal *"blast-cell leukemia,"* which GALTON observed as a fulminating end phase after a course of many years with few symptoms. He compared it to the blast crisis in chronic myeloid leukemia.[604] Histologically, it corresponds to a transformation of M.L. centroblastic/centrocytic into M.L. centroblastic (see p. 359f.).

---

[600] 1956.

[601] RAPPAPORT, WINTER and HICKS, 1956.

[602] ROSENBERG, DIAMOND, JASLOWITZ and CRAVER, 1961.

[603] GALTON, 1964; SPIRO, GALTON, WILTSHAW and LOHMANN, 1975.

[604] SPIRO, GALTON, WILTSHAW and LOHMANN, 1975.

# II. Malignant Lymphomas of High-Grade Malignancy

## A. Malignant Lymphoma, Centroblastic

*Synonyms:* Germinoblastic sarcoma
Malignant lymphoma, FCC, large noncleaved
In some instances:
Malignant lymphoma, lymphoblastic
Malignant lymphoma, lymphocytic, poorly differentiated
Malignant lymphoma, undifferentiated
Reticulosarcoma arising from follicular lymphoma, etc.

**History, Definition.** On the basis of their studies with a camera lucida, LUKES and COLLINS[605] have distinguished a lymphoma in which the essential components are large noncleaved follicular center-cells (FCC), i.e., our centroblasts. They claimed that this tumor differs from centroblastic/centrocytic lymphoma in that it contains more than 25% centroblasts. The tumor was reported to be closely related to immunoblastic sarcoma, and, like the latter, it occasionally showed monoclonal Ig production. For LUKES and COLLINS, the distinction between the centroblastic tumor and immunoblastic sarcoma depended either upon the demonstration of an FCC tumor (e.g., M.L. centroblastic/centrocytic) in a previous biopsy or upon the finding of a proportion of cleaved FCC in the tumor.

The definition of LUKES and COLLINS therefore puts centroblasts (large noncleaved FCC) in the forefront, irrespective of the fact that the tumor may contain numerous immunoblasts. The diagnosis of centroblastic lymphoma is supported by the simultaneous or previous demonstration of a low-grade germinal center-cell tumor (in general M.L. centroblastic/centrocytic) or by the presence of centrocytes among the blast cells.

In the classification of our material, we originally placed only the following malignant lymphomas in the centroblastic group:

1. High-grade malignant lymphomas that developed subsequent to or together with M.L. centroblastic/centrocytic.

2. High-grade malignant lymphomas that consisted of pure populations of centroblasts.

The pure form of the second group is not very common. If one were to follow LUKES and COLLINS,[605] however, and use the term centroblastic for all lymphomas containing centroblasts, centrocytes and immunoblasts as well, then one would have to classify a considerable number of the cases that we originally diagnosed as immunoblastic lymphomas in this group. In fact, STEIN proved that immunoblastic lymphomas with centroblasts are actually derived from germinal-center cells (see Part Six) by demonstrating positivity in the EAC-rosette test. Therefore, we have now added a polymorphic subtype to the group

[605] 1974a, b, 1975a, b.

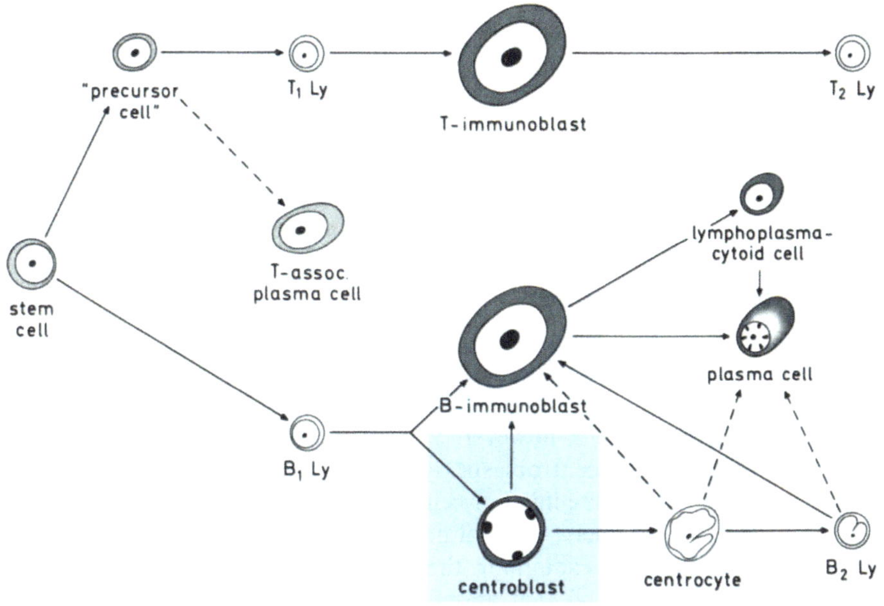


Fig. 170. Hypothetical origin of tumor cells of M.L. centroblastic. In the monomorphic subtype, virtually only centroblasts are found: dark blue area. In the polymorphic subtype, centrocytes and immunoblasts can be found as well: light blue area

of "pure" centroblastic lymphomas in order to accommodate the formerly "immunoblastic" lymphomas that contain immunoblasts, centroblasts, and (atypical) centrocytes. The close relationship between centroblastic and immunoblastic lymphomas is evident from this polymorphic subtype. It also sheds light on the normal development of cells in germinal centers.

In the following account we shall distinguish primary from secondary centroblastic lymphomas. The distinction is based on whether or not a centroblastic/centrocytic lymphoma was demonstrated previously or at the same time.

### *1. Primary Centroblastic Lymphoma*

**Origin of the Neoplastic Cells.** Based on light- and electron-microscopic as well as cytochemical findings, the chief tumor cells are unquestionably centroblasts. That is also supported by the demonstration of dendritic reticulum cells on electron microscopy.[606] In addition to the centroblasts, a variable number of immunoblasts and centrocytes may be present (see Fig. 170).

**Occurrence.** The tumor did not appear to be very common in our first series (Table 70). We encountered it seven times among 9083 routine lymph-node biopsies, or 0.5% of all malignant lymphomas and 0.8% of the non-Hodgkin's

[606] Kaiserling, 1975.

Table 70. M.L. centroblastic. Material and incidence

| | Primary | Secondary |
|---|---|---|
| Total No. of cases | –[a] | 48 |
| Biopsy | – | 31 |
| Autopsy | – | 17 |
| Incidence in routine lymph-node material | 7 cases | 3 cases |
| = % of malignant lymphomas | 0.5 | 0.2 |
| % of non-Hodgkin's lymphomas | 0.8 | 0.35 |

[a] Primary centroblastic lymphoma was not diagnosed when the lists were made. Thus, the figures cannot be given here; they are included in those for M.L. lymphoblastic, unclassified and M.L. immunoblastic

lymphomas. We must add, however, that, at the time we reviewed our slides, we did not classify the centroblastic lymphomas containing immunoblasts in this group. Thus, the percentage of centroblastic lymphomas was much higher in our second series, namely, 5.5% of non-Hodgkin's lymphomas. We have also had the opportunity of examining the extensive lymphoma material of VAN UNNIK, in which we found that about 5% of 295 non-Hodgkin's lymphomas were primary centroblastic lymphomas.

Although the tumor usually affects people of advanced years, it does occur in children. Our youngest patient was 6 years old, our oldest was 97. In the cases seen so far, males were affected somewhat more commonly than females (1.3:1).

**Clinical Manifestations.** Whereas in our cases the tissue extract revealed a considerable increase in IgM, the blood generally showed clearly reduced IgM values and no paraproteinemia. LUKES and COLLINS[607] reported on several cases showing monoclonal Ig production. One of our 17 patients had a leukemic blood picture.

Another patient in our series had cold-hemagglutination disease for many years and was finally treated with 50 mg azathioprine (Imurek®) daily for one year.[608] At the end of treatment, she developed M.L. immunoblastic with many centroblasts and with dendritic reticulum cells. STEIN demonstrated a marked increase in μ-chains in a tissue homogenate.

**Localization.** Most of the lymph nodes we received for study came from the cervical region (10 nodes). Three were removed from the inguinal region and one from the axilla.

**Histology.** The lymph-node architecture is replaced by either a follicular (Fig. 171) or a diffuse (Fig. 172) proliferation of large basophilic cells. The follicular pattern is much rarer than the diffuse one. There are two cytologic subtypes. In the monomorphic subtype ("pure form"; Figs. 172 and 173) the proliferating cells are large centroblasts. The polymorphic subtype (Fig. 174)

[607] 1975a, b.

[608] We wish to thank Dr. NASSIF, Landkrankenhaus Coburg, for providing the clinical data on this case.

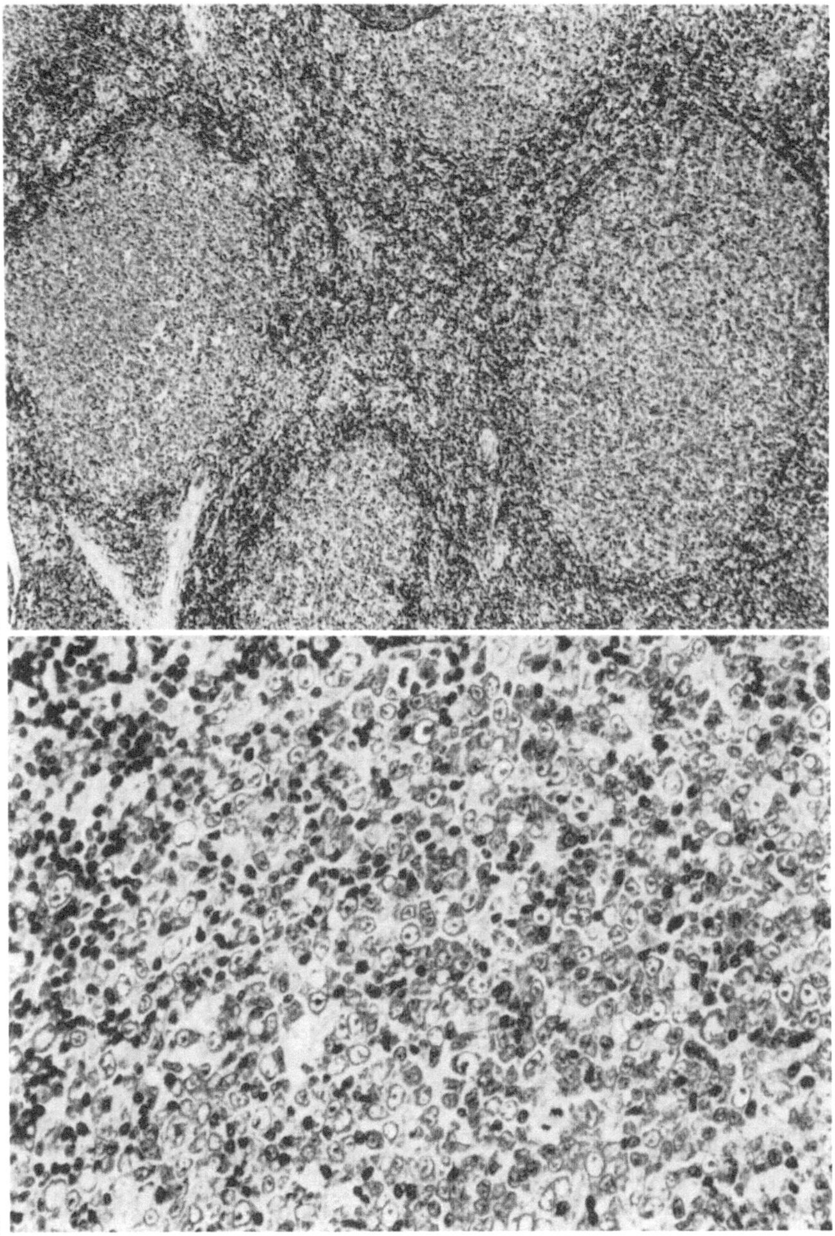

(a)

(b)

Fig. 171a and b. M.L. centroblastic with follicular growth pattern. The follicles contain more than 90% centroblasts and immunoblasts. ♀, 63 years, Lymph node. Giemsa. (a) ×70, (b) ×440

is composed of medium-sized to large cells. Only some of these cells are centroblasts; the others are large immunoblasts and smaller centrocyte-like cells. As usual, the centroblasts are strongly basophilic and have round or oval nuclei containing multiple medium-sized nucleoli located chiefly at the nuclear mem-

(a)

(b)

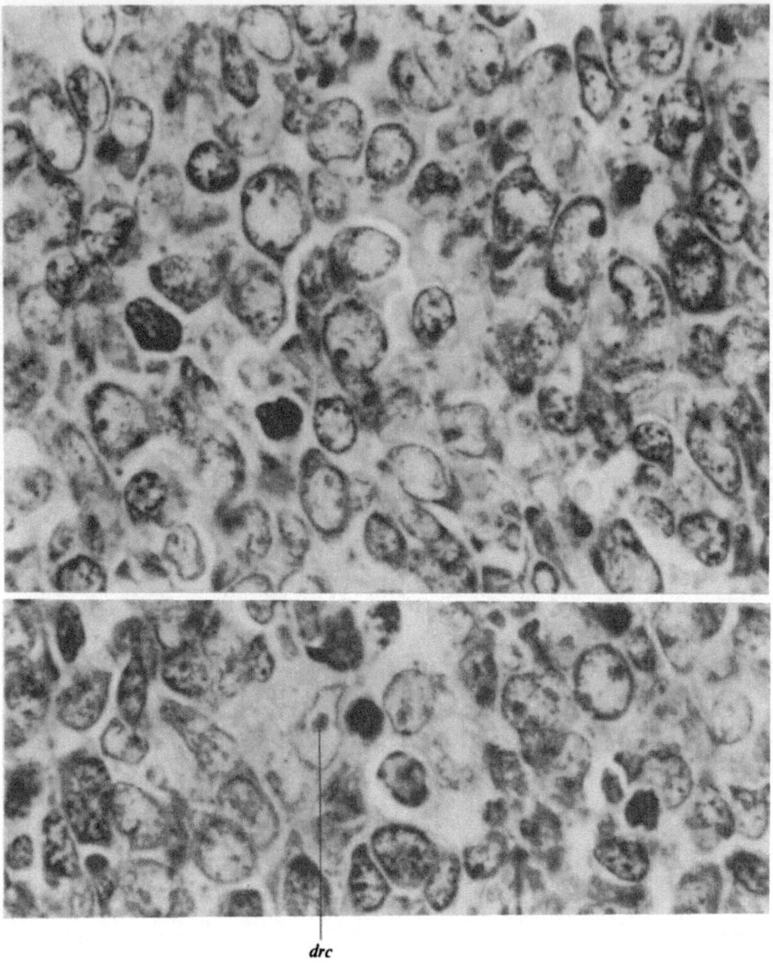


Fig. 172a and b. M.L. centroblastic. There is a relatively monomorphic appearance. Most of the cells are medium-sized to large centroblasts. The growth pattern was diffuse. A dendritic reticulum cell (*drc*) is seen in (b). ♀, 75 years. Cervical node. Giemsa. ×1,550

brane. The rim of cytoplasm is narrow and sharply defined. The tumor cells appear less cohesive than those seen in lymphoblastic lymphoma of the Burkitt type. Multinucleate giant cells were found in some cases. They showed some similarity to Sternberg-Reed cells, but the rim of cytoplasm and the nucleoli were more basophilic and not as large as in Sternberg-Reed cells. Mitotic figures are numerous. Among the characteristic centroblasts one can often identify a few, sometimes moderately abundant centrocyte-like cells whose polymorphic nuclei contain small nucleoli and whose lightly staining cytoplasm can hardly be seen. These centrocyte-like cells often differ from the centrocytes of centroblastic/centrocytic lymphoma: they are more atypical and have larger, more "succulent" nuclei than the latter. Through transitional forms, the centrocyte-

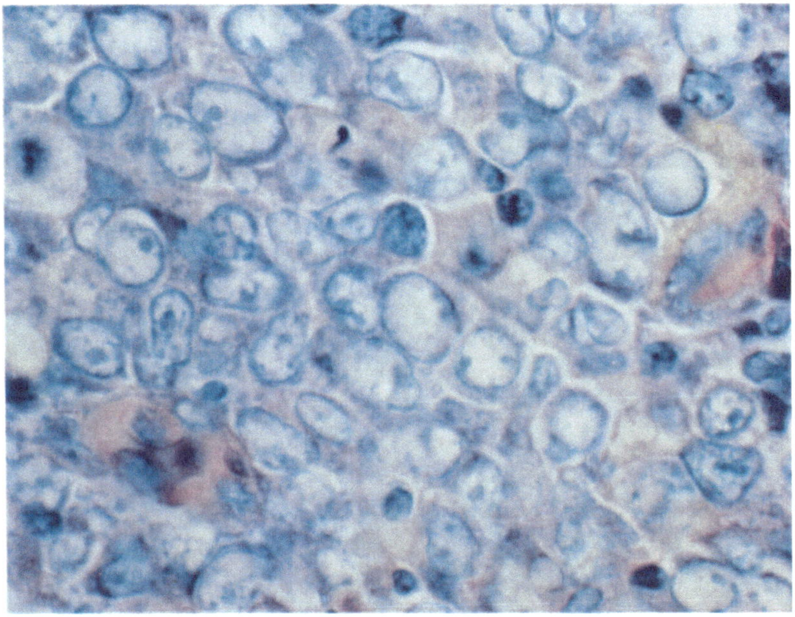

Fig. 173. M.L. centroblastic, monomorphic variant, with Giemsa staining. Note the relative monomorphism of medium-sized to large centroblast-like cells. Nucleoli often lie at the nuclear membrane. ♀, 78 years. Cervical node. × 1,550

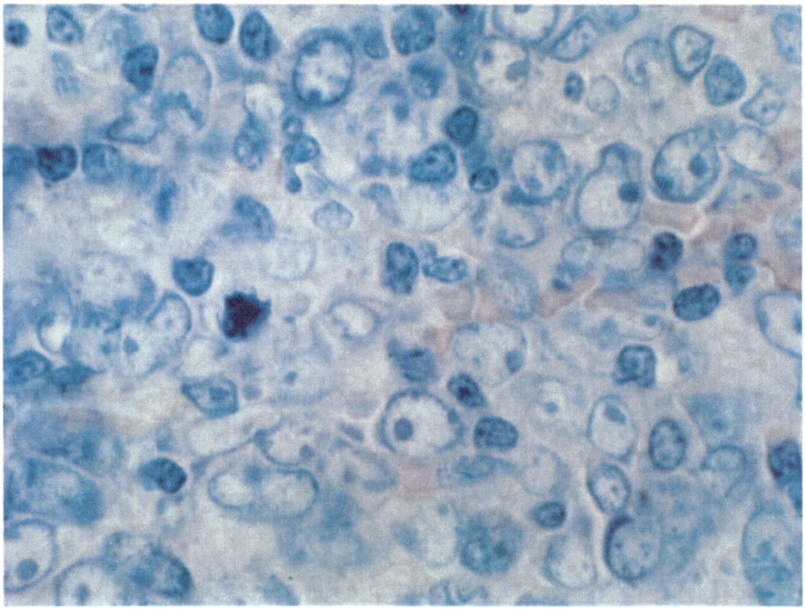

Fig. 174. M.L. centroblastic, polymorphic variant, with Giemsa staining. Because of the occurrence of large immunoblasts, this tumor was originally listed as an immunoblastic lymphoma; however, the tumor cells formed EAC rosettes. Note the great variations in size and shape of the cells. There are cells that are similar to centroblasts (nucleoli at the membrane, basophilic cytoplasm), centrocytes (small central nucleoli; cytoplasm is not visible), or immunoblasts (large central nucleoli, basophilic cytoplasm). Among the small and large cells there are many intermediate types. ♀, age unknown. Inguinal node. × 1,550

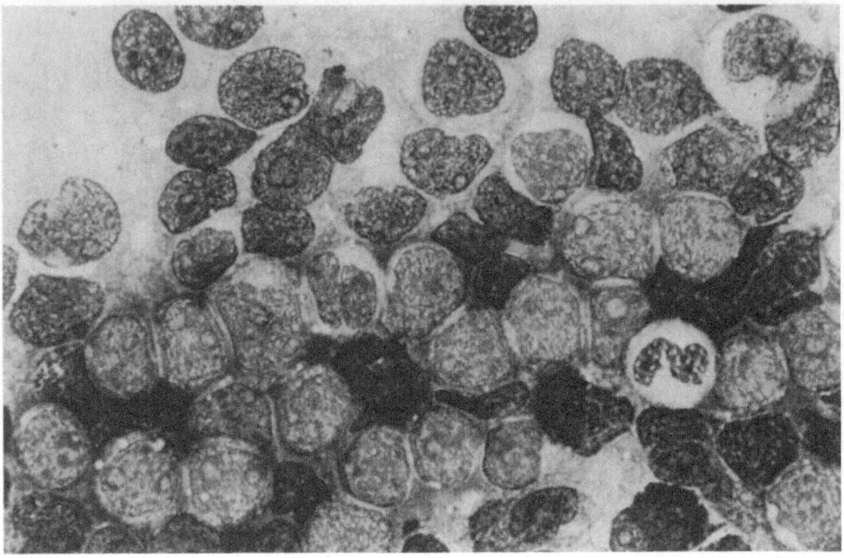

Fig. 175. M.L. centroblastic, monomorphic variant, in imprint. Most of the blast cells show multiple medium-sized distinct nucleoli. Cytoplasm is scanty and basophilic. ♂, 54 years. Axillary node. Pappenheim. ×875

like cells of centroblastic lymphoma are related to centroblasts. All of these cells appear to be variations of the same tumor cell. The same is true for the immunoblasts found in the polymorphic type of centroblastic lymphoma. They are also related to centroblasts through transitional forms. The immunoblasts, however, are usually larger than centroblasts and have more abundant cytoplasm and large central nucleoli. Macrophages are also present, but do not form the typical starry-sky picture seen in Burkitt's tumor. Occasionally, a large number of epithelioid cells are intermingled. There is a small amount of fiber. BENNETT,[609] however, described sclerosis in 31% of his cases.

**Smear/Imprint.** Medium-sized to large, strongly basophilic cells with round or oval nuclei and fine chromatin predominate (Fig. 175). Sometimes one can easily recognize multiple medium-sized light nucleoli in the nucleus. The rim of cytoplasm varies from narrow to moderately broad and may contain some vacuoles.

**Histochemistry and Cytochemistry.** In sections the tumor cells occasionally show globular PAS-positive inclusions in the cytoplasm. In smears the cells never give the coarse granular PAS-positive reaction seen in the cells of the PAS type of acute lymphoblastic leukemia. In smears there is a weakly positive granular reaction for acid phosphatase. The nonspecific esterase reaction is negative.

[609] 1975b.

Table 71. Diagnostic criteria of primary M.L. centroblastic

1. All ages. Peak in later life
2. Monotonous or polymorphic proliferation of medium-sized to large cells
3. Always centroblasts (25–100%): medium-sized or large, nucleoli at the membrane
4. Often anaplastic centrocytes and immunoblasts
5. PAS-negative in most cases

**Diagnosis** (see Table 72). The diagnostic cell is the basophilic, medium-sized to large centroblast, i.e., a cell whose nucleoli are chiefly found at the nuclear membrane. Among the centroblasts there may be a few or moderately abundant anaplastic centrocytes. In many cases a moderate number of immunoblasts can be found. The centroblasts, centrocytes, and immunoblasts are not clearly distinguishable from one another. They appear to be variants derived from the same tumor blastema.

**Differential Diagnosis.** Centroblastic lymphoma must be distinguished from centroblastic/centrocytic lymphoma, immunoblastic lymphoma, and M.L. of Burkitt type. In centroblastic lymphoma the predominant cells are centroblasts or centroblasts and immunoblasts. In centroblastic/centrocytic lymphoma centrocytes clearly predominate, while centroblasts generally make up less than a quarter of the cells (cf., borderline cases, pp. 332 and 359). When there is a follicular picture, a large proportion of centroblasts means a relatively poor prognosis, but does not necessarily mean a transition into a blastic high-grade malignant lymphoma. When transition into a high-grade malignant lymphoma does occur, there is also generally a change in the cell type. The follicles or the interfollicular tissue are then filled with pure populations of this newly formed, more malignant type of cell. In our opinion, only such a change justifies a diagnosis of M.L. centroblastic.

The border between centroblastic lymphoma and immunoblastic lymphoma is not sharp, as LUKES and COLLINS[610] also emphasized. That is demonstrated by the occurrence of centroblastic lymphomas with numerous immunoblasts.

M.L. of Burkitt type consists of strongly cohesive, basophilic cells. Their nuclei contain multiple, medium-sized nucleoli, which generally lie in the middle of the nucleus and not at the nuclear membrane. A starry-sky picture gives further support to the diagnosis of Burkitt's tumor. The size of the tumor cells is of no help in making a clear distinction between M.L. centroblastic and M.L. of Burkitt type, contrary to the conclusion that might be drawn from the studies of LUKES and COLLINS.[610] We have seen cases of EBV-positive Burkitt's tumor in which the tumor cells were not smaller than typical centroblastic lymphoma cells.

**Prognosis.** The prognosis is probably poor.

---

[610] 1975a, b.

### 2. Secondary Centroblastic Lymphoma

**Definition.** Many cases of M.L. centroblastic/centrocytic develop into "sarcomas." This fact had long been recognized and led to the unfortunate term "preblastomatosis" for follicular lymphoma. Actually, the process is malignant from the very beginning. It is merely that the degree of malignancy is low at first; but later there is often transformation into a highly malignant lymphoma, which we used to call sarcoma. This transformation is coupled with a basic change in the type of cells composing the tumor. The *mixed-cell* type of germinal-center tumor, in which centrocytes are always found together with centroblasts, gives rise to an anaplastic tumor of *pure-cell* type, which we previously referred to as germinoblastic sarcoma. It consists chiefly of centroblasts. We call this tumor secondary M.L. centroblastic, irrespective of whether or not the anaplastic germinal-center cells have the exact same morphology as centroblasts. In contrast to primary M.L. centroblastic, it arises either following a definite M.L. centroblastic/centrocytic, or at the same time but at another site. Recently, we also found a secondary centroblastic lymphoma in a case of LP immunocytoma (see p. 243).

**Occurrence.** The frequency with which the anaplastic germinal-center tumor is encountered partly depends on when the biopsy is made during the course of the disease. One rarely finds "sarcomatous transformation" of M.L. centroblastic/centrocytic in the first biopsy (1.4% of our centroblastic/centrocytic lymphomas), but somewhat more often in a second biopsy (3.9% of our centroblastic/centrocytic lymphomas). In addition, our material contained borderline cases between centroblastic/centrocytic lymphoma and centroblastic lymphoma that we could not definitely put into one or the other category. Such borderline cases made up 3.2% of the centroblastic/centrocytic lymphomas.

The clear-cut centroblastic lymphomas developed from the following subtypes of centroblastic/centrocytic lymphoma (biopsy and autopsy material):

1. Follicular without sclerosis (24 cases).
2. Follicular with sclerosis (2 cases).
3. Follicular and diffuse without sclerosis (5 cases).
4. Follicular and diffuse with sclerosis (4 cases).

"Sarcoma" is more frequently seen in terminal stages of the disease. In 39 autopsies of follicular lymphoma we found 17 (44%) "sarcomas," in many instances together with remnants of the follicular lymphoma. Rappaport *et al.*[611] reported that of their 64 autopsied patients, the tumor had retained its follicular character in 14 (22%). In all the others, however, the tumor revealed a diffuse type of growth, which for the most part was probably equivalent to our sarcoma.

In unselected biopsy material, secondary "germinoblastic sarcoma" accounted for 0.2% of the malignant lymphomas, or 0.35% of the non-Hodgkin's lymphomas.

So far, we have not found that the age distribution differs significantly from that of M.L. centroblastic/centrocytic. There is, however, a preponderance of males with M.L. centroblastic (male-to-female ratio 1.4 :1).

[611] Rappaport, Winter and Hicks, 1956.

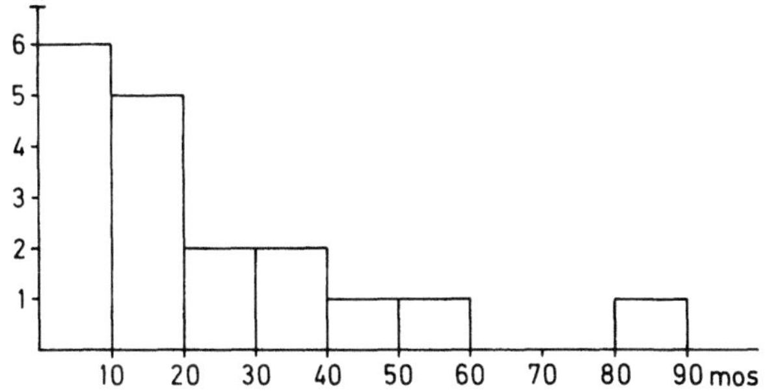


Fig. 176. Transition from M.L. centroblastic/centrocytic into M.L. centroblastic. Histogram showing time interval between first and second diagnoses. Eighteen patients of own series

**Clinical Manifestations.** GALTON[612] has had the most experience in studying the transformation of M.L. centroblastic/centrocytic into an anaplastic germinal-center tumor. SPIRO *et al.*[612] reported that in 12 (22%) of their patients, the disease suddenly changed from one characterized by an often indolent course of many years without symptoms to a rapidly progressing disease that led to death within 3 months. Of these 12 patients, seven disclosed "sarcomatous" transformation, and five, transition into "acute leukemia" (see p. 359). Six of the seven "sarcomatous" follicular lymphomas were noticed as local, invasive, therapy-resistant tumors that caused death because of their location (in the spinal canal or pelvis) or widespread metastases. In the seventh patient, firm enlargement of left cervical and inguinal lymph nodes was the first ominous sign.

An anaplastic germinal-center tumor often develops a short time after the initial manifestation of M.L. centroblastic/centrocytic. In our cases the development of "germinoblastic sarcoma" took from 0–87 months. In 50% of the cases "sarcomatous" transformation occurred during the first year (Fig. 176). That can also happen in the younger patients.

SPIRO *et al.*[612] reported that the duration of the illness in their twelve patients with "malignant transformation" varied from 1–$13^1/_2$ years. The lengths of survival in six patients were 6, $8^1/_2$, $9^5/_{12}$, $11^{10}/_{12}$, 12, and $13^1/_2$ years, measured from the time of the initial diagnosis.

**Localization.** Table 72 shows the sites at which the biopsies of our secondary centroblastic lymphomas were performed. The lymph-node regions do not differ significantly from those biopsied in centroblastic/centrocytic lymphoma. The list of extranodal sites reveals the notable finding that tumors were removed from the orbit in five cases.

**Histology.** The follicular structure of the preexistent M.L. centroblastic/centrocytic may remain intact, at least for a certain length of time. That was true in five out of 23 biopsy cases. We used to call such a picture "follicular germinoblastic sarcoma." Instead of the mixed population of centroblasts and

[612] SPIRO, GALTON, WILTSHAW and LOHMANN, 1975.

Table 72. Localization of 30 biopsies of secondary M.L. centroblastic

| Localization | n | | % |
|---|---|---|---|
| Lymph nodes | 23 | | 76.6 |
| Cervical | | 6 | |
| Axillary | | 3 | |
| Mediastinal | | – | |
| Abdominal | | 1 | |
| Inguinal | | 6 | |
| Unknown | | 7 | |
| Extranodal | 7 | | 23.3 |
| Orbit | | 5 | |
| Spleen | | 1 | |
| Bone marrow | | 1 | |
| Total | 30 | | |

centrocytes, one sees a uniform population of blast cells. In most cases the "sarcomatous" transformation is associated with a diffuse growth pattern (18 out of 23 cases). Sometimes the transformation into a centroblastic lymphoma can be recognized from the large number of starry-sky cells, since they signalize a high rate of cell turnover.

The detailed cell morphology varies from case to case. The most common type is the purely *centroblastic* variant (Fig. 177). It often presents a picture resembling that of Burkitt's tumor, namely, cohesive medium-sized basophilic cells intermingled with abundant starry-sky cells (Fig. 178). There are two other anaplastic variants of follicular lymphoma, however, which have a clearly different cytology, but which are also undoubtedly derived from germinal-center cells:

1. We have seen cases in which the tumor consisted of large *immunoblast*-like cells (Fig. 179). They contained large central nucleoli in oval nuclei and a moderately broad to broad rim of basophilic cytoplasm. With the PAS reaction, we could demonstrate in one case that these cells were truly immunoblasts: they showed strong diffuse PAS positivity in paraffin sections. Furthermore, among these cells there were plasma cells with Russell bodies. In another case the true immunoblastic nature of the anaplastic tumor was indicated by the many plasmacytoid cells with PAS-positive intranuclear inclusions seen in a previous biopsy.

This immunoblastic variant occasionally shows purely follicular growth for a time, which speaks for its germinal-center origin. In such cases silver staining clearly reveals that the proliferation of tumor cells occurs selectively in the almost fiber-free follicles, whereas the surrounding areas are rich in fibers and venules. When the same type of cell proliferates diffusely, there is only a small amount of fiber in the tumor.

On rare occasions, a relatively large number of multinucleate giant cells may appear among the immunoblast-like cells, producing a picture that has certain similarities to that of Hodgkin's sarcoma. Such giant cells are not specific

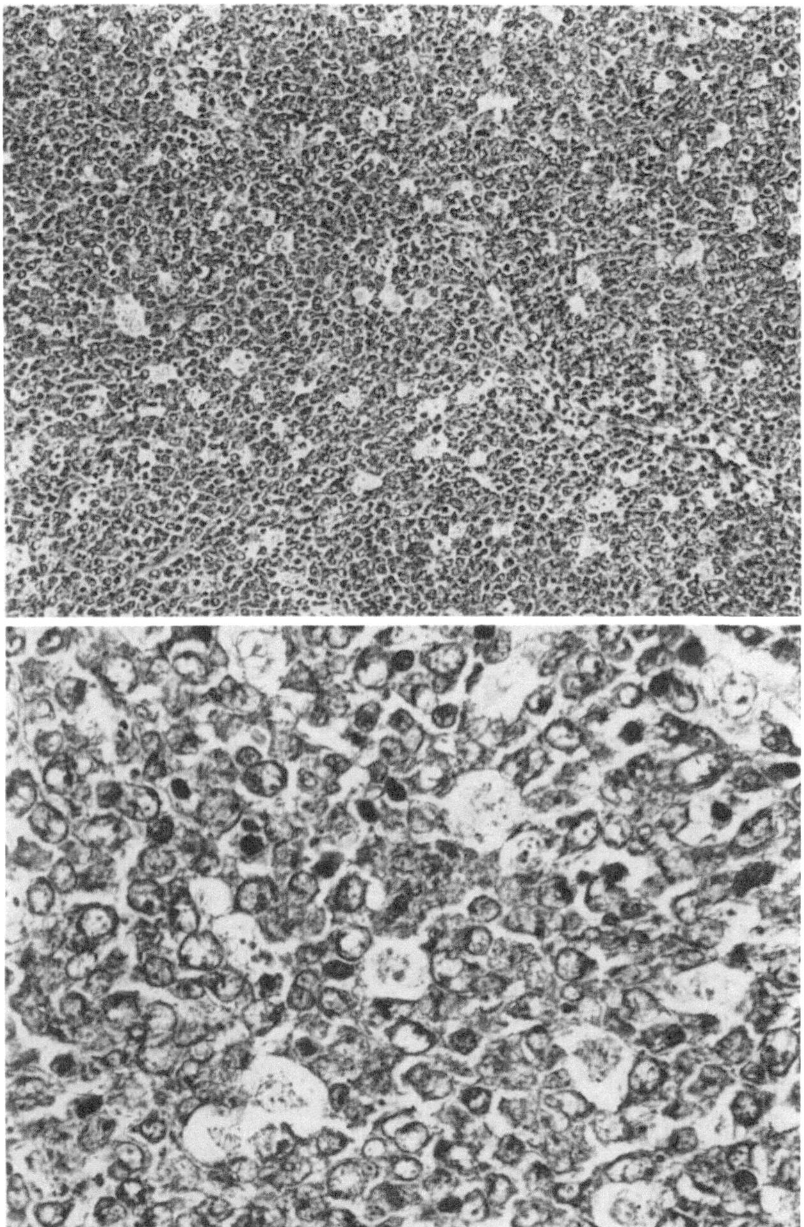

(a)

(b)

Fig. 177a and b. Secondary M.L. centroblastic. Diffuse growth pattern. Splenic hilar lymph node. In the spleen there was still a typical centroblastic/centrocytic lymphoma. Note the medium-sized nucleoli, mostly at the nuclear membrane. There are many histiocytes, giving some impression of a starry-sky pattern. ♀, 60 years. Giemsa. (a) × 140, (b) × 560

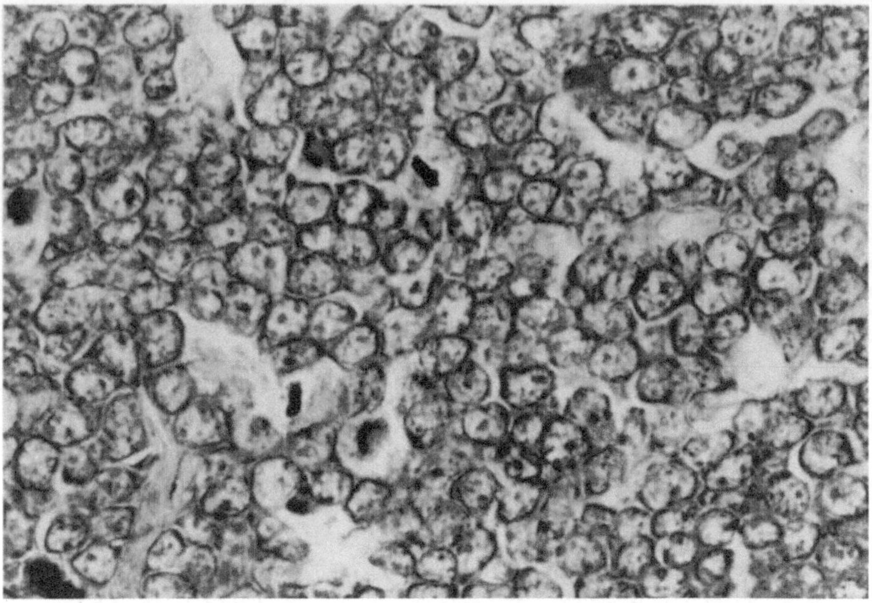

Fig. 178. Secondary M.L. "centroblastic," Burkitt's tumor-like. Multiple, mostly central nucleoli. Four mitotic figures. ♀, 49 years. Abdominal node. Giemsa. ×875

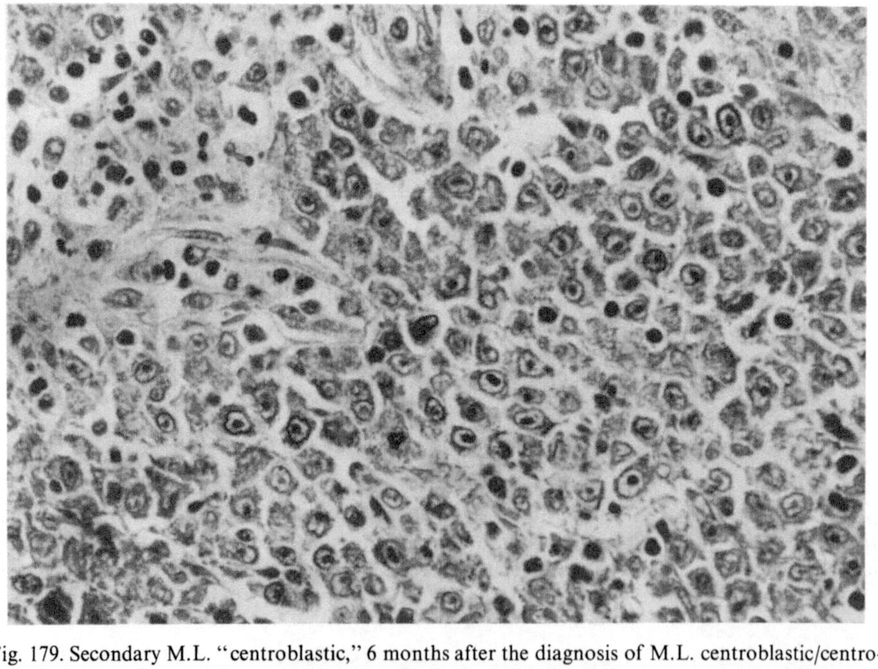

Fig. 179. Secondary M.L. "centroblastic," 6 months after the diagnosis of M.L. centroblastic/centrocytic. Follicular growth pattern. Predominantly immunoblast-like cells. ♀, 76 years. Inguinal node. Giemsa. ×560

to this type, however, for they may be found with variable frequency in all anaplastic germinal-center tumors.

2. There are also rare, uniform-appearing tumors composed of pure populations of *large anaplastic centrocytes*. These differ from the cells of centro*blastic* "sarcoma" by their light, barely recognizable cytoplasm and by their polymorphic nuclei, which contain relatively small nucleoli. Analogous to lymphoblastic lymphomas, we may classify these lymphomas consisting of anaplastic centro*cytes* as centroblastic lymphomas. In both the analogous lymphoblastic lymphomas and such centroblastic lymphomas, "-blast" would then stand for the anaplastic "-cyte."

**Diagnosis and Differential Diagnosis.** When M.L. centroblastic/centrocytic has been diagnosed previously or when it is found concurrently with a supervening monomorphic lymphoma, we may diagnose an anaplastic germinal-center tumor. The distinction between centroblastic lymphoma and centroblastic/centrocytic lymphoma is discussed on page 353.

**Borderline Cases.** When a follicular or follicular and diffuse lymphoma contained a very large number of centroblasts in some of the follicles or in parts of the lymphoma with a diffuse growth pattern, we diagnosed a borderline case between centroblastic/centrocytic and centroblastic lymphoma. In these borderline cases we did not see pure populations of blast cells, either typical centroblasts or the other variants described previously. The prognosis is certainly poor, irrespective of whether we call the tumor a follicular lymphoma with abundant centroblasts or a centroblastic lymphoma.

**Prognosis.** Once an anaplastic germinal-center tumor has developed, the prognosis becomes exceedingly poor. In our cases the mean life expectancy proved to be only 4.1 months. If we add to this interval the time since the diagnosis of M.L. centroblastic/centrocytic was first made, however, then the mean life expectancy of patients with tumors showing "sarcomatous transformation" is 25.4 months.

### *Addendum*
### *The Leukemic Variant of M.L. Centroblastic*

Leukemic variants of primary M.L. centroblastic are very rare. Perhaps a few of the cases of MATHÉ *et al.*[613] may be regarded as such. We have seen only one case.

Compared with the leukemic variant of primary M.L. centroblastic, blast-cell leukemia occurs more frequently in cases of the secondary type. SPIRO *et al.*[614] reported that "acute leukemia" suddenly developed terminally in about 7% of their patients with M.L. centroblastic/centrocytic. This leukemia corresponds histologically to our M.L. centroblastic. We have observed a few similar cases. The leukemic cells found circulating in the blood were large and had narrow to moderately broad rims of strongly basophilic cytoplasm. All of the patients of SPIRO *et al.*[614] with terminal "blast crisis" died within 3 months. Two of

[613] MATHÉ, BELPOMME, DANTCHEV, POUILLART *et al.*, 1974.

[614] SPIRO, GALTON, WILTSHAW and LOHMANN, 1975.

the four patients with "lymphosarcoma-cell leukemia" complained of considerable generalized bone pain. In the fifth patient the leukemic cells were large and intensely basophilic and contained irregular nuclei with two or more lobes. A few "notched-nucleus cells" could be identified among them, but transitional forms between these and the atypical blast cells could not be identified.

## B. Malignant Lymphoma, Lymphoblastic (Lymphoblastic Sarcoma, Including Acute Lymphoblastic Leukemia)

Under the heading M.L. lymphoblastic we include all those lymphomas that consist of rather small or, more often, medium-sized "blast cells." We are well aware, however, that the term lymphoblastic is somewhat confusing, since the lymphoblast may be understood to mean the normal precursor of lymphocytes. Nowadays the term lymphoblast is no longer used in this sense when we are speaking of cells in postfetal lymph nodes. We now assume that this postfetal production of lymphocytes is brought about by the transformation of lymphocytes through antigenic stimulation (see Part One). The stimulated B-lymphocyte transforms into a centroblast and the stimulated T-lymphocyte transforms into a T-immunoblast. It is these transformed blast cells that are the precursors of a new generation of lymphocytes.

The term lymphoblastic is not used to express the fact that the proliferating cells are precursors of lymphocytes, but instead that the lymphoma is composed of anaplastic lymphoid cells with basophilic cytoplasm and the capacity for mitotic division ("blast cells" in the hematologic sense). These cells are not identical with the "lymphoblasts" of B-CLL, which we interpret as underdeveloped B-immunoblasts ("paraimmunoblasts").

The lymphoblasts of lymphoblastic lymphomas have predominantly rounded nuclei with fine chromatin and a narrow rim of strongly or moderately basophilic cytoplasm. Three main groups of lymphoblastic lymphomas can be distinguished by cytologic and immunologic differences in the cells.

In group 1 the *strongly* basophilic lymphoblasts bear surface Ig but do not contain intracytoplasmic Ig. They do not form spontaneous sheep-erythrocyte rosettes (sheep-E rosettes) and do not show focal acid phosphatase positivity. These cells belong to the B-cell series and the tumors are thus classed as B-lymphoblastic lymphomas. This type is best exemplified by the Burkitt type.

If there is a positive reaction for intracytoplasmic Ig, the B-cell is in fact a plasmablast and therefore the tumor is classed as an immunoblastic lymphoma.

In group 2 the *moderately* basophilic lymphoblasts do not show surface Ig or intracytoplasmic Ig, but give a positive sheep-E rosette test. As a rule, we can demonstrate a focal acid phosphatase positivity in their cytoplasm. The immunologic and cytochemical features indicate a T-cell origin, and the tumor is thus classed as a T-lymphoblastic lymphoma. The predominant type of T-lymphoblastic lymphoma is the convoluted-cell type.

In group 3 the *moderately* basophilic lymphoblasts do not show any immunologic or specific cytochemical features, although they often show granular PAS positivity. The cells are called null lymphoblasts, but they may include hemopoietic stem cells. The tumors are called null-lymphoblastic lymphomas. They occur especially as (common) acute lymphoblastic leukemia (ALL).

It must be pointed out that no immunologic or cytochemical criterion is absolute in the sense that it has to be present in every case. We know, for example, that in B-CLL or M.L. centroblastic/centrocytic the specific immunologic marker may be lacking or expressed very weakly. The same is true for the acid phosphatase reaction—not only for technical reasons.

All subtypes of lymphoblastic lymphoma are negative for neutral nonspecific esterase, chloroacetate esterase, and peroxidase. They occur most frequently in childhood and adolescence. A number of reviews of non-Hodgkin's lymphomas in childhood have been published.[615]

## *1. B-Lymphoblastic Lymphoma*

### *a) M.L. Lymphoblastic, Burkitt Type*[616]

**History, Terminology.** In 1958, BURKITT published a report on a clinical tumor syndrome in African children (Uganda) and later, with O'CONOR,[617] he gave a detailed description. The first symptom was a tumor of the jaw or orbit, or a large abdominal tumor; peripheral lymph nodes were rarely involved. With or without tumors of the jaw or abdomen, the clinical picture was often characterized by paraplegia and tumors of the gonads, especially ovaries, and thyroid. The disease predominantly affected children (peak at age of 5 years) and occurred in a sharply defined geographic region of Central Africa, which indicated that one or more local factors play an etiologic role in the disease.

At the same time, O'CONOR and DAVIES[617a] recognized that the tumor is a morphologic entity, which they called "poorly differentiated lymphocytic lymphoma."

A year later O'CONOR[618] published the first detailed morphologic description of the tumor on the basis of 106 cases collected by BURKITT. O'CONOR studied

[615] ROSENBERG, DIAMOND, DARGEON and CRAVER, 1958; LENNERT and MOHRI, 1971; NEIDHARDT and FOLTIN, 1973; HUTTER, FAVARA, NELSON and HOLTON, 1975; LANDBERG, GARWICZ and ÅKERMAN, 1975; LEMERLE, GÉRARD-MARCHANT, SANCHO and SCHWEISGUTH, 1975; PINKEL, JOHNSON and AUR, 1975; LANDBECK, GAEDICKE, WINKLER and STEIN, 1976; WOLLNER, BURCHENAL, LIEBERMAN, EXELBY *et al.*, 1976.

[616] BURKITT, 1958/59, 1963, 1964a, b, 1967a–d, 1970a–e; BURKITT and O'CONOR, 1961; O'CONOR, 1961, 1963, 1970; BERNARD, 1963, 1966; CAMAIN, BAYLET, BRES and LAMBERT, 1964; CAMAIN and LAMBERT, 1964; DAVIES, 1964; EDINGTON and MACLEAN, 1964; EDINGTON, MACLEAN and OKUBADEJO, 1964; OETTLÉ, 1964a, b; PAYET, CAMAIN, PENE, SANKALE *et al.*, 1964; PULVERTAFT and PLATT, 1964; REYNAUD, QUÉRÉ and LAMBERT, 1964; WRIGHT, 1964a, b, 1970a, b; COX and WIDGREN, 1965; BURKITT and WRIGHT, 1966; BRABAND, 1967, 1968; BURCHENAL, 1967; HUTT, 1967, 1970; PULVERTAFT, 1967; WRIGHT, 1967; HENLE, 1968; MOHR and KINZEL, 1968; BERARD, O'CONOR, THOMAS and TORLONI, 1969; BURCHENAL and WOLLNER, 1969; HADDOW, 1970; HUTT, 1970; KLEIN, 1970; NGU, BURKITT and OSUNKOYA, 1970; STJERNSWÅRD, CLIFFORD and SVEDMYR, 1970; WAUBKE, 1970; LAMPERT, 1973.

[617] BURKITT and O'CONOR, 1961.

[617a] 1960.

[618] 1961.

the tumor in sections and imprints and regarded it as a malignant lymphoma in the broadest sense. He was the first to describe the starry-sky pattern, which has since been recognized as the most important histologic criterion. He also observed fat vacuoles and deposits of PAS-positive material in tumor cells. In addition, he reviewed the autopsy findings and stressed the absence of leukemic changes.

Further histologic, histochemical, and cytologic studies by WRIGHT[619] soon followed, as well as pathoanatomic studies of the disease in Africa[620] and New Guinea.[621]

Following the clinical and pathoanatomic identification of the tumor that has been named after BURKITT, a vast literature pertaining to the study of the disease has appeared, contributing much to fundamental research on tumors in general. From this great wealth of publications, the contribution of EPSTEIN *et al.*[622] stands out especially. These investigators succeeded in demonstrating a virus of the herpes group in cell cultures of Burkitt's tumor by means of electron microscopy—the Epstein-Barr virus (EBV). Subsequently, this DNA virus has been identified not only in nasopharyngeal carcinoma (lymphoepithelial carcinoma of Schmincke and Regaud[623]) but also as the agent causing infectious mononucleosis.[624]

Another great advance was the discovery by MINOWADA *et al.*[625] that the cells of Burkitt's tumor produce immunoglobulin (IgM, IgG) *in vitro*, but do not secrete it. This finding has now been confirmed by numerous investigators.[626] It is therefore certain that Burkitt's tumor is a B-cell lymphoma.

After BURKITT's publication, numerous reports appeared in all parts of the world describing similar lymphomas that were called Burkitt's tumors.[627] Some of these cases, however, do not pass a histologic reexamination. In the cases that were isomorphic with Burkitt's tumor, the authors found certain deviations from the typical picture of African lymphoma. For example, the age curve did not show a peak in the first decade (between the ages of 3 and 6) described by BURKITT. There was also a different pattern of organ involvement; in particular, involvement of the jaw bones was frequently absent, whereas involvement of peripheral lymph nodes was more frequently observed.

In contrast, DORFMAN[628] and OETTGEN and MURPHY[629] found that the age and sex distribution of lymphosarcoma (lymphoblastic sarcoma) of children in the USA was like that of African lymphoma. In addition, DORFMAN[628] reported that the clinical manifestations and course were identical when the histologic picture was the same. OETTGEN and MURPHY,[629] however, described differences in the pattern of organ involvement (more frequent involvement

---

[619] 1963.
[620] HARRIS, 1964.
[621] TEN SELDAM, COOKE and ATKINSON, 1966; BOOTH, BURKITT, BASSETT, COOKE *et al.*, 1967.
[622] EPSTEIN, ACHONG and BARR, 1964.
[623] KLEIN, GEERING, OLD, HENLE *et al.*, 1970; ZUR HAUSEN and SCHULTE-HOLTHAUSEN, 1970; WOLF, ZUR HAUSEN and BECKER, 1973.
[624] HENLE, HENLE and DIEHL, 1968; HENLE and HENLE, 1973; HENLE, HENLE and HORWITZ, 1974.
[625] MINOWADA, KLEIN, CLIFFORD, KLEIN *et al.*, 1967.
[626] E.g., OSUNKOYA, MCFARLANE, LUZZATTO, UDEOZO *et al.*, 1968; SHERR and UHR, 1971; VAN FURTH, GROTER, NADKARNI, NADKARNI *et al.*, 1972.
[627] Review: WILLEMIN-CLOG, CAVAROC, MENUT and RAYNAUD, 1967.
[628] 1965.
[629] 1967b.

of mediastinal and peripheral lymph nodes, very rarely tumors of the jaw). Sometimes, transformation into acute lymphoblastic leukemia was also observed, which does not occur in African lymphoma. O'CONOR *et al.*[630] stated that the only differences discovered in their American cases were the greater rarity of the disease and the less frequent involvement of facial bones.

Thus, the questions arose as to whether the isomorphic tumors occurring outside Africa are truly identical with Burkitt's tumor and which criteria really warrant the diagnosis of Burkitt's tumor. To answer these questions and to clarify the matter, the World Health Organization, in conjunction with the International Agency for Research on Cancer, organized a work session that took place in October, 1967, in Bethesda, U.S.A. The results of the meeting were published in 1969.[631] This report gives a precise description of all of the important pathoanatomic and histologic criteria, and, above all, it contains excellent illustrations.

Since then, virologic and serologic investigations have yielded significant new facts,[632] notably the discovery that Epstein-Barr virus-specific antigens[633] and nucleic acids[634] can be demonstrated in every tumor cell of African Burkitt's tumor and are therefore prerequisites for the diagnosis. For example, GUNVÉN *et al.*[635] showed that all patients with Burkitt's tumor had high serum titers of antibodies against EBV antigens. Finally, ZUR HAUSEN and SCHULTE-HOLTHAUSEN[636] were able to demonstrate persistent EBV genomes in hybridization studies, even in cells of Burkitt's tumor that did not yield virus in tissue cultures.

As a rule, EBV is demonstrated using immunofluorescence-serologic methods (indirect immunofluorescence,[637] anticomplementary immunofluorescence[633]), with which one can detect intracellular virus antigens as well as surface antigens. Complement-fixation tests[638] and methods of immunoprecipitation in agar gel[639] are usually not as sensitive for demonstrating virus antigens or their corresponding antibodies. Furthermore, it is possible to detect the virus biologically from its transforming activity.[640] The most accurate method is undoubtedly the hybridization technique.[636]

There is still no final answer to the question as to the significance of EBV in the tumor tissue. If EBV really does cause the tumor, then we must explain why this virus incites in one patient merely a harmless infectious disease (infectious mononucleosis), but in another a malignant lymphoma. The endemic coincidence of malaria and Burkitt's tumor is said to strongly suggest that malaria infection may play a role in the development of the tumor. It is presumed that the malaria infection overburdens or disturbs the lymphoreticular tissue; as a result, the EBV induces Burkitt's tumor. The various ideas on this problem are still hazy, however, and of a speculative nature.[641]

[630] O'CONOR, RAPPAPORT and SMITH, 1965.
[631] BERARD, O'CONOR, THOMAS and TORLONI, 1969.
[632] Review: ZUR HAUSEN, 1975.
[633] REEDMAN and KLEIN, 1973.
[634] ZUR HAUSEN, SCHULTE-HOLTHAUSEN, KLEIN, HENLE *et al.*, 1970.
[635] GUNVÉN, KLEIN, HENLE, HENLE *et al.*, 1970.
[636] ZUR HAUSEN and SCHULTE-HOLTHAUSEN, 1970.
[637] HENLE and HENLE, 1966.
[638] POPE, HORNE and WETTERS, 1969.
[639] OLD, BOYSE, OETTGEN, DE HARVEN *et al.*, 1966.
[640] HENLE, DIEHL, KOHN, ZUR HAUSEN *et al.*, 1967.
[641] BURKITT, 1970e; KLEIN, 1970; O'CONOR, 1970; KRÜGER and O'CONOR, 1972.

Since EBV can be detected in virtually all African Burkitt's tumors, the demonstration of EBV is essential for the diagnosis of this disease. The situation appears to be different outside Africa; at least, isomorphic tumors have been described in which EBV could not be demonstrated.[642] For example, for some years ZUR HAUSEN did not succeed in substantiating a single case of European "Burkitt's tumor" through the demonstration of EBV. The first EBV-positive case outside Africa, verified by hybridization, was not discovered until 1975 by BORNKAMM and ZUR HAUSEN[643] in one of our lymphomas of the Burkitt type. This proves that the Burkitt type of M.L. lymphoblastic found outside Africa may contain EBV or it may not. It also raises the question about the importance of demonstrating EBV. Since infection of the tumor cells with EBV appears to be essential for African lymphoma, it may be argued that one should speak of Burkitt's *tumor* only when an EBV infection has actually been demonstrated. As long as there is no proof of EBV in a particular case, one should speak of M.L. lymphoblastic of the Burkitt *type* when the histologic picture is isomorphic with that of Burkitt's tumor. Since EBV-negative Burkitt's lymphomas do occur with extreme rarity in Africa and EBV-positive Burkitt's lymphomas are reported quite rarely (the percentage is estimated at about 8–17% in the U.S.A.[644]) outside Africa, however, ZUR HAUSEN[645] proposed that one should simply speak of EBV-associated and EBV-negative lymphomas.

Chromosome analysis appears to be another way of defining Burkitt's tumor. MANOLOV and MANOLOVA[646] described a specific marker chromosome (14q+). This finding has now been confirmed several times.[647] The marker chromosome represents a translocation of chromosome 8 (8q−).[648] ZECH *et al.*[648] suggested that the 14q+ marker is lymphoma-associated rather than specific to Burkitt's tumor. It is by no means restricted to EBV-positive Burkitt's lymphomas. BEN-BASSAT *et al.*[649] found the same chromosome anomaly in an EBV-negative lymphoma of the Burkitt type in Israel. PRIGOGINA and FLEISCHMAN[650] reported this anomaly in a case of generalized "lymphosarcoma" and one of CLL.

It would be impossible to mention all of the important facts that have been established pertaining to Burkitt's tumor, including those worked on under the stimulating leadership of BURKITT himself. Several monographs provide eloquent testimony of the volume of research in recent years.[651]

**Origin of the Neoplastic Cells.** EBV induces malignant lymphomas in marmosets[652] and transforms B-lymphocytes *in vitro* into permanent cell lines. T-lymphocytes are not infected. From the transformation of B-lymphocytes into

642 ABLASHI, DE THÉ, EASTON, LIABEUF *et al.*, 1974.

643 BORNKAMM, STEIN, LENNERT, RÜGGEBERG *et al.*, 1976. Since then, two EBV-positive cases have been verified by hybridization in the U.S.A. (GRAVELL, LEVINE, MCINTYRE, LAND *et al.*, 1976; ZIEGLER, ANDERSSON, KLEIN and HENLE, 1976). We were informed of another case by GOLDBLUM in Israel.

644 ZIEGLER, ANDERSSON, KLEIN and HENLE, 1976.

645 ZUR HAUSEN, 1975, 1976.

646 1972.

647 JARVIS, BALL, RICKINSON and EPSTEIN, 1974; ZECH, HAGLUND, NILSSON and KLEIN, 1976.

648 ZECH, HAGLUND, NILSSON and KLEIN, 1976.

649 BEN-BASSAT, GOLDBLUM, MITRANI, GOLDBLUM *et al.*, 1977.

650 1975.

651 ROULET, 1964; BURCHENAL and BURKITT, 1967; BRABAND, 1968; BURKITT and WRIGHT, 1970.

652 EPSTEIN, HUNT and RABIN, 1973; SHOPE, DECHAIRO and MILLER, 1973; WERNER, WOLF, APODACA and ZUR HAUSEN, 1975; WOLF, WERNER and ZUR HAUSEN, 1975.

permanent cell lines, one could conclude not only that EBV might be one of the causes of Burkitt's tumor, but also that the *in-vitro* proliferation of B-lymphocytes is an analogue of germinal centers *in vivo*—proliferation of B-lymphocytes that have transformed into large blast cells occurs in both Burkitt's lymphoma and germinal centers. That may explain the morphologic similarity of Burkitt's tumor to germinal centers in certain phases of development. In highly active germinal centers in the early phases and in basal portions later on, one sees similar pure populations of blast cells, intermingled with abundant starry-sky cells. Years ago, O'CONOR[653] pointed out this similarity between germinal centers and Burkitt's tumor and has emphasized it since.[654] Correspondingly, LUKES and COLLINS[655] derive Burkitt's tumor from noncleaved follicular-center cells, specifically from their small variant. One must ask, however, why EBV does not induce formation of germinal centers in infectious mononucleosis, but instead leads to their disappearance.

The arguments suggesting that centroblasts and the cells of Burkitt's tumor are identical may be summarized as follows:

1. Electron microscopically, the tumor cells closely resemble centroblasts (their nucleus is round, with medium-sized or large nucleoli, and the narrow rim of cytoplasm is rich in polyribosomes) and some of the tumor cells are similar to centrocytes (polymorphic nuclei with nuclear pockets).[656]

2. The tumor cells of Burkitt's lymphoma bear immunoglobulin on their surfaces, usually IgM. Accordingly, the tissue homogenates of our malignant lymphomas of the Burkitt type usually contained increased amounts of IgM. Moreover, in tissue culture the cells of Burkitt's tumor may reveal complement receptors.[657] Surface Ig and complement receptors are characteristic of germinal-center cells. Further immunologic data are given in Part Six.

3. A high rate of proliferation[658] and a tendency to phagocytose intact cells undergoing DNA synthesis[659] are properties common to both germinal-center cells and the cells of Burkitt's tumor.

4. Follicular lymphoma, the tumor of germinal-center cells, often transforms into a "sarcoma" that is very similar to Burkitt's tumor.

5. MANN *et al.*[660] reported that in several American cases they observed the development of Burkitt's tumor in germinal centers in histologic sections from lymph nodes and Peyer's patches.

Despite these facts, there are differences between the cells of Burkitt's tumor and those of typical M.L. centroblastic. Indeed, at the meeting on Burkitt's tumor in Bethesda in 1967, one of us (K.L.) rejected the idea of Burkitt's tumor being centroblastic in origin, because he could not identify the Burkitt's tumor cells as centroblasts, with which he was very familiar from earlier studies. It is for this reason that we have so far not included Burkitt's tumor with M.L. centroblastic.

Because of the powerful arguments in favor of the centroblastic nature

[653] 1961.

[654] KRÜGER and O'CONOR, 1972.

[655] 1973.

[656] BERNHARD and LAMBERT, 1964; BERNHARD, 1970; KAISERLING, 1975.

[657] SHEVACH, HERBERMAN, FRANK and GREEN, 1972; SHEVACH, JAFFE and GREEN, 1973.

[658] COOPER, FRANK and WRIGHT, 1966; IVERSEN, IVERSEN, BLUMING, ZIEGLER *et al.*, 1972; IVERSEN, IVERSEN, ZIEGLER and BLUMING, 1974.

[659] KAISERLING, 1975.

[660] MANN, JAFFE, BRAYLAN, NANBA *et al.*, 1976.

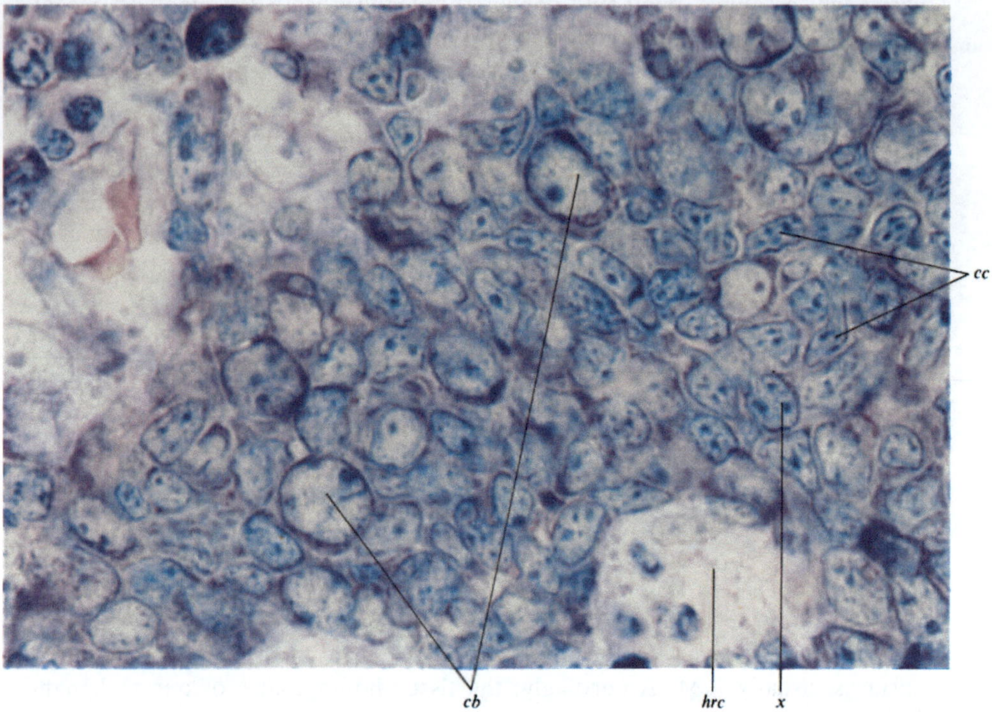


Fig. 180. Reactive germinal center with Giemsa staining. There are some large centroblasts (*cb*), small centrocytes (*cc*), a medium-sized cell (*x*) with multiple central nucleoli, and one starry-sky cell (*hrc*). The medium-sized cell with multiple nucleoli shows some resemblance to Burkitt's tumor cells. ♂, 7 years. Cervical node. ×1,120

of Burkitt's tumor cells, however, we have reexamined reactive germinal centers in Giemsa-stained sections to see whether there might be another cell type corresponding to the Burkitt's tumor cell. Our attention was caught by a cell that did not fit into any of the known categories (Fig. 180). It was medium-sized and had a round nucleus with two or three medium-sized nucleoli that were distributed about the interior of the nucleus and were usually not found at the nuclear membrane. The rim of cytoplasm was narrow and basophilic, but could hardly be identified in sections. We consider it possible that this cell serves as an intermediate stage between the B-lymphocytes that have reached the stage of transformation and the ultimate centroblasts. Burkitt's tumor might be derived from this cell, whose nuclear structure and nucleolar distribution would agree with the cells of Burkitt's tumor. Nevertheless, one must differentiate this cell from the classic centroblast that proliferates in M.L. centroblastic. Only the latter forms noncohesive sheets and has the characteristic membrane-associated nucleoli together with a clearly defined rim of cytoplasm.

In any event, Burkitt's tumor cells are definitely transformed B-lymphocytes. The transformation normally occurs in germinal centers and probably outside them as well. One might expect the transformed lymphocytes to have a similar morphology, whether one uses the term centroblast or not.

It is generally accepted that the cells of African Burkitt's tumor and of lymphoblastic lymphoma of the Burkitt type outside Africa[661] are derived from B-lymphocytes. MAGRATH[662] recently reported that he was able to demonstrate *in vitro* that the tumor cells of a few African Burkitt's tumors had both B- *and* T-cell characteristics. STEIN recently obtained the same results in cell suspensions from a European lymphoma of the Burkitt type: all of the tumor cells bore surface Ig, but some formed sheep-E rosettes. These tumor cells were clearly distinguishable from intermingled T-lymphocytes, which have been demonstrated in varying numbers in Burkitt's tumor.[663]

**Definition.** African Burkitt's tumor is a "lymphoblastic" lymphoma whose cells are medium-sized. Histologically, it usually reveals the characteristic starry-sky picture. It shows a predilection for extranodal tissues. Clinically, the tumor frequently presents as a large tumor of the jawbones. Children in the first decade of life develop the disease most often. The patient's blood and tumor virtually always show signs of infection with EBV.

In contrast, EBV cannot be demonstrated in many non-African cases, in which the sites of involvement and age distribution are also different.

A morphologist should only make the diagnosis of M.L. lymphoblastic of the Burkitt *type*. To diagnose the true Burkitt's *tumor*, one needs the characteristic features of African lymphoma, in particular the demonstration of EBV infection.

**Occurrence.** Burkitt's tumor is endemic in Central Africa, New Guinea, and perhaps a few other regions.[664] In Africa the tumor is limited almost exclusively to the region between the 20th latitudes north and south of the Equator. The disease affects mainly, but not exclusively, the native African population. When compared with the incidence in other parts of the world, the increased incidence of Burkitt's tumor in Africa is not only relative, but also absolute. In Ibadan, for example, the incidence of lymphomas in children is at least 12 times that in Norway.[665] In addition, malignant lymphomas in Africa account for a much higher percentage of the total number of cancer cases than they do elsewhere in the world.[666] In Ibadan about 12.6/100,000 children develop cancer each year; in Norway, 12.1/100,000. In Ibadan, however, the number of malignant lymphomas is 8.9/100,000 each year, whereas in Norway the figure is 0.7/100,000.[666] O'CONOR[667] also called attention to the fact that malignant lymphoma in childhood is much less common outside of Africa. In the Mengo district of Kampala, which is provided with the best medical care of all the local districts, the incidence of Burkitt's tumor steadily decreased from 3 cases/100,000 in 1959 to 0.9 cases/100,000 in 1968.[668] In Europe only a very few cases have been reported that were positive for EBV. GALLMEIER *et al.*[669] and GOETZ *et al.*[670] were the first to report such cases

[661] E.g., BINDER, JENCKS, CHUN and RATH, 1975; GAJL-PECZALSKA, BLOOMFIELD, COCCIA, SOSIN *et al.*, 1975.

[662] 1974.

[663] GROSS, STEEL, LEVIN, SINGH *et al.*, 1975.

[664] WILLIAMS, 1967; BURKITT, 1970e.

[665] EDINGTON and MACLEAN, 1964; IVERSEN and HARKET, 1968.

[666] IVERSEN and HARKET, 1968.

[667] 1963.

[668] MORROW, PIKE, SMITH and ZIEGLER, 1974.

[669] GALLMEIER, GÖBEL, HARTUNG and SCHMIDT, 1970.

[670] GOETZ, LAMPERT, PELLER and PRECHTEL, 1970.

Table 73. M.L. lymphoblastic, Burkitt type. Material and incidence

| | | |
|---|---|---|
| Total No. of biopsy cases | 29 | |
| Total No. of biopsies | 31 | |
| Lymph nodes | | 26 |
| Extranodal | | 5 |
| Incidence in routine lymph-node material | 6 | |
| =0.4% of malignant lymphomas | | |
| 0.7% of non-Hodgkin's lymphomas | | |

in Germany. We were also able to study two patients who had high titers of antibody against EBV. By means of hybridization techniques, ZUR HAUSEN proved that one of these tumors contained EBV.[670a]

In contrast, M.L. lymphoblastic of the Burkitt type that has not been substantiated virologically is not so rare. We found six among 9083 biopsies (Table 73). They represented 0.4% of the malignant lymphomas and 0.7% of the non-Hodgkin's lymphomas in our first series. In our second series the number of lymphomas of this type among the non-Hodgkin's lymphomas was higher (2.1%).

According to BURKITT,[671] the *age* distribution in Uganda shows a definite peak between the 4th and 7th years of life. For patients with jaw tumors the curve peaks somewhat earlier than that for patients without changes in the jaw. Burkitt's tumor virtually never develops during the first year of life, and after the age of 14 the disease is rare, although it does affect older patients on occasion. Where adult African settlers have moved in considerable numbers from nonendemic areas into regions where Burkitt's tumor is endemic, there has been an increased number of such cases and they have occurred in older people, in comparison with endemic regions without many settlers. That is consistent with the observation that Burkitt's tumor outside Africa and New Guinea shows a broader spectrum in the age distribution, even though a predilection for children is also obvious (see Fig. 181).

LEVINE *et al.*[672] calculated a mean age of 9.1 years for the African patients and a mean age of 12.2 years for the American patients. Our material shows a predominance in the first decade (Fig. 182); but there were several patients who were much older (maximum age 79 years).

The disease affects predominantly the male *sex*. According to BURKITT,[671] among more than 600 patients with involvement of the jawbones the male-to-female ratio was 3.2:1, whereas among patients without involvement of the jaw the ratio was 1:1. The probable reason for this difference is that girls frequently present with ovarian tumors instead of tumors of the jawbones. BURKITT calculated the overall sex ratio to be 2.1:1 (male-to-female). This corresponds to our male-to-female ratio of 2:1 (see Fig. 182) and also to the male-to-female ratio of American patients.[672]

**Clinical Manifestations.** According to WRIGHT,[672a] the main sites of Burkitt's tumor observed by clinicians in Africa are as follows. More than half the

[670a] BORNKAMM, STEIN, LENNERT, RÜGGEBERG *et al.*, 1976.
[671] 1970a.
[672] LEVINE, CHO, CONNELLY, BERARD *et al.*, 1975.
[672a] 1970a.

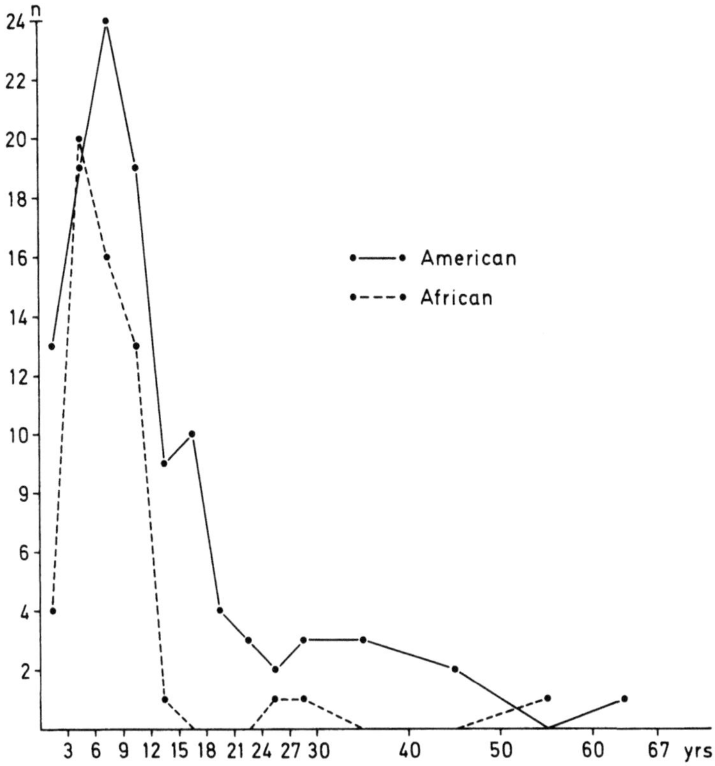


Fig. 181. Age distribution of an African and an American series of "Burkitt's tumor." Data from the African series obtained from ZIEGLER, MORROW, FASS, KYALWAZI *et al.* (1970), and data from the American series from LEVINE, CHO, CONNELLY, BERARD *et al.* (1975)

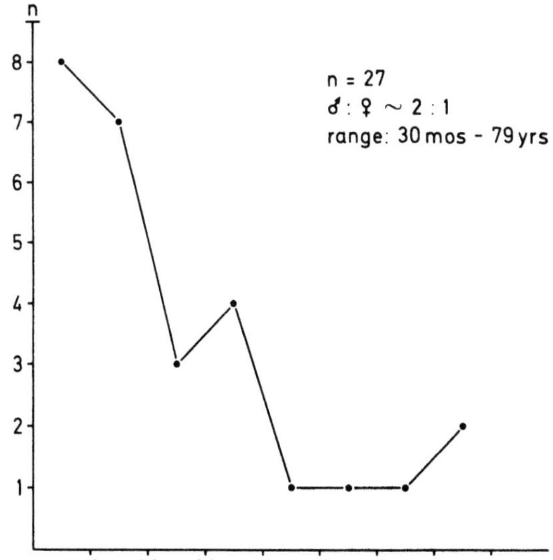


Fig. 182. Age distribution and sex ratio of M.L. lymphoblastic, Burkitt type, in our material (first series; 27 patients)

patients (55%) seek medial help because of tumors of the jaw. Those with abdominal tumors make up the second largest group (25%). Large ovarian tumors are often found in these patients (38% of female patients). Of all patients 6.8% present with paraplegia due to tumor growth in the spinal canal. Tumors in bones other than the jaw (femur, tibia, humerus, etc.) are found in 6.7% of cases, followed by tumors of the thyroid (4.3%), salivary glands (3%), and the breast (1.6%). In only 5.2% were superficial lymph nodes involved, most of which were cervical (3.4%), followed by inguinal lymph nodes (1.6%).

The figures for organ involvement collected by WRIGHT[673] from 88 autopsies reveal only slight variations between children and adults. The data for the lymph nodes, however, are of importance to us. WRIGHT found involvement of lymph nodes in 69% of the children and 70% of the adults. Autopsies performed in New Guinea disclosed a frequency of organ involvement identical with that of the African cases.[674]

Leukemic changes are not observed in cases of African Burkitt's tumor. That is remarkable in view of the fact that in countries outside Africa ALL of childhood is considerably more common that the corresponding lymphoblastic "sarcoma." In Africa the situation is just the opposite: ALL is only very rarely observed. Our series contains three cases in which numerous tumor cells were found in the blood. ALL of the Burkitt's tumor-cell type[675] is described on page 412f.

Outside Africa malignant lymphoma of the Burkitt type shows certain clinical features in common with the African tumor, but also variant features. That is especially apparent from a systematic study of 30 cases of American "Burkitt's lymphoma."[676] In 23 of these cases the initial presentation "was predominantly with abdominal tumor. In 19 instances abdominal disease primarily involved the gastrointestinal tract or presented as an abdominal tumor of uncertain anatomical origin. In the remaining four cases, the tumor appeared to have arisen primarily as ovarian masses. Lymph nodes (most frequently abdominal) were involved with tumor in 25 of 30 cases, but in only three was lymphadenopathy the sole presenting physical finding and in only one of these was lymphadenopathy generalized. Facial bones were involved in five cases ... Involvement of bone marrow was documented in five out of 26 patients at the time of the initial staging evaluation... The [lactic dehydrogenase] level of the serum was well correlated to the stage of disease, localized disease corresponded with low levels."[676]

In a new study, the American Burkitt's Lymphoma Registry[677] has carried out a systematic comparison of 114 American cases with the known data from Africa. The investigators found numerous common features, but also differences in the tumors of the two continents. One similarity was the abrupt clinical presentation with involvement of the gastrointestinal tract, jaw, gonads, or central nervous system. In American patients abdominal disease was prominent in 73%. Initial involvement of the central nervous system was found in 10%

---

[673] 1970a.

[674] TEN SELDAM, COOKE and ATKINSON, 1966; BOOTH, BURKITT, BASSETT, COOKE *et al.*, 1967.

[675] FLANDRIN, BROUET, DANIEL and PREUD'HOMME, 1975.

[676] ARSENEAU, CANELLOS, BANKS, BERARD *et al.*, 1975.

[677] LEVINE, CHO, CONNELLY, BERARD *et al.*, 1975.

Table 74. Localization of biopsies of M.L. lymphoblastic, Burkitt type

| Localization | n | | % | |
|---|---|---|---|---|
| Lymph nodes | 26 | | 83.9 | |
| Cervical | | 19 | | 79.2 |
| Axillary | | 1 | | 4.2 |
| Mediastinal | | — | | — |
| Abdominal | | 3 | | 12.5 |
| Inguinal | | 1 | | 4.2 |
| Cubital | | — | | — |
| Unknown | | 2 | | — |
| Extranodal | 5 | | 16.1 | |
| Tonsils | | 3 | | — |
| Ileum | | 1 | | — |
| Liver | | 1 | | — |
| | 31 | | 100 | |

of the American patients, mainly before 15 years of age, but involvement of the CNS during the clinical course was observed in 40%. Initial involvement of the nasopharynx was also found in 10% of the patients under 20 years of age. The incidence of bone-marrow and peripheral lymph-node involvement was clearly higher in American than in African patients.[678] Staging was performed in 61 cases: 15% of the patients were in stage I, 20% in stage II, 36% in stage III, and 29% in stage IV.

**Localization.** In African Burkitt's tumor the peripheral lymph nodes become involved only very rarely,[679] and even enlarged lymph nodes often reveal nothing but reactive changes. This finding is one of the most characteristic features of Burkitt's lymphoma. Even terminally, when the jaw tumor is enormous, enlargement of lymph nodes is extremely rare.[680] In contrast, WRIGHT[681] and BURKITT[682] very frequently found enlarged abdominal lymph nodes with massive infiltrates in the retroperitoneal tissue and with destruction of adjacent organs. WRIGHT reported such involvement in 80% of his autopsies. The involvement of retroperitoneal lymph nodes may have been primary in these cases. Mediastinal lymph nodes were rarely involved and also seldom caused clinical symptoms.[682] In contrast to lymphoblastic lymphoma of the convoluted-cell (T-cell) type, the thymus never becomes enlarged or involved by tumor.

Our material of M.L. lymphoblastic of the Burkitt type (Table 74) consists mostly of cervical lymph nodes (79%). Abdominal lymph nodes follow with a much lower frequency. Inguinal and axillary lymph nodes were rarely sent to us. We have never received a mediastinal lymphoma of this type. Extranodal specimens came from the tonsil three times, from the ileum once, and from a liver metastasis once.

[678] COHEN, BENNETT, BERARD, ZIEGLER *et al.*, 1969; LEVINE, CHO, CONNELLY, BERARD *et al.*, 1975.

[679] WRIGHT, 1970a; BURKITT, 1970b.

[680] CLIFFORD, 1961; KHAN, 1964.

[681] 1970a.

[682] BURKITT, 1970b.

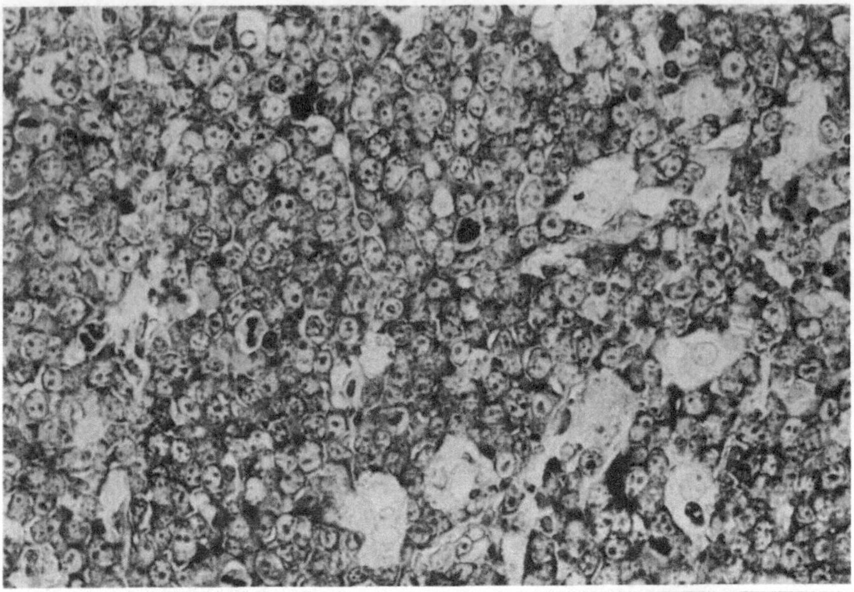

(a)

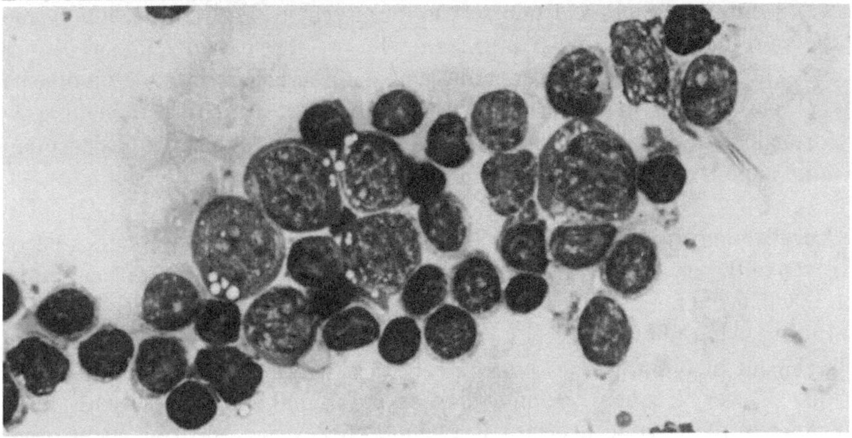

(b)

Fig. 183a and b. True Burkitt's tumor from West Germany in section (a) and imprint (b). EBV-positive, proved by means of hybridization by BORNKAMM and ZUR HAUSEN. (a) Relatively large, basophilic, cohesive cells and some starry-sky appearance. Note the difference from the cells in Fig. 185b, photographed at the same magnification. (b) Fat vacuoles in the hyperbasophilic large tumor cells. Note again the difference from the cells in Fig. 186. Compare the sizes of tumor cells and lymphocytes. Case published by BORNKAMM, STEIN, LENNERT, RÜGGEBERG *et al.* (1976). ♀, 6 years. Cervical node. (a) Giemsa. ×560. (b) Pappenheim. ×875

**Histology.** The tumor may infiltrate the whole lymph node and in some instances grow into surrounding tissue. In such cases doubt may arise as to whether the tumor has invaded the lymph node from outside, or has spread from the node into the neighboring tissue. At times only a few islets of tumor are found in the lymph-node parenchyma.

Cytologically, one sees closely packed, medium-sized, strongly basophilic (pyroninophilic) cells with multiple medium-sized nucleoli (Fig. 183). These

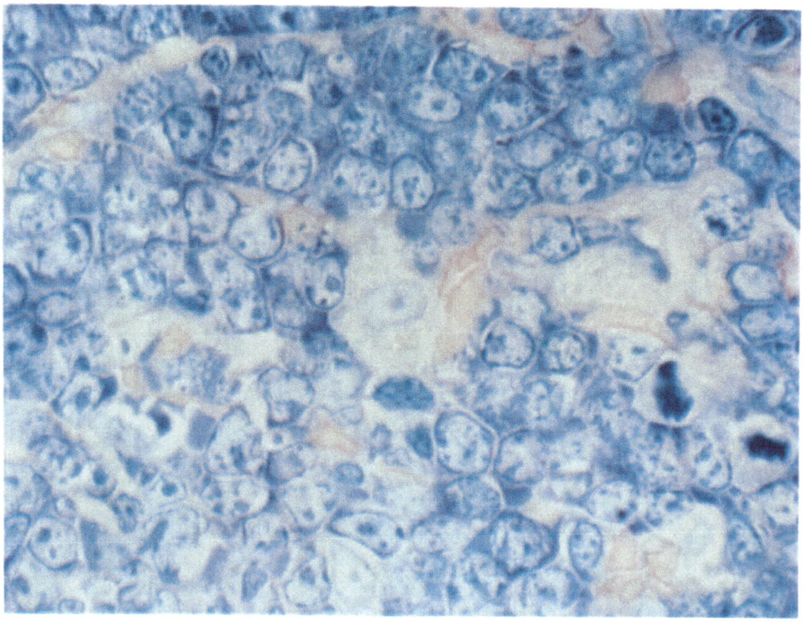

Fig. 184. True Burkitt's tumor from West Germany with Giemsa staining. Note the basophilic, cohesive, relatively large tumor cells with two mitoses. Most of the nucleoli are centrally located. In the center of the picture, a large histiocyte (starry-sky cell). Note the weakly stained nucleus with one medium-sized, weakly basophilic nucleolus, and the abundant light cytoplasm. Same case as Fig. 183. × 1,550

nucleoli are chiefly found away from the nuclear membrane; only a very small proportion of them are membrane-associated. Distributed among these cells in a fairly regular fashion are, as a rule, starry-sky cells. To be sure, this starry-sky picture is not an absolute criterion; in rare cases it is absent, and it can also appear in other hemopoietic neoplasms of high-grade malignancy, e.g., ALL or myelosarcoma.

The first case of EBV-positive Burkitt's tumor in Germany that was proved by hybridization[682a] showed the following morphology (Figs. 183 and 184). The monotonous cells were medium-sized, but relatively large, and cohesive in peripheral areas of the section; in the middle of the section they were separated from one another (artifact of fixation). The rim of cytoplasm was narrow and intensely basophilic. The nuclei contained up to three medium-sized or large nucleoli, which were usually found in the interior of the nucleus, very rarely at the nuclear membrane. Among these cells there were numerous starry-sky cells, which had phagocytosed apparently intact tumor cells and even one mitotic figure. In addition, the starry-sky cells contained many cells in all phases of cell death and lysis.

A second case of Burkitt's tumor in Germany,[682b] proved by indirect immunofluorescence, did not show a prominent starry-sky pattern, but revealed relatively large, strongly basophilic tumor cells.

[682a] Bornkamm, Stein, Lennert, Rüggeberg *et al.*, 1976.

[682b] Goetz, Lampert, Peller and Prechtel, 1970.

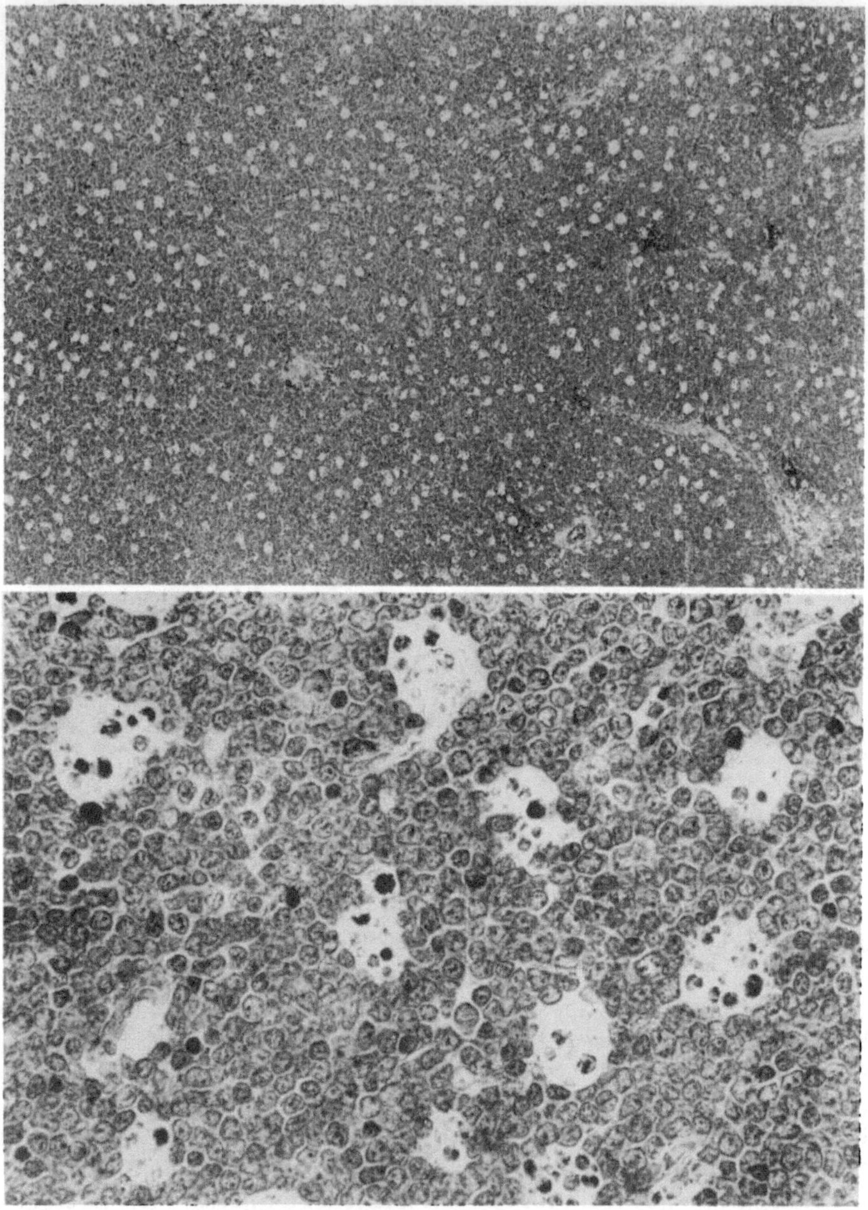

(a)

(b)

Fig. 185a and b. M.L. lymphoblastic, Burkitt type. Prominent starry-sky pattern. Relatively small tumor cells. The starry-sky cells contain much tumor-cell debris. ♂, 7 years. Patient had a high EBV-antibody titer. Axillary node. Giemsa. (a) × 56, (b) × 560

Whereas both of the EBV-positive Burkitt's tumors in our series contained relatively large blast cells, other lymphomas of the Burkitt type were composed of somewhat smaller cells (Fig. 185). These lymphomas might be equivalent to the kind of "Burkitt's tumor" that LUKES and COLLINS[683] claimed was

[683] 1975a, b.

derived from small "noncleaved follicular-center cells." The cells in the EBV-positive cases of our series were too large, however, to be described as "small" noncleaved FCC.

At the working conference in Bethesda[684] the members formulated a precise histologic and cytologic description of Burkitt's tumor, a part of which is quoted here:

> The growth pattern of Burkitt's tumor tends to be that of an expanding nodular mass rather than of diffusely infiltrating cells...
>
> Sections of tumour reflect a monotonous overgrowth of undifferentiated lymphoreticular cells with little variation in size and shape. Mitotic activity is high. Macrophages with abundant clear cytoplasm containing tumour cells or cell debris are almost invariably found scattered uniformly throughout the tumour, producing the characteristic "starry-sky" pattern... [In lymph nodes] reticulin is scanty and found as short thin strands between occasional groups of neoplastic cells.
>
> The cohesiveness of the principal tumour cells varies considerably in different portions of the same section and depends largely on fixation. In well-fixed areas they are generally cohesive. Each cell, however, has a narrow rim of cytoplasm which [has a high grade of basophilia in Giemsa-stained sections and is correspondingly highly pyroninophilic.] Use of an oil-immersion objective usually reveals a few of the cytoplasmic vacuoles that are such a prominent feature of most imprint preparations.
>
> The tumour cell nuclei are also very uniform in size and approximate to that of the nuclei of scattered macrophages. They are usually round but may occasionally be ovoid and show a slight indentation. The nuclear membrane is prominent. The coarsely reticulated chromatin is irregularly distributed in a relatively clear parachromatin. Nucleoli are prominent and are usually 2 to 5 in number.

In our experience the cohesiveness of the tumor cells is especially evident with silver staining. The tumor grows in large strands and sheets that are virtually free of fibers and in which the tumor cells appear to be cohesive. The same picture is seen when the tumor grows into surrounding connective tissue and fat.

**Smear/Imprint.** First, we shall mention our findings in the first proved European case of EBV-positive Burkitt's tumor mentioned previously. The tumor cells were medium-sized to large and deeply basophilic (Fig. 183b). They contained numerous cytoplasmic vacuoles that were negative for both PAS and acid phosphatase. The round nuclei revealed fine chromatin and up to three remarkably well-defined, light nucleoli. With PAS staining a considerable number of tumor cells showed a fine to coarse, granular, strongly positive reaction. The acid phosphatase reaction was virtually negative. The α-naphthyl acetate esterase reaction was completely negative.

The smaller-cell variant of the Burkitt type does not show the hyperbasophilia and lipid droplets that are seen in true Burkitt's tumor (Fig. 186). Instead, the cells have some resemblance to the centrocytes of M.L. centrocytic, especially the more anaplastic variants of that tumor (see Fig. 146).

The cytologic description of Burkitt's tumor that was formulated at the meeting in Bethesda is quoted here:

> In air-dried Romanovsky-stained imprints of tumour tissue the predominant cells again have very uniform nuclear and cytoplasmic qualities. There is often, however, a variation in cell size – from 10 μ to 25 μ – which is much greater than is usually appreciated in sections but which does not correspond to any apparent maturation. The cytoplasm is moderate in amount, well defined, deeply basophilic and usually contains a number of clear vacuoles 1 μ to 2 μ in diameter. The cytoplasm

[684] Berard, O'Conor, Thomas and Torloni, 1969.

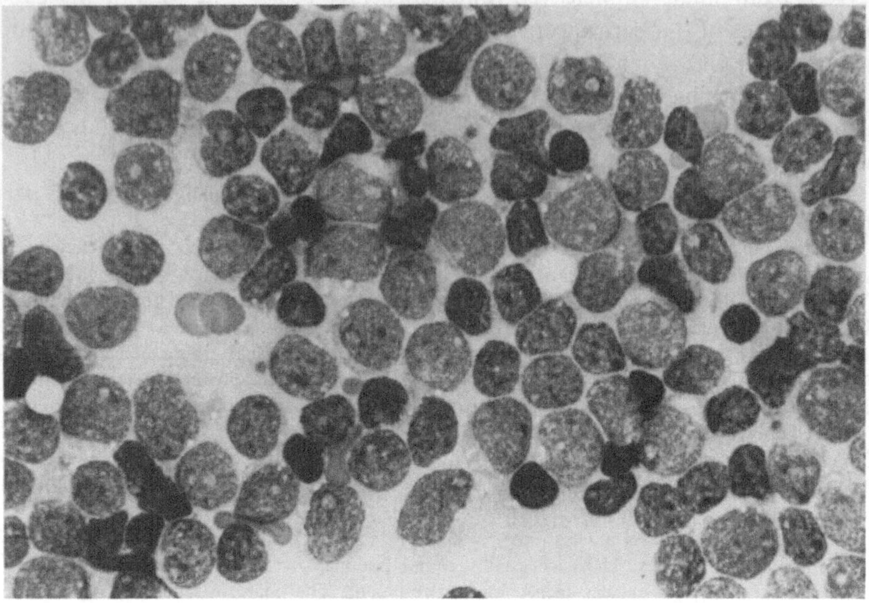

Fig. 186. M.L. lymphoblastic, Burkitt type. Relatively small tumor cells without vacuoles. Note some similarity to centrocytes. Same case as Fig. 183. Same magnification as Fig. 183b. Pappenheim. ×875

is non-granular and homogeneous apart from a pale-staining area at the nuclear indentation. In imprints the nuclei may also show more variation in shape than in sections and varying degrees of nuclear indentation are more commonly seen. The reticulated chromatin is more evenly distributed than in sections but the parachromatin remains fairly well defined and 2–5 nucleoli of moderate size are usually visible.

**Histochemistry and Cytochemistry.** The vacuoles of the tumor cells are sudanophilic and therefore represent fat droplets.[685] WRIGHT[686] found such vacuoles in 85% of his Burkitt's tumors and in more than 50% of the tumor cells of such cases. In addition, the tumor cells of smears occasionally reveal a few, and rarely massive numbers of PAS-positive granules. In electron-microscopic studies[687] these granules proved to be glycogen. In sections the tumor cells always give a negative PAS reaction, but macrophages may contain globular PAS-positive inclusions. Tumor cells of smears exhibit a weakly positive, granular reaction for acid phosphatase, whereas macrophages are strongly positive. The nonspecific esterase reaction proves to be negative in tumor cells, but intensely positive in starry-sky cells.

According to the results of semiquantitative studies of WRIGHT and MCALPINE,[688] the RNA content of the tumor cells is strikingly high. This corresponds to the large number of polyribosomes found in a large proportion of tumor cells.

---

[685] O'CONOR, 1961; WRIGHT, 1963, 1970b; PULVERTAFT and PLATT, 1964.

[686] 1970b.

[687] KAISERLING, 1975.

[688] 1966.

Table 75. Diagnostic criteria of M.L. lymphoblastic, Burkitt type, including Burkitt's tumor

1. Burkitt type = EBV − or? Burkitt's tumor = EBV +
2. All ages, but most patients younger than 20 years
3. Often cervical or abdominal mass
4. Leukemic variants very rare
5. Tumor cells "stuck" together like epithelium (outer part of slide)
6. Tumor cells medium-sized to large, intensely basophilic (pyroninophilic); some medium-sized to large nucleoli (not at the nuclear membrane); many fat vacuoles (in imprints)
7. High mitotic activity
8. Starry-sky pattern
9. Many remnants of tumor cells and even intact tumor cells in starry-sky cells (macrophages)

**Diagnosis.** The most important criteria of lymphoblastic lymphoma of the Burkitt type are summarized in Table 75. We diagnose this lymphoma on the basis of the morphologic picture alone. Closely packed (cohesive), intensely basophilic, medium-sized cells are more or less regularly intermingled with large light macrophages containing abundant phagocytosed cells and cellular debris (starry-sky picture). When EBV can be demonstrated in the tumor, we speak of Burkitt's tumor. When not, we merely call it malignant lymphoma of the Burkitt type.

In any event, we recommend that attempts be made to find out whether the patient's serum contains antibodies against EBV antigens. The titers for such antibodies are, as a rule, markedly elevated in patients with true Burkitt's tumor, but may vary within a wide range. If the serologic tests prove negative, then that rules out the possibility of African Burkitt's lymphoma. Nevertheless, positive findings may also result from an incidental infection with EBV that has appeared at the same time or a long time beforehand. Therefore, they have no absolute diagnostic value.

Antibodies against viral structural components can be demonstrated by indirect immunofluorescence (VCA test). Antibodies can also be detected by using the complement-fixation test. Furthermore, there are antibodies against an intranuclear EBV-specific antigen (EBNA), which can be relatively easily demonstrated in cells with EBV genomes by means of anticomplementary immunofluorescence.[689] Smears or imprints fixed in acetone are incubated with the patient's serum (anti-EBNA-positive), then layered with human complement, and finally stained with fluorescein isothiocyanate-coupled anti-human complement (anti-$\beta_{1C}/\beta_{1A}$). The demonstration of EBNA with the corresponding reference serum enables a quick and clear differentiation of the tumor cells.

Finally, patients with Burkitt's tumor often reveal antibodies against a further EBV-specific antigen, which can be induced after infection of B-lymphoblasts with a certain EBV strain (P3 HR-1). This antigen appears "early" after infection of the cells; it is not a viral structural protein, and it can be differentiated into two components using the EA (early antigen) test.[690]

Antibodies against virus-specific surface antigens, which are occasionally found on cells containing virus genomes, now have less practical significance (MA test).

[689] REEDMAN and KLEIN, 1973.

[690] HENLE, HENLE, ZAJAC, PEARSON *et al.*, 1970.

Antibodies against EBV were absent in about one third of the American patients.[691] A number of our patients with lymphoblastic lymphoma of the Burkitt type also revealed no antibodies. Antibodies (VCA and EA) were demonstrated in a few cases. In one of our cases the EBV genome was confirmed by hybridization[692] and in another case with the EBNA test.[693]

**Differential Diagnosis.** The differential diagnosis was discussed in detail at the meeting in Bethesda.[694] It was concluded that distinguishing other neoplasms from Burkitt's tumor is particularly difficult when one or more of the following features are present:

a) the disease presents as a solid tumour either in a lymph-node or in an extra-nodal location, particularly the latter;

b) the peripheral blood picture is not leukaemic;

c) a "starry-sky" pattern is a prominent feature in tissue sections;

d) differentiation or maturation of the tumour cells is not present or not readily apparent in routinely stained sections;

e) the tumour cells contain cytoplasmic vacuoles resembling those in the cells of Burkitt's tumour.

It was also stated that the following malignant neoplasms must be considered in the differential diagnosis: acute lymphoblastic leukemia (ALL), acute myeloblastic leukemia (AML), "reticulosarcoma," and "lymphosarcoma" (malignant lymphoma, poorly differentiated lymphocytic type).

According to the decision reached at the Bethesda conference, the diagnosis of *acute lymphoblastic leukemia* is favored when:[694]

a) the nuclei are smaller than those of the histiocytes [starry-sky cells] in the same sections [whereas they are of about the same size in Burkitt's tumor];

b) nuclear indentations and clefts are relatively frequent [whereas only slight indentations are observed in Burkitt's tumor];

c) nuclear chromatin is delicate, and evenly distributed [whereas in Burkitt's tumor the chromatin is coarsely reticulated and irregularly distributed in a relatively clear parachromatin];

d) the nucleoli are small and relatively inconspicuous [whereas they are prominent in Burkitt's tumor];

e) cytoplasmic pyroninophilia [basophilia] is not marked [whereas it is very distinct in Burkitt's tumor];

f) diastase-sensitive, PAS-positive granules are demonstrated in the cytoplasm [whereas they are found in only a few of the tumor cells in Burkitt's tumor].

In our opinion, the last criterion is useless, since ALL cells may be negative for PAS and since the cells of Burkitt's tumor may also contain many diastase-sensitive PAS-positive granules. On the other hand, a positive Sudan reaction appears to be quite a useful criterion. We found a negative reaction in ALL, as did HERTL,[695] whereas in Burkitt's tumor there was usually a positive Sudan staining. In addition, the regular infiltration of trabeculae and capsule without destruction often allows the identification of ALL and its distinction from

[691] LEVINE, CHO, CONNELLY, BERARD *et al.*, 1975.

[692] BORNKAMM, STEIN, LENNERT, RÜGGEBERG *et al.*, 1976.

[693] GOETZ, LAMPERT, PELLER and PRECHTEL, 1970.

[694] BERARD, O'CONOR, THOMAS and TORLONI, 1969.

[695] 1963.

Burkitt's tumor. In the latter we have never found this type of infiltrate, which is characteristic of leukemias.

The following criteria favor the diagnosis of *acute myeloblastic leukemia* or blastic crisis in chronic myelocytic leukemia:[696]

a) occasional eosinophilic myelocytes, with nuclear features similar to undifferentiated nongranular cells, are found;
b) a [positive reaction] in the cytoplasm of some [or many] of the neoplastic cells is demonstrable by the naphthol-AS-D-chloroacetate [esterase] method;
c) there is a marked PAS-positivity in the cytoplasm of the maturing abnormal granulocytes.

The following criteria support the diagnosis of *"reticulosarcoma"* (now called immunoblastic lymphoma):[696]

a) the tumour cells have a relatively abundant cytoplasm;
b) there are variations in the staining quality of the cytoplasm, particularly in the pyroninophilia [basophilia];
c) there is an absence of uniform sudanophilic vacuoles in the cytoplasm (when vacuoles are present they are larger than those in Burkitt's tumour cells);
d) the nuclei are larger and more pleomorphic than those of Burkitt's tumour cells;
e) the nuclear chromatin is relatively coarse and irregularly distributed;
f) the nucleoli are very large and eosinophilic.

The following criteria are said to favor the diagnosis of *"lymphosarcoma, poorly differentiated,"* which includes our unclassified lymphoblastic lymphoma and our centrocytic lymphoma:[696]

a) the nuclei are generally smaller than those of histiocytes [macrophages] in the same sections;
b) considerable variations in nuclear size and shape are evident and there are prominent nuclear indentations and clefts;
c) the nuclear chromatin is coarse and irregularly distributed;
d) pyroninophilia [basophilia] is not marked or is variable from cell to cell.

We have listed separately the criteria of the Bethesda conference even though some of them must be reexamined and revised. That is especially true for the differentiation of ALL and "lymphosarcoma."

**Prognosis.**[697] Without therapy *African* Burkitt's tumor grows so rapidly and unremittingly that, before chemotherapy was introduced, small children seldom survived more than 6 months after the onset of initial symptoms.[698] Worthy of note are the occasional spontaneous remissions, which may also occur after biopsy.[698]

Although Burkitt's tumor is very radiosensitive, chemotherapy is preferred, primarily because the generalized extent of the tumor is often not recognized. Cyclophosphamide in large doses is usually given as the sole agent and in 77% of 103 African patients this treatment led to complete remission.[699] Only two of the 24 therapy-resistant patients could be brought into complete remission with vincristine plus methotrexate or cytosine arabinoside. Of the patients with complete remission, 52% subsequently relapsed with tumor. This occurred more often in patients who presented in stages III–IV than in stages I–II. Details

---

696 Berard, O'Conor, Thomas and Torloni, 1969.
697 Burkitt, 1967d, 1970c; Oettgen and Murphy, 1967a; Burkitt, Hutt and Wright, 1965; Ngu, 1965; Pike, 1966; Morrow, Pike and Kisuule, 1967; Clifford, 1968, 1970.
698 Burkitt, 1970c.
699 Nkruhmah and Perkins, 1976a.

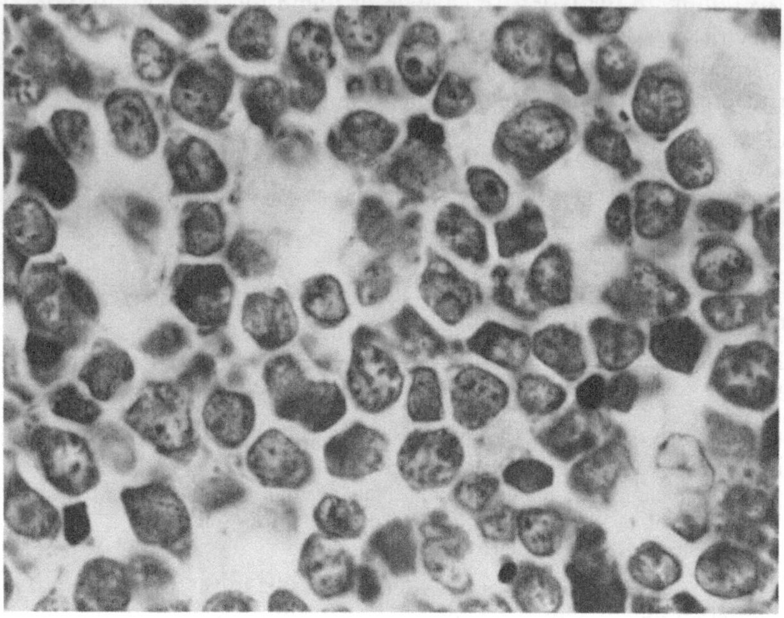

Fig. 187. B-lymphoblastic lymphoma other than Burkitt type with Giemsa staining. Strongly basophilic, medium-sized cells. Some medium-sized nucleoli in the rounded nuclei. ♀, 54 years. Cervical node. × 1,550

on early and late relapses, their localization, and their response to treatment are given by NKRUHMAH and PERKINS.[700] If no recurrence appears within 2 years after therapy, then in a majority of cases one may probably assume that the patient has been cured.

The prognosis depends on the stage of disease at the time of diagnosis, on the size of the tumor, on its localization, and on its sensitivity to cyclophosphamide. Burkitt's tumor of the lymph nodes has a poorer prognosis than that of the jawbones. Finally, the prognosis for small children is better than that for young adults, since instead of the readily visible tumors of the jaw, the young adults often develop deep-seated tumors, e.g., in the abdomen, which result in late clinical recognition of the disease.

The titer of the antibody against early antigen has prognostic value for the course of the disease. An increase in the titer after removal or irradiation of the primary tumor can probably be interpreted as an unfavorable prognostic sign.

The prognosis of *non-African* lymphoma of the Burkitt type was given as follows by ARSENEAU *et al.*[701] for 30 American cases. The first decisive factor was the stage of disease at the start of treatment. Sixty percent of the patients in stages I and II, 47% of those in stage III, and 17% of those in stage

[700] 1976b.

[701] ARSENEAU, CANELLOS, BANKS, BERARD *et al.*, 1975.

IV experienced complete remission. The remissions lasted for 37–80 months or longer in nine out of 13 patients without application of maintenance therapy. These American patients apparently did not have late relapses.

LEVINE *et al.*[702] reported that with large doses of cyclophosphamide, 59% of their American patients achieved a 2-year remission without maintenance chemotherapy. These 2-year survivors were probably cured, since no later relapses were observed.

The survival rate is critically dependent on the stage of disease at the time of diagnosis and also on sex (male patients generally have a shorter survival). Elevated VCA antibody titers might be a prognostically favorable sign.[703]

### *b) B-Lymphoblastic Lymphomas Other than Burkitt Type*

We have repeatedly found lymphomas composed of medium-sized, strongly *basophilic* cells (Fig. 187). These lymphomas were of similar cytology as the Burkitt type, but did not reveal a starry-sky picture or the typical cohesiveness of the tumor cells. They were chiefly abdominal and appeared predominantly in childhood. We do not yet have immunocytologic data that would prove that the tumor cells belong to the B-cell series. The B-cell nature of isomorphic cases of ALL has been proved, however, in a number of papers (see p. 412).

## *2. T-Lymphoblastic Lymphoma*

### *a) M.L. Lymphoblastic, Convoluted-Cell Type*

*Synonyms:* Leukosarcomatosis (STERNBERG)
Acute, extremely immature-cell erythremia (LEDER)
M.L. convoluted lymphocytic type (LUKES)
For leukemic cases:
acute lymphoblastic leukemia (ALL), T-type

**History.** For a long time the "leukosarcomatosis" described by STERNBERG in 1908 was poorly defined. It was considered to be more of an odd collection than an entity.[704] LINKE[705] was about the only one to insist for many years that it is a special type of malignant lymphoma. Subtle cytologic, cytochemical, and immunologic studies have now shown that it is indeed a tumor *sui generis*.

At the lymphoma workshop in Chicago, LUKES[706] reported a new entity of malignant lymphoma, which he called malignant lymphoma of convoluted lymphocytes. In 20 out of 27 patients it was associated with a mediastinal mass. Cytologically, the cells of the tumor were characterized by a peculiar nuclear form, although this feature was seen in only a small proportion of the cells.

---

[702] LEVINE, CHO, CONNELLY, BERARD *et al.*, 1975.

[703] ZIEGLER, ANDERSSON, KLEIN and HENLE, 1976.

[704] See COOKE, 1932, for earlier literature.

[705] E.g., LINKE and FREUDENBERGER, 1960.

[706] 1973.

The nuclei were "humped" or "convoluted," which means the same as the old pathologic term "gyriform" (gyrate), in other words, similar to cerebral gyri. The cells were not cohesive or pyroninophilic. They varied markedly in size; some were the size of lymphocytes, while the diameter of others was three to four times greater. In contrast to the chromatin of lymphocytes, that of these cells was very fine ("primitive nuclear structure"). Mitotic figures were found frequently. The prognosis was relatively poor. The tumor was radiosensitive and also responded well to corticosteroid therapy.

LUKES claimed that the tumor cells of "convoluted lymphocytic lymphoma" are the human counterparts of the "immunologically incompetent" thymic cortical lymphocytes in mice. His presentation at the meeting in Chicago was based on a study that he did with BARCOS and that unfortunately was not published until 1975.[707] This type of lymphoma had already been mentioned in 1974, however, and then in 1975 by LUKES and COLLINS.[708]

In our comparative cytochemical-histologic studies of malignant lymphomas, a type of lymphoma came to our attention that corresponded morphologically to the type described by LUKES. The cells of the tumor gave a focal paranuclear reaction for acid phosphatase. We presented this finding at the meetings in Chicago[709] and London[710] in 1973.

The same type of acid phosphatase reaction had been found by LEDER[711] and DRESCHER and LEDER[712] in neoplasms that they interpreted as extremely immature-cell erythremia. Among other criteria, they based their diagnosis on the normoblasts and macroblasts that they claimed to have found among the infiltrating cells. A striking autopsy finding in all three cases described by DRESCHER and LEDER, however, was the massive infiltration of the thymus. In the first case the thymic mass was so large that at the time of autopsy we diagnosed "thymic leukemia." BECKMANN *et al.*[713] studied eight children with this type of hemoblastosis. At first, they called the disease paraproerythroblastic leukemia. In some of their cases they performed the silver sulfide reaction. In contrast to cells of all other forms of childhood leukemia, the blast cells gave a positive reaction, indicating that they contained nonhemoglobin iron, which is said to be typical of erythropoietic cells. MEISTER and FUCHS[714] also agreed with the interpretation of LEDER and considered the acid phosphatase reaction to be proof of the diagnosis erythremia. LÖFFLER,[715] however, was of the opinion that this interpretation had not been proved on the basis of the acid phosphatase reaction. The course of the disease in the cases of DRESCHER and LEDER was very rapid. The nucleated-cell count in the blood was unusually high.

Since then, we have used immunologic methods in a study of a series of lymphomas whose cells showed the acid phosphatase reaction described above.[716] We found that the tumor cells did not bear surface Ig, that always

---

[707] BARCOS and LUKES, 1975.
[708] LUKES and COLLINS, 1974a, b, 1975a, b.
[709] LENNERT, 1973b.
[710] LENNERT, STEIN and KAISERLING, 1975.
[711] 1965, 1967b, 1969b, 1973.
[712] 1970.
[713] BECKMANN, LANDBECK, NETH and SCHMIDTKE, 1971.
[714] 1972.
[715] 1973.
[716] LENNERT, STEIN and KAISERLING, 1975; STEIN, PETERSEN, GAEDICKE, LENNERT *et al.*, 1976.

a high percentage formed sheep-E rosettes, but that several cells formed mixed E/EAC rosettes or EAC rosettes alone. The formation of sheep-E rosettes by T-derived "lymphoblasts" has been described by other authors.[717] The simultaneous occurrence of sheep-E and EAC rosettes as T- and B-cell markers, respectively, has also been reported several times.[718] Acid phosphatase-positive ALL was independently identified as a T-cell leukemia in London,[719] Paris,[720] and Kiel and Hamburg.[721]

Recently, RILKE *et al.*[722] published a review of 15 cases of M.L. lymphoblastic of the convoluted-cell type. They confirmed most of the findings of LUKES and agreed with the following description in all significant points. NATHWANI *et al.*[723] have also reported on lymphoblastic lymphomas with convoluted nuclei and distinguished these tumors from a lymphoblastic type without convoluted nuclei (see p. 399). HUANG *et al.*[724] have reported on cytogenetic studies of two cases of ALL of the T-cell type.

The tumor under discussion may therefore be defined in three ways:

1. Through the demonstration of convoluted nuclei.
2. Through the demonstration of focal paranuclear acid phosphatase reactivity.
3. Through the demonstration of sheep-E and mixed E/EAC rosettes.

The future must teach us which of the three characterisitics is the most reliable. Each of the three criteria may be absent or poorly developed. The nuclear convolution has the lowest diagnostic value, since it is often inconspicuous and since convolution-like irregularities are also occasionally seen in null-lymphoblastic lymphomas. In contrast, the acid phosphatase reaction is a much more reliable marker. Therefore, in every case one should first perform at least a cytologic analysis and the acid phosphatase reaction. The reaction for $\beta$-glucuronidase[725] might provide the same information and could be used in place of the acid phosphatase reaction.

**Terminology.** We prefer the term M.L. lympho*blastic,* convoluted-cell type to the term M.L. lympho*cytic* suggested by LUKES, since the tumor cells in the blood and in imprints look like undifferentiated blast cells. As a synonym, we preferably use the expression "acid phosphatase type" instead of "convoluted-cell type," because the demonstration of this indicative enzyme sometimes provides more significant and clearer information than do histologic studies and especially the detection of convoluted nuclei.

---

717 SMITH, BARKER, CLEIN and COLLINS, 1973; KAPLAN, MASTRANGELO and PETERSON, 1974; MANN, JAFFE, BRAYLAN, EGGLESTON *et al.*, 1975; PALUTKE and TRANCHIDA, 1975; for further papers, see NATHWANI, KIM and RAPPAPORT, 1976.

718 JONDAL, WIGZELL and AIUTI, 1973; KERSEY, GAJL-PECZALSKA and NESBIT, 1974; SANDILANDS, GRAY, COONEY, BROWNING *et al.*, 1974.

719 CATOVSKY, GALETTO, OKOS, MILIANI *et al.*, 1974; CATOVSKY, 1975; CATOVSKY, FRISCH and VAN NOORDEN, 1975.

720 FLANDRIN, 1975.

721 RITTER, GAEDICKE, WINKLER, BECKMANN *et al.*, 1975; RITTER, GAEDICKE, WINKLER and LANDBECK, 1975; LANDBECK, GAEDICKE, WINKLER and STEIN, 1976.

722 RILKE, CLEMENTE, PILOTTI and MUSUMECI, 1975.

723 NATHWANI, KIM and RAPPAPORT, 1976.

724 HUANG, HOU, WOODS, MOORE *et al.*, 1974.

725 LORBACHER, YAM and MITUS, 1967; BENNETT, 1975; FLANDRIN, 1975.

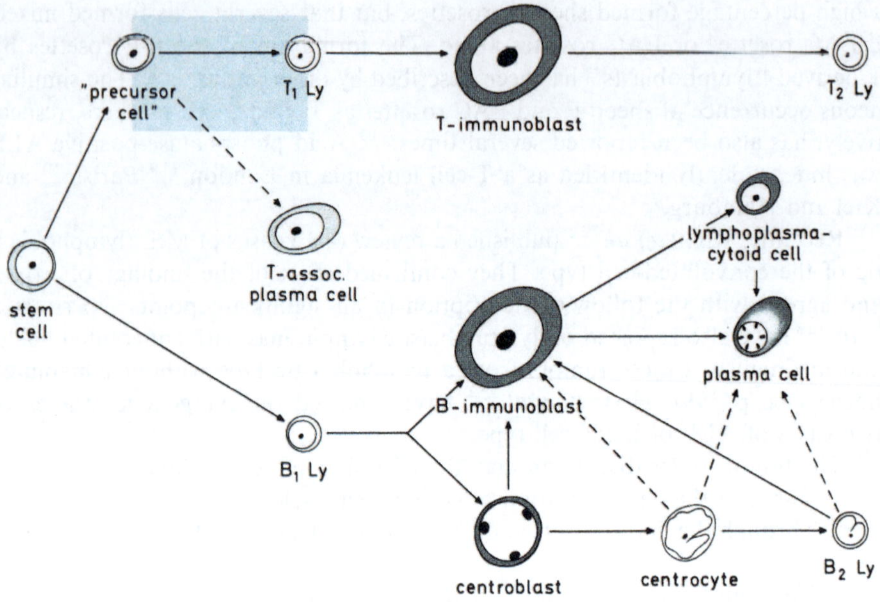


Fig. 188. Hypothetical origin of tumor cells of T-lymphoblastic lymphoma, convoluted-cell type

Table 76. M.L. lymphoblastic, convoluted-cell type. Material and incidence

| | | |
|---|---|---|
| Total No. of cases | 42 (+26[a]) | |
| Biopsy | | 39 (+26[a]) |
| Autopsy | | 3 |
| Total No. of biopsies | 39 (+26[a]) | |
| Incidence in routine lymph-node material | | 7 |
| =0.5% of malignant lymphomas | | |
| 0.8% of non-Hodgkin's lymphomas | | |

[a] Probable cases

**Origin of the Neoplastic Cells.** This type of lymphoma is definitely derived from the T-cell system (Fig. 188). The following features support this interpretation:

1. The thymus is frequently infiltrated, whereas the bone marrow may remain free of tumor infiltrates until death.

2. Thymocytes exhibit essentially the same type of acid phosphatase reactivity as the lymphoma cells (see p. 10).

3. The ATPase reaction is negative, as it is in normal T-dependent lymphatic tissue.

4. Sheep-E rosettes can be demonstrated.

5. Like those of the thymus, homogenates of tumor tissue from most cases do not contain significant amounts of Ig.

The formation of mixed E/EAC-rosettes and pure EAC rosettes (as well as sheep-E rosettes) shows that the cells are more or less immature T-cells.

From the studies of GATIEN *et al.*[726] one may assume that in the thymus EAC-negative, sheep-E-positive thymocytes develop from EAC-positive, sheep-E-negative precursor cells. The EAC-negative, sheep-E-positive cells have convoluted nuclei. Therefore, on the basis of the differentiation of the membrane, the tumor cells of lymphoblastic lymphoma of the convoluted-cell type can be interpreted as precursor cells or as transitional forms between the precursor cells and mature thymocytes.

**Occurrence.** Lymphoblastic lymphoma of the convoluted-cell type is rarer than the other types of lymphoblastic lymphoma (Table 76). Among our lymph-node biopsies, it was diagnosed in only 0.2%. Only 0.5% of all malignant lymphomas and 0.8% of the non-Hodgkin's lymphomas were lymphoblastic lymphomas of the convoluted-cell type.

These values from our first series are too low, as evident in our second series (Table 13). Because the acid phosphatase reaction had been applied more frequently and because we had had more experience in the diagnosis of lymphoblastic lymphomas, we were able to make a definite diagnosis of lymphoblastic lymphoma of the convoluted-cell type in 3.8% of the non-Hodgkin's lymphomas in our second series. In another 2.0% of the non-Hodgkin's lymphomas the diagnosis was merely probable and could not be proved. In 32 cases of lymphoblastic lymphoma in which we were able to apply enzyme reactions to imprints, we found that 13, or 41%, were acid phosphatase-positive and therefore of the convoluted-cell type. Thus, we estimate that this type of lymphoma makes up about 2% of all malignant lymphomas and about 3–5% of the non-Hodgkin's lymphomas. These values also depend, however, on a number of imponderables. In particular, the leukemic variants of the lymphoblastic lymphomas must also be included in the calculation. Leukemia is not as common in the convoluted-cell type as it is in the unclassified type, but it is more common than in the Burkitt type. Leukemic lymphomas are not biopsied as often, however, as aleukemic lymphomas.

BARCOS and LUKES[727] reported that the disease was predominant at the age of puberty (13–16 years). In our second series we also found more patients in the second decade than in the first. A peak in the first 5 years of life, which is characteristic of ALL of childhood, was not evident (Fig. 189). In patients in the first two decades of life, the disease occurred most frequently between the ages of 10 and 15 years. The tumor was less common after the age of 20, but it did occur in patients up to 74 years old. Our youngest patient was 11 months old.

Among their patients, BARCOS and LUKES[727] found twice as many males as females. Our material showed a similar predominance in boys and men (male-to-female ratio of 2.2:1).

**Clinical Manifestations.** A careful examination will disclose a mediastinal tumor (thymic tumor) in most patients at the onset of illness. In 54 of our

[726] GATIEN, SCHNEEBERGER and MERLER, 1975; GATIEN, SCHNEEBERGER, PARKMAN and MERLER, 1975.

[727] 1975.

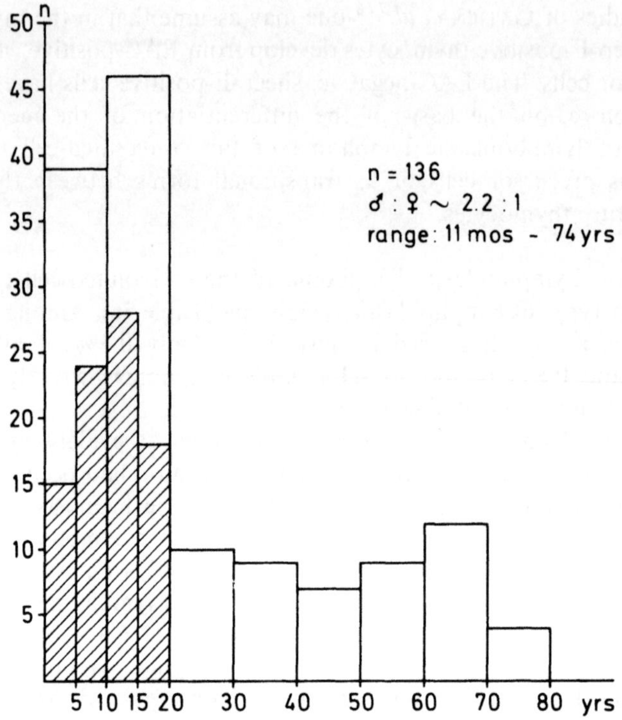


Fig. 189. Age distribution and sex ratio of T-lymphoblastic lymphoma, convoluted-cell type. 136 patients of our second series (1973–1976)

cases, the clinical records showed that 44 patients, or 81.5%, had a mediastinal tumor. It was found with about equal frequency in cases with a leukemic blood picture and those without leukemia.[728] The mediastinal tumor may appear primarily without a leukemic blood picture. It is frequently accompanied by leukemia at the onset, however, or it appears in the course of ALL of the acid phosphatase type.[729] The tumor sometimes leads to dyspnea and, through infiltration of the pleura, to pleural effusion, in which tumor cells can be identified best with the acid phosphatase reaction, but also with the rosette technique. Tumor cells can also be detected in the cerebrospinal fluid of patients with involvement of the central nervous system, which is not so rare. Clinically, LANDBECK *et al.*[729] found primary involvement of the central nervous system in one case. They also reported that tumor infiltration of the testes was relatively common.

Together with the mediastinal tumor there is often widespread enlargement of peripheral lymph nodes. The bone marrow may remain free of tumor for a long time. In a few cases we found merely very small disseminated infiltrates in the bone marrow at autopsy.

[728] SATODATE, unpublished data.

[729] LANDBECK, GAEDICKE, WINKLER and STEIN, 1976.

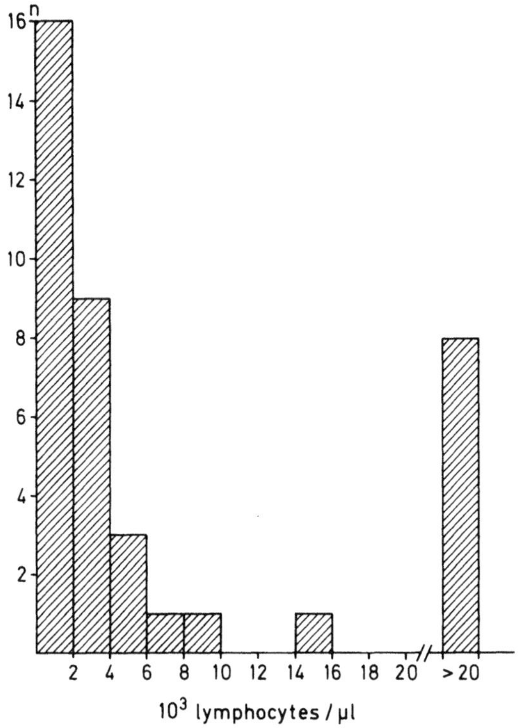


Fig. 190. Blood lymphocyte counts in T-lymphoblastic lymphoma, convoluted-cell type (n = 39 cases)

**Blood Picture.** In 20 out of 42 patients (48%) the leukocyte count was higher than 10,000/µl at the time of diagnosis. The lymphocyte count was higher than 4000/µl in 14 out of 39 patients (36%; see Fig. 190). The highest leukocyte count was 259,000/µl. The median leukocyte count lay at 7500/µl, the median lymphocyte count at 2462/µl. For our cases, we cannot say how frequently an initially aleukemic blood picture became leukemic in the further course of the disease. A moderate number of cases (estimated at about 20%), however, definitely remains aleukemic until death.

**Localization.** Most of our biopsy material (46%) came from cervical lymph nodes, and of that at least half were nodes from the supraclavicular region (Table 77). This suggests that the tumor had spread from the mediastinum. Twenty-four percent of our material came from the mediastinum and was usually described as lymph-node material. In two instances, however, it was clearly thymic tissue. Next in frequency were inguinal (15%), abdominal (12%), and axillary (9%) lymph nodes.

**Gross Appearance.** The lymph nodes are often greatly enlarged, and on section present a uniformly gray-white, soft, or even pulpy tissue.

Table 77. Localization of biopsies of M.L. lymphoblastic, convoluted-cell type

| Localization | With leukemia | Without leukemia | Blood picture unknown | Total n | Total % |
|---|---|---|---|---|---|
| Lymph nodes | | | | | |
| Cervical | 8 | 6 | 1 | 15 | 46 |
| Axillary | 3 | — | — | 3 | 9 |
| Mediastinal | 1 | 4 | 1 | 6 | 18 |
| Abdominal | — | 1 | 3 | 4 | 12 |
| Inguinal | 4 | 1 | — | 5 | 15 |
| Cubital | — | — | — | — | — |
| Unknown | — | 2 | 2 | 4 | — |
| Extranodal | | | | | |
| Thymus | 1 | 1 | — | 2 | — |
| | 17 | 15 | 7 | 39 | |

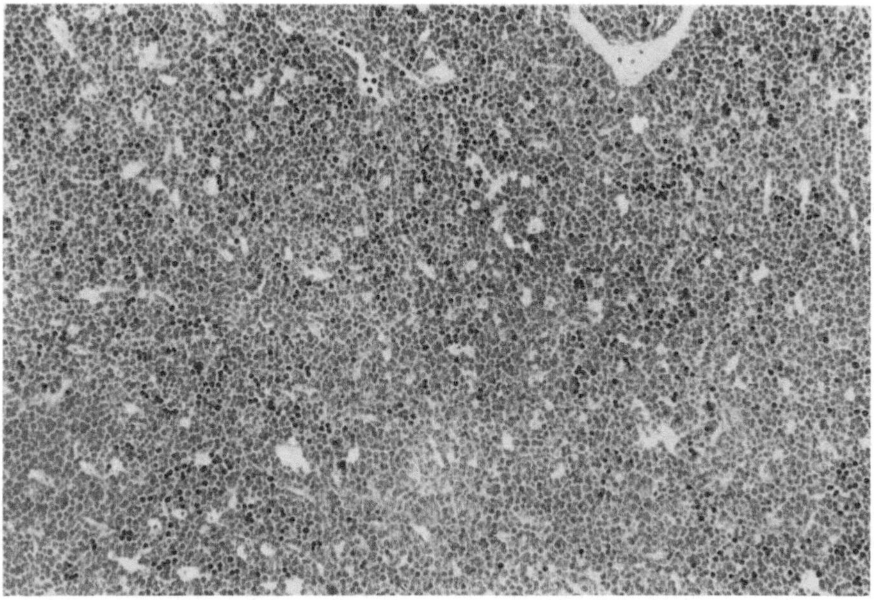

Fig. 191. T-lymphoblastic lymphoma, convoluted-cell type. Many large histiocytes are scattered throughout the section, but they are not as conspicuous as in the Burkitt type. No typical starry-sky pattern. Monotonous appearance of tumor cells. See Fig. 197 for cytology. There was a focally positive acid phosphatase reaction in imprints. ♀, 10 years. Patient had a mediastinal mass. Supraclavicular node. Giemsa. × 140

**Histology.** Small to medium-sized round cells uniformly infiltrate the lymph node, ultimately replacing the entire parenchyma (Fig. 191). The tumor cells are always isolated, that is, well separated from one another. They are not cohesive (Figs. 192–195). Most of the tumor cells are small, not much larger than lymphocytes. In contrast to lymphocytes, they have a finely dispersed

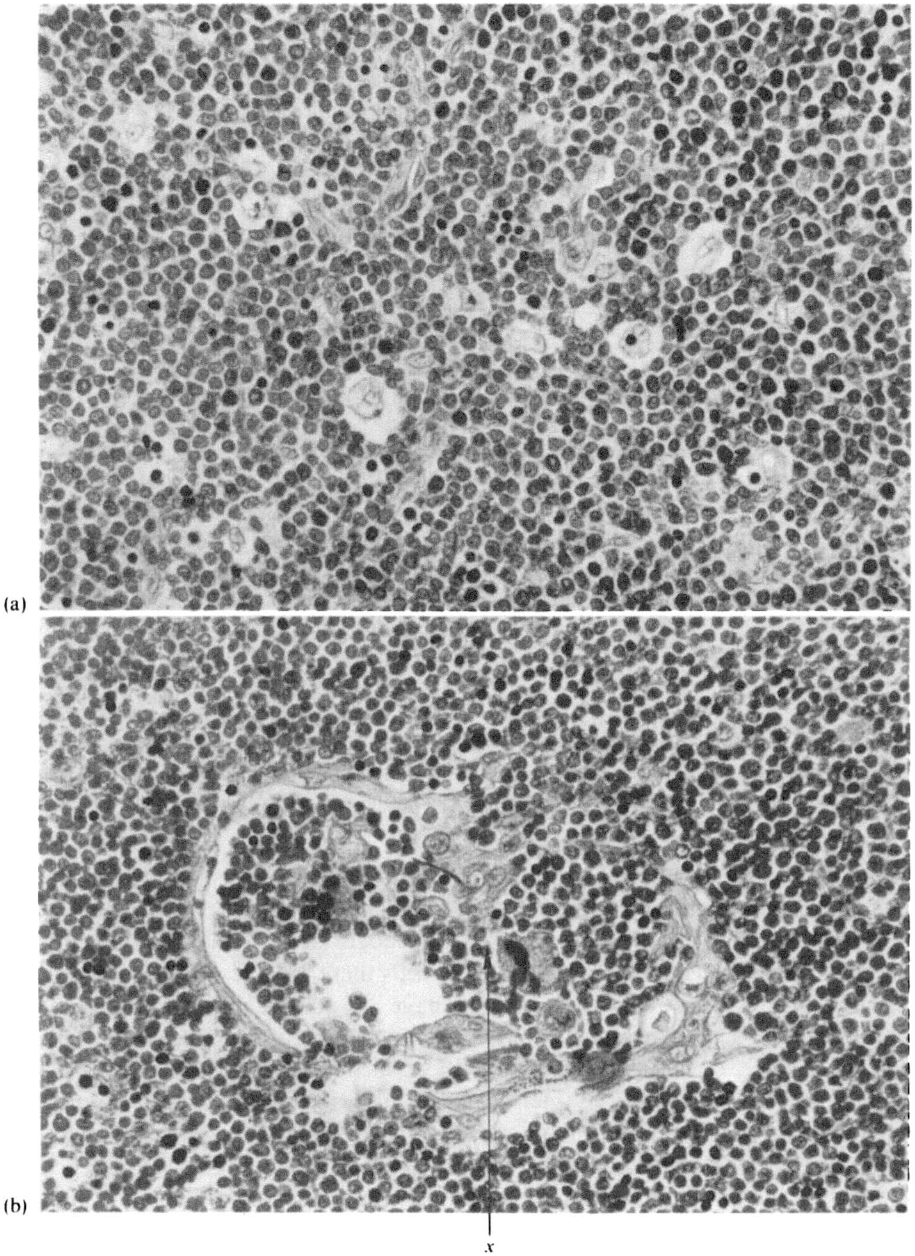


Fig. 192a and b. T-lymphoblastic lymphoma, convoluted-cell type. The cells are well separated from one another. Numerous pyknotic tumor cells. Some large histiocytes with moderate tumor-cell phagocytosis. In (b), a Hassall's corpuscle, infiltrated and partly destroyed by tumor cells (*x*). ♂, 14 years. Thymic tumor. (a) Giemsa. (b) Hematoxylin and eosin. (a, b) ×350

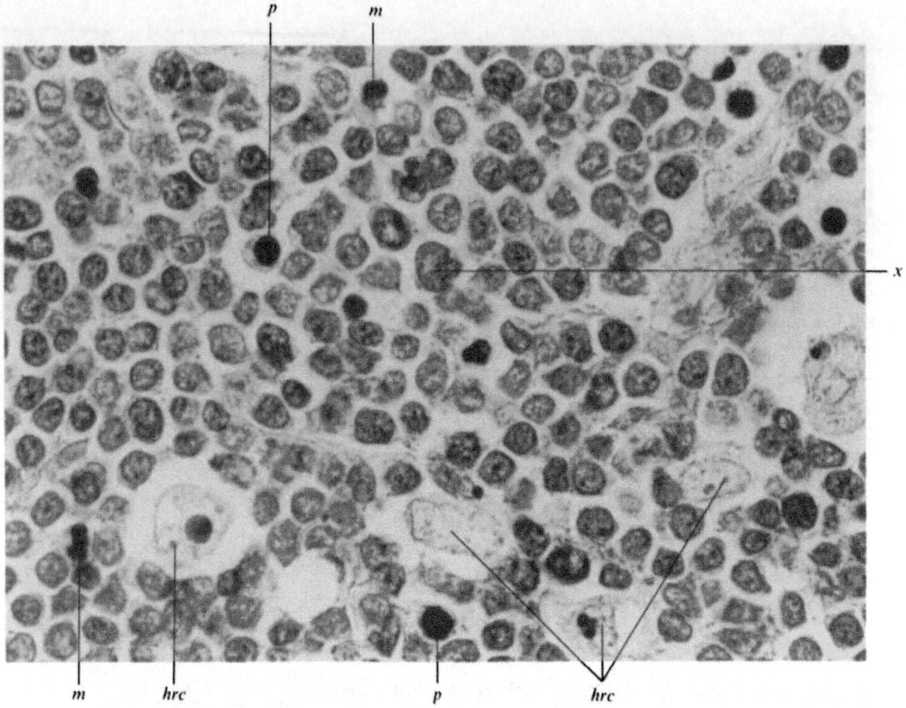


Fig. 193. T-lymphoblastic lymphoma, convoluted-cell type, with Giemsa staining. Note the pyknotic tumor cells (*p*) and the large histiocytes (*hrc*) with a few remnants of phagocytosed tumor cells. Only a few convoluted nuclei, most prominent in *x*. Some mitotic figures (*m*). Chromatin is finer than with hematoxylin and eosin staining (cf., Fig. 194). Same biopsy as Figs. 192 and 194. ×875

chromatin and small, often solitary nucleoli. Their nuclei are usually round, but may appear more oval or indented on one side. The rim of cytoplasm is narrow, moderately basophilic, and more or less clearly recognizable. With Giemsa staining it appears gray-blue (Fig. 195). Among these cells there are a few larger cells with diameters two to three times as great. They have a moderate amount of intensely basophilic cytoplasm. These cells contain large, round to oval nuclei and large nucleoli. Finally, one usually finds only a small number of the diagnostically crucial cells. They are clearly larger than the majority of cells and have nuclei with a gyrate surface, which LUKES considered to be characteristic ("convoluted lymphocytes"). These nuclei reveal multiple deformities, such as knob-like projections and bulging protrusions. Occasionally, they may appear lobed or binucleated. LUKES and COLLINS[730] described linear subdivisions of the nuclei, typically resembling a "chicken footprint." The nucleus contains one or two barely visible, medium-sized nucleoli. The cytoplasm of these cells forms a fairly broad rim and is moderately basophilic. Some of these large cells are probably polyploid.

On the whole, despite the overall impression of a monotonous small-cell picture, there is considerable anisocytosis and polymorphism, although this

[730] 1975a.

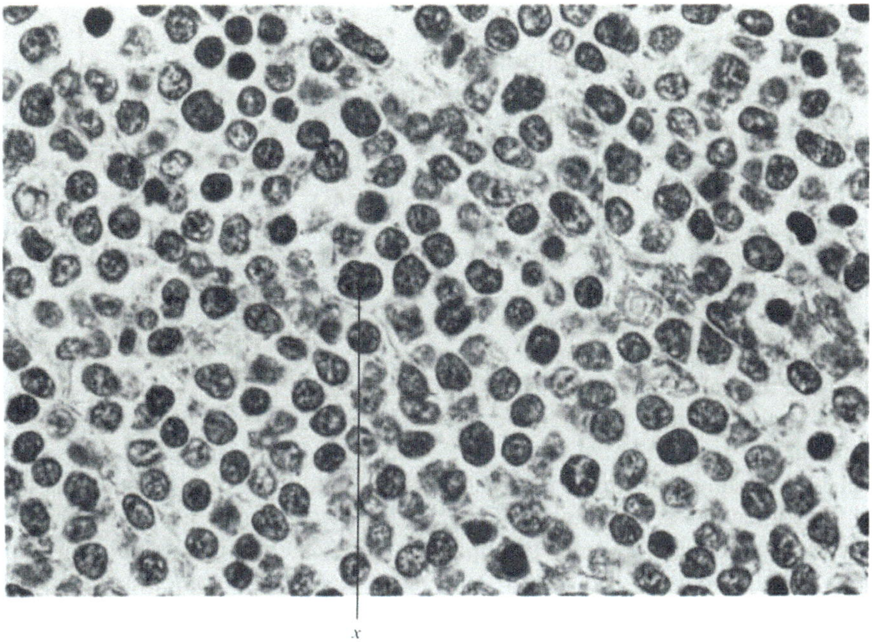


Fig. 194. T-lymphoblastic lymphoma, convoluted-cell type, with hematoxylin and eosin staining. Some convoluted nuclei, for instance, in *x*. Chromatin is somewhat coarser, and pyknotic cells and mitotic figures are less prominent than with Giemsa staining (cf., Fig. 193). Tumor cells are not cohesive. Same biopsy as Figs. 192 and 193. ×875

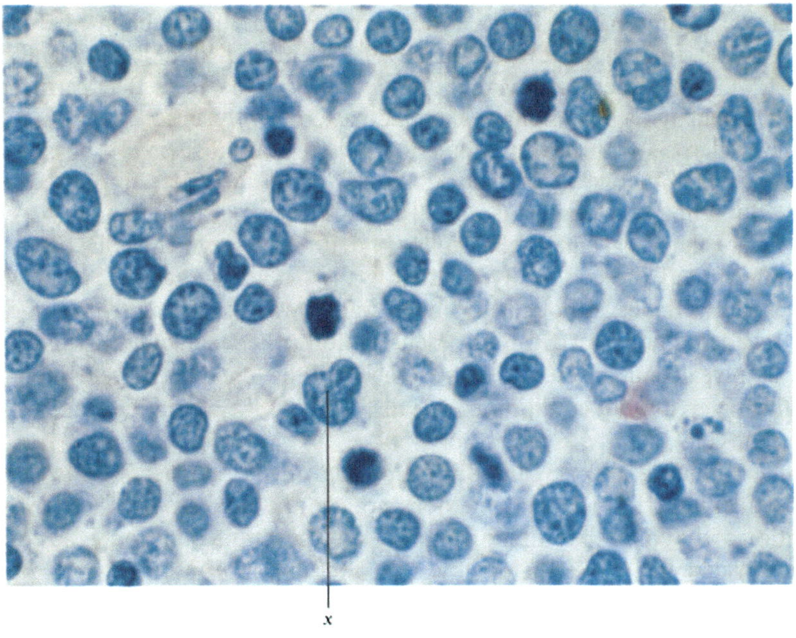


Fig. 195. T-lymphoblastic lymphoma, convoluted-cell type, with Giemsa staining. Some polymorphism with some convoluted nuclei (*x*). Cytoplasm is hardly visible. Well separated tumor cells. Multiple small nucleoli. A few mitotic figures. One pyknotic cell. Same biopsy as Figs. 192–194. ×1,550

is evident only at a high magnification. The number of mitotic figures is usually high or very high. According to LUKES and COLLINS,[731] the number of mitotic figures is correlated with the number of large (convoluted) cells. Sometimes some of the small cells are pyknotic (as in the thymus; see Fig. 193). In two cases we detected necrosis.

There are always a few reticulum cells mixed in among the actual tumor cells, and about half of our cases revealed starry-sky cells, i.e., prominent macrophages with some phagocytosed cell debris (Figs. 191, 192a, 193). These cells, however, are not as large or as evenly dispersed as those seen in Burkitt's tumor. Sometimes they produce a pseudo-starry-sky pattern that is not as pronounced as the one seen in Burkitt's tumor.[731a]

At times one may find some eosinophils. SATODATE[732] counted the eosinophils in 15 cases. In three cases, he found 176–706 eosinophils per section, i.e., 8–13 eosinophils/mm$^2$ of the slide. He counted 0.03–0.13 eosinophils/mm$^2$ in five other cases. Sections from seven cases contained no eosinophils. In one case there were several eosinophil myelocytes among eosinophil granulocytes. Lymphomas of the Burkitt type were studied for comparison, and the highest value SATODATE found was 2.8 eosinophils/mm$^2$. The median value was lower (0.10 compared with 0.83), but the difference was not quite statistically significant ($0.05 < p < 0.10$). In one case of M.L. lymphoblastic, convoluted-cell type, we saw a few mast cells together with eosinophils. Mast cells were very rare in all other cases.

We did not find any typical plasma cells. In contrast, BARCOS and LUKES[732a] reported that they saw a large number of them in five out of 27 cases.

Silver staining discloses only a very small number of reticulin fibers, which are often so fine that they can hardly be identified at a low magnification (Fig. 196). Sometimes, however, there are a few thick fibers that permeate the tumor parenchyma in a coarse alveolar pattern. Only once did we see band-forming sclerosis with hyalin deposition. There was no increase in epithelioid venules in all but one of our cases. In that tumor we were impressed by the unusually numerous venules, some of which appeared atypical. They were incompletely lined by endothelial cells, and in short segments the tumor cells had interrupted the continuity of their walls. In the larger veins the wall of the vessel was intact, although the lumen was sometimes packed with tumor cells that invaded the vessel from the densely infiltrated surrounding tissue. The arteries revealed a different picture; their intima and media remained intact and the lumen did not contain tumor cells, whereas the adventitia was populated by tumor cells.

Silver staining also reveals infiltration and often destructive growth in the connective-tissue framework. One does not see the uniform, nondestructive infiltration of the connective-tissue framework of the lymph node that is so common in acute leukemia. Nevertheless, there is often massive infiltration of the hilar connective tissue and of the capsule, especially in the triangular areas where trabeculae join the capsule. Usually, only one such region can be seen in a given slide. Within the collagenous-fiber bundles the sarcoma reveals the same type

[731] 1975a.
[731a] Also BARCOS and LUKES, 1975.
[732] Unpublished.
[732a] 1975.

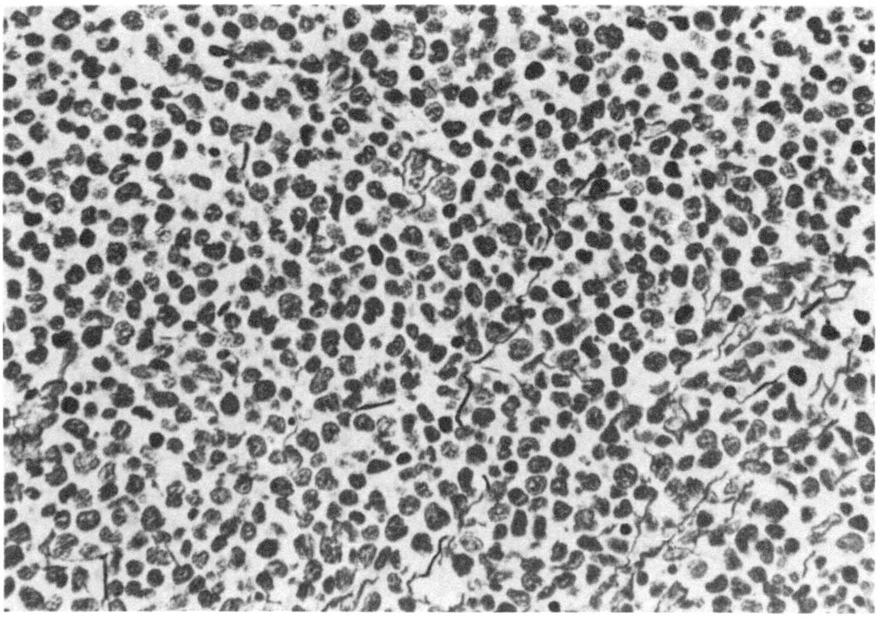

Fig. 196. T-lymphoblastic lymphoma, convoluted-cell type, with silver staining. Only very few fine reticulin fibers. Tumor cells are not cohesive. ♂, 60 years. Inguinal node. Gomori. ×350

of growth pattern as Burkitt's tumor. It forms solid cords and clusters that contain no fibers. Occasionally, there is focal destruction of preexistent fiber structures. The deeper trabeculae within the lymph node are usually free of tumor-cell infiltrates. The adipose tissue surrounding the lymph node usually shows widespread infiltration.

**Smear/Imprint.** In smears or imprints one notices extreme anisocytosis (Fig. 197). Most of the cells are relatively small. They have a slightly indented, but otherwise round nucleus. The cytoplasm forms a narrow, intensely basophilic rim that is lighter, however, at the nuclear indentation. It is here that the Golgi apparatus is located. Some cells have such a small rim of cytoplasm that it can hardly be recognized. Other cells, however, are damaged so greatly by the preparation of the slide that they appear to have no cytoplasm. The nuclei occasionally contain small, usually solitary, light nucleoli. The chromatin is finely dispersed ("primitive").

Then, there are the larger cells described in sections with relatively abundant cytoplasm and larger light nucleoli. These cells have large, at times giant, round or oval nuclei. Their cytoplasm is often wider on one side and varies from gray-blue to dark blue. Sometimes it contains small vacuoles.

In addition, there are the larger cells with polymorphic nuclei that are probably equivalent to the convoluted cells of LUKES. The polymorphic nuclei are most easily recognized in squashed cells, in which not only the nuclear contour, but also the chromatin pattern and sometimes the nucleoli are particularly

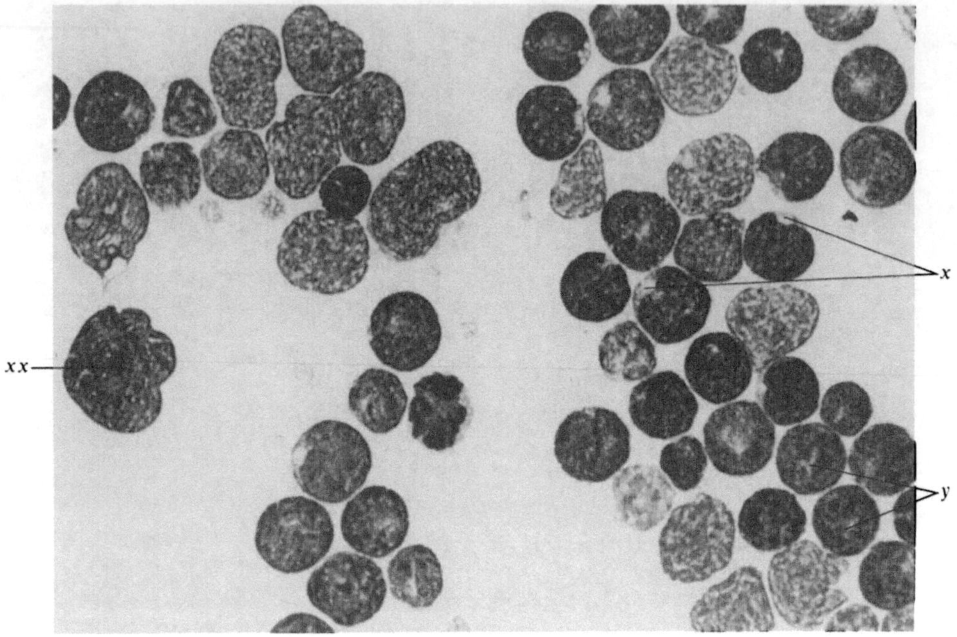


Fig. 197. T-lymphoblastic lymphoma, convoluted-cell type, in imprint. Most nuclei are medium-sized and show a shallow impression where a light area (*x*; Golgi body) is seen. This area would be acid phosphatase-positive. Sometimes the light area (Golgi body) is situated upon the nucleus (*y*). The large cells that have lost their cytoplasm reveal the "convolutions" especially well (*xx*). One mitotic figure near the center of the picture. Same node as Fig. 191. Pappenheim. ×875

prominent. The nuclei of these cells display all variations in shape, with protrusions and humps. The cytoplasm of intact cells is relatively sparse and basophilic. Occasionally, the nuclear protrusions extend beyond it.

**Histochemistry and Cytochemistry.** In six out of 16 cases the PAS reaction in sections revealed solitary clumped PAS-positive deposits in the cytoplasm of tumor cells. The reaction was diastase-resistant in four cases. In addition, there were occasional plump macrophages that contained abundant PAS-positive globules. The chloroacetate esterase reaction always proved to be negative in sections.

The most important cytochemical finding is the positive *acid phosphatase reaction* in imprints (Fig. 198) or cryostat sections. One finds strong focal activity in the paranuclear area, sometimes in a shallow recess of the nucleus. If the nucleus is, so to speak, lying on its back with the recess directed upward, then the acid phosphatase activity appears to lie in the middle of the cell and nucleus. Under low magnification this reaction is apparent as red, round to oval or disk-shaped spots. Under higher magnification, however, one can often make out small and larger granules. Usually each cell has only *one* such site of positive reaction. As electron-microscopic studies have disclosed, the site largely corresponds to the Golgi apparatus, which usually contains some

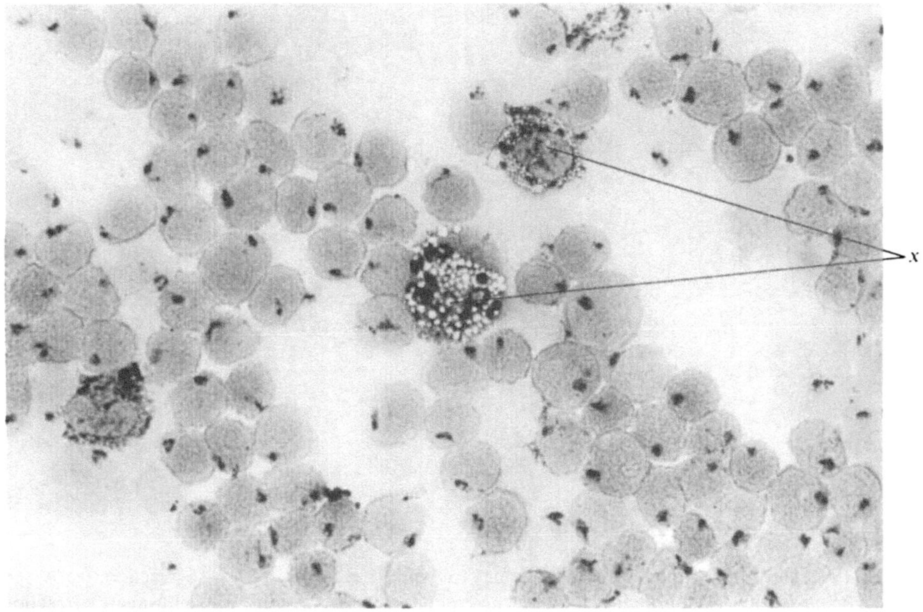


Fig. 198. T-lymphoblastic lymphoma, convoluted-cell type, with acid phosphatase reaction. Note the focal positivity in all tumor cells. Some macrophages (*x*) with lipid droplets and a strongly positive acid phosphatase reaction. ♀, 4 years. Patient had a mediastinal mass. Cerebrospinal fluid. ×560

lysosomes at the periphery.[732b] Besides this focal type of reaction, we occasionally found some cells with numerous small and larger positive granules that were dispersed throughout the whole cytoplasm (lysosomes). The appearance of the cytochemical reaction is generally so characteristic that even at low magnification the diagnosis is obvious at a glance. The acid phosphatase reaction is tartrate-sensitive. In a few of our cases, however, the acid phosphatase reaction was negative or weakly positive in imprints, but definitely positive in blood smears (when leukemic). We cannot yet say what a negative acid phosphatase reaction in this type of lymphoma means. The reason for the negative reaction may be merely a technical one. If, for example, the imprints are too fresh (less than 24 hours old) or too old (more than 7 days old), the acid phosphatase reaction may be negative or very weakly positive.

When the different types of cells seen in imprints are compared in slides stained for acid phosphatase, one finds that the strongly positive cells are the relatively small cells with a pale-staining area in the cytoplasm near the nuclear indentation. The larger forms, including the so-called convoluted cells, are generally negative.

LUKES[732c] did not find a positive paranuclear acid phosphatase reaction in about half of the cases he studied. He used a different technique, however:

[732b] CATOVSKY, FRISCH and VAN NOORDEN, 1975; KAISERLING, 1975.

[732c] Cited by NATHWANI, KIM and RAPPAPORT, 1976.

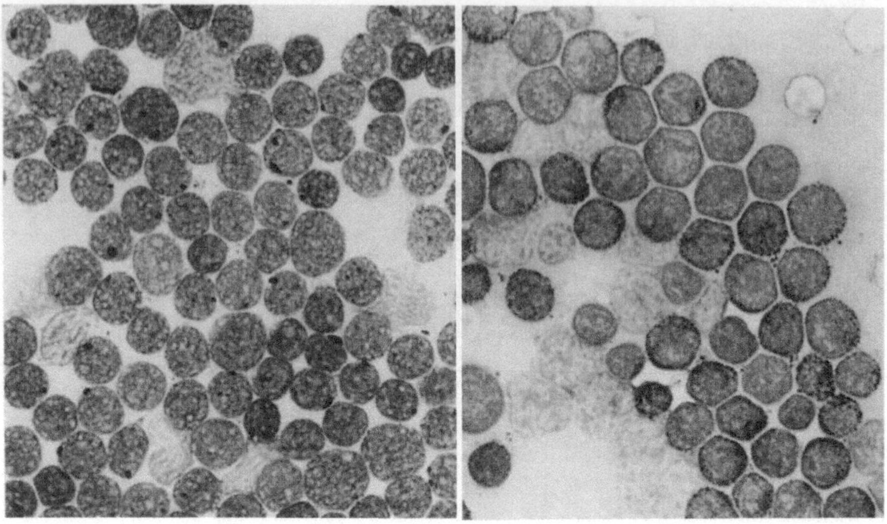

(a) (b)

Fig. 199a and b. T-lymphoblastic lymphoma, convoluted-cell type, with PAS reaction. (a) A spot of PAS positivity (glycoproteins) roughly corresponding to the positive acid phosphatase reaction. (b) Granular PAS positivity (glycogen) with no relation to acid phosphatase positivity. (a) ♂, 5 years. Cervical node. (b) Same case as Figs. 192—195. ×745

he performed the enzyme reaction after fixation, whereas we use unfixed material. Furthermore, we do not know how long the interval between preparation of the imprint and application of the enzyme was.

In place of the acid phosphatase reaction, the reaction for *acid* nonspecific esterase was proposed by HESS[732d] as a marker enzyme for ALL of the T-type. We have also applied this enzyme together with acid phosphatase and found equal reactions in five cases, a stronger acid phosphatase reaction in seven cases, and a stronger acid nonspecific esterase reaction in five cases. In four cases only the acid phosphatase reaction was positive.[732e] It appears that the β-glucuronidase reaction demonstrates the same structures as the acid phosphatase reaction,[732f] but it has to be compared with the results of the acid and neutral[732g] nonspecific esterase reactions.

The *PAS reaction* in imprints is of less value (Fig. 199). DRESCHER and LEDER[733] found the PAS reaction to be positive (coarse clumps) in five out of seven cases. The same was true for most of our cases. In four of our cases the reaction in both sections *and* smears was strongly positive, with coarse clumps in some of the (small) cells in each case. This PAS-positive material lay in the same part of the cell as the acid phosphatase reactivity (in part of the area containing the Golgi apparatus with associated lysosomes). The assumption that the PAS-positive material is glycoprotein and not glycogen receives support

[732d] 1975.

[732e] SUGIYAMA, MÜLLER-HERMELINK and SCHWARZE, to be published.

[732f] SHAW and ISHMAEL, 1975; WASASTJERNA, VUORINEN, LEHTINEN, IKKALA *et al.*, 1975.

[732g] See also SHAW and ISHMAEL, 1975.

[733] 1970; DRESCHER, HANSEN, ALTHOFF and GRAUCOB, 1969.

Table 78. Diagnostic criteria of M.L. lymphoblastic, convoluted-cell type

| | |
|---|---|
| 1. | All ages, but high peak in 1st and particularly in 2nd decade |
| 2. | Often mediastinal mass (thymus) |
| 3. | Bone marrow sometimes not infiltrated or not until late stages |
| 4. | Often is or becomes leukemic |
| 5. | No typical starry-sky pattern, but sometimes a number of large histiocytes with a few engulfed cells (pseudo-starry-sky pattern) |
| 6. | Tumor cells small to medium-sized, moderately basophilic. Narrow rim of cytoplasm. Nuclei of medium-sized cells sometimes convoluted (gyriform). Small nucleoli |
| 7. | High mitotic activity and often pyknotic nuclei |
| 8. | Fibers very fine and interspersed |
| 9. | Sometimes small solitary clumps of PAS positivity in sections |
| 10. | Focal acid phosphatase reaction in imprints and cryostat sections |

from the finding that it is diastase-resistant and is not dissolved when the tissue is embedded.

In addition to this PAS reaction at the same site as the acid phosphatase reaction, we noted that the positive PAS reaction in imprints from other cases appeared as quite uniformly distributed, fine to coarse granules. In one of these cases we observed that the large cells gave a negative PAS reaction, whereas the small cells were strongly positive. Undoubtedly what was stained was glycogen, as confirmed by electron microscopy.[734]

The reactions for neutral nonspecific esterase, chloroacetate esterase, peroxidase, and alkaline phosphatase were always negative in tumor cells in imprints.

**Diagnosis.** The diagnosis rests on the demonstration of a relatively monotonous proliferation of small round noncohesive cells, interspersed with a few convoluted cells. There may be a lumpy PAS-positive reaction in sections. In imprints the acid phosphatase reaction reveals uniform paranuclear positivity in the form of a solitary, round or oval spot composed of several coarse granules. This enzyme pattern is probably the most valuable criterion for making the diagnosis. The tumor cells of lymph nodes, blood, cerebrospinal fluid, etc., form sheep-E rosettes and also, as a rule, mixed rosettes (E/EAC). The demonstration of sheep-E rosettes suffices for confirming the diagnosis. Sometimes, however, only a few cells fulfill this criterion. The diagnosis receives further support from the clinical demonstration of a tumor in the anterior mediastinum. Additional diagnostic criteria are given in Table 78.

**Differential Diagnosis.** In practice, the most important tumor to be considered in the differential diagnosis is unclassified lymphoblastic lymphoma and all of the neoplasms mentioned in connection with it (see p. 406ff.).

Unclassified lymphoblastic lymphoma of the small-cell type is very similar to the convoluted-cell type of lymphoblastic lymphoma. The following four histologic/cytologic criteria are of help in the distinction of the unclassified type:

1. It does not contain the strikingly large cells that have convoluted nuclei.

2. The tumor cells are sometimes more closely packed and may appear to be cohesive, whereas in the convoluted-cell type the cells are isolated.

[734] Kaiserling, 1975.

3. In imprints the reaction for acid phosphatase is negative or, at most, there is a fine granular reaction.

4. The discovery of a large tumor in the anterior mediastinum points to a thymic lymphoma. Mediastinal lymphomas that cannot be distinguished clinically from thymogenic lymphomas can also be found, however, in cases of unclassified lymphoblastic lymphoma.

Centroblastic lymphoma should be easy to distinguish from lymphoblastic lymphoma of the convoluted-cell type by the size of the cells and nucleoli and by the basophilia of the tumor cells.

Centrocytic lymphoma shows certain cytologic similarities to the convoluted-cell type of lymphoblastic lymphoma, such as a fine chromatin and small nucleoli. What it lacks, however, are the convoluted nuclei. In lymphoblastic lymphoma of the convoluted-cell type it is easier to recognize the cytoplasm of the tumor cells. In centrocytic lymphoma the reaction for acid phosphatase is negative, or there is only a weakly positive, fine granular reaction. Furthermore, the fiber pattern is much coarser and occasionally somewhat nodular.

We can distinguish acute myeloid leukemia by its chloroacetate esterase-positive cells.

We should be able to recognize the lymphocytic neoplasms, such as B-CLL and LP immunocytoma, by their special cytologic characteristics. Lymphocytes have coarse chromatin, in contrast to the cells of lymphoblastic lymphoma of the convoluted-cell type. The "lymphoblasts" (paraimmunoblasts) of CLL are larger than the largest cells of lymphoblastic lymphoma of the convoluted-cell type and are unmistakable because of their moderately basophilic, gray-blue cytoplasm and their oval nuclei with large nucleoli. The plasmacytoid cells and immunoblasts should make it easy to distinguish LP immunocytoma from lymphoblastic lymphoma of the convoluted-cell type.

Metastases of neuroblastoma, juvenile rhabdomyosarcoma, Ewing's sarcoma, and small-cell bronchial carcinoma consist of tightly packed cell complexes. In contrast, the cells comprising lymphoblastic lymphoma of the convoluted-cell type are isolated from one another. Furthermore, the fiber network of the metastases is clearly distinguishable from that of convoluted-cell lymphoma by its coarse arrangement.

**Combination with Other Diseases.** LUKES[735] has observed a lymphoblastic lymphoma of the convoluted-cell type in a patient with ataxia telangiectasia. We also found this combination with ataxia telangiectasia in a boy with acid phosphatase-positive "lymphoblastic" lymphoma (see p. 400).

**Prognosis.** According to BARCOS and LUKES,[736] the prognosis is relatively poor. They estimated the median survival at 10 months. At the end of their study, however, two patients were still alive after 24 and 33 months, respectively. RILKE *et al.*[737] reported that four out of 15 patients died within 10 months and two survived for up to 17 months. Conventional lymphoma therapy, such as the Pinkel protocol, usually led merely to short remissions of a few months,

[735] LUKES and LENNERT, 1974.
[736] 1975.
[737] RILKE, CLEMENTE, PILOTTI and MUSUMECI, 1975.

whereas additional radiotherapy of the mediastinum with 2400 rad brought an average remission of 1 year.[738]

Many years ago, ROHR[739] stated that lymphosarcoma of the thymus, despite its radiosensitivity, rapidly generalized and soon led to death with a leukemic blood picture. JENKIN[740] reported that patients with lymphosarcoma and large mediastinal tumors survived on average only 0.85 years, whereas those without mediastinal tumors had a median survival of 2.6 years.

### *b) T-Lymphoblastic Lymphomas without Convoluted Nuclei*

The question as to whether there are other T-lymphoblastic lymphomas besides the convoluted-cell type may definitely be answered in the affirmative. On the one hand, the nuclear convolutions may be only partially developed or difficult to demonstrate. On the other hand, there are cases in which the nuclei do not show any convolutions, but which, in our opinion, can nevertheless be interpreted as T-lymphoblastic lymphomas. Some of them definitely correspond to the group of lymphoblastic lymphomas without convoluted nuclei described by NATHWANI *et al.*[740a] This is not the right time, however, to express a final opinion, since there have not yet been enough comparative studies of the morphology, cytochemistry, and immunology of such tumors. Nevertheless, we would like to present some examples of two variants of this type of lymphoma. The first variant is represented by apparently typical examples of the nonconvoluted T-type. The second variant is of special interest because of the presence of T-associated plasma cells.

The first example of the *first variant* is a case that the author (K.L.) observed in 1948. The patient was a 15-year-old boy whose condition was classified by LINKE as a classic example of leukosarcomatosis. This patient presented with generalized lymphadenopathy and moderate hepatosplenomegaly. He died within a few months. Histologically, the tumor cells were uniformly medium-sized and had oval nuclei with relatively fine chromatin and small nucleoli.[740b]

Since then, we have observed an identical histologic picture a number of times. Recently, we found it in a 21-year-old man. The nuclei of the lymphoma cells were oval like those of the cells described in the first case; they showed no convolutions at all. There were focal coarse positive reactions for acid nonspecific esterase and acid phosphatase, which then disappeared in the course of the disease. Immunoglobulin analyses of a tumor homogenate furnished normal values. Intracytoplasmic Ig could not be demonstrated. The histologic picture (Fig. 200) fully matched that illustrated by NATHWANI *et al.*[740a] in their Figure 12. Unfortunately, it was not possible to perform immunologic tests on fresh, living cells. Nevertheless, it is very probable that the focally positive acid phosphatase reaction may be considered proof of a T-lymphoblastic origin, as CATOVSKY *et al.*[740c] assumed for ALL. It would therefore be under-

---

[738] LANDBECK, GAEDICKE, WINKLER and STEIN, 1976.
[739] 1960.
[740] 1972.
[740a] NATHWANI, KIM and RAPPAPORT, 1976.
[740b] LENNERT, 1948; Fig. 4a
[740c] CATOVSKY, GALETTO, OKOS, MILIANI *et al.*, 1974

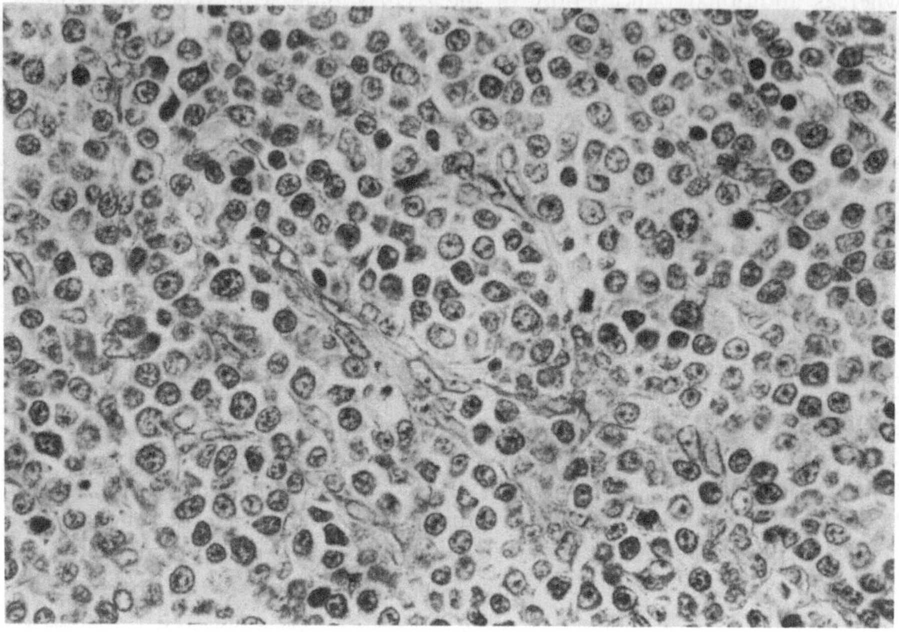

Fig. 200. T-lymphoblastic lymphoma without convoluted nuclei. Note the relatively uniform cells with oval nuclei. See text (p. 400f.) for clinical details. There was focal reactivity for acid phosphatase. ♂, 21 years. Inguinal node. Giemsa. × 560

standable that a number of the lymphoblastic lymphomas with nonconvoluted nuclei of the type described by NATHWANI *et al.*[740d] can show the same clinical behavior as lymphoblastic lymphomas with convoluted nuclei.

In another case with the same morphology, the cells in the first biopsy exhibited a strong focal acid phosphatase reaction, whereas those in the second biopsy were completely negative for acid phosphatase.

*In conclusion,* there is evidently a subtype of lymphoblastic lymphoma in which the tumor cells do not have convoluted nuclei, although they are essentially acid phosphatase-positive, and are probably derived from T-cells. Since the acid phosphatase positivity is not constant and may disappear in the course of the disease, the T-cell nature of the tumor cells cannot always be substantiated by cytochemistry. Further systematic studies with immunologic markers should be performed in such cases.

The patient with the *second variant* was a 3-year-old boy who had ataxia telangiectasia – a diagnosis that was supported by chromosome analysis.[741] Two weeks before diagnosis, the patient developed generalized lymphadenopathy, with the greatest enlargement of nodes in the cervical region. He also had a small mediastinal mass. Furthermore, he showed moderate splenomegaly

[740d] NATHWANI, KIM and RAPPAPORT, 1976.

[741] We wish to thank Dr. VON PAWEL, Department of Pediatrics (Head: Professor Dr. WOLF), Kassel City Hospital, for providing the clinical data.

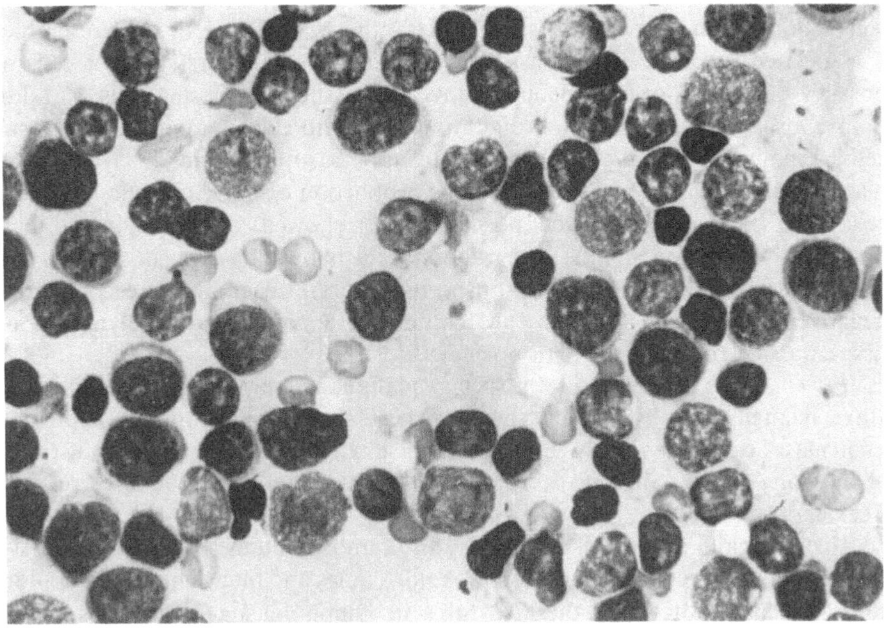

Fig. 201. T-lymphoblastic lymphoma without convoluted nuclei, but containing many T-associated plasma cells. Clinically, there was a mediastinal mass and ataxia telangiectasia. See text (pp. 400–402) for further clinical details. ♂, 3 years. Imprint of a cervical node. Pappenheim. ×875

and enlarged tonsils. The erythrocyte sedimentation rate was highly accelerated (140/180 mm/Hg). There was a polyclonal increase in serum IgM (the value was 1.6 times higher than normal). The blood picture was not leukemic and the bone marrow did not show infiltration by tumor cells. After high doses of prednisone, vincristine, and cyclophosphamide, the lymphadenopathy receded and the patient's general condition improved. Nevertheless, the cytostatic therapy was continued for 3 years. At the end of that period, there were no clinical signs of the lymphoma, so therapy was discontinued. Thereupon, the patient's condition quickly worsened, with development of abdominal masses that led to ileus-like symptoms. The child died immediately after abdominal surgery. At autopsy, abdominal lymph nodes (mesenteric, splenic hilar, hepatic, and para-aortic) were greatly enlarged. The spleen, bone marrow, and Waldeyer's tonsillar ring were also infiltrated.

Histologically, the normal lymph-node structure was effaced. Epithelioid venules were unusually numerous. Apart from remnants of lymphatic tissue with germinal centers, the normal structure was obliterated by polymorphic medium-sized cells. The capsule did not show the type of infiltration seen in acute leukemia. Imprints (see Fig. 201) revealed two principal types of cell. First, there were tumor cells with round, somewhat variable nuclei that did not have pronounced convolutions, but that contained large light nucleoli. Secondly, there were medium-sized cells with round nuclei and deep gray-blue cytoplasm, which was somewhat more abundant than that of the lymphoid cells. On electron microscopy (see p. 517ff.) the second type of cells resembled T-associated plasma cells. KAISERLING[742] interpreted the first type of cells as possible precursors or anaplastic variants of T-associated plasma cells. In addition, KAISERLING identified interdigitating reticulum cells among the neoplastic cells. Finally, there were also a few strongly basophilic, small "lymphatic" plasma cells and a few mast cells. A large proportion of the neoplastic lymphoid cells (and of the T-associated plasma cells?) showed a focal clumped acid phosphatase reaction. Diffuse or granular acid phosphatase positivity was not observed. The PAS and neutral nonspecific esterase reactions were completely negative. STEIN found that the IgM content of a homogenate of lymph-node tissue was 4.4 times higher than normal.

*In conclusion,* this was a very special malignant lymphoma in a child with ataxia telangiectasia. The patient showed generalized lymphadenopathy, a mediastinal mass, enlarged tonsils, and splenomegaly, but no leukemia. Infiltration of the bone marrow did not occur until the final stage, i.e., after three relapse-free years.

Histologically and ultrastructurally, the tumor contained two characteristic elements of the T-region, namely, epithelioid venules and interdigitating reticulum cells. We have not found these features in lymphoblastic lymphomas of the convoluted-cell type. The focal acid phosphatase reaction in numerous tumor cells and the occurrence of a mediastinal mass provided further arguments for the assumed T-cell nature of the lymphoma. The special feature of this case is the large number of T-associated plasma cells found in the tumor tissue.

We have observed two other cases of malignant lymphoma that should be mentioned in this context. The tumors apparently consisted of a pure population of T-associated plasma cells. One of these lymphomas developed in the final stage of mycosis fungoides. So far, however, we have not been able to provide any further (electron-microscopic or immunologic) proof supporting the interpretation of the tumor cells as T-associated plasma cells. For this reason, we must still be cautious in our interpretation of the tumors.

### *3. M.L. Lymphoblastic, Unclassified, Including Null-Lymphoblastic Lymphomas*

*Synonyms:* M.L. lymphocytic, poorly differentiated
Lymphoblastic lymphosarcoma and lymphoblastic leukemia (ALL)
Paraleukoblastic sarcoma and paraleukoblastic leukemia

In this group we include all medium-sized "blast-cell" lymphomas that we are still unable to classify precisely as B- or T-cell-derived because they lack immunologic markers or do not fulfill the necessary morphologic or cytochemical criteria. Practically speaking, we must also include cases in which immunologic and cytochemical data are not available and the morphology alone is not conclusive. Most cases of acute lymphoblastic leukemia (ALL) belong to this group (see p. 410ff.). We assume that a small number of the tumors

[742] 1975.

Table 79. M.L. lymphoblastic, unclassified. Material and incidence

| | | |
|---|---|---|
| Total No. of biopsy cases | 162 | |
| Total No. of biopsies | 203 | |
| Lymph nodes | | 161 |
| Extranodal | | 42 |
| Incidence in routine lymph-node material | | 94 |
| = 6.3% of malignant lymphomas | | |
| 11.2% of non-Hodgkin's lymphomas | | |

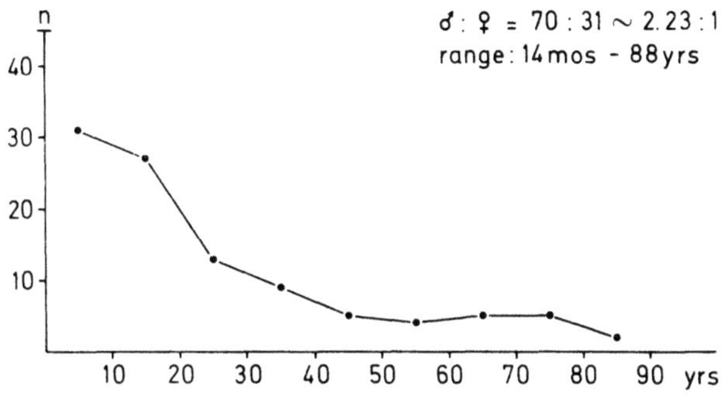


Fig. 202. Age distribution and sex ratio of M.L. lymphoblastic, unclassified. 101 patients of our first series

of the "unclassified lymphoblastic type" are derived from the B-cell system and a somewhat larger number from the T-cell system. The largest proportion of tumors, however, are probably neither B- nor T-cell-derived. They may be called Null-lymphoblastic lymphomas. At least some of them might be derived from stem cells of the bone marrow.

**Occurrence.** In our first series the unclassified lymphoblastic lymphomas accounted for 1% of the lymph-node biopsies and represented 6.3% of all malignant lymphomas and 11.2% of the non-Hodgkin's lymphomas (Table 79), whereas in our second series they made up only 4.2% of the non-Hodgkin's lymphomas (see Table 13).

Almost 60% of the tumors developed before the age of 20 (Fig. 202). The lymphoma appears most commonly in children, as is usual for ALL. As a matter of fact, our data were influenced to a great extent by the leukemias: in 14.7% of our cases the clinicians reported that the blood picture was leukemic, although we assume the true percentage is much higher. The male-to-female ratio was 2.2:1.

**Clinical Manifestations.** According to LANDBECK,[743] about 27% of the "lymphoblastic sarcomas" of childhood transform into leukemias. MITUS[744] reported transformation into ALL in 50% of cases. These values need to be reexamined now that the diagnosis of lymphomas is more differentiated, and they especially need to be specified for the different types of lymphoma of childhood.

[743] 1973. [744] 1972.

Table 80. Localization of biopsies of M.L. lymphoblastic, unclassified

| Localization | n | | % |
|---|---|---|---|
| Lymph nodes | 161 | | |
| Cervical | | 94 | 66.7 |
| Axillary | | 22 | 15.6 |
| Mediastinal | | 3 | 2.1 |
| Abdominal | | 7 | 5.0 |
| Inguinal | | 15 | 10.6 |
| Cubital | | — | — |
| Unknown | | 20 | — |
| Extranodal | 42 | | |
| Skin and subcutis | | 14 | — |
| Intestine | | 8 | — |
| Tonsils | | 5 | — |
| Stomach | | 3 | — |
| Diverse | | 12 | — |

**Stage.** If we consider only the nonleukemic cases of lymphoblastic lymphoma, which were previously referred to as lymphoblastic lymphosarcoma, then a fairly large percentage of the patients presented with localized tumors. According to the records available to us, of our 22 children with "lymphoblastic lymphosarcoma," in 16 the tumor was still localized (stages I and II) at the time of diagnosis, whereas in four children the tumor was already generalized. No information was available for the other two patients.[745]

**Localization.** According to Table 80, 66.7% of the lymph nodes we studied came from the cervical region. Of those, 13.5% were supraclavicular nodes. The axillary and superficial thoracic lymph nodes made up 15.6%, the inguinal lymph nodes accounted for 10.6%. Five percent of the lymph nodes were from the abdominal region and only 2.1% from the thorax. The most common extranodal sites were the skin and subcutis (14 cases), the intestine (8 cases), and the tonsils (5 cases).

**Gross Appearance.** In the nonleukemic forms the lymph nodes are often excessively enlarged. When sectioned, the fresh surface of the soft pulpy tissue appears uniformly gray-white.

**Histology.** The lymph nodes are usually completely replaced by tumor tissue and their structure is therefore effaced. Occasionally, however, remnants of normal lymphatic tissue persist with its characteristic structural features, contrasting sharply with the tumor. That is immediately evident from the differences in size and staining of the cells. The nuclei of the tumor cells are larger and with Giemsa staining are paler than those of lymphocytes.

On the one hand, the neoplastic cells may show infiltrative and destructive growth, revealing the same macroscopic behavior as is seen in "sarcoma" (nodularity or tumor masses). The cells then destroy the preexistent fiber structures,

[745] Lennert and Mohri, 1971.

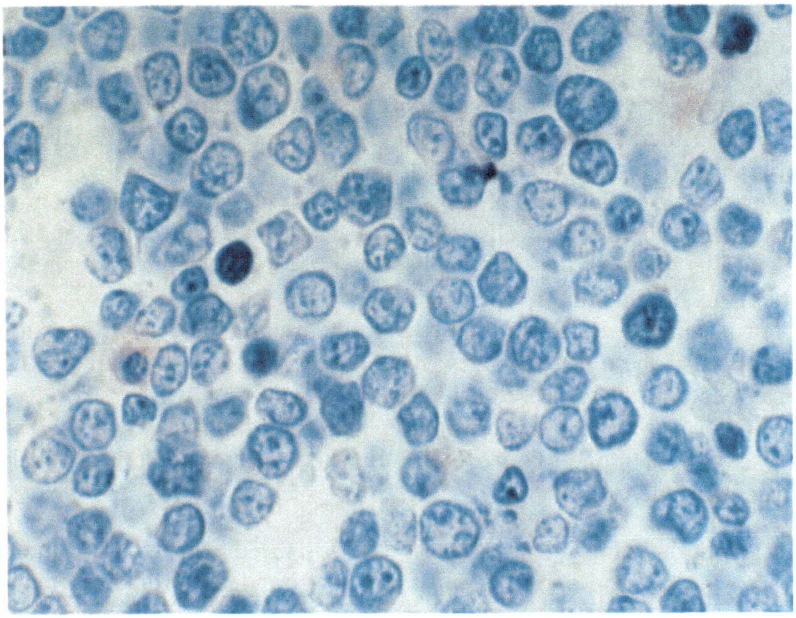

Fig. 203. M.L. lymphoblastic, unclassified, with Giemsa staining. Relatively small cells with a narrow rim of moderately basophilic cytoplasm. There is some similarity to T-lymphoblastic lymphoma, but the acid phosphatase reaction was negative. ♂, 11 years. Mediastinal node. × 1,550

such as capsule and trabeculae, and may penetrate deep into the surrounding adipose tissue.

On the other hand, the cells of some tumors show only infiltrative growth. They extensively infiltrate the connective-tissue network (capsule and trabeculae) of the lymph node, without destroying it, although it is distended by the tumor cells. This picture is predominant in the leukemic variant of lymphoblastic lymphoma.

The tumor consists of relatively small cells that are somewhat larger than lymphocytes or of medium-sized cells. The smaller cells (Fig. 203) have a narrow rim of moderately basophilic cytoplasm, whereas the larger cells show a more distinct, clearly basophilic cytoplasm. The size of the nucleoli is largely correlated with that of the cells: the nucleoli of smaller cells are small and often difficult to recognize, and the nucleoli of larger cells are larger and more prominent. They number between two and five. The nuclei of the tumor cells are usually rounded, but they are occasionally deformed by clefts or indentations. They have fine chromatin. As Wright[746] has justly stressed, tumor cells of this appearance are often seen only at the periphery of the section. In the center of the section the tumor cells may show more vesicular nuclei with coarser chromatin and, in particular, larger nucleoli. One reason for this is that fixation of the tissue is often inadequate. Another reason is the unusually delicate nature of the blast cells, which are very easily injured by even the slightest irregularity occurring during the preparation of the slides, from the

[746] 1970b.

initial fixation, embedding, and staining to the final mounting. Like the nuclei, the cytoplasm often reveals certain differences in the cells of peripheral and central parts of the lymph node. At the periphery the tumor cells are sometimes more clearly demarcated from one another than the cells in the central parts; consequently, their narrow rim of cytoplasm is more distinct. In the central parts the cells often appear to stick so close together that under low magnification they suggest a syncytial mass of cells. Sometimes, however, the peripheral cells stick together, whereas the cells in central parts are spread apart and appear shrunken. The nuclei of the tumor cells vary only moderately in size and shape. Mitotic figures are common.

A few macrophages can frequently be found among the monotonous-appearing tumor cells. These macrophages have abundant, often vacuolated cytoplasm that may contain phagocytosed cells and cell debris.

The preexistent fibers are destroyed and the tumor itself contains only a few thick fibers. In one tumor we found marked sclerosis like that of sclerotic M.L. centroblastic/centrocytic.

**Smear/Imprint.** Imprints are quite useful for the diagnosis. The tumor cells appear relatively monotonous. Their nuclei are rounded or somewhat polymorphic and sometimes reveal small to medium-sized nucleoli. The chromatin is fine. The rim of cytoplasm is narrow and intensely basophilic and contains no granules.

**Histochemistry and Cytochemistry.** In paraffin sections the tumor cells always give a negative PAS reaction. In contrast, in cryostat sections one sometimes finds coarse granular PAS reactivity. The chloroacetate esterase reaction should be performed in every case and must be negative in all tumor cells to exclude myeloblastic leukemia (see p. 408).

In imprints there is often a fine to moderately coarse, granular PAS reaction in a few or even numerous tumor cells of lymphoblastic lymphoma of the unclassified type. After pretreatment with diastase there is no PAS positivity. The PAS-positive material is therefore glycogen. Fat vacuoles are seen only rarely.

The acid phosphatase reaction reveals only occasional positive granules. In essence, therefore, the tumor cells are negative for this enzyme as well as for nonspecific esterase. The peroxidase reaction is also negative in smears.

**Diagnosis.** The diagnosis rests on the monotonous appearance of the proliferating basophilic cells. The chloroacetate esterase reaction is negative. In imprints the PAS reaction is often positive. There are never follicle-like structures, even with silver staining. Centrocytes, plasma cells, and mast cells are not found. Further criteria are listed in Table 81.

**Differential Diagnosis.** Previously, when a pathologist examined a lymphoblastic proliferation, the first question he had to answer was whether the process was a sarcoma or a leukemia. This leads us to consider more basic questions: is it fundamentally possible to make this distinction when the cytology is the same? Have we not concocted an artificial alternative that disregards the true

Table 81. Diagnostic criteria of M.L. lymphoblastic, unclassified

| |
|---|
| 1. Most patients are children or adolescents |
| 2. In most cases leukemic blood picture (ALL) and infiltration of bone marrow |
| 3. Small or medium-sized cell type neither Burkitt nor convoluted type |
| 4. In most leukemic cases infiltration and expansion of capsule and trabeculae without destruction |
| 5. In most nonleukemic cases ("sarcomas") capsule intact or destroyed (not ~4) |

nature of the disease and merely describes varieties of the same process? The first question also has practical implications: does the postulated sarcoma type of the disease show a different age distribution, does it affect different sites, or does it run a different clinical course?

The questions we have just asked are irrelevant to the Kiel Classification, because it does not make a distinction between sarcoma and leukemia. Nevertheless, we shall discuss these questions, since the compromises in terminology made in the Kiel Classification have not eliminated the underlying problem of sarcoma/leukemia. We shall present the discussion we had already written before the Kiel meeting:

We fully agree with GALTON[747] that there are weighty arguments against the viewpoint of APITZ,[748] who was unwilling to accept a basic distinction between leukemia and sarcoma. The cells of sarcoma apparently have one more criterion of malignancy than the cells of leukemia, i.e., they show not only infiltrative but also destructive growth. In contrast, the cells of leukemia have merely the capacity to break loose and actively migrate, eventually entering the bloodstream. It is perhaps too much of a simplification to say that the cells of sarcoma are more cohesive than those of leukemia, whereas in a leukemic proliferation the cells are not stuck together and do not form groups, but instead penetrate separately into the preexistent structures without destroying them. When there is destructive growth, a tumor nodule or mass is produced that can easily be recognized grossly. When growth is infiltrative, there is diffuse infiltration that may spread to certain specific areas of an organ without endangering the basic structure (see, for example, the infiltration of the liver).

The proliferating cells of sarcoma therefore lack a quality possessed by leukemic cells: unlike their normal counterparts, they are unable to migrate, but they can acquire this quality during the course of the disease. We must ask the following question, though: is this later acquired ability to migrate of the same nature as that inherent in cells of primary leukemia? GALTON[747] refers to "overflowing" of the tissue, in contrast to the higher grade of differentiation of "true" leukemic cells. Conversely, leukemic cells may lose their ability to migrate. This may be associated with a change in the cell picture. Nodular infiltrates and/or tumor masses then develop and efface the lymph-node boundaries. It therefore seems as if qualities exist that on one occasion enable a "sarcoma" to develop, at another time a "leukemia," or a combination of both types of neoplasm.

The reasons already given induced us to try to distinguish lymphoblastic "sarcoma" from lymphoblastic leukemia by means of histologic methods. From our efforts we discovered that indeed in lymph nodes there is a criterion that enables one to differentiate purely infiltrative growth from infiltrative-destructive growth. This criterion is the behavior of the neoplastic cells toward the connective-tissue structures of the lymph node (Fig. 207). The leukemic cells infiltrate the capsule and trabeculae diffusely and often in a relatively uniform manner, causing expansion of these structures to a greater or lesser degree. The fiber network, however, is basically preserved and the outlines of the capsule and trabeculae are maintained. The sinuses and lymph-node parenchyma are clearly distinct from the capsule and trabeculae, often with a cleft separating them, which is merely an artifact due to shrinkage. In contrast, although the cells of lymphoblastic "sarcoma" may grow into regions of the capsule and trabeculae in an infiltrating manner, they often destroy parts of these structures as well. They also grow out of the lymphatic parenchyma

[747] 1964. [748] 1937a, 1940.

directly into the capsule, thereby obliterating the sinus, so that often it becomes impossible to distinguish sharply the lymphatic parenchyma from the capsule, in contrast to the situation in ALL.

From these differences in proliferation we distinguished histologically a leukemic type of lymphoblastic neoplasm from a sarcoma type. In addition, we were able to detect corresponding differences in the pattern of lymph-node involvement, in the behavior of the blood picture, and in other properties.[749] We observed, for example, that in the leukemic type there was usually generalized lymphadenopathy, rarely a local tumor. On the other hand, the sarcoma type was regularly associated with a localized neoplastic process that gave rise to large tumors of lymph nodes. Whereas most of the lymph nodes we studied from the leukemic type originated from the neck, those from the sarcoma type often came from the abdomen (mesenteric and intestinal, retroperitoneal) and mediastinum. In those cases in which we had made a histologic diagnosis of "leukemic type," the blood picture was leukemic in 22 patients and nonleukemic in 12. In contrast, in 22 patients in whom we had diagnosed the sarcoma type, we found no evidence of leukemic changes in the blood at the time of biopsy. That of course does not exclude the possibility of finding tumor cells in the blood later.

We have systematically used the given criterion for differentiating lymphoblastic leukemia from "sarcoma" since 1971 and must admit that it sometimes fails. It is definitely not an absolute criterion; it merely enables us to suspect a "leukemia" or "sarcoma" with a certain degree of probability.

At times it proves difficult to distinguish the unclassified type of lymphoblastic lymphoma from the *convoluted-cell type* (acid phosphatase type), since the cells of the unclassified type may be small and isolated. They usually do not reveal distinct convoluted nuclei, however, and above all they fail to give the typical acid phosphatase reaction seen in the convoluted-cell type. A positive PAS reaction in paraffin sections is always presumptive evidence of a convoluted-cell lymphoma, since it never occurs in the unclassified type. In imprints, however, the tumor cells of both types of lymphoblastic lymphoma may contain abundant PAS-positive granules (glycogen).

Besides ALL, every other type of blastic leukemia, including *acute myeloid leukemia* (AML; myeloblastic leukemia) should be considered in the differential diagnosis. The latter may be of the small-cell or medium-sized-cell varieties. Slides stained with Giemsa or hematoxylin and eosin occasionally reveal a few granulocytic cells, for example, eosinophils and their precursors. Often it is also possible to demonstrate a few myeloid precursors (with round or oval nuclei), as well as more mature granulocytic cells, that are positive for chloroacetate esterase. There are rare cases of AML in which the tumor cells are completely negative for this enzyme. Such variants, however, may occasionally be identified by electron microscopy.

The sarcomatous variant of AML, *myelosarcoma,* must be differentiated from (medium-sized cell) lymphoblastic sarcoma in which the tumor cells, have strongly basophilic cytoplasm (probably B-cell type).[750] As a rule, this distinction can be made with the reaction for chloroacetate esterase, since abundant, or at least some, positive cells are present in myelosarcoma.

Occasionally, the distinction between unclassified lymphoblastic lymphoma and *immunoblastic lymphoma* proves difficult, although it is usually possible just from the differences in cell size. Immunoblastic lymphoma is composed of larger, strongly basophilic cells containing more oval nuclei and large central nucleoli.

Lymph-node *metastases* may also appear similar to lymphoblastic lym-

---

[749] LENNERT and MOHRI, 1971.

[750] WRIGHT, 1970b.

phoma. The tumors of childhood or youth that need to be considered are: neuroblastoma, including retinoblastoma; juvenile rhabdomyosarcoma (especially alveolar rhabdomyosarcoma); and Ewing's sarcoma. In adults one should also keep in mind anaplastic small-cell bronchial carcinoma.

The cells of neuroblastoma are small and uniform, and at times form pseudorosettes. They grow in solid complexes and/or cords. In between these groups there are thick connective-tissue fibers that surround the tumor-cell masses, but are not intermingled with them. The PAS reaction is negative. In imprints, on the other hand, there may be a weakly to moderately positive (diffuse) reaction for acid phosphatase.

The cells of juvenile rhabdomyosarcoma and Ewing's sarcoma contain abundant PAS-positive material, probably glycogen, which partially dissolves away in the process of tissue embedding. The PAS-positive material is *diffusely* scattered in the cytoplasm, whereas in unclassified lymphoblastic lymphoma the PAS reaction in paraffin sections is negative. In rhabdomyosarcoma and Ewing's sarcoma the tumor cells and fiber network are sharply demarcated from one another. That is especially true in rhabdomyosarcoma, in which the tumor parenchyma can usually be distinguished from the stroma without difficulty.

The cells of anaplastic small-cell bronchial carcinoma are negative for PAS. They reveal neither nucleoli nor cytoplasm. The nuclei are sometimes of an elongate shape ("oat-cell carcinoma"). In between the solid tumor masses there is a slightly or moderately developed stroma that often shows metachromatic staining. No neoplasm of lymphoreticular tissue ever has a stroma.

**Prognosis.**[751] The prognosis of nonleukemic unclassified lymphoblastic lymphoma ("sarcoma") is usually poor. In the group of patients studied by MARSDEN and STEWARD,[752] which included only children, 25 out of 34 died of the disease within 6 months after the onset of symptoms. The longest period of observation was 3 years (one child). Six children, however, survived. Their tumors had been localized in either the neck or the ileocecal region. These data indicate that the prognosis of lymphoblastic "lymphosarcoma" depends to a great extent on the localization of the tumor. If it arises in a region that makes its early detection and surgical removal easy (superficial lymph nodes, ileocecal region), then a cure is possible.

At Stanford[753] 32 non-Hodgkin's lymphomas of children were analyzed. It was found that a high percentage of the patients with disease in stages I–III remained well and free of recurrence for more than 4 years. Those in stage IV never survived more than 12 months. Unfortunately, the classification used by those investigators is not directly comparable with ours.

Of the 30 patients with lymphoblastic lymphosarcoma reported by MILLETT *et al.*,[754] eight were in stages I or II at the time they first sought medical care. Three of these lived more than 5 years without recurrences (up to 17 years). None of the patients with generalized disease (22) survived until the end of the second year, and 90% died during the first year after diagnosis.

---

[751] E.g., GARWICZ, LANDBERG and ÅKERMAN, 1974.

[752] 1968.

[753] GLATSTEIN, KIM, DONALDSON, DORFMAN *et al.*, 1974.

[754] MILLETT, BENNETT, JELLIFFE and FARRER-BROWN, 1969.

### *Addendum (to 1–3)*
### *The Leukemic Variants of Malignant Lymphoma, Lymphoblastic: Lymphoblastic Leukemias (ALL)*

*Synonyms:* Paraleukoblastic leukemia
Acute lymphatic leukemia
Acute lymphocytic leukemia
Stem-cell leukemia

**Terminology/Origin of the Neoplastic Cells** (Fig. 204). In Germany, acute lymphoblastic leukemia (ALL) has often been referred to as paraleukoblastic leukemia, because the lymphocytic nature of the cells remains unproved, at least for some of the cases. The disease could just as well arise from very immature cells, such as stem cells of the bone marrow. Nonetheless, for practical reasons, we accept the much more popular term ALL, since most of these leukemias are definitely lymphatic in nature. We are well aware, however, that the term ALL is a simplification and that new labeling techniques will help us someday to define the disease better and to divide it into appropriate subgroups.

The subclassification of ALL into four or five types given by MATHÉ *et al.*[755] is hardly reproducible and apparently includes types of malignant lymphoma other than the lymphoblastic varieties (e.g., M.L. centrocytic). In contrast to such morphologic approaches, modern immunologic and cytochemical methods have proved useful in determining whether the "lymphoblasts" of ALL are derived from B-cells or from T-cells (see also p. 360).

Only a small number of cases of ALL disclose markers of B-lymphocytes, in particular surface Ig. Of the 69 cases of ALL studied by BROUET *et al.*,[756] only *one* was definitely of the B-cell type, with cells bearing monoclonal IgM on their surfaces. In seven other cases the authors were unable to exclude secondary binding of Ig to the cell surfaces. Among 35 cases of ALL, GAJL-PECZALSKA *et al.*[757] found one patient (a 75-year-old man) in whom the blast cells bore monoclonal Ig.

In 1975, BROUET *et al.*[758] reported on immunologic studies of 90 patients with ALL. Eleven of them showed a monoclonal B-cell proliferation. Of these 11, six cases corresponded to the leukemic variant of Burkitt's tumor,[759] three cases represented a lymphoblastic transformation from typical B-CLL, and only two cases corresponded to "common ALL."

By means of the rosette technique (sheep-E rosettes), it has been shown that a number of cases of ALL can be considered to be T-cell-derived.[760]

---

[755] MATHÉ, POUILLART, STERESCU, AMIEL *et al.*, 1971; MATHÉ, BELPOMME, DANTCHEV, POUILLART *et al.*, 1975.

[756] BROUET, TOBEN, CHEVALIER and SELIGMANN, 1974; see also SELIGMANN, PREUD'HOMME and BROUET, 1973.

[757] GAJL-PECZALSKA, BLOOMFIELD, NESBIT and KERSEY, 1974.

[758] BROUET, PREUD'HOMME and SELIGMANN, 1975.

[759] See also FLANDRIN, BROUET, DANIEL and PREUD'HOMME, 1975; FLANDRIN and BERNARD, 1975.

[760] BORELLA and SEN, 1973, 1974; JONDAL, WIGZELL and AIUTI, 1973; CATOVSKY, GOLDMAN, OKOS, FRISCH *et al.*, 1974; HUBER, MICHLMAYR and HUBER, 1974; HUHN, 1974, personal communication; MICHLMAYR, HUBER, FINK, FALKENSAMMER *et al.*, 1974; SCHWENK, 1974.

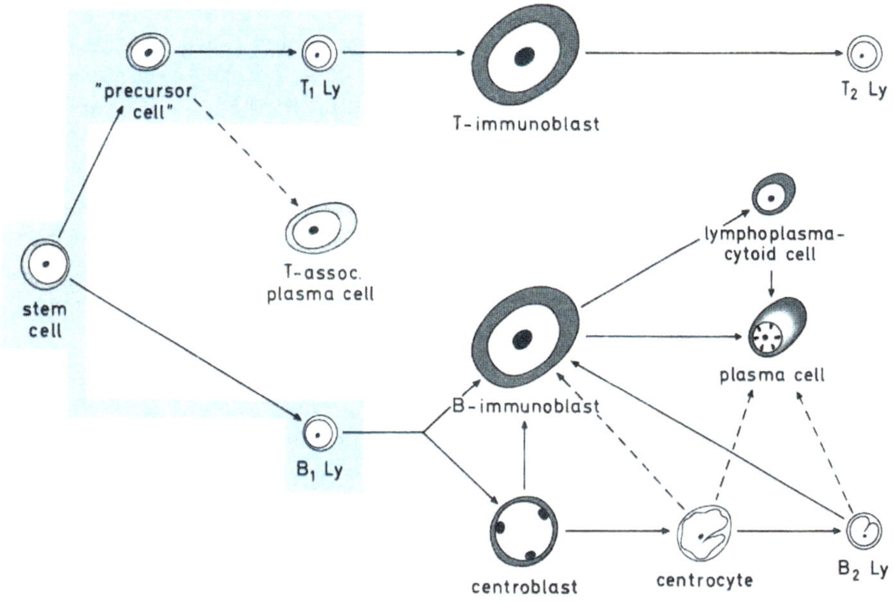


Fig. 204. Hypothetical origin of tumor cells of the different subtypes of ALL

These probably make up about 25% of the cases of ALL (17/69,[756] 1/6,[761] 4/24,[757] 5/20,[762] 7/20,[763] 11/48[764]). The tumor cells are negative for surface Ig. The blast cells of most cases of ALL (about 70%) lack all markers on their surfaces.[765] When anti-T-serum[766] is used to identify the cells from such cases, the percentage of cases of ALL derived from T-cells increases considerably. For example, KERSEY *et al.*[763] found that, among 20 children with ALL, the leukemic blast cells of five did not form sheep-E rosettes, but were killed by anti-T-serum. Later, KERSEY *et al.*[767] identified a total of 14 out of 22 cases of ALL in children as T-cell-derived.

The remaining cases of sheep-E rosette-negative and T-lymphocyte antigen-negative ALL that are also surface Ig-negative are called null-cell ALL; they may perhaps be interpreted as stem-cell leukemias. The studies of GREAVES[768] supported this interpretation. He was able to prepare a rabbit antiserum against membrane antigen on human ALL cells. This serum reacted with the cells from 102 out of 117 cases of non-B/non-T ALL, but there were no positive reactions in 21 T-like and six B-like ALL cases. Clinically, the prognosis was better for the leukemias with membrane antigen.

---

[761] GREENWOOD and HOLLAND, 1974.
[762] BELPOMME, DANTCHEV, DU RUSQUEC, GRANDJON *et al.*, 1974.
[763] KERSEY, NESBIT, LUCKASEN, HALLGREN *et al.*, 1974.
[764] SEN and BORELLA, 1975.
[765] See also KAPLAN, MASTRANGELO and PETERSON, 1974.
[766] CHIN, SAIKI, TRUJILLO and WILLIAMS, 1973.
[767] KERSEY, NESBIT, HALLGREN, SABAD *et al.*, 1975.
[768] 1976; GREAVES, CAPELLARO, BROWN, REVESZ *et al.*, 1976.

In addition to T-cell ALL, including the cases with cells forming mixed rosettes, we should mention one peculiar case that was characterized by two cell populations (T-cells forming sheep-E rosettes and B-cells bearing surface Ig). This patient had a large thymic tumor and very high WBC counts.[771]

We should also mention the occurrence of *paraproteinemia* in ALL of childhood.[772] There are several reports in the literature of increased serum levels of IgG or IgM in ALL. We also have occasionally observed an increase in IgM (probably monoclonal) in the blood of patients with ALL. Such paraproteinemias suggest the presence of a B-cell lymphoma. Unfortunately, the cases reported in the literature cannot be evaluated in this respect owing to lack of information.

**Definition.** We define ALL as the leukemia that, if left untreated, runs a rapid course and is characterized by a systemic proliferation of undifferentiated lymphoid cells ("lymphoblasts") in lymphatic and other hemopoietic tissues. In blood smears these lymphoblasts account for more than 1% of the leukocytes. As a rule, the bone marrow is infiltrated. We use the term leukemia, however, only when the blood reveals a moderate to large number of neoplastic cells. The peroxidase, chloroacetate esterase, and nonspecific esterase reactions are negative. When the cells in smears show a focal paranuclear acid phosphatase reaction, we consider the neoplasm to be T-cell-derived; this is ALL of the convoluted-cell type (acid phosphatase type). In many cases of lymphoblastic leukemia, however, the morphologic and cytochemical characteristics do now allow an exact characterization of the leukemic cells.

We distinguish three morphologically and cytochemically different types of ALL that largely correspond to the respective types of nonleukemic lymphoblastic lymphoma:

1. The B-lymphoblastic type, including the Burkitt type (not focally positive for acid phosphatase, mostly PAS-negative).
2. The T-lymphoblastic type, morphologically defined as the convoluted-cell type and cytochemically defined as the acid phosphatase type (focally positive for acid phosphatase, sometimes PAS-positive).
3. The null-lymphoblastic type, in most cases morphologically registered as unclassified lymphoblastic lymphoma (not focally positive for acid phosphatase, sometimes PAS-positive).

*1. ALL of the B-Lymphoblastic Type, Including the Burkitt Type.* In 1975, Flandrin *et al.*[773] described an acute leukemia with Burkitt's tumor cells in six patients. The blast cells of the blood and bone marrow showed all the cytologic, cytochemical, and electron-microscopic features of Burkitt's tumor cells. They were usually devoid of PAS-positive material. Immunologically, they

---

[771] Haegert, Cawley, Karpas and Goldstone, 1974.

[772] Märki and Siegenthaler, 1964; Stoop, Zegers, van der Heiden and Ballieux, 1968; Lindqvist, Ragab and Osterland, 1970; Čejka, Bollinger, Schuit, Lusher *et al.*, 1974; Karitzky and Jacobi, 1974.

[773] Flandrin, Brouet, Daniel and Preud'Homme, 1975; Flandrin and Bernard, 1975.

bore monoclonal surface Ig and formed EA rosettes but no sheep-E rosettes. Therefore, the cells were definitely B-cells. The clinical course was usually rapidly fatal. In the extensive material of FLANDRIN and BERNARD[774] this type of ALL was rare (<2% of ALL). Further cases of leukemic Burkitt's lymphoma have been published.[775]

In our material we found that 8.8% of the cases of ALL corresponded morphologically to lymphoblastic lymphoma of the Burkitt type. Although we have not performed immunologic studies of these cases, there is no doubt in our mind that they are morphologically identical with the cases of FLANDRIN *et al.* and are therefore B-cell leukemias.

In addition to these ALL cases of the Burkitt type, there are a few cases that are defined immunologically as B-cell leukemias, but are not very well defined histologically.

*2. ALL of the T-Lymphoblastic Type (Convoluted-Cell Type, Acid Phosphatase Type).* This form of leukemia is related to, but clearly distinguishable from T-CLL. It is equivalent to the "extremely immature-cell erythremia" distinguished by LEDER[776] and DRESCHER and LEDER,[777] and to the "paraerythroblastic leukemia" of BECKMANN *et al.*[778] It is histologically identical with the malignant lymphoma of the "convoluted lymphocytic type" described by LUKES (see p. 381 ff.). Since the nuclear convolutions are not always clearly recognizable, or even absent, however, the acid phosphatase reaction is a more reliable marker of this type of ALL. Another reason the acid phosphatase reaction is a useful criterion is that blood smears can be easily obtained at any time without burdening the patient.

The clinical picture differs from that of common ALL of childhood.[779] The leukemia is often accompanied by a thymic tumor and may manifest very high leukocyte counts as well as unusually severe hepatosplenomegaly. The bone marrow apparently becomes involved secondarily. Accordingly, there is often no reduction in blood platelets or erythrocytes for a long time, in contrast to common ALL of childhood.[780] In addition, the mean age is higher, and boys are more frequently affected than girls.[781] The disease responds poorly to the customary therapy used for ALL. Consequently, the prognosis is worse than that of common ALL (null ALL).

We define this T-lymphoblastic leukemia on the basis of the focal paranuclear acid phosphatase reaction in blood smears or lymph-node imprints. The cytology in sections—polymorphism and the so-called convoluted cells—and the noncohesion of the cells support the diagnosis.

---

[774] 1975.

[775] GUTTERMAN, RODRIGUEZ and MCMULLAN, 1972; KERSEY, GAJL-PECZALSKA and NESBIT, 1974; JAIYESIMI, OLUBOYEDE, TAYLOR and FAMILUSI, 1975.

[776] 1965, 1967b, 1969b.

[777] 1970; DRESCHER, HANSEN, ALTHOFF and GRAUCOB, 1969.

[778] BECKMANN, LANDBECK, NETH and SCHMIDTKE, 1971.

[779] DRESCHER and LEDER, 1970; BECKMANN, LANDBECK, NETH and SCHMIDTKE, 1971; CATOVSKY, GALETTO, OKOS, MILIANI *et al.*, 1974; CATOVSKY, 1975; SEN and BORELLA, 1975; LANDBECK, GAEDICKE, WINKLER and STEIN, 1976.

[780] LANDBECK, GAEDICKE, WINKLER and STEIN, 1976.

[781] SEN and BORELLA, 1975; LANDBECK, GAEDICKE, WINKLER and STEIN, 1976.

The cells of acid phosphatase-positive ALL bear T-cell markers.[782] They form sheep-E rosettes, often EAC rosettes, and mixed E/EAC rosettes.[783] This does not mean that all cases of T-cell ALL have to be positive for acid phosphatase, as might be concluded from the paper of CATOVSKY *et al.*[783a] On the contrary, we cannot exclude the possibility that there are cases of ALL derived from T-cells in which the cells are acid phosphatase-negative.

*3. ALL of the Null-Lymphoblastic Type, "Common ALL."* These leukemias do not reveal any immunologic markers that would enable us to classify them as T- or B-cell neoplasms. Like unclassified lymphoblastic lymphomas, they are morphologically and cytochemically defined by small to medium-sized tumor cells, which in smears or cryostat sections are enzyme-negative, but often show a granular PAS reaction (glycogen). Especially significant is the absence of the characteristic focal acid phosphatase activity seen in the convoluted-cell type.

**Occurrence.** ALL accounted for about three lymph nodes out of every 1000 in our first series; that represents 1.7% of all malignant lymphomas and 2.8% of the non-Hodgkin's lymphomas. This number of lymph nodes certainly does not represent the true incidence of the disease, however, since in some of the patients with ALL biopsies of lymph nodes are not made. In Germany the incidence of the disease is about four cases a year per 100,000 population. In Japan ALL is very rare.[784]

The age curve for our biopsy material reproduces the known rise in the first decade of life with a gradual fall thereafter until the age of 30 (Fig. 205). Within the first decade there is a distinct peak around the third to fourth years. We are unable to give any exact statistical data about the occurrence of ALL in adult life. Therefore, we used the data given by CUTLER *et al.*[785] (Fig. 206). The curves show that there is apparently a second slight rise in advanced ages. We must remember, however, that the diagnosis of this leukemia in the precytochemical era rested on morphologic methods alone. Consequently, we cannot be sure whether these cases were truly acute *lymphoblastic* leukemias. Nevertheless, other statistics (e.g., those of JACQUILLAT *et al.*[786]) and our own observations indicate that acute lymphoblastic leukemias do occur in older adults, although such leukemias are rare at these ages.

In our material 65% of the lymph nodes came from males, an incidence almost twice that for females. In the very large series of CUTLER *et al.*[787] the male sex accounted for 55.9%.

**Localization.** The percentage of lymph nodes removed from the neck exceeds that for lymphoblastic "sarcoma" (75.9:59.5%). On the other hand, mediastinal

[782] CATOVSKY, GALETTO, OKOS, MILIANI *et al.*, 1974; RITTER, GAEDICKE, WINKLER and LANDBECK, 1975; LANDBECK, GAEDICKE, WINKLER and STEIN, 1976; STEIN, PETERSEN, GAEDICKE, LENNERT *et al.*, 1976.

[783] STEIN, PETERSEN, GAEDICKE, LENNERT *et al.*, 1976.

[783a] CATOVSKY, GALETTO, OKOS, MILIANI *et al.*, 1974.

[784] SENO, MONDEN, SHIBATA, SEKI *et al.*, 1964.

[785] CUTLER, AXTELL and HEISE, 1967; see Fig. 3 in LENNERT and MOHRI, 1971; see also ROATH, ISRAËLS and WILKINSON, 1964.

[786] JACQUILLAT, WEIL, GEMON, AUCLERC *et al.*, 1973.

[787] CUTLER, AXTELL and HEISE, 1967.

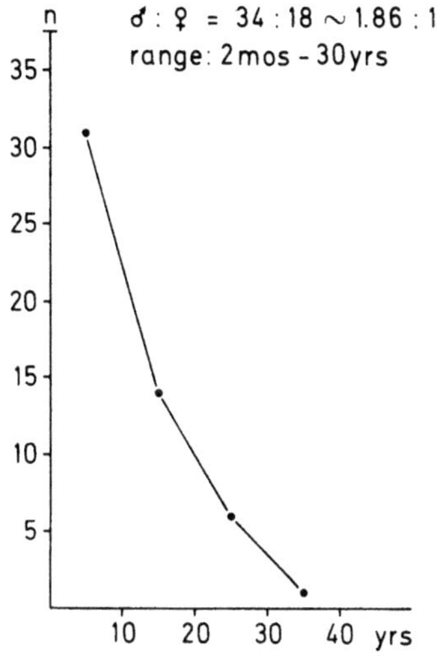


Fig. 205. Age distribution and sex ratio of ALL, null-type (common ALL). Lymph-node biopsies from 52 patients in our first series

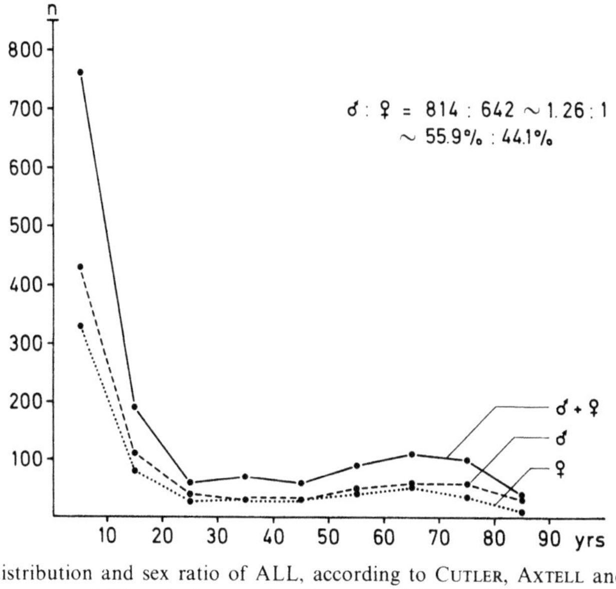


Fig. 206. Age distribution and sex ratio of ALL, according to CUTLER, AXTELL and HEISE (1967). 1456 patients, examined between 1940 and 1962

lymph nodes are less commonly represented than in lymphoblastic "sarcoma." We have no abdominal lymph nodes in our collection of ALL biopsies.

Of the 10 extranodal biopsies, three were from the skin and two from the tonsils. No biopsies came from the intestinal tract.

**Gross Appearance.** The lymph nodes may be slightly, moderately, or even greatly enlarged, although they generally remain discrete. They are soft and

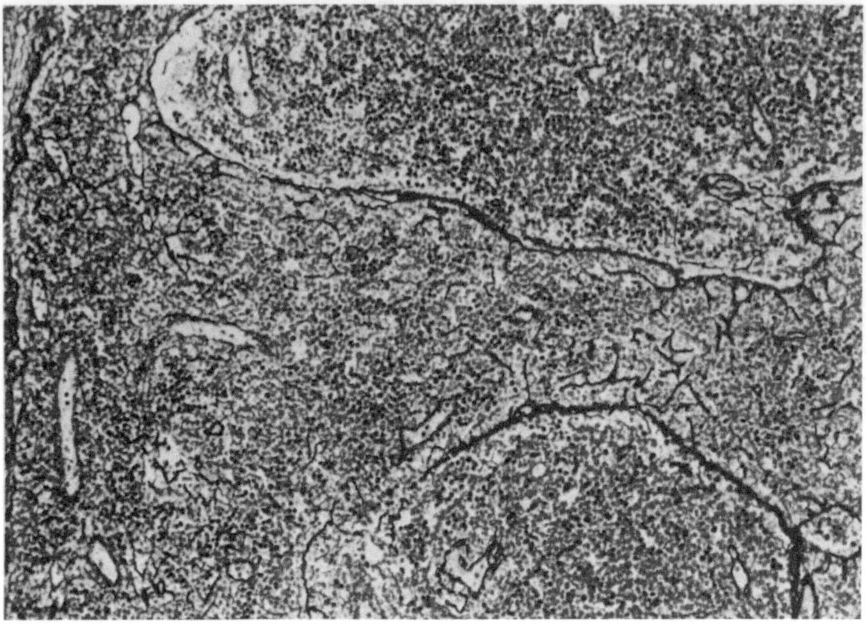

Fig. 207. ALL, unclassified (common type) with silver staining. Note the expanded, but not destroyed, trabecula and adjacent capsule, which in most parts are sharply demarcated from the sinuses and the infiltrated pulp. ♀, 4 years. Supraclavicular node. Gomori. ×140

pulpy. A section through the node discloses a light gray to gray-red tissue, occasionally flecked with small hemorrhages. Areas of necrosis are virtually never seen.

**Histology.** The histologic pictures correspond to those of the respective subtypes of lymphoblastic lymphoma. In contrast to the nonleukemic lymphomas, however, the capsule and trabeculae are massively infiltrated and expanded, but despite that are not destroyed (Fig. 207). The uniform leukemic infiltration of the lymph-node parenchyma is often sharply separated from the capsule and trabeculae by clefts, which are actually artifacts due to shrinkage. This criterion for leukemic variants of lymphoblastic lymphoma cannot be used for the convoluted-cell type. Furthermore, in that type even massive infiltration of veins by tumor cells does not denote a leukemic blood picture. Mitotic figures are usually abundant in all subtypes. The starry-sky pattern of Burkitt's tumor is rarely seen (Fig. 208). Reticulin fibers are always scanty and usually fine.

A number of reports in the literature maintain that the nuclear chromatin of the cells of ALL is finer and their nucleoli are smaller than the equivalent components of lymphoblastic sarcoma cells.[788] So far, however, we have been unable to distinguish with certainty ALL and unclassified lymphoblastic lymphoma on the basis of these cytologic criteria, particularly since we also find

[788] E.g., Rappaport, 1966; Wright, 1970b.

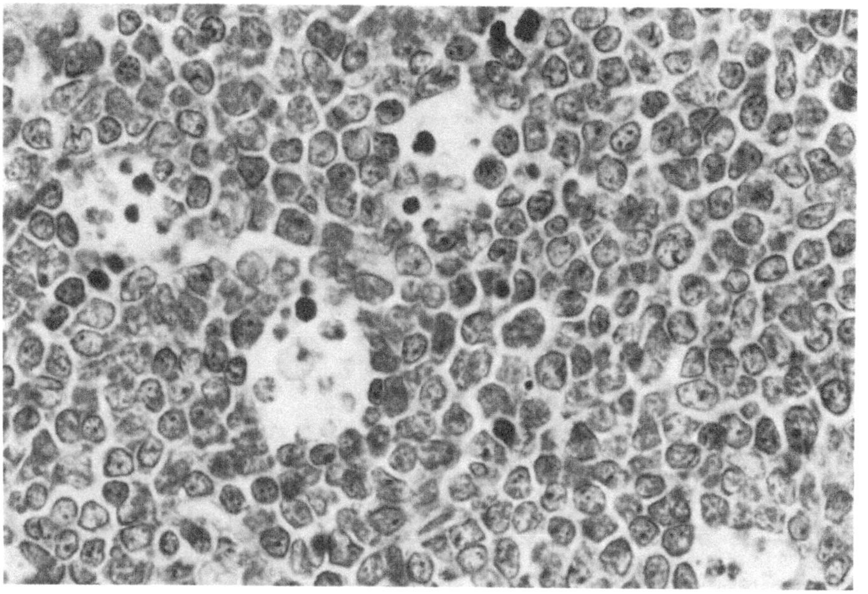

Fig. 208. ALL. Starry-sky pattern, but tumor cells are not cohesive. There is some similarity to the Burkitt type. Age, sex, and site of lymph node unknown. Giemsa. ×875

leukemias of medium-sized-cell types that have conspicuous nucleoli and a coarser chromatin than is usual.

If we roughly distinguish two subtypes of ALL according to the size of the cells, we find that about two thirds of the cases are of a relatively small-cell type and that the other third of the neoplasms are composed of medium-sized cells. Such a division of ALL into a small-cell type and a medium-sized-cell type merely indicates a general tendency. Not only are there transitional forms between the two types, but variations in cell size may also be seen in any given case. Only rarely are *all* the cells of a particular leukemia of a uniform size, either small or medium-sized. No correspondence exists between the cell size and a positive PAS reaction (see below); that is, the size of the cells is no indication of how the PAS reaction will behave.

**Smear/Imprint.** The cytology of a lymph-node smear or imprint (Fig. 209) corresponds to that of the three subtypes of lymphoblastic lymphoma.[789] When the cells are small, the chromatin is very fine and the nucleolus is barely visible. When the cells are medium-sized, the chromatin is coarser, the nucleoli are larger, and the rim of cytoplasm is broader. In all cells, regardless of size, the cytoplasm is more or less intensely basophilic.

**Histochemistry and Cytochemistry.** In a number of cases we found a diastase-sensitive positive *PAS reaction*, which could be demonstrated as granular depo-

[789] Cf., STEGAGNO, 1950.

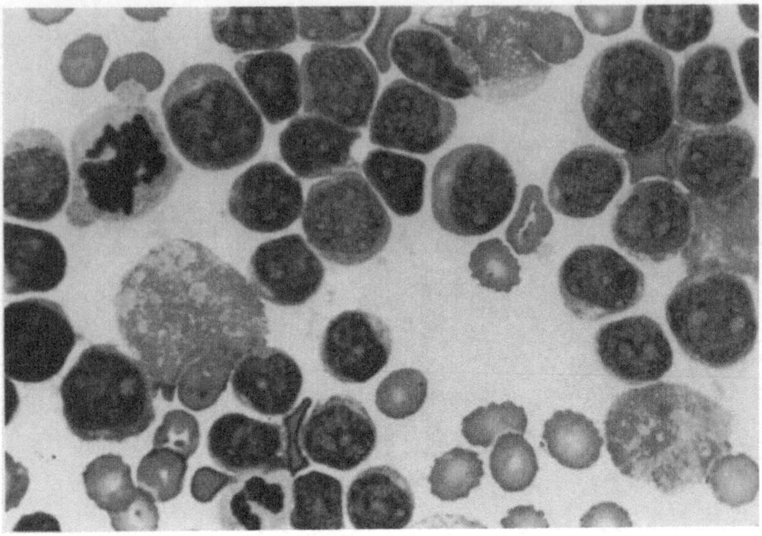

Fig. 209. ALL, unclassified. Bone-marrow smear. Note the multiple, distinct nucleoli and the moderately basophilic cytoplasm. Mitotic figure at the upper left. Some cell ghosts. ♀, 12 years. Pappenheim. × 1,250

sits only in imprints and cryostat sections. In electron-microscopic studies these deposits proved to be glycogen.[790] HAYHOE[791] described the PAS positivity as "coarse granularity or block deposits against a clear background." This type of positivity was said to be more important than the number of positive cells. According to HAYHOE *et al.*,[792] the blast-cell leukemias that are PAS-positive, but negative for fat and enzymes, should be regarded as lymphatic in type. LÖFFLER[793] used the term "PAS type" of acute leukemia for all those cases that revealed a granular or lumpy (diastase-sensitive) PAS reaction, but negative peroxidase and nonspecific esterase reactions. He differentiated this type from the (completely) undifferentiated leukemias that show neither positive PAS nor positive enzyme reactions. Among other characteristics, he based this classification on the differences in response to therapy.[794] The mean survival of children (20 patients) with the PAS type was about the same (376 days) as that of adults with the PAS type (15 patients, 364 days), and complete remissions were about equally frequent (90% and 87%, respectively). In contrast, the admittedly very rare cases of undifferentiated leukemia (four patients) showed a mean survival of 151 days and no complete remissions.

DESAGA *et al.*[795] said that they were able to confirm the lower proliferative activity of PAS-positive ALL after studies using short-term cultures and $^{3}$H-thymidine incubation. PAS-positive blast cells were found to show a significantly lower labeling index than PAS-negative blast cells.

790 MORI and LENNERT, 1969.

791 1969.

792 HAYHOE, QUAGLINO and DOLL, 1964.

793 1963, 1969a, b.

794 LÖFFLER, PRALLE, LÜCK, FISCHER *et al.*, 1973.

795 DESAGA, SCHMIDT, SCHMIDT-MENARD, LÜCK *et al.*, 1974.

Among the leukemias of childhood, BECKMANN *et al.*[796] also distinguish, in addition to the enzyme-positive blast-cell leukemias, a PAS type from the undifferentiated type.

LEDER[797] doubted whether a positive PAS reaction alone serves as sufficient proof for the lymphatic nature of a blast-cell leukemia. We[798] have also expressed our reluctance to consider the PAS type as a homogeneous entity. The great majority are probably of a lymphatic (or stem-cell?) nature—if the reactions for peroxidase and nonspecific esterase are performed and prove to be negative. There are certainly very immature myeloid leukemias, however, that are PAS-positive, but either cannot be recognized or can be identified only by electron-microscopic evidence of a small number of granules.

When using cytochemical methods for the diagnosis of acute leukemias, a practice that we, as well as FISCHER,[799] LEDER, LÖFFLER, and others, value highly,[800] a basic principle is that only definitely positive findings should be utilized. Above all, these methods include enzyme cytochemical reactions; each positive enzyme reaction, taken in conjunction with the degree and site of activity, yields specific information that is of significant diagnostic relevance. Enzyme-negative leukemias are ambiguous and, strictly speaking, should not be classified as *lymphatic* without further evidence. We should like to cite the following case as an example.

A 10-year-old boy first developed a tumor of the cranium, then a skin tumor, and finally infiltration of the bone marrow. All enzyme reactions and the PAS reaction were negative. Initially, the blood picture also disclosed no leukemic cells. After a period of 7 months, lymph nodes became enlarged. In these we were able to demonstrate both undifferentiated blast cells and numerous chloroacetate esterase-positive cells. Thus, we could establish unequivocally the myeloid nature of the neoplasm. Accordingly, the cells that appeared originally to be undifferentiated could be interpreted as myeloblasts or hemopoietic stem cells.

**Differences between ALL in Children and Adults.**[801] The main anatomic difference lies in the changes in the skeleton. As to be expected in the child, whose bones are growing and undergoing active remodeling, the skeleton reveals great changes when the marrow is infiltrated. Moreover, the infiltrates in nonhematopoietic organs, such as the kidneys, lungs, and gonads, are more extensive in the child.

Above all, it is said that therapy in children is more successful than in adults, probably because children tolerate higher doses of chemotherapeutic agents than adults do.[802]

**Diagnosis.** The lymph-node parenchyma is infiltrated by small to medium-sized cells that are moderately to strongly basophilic. The capsule and trabeculae

[796] BECKMANN, LANDBECK, NETH and SCHMIDTKE, 1971.

[797] 1970.

[798] MORI and LENNERT, 1969.

[799] E.g., FISCHER, LORBACHER and KÄUFER, 1964.

[800] Also HERTL, 1963, 1966; GORDON, 1974; KURZ and HAAS, 1974; BENNETT and REED, 1975.

[801] GUNZ and HOUGH, 1956; OEHME, 1957; OEHME, JANSSEN and HAGITTE, 1958; HERTL and LANDBECK, 1969, LENNERT and MOHRI, 1971, Lit.

[802] JACQUILLAT, WEIL, GEMON, AUCLERC *et al.*, 1973; GEE, HAGHBIN, DOWLING, CUNNINGHAM *et al.*, 1976.

show widespread infiltration and expansion. Clinically, there is often generalized enlargement of lymph nodes, hepatosplenomegaly, and leukemic infiltration of the bone marrow. The blood picture shows at least 1% blast cells. Smears in many cases reveal a fine to coarse, granular PAS reaction. With the exception of the convoluted-cell type, ALL reveals either a negative acid phosphatase reaction or only a few, very fine, positive granules. In smears the reactions for peroxidase, chloroacetate esterase, and nonspecific esterase are negative. In sections the chloroacetate esterase reaction is also negative in the blast cells.

**Differential Diagnosis.** The subject is discussed under the various types of lymphoblastic lymphoma, particularly the unclassified type (p. 406ff.).

**Prognosis.** Until a few years ago, the prognosis of ALL was very poor. This type of leukemia was classed as an "acute leukemia." In 1964, ROATH *et al.*[804] published a review of cases in Manchester. The mean survival for patients treated until 1950 was only 2.85 months, for those treated between 1950 and 1955 it was 4.3 months, and for those treated between 1956 and 1963 it was 7.0 months. CUTLER *et al.*[805] in America reported similar data on their large series of patients.

In the meantime, the situation has continued to improve.[806] Through the introduction of new treatment regimes and the systematic evaluation of their efficacy by PINKEL[807] and by other leukemia centers and study groups, the number of long-lasting remissions has undoubtedly been greatly increased. The number of cures, formerly extremely small, has also risen. PINKEL and coworkers[808] succeeded in reaching a 7-year cure rate of 17% of their children with ALL; all of these patients were no longer under treatment, some for as long as 5 years. Similarly good results have been reported by many other groups, e.g., RIEHM *et al.*[808a] and WINKLER *et al.*[808b] Consequently, ALL has lost some of the feeling of absolute hopelessness and inevitable fate that characterized it for so long.

JACQUILLAT *et al.*[808c] reported that their program of therapy produced more frequent complete remissions in patients under 15 years of age and in females than in patients older than 15 and in males. The median duration of remission was 34 months for the younger patients and 11 months for the older ones. In addition, the prognosis depends on the initial leukocyte counts[809] and on the dose of medication needed to produce a complete remission. The prognosis is worse for patients with massive hepatosplenomegaly[809] or widespread involvement of the viscera,[809] and for Negro children.[810] Finally, the medium-sized-cell

[804] ROATH, ISRAËLS and WILKINSON, 1964.
[805] CUTLER, AXTELL and HEISE, 1967; see also WOLFF, BRUBAKER, MURPHY, PIERCE *et al.*, 1967.
[806] O'GORMAN HUGHES, 1974.
[807] 1971; AUR and PINKEL, 1973.
[808] AUR and PINKEL, 1973.
[808a] RIEHM, GADNER and WELTE, 1977.
[808b] WINKLER, GAEDICKE, GROSCH-WÖRNER, MARSMANN *et al.*, 1977.
[808c] JACQUILLAT, WEIL, GEMON, AUCLERC *et al.*, 1973; GEE, HAGHBIN, DOWLING, CUNNINGHAM *et al.*, 1976.
[809] Also WOLFF, BRUBAKER, MURPHY, PIERCE *et al.*, 1967; HENDERSON, 1969.
[810] HOLTON, VIETTI, NORA, DONALDSON *et al.*, 1969.

type seems to have a poorer prognosis than the small-cell type.[811] The PAS-positive leukemias are also said to respond more favorably to therapy than PAS-negative ALL.[812]

## C. Malignant Lymphoma, Immunoblastic (Immunoblastic Sarcoma)

*Synonyms:* Reticulosarcoma and numerous synonyms of reticulosarcoma (see p. 451 ff.)

**History and Terminology.** The history of M.L. immunoblastic is chiefly that of reticulosarcoma (see p. 452 ff.). In 1966, we[813] first presented the term immunoblastic sarcoma for discussion, having found abundant rough endoplasmic reticulum in a basophilic large-cell lymphoma on electron microscopy. We suggested the term at the Lymphoma Conference in Nagoya again in 1971, after demonstrating abundant IgM in the tumor homogenates of four so-called reticulosarcomas studied jointly with STEIN and KAISERLING. LUKES and COLLINS[814] were the first to accept this term and described the morphology of the tumor in detail.

For understandable reasons, our new interpretation of "reticulosarcoma" as "immunoblastic sarcoma" was at first received with astonishment and skepticism. In particular, the analysis of Ig in tissue homogenates[815] was not considered to provide sufficient proof. We have not based our conclusions only on the analysis of Ig in tissue homogenates, however, and in 1974 we set down in detail our arguments supporting the interpretation of reticulosarcoma as an immunoblastic sarcoma.[816]

As a rule, immunoblastic sarcomas revealing a great increase in Ig in the tumor tissue and/or blood are derived from B-immunoblasts, i.e., transformed B-lymphocytes, or from precursors of the plasma-cell series ("plasmablasts"). Indeed, it is not unusual to find signs of plasmacytic differentiation on light and electron microscopy.

Immunoblastic sarcomas that do not show significant increases in tissue Ig might well be very anaplastic tumors of the same B-immunoblasts. Theoretically, however, they might be derived from T-immunoblasts. Finally, we cannot in principle exclude the possibility that anaplastic reticulum cells can assume a morphology similar to that of immunoblasts.

In 1974, LUKES briefly reported on two immunoblastic sarcomas that he thought to be of T-cell origin. He found that the tumor cells had $\beta$-glucuronidase activity and regarded that as an important indication of their T-cell nature. We have observed a basophilic large-cell sarcoma in the terminal stage of a

---

811 RIND, 1969; BOIRON, JACQUILLAT and LÉVY, 1970.

812 LÖFFLER, PRALLE, LÜCK, FISCHER *et al.*, 1973, 1974; DESAGA, SCHMIDT, SCHMIDT-MENARD, LÜCK *et al.*, 1974; FELDGES, AUR, VERZOSA and DANIELS, 1974.

813 LENNERT, 1967.

814 1974a, b, 1975a, b.

815 STEIN, LENNERT and PARWARESCH, 1972; STEIN, KAISERLING and LENNERT, 1973.

816 STEIN, KAISERLING and LENNERT, 1974a, b.

case of mycosis fungoides. This sarcoma did not differ morphologically from other immunoblastic sarcomas, and it is possible that it was a T-immunoblastic sarcoma. The cells of another tumor with the same morphology formed almost exclusively sheep-E rosettes and did not bear surface Ig.[816a] Therefore, we can be sure that there are T-immunoblastic sarcomas, but that they are much rarer than B-immunoblastic sarcomas. Such cases have to be substantiated, above all by demonstrating specific T-cell markers.

More recently, RAPPAPORT and BRAYLAN[817] and SELIGMANN[817a] have also demonstrated immunoblastic lymphomas of B- and T-types in immunologic studies and have therefore revised the old concept of histiocytic lymphoma. The cases described in the literature, however, are not morphologically uniform. Some of the so-called T-immunoblastic sarcomas might belong to our group of T-zone lymphomas. It is still too early to make a final statement about such T-cell-derived cases.

From the numerous case reports published previously in the literature, the existence of B-immunoblastic sarcomas could have been predicted long ago. Time and again papers appeared describing malignant lymphomas, especially "reticulosarcomas," in cases of macroglobulinemia of Waldenström and multiple myeloma,[818] either combined from the beginning, or the former tumors developed in the course of the latter diseases. In his report on 420 malignant immunocytomas with a monoclonal increase in serum Ig, HOBBS[819] mentioned six "reticulosarcomas (including five atypical Hodgkin's)."

The occurrence of "reticulosarcomas" during chronic immune disorders,[820] such as Sjögren's syndrome,[821] or in patients treated with immunosuppressives after organ transplantation,[822] in patients treated with diphenylhydantoin,[823] in immune-deficiency syndromes,[824] and in graft-versus-host reactions[825] is also more readily explained if, in all such cases, we assume that the tumors are derived from immunologically active and proliferating cells and not from reticulum cells.

We describe M.L. immunoblastic below, basing our account chiefly on the experience we have had in studying definite cases of this lymphoma by means of cytologic, electron-microscopic, and immunologic methods. The statistical data on the occurrence, etc., of immunoblastic lymphoma are not yet ample enough. We commit only a small error, however, when we extrapolate the data we have now accumulated to our earlier cases, which we studied chiefly

---

[816a] This case was kindly shown to us and published by OEHMICHEN, GÄRTNER and KNITTEL-JUNG, 1977.

[817] 1975.

[817a] 1975.

[818] SCHAUB, 1952; HEUCHEL and EITNER, 1954; MIELKE, 1956; AZAR, HILL and OSSERMAN, 1957; BRECHER, TANAKA, MALMGREN and FAHEY, 1963; KRAUSS and SOKAL, 1966; OKANO, AZAR and OSSERMAN, 1966; WALDENSTRÖM, 1968; MICHAUX and HEREMANS, 1969; MOORE, MIGLIORE, SHULLENBERGER and ALEXANIAN, 1970; BRAUN, BRUCHHAUS and ALY, 1973; KIM, HELLER and RAPPAPORT, 1973.

[819] 1971.

[820] MILLER, 1967b; JONES, 1973.

[821] TALAL and BUNIM, 1964; TALAL, SOKOLOFF and BARTH, 1967.

[822] E.g., PENN, HALGRIMSON and STARZL, 1971; KRÜGER, 1972; PENN and STARZL, 1972; REIS, 1972; BROWN, SCHIFF and MITCHELL, 1974.

[823] LI, WILLARD, GOODMAN and VAWTER, 1975.

[824] MILLER, 1967a; KRÜGER, 1972; WALDMANN, STROBER and BLAESE, 1972; BRUCE and BLAESE, 1974; COTTIER, HESS, KELLER, LUSCIETI *et al.*, 1974; HEIDELBERGER and LEGOLVAN, 1974.

[825] GRUNDMANN and HOBIK, 1973.

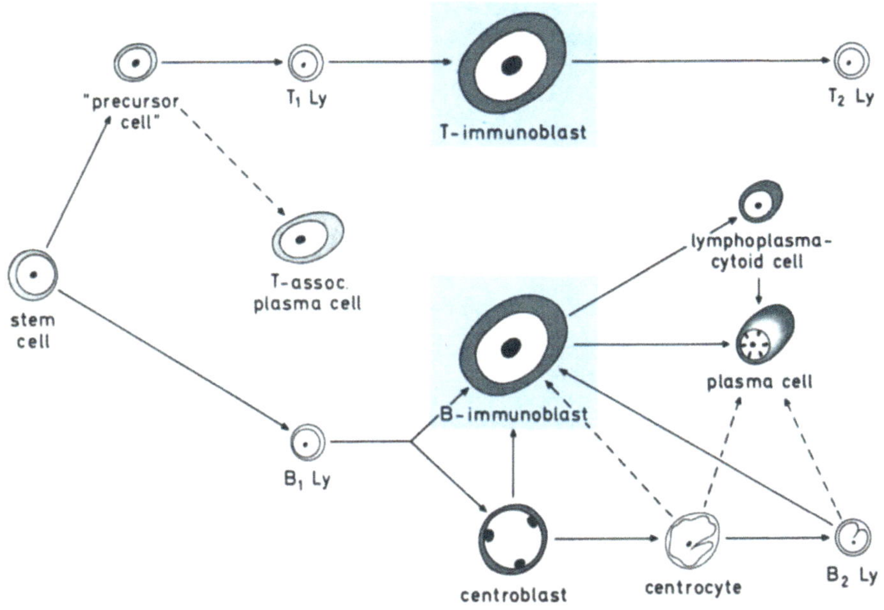


Fig. 210. Hypothetical origin of tumor cells of M.L. immunoblastic. Dark blue: pure T- and B-immunoblastic types. Light blue: differentiation of plasma-cell series seen in some cases of B-immunoblastic lymphoma

with cytologic and histologic methods, and include the cases diagnosed previously as reticulosarcoma. Likewise, we may utilize the data from the literature for calculating the incidence of immunoblastic lymphoma. We may start by taking the figures given for reticulosarcoma, since most cases probably represent immunoblastic lymphomas. It soon becomes evident, however, that such calculations contain large errors when we begin to make comparisons, e.g., between age distribution curves (Fig. 211). The definition of reticulosarcoma has always been unsatisfactory and in no way uniform.

**Origin of the Tumor Cells.** From the meager data provided in the recent literature, it appears that there are both immunoblastic lymphomas derived from the B-cell series[826] (SIg- and/or CIg-positive) and those derived from the T-cell series[827] (sheep-E rosette-positive; Fig. 210). According to SELIGMANN *et al.*,[828] about 50–60% of immunoblastic lymphomas are derived from B-cells, less than 10% are derived from T-cells, and about 30% apparently show no surface markers. That does not mean, however, that the negative tumor cells are not immunoblasts, since the cells might be so anaplastic that they lack both B- and T-antigens.[827] Furthermore, we may assume that a small proportion of the "immuno-

[826] STEIN, KAISERLING and LENNERT, 1974 a; MATHÉ, BELPOMME, DANTCHEV, KHALIL *et al.*, 1975; BROUET, PREUD'HOMME, FLANDRIN, CHELLOUL *et al.*, 1976.

[827] MATHÉ, BELPOMME, DANTCHEV, KHALIL *et al.*, 1975; BROUET, PREUD'HOMME, FLANDRIN CHELLOUL *et al.*, 1976.

[828] SELIGMANN, BROUET and PREUD'HOMME, 1977.

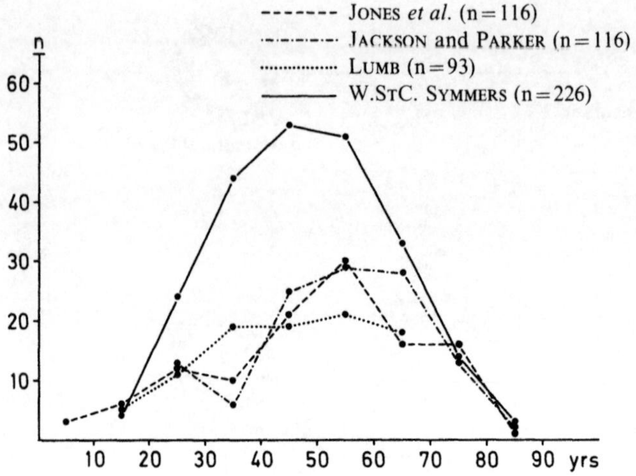


Fig. 211. Age distribution of four reticulosarcoma series given in the literature: JONES, FUKS, BULL, KADIN *et al.* (1973); JACKSON and PARKER (1947); LUMB (1954); and W.STC. SYMMERS (1958)

blastic lymphomas" were in fact undifferentiated carcinomas, e.g., lymphoepithelial carcinoma (nasopharyngeal carcinoma), because it is sometimes very difficult to distinguish these neoplasms from immunoblastic lymphoma. Indeed, that was the reason we started our immunologic analyses of malignant lymphomas. In the first case we studied, we could not decide whether the tumor was a lymphoepithelial carcinoma or a "blastic" lymphoid neoplasm. Ig analysis of the tumor revealed a very large amount of IgM; thus, we interpreted it as an immunoblastic lymphoma. We therefore realize that, without special techniques, it may be impossible to distinguish immunoblastic lymphoma from lymphoepithelial carcinoma. Finally, immunologic analysis has also uncovered a few cases of true reticulosarcoma in which the cells were able to phagocytose and to form EA rosettes.[829]

According to the results of our studies, the B-immunoblastic lymphomas appear to predominate, even if one takes out the EAC-positive tumors containing centroblasts (see p. 346 ff.). In any event, the immunoblastic lymphomas with plasmablastic and/or plasmacytic differentiation, which reveal rough endoplasmic reticulum on electron microscopy, are definitely B-immunoblastic lymphomas. The cells of immunoblastic lymphomas without plasmablastic and/or plasmacytic differentiation and without centroblasts may be B- or T-immunoblasts or undefinable immunoblasts ("null immunoblasts").

**Occurrence.** Among every 1000 lymph-node biopsies in our first series, about 15 fulfilled our morphologic criteria for immunoblastic lymphoma. This means that about 9.0% of our malignant lymphomas and about 15.9% of our non-Hodgkin's lymphomas were immunoblastic lymphomas (Table 82). We were able to define the immunoblastic lymphomas in our second series more precisely because of the better definition by immunologic techniques. Some of the cases

[829] E.g., HABESHAW and STUART, 1975.

Table 82. M.L. immunoblastic. Material and incidence

| | | |
|---|---|---|
| Total No. of cases | 193 | |
| Biopsy | | 187 |
| Autopsy | | 6 |
| Total No. of biopsies | 223 | |
| Lymph nodes | | 193 |
| Extranodal | | 30 |
| Incidence in routine lymph-node material | | 134 |
| = 9.0% of malignant lymphomas | | |
| 15.9% of non-Hodgkin's lymphomas | | |

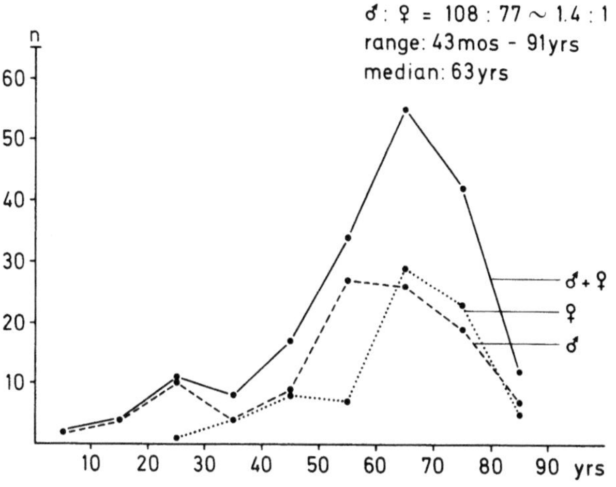


Fig. 212. Age distribution and sex ratio of M.L. immunoblastic. 185 patients of our first series

originally classified as immunoblastic lymphomas are now listed under M.L. centroblastic. Thus, the percentage of immunoblastic lymphomas has been lowered to 10.3% of non-Hodgkin's lymphomas.

From these figures and our previous inquiry in Schleswig-Holstein, we calculated the morbidity rate for immunoblastic lymphoma in Northern Germany to be 0.4–0.5/100,000 inhabitants per year.[830]

Figure 212 presents the age distribution. A sharp peak is found in the 7th decade, although it applies only to women (and to both sexes together), whereas men appear to be affected somewhat more commonly in the 6th decade. Our youngest patient was 43 months old; our oldest, 91 years old. Immunoblastic lymphomas in childhood and adolescence are extremely rare. That the curve shown does not reflect the true morbidity rate for the various ages is evident from our survey in Schleswig-Holstein:[830] we compared the number of cases of reticulosarcoma to the number of inhabitants in the different age groups and found that, relative to age, the highest incidence of reticulosarcoma is in the 8th and 9th decades.

[830] Lennert, 1969b.

Table 83. Incidence of reticulosarcoma (and immunoblastic lymphoma) in various countries

| Author | Country | Percentage of lymphomas | | Percentage of non-Hodgkin's lymphomas | |
|---|---|---|---|---|---|
| LUMB, 1954 | Great Britain | | | | |
| reticulosarcoma | | 5.6 | 22.5 | 10.5 | 45.7 |
| anaplastic sarcoma | | 16.9 | | 35.2 | |
| LUMB and NEWTON, 1957 | USA | | | | |
| reticulosarcoma | | 7.7 | 17.0 | – | |
| anaplastic sarcoma | | 9.3 | | | |
| SYMMERS, 1958 | Great Britain | 26.2 | | 47.1 | |
| ROSENBERG *et al.*, 1961 | USA | – | | 43.6 | |
| KIMURA, 1964 | Japan | 55 | | – | |
| DESAI *et al.*, 1965 | India | 14 | | – | |
| TALERMAN, 1970 | Jamaica | 14.2 | | – | |
| KAHN, 1972 | South Africa | 20 | | – | |
| AKAZAKI, 1973 | Japan | | | | |
| Japan Lymphoma Study Group | | 66.8[a] | | – | |
| Aichi Cancer Center | | 74.8[a] | | – | |
| JONES *et al.*, 1973 | USA | | | | |
| histiocytic | | – | | 28.7 | 32.2 |
| undifferentiated | | – | | 3.5 | |
| Our first series (immunoblastic lymphoma) | West Germany | 9.0 | | 15.9 | |

[a] Autopsies and biopsies. All other values are based on biopsies

The disease is slightly more prevalent in males. The male-to-female ratio is 1.4:1.

If we compare the frequency of "reticulosarcoma" in various countries and as reported by various investigators, then the range of variation proves to be broad (see Table 83). So-called reticulosarcomas, including the poorly differentiated and anaplastic sarcomas, constitute between 9% and 75% of all malignant lymphomas, and between 16% and 47% of the non-Hodgkin's lymphomas. At the top of the list is Japan, where low-grade malignant lymphomas (B-CLL, follicular lymphoma, lymphocytic lymphosarcoma) and Hodgkin's disease are much rarer than in Europe or the United States.

The morbidity or mortality rate according to the world literature lies between 1 and 3 cases per 100,000 inhabitants per year (in contrast to 0.5 in our material). In Japan the rate is only one-third higher than that of the United States. This indicates that the lymphomas of low-grade malignancy just mentioned, including Hodgkin's disease, have a lower incidence in the United States than in white races elsewhere. Reticulosarcoma appears to be less common in Negroes,[831] although the figures of KAHN[832] seem to suggest otherwise. For South Africa he calculated a white-to-black ratio of 1.3:1.

A comparison of the age curves clearly reveals just how much the definition of reticulosarcoma varies among the different large series reported in the literature. Figure 211 presents the age distribution calculated from data supplied by JACKSON and PARKER,[833] LUMB,[834] W.StC. SYMMERS,[835] and JONES *et al.*[836]

We find the same variation in the statistics covering the sex distribution. Although all indicate that the male sex is affected more frequently, the male-to-female ratios vary from 3:1 to 1.2:1.

[831] ROSENBERG, DIAMOND, JASLOWITZ and CRAVER, 1961.
[832] 1972.
[833] 1947.
[834] 1954.
[835] 1958.
[836] JONES, FUKS, BULL, KADIN *et al.*, 1973.

**Clinical Manifestations.** On the basis of 20 cases of immunoblastic lymphoma, MATHÉ *et al.*[837] presented the clinical picture of this tumor. They were convinced that this lymphoma is a characteristic clinical entity. In 85% of the cases, the patients were men. Eight patients came from Central America. Two patients had a previous history of chronic rheumatoid arthritis. In 10 patients the disease was already in stage IV at the first presentation. Twelve patients showed involvement of deep (mediastinal or abdominal) lymph nodes. Eight out of 13 patients had hypogammaglobulinemia. Chemotherapy like that used in other "lymphosarcomas" did not lead to remission in six out of 15 cases. The prognosis was poorer than for other "lymphosarcomas" (median survival for all stages: 8 months). The tumor led to death after conversion into a leukemia (nine out of 20 patients) or because of infiltration of vital organs (brain, kidney).

The earlier literature on the clinical features of "reticulosarcoma" includes a review by JACKSON and PARKER,[838] to which the reader may wish to refer.

Among the clinical data, the *blood protein values* are of particular interest. In a small number of immunoblastic lymphomas there is a monoclonal increase in serum Ig.[839] Usually IgM is increased, occasionally IgA or IgG. In the cases we studied with STEIN and KAISERLING,[840] we found in two a monoclonal increase in serum IgM, whereas the serum IgM values were normal or below normal in most cases. The monoclonal increase in Ig in the blood is, however, only the tip of the iceberg. Although the levels of IgM in tumor homogenates of about two thirds of our immunoblastic sarcomas were considerably increased, the IgM was not secreted into the blood. That might have been related to disturbances in the production mechanism. For example, in some cases only the monomer 8 S IgM and not the pentamer 19 S IgM was formed. That perhaps impeded the secretion of the IgM into the blood.

In addition to these tumors, which we studied with immunologic and electron-microscopic methods, there were among our total of 220 cases in recent years four further cases that revealed a monoclonal increase in serum Ig. These lymphomas all showed plasmablastic/plasmacytic differentiation. Two were associated with an increase in IgM and the other two with a monoclonal increase in IgG in the blood.

From our own studies we estimate that the frequency of paraproteinemia in immunoblastic lymphoma is between 5 and 10%.

**Stage of Disease When First Diagnosed.** Of the 116 patients with diffuse histiocytic lymphoma studied by JONES *et al.*,[841] at the time therapy was started 11.2% were in stage I (9 in I, 4 in $I_E$), 32.8% were in stage II (20 in II, 18 in $II_E$), 17.2% in stage III (18 in III, 2 in $III_E$), and 38.8% in stage IV. Of the patients in stages II–IV, 27.6% presented with constitutional symptoms (fever of unknown origin, night sweats). Poorly differentiated lymphoma was diagnosed in stage I in three patients, in stage II in two patients, and in stage IV in nine patients.

---

[837] MATHÉ, BELPOMME, DANTCHEV, KHALIL *et al.*, 1975.

[838] 1947; cf., MUNDT, 1952; MIELKE, 1956; SCHEURLEN and SCHWARZ, 1973.

[839] SCHAUB, 1952; HEUCHEL and EITNER, 1954; MIELKE, 1956; AZAR, HILL and OSSERMAN, 1957; KRAUSS and SOKAL, 1966; OKANO, AZAR and OSSERMAN, 1966; WALDENSTRÖM, 1968; MICHAUX and HEREMANS, 1969; MOORE, MIGLIORE, SHULLENBERGER and ALEXANIAN, 1970; BRAUN, BRUCHHAUS and ALY, 1973; KIM, HELLER and RAPPAPORT, 1973.

[840] STEIN, KAISERLING and LENNERT, 1974a.

[841] JONES, FUKS, BULL, KADIN *et al.*, 1973.

Table 84. Localization of biopsies of M.L. immunoblastic

| Localization | n | | % | |
|---|---|---|---|---|
| Lymph nodes | 193 | | 86.5 | |
| Cervical | | 89 | | 50.6 |
| Axillary | | 40 | | 22.7 |
| Mediastinal | | 2 | | 1.1 |
| Abdominal | | 5 | | 2.8 |
| Inguinal | | 40 | | 22.7 |
| Cubital | | — | | — |
| Unknown | | 17 | | — |
| Extranodal | 30 | | 13.5 | |
| Tonsils | | 12 | | — |
| Stomach and intestine | | 4 | | — |
| Skin and subcutis | | 10 | | — |
| Others | | 4 | | — |

Involvement of the gastrointestinal tract was diagnosed before therapy in 24% of the patients with histiocytic lymphoma and in 43% of the patients with poorly differentiated tumors. In contrast, only 9% of the patients with histiocytic lymphomas and none of those with the undifferentiated type initially showed infiltration of the bone marrow.

In the series reported by JONES *et al.*[842] the mediastinum was involved from the beginning in 25.2% of the patients with (diffuse) histiocytic lymphoma, whereas the mediastinum was bypassed in 16%, i.e., the tumor involved the upper para-aortic and lower cervical lymph nodes, but avoided the mediastinal lymph nodes. Ninety-three percent of the histiocytic lymphomas spread by continuous infiltration. The number of observations made of *un*differentiated lymphomas was too small to allow a statistical analysis.

**Blood Picture.** Besides the nonspecific changes occurring in the blood picture, reports indicate that cells of "reticulosarcoma" may appear in the blood. It is not so uncommon to find a few tumor cells in the blood, particularly in leukocyte concentrates.[843] A pronounced leukemic blood picture develops only rarely (see *Addendum*, p. 448). JACKSON and PARKER[844] described a fulminating acute leukemia that appeared in a patient with reticulosarcoma of the breast. SHIMOYAMA and MIKUNI[845] observed leukemic transformation in 13% of their patients with reticulosarcoma. They said that it generally appeared in preterminal stages. In our material we found that 4.7% of the cases (5 out of 107 patients) were associated with leukemic or subleukemic blood pictures. One of these five cases was a leukemic immunocytoma with secondary M.L. immunoblastic.

**Localization.** In our collection of 176 lymph-node biopsies of known localization, one half (50.6%) came from the neck. Most of the others came from the axillary and inguinal regions (22.7% each), whereas abdominal and mediastinal lymph nodes were rarely removed for study (2.8% and 1.1%, respectively; Table 84). Of the extranodal sources, 12 biopsies were from the tonsils and ten from the skin and subcutis. Four biopsies came from the gastrointestinal tract. There were single instances of biopsies from numerous other organs.

[842] JONES, FUKS, BULL, KADIN *et al.*, 1973.
[843] E.g., DA SILVA PARREIRA and SALVIDIO, 1952.
[844] 1947.
[845] 1973.

Table 85. Involvement of various lymph-node regions and organs in the course of 102 cases of reticulosarcoma according to JACKSON and PARKER, 1947

| Organ | n | |
|---|---|---|
| Superficial lymph nodes | 71 | |
| Mediastinal lymph nodes | 15 | |
| Pharynx (especially tonsils) | 33 | |
| Gastrointestinal tract | 23 | |
| Stomach | | 10 |
| Spleen | 15 | |
| Bone | 15 | |
| Skin | 13 | |
| Liver | 10 | |
| Nervous system | 10 | |
| Lungs | 7 | |
| Breasts | 5 | |
| Urogenital tract | 2 | |
| Thyroid gland | 1 | |

Table 86. Frequency of localization of reticulosarcoma in the thorax according to ROSENBERG *et al.*, 1961

| Localization | Initial involvement % | Clinical total % | Involvement at autopsy % |
|---|---|---|---|
| Mediastinal and bronchopulmonary lymph nodes | 3.4 | 33.9 | 56.6 |
| Lung parenchyma | 0.4 | 24.3 | 45.3 |
| Pleura | 0.4 | 27.6 | 14.7 |

JACKSON and PARKER[846] have provided detailed information on the involvement of the different organs and lymph-node regions by reticulosarcoma. In their study of 102 patients they recorded the distribution of organ and lymph-node involvement shown in Table 85. The frequency of thoracic involvement found by ROSENBERG *et al.*[846a] is given in Table 86.

**Gross Appearance.** The lymph nodes are often greatly enlarged. They vary from moderately firm to pulpy. The freshly sectioned tissue is gray-red to gray-white. Necrosis and hemorrhages are rare.[847] The lymph nodes are firmly adherent to one another.

**Histology.** With Giemsa staining the majority of cells are large to very large and intensely basophilic. Their usually oval or round nuclei contain very large basophilic nucleoli. These nucleoli are mostly solitary; but sometimes there are two or three medium-sized or large nucleoli that generally lie in the center of the nucleus and not at the nuclear membrane. The chromatin is clearly coarser and more intensely stained than that of macrophages. The nuclear membrane stains deep blue. The rim of cytoplasm is narrow to moder-

[846] 1947.

[846a] ROSENBERG, DIAMOND, JASLOWITZ and CRAVER, 1961.

[847] RÖSSLE, 1939; W.STC. SYMMERS, 1958.

ately broad, only rarely broad. With Giemsa staining it is usually basophilic or strongly basophilic, colored bluc or sometimes blue-violet (like that of plasma cells). Mitotic figures usually abound.

In many cases the basophilic cells are present in "pure culture," often forming cohesive cell clusters. Mono- or polynuclear giant cells are found only occasionally. In rare cases (2 out of 185), however, we found numerous giant cells; thus, the picture resembled what one previously would certainly have called Hodgkin's sarcoma. Occasionally, the anisocytosis of the tumor cells is considerable. In such instances the smaller cells of the tumor may show a nuclear chromatin structure and cytoplasmic features that are somewhat reminiscent of plasma cells.

In addition to such plasma cell-like forms, but more frequently, a larger number of tumor cells reveal a plasmablastic aspect. The rim of cytoplasm is relatively broad and displaced more to one side of the nucleus. It contains vacuoles and an enlarged Golgi body (light perinuclear halo). The nuclei are much larger than those of plasma cells and have multiple, medium-sized or large nucleoli that in general do not lie at the nuclear membrane. Cells in imprints of this tumor variant display a morphology like that known for the plasmablasts of reactive lymph nodes. On electron microscopy, the cells have moderately abundant to abundant rough endoplasmic reticulum. We call tumors with this morphology "immunoblastic lymphomas with plasmablastic differentiation." In 26.7% of our cases we found slight plasmablastic differentiation and in 14.4% it was well developed, so we referred to these cases at first as "plasmablastic sarcomas."[848]

As mentioned in the chapter on centroblastic lymphoma, our group of immunoblastic lymphomas originally contained a number of cases that revealed some or numerous centroblasts and centrocytes in addition to immunoblasts (see p. 346).

We now distinguish the following variants of immunoblastic lymphoma:

1. Immunoblastic with plasmablastic or plasmacytic differentiation (Figs. 213–216).

2. Purely immunoblastic without plasmablastic or plasmacytic differentiation (Figs. 217–219).

Whereas the second variant may be of either B- or T-cell origin, the first variant is of B-cell origin without exception.

The following description of the histologic features of immunoblastic lymphoma is given without regard to the specific cytologic subtype. The data given in this account apply to our original series of immunoblastic lymphomas, which contained a number of cases that showed germinal-center cells and that are now included in the group of centroblastic lymphomas (see p. 346).

A few *macrophages* can always be found among the basophilic tumor cells of immunoblastic lymphoma (Table 87). In a few cases (5.4%) the macrophages are extremely numerous. They usually contain remnants of phagocytosed tumor cells. Only rarely does a starry sky-like pattern develop like that in Burkitt's tumor.

---

[848] See also LENNERT, 1967; MORI and LENNERT, 1969.

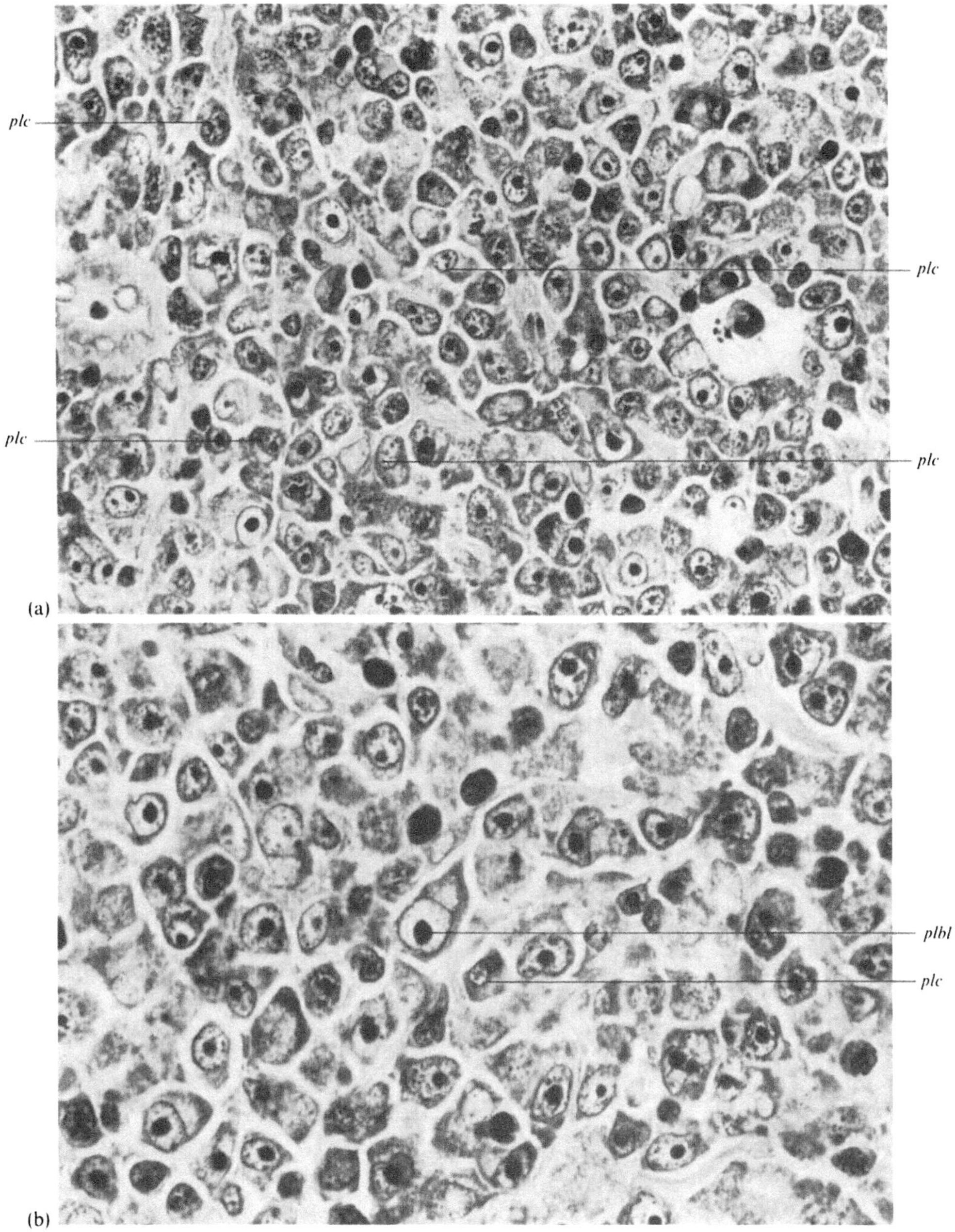


Fig. 213a and b. M.L. immunoblastic with plasmacytic differentiation. The immunoblasts are large and contain solitary large central nucleoli of high basophilia. Note a very large plasmablastoid cell (*plbl*) with a large perinuclear halo (Golgi body). Some plasmacytoid cells (*plc*). ♂, 42 years. Supraclavicular node. Giemsa. (a) ×560, (b) ×875

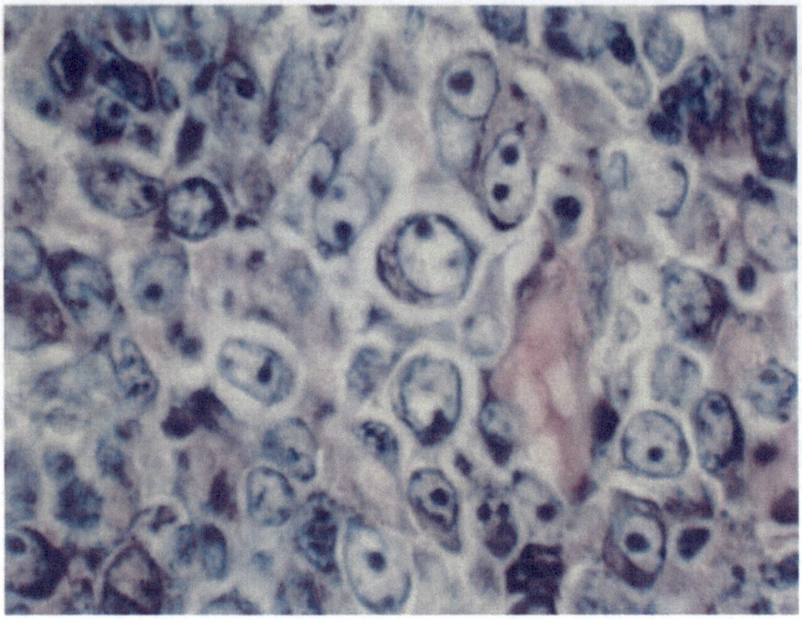

Fig. 214. M.L. immunoblastic with plasmablastic differentiation with Giemsa staining. One or two large central basophilic nucleoli. Cytoplasm is strongly basophilic with a violet tinge and some lighter areas representing Golgi bodies, etc. ♀, 67 years. Cervical node. ×1,550

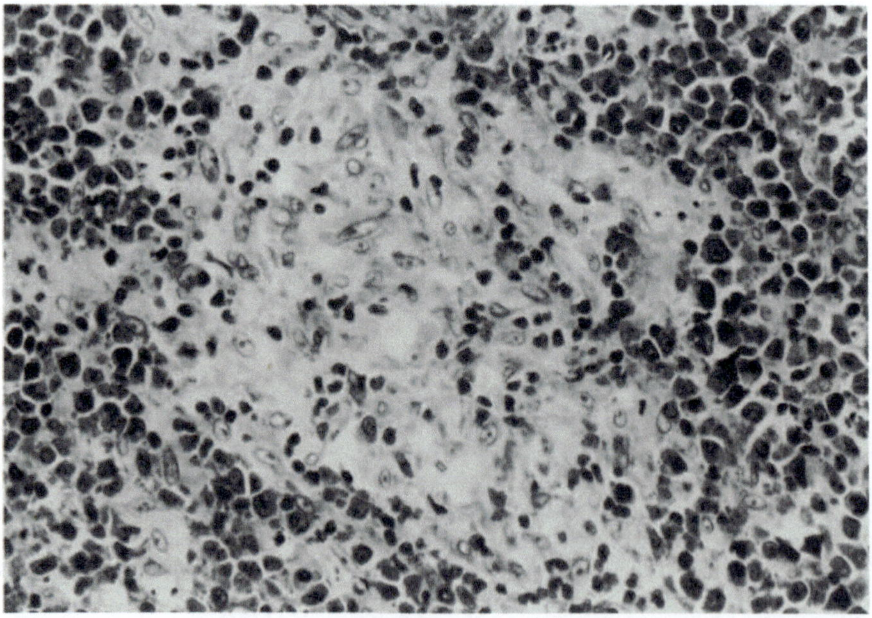

Fig. 215. M.L. immunoblastic with plasmablastic differentiation and epithelioid-cell cluster. Note the difference in staining between the oxyphilic epithelioid cells and the basophilic tumor cells around them. ♂, 75 years. Axillary node. Giemsa. ×350

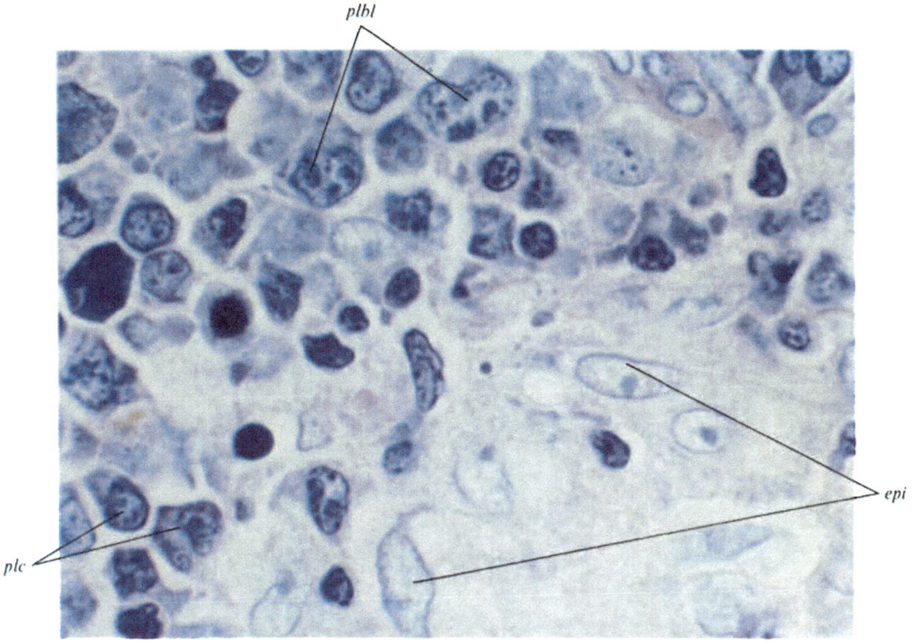


Fig. 216. M.L. immunoblastic with plasmacytic differentiation and part of an epithelioid-cell cluster. Giemsa staining. At the top and on the left, basophilic tumor cells, including plasmablasts (*plbl*) and plasmacytoid cells (*plc*). The cytoplasm of epithelioid cells (*epi*) is oxyphilic. Their nuclei show a fine chromatin and a large nonbasophilic nucleolus. The nuclear membrane is stained more gray-blue, in contrast to the blue of tumor cells and intermingled lymphocytes. Same slide as Fig. 215. ×1,550

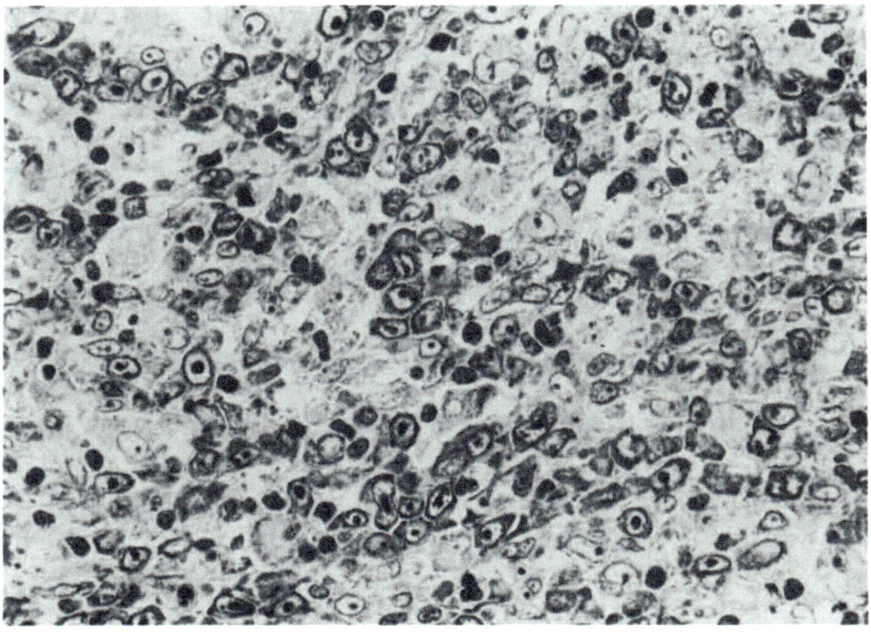

Fig. 217. M.L. immunoblastic without plasmablastic/plasmacytic differentiation. The tumor cells are large and strongly basophilic. They have large solitary central nucleoli. Among the tumor cells there are many nonneoplastic histiocytes with abundant light cytoplasm and small nucleoli. ♀, 66 years. Inguinal node. Giemsa. ×560

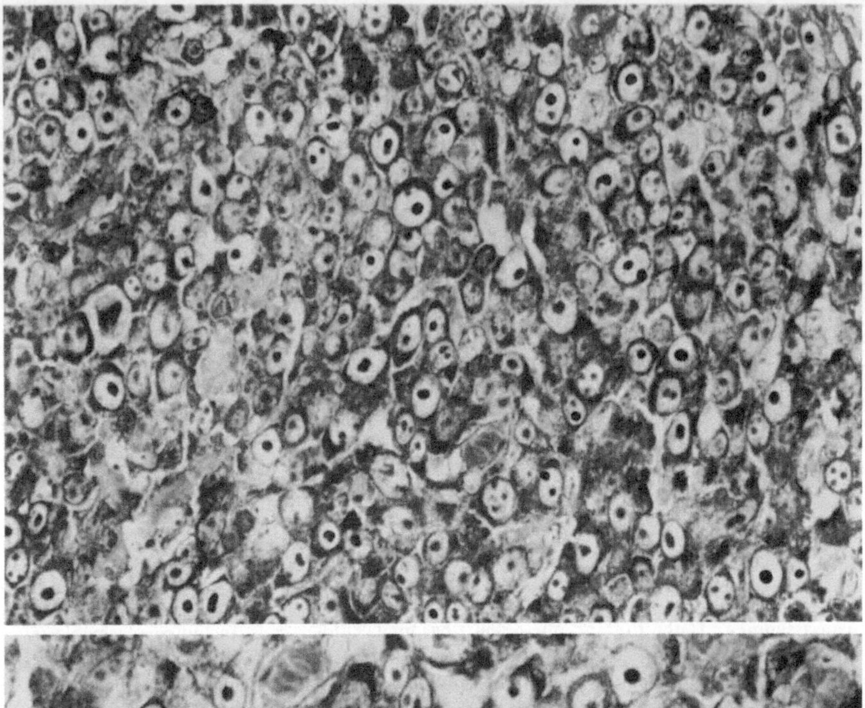

(a)

(b)

Fig. 218a and b. M.L. immunoblastic without plasmablastic/plasmacytic differentiation. The strongly basophilic tumor cells are cohesive and contain large, mostly solitary, basophilic nucleoli in the center of the nuclei. Nonneoplastic histiocytes are almost absent. ♀, 81 years. Inguinal node. Giemsa. (a) ×560, (b) ×875

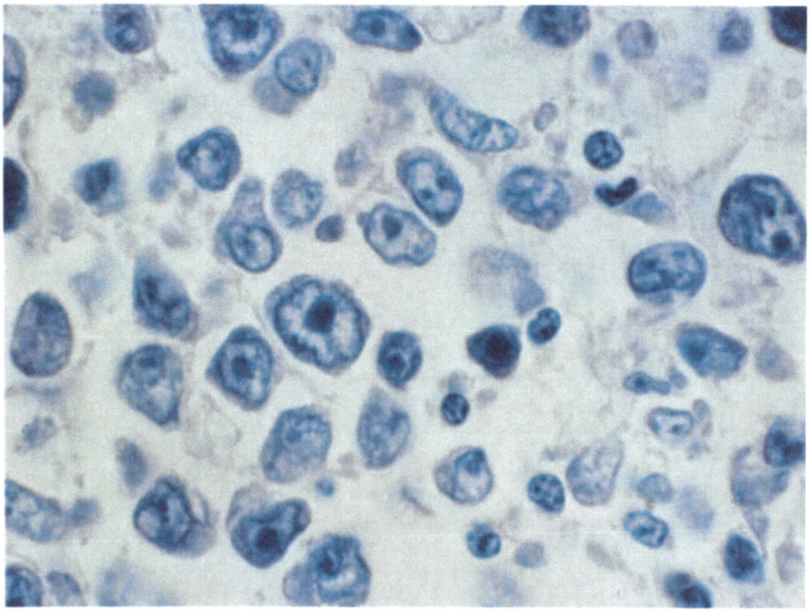

Fig. 219. T-immunoblastic lymphoma with Giemsa staining. Strongly basophilic tumor cells with large, mostly solitary nucleoli. Autopsy case, therefore the cells are shrunken. Case of OEHMICHEN, GÄRTNER and KNITTEL-JUNG (1977). ♀, 65 years. Abdominal node. ×1,550

In addition to the macrophages of typical morphology, there are sometimes *epithelioid cells*. On light microscopy, these cells differ from macrophages by the oxyphilia of their cytoplasm, the absence of phagocytosis, and other features (see p. 55ff.). If the lymph-node tissue is not fixed or embedded well enough, or if histologic sections are not optimally thin, then the distinctions between epithelioid cells and macrophages are not always clear. As Table 88 shows, moderate numbers of epithelioid cells were present in 22.4% of the tumors studied, and in a further 4.3% they were very numerous. Thus, 26.7% of the tumors proved beyond all doubt to contain epithelioid cells. These sometimes lay separately, sometimes together in small groups. In the latter instance there may be a certain similarity to *epitheloidzellige Lymphogranulomatose* (lymphoepithelioid-cell lymphoma). The epithelioid-cell reaction is sometimes especially prominant at the border between the tumor and residual lymphatic tissue. In a few cases we found typical epithelioid-cell tubercles without caseation but with characteristic Langhans' giant cells (Figs. 215 and 216). There was no other indication of tuberculosis.

*Silver staining* reveals mostly fine to moderately thick fibers that entwine the tumor cells (see Table 89 and Fig. 220). When there is an extremely large number of fibers, they separate the tumor cells from one another. There were so few fibers in 41.8% of the tumors that it proved difficult at times to differentiate these tumors from large-cell anaplastic carcinoma, and in particular from

Table 87. Number of macrophages in M.L. immunoblastic (187 biopsies)

| Macrophages | n | % |
|---|---|---|
| Very few | 24 | 12.8 |
| Few | 49 | 26.2 |
| Many | 104 | 55.6 |
| Very numerous | 10 | 5.4 |
| | 187 | 100 |

Table 88. Number of epithelioid cells in M.L. immunoblastic (187 biopsies)

| Epithelioid cells | n | % | |
|---|---|---|---|
| None | 91 | 48.7 | 73.3 |
| Questionable[a] | 46 | 24.6 | |
| Moderately abundant | 42 | 22.4 | 26.7 |
| Abundant | 8[b] | 4.3 | |
| | 187 | 100 | |

[a] In these cases, several macrophages were found, some of which could perhaps be interpreted as epithelioid cells but could not be *definitely* classified as such

[b] One of these slides revealed typical epithelioid-cell tubercles

Table 89. Number of fibers in M.L. immunoblastic (182 biopsies)

| Fibers | n | % | |
|---|---|---|---|
| Very sparse | 76 | 41.8 | |
| Moderately abundant | 60 | 33.0 | 58.2 |
| Abundant | 45 | 24.7 | |
| Highly abundant | 1 | 0.5 | |
| | 182 | 100 | |

the lymphoepithelial carcinoma of Schmincke and Regaud (nasopharyngeal carcinoma). The number of fibers found in this group was much smaller than the number of reticulin fibers in diffuse lymphatic parenchyma. The fibers lay far apart. The tumor-cell masses in between the fibers appeared either free of fibers or very poor in them. In 58% of the cases the reticulin fibers were increased—in 33% to a moderate degree, in 24.7% to a high degree, and in 0.5% to a very high degree. There were no corresponding differences in the cell pictures. BENNETT[848a] found sclerosis in 13 out of 41 cases. In a few cases with

[848a] 1975b.

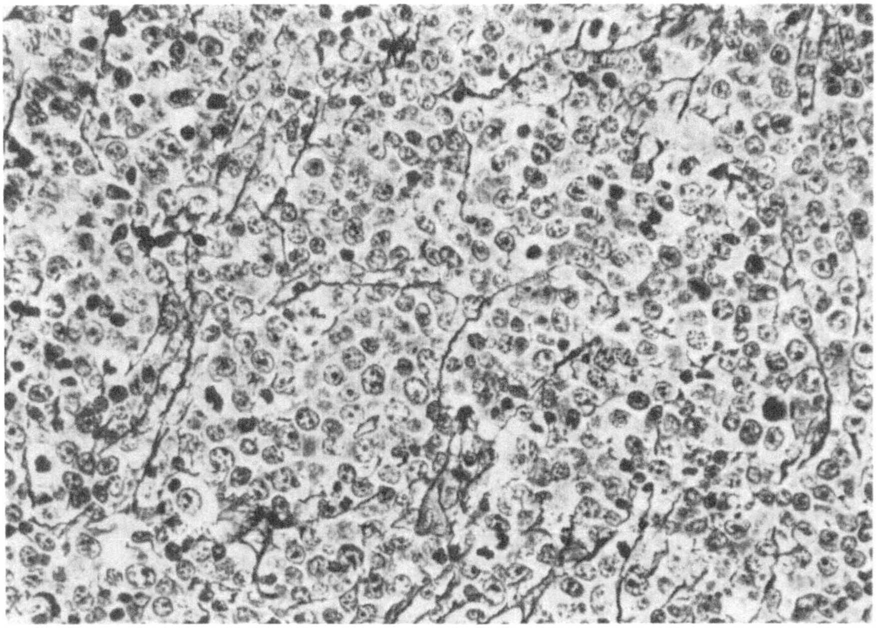

Fig. 220. M.L. immunoblastic with plasmacytic differentiation with silver staining. A moderate number of reticulin fibers among the tumor cells. Same node as Fig. 213. Gomori. ×350

very high fiber content ("dictyocytic reticulosarcoma") electron-microscopic and cytochemical studies and Ig analyses enabled us to clearly establish the immunoblastic nature of the tumor cells.

**Smear/Imprint.** Immunoblastic lymphoma chiefly consists of large basophilic cells with a moderately wide to wide rim of dark blue cytoplasm (Fig. 221). Only occasionally are there also a few medium-sized cells with gray-blue, i.e., less basophilic cytoplasm. Occasionally, we found numerous vacuoles in the basophilic cells, and these proved to be fat on electron microscopy. These cases closely resembled Burkitt's tumor in other characteristics as well, except that the cells were considerably larger than those of typical Burkitt's lymphoma (Fig. 222). The nuclei are round or oval and have a distinct reticular chromatin network. The nucleoli are conspicuous as large, bright blue bodies that often stand out sharply. The similarity of these cells to those we previously described as basophilic stem cells[849] is often striking. Rarely, basophilic giant cells with one or more nuclei occur.

Reference is made in the footnote[850] to the numerous older studies of the cytology of reticulosarcoma in smears.

---

[849] LENNERT, 1961.

[850] STAHEL, 1939; BESSIS, 1946; DREYFUS and ANDRÉ, 1950; TISCHENDORF, 1951, 1957; MUNDT, 1952; BERMAN, 1953; HECKNER and VOTH, 1954; MALLARMÉ, 1955; PAVLOVSKY, 1966.

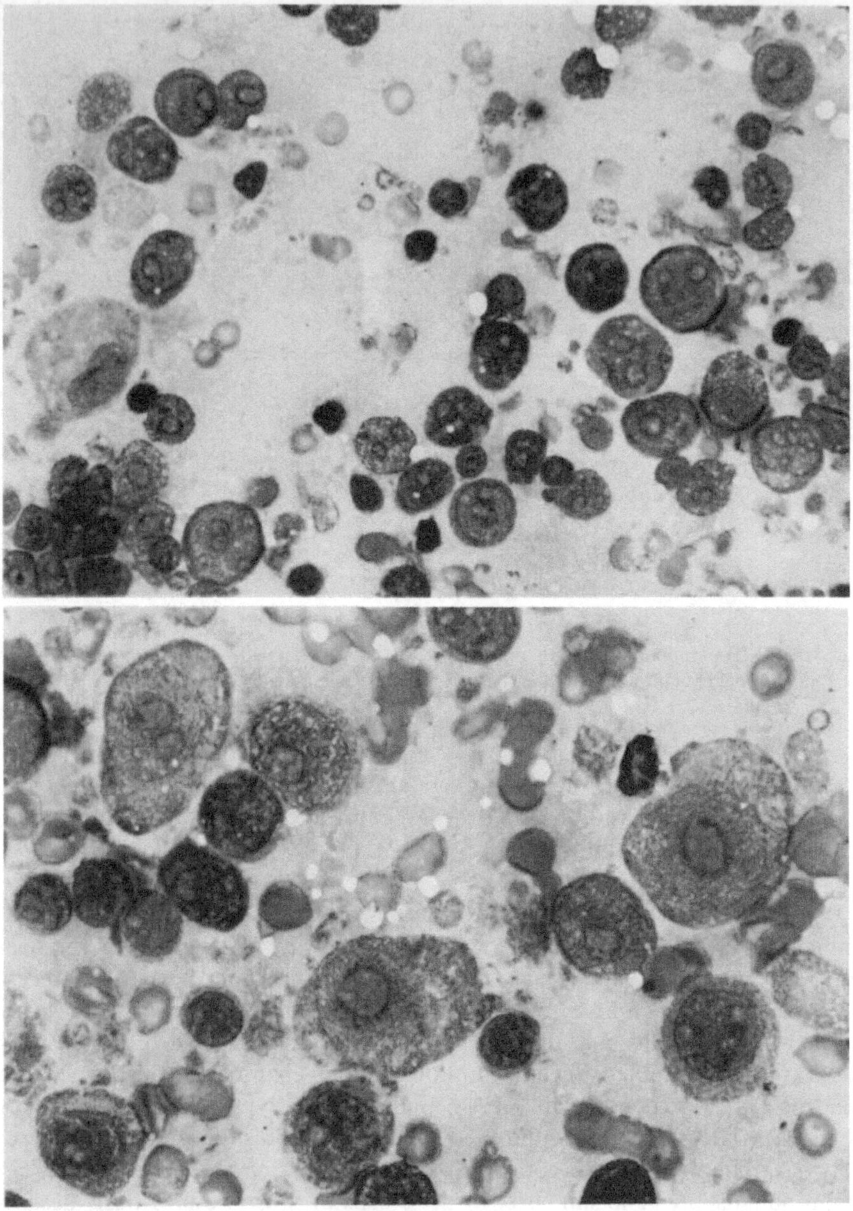

(a)

(b)

Fig. 221 a and b. M.L. immunoblastic with plasmablastic differentiation in imprint. The strongly basophilic cells are of different sizes. The smaller cells are somewhat like plasma cells and plasmablasts. In the large cells note the very distinct large nucleoli with sharp edges. On the left in (a), an epithelioid cell with abundant nonbasophilic cytoplasm. Same node as Fig. 214. Pappenheim. (a) ×560, (b) ×875

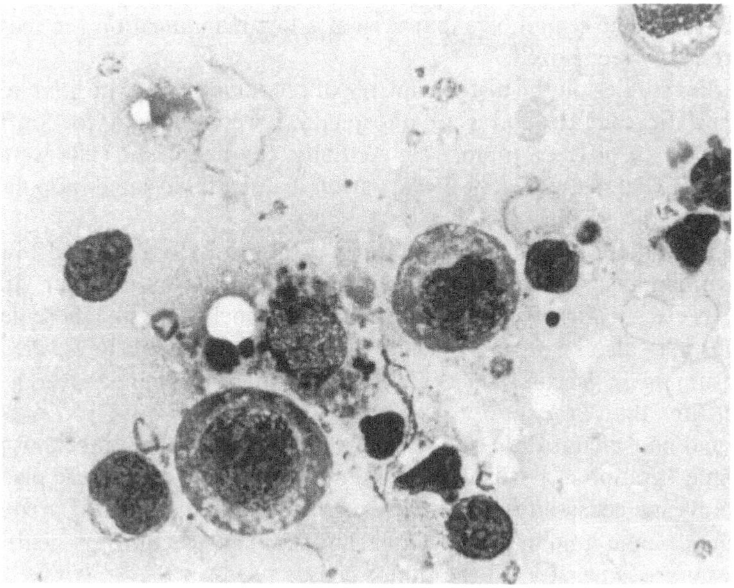

Fig. 222. M.L. immunoblastic without plasmablastic/plasmacytic differentiation in imprint. The large hyperbasophilic tumor cell seen at the lower left shows some resemblance to a Burkitt's tumor cell, but it is somewhat larger. In the center, a histiocyte containing nuclear debris. ♀, 76 years. Pappenheim. ×875

**Histochemistry and Cytochemistry.** In paraffin *sections* we always apply the PAS reaction, which demonstrates diastase-resistant inclusions in the cytoplasm and sometimes also in the nucleus of tumor cells. In 54.5% of the cases we detected deposits of PAS-positive material, which certainly represented mostly Ig. Occasionally, the PAS-positive material was evident in the nuclei as globules. In the cytoplasm the deposits were sometimes small (coarsely granular) and sometimes medium-sized to large (globular). At times the PAS positivity was diffusely dispersed throughout the cytoplasm. The first case of so-called reticulosarcoma with PAS-positive inclusions in the cells was reported in 1955 by RAPPAPORT and JOHNSON.

Table 90 provides information about the intensity and the frequency of PAS positivity in M.L. immunoblastic. As is indicated, the intensity of the PAS

Table 90. PAS reaction in M.L. immunoblastic (90 biopsies)

| Degree of PAS positivity | n | % | |
|---|---|---|---|
| None | 27 | 30.0 | 45.5 |
| Questionable | 14 | 15.5 | |
| Slight/moderately intense | 44 | 49.0 | 54.5 |
| Intense | 5 | 5.5 | |
| | 90 | 100 | |

reaction varies greatly. In a few tumors the globular PAS-positive inclusions appeared in such large numbers that even at a low magnification the red-stained cells were easily recognized.

In earlier studies on the histochemistry of reticulosarcoma, positive reactions for nonspecific esterase and acid phosphatase were thought to confirm the histiocytic origin of these tumors.[851] Actually, the neoplastic cells were essentially negative, and the reaction was given by the associated population of macrophages and epithelioid cells.

In *imprints* the PAS reaction was clearly positive in seven out of 12 immunoblastic lymphomas. The positivity may be diffuse and/or granular. In a few cases it was extraordinarily intense. Large globular inclusions like those described in sections may also be seen in smears. Their demonstration, however, is more time-consuming in smears, since fewer cells can be examined over a certain period of time than in sections.

The acid phosphatase reaction reveals a few to moderate numbers of positive cytoplasmic "granules" (lysosomes) in immunoblasts and cells of the plasma-cell series. In plasma cells and precursors, a circumscribed paranuclear area is often also positive (area containing the Golgi body?). The reaction for neutral nonspecific esterase is negative in the tumor cells.

For cytochemical studies of reticulosarcoma the reader may wish to refer to the literature.[852]

**Diagnosis.** The diagnosis of immunoblastic sarcoma is best made with Giemsa-stained slides. In these most of the tumor cells appear large and intensely basophilic. The nucleoli stand out sharply. Macrophages with a clear "neutrophilic" cytoplasm and signs of phagocytosis, and oxyphilic nonphagocytic epithelioid cells may be found among the tumor cells. The reticulin fibers are either scanty or abundant and sometimes enclose individual tumor cells. When there is a globular diastase-resistant PAS reaction, one may be sure that the tumor is an Ig-producing immunoblastic lymphoma, that is, an immunoblastic lymphoma of the B-cell type. The diagnostic criteria of M.L. immunoblastic are summarized in Table 91.

**Differential Diagnosis.** W.StC. Symmers[853] published a helpful study of the histologic differential diagnosis. One can gather from this study which diseases have been misinterpreted as reticulosarcoma and in which diseases the reticulosarcomatous nature of the tumor was not recognized. We have recorded the data for both groups in Table 92. As can be seen, the majority of false diagnoses concern other malignant lymphomas, namely, Hodgkin's disease and lymphosarcoma (61.4% of the cases). The next most common group causing mistakes in identification are tumor metastases with 32.3%. In this group the most important example is anaplastic carcinoma, including lymphoepithelial carci-

[851] Dorfman, 1961, 1964a; Lennert, Löffler and Leder, 1961, 1963; Braunstein, Freiman, Thomas and Gall, 1962b; Lennert, Löffler and Grabner, 1962; Lennert, Leder and Löffler, 1965; Wright, 1970b.

[852] Lennert, Löffler and Leder, 1961; Rinneberg and Lennert, 1961; Braunstein, Freiman, Thomas and Gall, 1962b; Lennert, Löffler and Grabner, 1962; Lennert, Leder and Löffler, 1965; Wright, 1970b.

[853] 1968.

Table 91. Diagnostic criteria of M.L. immunoblastic

1. All ages, peak in 7th decade
2. ~5% leukemic
3. More or less monotonous infiltration with large basophilic (pyroninophilic) cells
4. Cytologically two possibilities:
   a) Without plasmablastic/plasmacytic differentiation:
      pure population of immunoblasts (B- or T-type):
      oval nuclei, large central nucleoli
   b) With plasmablastic/plasmacytic differentiation (B-type):
      plasmablasts:
         somewhat smaller;
         rim of cytoplasm broader, intensely basophilic;
         multiple medium-sized to large nucleoli, centrally located in round nuclei
      or plasmacytoid cells:
         relatively small;
         nuclei eccentrically located in relatively abundant, strongly basophilic cytoplasm
5. Epithelioid cells in ~25% of cases
6. ~50% of cases PAS+(diffuse or globular reaction)
7. Few or numerous fibers

Table 92. Diseases most often confused with reticulum-cell sarcoma (according to W.StC. Symmers, 1968)

| Other diseases | Reticulosarcomas misdiagnosed as other diseases n | | Other diseases misdiagnosed as reticulosarcoma n | |
|---|---|---|---|---|
| Hodgkin's disease | 34 | | 24 | |
| Lymphosarcoma | 12 | | 8 | |
| Metastatic tumors | 18 | | 23 | |
| Squamous and anaplastic carcinoma | | 14 | | 10 |
| Melanoma | | 1 | | 3 |
| Lymphoepithelioma | | 2 | | 2 |
| Seminoma/dysgerminoma | | – | | 3 |
| Malignant glioma | | – | | 2 |
| Hepatoma | | – | | 1 |
| Granular-cell myoblastoma | | – | | 1 |
| Nonchromaffin paraganglioma | | – | | 1 |
| Choriocarcinoma | | 1 | | – |
| Lymphadenitis and immunologic reactions | 2 | | 6 | |
| Total | 66 | | 61 (out of 226 cases) | |

noma of Schmincke. Here a correct differential diagnosis may be exceedingly difficult and for the patient of greatest significance. Malignant melanoma and seminoma or dysgerminoma make up the next most frequent group. All other tumors in this list are rarities. The few cases of lymphadenitis that were mistaken for reticulosarcoma or vice versa were of little account (6.3%).

The differential diagnosis from *Hodgkin's disease*[854] is sometimes difficult, especially if the immunoblastic lymphoma contains abundant epithelioid cells and macrophages. To identify the tumor then as immunoblastic lymphoma, the predominating, *relatively* monomorphic, intensely basophilic cells serve as the important criterion. The presence of giant cells is neither proof of Hodgkin's disease nor evidence against immunoblastic lymphoma. Large numbers of lymphocytes and eosinophils speak against immunoblastic lymphoma, although eosinophils are rarely found (without a large number of lymphocytes) in immunoblastic lymphomas. Plasma cells or plasma-cell precursors may be found in the spectrum of immunoblastic lymphoma as well as in Hodgkin's disease.

Of the *tumor metastases,* it is most important to differentiate those from large-cell anaplastic carcinomas. They are best recognized with silver staining. The cells of anaplastic carcinoma grow in solid cords and larger groups that are enclosed by fibers. These fibers are often thick or they form small networks. Sometimes a conspicuous stroma is evident.

In *lymphoepithelial carcinoma* (nasopharyngeal carcinoma, Schmincke's tumor; Fig. 223) the large basophilic tumor cells that are often seen in the lymph sinuses and the intense inflammatory reaction in the surrounding tissue serve as helpful criteria. One finds masses of very cohesive tumor cells with abundant, homogeneously deep gray-blue cytoplasm and conspicuous *clear* nuclei containing one or more very *prominent* nucleoli. These features are best seen in Giemsa-stained sections, which, as a rule, allow the almost certain conclusion that there is a primary tumor in the nasopharynx or tonsils. The remnants of lymph-node parenchyma left between the tumor complexes contain chiefly numerous plasma cells and often some eosinophils. There are sometimes clusters of epithelioid cells and occasionally caseation necrosis.[854a] In sections lymphoepithelial carcinoma always gives a negative PAS reaction, whereas fine granular to diffuse PAS positivity (glycogen) is occasionally found in the cytoplasm of tumor cells in anaplastic carcinomas, which show slight squamous differentiation. In imprints, on the other hand, many tumor cells of lymphoepithelial carcinoma show granular PAS positivity, which is seen as glycogen in electron micrographs;[854b] sometimes there is predominantly focal acid phosphatase and nonspecific esterase positivity. The enzyme activity is evident as small or large granules, often accumulated on one side of the nucleus (Golgi body with lysosomes?). Since the carcinoma cells of lymphoepithelial carcinoma always contain genomes of Epstein-Barr virus, this tumor can be successfully differentiated from other undifferentiated carcinomas and from immunoblastic lymphoma by means of serologic methods. All patients with lymphoepithelial carcinoma have increased titers of antibody against EBV-antigens in the blood. The level

[854] The study of the differential diagnosis of reticulosarcoma and Hodgkin's disease published by WAKASA (1958) is worth reading.

[854a] RENNKE and LENNERT, 1973.

[854b] KAISERLING, unpublished data.

(a)

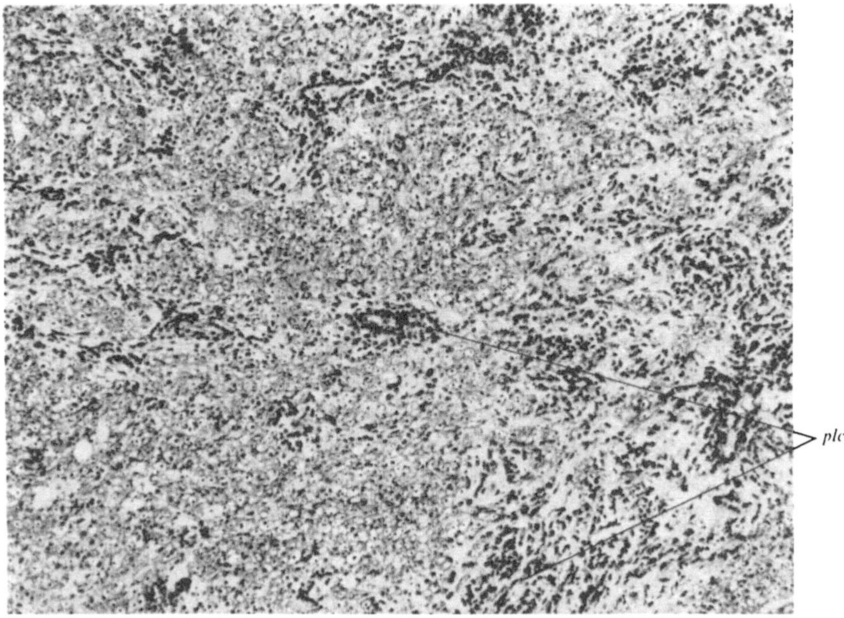


(b)

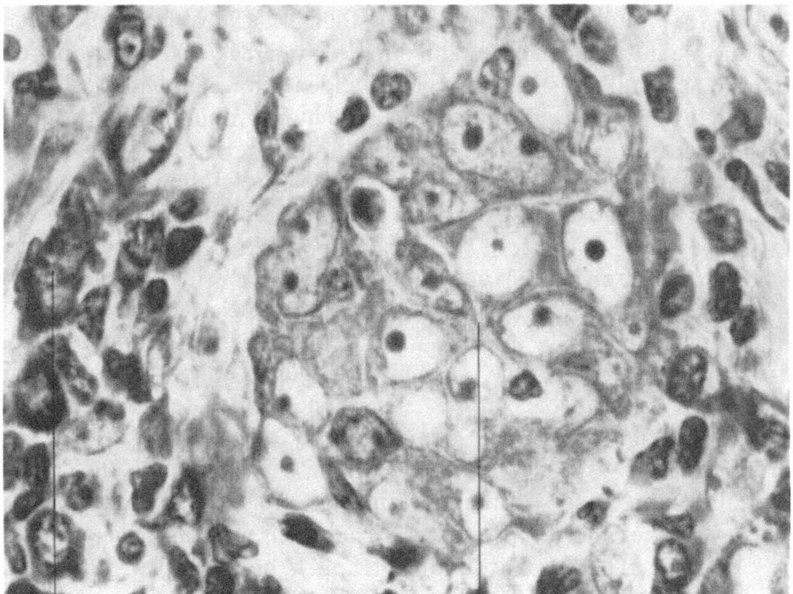


Fig. 223a and b. Lymphoepithelial carcinoma (Schmincke's tumor, nasopharyngeal carcinoma). The tumor cells (*tu*) have a clear nucleus with very conspicuous basophilic nucleoli and are mutually adherent. Among the tumor cells there are strands and sheets of plasma cells (*plc*) that are even more basophilic than the tumor cells (dark blue versus deep gray-blue). ♀, 62 years. Cervical node. Giemsa. (a) × 140, (b) × 1,550 of the antibody titers (especially those against certain antigens) even allows certain conclusions to be drawn about the course of the disease. In other respects, everything that was said on page 377f. about the demonstration of EBV infection is also true here.

The cells of malignant *melanoma* generally have larger nuclei and, above all, a much broader rim of cytoplasm, which with Giemsa staining appears a deep reddish violet and often bluish at the margins. Usually the tumor-cell masses are also well defined. The polymorphism is sometimes striking, and the nucleoli are often unusually conspicuous because of their size. Occasionally, the cytoplasm contains fine PAS-positive granules, but never diffuse or globular PAS positivity. In any event, to identify traces of melanin, we carry out the Prussian blue reaction, which best demonstrates small numbers of iron-negative pigment granules. With Giemsa staining melanin appears green and, when detected on scrutinizing Giemsa-stained sections, this serves as an important diagnostic indicator. The fiber network of malignant melanoma is sparse and coarsely alveolar. Frequently, mitotic figures are particularly numerous.

In *seminoma* of the testes and mediastinum and in the morphologically identical dysgerminoma the PAS reaction is generally positive; in that case it is the best way to identify these tumors. With this reaction they show an intense diffuse red staining, which represents glycogen and not glycoproteins. Because of the solubility of glycogen ("flight" of glycogen), however, the staining may be missing or accumulated in certain areas of the section. Another very important feature of seminoma is the tendency for epithelioid-cell reactions to occur. The epithelioid cells often form tuberculoid granulomas with Langhans' giant cells and are predominantly found in a delicate stroma (not seen in immunoblastic lymphoma), which also contains relatively abundant lymphocytes. Finally, there is almost always sparse lymphocytic infiltration between the tumor-cell masses.

Another important malignant tumor we should consider in the differential diagnosis that was not included in SYMMERS'[855] article is *myelosarcoma*.[856] This tumor, which usually appears in the course of a myeloid leukemia, is likewise characterized by large, strongly basophilic cells with large nucleoli. If the reaction for chloroacetate esterase is performed, however, then some or many of the tumor cells will give a strongly positive reaction.[857] Further support for the diagnosis, best achieved with the Giemsa stain, is the demonstration of granular precursors of the myelopoietic series (eosinophil or neutrophil granular myelocytes and promyelocytes). These cells may also give a fine granular PAS reaction. That usually does not apply, however, to the (basophilic) myelosarcoma cells, which generally dominate the picture of these tumors.

Besides malignant tumors, all "inflammatory" lymph-node lesions that reveal relatively marked immunoblastic hyperplasia must also be considered in the differential diagnosis. *Infectious mononucleosis* is the most important of these conditions. In this disease there are often areas of rather monotonous infiltration by immunoblasts with numerous mitotic figures. These cells are easily confused with the cells of M.L. immunoblastic. If one examines the tissue at a

[855] 1968.

[856] See also JOSEPH, ZARAFONETIS and DURANT, 1966; PASCOE, 1970; SUCHI and OTA, 1973.

[857] LEDER, 1965.

high magnification, preferably with oil immersion, however, one will find a cytologic spectrum with some smaller basophilic cells, ranging as far as "lymphatic" plasma cells, among the immunoblasts. There are also numerous transitional stages, starting with lymphocytes and going through larger lymphoid cells to immunoblasts, among the immunoblasts or around sheets of them. We know of several instances in which immunoblastic sarcoma was falsely diagnosed in biopsies of the tonsils and in which the patients were subjected to radiotherapy. In reality, these were cases of infectious mononucleosis, as the blood picture and serologic reactions for EBV showed. In doubtful cases one should therefore consider the clinical manifestations (bilateral tonsillitis, fever), the blood picture, and the age of the patient (young adults), and one should not forget to look for evidence of EBV infection. When positive EBV titers are found, one must also consider the possibility of lymphoepithelial carcinoma (nasopharyngeal carcinoma).

Most other *immunologic disorders* and *virus diseases* (e.g., rubella, herpes zoster) less often present a problem in differential diagnoses. In toxoplasmosis (Piringer's lymphadenitis) there may also be a great increase in immunoblasts in the pulp with some effacement of the normal structure and small focal clusters of epithelioid cells. The presence of so-called immature sinus histiocytosis, however, is a reliable criterion for easily distinguishing Piringer's lymphadenitis from immunoblastic lymphoma.

**Borderline Cases.** It is not always easy to draw a line between M.L. immunoblastic and *M.L. centroblastic* or LP immunocytoma. Large-cell centroblastic lymphoma, in particular, occasionally causes difficulty, no doubt because immunoblasts and centroblasts are closely related. As discussed earlier, we have now reclassified as M.L. centroblastic some tumors composed of a mixture of immunoblasts and germinal-center cells. The problem is not a simple one, however, and will have to be clarified in the future by means of immunologic techniques. It will be particularly important to determine whether centroblastic lymphomas in which the cells form EAC rosettes contain immunoblasts with intracytoplasmic Ig. If that should be the case, one would have to decide whether to classify such tumors as centroblastic or immunoblastic lymphomas.

The same difficulties arise when we try to draw a line between M.L. immunoblastic and *immunocytoma.* Since the latter occasionally shows dedifferentiation and transforms into an immunoblastic lymphoma, it is inevitable that one will find transitional cases in which one cannot yet speak of a fully developed immunoblastic lymphoma and which contain abundant remnants of the original immunocytoma (lymphocytes, plasma cells, plasmacytoid cells, and perhaps centroblasts and centrocytes) as well as immunoblasts.

**Combination with Other Diseases.** A combination with other infectious or neoplastic diseases has not been found in our material. In four out of 187 cases (=2.1%) immunocytoma either preceded or was demonstrated simultaneously with the immunoblastic lymphoma, which was therefore a secondary M.L. immunoblastic of the B-cell type. In one case of secondary immunoblastic lymphoma a leukemic immunocytoma with macroglobulinemia had been observed in the patient for 7 years. The homogenate of an immunoblastic tumor

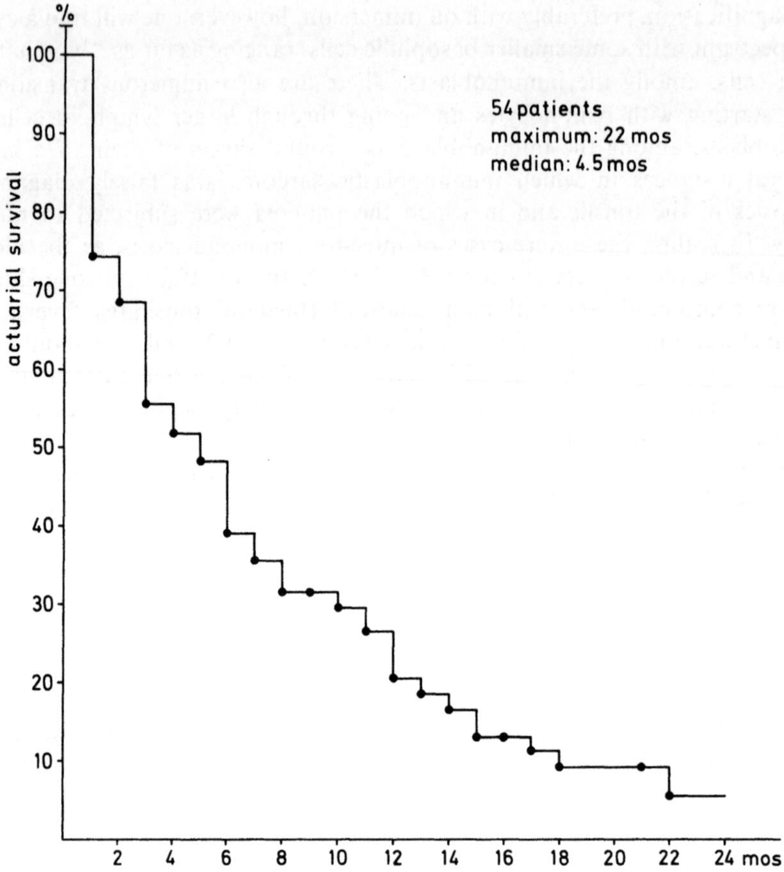


Fig. 224. Actuarial survival of patients with M.L. immunoblastic. 54 patients of our first series

excised from the patient's thigh contained increased amounts of IgM, about 2.5 times that of normal lymph nodes.

We have already pointed out that immunoblastic lymphoma may develop in immune-deficiency states. To that extent, one may say that certain immunologic disorders or forms of therapy may predispose the patient to develop M.L. immunoblastic.

**Prognosis.** Figure 224 indicates the survival data for 54 of our own cases. From the data one can see that the median survival was 4.5 months and that only very few patients survived 24 months. In addition to the patients included in Figure 224, we have studied three patients who remained healthy and free of recurrence for 9, 13, and 22 years, respectively, after the localized tumor (probably stage I) had been removed and after the patients had received postoperative radiotherapy; one of them also received additional treatment with cyclophosphamide. It is noteworthy that the initially examined tumors from the two patients with remissions lasting 13 and 22 years were markedly pleomorphic and contained numerous giant cells. Originally, these tumors had been diagnosed as Hodgkin's sarcoma. At recurrence they were replaced by monomorphic immunoblastic tumors.

BENNETT[858] reported on the prognosis of immunoblastic sarcoma with respect to stage and sclerosis in 41 cases. Of 24 patients with localized tumors, 37% survived 5 years. The generalized tumors led to death within 4 years after therapy was begun. The sclerotic immunoblastic lymphomas showed a 5-year survival rate of 23%. The nonsclerotic lymphomas had already led to death in the second year after the start of therapy. The 5-year survival rate for all 41 patients was 7%.

One finds time and again reports in the literature citing the relatively favorable prognosis of "reticulosarcoma" of the tonsil. Although we are unable to express a definite opinion on this matter, we should like to point out that the allegedly favorable prognosis of tonsillar "reticulosarcoma" is not necessarily attributable to reticulosarcoma; it may also result from a misinterpretation: lymphoepithelial carcinoma of the tonsils and nasopharynx, which is known to have a favorable prognosis, is sometimes misdiagnosed as reticulosarcoma.

In older statistics the prognosis of reticulosarcoma is judged differently, but on the whole it was thought to be poor.[859] According to GALL and MALLORY,[860] the average survival of patients with stem-cell lymphoma is 1.7 years (median: 1.1 years) and that of those with clasmatocytic lymphoma is 2.1 years (median: 1.1 years). These authors reported that 14% of their patients with stem-cell lymphoma and 11% with clasmatocytic lymphoma survived 5 years. In JACKSON and PARKER's series[861] 6% of the patients with reticulosarcoma lived longer than 5 years. LUMB and NEWTON[862] found that 13.8% of their patients with "reticulosarcoma" survived 5 years, as did 5.7% with "anaplastic sarcoma." Fifty-two percent of the patients of JACKSON and PARKER died within the first year after appearance of the tumor. In contrast, 47% of the patients of HOHL and GRETENER[863] survived 5 years, an unusually high percentage. In a series of 554 patients with reticulosarcoma, ROSENBERG *et al.*[864] observed that the median survival was 21.4 months and the 5-year survival rate was 13.9%. NEWALL and FRIEDMAN,[865] on the other hand, reported a 5-year survival rate of 39.8%.

JONES *et al.*[866] graphically plotted the survival rate of their patients with diffuse histiocytic, and poorly differentiated lymphomas. The longest time a patient with histiocytic lymphoma survived was 6 years. Most patients died, however, in the first 2 years after the start of therapy. Patients with poorly differentiated lymphoma never survived more than 2 years according to the graph, but, from the text of the paper, never longer than 8 months, with a median survival of 6 months. The prognosis was not influenced by age, sex, or general symptoms. When the bone marrow was already infiltrated at the start of treatment (stage IV), all patients died within the first year.

As far as we know, MUSSHOFF[867] is the only investigator who presented exact data on a large series of patients showing how the life expectancy depends on the stage of the disease at the time therapy is started. To be sure, his series was not quite homogeneous; his 224 cases included 33 "lymphoreticular sarcomas." Nonetheless, the results of his studies are impressive. Of the patients with reticulosarcoma confined to one organ or lymph-node region, 60% and 55%, respectively, were still alive after 20 years and could therefore be considered cured. The prognosis for patients in stages II and III with lymph-node involvement was, however, appreciably worse,

858 1975b.

859 ROULET, 1932; RÖSSLE, 1939; GALL and MALLORY, 1942; JACKSON and PARKER, 1947; LUMB, 1954; HOHL and GRETENER, 1956; LUMB and NEWTON, 1957; ROSENBERG, DIAMOND, JASLOWITZ and CRAVER, 1961; MUSSHOFF, 1970.

860 1942.

861 1947.

862 1957.

863 1956.

864 ROSENBERG, DIAMOND, JASLOWITZ and CRAVER, 1961.

865 1970.

866 JONES, FUKS, BULL, KADIN *et al.*, 1973.

867 1970.

whereas of the patients with disseminated organ involvement (corresponding to stage IV) 60% died after only 1 year and none survived 5 years.

DeVita *et al.*[868] have now reported that with combination chemotherapy, 41% of their patients with reticulosarcoma had complete remissions. Only one of the tumors recurred in these cases. Whereas most of the responders could be considered cured 2 years after the end of therapy, all of the nonresponders and partial responders died within a short time.

## *Addenda*

### *a) The Leukemic Variant of M.L. Immunoblastic: Immunoblastic Leukemia*

*Synonyms:* Large-cell reticulosis (basophilic type)
Immunoblastic acute lymphoid leukemia
Leukemic phase of histiocytic lymphoma

**History and Terminology.** Leukemias with large "reticulum cell-like" cells in the blood have been described since 1935. Early cases were referred to as monoblastoma, reticulosarcoma with transition into acute leukemia, and the like.[869] The first such observation was published by Mitchell.[870] In 1971, Lowenbraun *et al.*[871] reviewed all such cases known in the American literature and added two case reports of their own. They concluded that reticulosarcoma with transition to leukemia was a hyperacute process that appeared "explosively," leading to death within a few weeks. They said that the disease could appear in the second decade; their youngest patient was 16 years old, their oldest, 75. Shortly before Lowenbraun *et al.* published their paper, Mathé *et al.*[872] reported on the same neoplasm, calling it histioblastic reticulosarcoma with transformation into leukemia. They said that this transformation occurred in 17.5% of the cases, whereas the histiocytic type never became leukemic. Flandrin *et al.*[873] described two leukemic reticulosarcomas, which, like monocytic leukemia, were reported to show a positive nonspecific AS-esterase reaction. The recently published cases of Schnitzer and Kass[874] cannot be classified with this group, but belong instead to the group of M.L. centroblastic/centrocytic or M.L. centroblastic.

As we pointed out previously,[875] these large-cell "leukemias" must be clearly separated into two types, namely, (1) a "neutrophilic" (nonbasophilic) and (2) a basophilic form. They probably differ in origin and nature, although they reveal great morphologic similarities in the blood. Previously, we called these

[868] DeVita, Canellos, Chabner, Schein *et al.*, 1975.

[869] Mitchell, 1935; Zeffren and Ultmann, 1960; Marin-Padilla, Fahimi and Moloney, 1964; Mathé, Gérard-Marchant, Texier, Schlumberger *et al.*, 1970; Lowenbraun, Sutherland, Feldman and Serpick, 1971; Shimoyama and Mikuni, 1973; Rehman, Rosner and Grünwald, 1974.

[870] 1935.

[871] Lowenbraun, Sutherland, Feldman and Serpick, 1971.

[872] Mathé, Gérard-Marchant, Texier, Schlumberger *et al.*, 1970.

[873] Flandrin, Daniel, Blanchet, Brière *et al.*, 1971.

[874] 1973.

[875] Lennert, 1964a, 1974c.

neutrophilic and basophilic types "large-cell reticuloses" and accordingly distinguished a neutrophilic large-cell reticulosis from a basophilic large-cell reticulosis.

*Neutrophilic large-cell "reticulosis"* is characterized by a large amount of nonspecific esterase and acid phosphatase in the very large, reticulum cell-like elements found in the blood. In Giemsa-stained sections and smears the cytoplasm appears reddish-violet. It forms a very wide rim and often contains numerous small vacuoles. The nuclei are round or oval and reveal a distinctly reticular structure. This type of large-cell reticulosis is *closely related to monocytic leukemia* and is perhaps a variant of that type of leukemia,[876] especially since sections of such cases often reveal monocytoid cells with reniform nuclei. Moreover, the blood picture shows further signs of a myeloid process, such as pseudo-Pelger cells,[877] some normoblasts, etc.

So-called *basophilic large-cell "reticulosis"* may appear at the same time as a "reticulosarcoma" develops or later, after the latter has existed for some time. The cells characterizing this type of reticulosis are large and intensely basophilic and have "reticular," round or oval nuclei. Their rim of cytoplasm is somewhat narrower than that of the cells of the preceding type and it is enzyme-negative. This basophilic type is equivalent to the histioblastic reticulosarcoma of MATHÉ *et al.*[878] and, according to our present knowledge, is to be interpreted as *immunoblastic lymphoma with a leukemic blood picture* ("immunoblastic leukemia"; Fig. 225).

Apparently, MATHÉ *et al.*[879] have now come to the same conclusion. They described as "immunoblastic acute lymphoid leukemia" an acute form of leukemia that they observed seven times among 200 patients with acute lymphoid leukemia. These authors said that the leukemia may be "primary," meaning that the bone marrow when first examined is infiltrated by immunoblasts ("primary immunoblastic acute lymphoid leukemia"). On the other hand, infiltration of the bone marrow may first become detectable a few weeks after discovery of a lymphoid mass ("early leukemic immunoblastic lymphosarcoma"). We are not sure, however, whether all of the cases described by MATHÉ *et al.*[879] correspond exactly to the basophilic type we have defined. Perhaps some of their cases represent Burkitt's tumor-like lymphomas.

**Origin of the Neoplastic Cells.** It is clear that the cells are derived from immunoblasts. The only question to be raised is whether they are B-immunoblasts or T-immunoblasts. Here, the findings of MATHÉ *et al.*[880] should be mentioned. In one patient the leukemic cells bore B-cell markers (they were SIg-positive, IgG-Fc receptor-positive, complement receptor-positive, and sheep-E receptor-negative). In two patients the tumor cells bore T-cell markers (sheep-E receptors) and were IgG-Fc receptor-positive, and in one patient the cells lacked both types of markers. The monoclonal increase in serum IgM

---

876 LEDER, personal communication.

877 E.g., MARIN-PADILLA, FAHIMI and MOLONEY, 1964.

878 MATHÉ, GÉRARD-MARCHANT, TEXIER, SCHLUMBERGER *et al.*, 1970.

879 MATHÉ, BELPOMME, DANTCHEV, POUILLART *et al.*, 1974; MATHÉ, BELPOMME, DANTCHEV, KHALIL *et al.*, 1975.

880 MATHÉ, BELPOMME, DANTCHEV, POUILLART *et al.*, 1974.

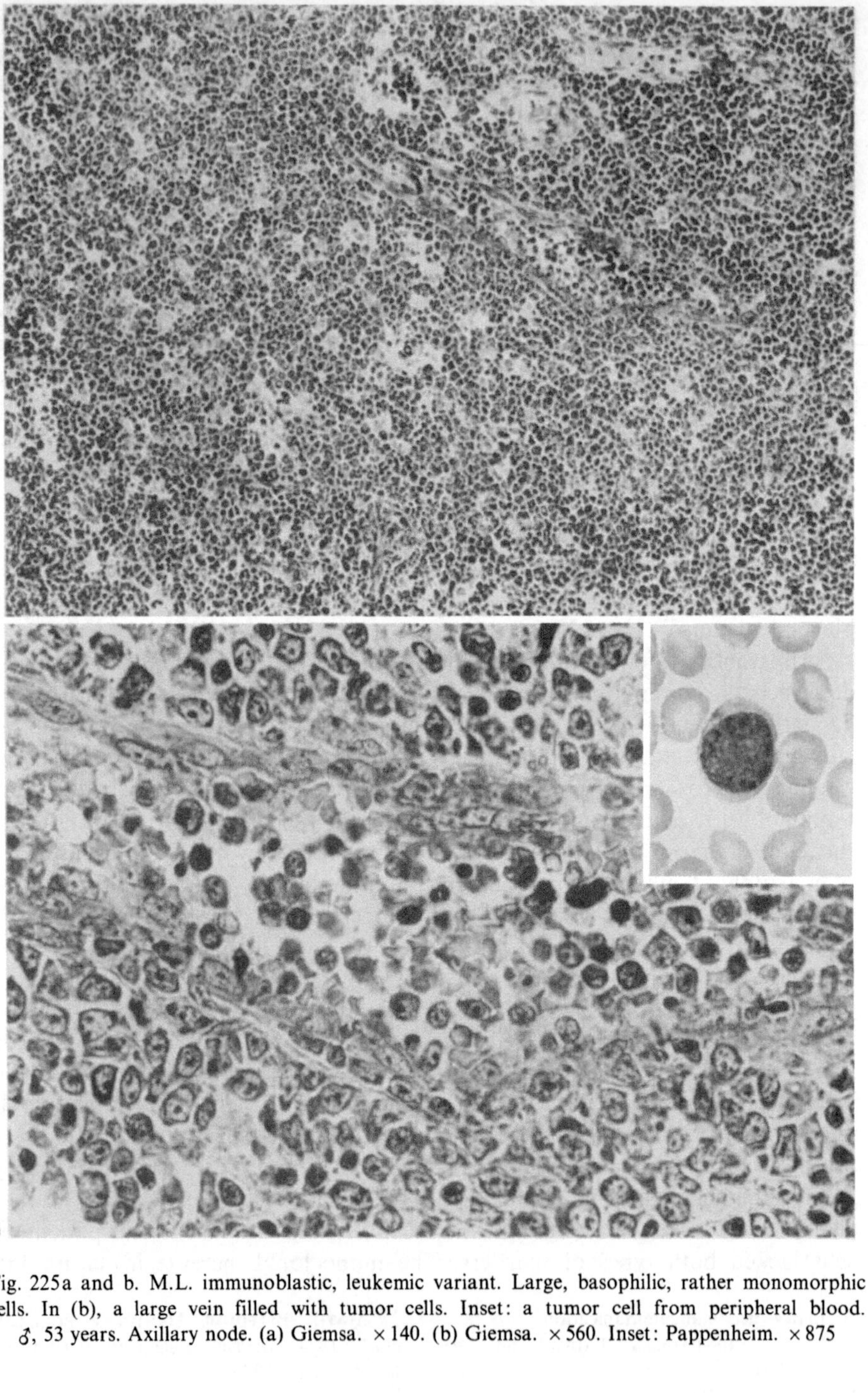

(a)

(b)

Fig. 225a and b. M.L. immunoblastic, leukemic variant. Large, basophilic, rather monomorphic cells. In (b), a large vein filled with tumor cells. Inset: a tumor cell from peripheral blood. ♂, 53 years. Axillary node. (a) Giemsa. ×140. (b) Giemsa. ×560. Inset: Pappenheim. ×875 found in one of our cases[881] spoke for the B-immunoblastic nature of the tumor cells in this case.

**Occurrence.** From our material we have calculated that immunoblastic leukemia is found in almost 5% of the cases of M.L. immunoblastic.

**Histology.** The histologic picture is largely identical with that of M.L. immunoblastic. Since there is usually massive infiltration and expansion of the capsule and trabeculae, however, in many cases we were able to predict a leukemic blood picture on the basis of the histologic pattern. This assumption was supported by the presence of numerous basophilic tumor cells in large blood vessels (Fig. 225). Occasionally, one finds residual infiltrates of a preexistent immunocytoma (lymphocytes, plasmacytoid cells, etc.) that also may have been leukemic.

**Smear/Imprint.** The cytologic picture fully corresponds to that of nonleukemic immunoblastic lymphoma. MATHÉ *et al.*[881a] attached great importance to the presence of numerous vacuoles, which is also typical of the tumor cells of Burkitt's lymphoma.

**Histochemistry and Cytochemistry.** See M.L. immunoblastic (p. 439f.).

**Diagnosis and Differential Diagnosis.** The same considerations apply as in the case of M.L. immunoblastic. Infiltration and widening of the lymph-node capsule and trabeculae, however, should always arouse suspicion of a leukemic process.

**Prognosis.** The prognosis is very poor. Patients with this disease usually die within a few weeks or months.

### *b) Reticulosarcoma*[882]

*Synonyms:* Retotheliosarcoma
Reticulum-cell sarcoma
Reticuloendothelial sarcoma
Reticuloendothelioma
Malignant lymphoma, histiocytic

---

[881] Prof. Dr. A. LINKE, Ludwigshafen, kindly provided this finding.

[881a] MATHÉ, BELPOMME, DANTCHEV, POUILLART *et al.*, 1974.

[882] ROULET, 1930, 1932, 1947, 1953; DE OLIVEIRA, 1936; ROBB-SMITH, 1938, 1947, 1964; RÖSSLE, 1939; GALL and MALLORY, 1942; AKAZAKI, 1943, 1953, 1973; JACKSON and PARKER, 1947; CUSTER and BERNHARD, 1948; SCHILD, 1949; BERMAN, 1953; FRESEN, 1953; LUMB, 1954; OTANI, MARUYA and SHIBUE, 1954; DOMENICI, 1956; W.STC. SYMMERS, 1958; AKAZAKI and WAKASA, 1964; LENNERT, 1964a, 1967; LUKES, 1964, 1967, 1968; RAPPAPORT, 1964a, b, 1966; EVANS, 1966; KELLNER, LAPIS and ECKHARDT, 1966; JACOBS, 1968; SHTERN, 1968, 1970; DUHAMEL, 1969; BERARD, 1972.

1. Undifferentiated (stem cells):
Retothelsarcoma, immature form (ROULET, RÖSSLE)
Stem-cell lymphoma (GALL and MALLORY)
Stem-cell sarcoma
Malignant lymphoma, reticulum-cell type, undifferentiated (RAPPAPORT, 1964)
Malignant lymphoma, undifferentiated (RAPPAPORT, 1966)
Malignant lymphoma, stem-cell type
*Reticulo-sarcoma indifferencié* (DUHAMEL)
Histio-blasto sarcoma (MATHÉ *et al.*)

2. Differentiated:
Retothelsarcoma, mature form (ROULET, RÖSSLE)
Clasmatocytic lymphoma (GALL and MALLORY)
Dictyocytic reticulosarcoma
Dictyosyncytial reticulosarcoma
Fibrillar reticulosarcoma
Fibrosyncytial reticulosarcoma
Malignant lymphoma, reticulum-cell type, histiocytic (RAPPAPORT, 1964)
Malignant lymphoma, histiocytic (RAPPAPORT, 1966)
*Reticulo-sarcoma differencié* (DUHAMEL)
Histio-cyto sarcoma (MATHÉ *et al.*)

3. Further related tumor:
Anaplastic sarcoma (LUMB)

**History.** VIRCHOW[883] created not only the term lymphoma, but also the term lymphosarcoma. He applied these terms to the sarcomas of the lymphatic tissue, including lymphogranulomatosis, which was not differentiated from lymphosarcoma until later by KUNDRAT.[884] The latter investigator also distinguished lymphosarcoma from the so-called pseudoleukemia of COHNHEIM,[885] as DRESCHFELD[886] had a year earlier. The first paper describing most of the essential entities of malignant lymphoma distinguished today, including reticulosarcoma, was published by GHON and ROMAN.[887]

It is mentioned time and again in Anglo-American literature, most pointedly by JACKSON and PARKER,[888] that EWING had already recognized this tumor as an entity in 1913/14 and that he later—for instance, in the 3rd edition of his monograph *Neoplastic Diseases* (1928)—described it correctly. In fact, however, even in the 4th and last edition of his tumor monograph, one looks in vain for a clear definition of reticulosarcoma.

Several case reports published in the 1920's then described malignant lymphomas that would now be included with reticulosarcoma.[889] The paper by

883 1864/65.
884 1893.
885 1865.
886 1892.
887 1916.
888 1947.
889 FOOT, 1924; KOMOCKI, 1924; SILHOL and ROUSLACROIX, 1924; GOORMAGHTIGH, 1925; ORSÓS, 1926; POUJOL, 1927; NAGAYO, 1929.

ARESU and SCALABRINO[890] stands out particularly: they coined the term "dictyosarcoma" ($\delta\iota\kappa\tau\upsilon o\nu$=net) because of the high content of reticulin fibers. The term dictyocytic (reticulo-) sarcoma was used for a time by many authors in England and France, and it is even still in use in a few places.

OBERLING[891] then created the term *reticulosarcoma* for the tumors of the bone or bone marrow and supposed that there must also be corresponding tumors in the lymph nodes.

This type of tumor had also been noticed by RÖSSLE, and for more than two decades he collected lymph-node tumors, which he called *retothelsarcoma*. He gave his collection to ROULET, who described and defined retothelsarcoma as an independent tumor of the lymph nodes in two highly regarded papers published in 1930 and 1932. Later, DE OLIVEIRA,[892] a pupil of RÖSSLE, followed with a comprehensive study, and RÖSSLE[893] himself published a final summary.

RÖSSLE and ROULET used the term retothelsarcoma not because they wanted to express the fact that reticulum cells *and* endothelial cells are involved. The word retothelium is not composed of the first syllable of reticulum cell (ret-) and the last syllables of endothelium (-othelium). Instead, retothelium meant to them the cells that cover (thelium ~ covering) the reticulum network (reto-).

ROULET[894] distinguished an immature large-cell form without fiber formation (which does not correspond to the stem-cell lymphoma of the present day) and a mature form with abundant fibers. The cells of the latter form were oval, stellate, or spindle-shaped and often included giant cells. A third "combined" form was to be found in Hodgkin's disease and leukemia. In 1932, ROULET then described systematized forms of retothelsarcoma ("retothelsarcomatosis"). Later, he gave two reports on retothelsarcoma: in 1947 on that of the spleen and in 1953 as part of a lecture on reticulosis.

AHLSTRÖM[895] added a special variant to the retothelsarcoma of ROULET: polymorphocellular retothelsarcoma, which was characterized by a particularly high content of giant cells.

DE OLIVEIRA[892] studied retothelsarcoma in two aspects: first, with regard to the embryogenesis of the lymphoreticular tissue and, second, to detailed study of reticulin fibers. DE OLIVEIRA distinguished six types, which RÖSSLE[893] evidently did not accept or at least did not specify in detail in his review. ROBB-SMITH,[895a] on the other hand, put great value on these types, but did not even mention the work of ROULET. DE OLIVEIRA discriminated (1) a cytoplasmic-syncytial afibrillar form, (2) a cytoplasmic-syncytial fibrillar form, (3) a fibro-reticulosyncytial form, (4) a fibro-cellular differentiated form with abundant reticulin fibers, and (5) a polymorphocellular form like AHLSTRÖM'S[895] variant. A special sixth type was introduced by DE OLIVEIRA. It was called "retothelsarcoma with hematopoietic differentiation" and described as a reticular tumor with lymphocytes and lymphoblasts or with plasma cells or plasmacytoid elements. This tumor type is probably equivalent to what we now call LP immunocytoma.

---

[890] 1927.
[891] 1928.
[892] 1936.
[893] 1939.
[894] 1930.
[895] 1938.
[895a] 1938.

The term retothelsarcoma was widely accepted in Germany and Japan, whereas the term reticulosarcoma was used in English- and French-speaking countries.

The first extensive studies of reticulosarcoma in England were published by DAWSON *et al.*[896] and by ROBB-SMITH.[896a] The latter author distinguished (1) a differentiated syncytial reticulosarcoma that showed no formation of fibers and that consisted of neutrophilic to weakly basophilic cells, (2) a dictyocytic reticulosarcoma that produced abundant fibers and that was composed of free or fiber-associated reticulum cells, and (3) a mixed type (polymorphocellular reticulosarcoma) that was rich in giant cells and that was at least closely related to Hodgkin's disease. ROBB-SMITH also used the term "lymphoblastic *reticulo-sarcoma*" for lymphoblastic lymphosarcoma. During this period further papers on reticulosarcoma were published by SJOEVALL[898] and DÖRING.[899]

In 1939, RÖSSLE presented a first systematic review of a large number of cases, unfortunately without giving exact numerical data. He reported that retothelsarcoma affects all age groups equally (youngest patient: 7 months old, oldest patient: 85 years old) and both sexes with about equal frequency. The order in which different sites were involved was said to go from the cervical lymph nodes to Waldeyer's tonsillar ring and the mediastinal, abdominal, and axillary lymph nodes. The other lymph-node regions were affected less often. The prognosis was reported to be always poor, but the tumor was said to be radiosensitive. Histologically, RÖSSLE essentially distinguished three types: (1) an immature-cellular form (roundish to oval cells with frequently large nucleoli, no formation of fibers), (2) a mature, fibril-producing form, and (3) a mixed-cell form (with round cells, monocytoid cells, giant cells).

This histologic subclassification agrees in basic principle with that of GALL and MALLORY[897]—they were the first to discriminate between *stem-cell lymphoma,* which they said was derived from undifferentiated, probably pluripotent cells of the hemopoietic tissue—lymphoid stem cells; and *clasmatocytic lymphoma,* which they attributed to the relatively highly differentiated wandering cells with phagocytic properties. Stem-cell lymphoma was said to be composed of large cells with a large solitary nucleolus, and the tumor did not form fibers. Clasmatocytic lymphoma consisted of cells that corresponded to normal clasmatocytes (histiocytes) or were highly reminiscent of monocytes. These cells were smaller, had abundant cytoplasm, and showed phagocytic properties. The nucleoli were small. The distinction between less differentiated forms and stem-cell lymphoma was thought to be difficult. The reticulin-fiber content was relatively low; at least there was hardly any proof that the reticulin fibers came from the tumor cells.

GALL and MALLORY then gave further copious data on the two types of lymphoma with respect to age, sex, clinical course, histology, etc. Stem-cell lymphoma is probably equivalent to the immature form of retothelsarcoma of RÖSSLE. But what has happened to the fiber-producing retothelsarcoma of RÖSSLE and his group?

---

[896] DAWSON, INNES and HARVEY, 1937.
[896a] 1938.
[897] 1942.
[898] 1936.
[899] 1938.

In Japan, after a large study by OGATA,[900] reticulosarcoma has been subjected to exhaustive study by AKAZAKI and his school since 1942.[901] After numerous attempts at subclassification, AKAZAKI concluded that in principle one should distinguish an undifferentiated and a differentiated reticulosarcoma. According to AKAZAKI, undifferentiated reticulosarcoma was composed of large, basophilic, closely packed cells that were not able either to phagocytose or to produce reticulin fibers. Therefore, this type corresponds to the stem-cell lymphoma of GALL and MALLORY and no doubt to the immature form of retothelsarcoma of RÖSSLE. Differentiated reticulosarcoma was said to consist of smaller, stellate cells with abundant cytoplasmic organelles, which were thought to be characteristic of reticulum cells. The tumor cells were capable of phagocytosis. AKAZAKI subclassified this differentiated reticulosarcoma into (1) a reticular type rich in reticulin fibers, (2) a histiocytic type, in which the cells were rounded and often showed erythrophagocytosis, but in which fiber formation was absent, (3) a pleomorphic type like that of AHLSTRÖM with numerous giant cells, (4) a mixed type, composed of stellate cells and immature rounded cells ("stem cells"), and (5) a small-cell type, which allegedly resembled lymphosarcoma.

It is not easy to relate these five subgroups to equivalent tumor entities described by other authors. One could compare the reticular type to the differentiated type of RÖSSLE and perhaps to the clasmatocytic type of GALL and MALLORY. The histiocytic type is highly reminiscent of the histiocytic medullary reticulosis of ROBB-SMITH.[902] The pleomorphic type is similar to Hodgkin's disease with lymphocytic predominance.

In the 1950s, FRESEN[903] did intensive work on the reticular neoplasms and paid particular attention to fiber content and arrangement. When associated with the appropriate morphology, the formation of reticulin fibers was indicative for FRESEN of the reticular nature of a neoplasm.

In 1956, the highly regarded, new classification of malignant lymphomas of RAPPAPORT *et al.*[904] appeared. It distinguished nodular and diffuse variants of each cell type, including the reticulum-cell type of lymphoma. In 1964, RAPPAPORT wrote further articles, and in 1966, he presented his final classification. It agreed with the concept of GALL and MALLORY in that RAPPAPORT also distinguished an undifferentiated and a differentiated reticulum-cell (histiocytic) type. There is no uncertainty about the first form, which was no longer called histiocytic or reticulum-cell type in the *Tumor Atlas*, but, instead, malignant lymphoma, undifferentiated. The second, differentiated, or histiocytic form, however, also included some tumors of germinal-center cells, in particular centrocytes. The term histiocytic or reticulum-cell is certainly not appropriate for all of the tumors included in this group.

RAPPAPORT's concept was accepted, at times with small variations, by numerous authors, particularly in North America.[905] LUKES[906] differentiated a stem-cell and a histiocytic type of malignant lymphoma and clearly rejected

---

[900] 1939.
[901] Reviews: 1953, 1973.
[902] 1938, 1947.
[903] 1949/1950, 1953.
[904] RAPPAPORT, WINTER and HICKS, 1956.
[905] E.g., LUKES, 1964, 1967, 1968; BERARD, 1972; DORFMAN, 1975.
[906] 1964, 1967.

the term reticulosarcoma. French, English, and German investigators in general held to the old distinction of (lymphocytic and lymphoblastic) lymphosarcoma and reticulosarcoma.[907] In 1964, MATHÉ suggested separating reticulosarcoma (consisting of stationary cells) from histiocytic sarcoma (consisting of mobile cells). Later, MATHÉ *et al.*[908] differentiated a histiocytic and a histioblastic type of reticulosarcoma. The histiocytic type always contained abundant fibers. The histioblastic type was said to be more frequent in males. Involvement of the skin was reported to appear in 27.7% of the cases of the histiocytic type and in only 2.6% of the cases of the histioblastic type. Only the histioblastic type could become leukemic.

A new perspective was provided by the electron microscopic,[909] immunochemical, and immunocytologic studies[910] of our research group (see p. 421 ff.). From their electron-microscopic studies, SUCHI *et al.*[911] also reported that reticulosarcoma cells have the power of Ig production (in particular IgM production). The cases they studied, however, appear to be of heterogeneous nature. In addition, the methods then used for demonstrating Ig are open to criticism.

At this stage, we must enquire again into the identity (or identities) of *true* reticulosarcoma. As recounted in Part One (p. 51 ff.), we distinguish four types of reticulum cells: histiocytic, fibroblastic, dendritic, and interdigitating reticulum cells. Of these, only the histiocytic reticulum cells are listed in the mononuclear phagocyte system (MPS), whose central cell is the monocyte.[912] Epithelioid cells, which are monocyte-derived, may also be seen in the scope of the MPS. Furthermore, sinus endothelial cells (littoral cells) must be considered. Theoretically, each of these cells should be capable of giving rise to malignant tumors. We are confronted, however, with the question of how to recognize and distinguish such tumors. Cytochemical, electron-microscopic, and immunologic analyses should be of help here.

### 1. *Sarcomas of Histiocytic Reticulum Cells*

Histiocytic (phagocytosing) reticulum cells are chiefly characterized by very high nonspecific esterase and acid phosphatase contents. Therefore, one would expect that tumors of this cell type would be recognizable by the high activity of these enzymes. Another indication would be the demonstration of active phagocytosis by the tumor cells.

In our material these two criteria were fulfilled in only one type of tumor, which cytologically corresponded to the malignant histiocytosis of RAPPAPORT.[913] Clinically, this sarcoma sometimes appeared as a large tumor confined to one or several lymph-node regions, without the typical general symptoms

---

[907] E.g., FRESEN, 1953; LENNERT, 1964a.

[908] MATHÉ, GÉRARD-MARCHANT, TEXIER, SCHLUMBERGER *et al.*, 1970.

[909] LENNERT, 1967; MORI and LENNERT, 1969.

[910] LENNERT, 1972; STEIN, LENNERT and PARWARESCH, 1972; STEIN, KAISERLING and LENNERT, 1973; LENNERT, STEIN and KAISERLING, 1974, 1975; STEIN, KAISERLING and LENNERT, 1974a.

[911] SUCHI, SATO, KOBAYASHI, AKATSUKA *et al.*, 1973.

[912] VAN FURTH, COHN, HIRSCH, HUMPHREY *et al.*, 1972.

[913] 1966; BYRNE and RAPPAPORT, 1973, Lit.

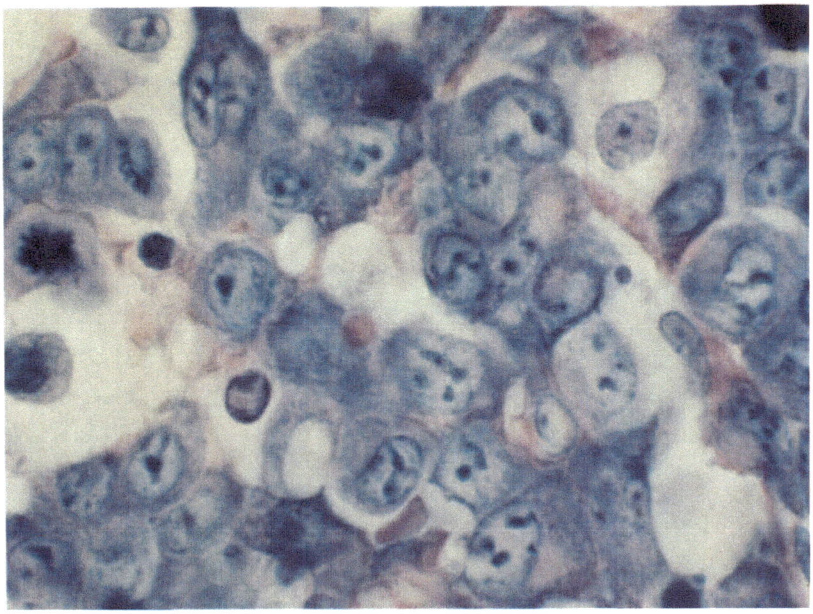

Fig. 226. Histiocytic reticulosarcoma ("malignant histiocytosis") with Giemsa staining. The tumor cells have quite abundant basophilic cytoplasm that is more gray than blue. The nuclei contain some medium-sized, polymorphic, irregularly situated nucleoli. Among the cohesive tumor cells there are some large nonneoplastic histiocytes, which are seen better at lower magnification (Fig. 227). ♂, 13 years. Subcutaneous tumor mass. × 1,550

of malignant histiocytosis, first described by SCOTT and ROBB-SMITH[914] under the term histiocytic medullary reticulosis.

Since the reticular neoplasms are not a subject of this book, this entity will not be discussed in detail. It is mentioned here merely because, at the moment, it represents the only proved histiocytic malignant neoplasm, which might be derived from histiocytic reticulum cells, and because it must be distinguished, as a differential diagnosis, from immunoblastic sarcoma.

We shall not discuss below the histologic picture of histiocytic medullary reticulosis or malignant histiocytosis described in detail by ROBB-SMITH and RAPPAPORT[915] as a more or less systemic disorder. We shall confine our description to that of the sarcomatous variants of this neoplasm. They show complete replacement of the lymph node by characteristic tumor tissue. The tumor often does not reveal a single plasma cell and may exhibit infiltrative and destructive growth in the capsule. Cytostatic therapy may lead to remissions of many years (and perhaps to cure?). The patients in our series were almost exclusively children.

Cytologically, this neoplasm consists of medium-sized to large cells. Their cytoplasm is more abundant than that of immunoblastic lymphoma cells (Fig. 226). These cells are relatively uniformly interspersed with nonneoplastic

[914] 1939; ROBB-SMITH, 1964.

[915] See also SERCK-HANSSEN and PUROHIT, 1968; SERCK-HANSSEN, 1973.

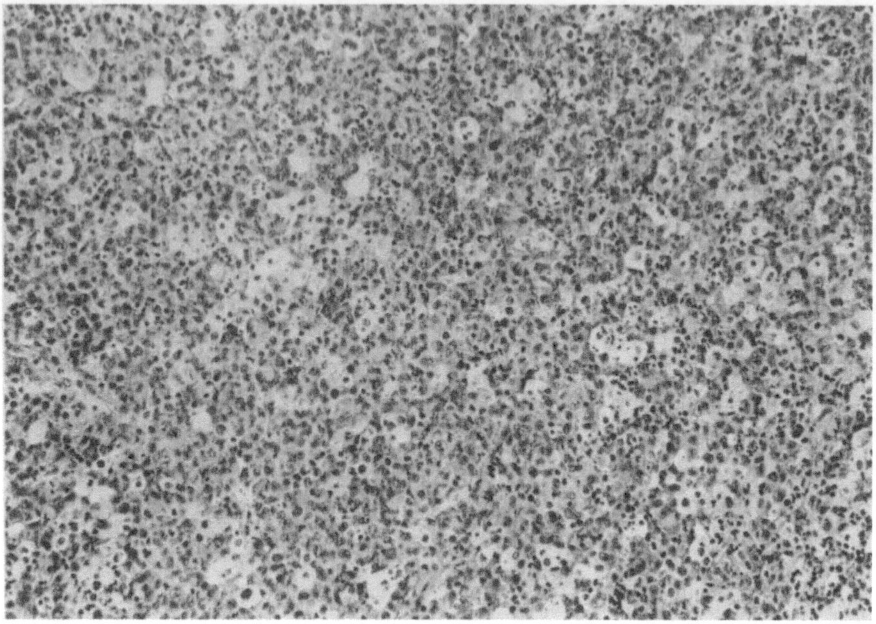

Fig. 227. Histiocytic reticulosarcoma ("malignant histiocytosis"). Note the cribriform appearance, conditioned by intermingled nonneoplastic histiocytes. ♀, 3 years. Axillary node. Hematoxylin and eosin. ×140

plump macrophages (Figs. 227 and 228). Since the cytoplasm of the normal macrophages is either very light (pink with Giemsa staining) or shrunken, leaving a gap around the cell, the dense sheets of tumor cells appear to be perforated by these normal cells. In Giemsa-stained sections the tumor cells usually have a gray-blue, sometimes a deep blue cytoplasm. They are cohesive in sarcomatous cases. The nuclei are round or oval, but occasionally polymorphic. They usually have several medium-sized, irregular, central nucleoli. The chromatin is somewhat irregularly clumped and not as uniformly fine as that of the normal macrophages lying among the tumor cells.

The tumor cells show very great differences in size. There are also more or less abundant binucleate and multinucleate giant cells. The nuclei are central or eccentric and very variable in size and shape. There are always a large number of mitotic figures. Polyploid mitotic figures are also found. Among the tumor cells one sees an increase in erythrocytes, which is pronounced in some cases but only slight in others.

A very small or even considerable number of tumor cells generally show erythrophagocytosis and occasionally leukophagocytosis. This can be recognized more easily in imprints than in sections (Fig. 229). The normal histiocytes lying among the tumor cells phagocytose almost exclusively perishing tumor cells and therefore largely correspond to the starry-sky cells of Burkitt's lymphoma.

(a)

(b)

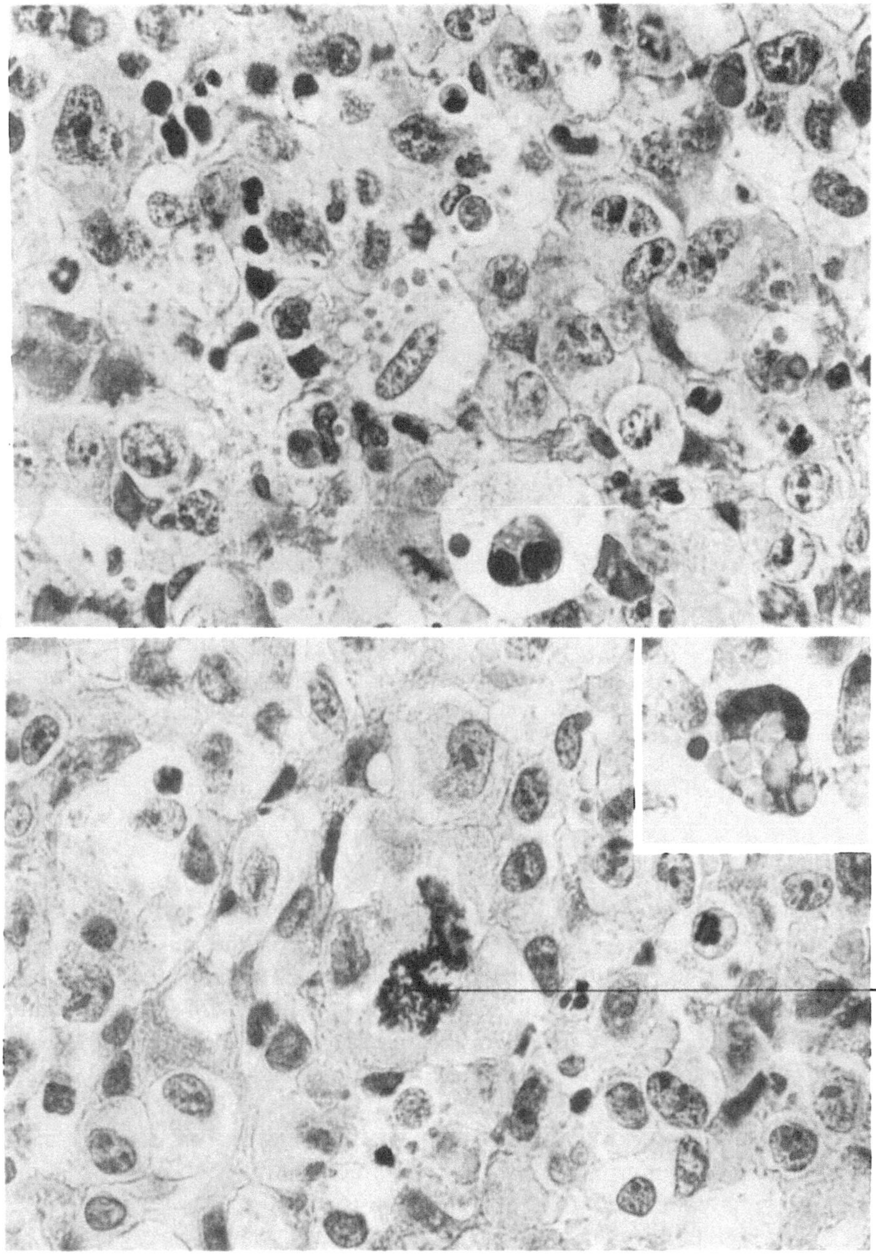


Fig. 228a and b. Histiocytic reticulosarcoma ("malignant histiocytosis"). Note the nuclear structure of the nonneoplastic histiocytes—well shown in the center of (a)—which differs from that of the irregularly shaped nuclei of the tumor cells. The chromatin is finer and the nucleoli are smaller than in the tumor cells. The nonneoplastic histiocytes contain remnants of tumor cells, not erythrocytes (!). In the center of (b), an atypical polyploid mitosis (*m*). Inset: a large tumor cell containing many erythrocytes. Same slide as Fig. 227. Hematoxylin and eosin. ×875

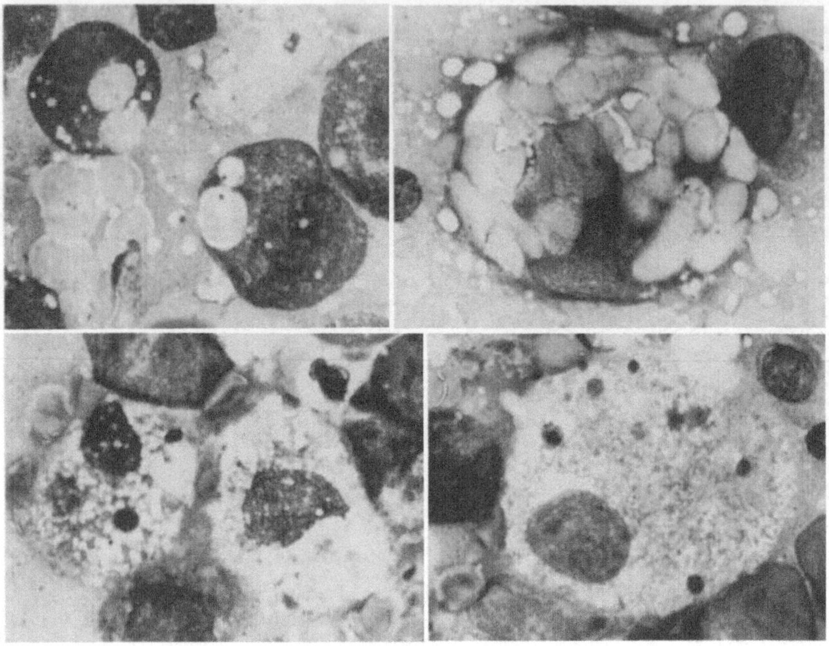


Fig. 229a–d. Histiocytic reticulosarcoma ("malignant histiocytosis"). Imprint from the same case as Figs. 227 and 228. (a, b) Tumor cells showing marked erythrophagocytosis. Tumor cells are very basophilic. In (a), vacuoles with and without remnants of erythrocytes. In (b), very large tumor cell filled with a huge number of erythrocytes. (c, d) Nonneoplastic histiocytes showing tumor-cell phagocytosis. In (c), relatively small histiocytes, probably monocytogenous, with many vacuoles and some cell debris. In (d), a very large histiocyte with remnants of tumor cells in the abundant cytoplasm. Pappenheim. ×875

In *imprints* the tumor cells are remarkably strongly basophilic (Fig. 230a). Thus, we were at first tempted to diagnose a tumor of the plasma-cell series. This assumption was supported by the finding of a narrow perinuclear halo in some cells. The nuclei are usually round or oval. They contain several medium-sized nucleoli, which are often hardly visible, and finely reticular chromatin. The rim of cytoplasm is moderately wide, but sometimes wide and then usually somewhat less basophilic. It often contains a few or even numerous vacuoles (similar to those in Burkitt's tumor cells). The tumor cells form strongly basophilic and very polymorphic giant cells, in which the nucleoli are only dimly recognizable, in contrast to those of Sternberg-Reed giant cells.

The degree of erythrophagocytosis by the tumor cells varies greatly (Fig. 229). A single cell often contains only one erythrocyte. In some cells there is a relatively large pale area, which corresponds to a digested erythrocyte. In other tumor cells there are several, sometimes huge numbers of erythrocytes. These erythrocytes occasionally lie in large cytoplasmic cavities. The latter may also be empty, indicating that an erythrocyte has disintegrated at this site. Occasionally, one sees degenerate tumor cells that are stuffed with erythrocytes. In the tumor cells we rarely found phagocytosed nuclei; some of these nuclei

(a)

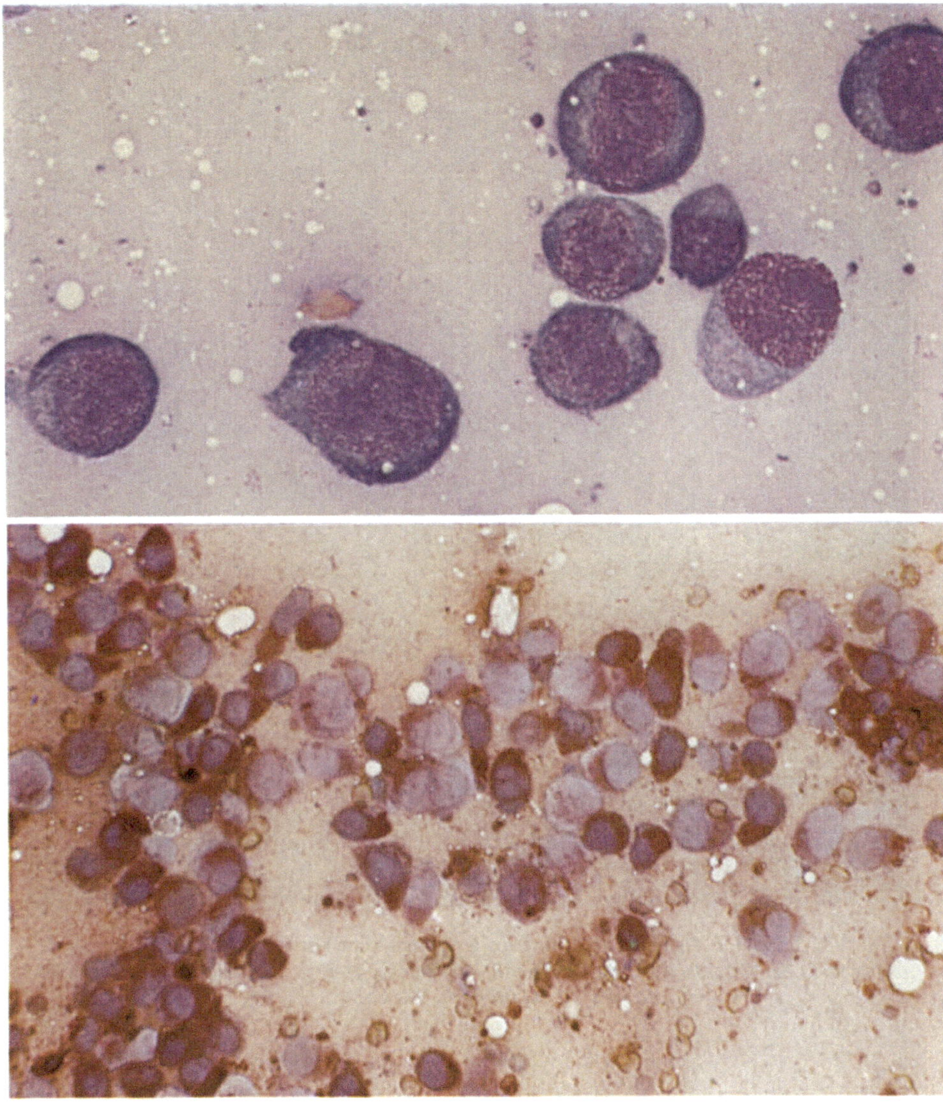

(b)

Fig. 230a and b. Histiocytic reticulosarcoma ("malignant histiocytosis"). Imprint from the same case as Fig. 226. (a) With Pappenheim staining there is strong basophilia of tumor cells that are reminiscent of the plasma-cell series. Fine chromatin. Large, light blue nucleoli are hardly visible. (b) Same imprint with neutral nonspecific esterase reaction. The tumor cells show a diffuse, moderately to strongly positive reaction. (a) ×875, (b) ×350

definitely originated from neutrophil granulocytes, whereas others gave no indication of their origin, although most of them probably originated from neutrophil granulocytes. The mitotic figures sometimes reveal fine, sometimes somewhat thicker chromosomes. Several times we saw phagocytosed erythrocytes in cells undergoing mitosis.

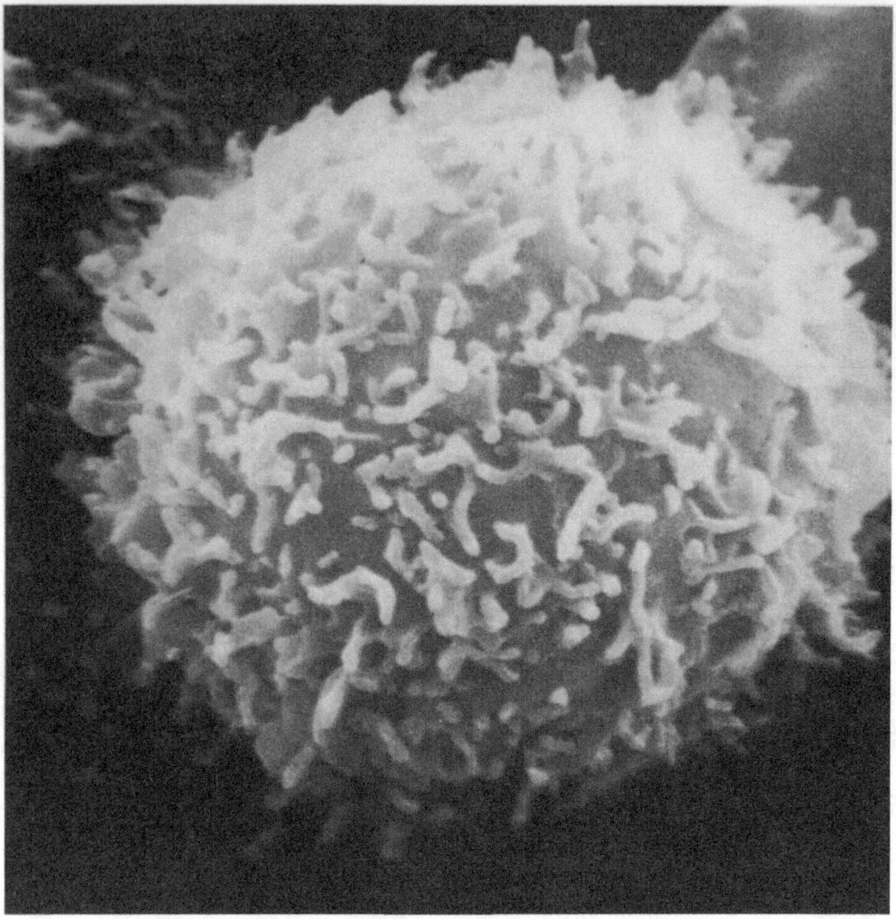

Fig. 231. Tumor cell of histiocytic reticulosarcoma ("malignant histiocytosis") with scanning electron microscope. Note the numerous surface villi. Same case as Figs. 226 and 230. Cell suspension. Photographed by U. MÜLLER-HERMELINK. ×8,100

Among the tumor cells there are moderately abundant normal macrophages, including all transitional forms up to small monocytes. The smaller macrophages have bean-shaped or polymorphic nuclei. Later forms have round or oval nuclei with fine chromatin and a solitary small nucleolus. The rim of cytoplasm of the large forms is extremely broad, stains a weak pink, and shows a uniform coarse vacuolation like that of lipophages. As a rule, one finds more or less abundant remnants of disintegrated nucleated cells and very occasional erythrocytes among the vacuoles. It is also noticeable in imprints that there is an increase in erythrocytes and sometimes in granulocytes among the tumor cells. Plasma cells were not demonstrated in imprints of the cases we studied.

On cytochemical analysis the tumor cells showed slight to moderately strong reactivity for nonspecific esterase (acid and neutral variants; Fig. 230b). The activity was usually seen in large areas of the cytoplasm or else it was diffuse and homogeneous. In comparison, the normal macrophages exhibited very strong activity and transition into small, moderately positive forms, which proved to be morphologically identical with monocytes. In the enzyme-cytochemistry preparations, however, there were no transitional forms between macrophages and tumor cells. The tumor cells revealed a focal or diffuse, strong, granular acid phosphatase reaction. In the macrophages the reaction was much stronger and more diffuse. The ATPase reaction was negative in the one case studied. In the tumor cells the PAS reaction was also negative. There was sometimes a slightly positive, granular PAS reaction in the macrophages. Stains for fat were not performed. U. MÜLLER-HERMELINK[916] studied one of our cases with the scanning electron microscope and found that the surface of the tumor cells showed an immense number of plump microvilli (Fig. 231).

All the cytologic data presented above leave no doubt that this is a malignant tumor of histiocytes (histiocytic reticulum cells?). Remarkably, it also contains normal histiocytic components, which are probably derived from immigrant monocytes. The tumor can be clearly distinguished from immunoblastic and lymphoblastic lymphomas on the basis of cytologic (gray-blue to blue cytoplasm, multiple medium-sized irregular nucleoli), cytochemical (positive nonspecific esterase reaction), and functional (erythrophagocytosis) criteria.

It is not yet clear whether there are still other types of tumors to be included under "histiocytic reticulosarcoma" besides the malignant histiocytic tumor described here. We have seen several cases, however, with a strong nonspecific esterase reaction in the cells, but with a different morphology. This indicates that it is advisable to continue looking for malignant tumors of these cells using all available methods. Electron-microscopic studies on their own have so far not brought us the degree of certainty in the identification of the tumor reported by HENRY.[917]

## 2. *Sarcomas of Fibroblastic Reticulum Cells*

As far as we know, pure populations of fibroblastic reticulum cells have not yet been found in reticulosarcoma, or at least not demonstrated with the alkaline phosphatase reaction. By itself, the reticulin-fiber content of a sarcoma is, in our opinion, insufficient evidence that the tumor has arisen from fibroblastic reticulum cells. We think it is unwise to draw any histogenetic conclusions from the *number* of fibers.

In our opinion, the fibroblastic reticulum cell is an integral part of lymphoreticular tissue. All tumors of this tissue contain at least a few fibers. The amount of fiber may depend on several factors: on the speed of growth of the actual tumor cells and especially on the inductive effect of the tumor cells. If they grow so fast that the "stroma cells" do not keep up, then fiber

[916] Unpublished data. [917] 1975.

production may be absent. On the other hand, if the tumor cells grow very slowly, the fiber-producing partner cell may contribute a correspondingly larger number of fibers. The fiber-inducing effect of the tumor cells, however, is probably of greater significance than the rate of growth. By producing some mediator substance, such as immunoglobulin, they might stimulate fibrogenesis.

The last possibility is worthy of serious consideration in the case of "reticulosarcomas" rich in fibers. This thesis is supported by measurements that we performed with NAGAI on the reticulin-fiber content of malignant neoplasms of the bone marrow.[918] To our amazement, we found that plasmacytoma of the bone marrow showed the highest fiber content next to osteomyelosclerosis, namely, $133.5 \pm 6.0$ mm/mm$^3$ fibers compared with $43.1 \pm 1.7$ mm/mm$^3$ in normal bone marrow. Here the slow growth or the long life of the plasmacytoma cells may be as important as the immunoglobulin secretion by the tumor cells. The high fiber content of plasmacytoma certainly does not indicate, however, that the tumor cells themselves produce fibers. Similar fibrosing effects may be found in plasma cell-rich inflammatory processes, for instance, in the liver or thyroid.

Therefore, the *number* of fibers is of little value in deciding whether or not a given tumor is a sarcoma of fibroblastic reticulum cells. It is undecided whether the *arrangement* of the fibers—for instance, the direct contact of cells with the fibers ("like pussy willows")—is more meaningful. One reason why we are so critical is that we have always seen the often cited "pussy willows" best in autopsy sections, i.e., in autolysed tissue.

Now one might ask whether a fibroblastic reticulosarcoma can perhaps be identified by electron microscopy. In fact, HENRY[918a] described such a case as follows: "It was composed of spindle-shaped cells exhibiting marked mitotic activity and associated with much reticulin formation. The fine structure of this lymphoma showed the features of the true reticular or fibre forming cells, with innumerable transitions between fibroblasts and reticular cells, even to the extent of desmosomal attachments."

Finally, one might ask whether a primary fiber-producing sarcoma of true fibroblasts (fibrosarcoma, spindle-cell sarcoma) can develop in lymph nodes. So far, we have not seen such a case, although we cannot exclude this possibility.

### *3. Sarcomas of Dendritic Reticulum Cells*

Dendritic reticulum cells are characterized in particular by their desmosomal junctions and are thereby recognizable in malignant lymphomas. In the search for malignant lymphomas containing this type of reticulum cell, it has become evident that dendritic reticulum cells appear only in tumors of germinal-center cells (M.L. centrocytic, M.L. centroblastic/centrocytic, M.L. centroblastic). Sarcomas composed purely of reticulum cells connected by desmosomes have not been described. Furthermore, we do not know whether such a tumor would necessarily retain the specific feature of dendritic reticulum cells, namely,

[918] LENNERT, NAGAI and SCHWARZE, 1975. [918a] 1975.

the development of desmosomes. Perhaps the demonstration of 5-nucleotidase will one day help us in the identification or exclusion of this hypothetical type of tumor.

### *4. Sarcomas of Interdigitating Reticulum Cells*

We do not know of any definite tumors composed exclusively of interdigitating reticulum cells from reports in the literature. It is possible, however, that MOLLO[919] demonstrated such a tumor by electron microscopy.

Recently, we observed a monomorphic malignant proliferation of interdigitating reticulum cells in a 69-year-old woman with mycosis fungoides in the tumor stage. The patient had been treated for classic M.F. with erythroderma and ultimately melanoderma over a period of 9 months with overdoses of radiotherapy and corticosteroids.

Large lymph-node tumors developed and a biopsy was obtained from one of them. The structure of the lymph node was destroyed. Two different types of neoplastic cell proliferation coexisted: (1) a proliferation of medium-sized anaplastic lymphoid cells (Lutzner cells), which fit the picture of the tumor stage of M.F. and which infiltrated the greater part of the lymph node, and (2) a large-cell proliferation of interdigitating reticulum cells. The reticulum cells were closely packed in many parts of the outer cortex, in the neighboring marginal and intermediate sinuses, and in the capsule. They also penetrated into the adjacent adipose tissue. In the sinuses, they grew in the manner of lymphangiosis carcinomatosa (Fig. 232). These interdigitating reticulum cells showing tumorous proliferation were easily identifiable by their polymorphic nuclear contour with manifold indentations and foldings and by the relatively wide rim of gray-blue cytoplasm (Fig. 233). The chromatin was fine. Nucleoli were small or undetectable. Occasionally, the interdigitating reticulum cells were atypical and had oval giant nuclei with a few marginal clefts. They also showed several definite mitotic figures. There was no increase in reticulin fibers in the sheets of reticulum cells. Unfortunately, cytochemical and electron-microscopic investigations were not possible because the lymph node had been fixed.

We have no doubt that the interdigitating reticulum cells proliferating in this case were malignant cells. They revealed several, sometimes atypical mitotic figures and infiltrative growth in the lymph-node parenchyma and surrounding tissue. Interdigitating reticulum cells also extended along the sinuses in the manner of lymphangiosis carcinomatosa.

### *5. Sarcomas of Sinus Endothelial Cells*

The existence of sarcomas of sinus endothelial cells[920] has been maintained for decades, for instance, by EWING.[921] According to RÖSSLE,[922] the cases

---

919 MOLLO, MONGA, CODA and PALESTRO, 1975.

920 Lit.: ROULET, 1930; RÖSSLE, 1939; EWING, 1940.

921 1928, 1940.

922 1939.

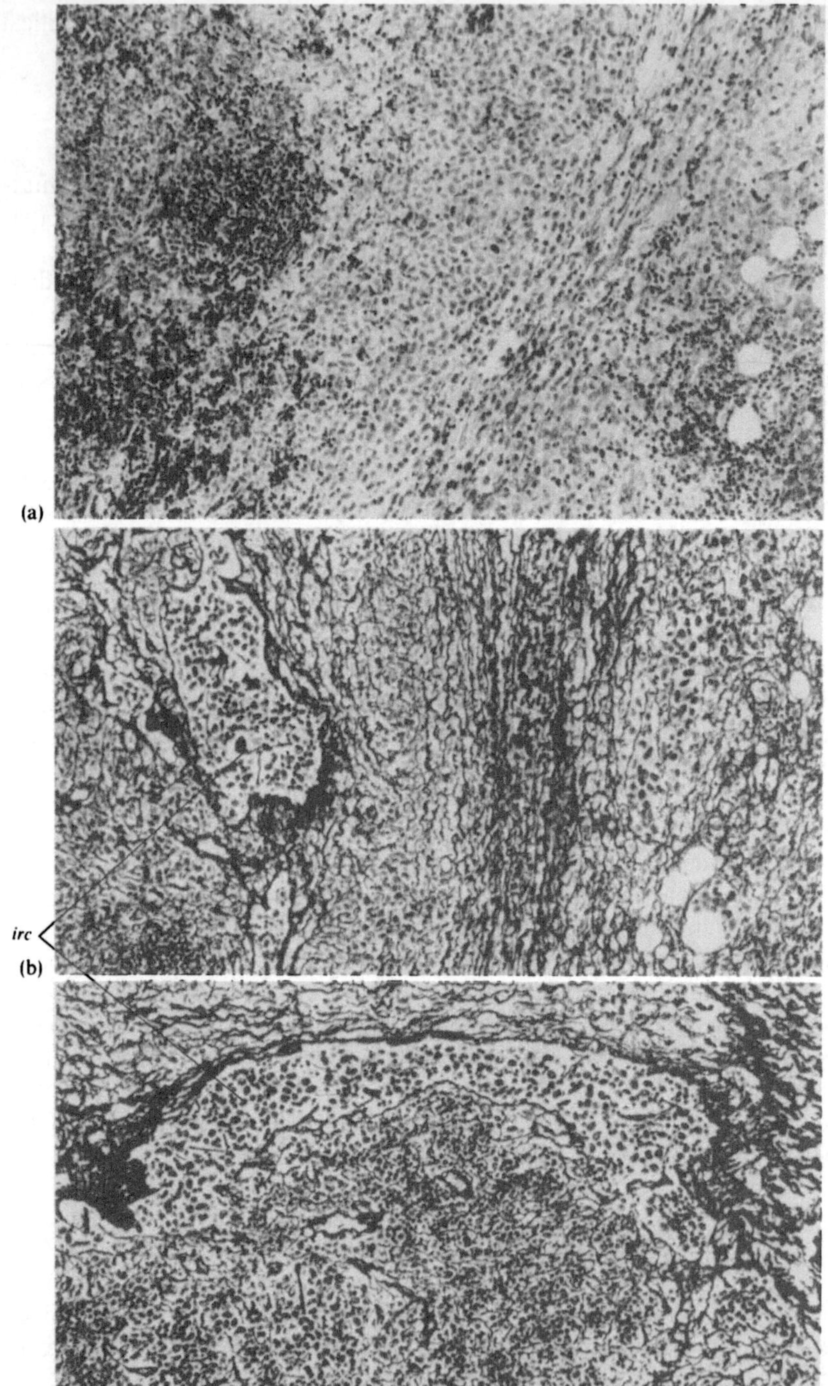
(a)
irc
(b)
(c)

of CRACIUN and URSU[923] and DA GRADI and DE AMICIS[924] are supposed to have been proved through the demonstration of "endothelial pearls." On the other hand, WILLIS[925] and JACKSON and PARKER[926] reject endothelioma of the sinus endothelial cells, unless the autopsy definitely establishes that there is not a primary tumor, such as an undifferentiated carcinoma, elsewhere in the body. That is particularly applicable to so-called endothelioma of the cervical lymph nodes; lymphoepithelial carcinoma (Schmincke's tumor) in particular has been misinterpreted as endothelioma (e.g., see Fig. 143 of EWING[927]): it often grows chiefly within the sinuses and forms foci of undifferentiated cells that can readily be mistaken for sinus endothelial cells. Such false diagnoses are, however, fateful for the patients; the correct diagnosis of Schmincke's tumor would give them a chance of recovery.

AKAZAKI[928] has also never seen an endothelioma of the lymph sinuses in lymph nodes. At least he emphasizes that Kupffer-cell sarcoma of the liver, which might be equivalent to lymph-node endothelioma, has an entirely different appearance from that of the previously described endotheliomas of the lymph node.

For the moment, we cannot yet conclusively determine whether or not there are sarcomas of sinus endothelial cells in lymph nodes. In any case, we know of no criterion that proves their existence and enables us to recognize them. Therefore, we do not make this diagnosis.

### 6. *Malignant Neoplasms of Monocytes and Their Derivatives*

We shall not discuss the neoplasms of monocytes here. They belong to the myeloproliferative diseases,[928a] since the monocyte definitely originates from precursor cells of the bone marrow and not from the RES or lymphatic system.

We shall also not present a detailed discussion of *epithelioid-cell lymphogranulomatosis*[929] (lymphoepithelioid-cell lymphoma). In this neoplasm the lymphocyte, and occasional larger basophilic lymphocyte-derived forms, might be considered the leading cell. It might produce one or more factors (i.e., migration inhibitory factor) that attract monocytes and cause their transformation into epithelioid cells.

923 1933.
924 1912.
925 1960.
926 1947.
927 1940.
928 1973.
928a RICHTER, 1956; LEDER, 1967a, 1969a.
929 LENNERT, 1952b, 1967; LENNERT and MESTDAGH, 1968.

◁ Fig. 232a–c. Sarcoma of interdigitating reticulum cells in mycosis fungoides. (a) Giemsa staining. On the left, residual normal lymphatic tissue and anaplastic Lutzner cells. Across the center, neoplastic interdigitating reticulum cells spreading through the capsule into the adjacent adipose tissue (right). (b, c) Silver stain showing dilated sinuses filled with neoplastic interdigitating reticulum cells (*irc*). In (b), infiltration of the adjacent adipose tissue is shown. Near the middle, remnants of the capsule. In (c), the tumor cells have infiltrated the subsinusoidal lymphoid tissue. ♀, 69 years. Inguinal node. ×125

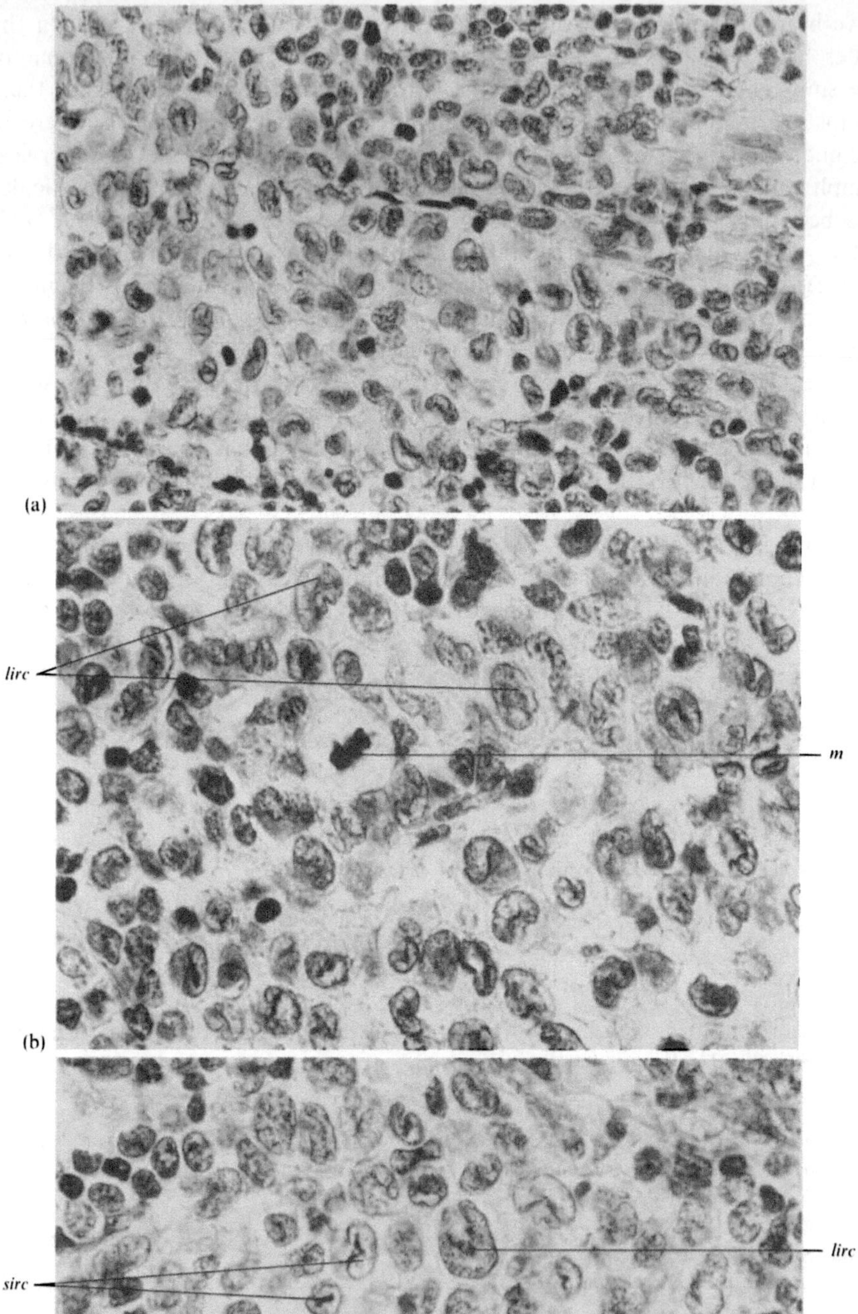
(a)
lirc
m
(b)
sirc
lirc
(c)

## *Conclusions*

At the end of this discussion all we can say is that the unequivocal identification of reticulosarcomas, particularly tumors of fiber-producing reticulum cells, is not yet possible. Earlier descriptions of reticulosarcoma, for instance, those of AKAZAKI,[930] were indeed very convincing on the basis of the methods available at the time. Nevertheless, we were made all the more skeptical by the results of studies using new methods. Therefore, we must rediscover what a reticulosarcoma really is and then from which type of reticulum cell it is derived.

The same question should also be posed for so-called reticulosis. We would prefer, however, to forego a presentation of this confusing subject here. We shall also leave out a description of histiocytosis X and ask the reader to refer to the comprehensive presentation of NEZELOF *et al.*[931]

[930] 1973 and earlier.

[931] NEZELOF, BASSET and ROUSSEAU, 1973.

◁ Fig. 233a–c. Sarcoma of interdigitating reticulum cells in mycosis fungoides. (a) Tumor cells in a sinus destroying the wall at the upper left. (b) Note the polymorphism of the nuclei. Some very large interdigitating reticulum cells (*lirc*). One mitosis (*m*) of an interdigitating reticulum cell. (c) Small (sirc) and large (*lirc*) interdigitating reticulum cells with contorted nuclei. Same case as Fig. 232. Hematoxylin and eosin. (a) ×492. (b, c) ×770

Part Five

# Ultrastructure of Non-Hodgkin's Lymphomas

E. KAISERLING

## Introduction

The previous development of ultrastructural studies of non-Hodgkin's lymphomas can be divided into three phases. The first phase was stimulated by the idea that it might be possible to find ultrastructural features that are specific to malignant cells. It appeared that it might also be possible to gain insight into the genesis of tumors. This hope has not been fulfilled, as BERNHARD anticipated as early as 1961.

The second phase was significantly molded by the studies of BERNHARD and LEPLUS[1] and MORI and LENNERT.[2] The foremost objects of interest were the ultrastructure of normal lymphoid cells and the correlation between the light- and electron-microscopic cytology of malignant lymphomas. These studies showed that malignant lymphomas have heterogeneous ultrastructures and that most lymphomas can be differentiated on electron microscopy. The question as to the cytologic relationships between normal and neoplastic cells could not be answered satisfactorily. The one exception is follicular lymphoma, now called centroblastic/centrocytic lymphoma, since it could be identified on electron microscopy as a germinal-center tumor.[3]

In the third phase we are now attempting to develop a new classification that takes the cytologic and functional features of normal lymphatic tissue into account. As mentioned previously, many experimental findings, but especially those of VELDMAN,[4] have contributed significantly to better understanding and precise knowledge of the ultrastructural features of normal lymphatic tissue, including its various reactions. Whereas results of exhaustive studies of the germinal-center reaction had already been available for a long time, VELDMAN presented the first detailed electron-microscopic studies of the reactions belonging to the "plasma-cell reaction," known since the publication of FAGRAEUS,[5] and, in particular, of the thymus-dependent reactions. VELDMAN showed that the

---

[1] 1964.
[2] 1969.
[3] MORI and LENNERT, 1969; LENNERT, 1973.
[4] 1970.
[5] 1948.

morphology of the thymus-dependent lymphatic system, which is represented by the T-nodules in lymph nodes, is very different from that of the B-dependent lymphatic system (germinal centers and the plasma-cell reaction). There are differences not only in the morphology of the lymphoid cells, but also in the nonlymphoid cells, above all dendritic and interdigitating reticulum cells. We have confirmed these findings, which VELDMAN obtained in rabbits, in normal human lymphatic tissue in all important respects.[5a]

The thymus-dependent lymph-node region (T-nodules) contains small lymphocytes with an oval, often irregularly shaped, occasionally cerebriform nucleus, and blast cells with abundant polyribosomes. Some of the small lymphocytes and blast cells have an electron-transparent, others an electron-dense cytoplasm. Regular components of T-nodules are, furthermore, interdigitating reticulum cells and epithelioid venules. T-associated plasma cells are also usually found in T-regions.[5b]

The B-regions of the lymph node show a completely different picture. Centrocytes and centroblasts are found exclusively in germinal centers. Centrocytes have a characteristic, irregularly shaped nucleus. Their cytoplasm contains monoribosomes, sometimes polyribosomes, and occasionally rough endoplasmic reticulum. The cytoplasm of centroblasts contains abundant polyribosomes; their nuclei show several marginal nucleoli. Immunoblasts are somewhat larger than centroblasts and have larger nucleoli with clearly visible nucleolonemata. Usually, plasma cells and plasma-cell precursors are also seen in germinal centers. Dendritic reticulum cells are regularly found in germinal centers. Occasionally, however, they are also seen in extrafollicular areas, namely, in the marginal zone, which is the site of the actual plasma-cell reaction. This region, especially the area near the marginal sinus, consists chiefly of small lymphocytes with a round nucleus containing abundant chromatin and of medium-sized cells with an oval or round nucleus containing moderately abundant chromatin and with cytoplasm revealing mono- and polyribosomes, several profiles of ergastoplasm, and a Golgi field with abundant vesicles. The medium-sized cells are reminiscent of the marginal-zone cells described by VELDMAN.[5c] In addition, one finds blast cells with abundant polyribosomes and plasma-cell precursors. The cytogenetic relationships between the various cells have already been described in Part One.

Our ultrastructural characterization of malignant lymphomas will be based on the findings in normal lymphatic tissue. We are most interested in the cytologic and histologic correlations between normal and neoplastic lymphatic tissue. Therefore, our attention will be drawn first to the cytologic features of the individual lymphoid cell. No less significant is the cytologic spectrum of the tumor cells, especially considering the findings on the different areas of normal lymphatic tissue. Finally, there is the question whether it might be possible to define the tumor cells more clearly on the basis of their relationship to the dendritic reticulum cells specific to the B-cell area and to the interdigitating reticulum cells that characterize the T-cell area.

---

[5a] KAISERLING, 1975, 1976, 1977; KAISERLING and LENNERT, 1974.

[5b] MÜLLER-HERMELINK, KAISERLING and LENNERT, 1973; LENNERT, KAISERLING and MÜLLER-HERMELINK, 1975.

[5c] 1970.

## *Remarks on Methods*

Primary fixation for 2 h at 4° C in buffered 4% glutaraldehyde (0.1 M cacodylate buffer, pH 7.3) and postfixation in 1% $OsO_4$ (Rhodin buffer) have proved to be particularly suitable for the ultrastructural study of malignant lymphomas (glutaraldehyde *reinst* in 25% aqueous solution—Serva, Fed. Rep. Germany—stored in nitrogen atmosphere at 4° C). Primary glutaraldehyde fixation offers the advantage over primary $OsO_4$ fixation in that the chromatin pattern of the nucleus, which is important for the differentiation of lymphoid cells, stands out more clearly. Moreover, the comparison of light- and electron-microscopic findings is easier. We use uranyl acetate[6] and lead citrate[7] staining.

In the classification of malignant lymphomas, the PAS reaction has proved to be a particularly easy method for the (nonspecific) demonstration of intracytoplasmic immunoglobulin (Ig), i.e., of so-called Russell bodies. The periodic-acid silver-methenamine reaction is based on the same chemical reactions as the PAS reaction. We use the method of DE MARTINO and ZAMBONI[8] in modification III. With this method, both the histologic structure of the lymphatic tissue and the cytology of the individual cells can be evaluated well. Insight into the histologic structure of the lymph node is made possible by the high electron density of the collagenous fibers and by the positive reaction of the basement membrane. The reaction is not specific, since heterochromatin and the nucleolus, as well as numerous other structures (ribosomes, lysosomes, centrioles, and the specific granules of monocytes, neutrophil and eosinophil granulocytes, and tissue mast cells), show a positive reaction. Besides Ig inclusions, extracellular Ig precipitates are also demonstrated. They can be more clearly distinguished than is possible with conventional uranyl acetate and lead citrate staining. When sections are not pretreated with periodic acid, the reaction of glycogen is considerably intensified. Sometimes glycogen is visible only when this procedure is followed.

# I. Low-Grade Malignant Lymphomas

## A. Malignant Lymphoma, Lymphocytic

### *1. Chronic Lymphocytic Leukemia*

#### *a) B-Type*

Most of the ultrastructural studies of chronic lymphocytic leukemia (CLL) have been performed on lymphocytes of peripheral blood.[9] In contrast, there

6 STEMPAK and WARD, 1964.
7 VENABLE and COGGESHALL, 1965.
8 1967.
9 ANDERSON, 1966; SMETANA, HEŘMANSY, JANELE and BUSCH, 1968; FOA, FOA and MURATORE, 1970; HUHN, 1970; SCHUMACHER, MAUGEL and DAVIS, 1970; SCHREK, 1972; BESSIS, 1973; LITOVITZ and LUTZNER, 1974; COHNEN, 1975; BRITTINGER, AUGNER, BREMER, COHNEN *et al.*, 1975; SCHAEFER, KRÜGER and FISCHER, 1975.

have been few investigations of the morphology of lymphatic tissue,[10] and these were mostly of the cytology of small lymphocytes.

The essential characteristic of CLL is the monotonous cytology. The peripheral blood reveals a uniform population of lymphocytes, which are difficult to distinguish from normal blood lymphocytes. CLL lymphocytes have a round or oval nucleus, which contains one, or rarely two ring-shaped nucleoli. There are triangular condensations of heterochromatin based at the nuclear membrane and a rim of nucleolus-associated chromatin. The cytoplasm is sparse and contains a small Golgi field, some mitochondria, and a few lysosome-like granules. There are many monoribosomes, but no polyribosomes and only a few profiles of rough endoplasmic reticulum. The cell surface may have many projections. This finding can be correlated with the villous surface structure of CLL lymphocytes seen with the scanning microscope.[11] Since in some cases CLL lymphocytes may have only a few microvilli and in rare cases they show no microvilli at all,[12] however, the surface structure of CLL lymphocytes has no great diagnostic value.

According to morphometric findings, CLL lymphocytes differ from normal blood lymphocytes by a smaller rim of cytoplasm, which results in a smaller total cell area than that of normal lymphocytes,[13] by abundant heterochromatin,[14] and by a significantly smaller number of lysosome-like granules.[15] According to studies of HUHN,[16] the number of cytoplasmic organelles and the amount of ergastoplasm are considerably greater in CLL lymphocytes of peripheral blood than in normal blood lymphocytes.

Cells with the same ultrastructural features as those seen in the blood also predominate in lymphatic tissue (Fig. 234). Besides small lymphocytes, two further types of lymphoid cells can be regularly found in lymphatic tissue: prolymphocytes (Fig. 234) and paraimmunoblasts (Fig. 235). These cells are not difficult to distinguish from the small lymphocytes on the basis of their size, the distribution of their chromatin, and their cytoplasmic organelles. The paraimmunoblasts have a large, round or oval nucleus. The nucleolus, which is chiefly found in the middle of the nucleus, is clearly contrasted with the nucleoplasm, in which chromatin is scarce. Nucleolus-associated heterochromatin is usually not found. The nucleolus is round or band-shaped and consists of loosely joined nucleolonemata. The cytoplasm contains a few rough membrane profiles concentric to the nucleus, a medium-sized Golgi field, and numerous mono- and polyribosomes. The mitochondria are usually electron-transparent and swollen. A giant mitochondrion is rarely found. The number of lysosome-like granules is small. The cytology of the prolymphocytes is between that of the small lymphocytes and the paraimmunoblasts. The cytoplasm contains chiefly monoribosomes, but also many polyribosomes and a few profiles of ergastoplasm. The Golgi field is sometimes well developed. The nucleus reveals a narrow

[10] BERNHARD and LEPLUS, 1964; MORI and LENNERT, 1969; SMETANA, GYORKEY, GYORKEY and BUSCH, 1970; MOLLO, MONGA and STRAMIGNONI, 1971; HENRY, 1975; KAISERLING, 1975, 1977.

[11] POLLIACK, SIEGAL, CLARKSON, FU *et al.*, 1975.

[12] COHNEN, FISCHER, LUDWIG and BRITTINGER, 1975.

[13] COHNEN, 1975.

[14] SCHUMACHER, MAUGEL and DAVIS, 1970.

[15] DOUGLAS, COHNEN, KÖNIG, BRITTINGER *et al.*, 1972; COHNEN, 1975.

[16] 1976, personal communication.

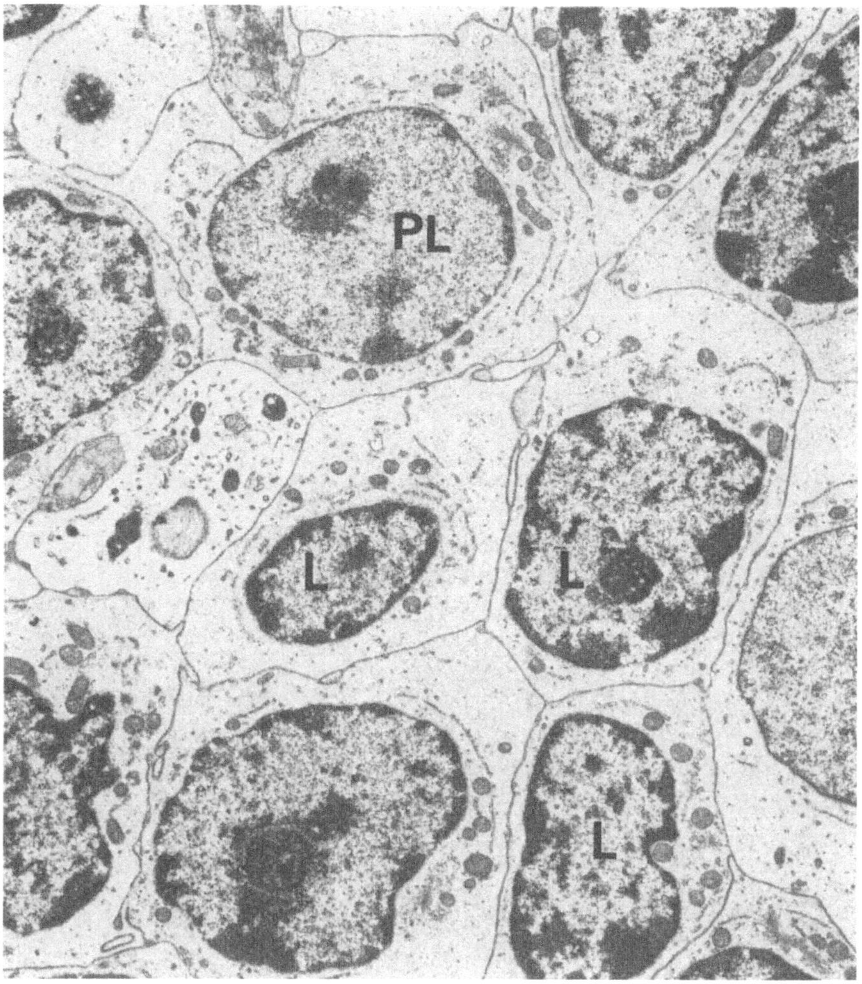


Fig. 234. Chronic lymphocytic leukemia (B-type). Typical CLL lymphocytes (*L*), characterized by marginally condensed heterochromatin and a small central ring-shaped nucleolus with nucleolus-associated chromatin. There are only a few rough membrane profiles in the cytoplasm. Furthermore, a somewhat larger lymphocyte (prolymphocyte; *PL*) with several rough membrane profiles in the cytoplasm. In contrast to the heterochromatin of the small lymphocytes, that of the larger cell shows a relatively uniform distribution in the nucleus. × 8,400

marginal rim of chromatin; sometimes the heterochromatin shows a patchy distribution. The nucleolus either consists of tightly joined nucleolonemata or is ring-shaped.

The mitochondria of CLL lymphocytes are sometimes vacuolated. They may reveal rarefaction of mitochondrial cristae or contain myelin figures or electron-dense intramitochondrial bodies. Since all of these structures can be seen in other lymphomas, they are of no diagnostic significance. The presence of giant mitochondria probably has no specific meaning, either. Ribosome-

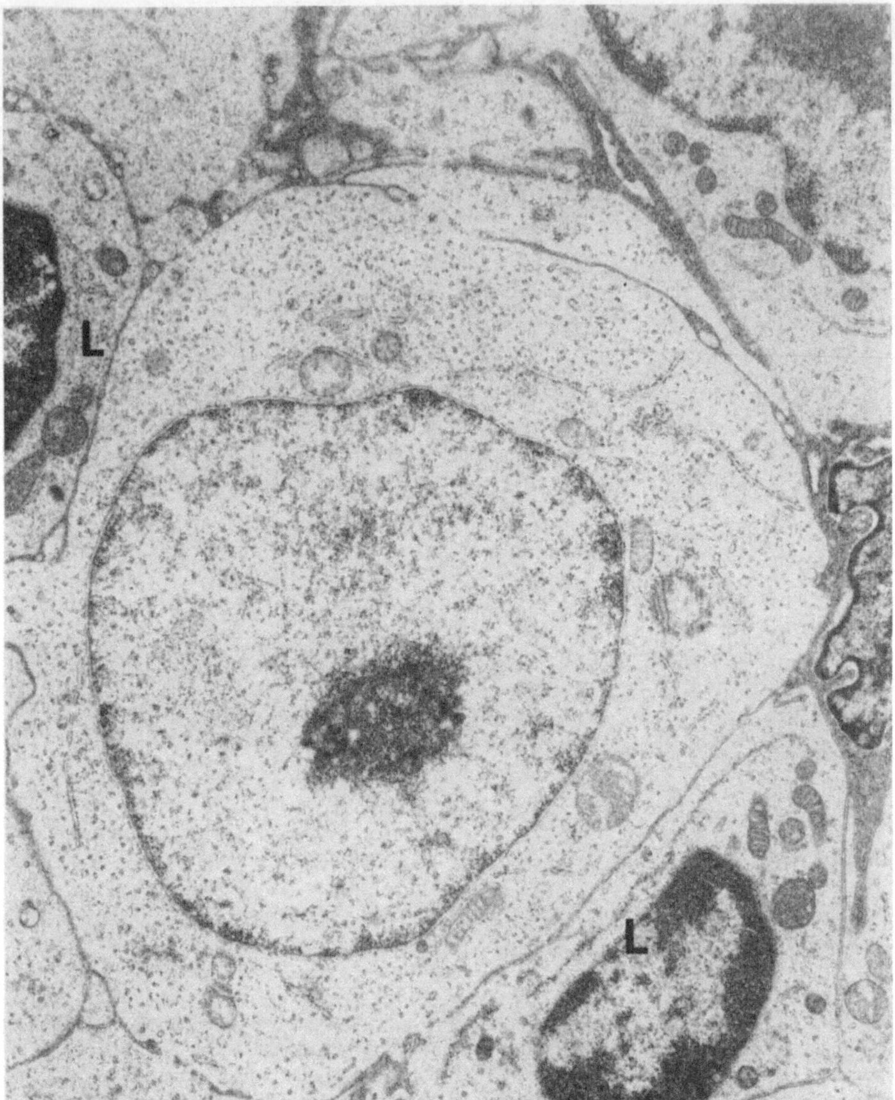


Fig. 235. Chronic lymphocytic leukemia (B-type). Blast cell (paraimmunoblast) with numerous polyribosomes and a few strands of rough endoplasmic reticulum. Lymphocytes (*L*). ×6,400

lamella complexes, which have been described in hairy-cell leukemia,[17] occasionally occur in CLL.[18] The literature contains several reports of crystalline or

[17] SCHREK and DONNELLY, 1966; KATAYAMA, LI and YAM, 1972; KATAYAMA, NAGY and BALOGH, 1973; SCHMALZL, HUHN, ASAMER and BRAUNSTEINER, 1975.

[18] ZUCKER-FRANKLIN, 1963; BRUNNING and PARKIN, 1975; CAWLEY, EMMINES, GOLDSTONE, HAMBLIN *et al.*, 1975; KAISERLING, 1975; WOESSNER and ROZMAN, 1976.

homogeneous Ig inclusions in CLL lymphocytes.[19] As a rule, the Ig inclusions were situated in cisterns of rough endoplasmic reticulum. In one case they were also seen in the perinuclear space,[19a] which suggested plasmacytic differentiation of the lymphoma as shown by LP immunocytoma. We have found no such Ig inclusions in any of our cases. Our studies of tumor cells in lymph nodes showed that CLL lymphocytes have only poorly developed rough endoplasmic reticulum, which is often seen as remarkably narrow profiles. There was no clear evidence of plasmacytic differentiation of CLL lymphocytes in the cases we have seen so far.

In agreement with the ultrastructural findings of other authors,[20] our studies showed that the acid phosphatase activity of CLL lymphocytes is extremely weak: only very few enzyme-positive lysosomes are found. In contrast, the reaction for ATPase is strongly positive.[21] As in other B-cell lymphomas, a broad ATPase-positive rim can be demonstrated at the surface membrane of the tumor cells (Fig. 236).

The presence of surface Ig on CLL lymphocytes is mentioned on page 565ff. In labeling experiments using the indirect immunoperoxidase method on three cases studied by electron microscopy, we found tumor cells that were labeled at several sites of the cytoplasmic periphery simultaneously, those that revealed pronounced capping (Fig. 237a), and those that showed a chiefly intracytoplasmic reaction as a result of internalization of labeled cytoplasmic membranes (Fig. 237b). According to the literature, cap formation on CLL lymphocytes is delayed[22] or it is missing entirely.[23] We found that when capping occurs, it does so chiefly at the cytoplasmic membrane near the Golgi field, as found in normal lymphocytes.[24]

In contrast to other malignant lymphomas, lymph nodes infiltrated by CLL lymphocytes contain only a few reticulum cells. One regularly finds some histiocytic and so-called dark reticulum cells.[25] Both types of reticulum cells may contain phagosomes, rarely tumor cells, and sometimes erythrocytes or erythrocyte fragments. Some of the reticulum cells can be interpreted as subsinus histiocytic reticulum cells (phagocytes)[26] due to their proximity to sinus endothelial cells. These reticulum cells show active phagocytosis, as seen in normal lymph nodes.

As may also be observed on light microscopy, small remnants of T-areas are sometimes seen in infiltrated lymph nodes. They consist of typical interdigi-

---

[19] Bessis, 1951, 1973; Bernard, Bessis, Soulier and Thiéry, 1959; deMan and Meiners, 1962; Hurez, Flandrin, Preud'Homme and Seligmann, 1972; Cawley, Barker, Britchford and Smith, 1973; Clark, Rydell and Kaplan, 1973; Smith, Cawley and Barker, 1973; Knapp, Schuit, Bolhuis and Hijmans, 1974; Brunning and Parkin, 1975; Cohnen, 1975; Huhn, Thiel and Rodt, 1975; Schaefer, Krüger and Fischer, 1975; Cawley, Smith, Goldstone, Emmines *et al.*, 1976; Nies, Marshall, Oberlin, Halpern *et al.*, 1976; Schaefer, 1976.

[19a] Huhn, Thiel and Rodt, 1975.

[20] Douglas, Cohnen, König, Brittinger *et al.*, 1972; Douglas, Cohnen and Brittinger, 1973; Cohnen, 1975.

[21] Kaiserling, 1975; Müller-Hermelink and Kaiserling, 1975.

[22] Flad, Huber, Bremer, Menne *et al.*, 1973.

[23] McLaughlin, Wetherly-Mein, Pitcher and Hobbs, 1973.

[24] Rosenthal, Davie, Rosenstreich and Cehrs, 1973.

[25] Mollo, Monga and Stramignoni, 1969.

[26] Ada, Nossal and Austin, 1964.

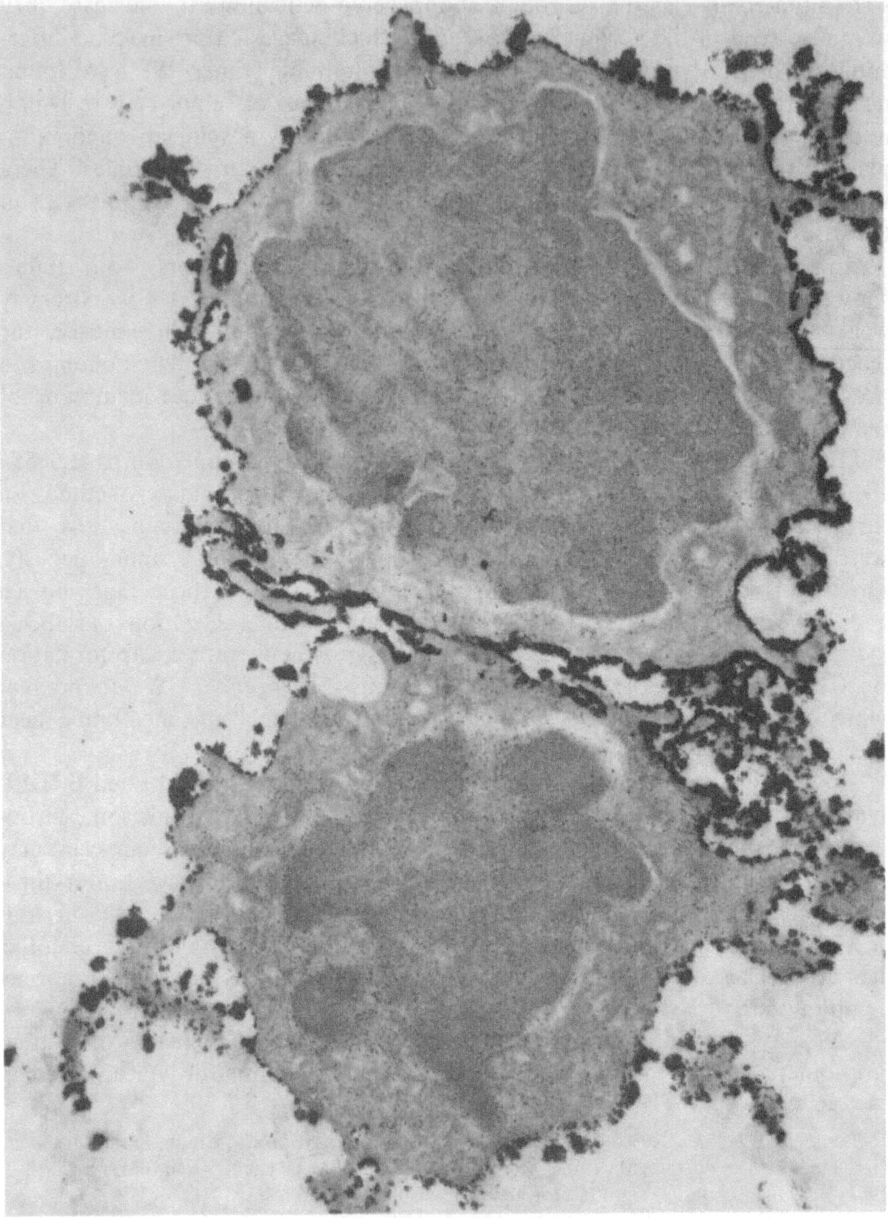

Fig. 236. Two CLL lymphocytes of the lymph node with a strongly positive ATPase reaction at the cell membrane. Unstained. ×18,000

tating reticulum cells in close contact with small lymphocytes and sometimes with blast cells containing numerous polyribosomes. The T-areas also contain epithelioid venules that reveal no ultrastructural particularities. In cases in which T-areas are not observed, there are usually a few epithelioid venules. As reported

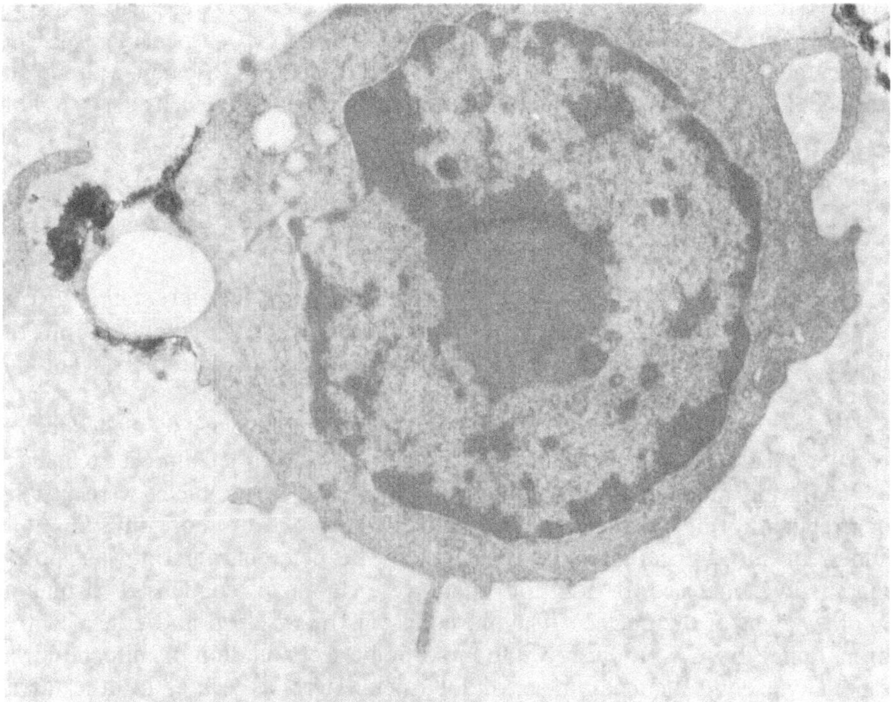
(a)

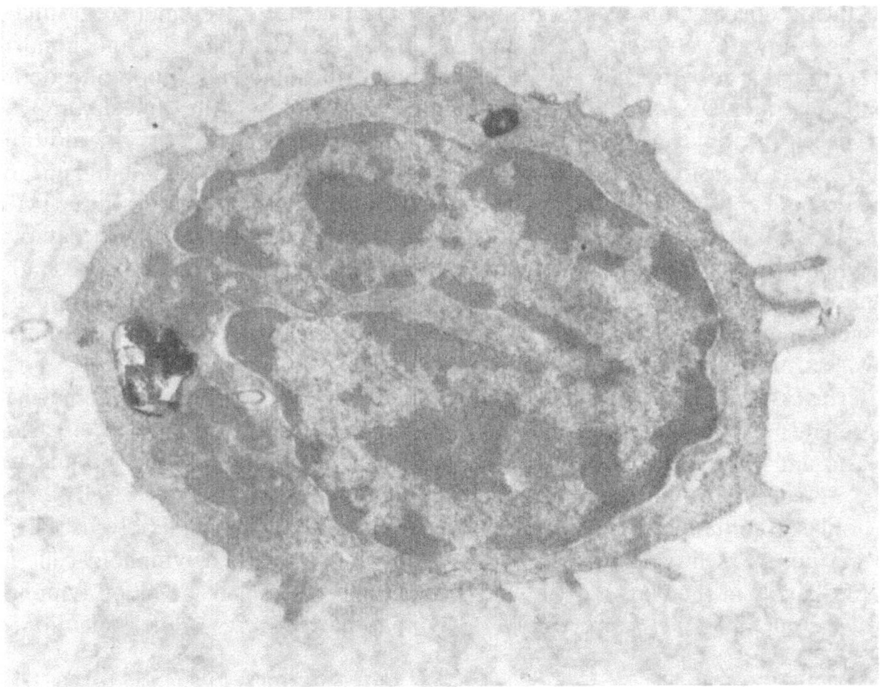
(b)

Fig. 237a and b. CLL lymphocytes labeled with peroxidase-coupled antibodies for surface IgM. (a) Lymphocyte showing cap formation. (b) Lymphocyte that has internalized labeled membranes. Unstained. (a) × 16,000, (b) × 12,000 by SÖDERSTRÖM and NORBERG,[27] however, there are sometimes no epithelioid venules at all. The lymphocytes and blast cells found in T-areas can probably be interpreted as T-cells, which make up 2–5% of cell suspensions of CLL lymph nodes, as we found in rosette tests. Within the vascular wall of the epithelioid venules there are chiefly small lymphocytes. These cells are probably T-cells in the stage of recirculation.

### *b) T-Type*

Although cases of T-CLL have been described by BROUET *et al.*,[28] RODT *et al.*,[29] THIEL *et al.*,[30] INSEL *et al.*,[31] and HUHN *et al.*,[32] the data on the ultrastructure of T-CLL are not consistent. So we shall describe one of our own cases[33] (case 1; see p. 140) in this section.

In that case 98% of the peripheral blood lymphocytes formed sheep-E rosettes. All areas of the lymph node were diffusely infiltrated almost exclusively by small and medium-sized lymphocytes (Fig. 238). Their nuclei were usually of irregular form. They were deeply indented by one or more invaginations and frequently appeared to be segmented. The heterochromatin was mostly marginally condensed. In addition, there were clumps of condensed chromatin in other areas of the nucleus. The nucleolus was ring-shaped and either central or marginal. In the cytoplasm we found a polar accumulation of mitochondria, especially around the medium-sized Golgi field. Here, as well as in other areas of the cytoplasm, there were groups of electron-dense lysosome-like granules, as also shown by BROUET *et al.*[28] in cases of T-CLL. Occasionally, lipochondria were found. The cytoplasm also contained monoribosomes, a few polyribosomes, and only rarely a few rough membrane profiles. Moreover, the almost complete absence of cytoplasmic projections was characteristic of these cells. In addition, there were occasionally a few blast cells with large nuclei containing one or two prominent nucleoli and irregularly distributed heterochromatin. In the cytoplasm we found a moderate number of polyribosomes, a medium-sized Golgi field, numerous mitochondria, and occasional lipid droplets. In between the tumor cells there was a wide intercellular space. Interdigitating reticulum cells, which were observed by LENNERT, were not evident in the slides we examined by electron microscopy.

The cases described by THIEL *et al.*[30] and HUHN *et al.*[32] presented a somewhat different morphologic picture. Apart from a clearly smaller amount of ergastoplasm and fewer cell organelles,[32] the ultrastructure of the blood lymphocytes did not differ from that of lymphocytes in other cases of typical CLL. The cytoplasm contained deposits of glycogen that were partly dissolved. There were numerous large mitochondria. A skin biopsy revealed lymphoid cells in a focal array in the dermis. These cells sometimes resembled the blood lymphocytes, sometimes they were similar to lymphoblasts. HUHN *et al.*[32] mentioned

[27] 1974.
[28] BROUET, FLANDRIN, SASPORTES, PREUD'HOMME *et al.*, 1975.
[29] RODT, THIEL, THIERFELDER, HUHN *et al.*, 1976.
[30] THIEL, RODT, HUHN and THIERFELDER, 1976.
[31] INSEL, MELEWICZ, LA VIA and BALCH, 1975.
[32] HUHN, RODT, THIEL, GROSSE-WILDE *et al.*, 1976.
[33] KAISERLING, 1977.

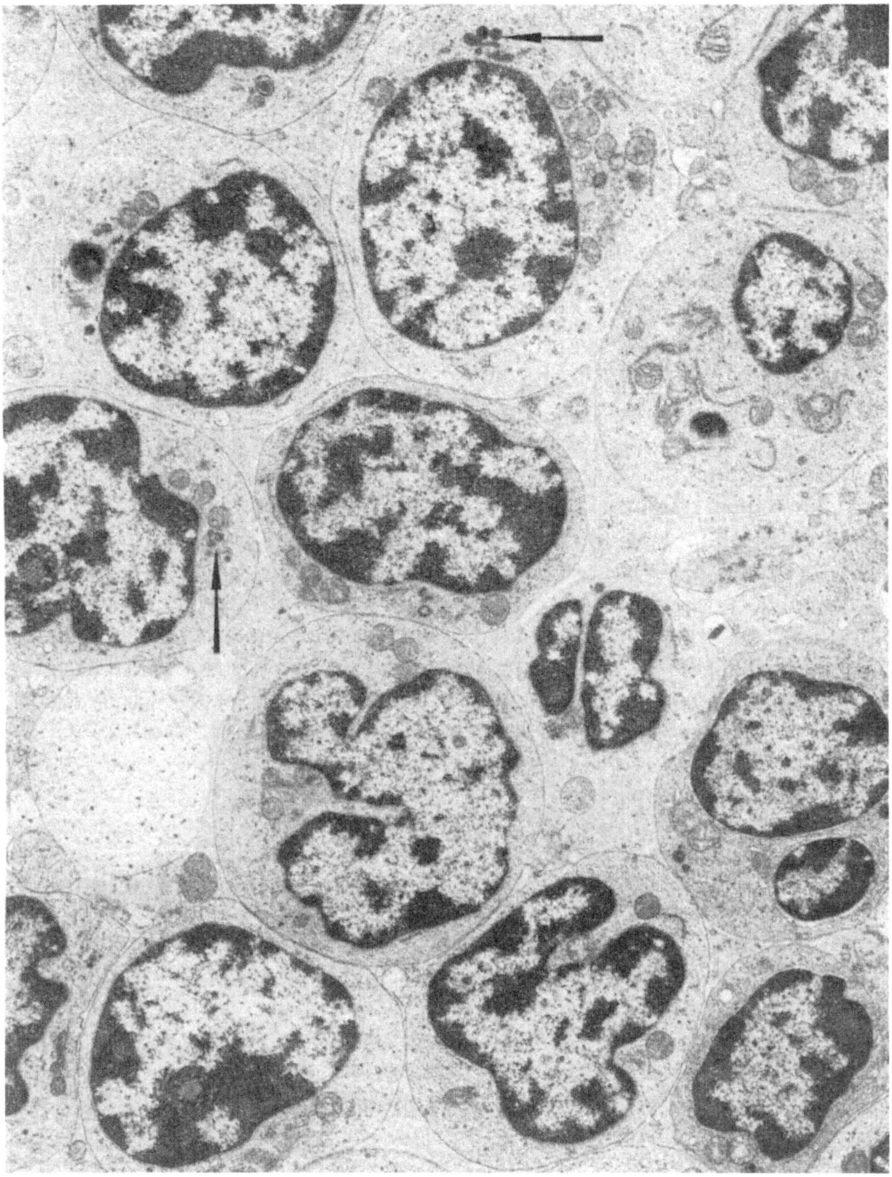

Fig. 238. Chronic lymphocytic leukemia (T-type). Tumor cells have a sometimes oval, sometimes irregularly shaped nucleus with a ring-shaped nucleolus and marginal chromatin condensation. The cytoplasm contains solitary lysosomes and groups of them (arrows). There are almost no cytoplasmic projections. × 9,600

that in one of their cases of T-CLL, 3% of peripheral blood lymphocytes had gyriform nuclei and could not be distinguished from Sézary cells.

INSEL *et al.*[34] described the tumor cells in the peripheral blood of their case of T-CLL as typical small lymphocytes with a high nuclear/cytoplasmic

[34] INSEL, MELEWICZ, LA VIA and BALCH, 1975.

ratio, a round or slightly indented nucleus, a few cytoplasmic organelles, and microvilli. The cells revealed the typical morphology of CLL lymphocytes.

In contrast to the cases described by THIEL *et al.*[35] and INSEL *et al.*,[35a] our case of T-CLL was not difficult to distinguish from B-CLL. For example, owing to the irregular shape of the nuclei and the very small amount of ergastoplasm, the ultrastructure of the tumor cells was much more polymorphic than in typical CLL of the B-cell type. The large number of lysosomes, which probably correspond to a positive acid phosphatase reaction on light microscopy, seems to be a further diagnostic feature of T-CLL. In contrast to the paraimmunoblasts of B-CLL, the blast cells of T-CLL contained a considerably smaller amount of polysomes. These blast cells were also not difficult to distinguish from the prolymphocytes of B-CLL by the irregular chromatin condensations. Finally, the wide intercellular spaces and the lack of cytoplasmic projections were characteristic in our case of T-CLL.

In some cases it would probably be difficult or even impossible to distinguish T-CLL from lymphoblastic lymphoma of the convoluted-cell type (acid phosphatase type) by their cytologic features on electron microscopy. If, however, interdigitating reticulum cells and epithelioid venules were regular components of T-CLL, as indicated by the findings of LENNERT, then it would be possible to distinguish between these two neoplasms—interdigitating reticulum cells and epithelioid venules are not found in lymphoblastic lymphoma of the convoluted-cell type on light or electron microscopy. A distinction between T-CLL and Sézary's syndrome or mycosis fungoides is not difficult, since typical Sézary or Lutzner cells are present in only small numbers, or are not seen at all in T-CLL.

### 2. *Hairy-Cell Leukemia*

The data on the ultrastructure of hairy-cell leukemia[36] reported so far in the literature yield an essentially uniform cytologic picture of the tumor cells. They are chiefly characterized by delicate, sometimes branched cytoplasmic projections, which appear as a villous surface structure when viewed with a scanning microscope.[37] The nucleus is oval or indented, contains a small nucleolus, and shows marginally condensed heterochromatin. Cytoplasm is abundant and reveals a few rough, as a rule narrow membrane profiles, monoribosomes, and numerous, often swollen mitochondria. The cytoplasm also contains

---

[35] THIEL, RODT, HUHN and THIERFELDER, 1976.

[35a] INSEL, MELEWICZ, LA VIA and BALCH, 1975.

[36] BEACHEY, HASHIMOTO and BURKETT, 1969; PADILLA and SOLOFF, 1969, 1971; RUBIN, DOUGLAS, CHESSIN, GLADE *et al.*, 1969; TRUBOWITZ, MASEK and FRASCA, 1971; GHADIALLY and SKINNIDER, 1972; KATAYAMA, LI and YAM, 1972a, b; KATAYAMA, NAGY and BALOGH, 1973; DANIEL and FLANDRIN, 1974; FLANDRIN and DANIEL, 1974; HAAK, DE MAN, HIJMANS, KNAPP *et al.*, 1974; HAEGERT, CAWLEY, COLLINS, FLEMANS *et al.*, 1974; SCHNITZER and KASS, 1974; DEBUSSCHER, BERNHEIM, COLLARD-RONGÉ, GOVAERTS *et al.*, 1975; KING, HURTUBISE, SAGONE, LOBUGLIO *et al.*, 1975; PEDIO, RÜTTNER, SPYCHER and GUT, 1975; SCHMALZL, HUHN, ASAMER and BRAUNSTEINER, 1975; BURKE, MACKAY and RAPPAPORT, 1976; LÖFFLER, ROUX, FISCHER, DESAGA *et al.*, 1976; ROZENSZAJN, GUTMAN, RADNAY, BEN DAVID *et al.*, 1976; VYKOUPIL, THIELE and GEORGII, 1976.

[37] TRUBOWITZ, MASEK and FRASCA, 1971; SCHNITZER and HAMMACK, 1974, 1975; DEBUSSCHER, BERNHEIM, COLLARD-RONGÉ, GOVAERTS *et al.*, 1975; GOLOMB, BRAYLAN and POLLIACK, 1975.

a sometimes well-developed Golgi field and lysosomes. There is a remarkably large number of variable-sized intracytoplasmic vesicles. Some of them are smooth, some are coated vesicles. Multivesicular bodies appear occasionally. Sometimes one finds coated vesicles that are in contact with the cell membrane and smooth vesicles that can probably be interpreted as pinocytotic vesicles.[38] On electron microscopy, a positive acid phosphatase reaction was localized in small and large profiles of endoplasmic reticulum, in some vesicles, in lysosomes, and in the perinuclear space.[39]

The presence of so-called ribosome-lamella complexes in hairy cells was first described by KATAYAMA *et al.*[40] These cytoplasmic structures consist of multiple parallel membranes that appear concentrically layered in cross section; ribosomes are strung between them. Segments of rough endoplasmic reticulum sometimes lie near such complexes. Ribosome-lamella complexes are not, however, specific features of hairy cells. They are also found in rare cases of CLL.[41] Furthermore, they have been observed in cases of lymphosarcoma-cell leukemia that were not classified further,[42] in two cases of macroglobulinemia,[43] in one case of immunocytoma,[44] and in a case of plasmacytoma.[44a] The nature of the ribosome-lamella complexes has not yet been clarified.

Other special ultrastructural features of hairy-cell leukemia, such as the virus-like particles in atypical plasma cells from peripheral blood described by PEDIO *et al.*,[45] the zipper-like junctions described by DANIEL and FLANDRIN,[46] or Langerhans-like granules,[47] are not constant findings. As far as we know, typical Langerhans granules have not been seen in hairy cells.

According to our findings, there is no principal difference between the leukemic cells of peripheral blood and the tumor cells in lymph nodes and spleen. There were only a few hairy cells in two lymph nodes we examined; most of them contained a large number of intracytoplasmic vesicles and were located in the sinuses. Hairy cells with a cytology similar to that of hairy cells observed in lymph nodes are found in Billroth's cords of the spleen (Fig. 239). The cytoplasm of most splenic hairy cells contains numerous vesicles and diffusely distributed lysosome-like granules. In a few hairy cells, however, there are almost no vesicles and the lysosome-like granules are found predominantly in groups near the nucleus. In lymph nodes we observed that the hairy cells were in close contact through their interdigitated cytoplasmic projections. This is much more prominent in the spleen (Fig. 239b), as also described by BURKE *et al.*[48] Hairy cells have another characteristic feature, namely, narrow cytoplasmic invaginations that contain amorphous, moderately electron-dense material. As

[38] HAAK, DE MAN, HIJMANS, KNAPP *et al.*, 1974.
[39] KATAYAMA, LI and YAM, 1972b; DEBUSSCHER, BERNHEIM, COLLARD-RONGÉ, GOVAERTS *et al.*, 1975; SCHMALZL, HUHN, ASAMER and BRAUNSTEINER, 1975; ROZENSZAJN, GUTMAN, RADNAY, BEN DAVID *et al.*, 1976.
[40] KATAYAMA, LI and YAM, 1972a.
[41] ZUCKER-FRANKLIN, 1963; ITO, 1974; KAISERLING, 1975, 1977; WOESSNER and ROZMAN, 1976.
[42] ANDAY, GOODMAN and TISHKOFF, 1973; DJALDETTI, LANDAU, MANDEL, HAR-ZAAV *et al.*, 1974.
[43] BRUNNING and PARKIN, 1975; HENRY, 1975.
[44] KAISERLING, 1975, 1977.
[44a] SCHAEFER, 1976.
[45] PEDIO, RÜTTNER, SPYCHER and GUT, 1975.
[46] 1974.
[47] BEACHEY, HASHIMOTO and BURKETT, 1969; PADILLA and SOLOFF, 1969, 1971; DANIEL and FLANDRIN, 1974.
[48] BURKE, MACKAY and RAPPAPORT, 1976.

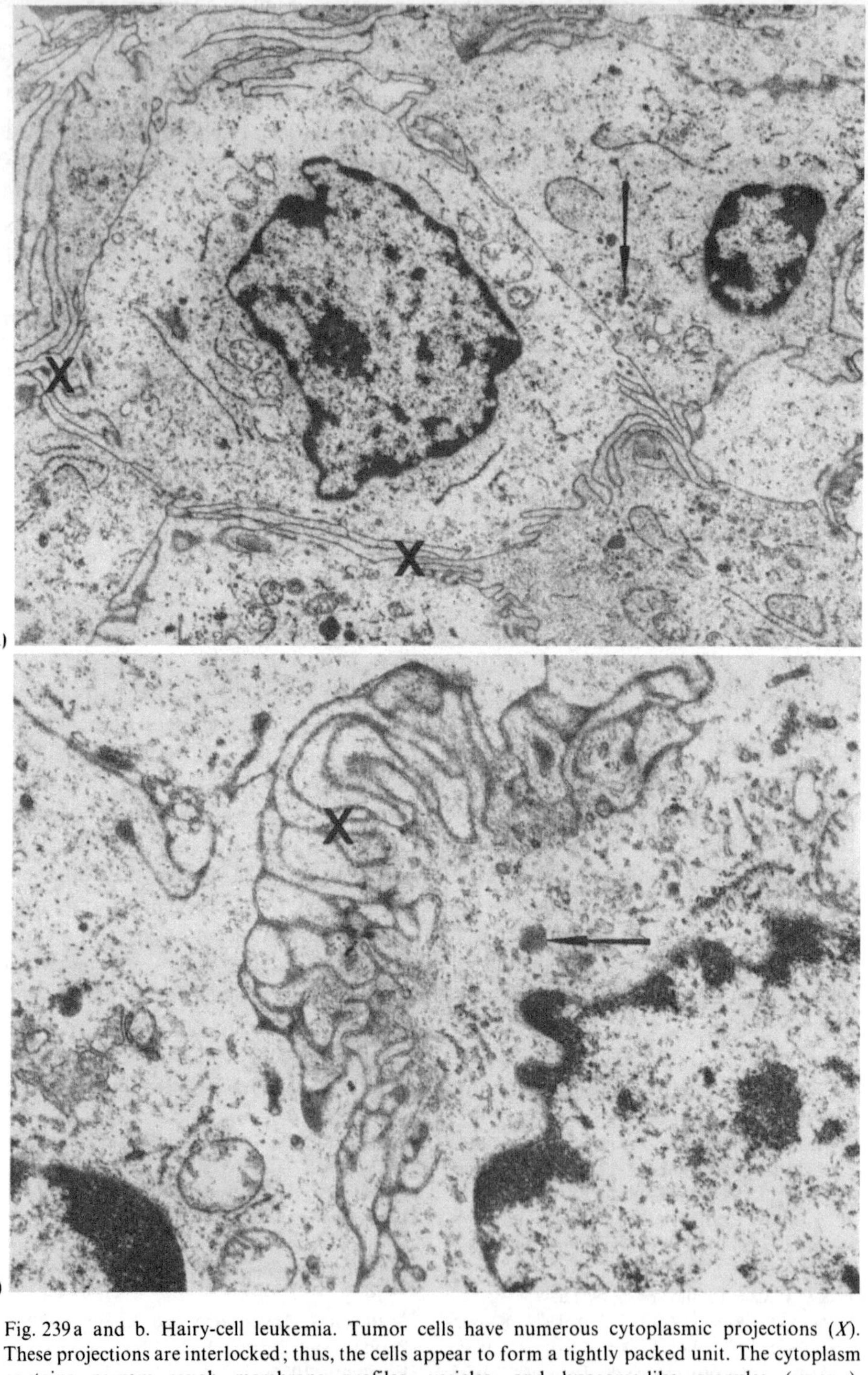

(a)

(b)

Fig. 239a and b. Hairy-cell leukemia. Tumor cells have numerous cytoplasmic projections (*X*). These projections are interlocked; thus, the cells appear to form a tightly packed unit. The cytoplasm contains narrow rough membrane profiles, vesicles, and lysosome-like granules (arrows). (a) ×13,000, (b) ×22,000

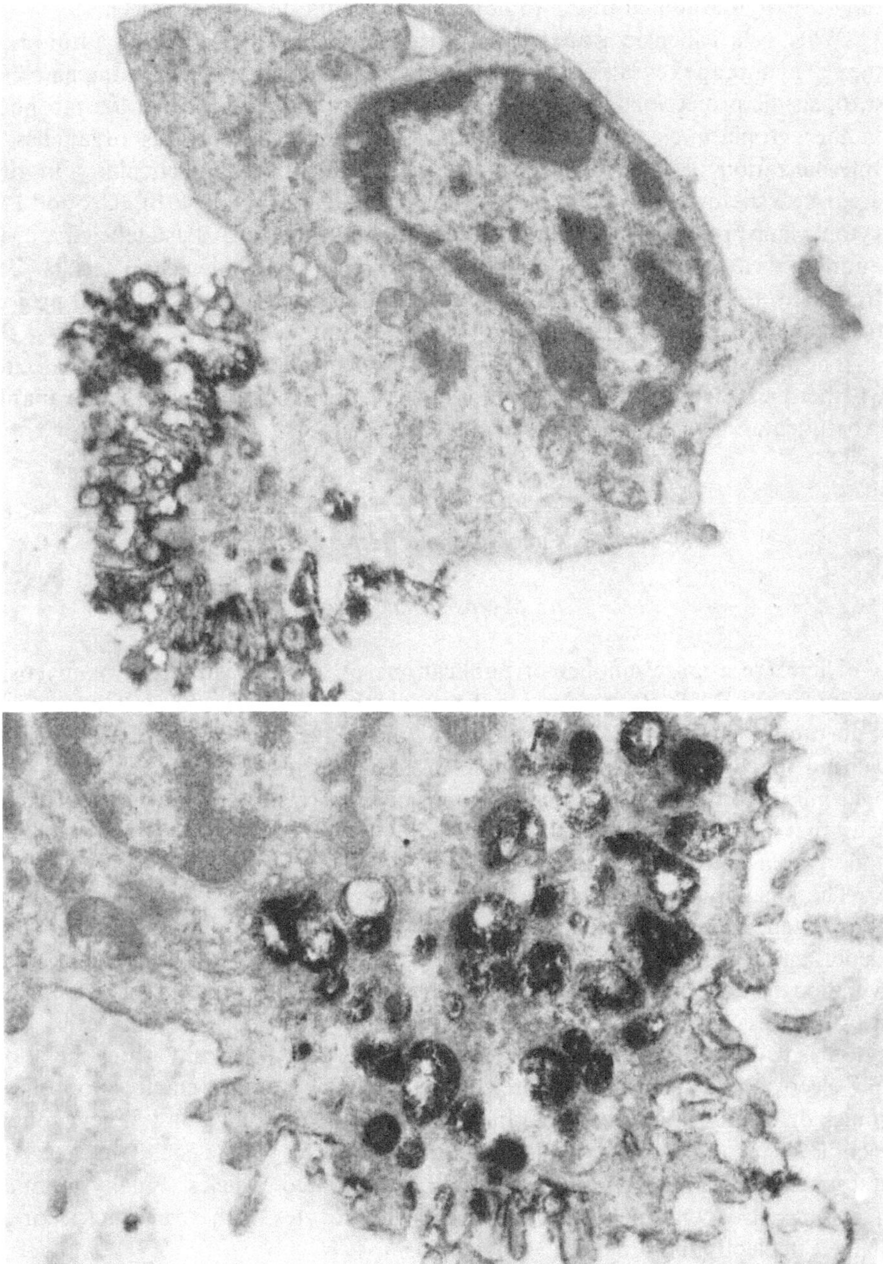

(a)

(b)

Fig. 240a and b. Hairy-cell leukemia. Two cells labeled with peroxidase-coupled anti-Ig antibodies for surface Ig. There is a strong positive reaction at the polar groups of uropod-like cytoplasmic projections (a). As shown in (b), peroxidase-positive aggregates and labeled membranes are internalized at this site. Unstained. (a) ×13,000, (b) ×25,000 in the leukemic cells of peripheral blood, rough endoplasmic reticulum was only slightly developed in the tumor cells of lymph nodes and spleen.

When cell suspensions are treated with peroxidase-labeled anti-Ig antibodies, the cell membrane reveals a strongly positive reaction, particularly at the hair-like cytoplasmic projections (Fig. 240a). These projections are formed like uropods in the cytoplasmic area containing the Golgi field and various organelles.[49] Internalization of labeled parts of the membrane occurs particularly in this area, i.e., the cytoplasmic area near the Golgi field (Fig. 240b). Uropod-like cytoplasmic projections like those of cells treated with peroxidase-labeled anti-Ig antibodies can also be found in untreated suspensions of splenic hairy cells. Cell fragments and amorphous condensates sometimes accumulate at the cell projections and are occasionally found in the cytoplasm.

The ultrastructural findings in hairy-cell leukemia have not helped us to decide whether hairy cells are derived from lymphoid or histiocytic cells. The available experimental data are still contradictory (see p. 153).

### *3. Mycosis Fungoides and Sézary's Syndrome*

#### *a) Mycosis Fungoides*

There are a large number of publications on the ultrastructure of mycosis fungoides (M.F.).[50] If we compare, however, the light-microscopic features described on page 168ff. with the ultrastructural data provided by the literature, we find that it is not always possible to draw correlations between them. On light microscopy, M.F. reveals small and medium-sized lymphocytes, and large cells that can be subclassified into several types according to nuclear shape and cytoplasmic basophilia (see p. 173).

The small lymphocytes, also called Lutzner cells, are characterized by a convoluted, deeply indented, often cerebriform nucleus containing a small nucleolus and marginally condensed heterochromatin (Fig. 241). The medium-sized lymphocytes exhibit a largely similar ultrastructure. The nucleus of these cells is usually less convoluted, however, than that of the small lymphoid cells. The cytoplasm of both the small and the medium-sized cells may show high or low electron density. Furthermore, both types may contain chiefly monoribosomes or chiefly polyribosomes. In the cytoplasm there are only a few rough membrane profiles and a medium-sized Golgi field with a small number of lysosome-like granules and a few smooth and coated vesicles. Finally, dermal infiltrates also contain occasional small lymphocytes with oval nuclei, ring-shaped nucleoli, and almost no ergastoplasm.

---

[49] Stein, Kaiserling and Lennert, 1974; Stein, Kaiserling and Stein, 1974.

[50] Orfanos and Stüttgen, 1963; Bonneau and Cesarini, 1967; Brownlee and Murad, 1970; Flaxman, Zelazny and van Scott, 1971; Lutzner, Hobbs and Horvath, 1971; Sandbank, 1971; Sandbank and Ben-Bassat, 1971; Gomez Orbaneja, Sanchez Yus, Diaz-Flores and Simon Huarte, 1972; Ryan, Sanderson, Barták and Samman, 1973; Rosas-Uribe, Variakojis, Molnar and Rappaport, 1974; Variakojis, Rosas-Uribe and Rappaport, 1974; Hamburg, Brynes, Reese and Golomb, 1976; Robinowitz, Noguchi and Roenigk, 1976.

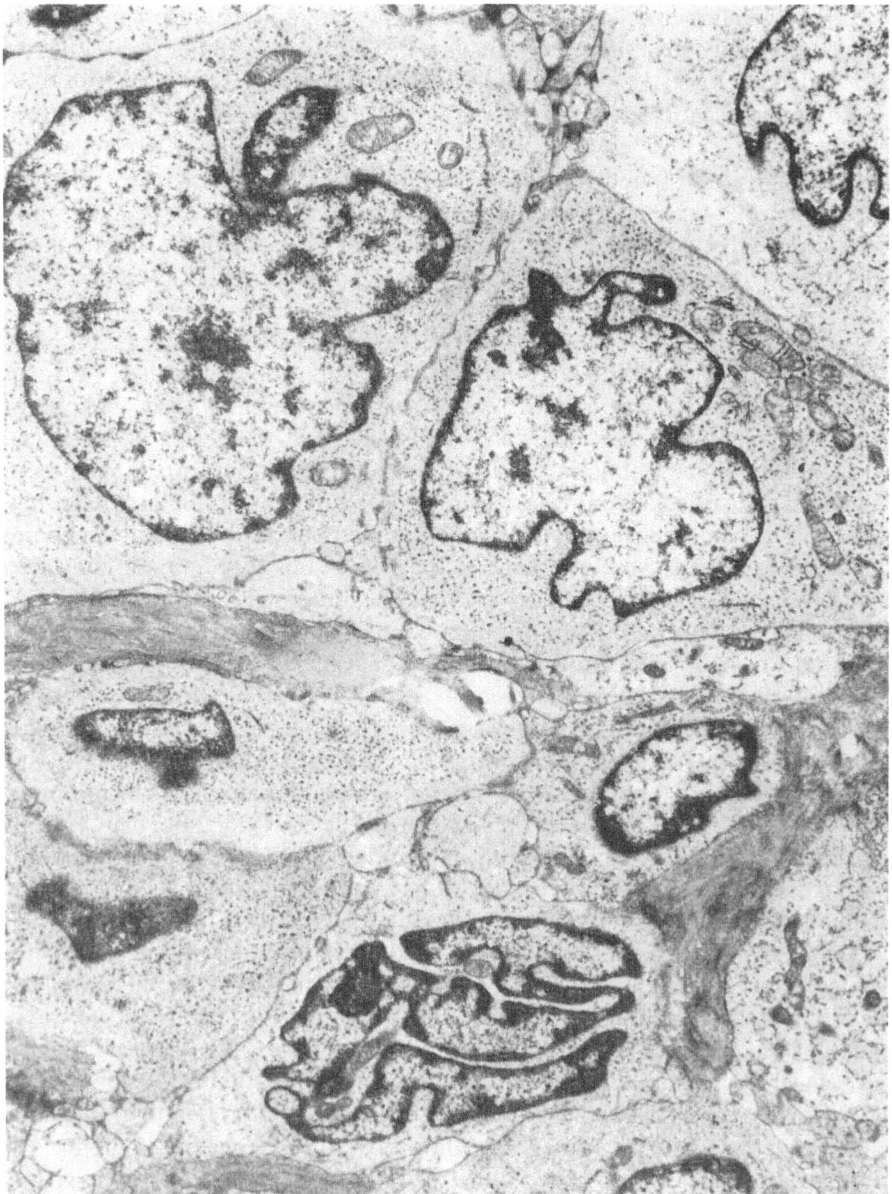

Fig. 241. Mycosis fungoides. Skin. At the lower edge of the picture, a tumor cell with a cerebriform nucleus. There are also several large blast cells containing abundant polyribosomes and an irregularly shaped nucleus with a moderate amount of heterochromatin. ×9,000

It is now known that the cells with convoluted or cerebriform nuclei in M.F. have T-cell membrane characteristics: they are able to form spontaneous rosettes with uncoated sheep erythrocytes.[51] The small lymphocytes with oval nuclei have not yet been characterized immunologically.

Numerous authors have pointed out that the lymphoid cells with cerebriform nuclei cannot be considered specific to M.F. Cells of similar or even identical morphology can be found in Sézary's syndrome and have also been observed in a tumor that was interpreted as reticulosarcoma, in lichen planus,[52] and in various nonlymphomatous dermatoses.[53] Cells that cannot be differentiated from Lutzner cells may also be present in cases of dermatopathic and nonspecific lymphadenitis, in which these cells are found in T-nodules.

As far as we know, none of the electron-microscopic analyses of M.F. include a description of the large mononuclear cells with a diameter 3–5 times as great as that of Lutzner cells. According to the unpublished findings of Goos, two types of large cells can be distinguished and each of these can be divided into two subtypes. The first type of cell, which predominates in number, has a large convoluted nucleus with one or more prominent marginal nucleoli. The heterochromatin is usually marginally condensed; but sometimes it shows a patchy distribution. Some of the cells of this type contain numerous polyribosomes. These cells can be distinguished from cells of similar size and with a similar nuclear configuration that contain almost exclusively monoribosomes and have an electron-transparent cytoplasm. On light microscopy, the cells containing polyribosomes reveal a narrow rim of basophilic cytoplasm. The cells containing monoribosomes have a pale cytoplasm. Because of their nuclear configuration, these two subtypes are reminiscent of Lutzner cells and might be of lymphatic nature. The second type of large cell, which is found much less often, has a merely slightly indented nucleus (Fig. 241). This type of cell can be subdivided into cells with numerous polyribosomes and those with few polyribosomes. Both subtypes are reminiscent of immunoblasts of normal lymphatic tissue.

The nonlymphoid cells found in M.F. infiltrates in the dermis include chiefly histiocytic reticulum cells that rarely contain phagosomes; neutrophil and eosinophil granulocytes are seen occasionally. In some cases we also observed interdigitating reticulum cells in the infiltrated dermis (Fig. 242). These cells have an irregularly shaped nucleus, a moderately developed tubulovesicular system, and narrow cytoplasmic invaginations. Besides typical interdigitating reticulum cells, there are sometimes cells that might represent emigrant blood monocytes in the process of transforming into interdigitating reticulum cells. As described elsewhere,[54] the interdigitating reticulum cells are in close membrane contact, sometimes with small and medium-sized lymphoid cells, sometimes with large blast cells containing polyribosomes (immunoblasts). Mitotic figures of lymphoid cells are occasionally found in this area. According to the unpublished findings

[51] Edelson, Kirkpatrick, Shevach, Schein *et al.*, 1974; van Leeuwen, Meijer and de Man, 1975; van Leeuwen, Meijer, van Vloten, Scheffer *et al.*, 1976; Robinowitz, Noguchi and Roenigk, 1976.

[52] Lutzner, Hobbs and Horvath, 1971.

[53] Flaxman, Zelazny and van Scott, 1971.

[54] Goos, Kaiserling and Lennert, 1976.

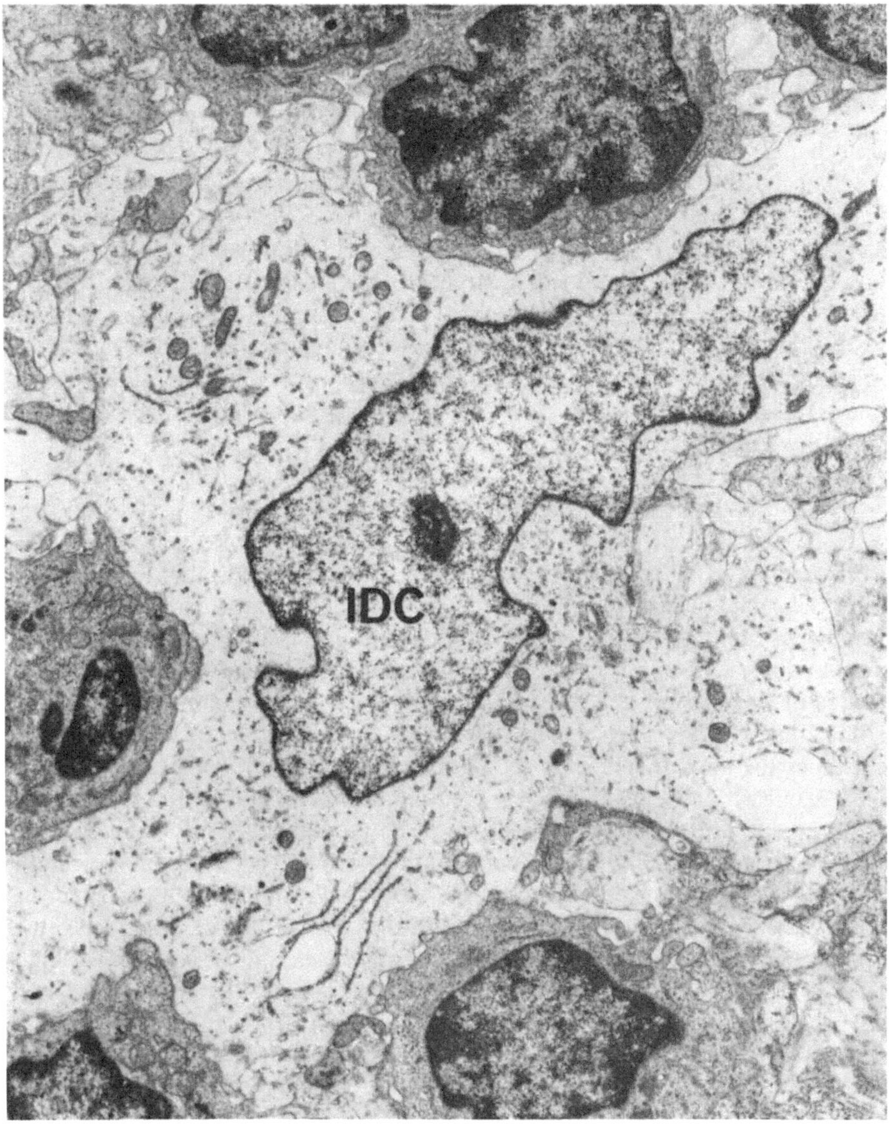


Fig. 242. Mycosis fungoides. Interdigitating reticulum cell (*IDC*) in the dermis. The cytoplasm of this cell contains numerous smooth and rough membrane profiles. The nucleus has an irregular shape. Tumor cells (lymphocytes) are in close membrane contact with the reticulum cell. Photograph kindly contributed by Dr. Goos, Kiel. × 7,700

of Goos, T-associated plasma cells and epithelioid venules are also occasionally seen in the dermis. Interdigitating reticulum cells, T-associated plasma cells, and epithelioid venules are essential components of thymus-dependent areas of normal lymphatic tissue and are not normally seen in the dermis. The occurrence of such structures in this lymphoma indicates that a T-cell-specific microenvironment is established in M.F. This assumption is also supported by the observation of VAN LEEUWEN *et al.*[55] We would also like to mention that dermal infiltrates in one of our cases revealed Langerhans cells surrounded on all sides by lymphocytes with irregularly shaped nuclei.

So far, we know only of the unpublished findings of GOOS on the ultrastructural changes in the tumor stage of M.F. Recently, he observed a case that was clinically characterized by a rapid course and extensive lymph-node involvement. Electron-microscopic study of dermal infiltrates and lymph nodes revealed chiefly large blast cells with abundant polyribosomes and an irregularly shaped nucleus. The nucleus contained a large central nucleolus with clearly visible nucleolonemata. Among these cells there were medium-sized lymphocytes with mostly irregularly shaped nuclei; the cytoplasm sometimes contained monoribosomes, sometimes polyribosomes. Cells with a cerebriform nucleus were extremely rare. In another case the histologic picture was dominated by medium-sized cells with cerebriform nuclei.

### *b) Sézary's Syndrome*

The tumor cells of Sézary's syndrome (Sézary cells) show the same, or nearly the same, ultrastructural features as the Lutzner cells described in M.F. The nucleus of Sézary cells is irregularly shaped, deeply invaginated, or cerebriform, looking like a serpentine in cross section (Fig. 243a). Several special features of this type of cell have been emphasized in the literature,[56] but they do not allow a distinction between Sézary cells and the Lutzner cells of M.F. Sometimes the nuclear segments are joined only by narrow bridges that consist of coarse nuclear particles and nuclear membranes.[57] The nucleoli are not remarkably large and are rarely seen. The cytoplasm contains monoribosomes, a few polyribosomes, and an extremely small amount of rough endoplasmic reticulum. Near the Golgi field there are a few lysosome-like granules and numerous coated and smooth vesicles. Furthermore, ZUCKER-FRANKLIN[58] described intracytoplasmic structures that were reminiscent of viruses, and fibrils with a diameter of 80 Å, which, however, are not specific to Sézary's syndrome and may also occur in M.F. and other diseases.[59] The presence of diastase-soluble glycogen (Fig. 243b) is an important characteristic of the tumor cells, although it is not seen in all cases. Electron microscopy reveals variable-sized cytoplasmic

[55] VAN LEEUWEN, MEIJER, VAN VLOTEN, SCHEFFER *et al.*, 1976.

[56] LUTZNER and JORDAN, 1968; LUTZNER, HOBBS and HORVATH, 1971; HUHN, DOBBELSTEIN and ENGELHARDT, 1972; LABAZE, MOSCOVIC, PHAM and AZAR, 1972; LUTZNER, EMERIT, DUREPAIRE, FLANDRIN *et al.*, 1973; EDELSON, LUTZNER, KIRKPATRICK, SHEVACH *et al.*, 1974; LITOVITZ and LUTZNER, 1974; LÖFFLER, MEYHÖFER, LANGE, EHLERS *et al.*, 1974; ZUCKER-FRANKLIN, 1974; ZUCKER-FRANKLIN, MELTON III and QUAGLIATA, 1974; BOSMAN and VAN VLOTEN, 1976; CHELLOUL, DAUMAS-DUPORT, BONVALLET, BRIERE *et al.*, 1976.

[57] LUTZNER and JORDAN, 1968.

[58] 1974.

[59] SANDBANK and BEN-BASSAT, 1971.

Fig. 243a and b. Sézary's syndrome. (a) Sézary cell of peripheral blood with a twisted nucleus containing abundant chromatin. (b) Tumor cell with widespread areas of glycogen (*X*). (a) ×17,000, (b) ×43,000 ▷

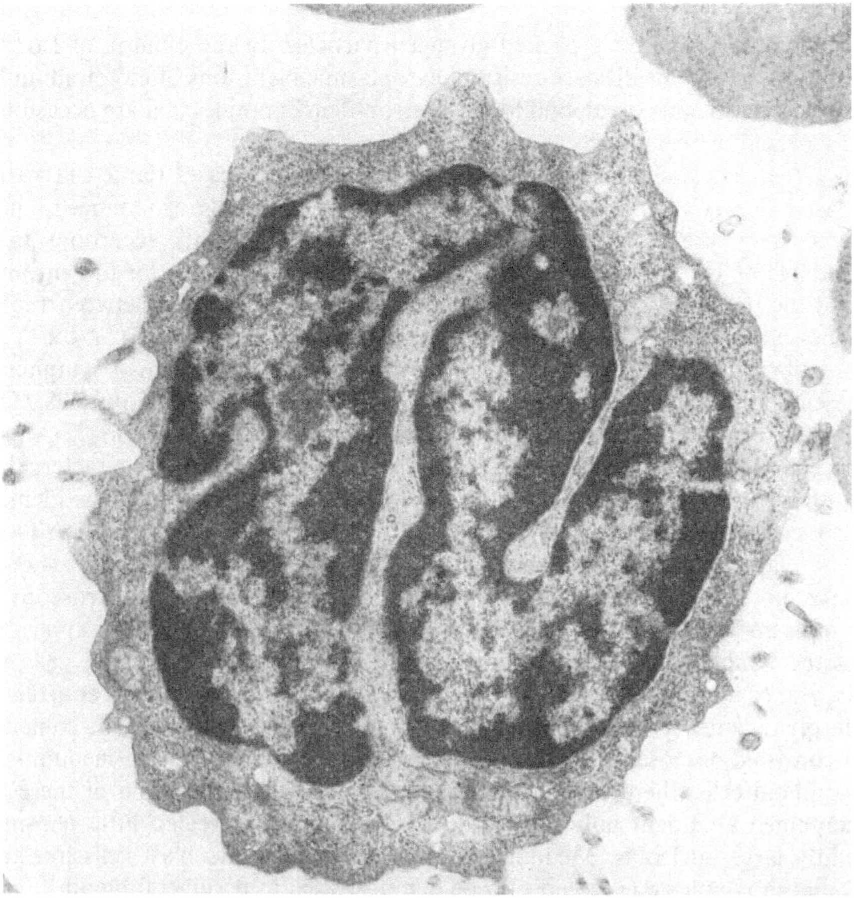
(a)

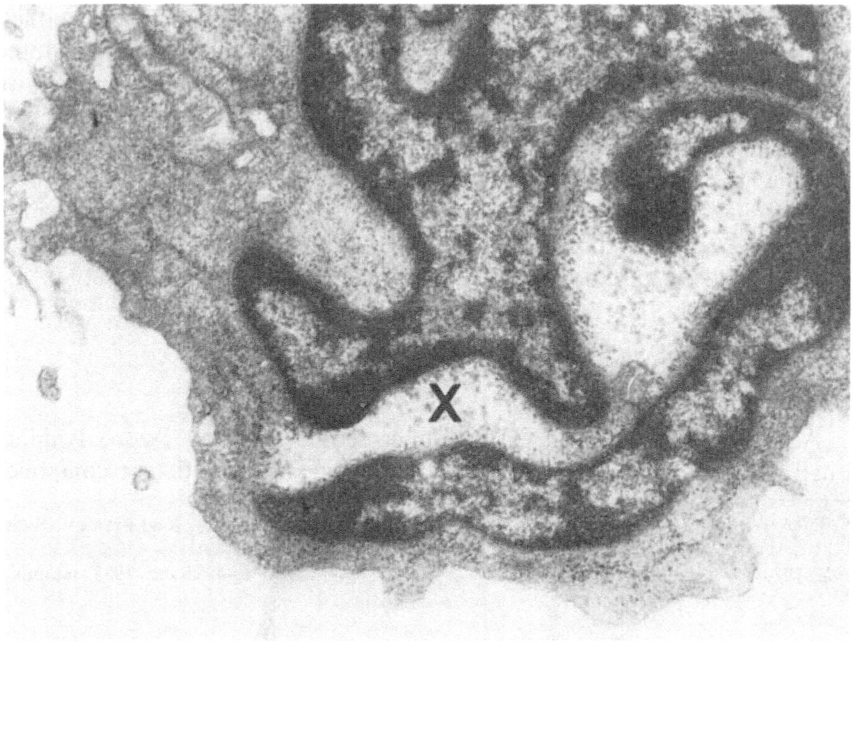

(b)

areas containing closely packed glycogen particles. In the opinion of LUTZNER and JORDAN,[59a] the diastase-resistant cytoplasmic inclusions often found on light microscopy might correspond to the electron-dense granules that are occasionally discovered in Sézary cells.

Whereas classic Sézary cells predominate in some cases (large-cell variant, classic Sézary's syndrome), small lymphocytes with less pronounced nuclear irregularity are found in other cases (small-cell variant) according to the findings of LUTZNER *et al.*[60] With respect to the distribution of the chromatin and the organization of the cytoplasm, there is no difference between the two types of cells. There might also be a third type of Sézary cell: EDELSON *et al.*[61] described a case in which the neoplasm was composed of small lymphocytes resembling CLL lymphocytes with a generally oval or round nucleus. These cells were usually characterized by cytoplasmic extensions or uropods.[61] Another special finding in this case was that the cells had features characteristic of both T- and B-cells, whereas the cells from the other cases could be identified as T-cells. As mentioned previously (p. 137), this case was closely related to T-CLL.

So far, electron-microscopic findings in lymph nodes from Sézary's syndrome have not been published. In the case we studied by electron microscopy the lymph node was diffusely infiltrated by tumor cells. The cytologic appearance of the lymphoid cells was quite uniform. Medium-sized lymphoid cells with an oval or invaginated nucleus predominated. Some of the cells had an irregular, deeply indented nucleus. The nucleolus was sometimes ring-shaped; sometimes it consisted of closely packed nucleolonemata. In addition to the medium-sized lymphoid cells, there were a few large blast cells. The cytoplasm of these cells contained abundant polyribosomes, and the nucleus revealed little chromatin and a large nucleolus. Medium-sized lymphoid cells and blast cells like those found in lymph nodes could also be demonstrated in peripheral blood.

As in M.F., we also identified interdigitating reticulum cells and epithelioid venules in Sézary's syndrome.[62] Tumor cells were often found among endothelial cells of the epithelioid venules, indicating that the tumor cells were in a stage of recirculation. Interdigitating reticulum cells were seen very often. They revealed a characteristic, irregularly shaped nucleus and were lying in close contact with the lymphoid cells. These findings show that a T-cell-specific microenvironment similar to that of M.F. also belongs to Sézary's syndrome. Again, the close topographic relationship between the tumor cells and the interdigitating reticulum cells is another, morphologic indication of the T-cell nature of this lymphoma.

### *4. T-Zone Lymphoma*

According to light- and electron-microscopic findings, T-zone lymphoma usually consists of two histologically and cytologically different components,

---

[59a] 1968.

[60] LUTZNER, EMERIT, DUREPAIRE, FLANDRIN *et al.*, 1973.

[61] EDELSON, LUTZNER, KIRKPATRICK, SHEVACH *et al.*, 1974.

[62] KAISERLING and GOOS, 1975, unpublished data.

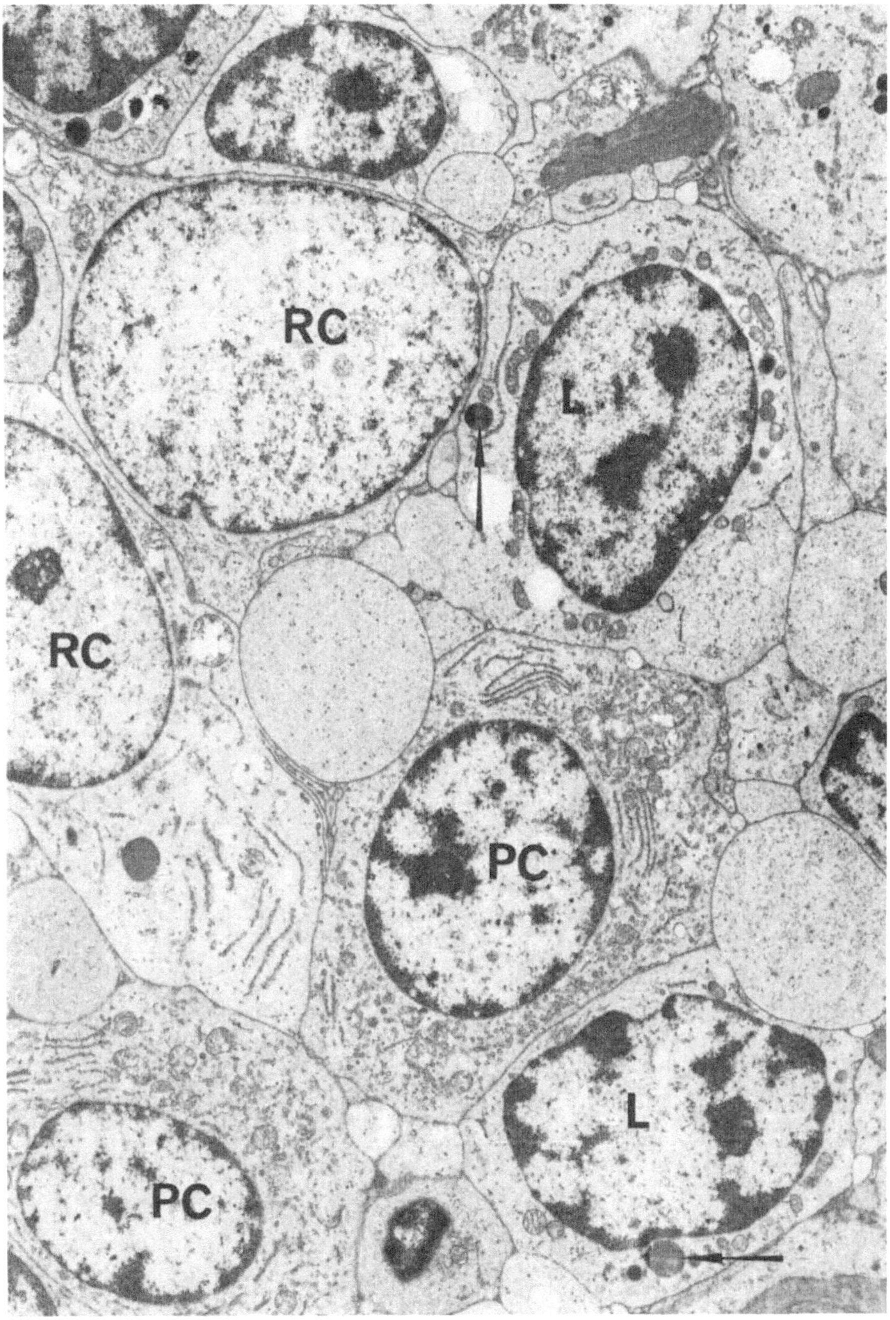


Fig. 244. T-zone lymphoma. Two histiocytic reticulum cells (*RC*), two T-associated plasma cells (*PC*), and medium-sized tumor cells (*L*) that proved to be T-cells in rosette tests. The cytoplasm contains a few osmiophilic lipid droplets (arrows). At the upper edge of the picture, part of an eosinophil granulocyte. ×9,600

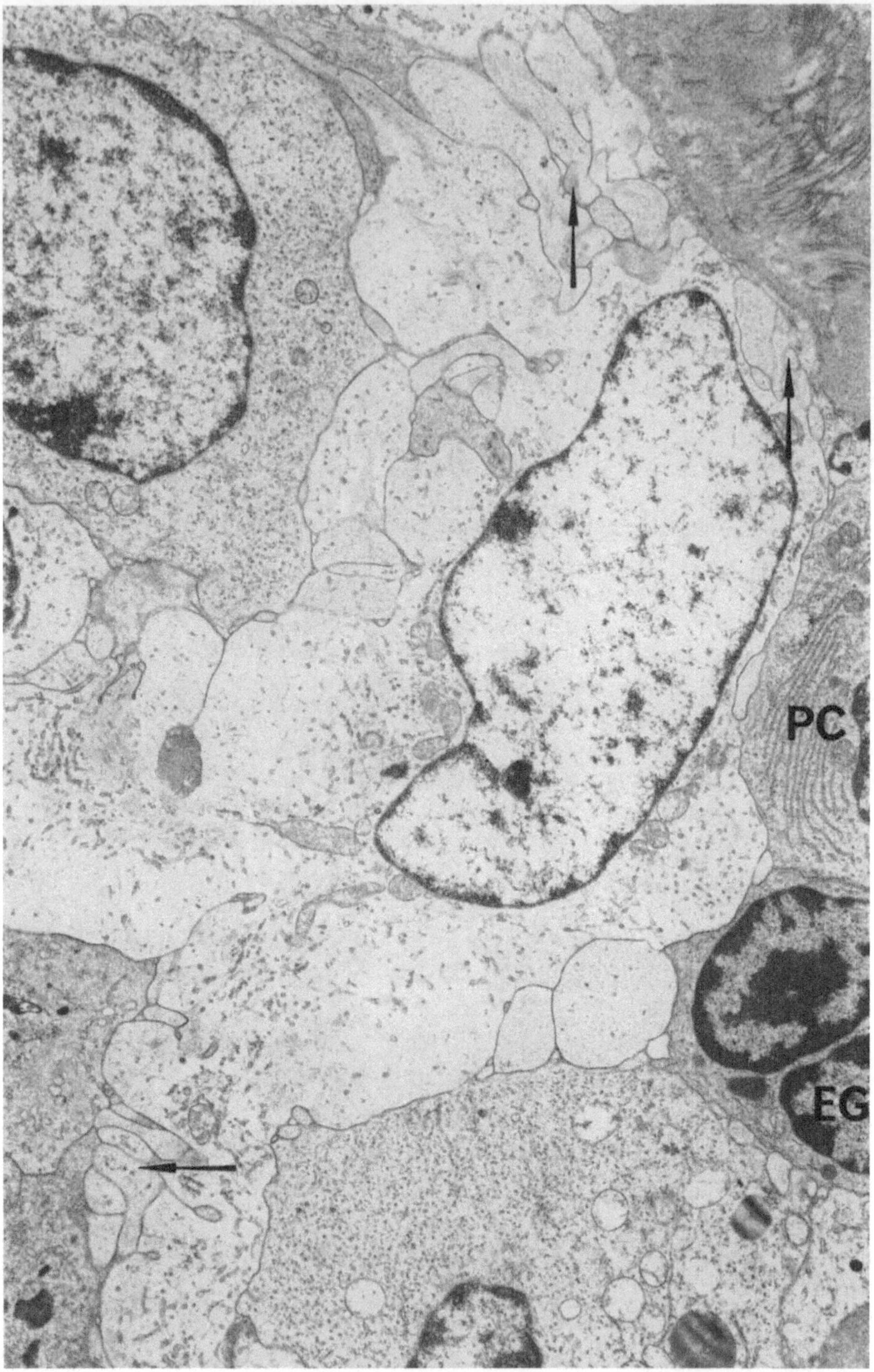


Fig. 245. T-zone lymphoma. Interdigitating reticulum cell with branched cytoplasmic projections (arrows) and numerous, chiefly smooth membrane profiles. In the direct vicinity of this cell, two tumor cells with numerous polyribosomes and parts of an eosinophil granulocyte (*EG*) and a T-associated plasma cell (*PC*). ×6,600

namely, follicles and a broad interfollicular area.[63] In this area one finds atypical medium-sized lymphocytes with a round or oval nucleus containing a large central nucleolus (Fig. 244). The heterochromatin reveals marginal condensation. Monoribosomes predominate in the cytoplasm. Occasionally, large blast cells (Fig. 245) with an oval or irregularly shaped nucleus are seen. The cytoplasm of these cells contains many polyribosomes. In one case we found osmiophilic lipid droplets in almost all of the tumor cells. In cell suspensions the medium-sized lymphoid cells can be clearly identified as T-cells in rosette tests with unsensitized sheep erythrocytes. The T-cell nature of the tumor cells is given further support by their presence in an area that shows essential features of a thymus-dependent area, namely, epithelioid venules and interdigitating reticulum cells (Fig. 245). In addition, there are T-associated plasma cells, which are also found in T-regions. Furthermore, the interdigitating reticulum cells, characterized by a bizarrely shaped nucleus, a so-called tubulovesicular system, and electron-dense cytoplasmic invaginations, are in close membrane contact with T-lymphocytes and sometimes with T-associated plasma cells (Fig. 245).

The follicles of T-zone lymphoma contain germinal centers that do not reveal any atypical cells and are composed of typical centrocytes, centroblasts, and dendritic reticulum cells. Sometimes, they are surrounded by a narrow wall of lymphocytes. The large number of closely packed dendritic reticulum cells in some of the germinal centers indicates that these are regressively altered germinal centers.

Interaction between the tumor cells and the interdigitating reticulum cells might be conjectured from the close topographic relationship between these two types of cells in T-zone lymphoma. We do not know the nature of this interaction. Similar findings with respect to a T-cell-specific microenvironment have already been mentioned in M.F. and Sézary's syndrome; but these morphologic findings also do not allow any conclusions that can be interpreted functionally. Since mitotic figures are occasionally found in the direct vicinity of interdigitating reticulum cells, one might presume that the tumor-cell proliferation is influenced by the interdigitating reticulum cells, although there is no proof of this.

## B. Malignant Lymphoma, Lymphoplasmacytic/Lymphoplasmacytoid (LP Immunocytoma)

Under the term Waldenström's disease or malignant lymphoma with dysproteinemia or paraproteinemia there have been many ultrastructural descriptions of tumors that we now call LP immunocytoma.[64] Corresponding to the

[63] Kaiserling, 1975, 1976, 1977; Lennert, 1976.

[64] Bessis, 1961; Stockinger, 1962; Zucker-Franklin, 1964; Argani and Kipkie, 1965; Kuhn, 1967; Laszlo, Gerber and Sommer, 1967; Mori and Lennert, 1969; Shigematsu, Kozuru and Hattori, 1970; Ward, Shortland and Darke, 1971; Akasaka, 1973; Kim, Heller and Rappaport, 1973; Diebold, Reynes, Kalifat and Tricot, 1974, 1975; Ottó, Balogh and Jákó, 1974; Henry, 1975.

light-microscopic findings, three subtypes can be distinguished on electron microscopy: a lymphoplasmacytic, a lymphoplasmacytoid, and a polymorphic subtype.

The lymphoplasmacytic subtype (Fig. 246) is composed of medium-sized lymphoid cells with a more or less well-developed rough endoplasmic reticulum and of small lymphocytes and plasma cells, which vary in number. There are sometimes a few intracytoplasmic globular Ig inclusions in the cisterns of rough endoplasmic reticulum. Globular inclusions may occur in large numbers in mature plasma cells, sometimes within the nucleus. A few globular inclusions may also be seen in the medium-sized lymphoid cells.

The picture of lymphoplasmacytoid immunocytoma (Fig. 247) is dominated by small and medium-sized lymphocytoid cells.[64a] The medium-sized cells sometimes have narrow strands, sometimes cisterns of rough endoplasmic reticulum. Cells that look like small lymphocytes on light microscopy also occasionally contain strands of rough endoplasmic reticulum, some of which are filled with amorphous precipitates (immunoglobulin). The chromatin is marginally condensed, similar to that of the small lymphocytes. In some cases there are numerous intracytoplasmic Ig inclusions. Typical plasma cells of the Marschalkó type are absent.

In the polymorphic subtype (Fig. 248) one finds a large number of cytologically different tumor cells. A few mature plasma cells are always found. Again, they occasionally contain globular intracytoplasmic or intranuclear amorphous Ig inclusions. In some cases the medium-sized lymphoid cells turn out to be typical centrocytes with an irregularly shaped nucleus that occasionally has nuclear pockets. There are also cells whose ultrastructure is reminiscent of that of centroblasts of germinal centers and that show marginal nucleoli. Immunoblasts with central nucleoli are found as well. The cytoplasm of both types of cells abounds in polyribosomes. Rough endoplasmic reticulum is hardly developed. In addition, one finds immature plasma cells, which vary in number from case to case.

PAS-positive cytoplasmic inclusions belong to the typical picture of LP immunocytoma. With silver methenamine staining they are highly electron-dense. These inclusions represent Ig condensates and are usually found in the cisterns of rough endoplasmic reticulum. At times they seem to displace the nucleus into the cytoplasmic periphery; the nucleus sometimes appears deformed. Occasionally, Ig condensates are found in the perinuclear space or within the nucleus. Sometimes it can be shown that the intranuclear inclusions are derived from the Ig formed in the perinuclear space and extrude from there into the nucleus. In cases of LP immunocytoma with macroglobulinemia the intercellular space sometimes shows a strong silver methenamine reaction (Fig. 246). Ig-retaining tumor cells that reveal great degeneration and contain extracellular amorphous precipitates are occasionally found in tumors in which immunochemical studies have demonstrated that the tumor cells have lost the capability to secrete Ig. The fine granular precipitates accumulate between collagenous fibers surrounding small vessels, as seen especially with silver methenamine staining (Fig. 249).

[64a] Kaiserling, 1975; Schwarze, Radaszkiewicz, Pülhorn, Goos *et al.*, 1976.

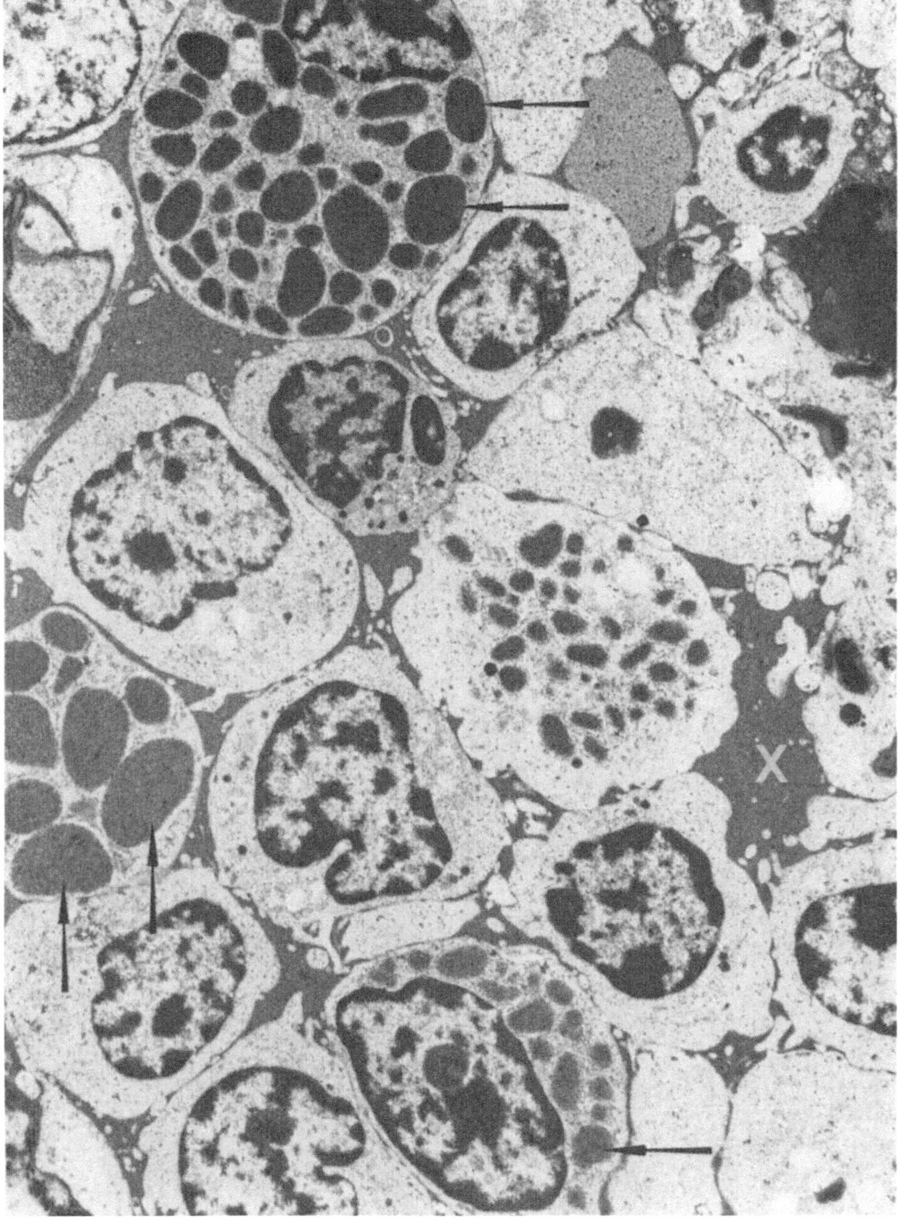


Fig. 246. Lymphoplasmacytic immunocytoma. Several small and medium-sized lymphoid cells. Some of them contain numerous globular intracytoplasmic (Ig) inclusions (arrows). With silver methenamine staining these inclusions are seen as electron-dense bodies. The amorphous material in the intercellular space (*X*), which is as electron-dense as the globular inclusions, suggests an increase in serum Ig. $\times$ 8,400

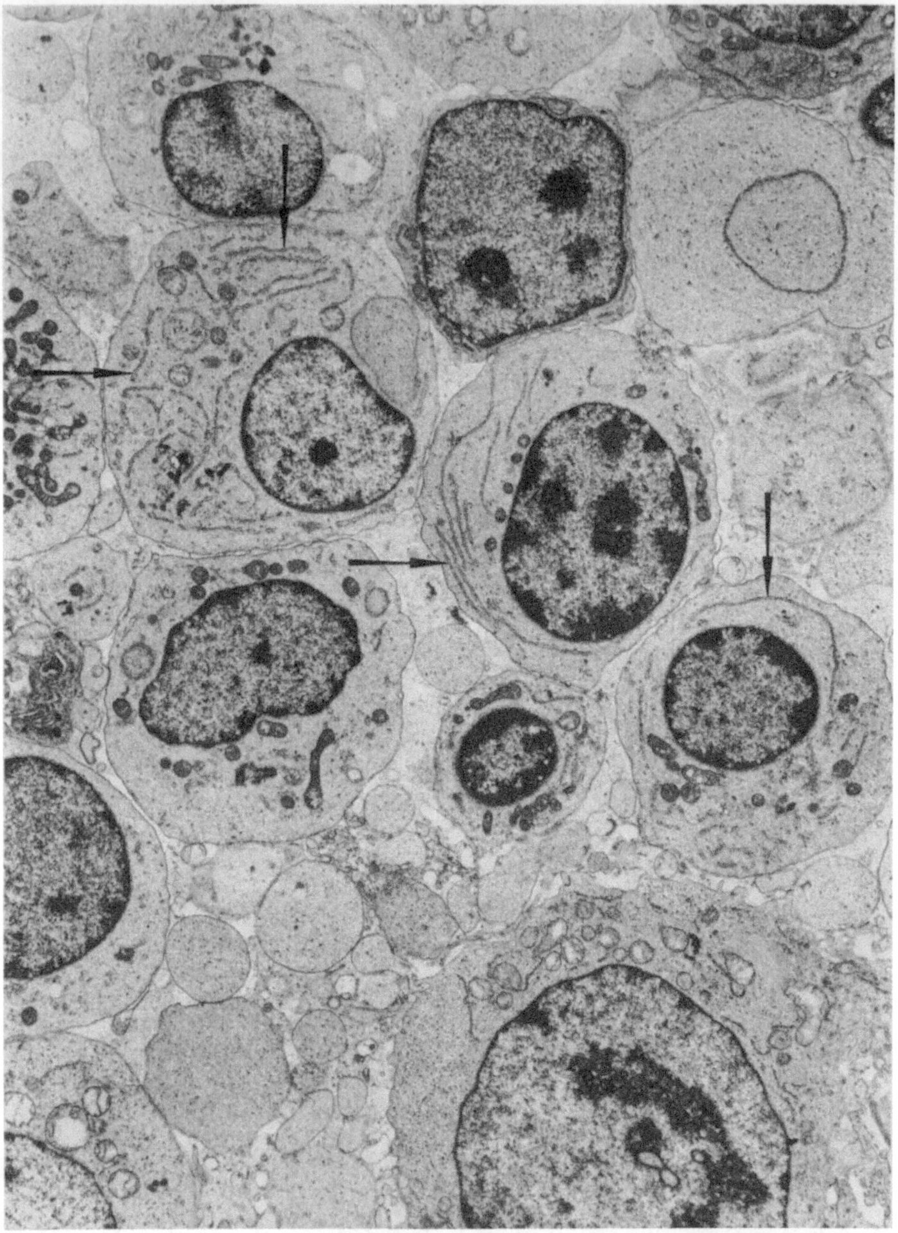

Fig. 247. Lymphoplasmacytoid immunocytoma. Medium-sized lymphoid cells with variably long, sometimes concentric profiles of rough endoplasmic reticulum (arrows). ×7,000

As in other non-Hodgkin's lymphomas, glycogen is observed only occasionally in LP immunocytoma. In one case, however, we found an extreme increase in glycogen (Fig. 250). Almost all of the tumor cells revealed large cytoplasmic areas containing this substance; in many cells more than 50% of the cytoplasm

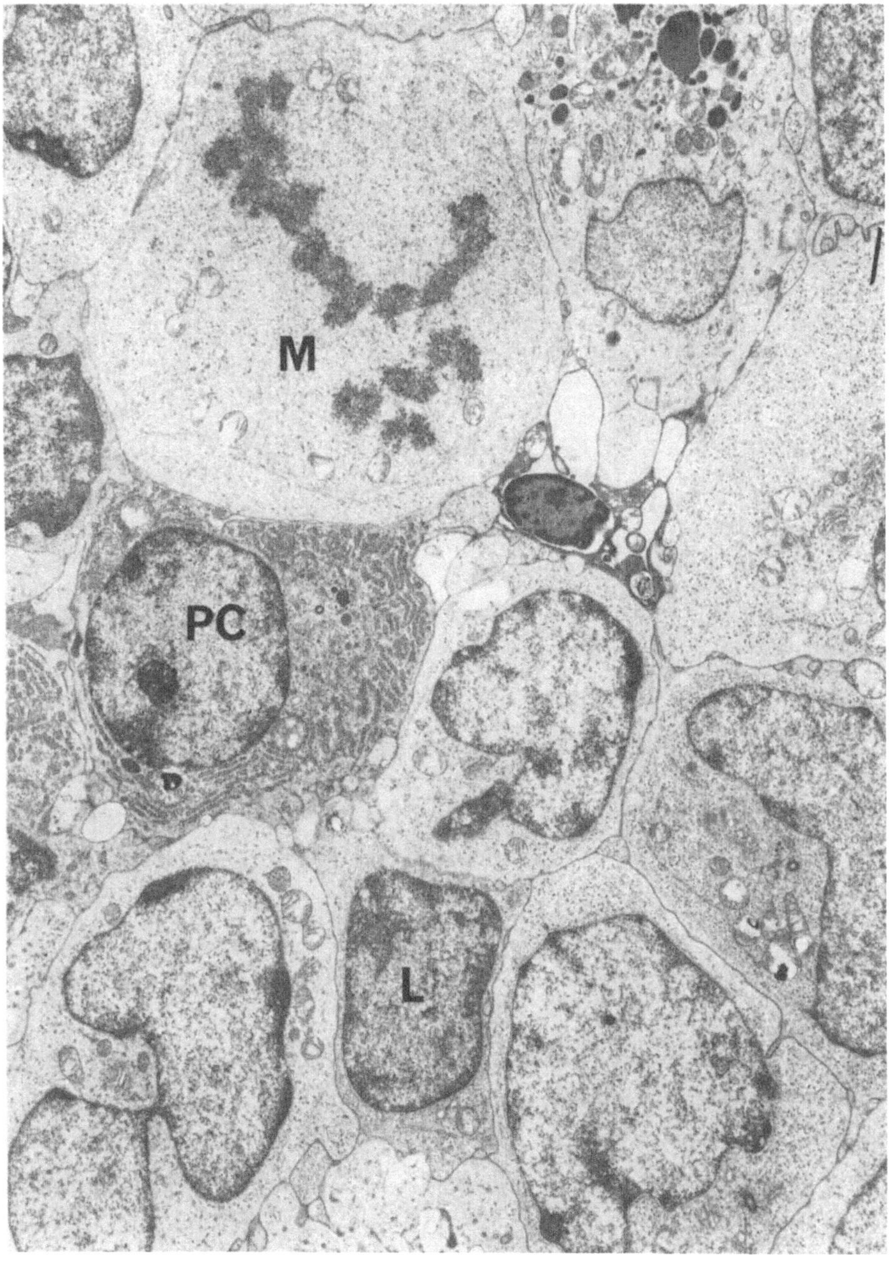


Fig. 248. Polymorphic immunocytoma. One plasma cell (*PC*), one lymphocyte (*L*), and several centrocyte-like cells. Mitotic figure (*M*). × 7,000

was filled with glycogen. The cause of this glycogen accumulation could not be clarified; perhaps there was an enzyme defect.

As mentioned in Part Six, in many cases of LP immunocytoma an increase

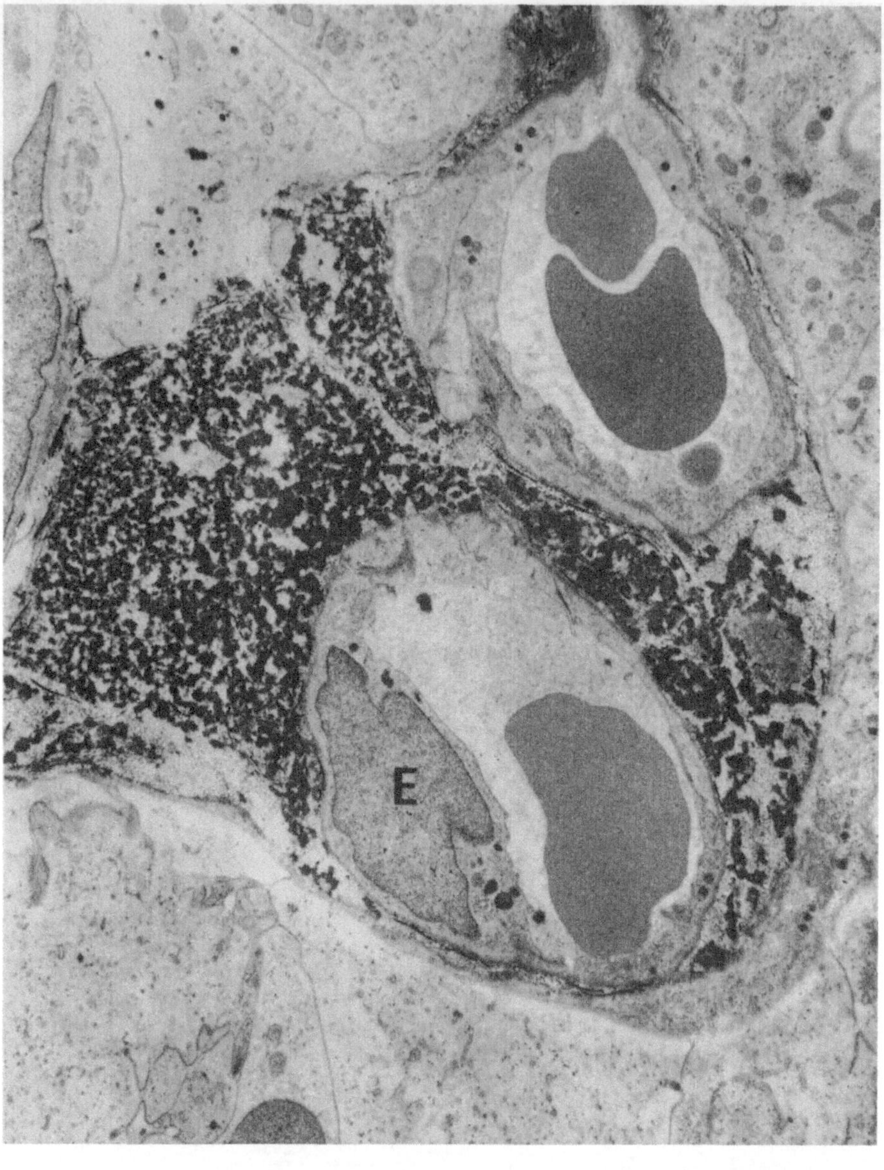


Fig. 249. LP immunocytoma. Widespread perivascular Ig precipitates in the lymph node. Endothelial cell (*E*). ×6,600

in serum Ig is absent, in spite of the large number of plasma cells and a sometimes extreme increase in tissue Ig. This finding, which suggests reduced or blocked Ig secretion, cannot be explained on the basis of ultrastructural findings. The cell organelles responsible for Ig secretion do not show any irregularities. Even in immunocytomas with completely blocked Ig secretion (the

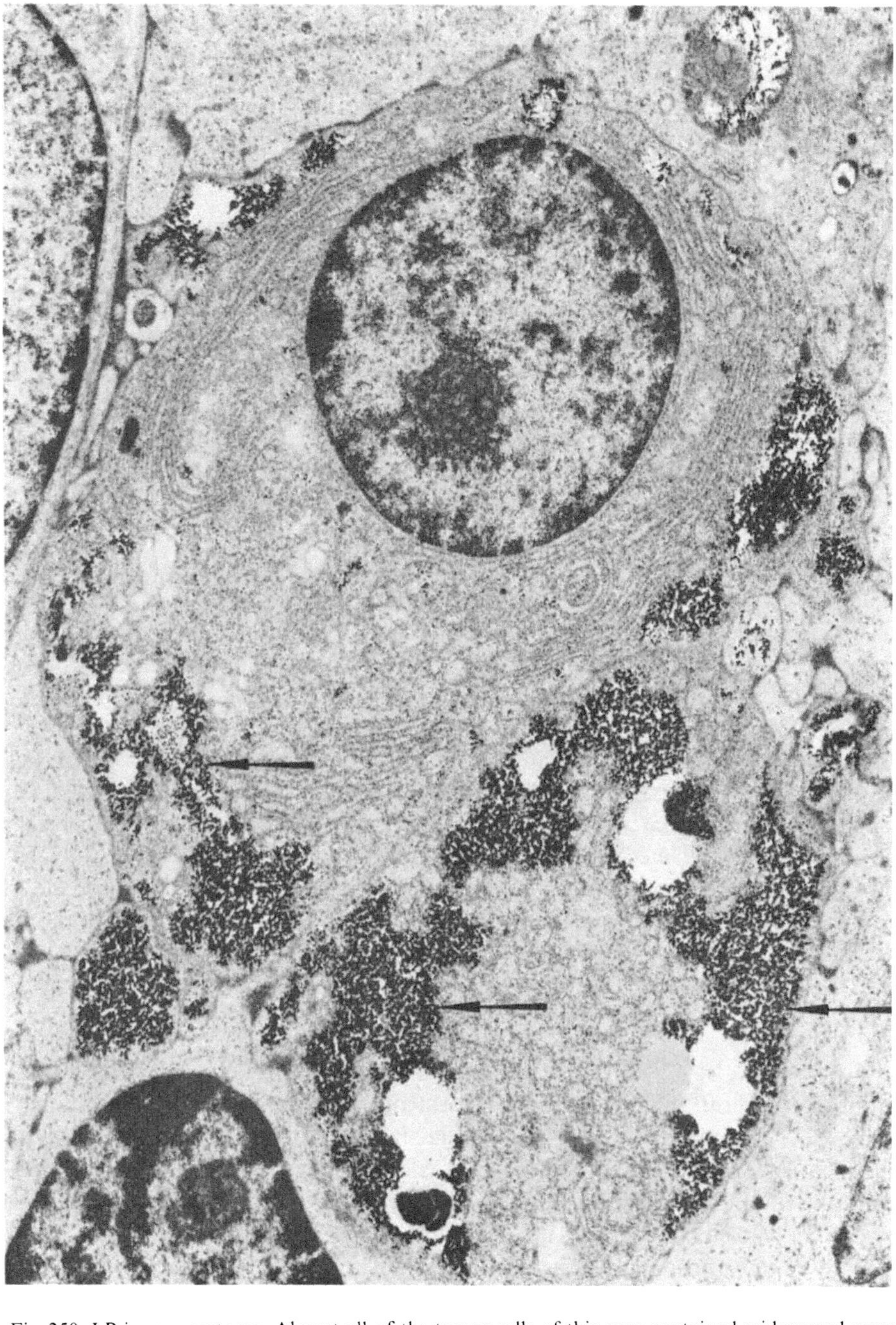

Fig. 250. LP immunocytoma. Almost all of the tumor cells of this case contained widespread areas of glycogen (arrows), which is highly electron-dense with silver methenamine staining. ×12,000

tumor cells may contain a large or a small number of globular intracytoplasmic inclusions), the Golgi field appears to be normally developed. Only the tumor cells that show an extreme accumulation of Ig sometimes contain sparse remnants of Golgi lamellae.

## C. Malignant Lymphomas of Germinal-Center Cells

Germinal centers contain a large number of different lymphoid cells (lymphocytes, centrocytes, centroblasts, immunoblasts, plasma-cell precursors, and plasma cells); thus, one might expect germinal-center neoplasms to be heterogeneous entities. So far, however, only tumors that may be considered to be neoplasms of centrocytes and those of centrocytes and centroblasts have been identified. The Kiel Classification distinguishes two germinal-center tumors among the non-Hodgkin's lymphomas of low-grade malignancy: centrocytic lymphoma and centroblastic/centrocytic lymphoma. In principle, however, we cannot exclude the possibility that the other types of lymphoma include tumors that are cytogenetically derived from germinal-center cells. That is probably true for a few cases of LP immunocytoma in which we found dendritic reticulum cells and for cases, especially of the polymorphic subtype, in which centrocytes and centroblasts may be found.

Our recent findings[64b] indicate that so-called nodular paragranuloma, a subtype of the lymphocytic and histiocytic type of Hodgkin's lymphoma differentiated by LUKES *et al.*[64c] that contains numerous lymphocytes, takes place in germinal centers. On electron microscopy, we found in the nodules not only small and medium-sized lymphocytes and a few germinal-center cells (centrocytes and centroblasts), but also numerous dendritic reticulum cells, occasionally with desmosomal junctions. The other types of Hodgkin's lymphoma did not show dendritic reticulum cells.

### *1. Malignant Lymphoma, Centrocytic*

Ultrastructurally, the cytology of centrocytic lymphoma is quite monotonous.[65] The tumor consists of medium-sized lymphoid cells (Fig. 251) with an irregularly shaped nucleus, which occasionally has nuclear pockets and contains a medium-sized nucleolus. The chromatin is sometimes uniformly distributed in the nucleus; sometimes it is clearly marginally condensed. The cytoplasm contains monoribosomes. Rough endoplasmic reticulum is only poorly developed. The Golgi field consists of a few parallel lamellae and a few mostly smooth, occasionally coated vesicles. The number of lysosomes is small. These medium-sized lymphoid cells are by far the most dominant in number and show all of the essential ultrastructural features of centrocytes. In addition,

[64b] LENNERT, KAISERLING and MÜLLER-HERMELINK, in press.

[64c] LUKES, BUTLER and HICKS, 1966.

[65] KAISERLING, 1976, 1977.

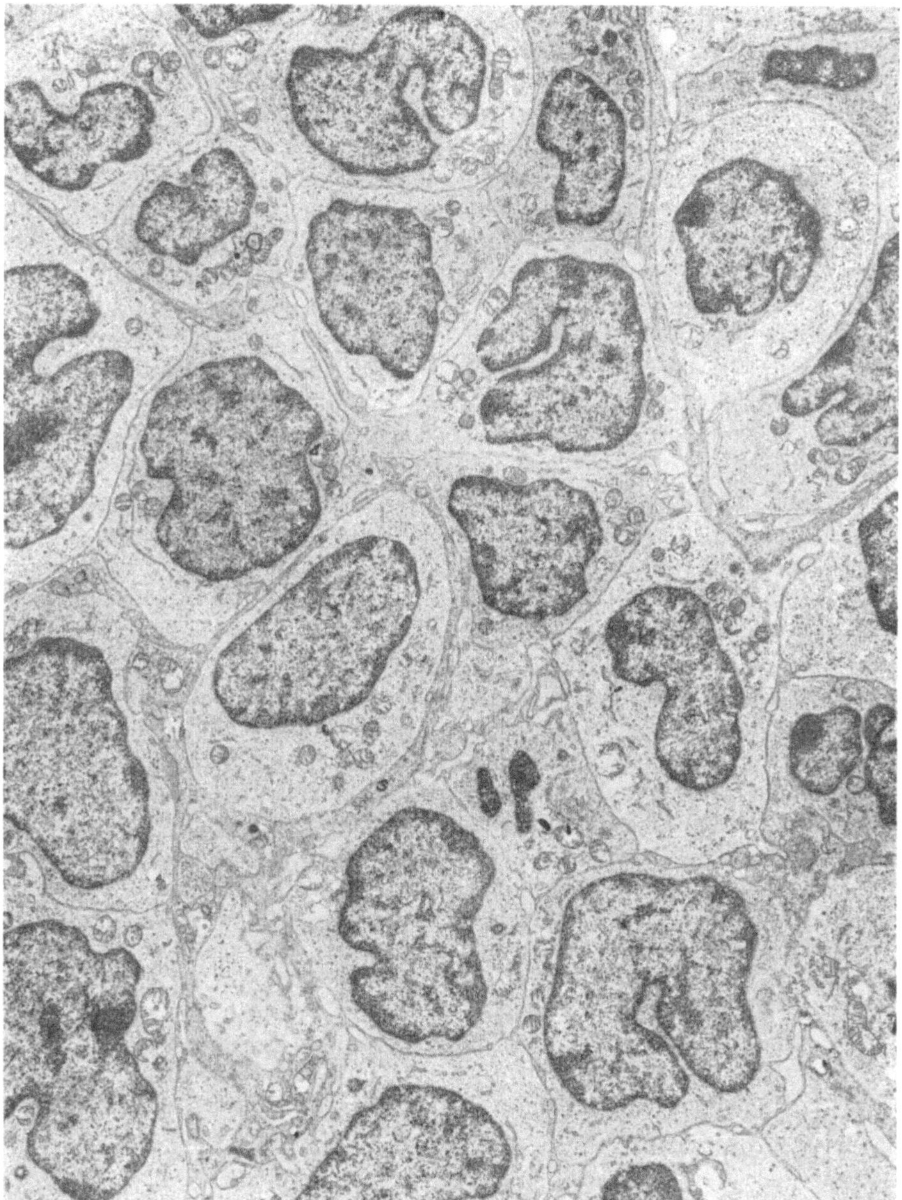

Fig. 251. Malignant lymphoma, centrocytic. Tumor consists of a cytologically uniform cell population. The cells are characterized by irregularly shaped nuclei. ×6,000

there are regularly a few small lymphocytes. In a few cases one finds occasional cells with large oval nuclei and polyribosomes. The nucleus reveals little chromatin and a usually prominent, central or marginal nucleolus. These cells are reminiscent of small centroblasts. In a small number of cases the tumor cells prove to be larger than normal centrocytes. These cells contain abundant polyribosomes and are characterized by prominent nucleoli with clearly visible nucleolonemata.

Some histiocytic reticulum cells with electron-transparent cytoplasm belong to the typical picture of most cases of centrocytic lymphoma. They have a sometimes round, sometimes bizarrely shaped nucleus. There are abundant intracytoplasmic lysosome-like granules and phagosomes of variable morphology.

Further components of centrocytic lymphoma are dendritic reticulum cells, which we could demonstrate by electron microscopy in 12 out of 20 cases. They can be identified by their desmosomes and/or characteristically narrow marginal chromatin condensations, and by widened short strands of rough endoplasmic reticulum and osmiophobic fat droplets, which often occur in this type of cell. The dendritic reticulum cells are in close contact with tumor cells *via* their branched cytoplasmic projections. In addition, one occasionally finds fibroblastic reticulum cells and so-called dark reticulum cells. We sometimes found remnants of typical T-nodules, which, according to comparative light-microscopic findings, are located exclusively in the lymph-node cortex. They consist of interdigitating reticulum cells, epithelioid venules, cytologically uniform small lymphocytes, and T-associated plasma cells.

The results of our light-microscopic, electron-microscopic, enzyme-cytochemical, and immunologic studies indicate that centrocytic lymphoma is a B-cell neoplasm. The relevant findings are discussed in detail on page 284ff. Our ultrastructural data are particularly important for demonstrating the cytologic relationship between the tumor cells of this lymphoma and the centrocytes of germinal centers. Although we could not find centrocytes containing ergastoplasm on electron microscopy, centrocytic lymphomas with plasmacytic differentiation, and occasionally with globular Ig inclusions, have now been observed on light microscopy. The tumor cells also bore surface Ig, which we demonstrated by electron microscopy. Furthermore, in two cases there was a membrane-bound ATPase reaction on both light and electron microscopy, which is another indication of the B-cell nature of centrocytic lymphoma.

## 2. *Malignant Lymphoma, Centroblastic/Centrocytic*

In its classic form, centroblastic/centrocytic lymphoma is a follicular lymphoma. It is composed of follicles containing tumor cells and of an interfollicular area in which tumor cells are found only in small numbers. As described by many authors,[66] the follicles consist chiefly of medium-sized lymphoid cells with an irregularly shaped nucleus (Fig. 252). These cells correspond to the centrocytes of germinal centers. The nucleus has sometimes uniformly distributed, sometimes marginally condensed chromatin, and at times it reveals nuclear pockets. As a rule, the cytoplasm contains only a few rough membrane profiles

[66] Kojima, 1969; Lennert and Niedorf, 1969; Mori and Lennert, 1969; Kojima, Imai and Mori, 1973; Lennert, 1973; Moragas, Guardia, Martinez-Vazquez, Vilaseca *et al.*, 1973; Glick, Leech, Waldron, Flexner *et al.*, 1975; Levine and Dorfman, 1975; Henry, 1975; Rivas and Oliva, 1975.

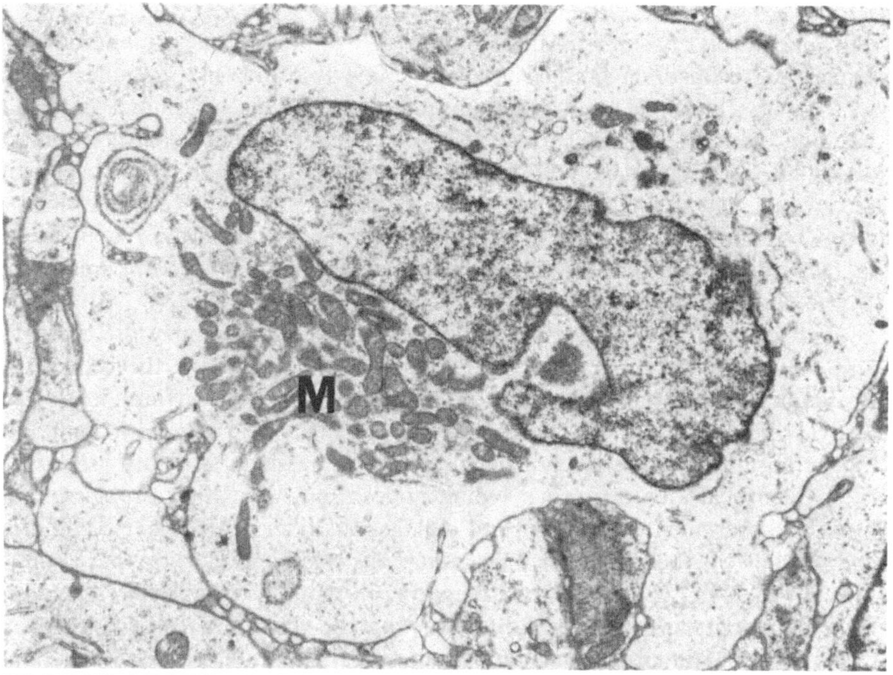


(a)

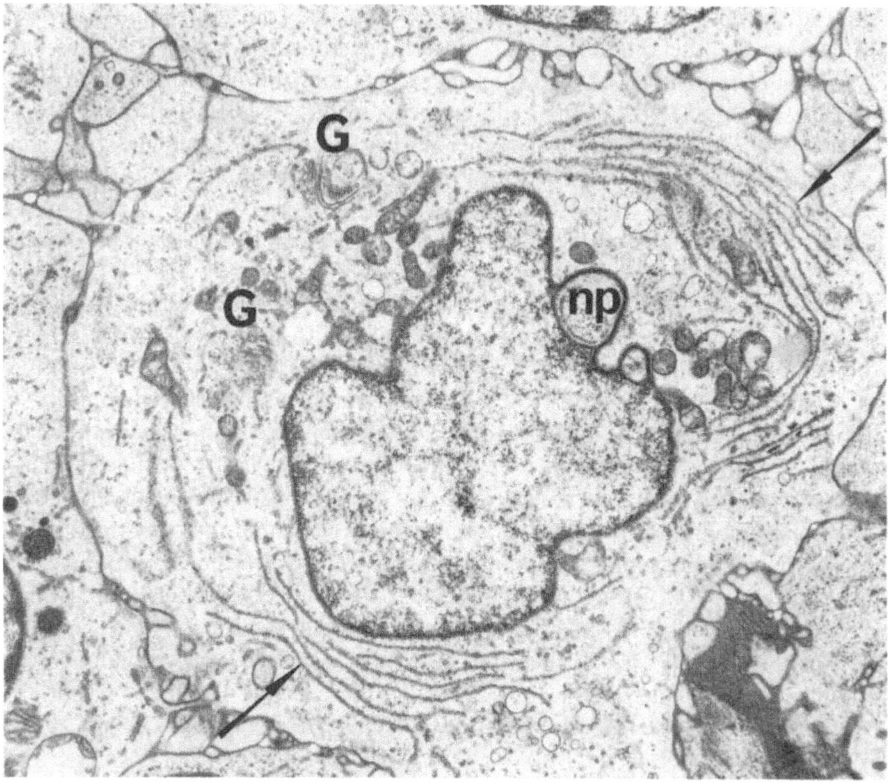


(b)

Fig. 252a and b. Malignant lymphoma, centroblastic/centrocytic. (a) Centrocyte with an irregularly shaped nucleus and abundant mitochondria (*M*). (b) Centrocyte with nuclear pockets (*np*), which are frequently seen in this type of cell, and several rough membrane profiles (arrows). Golgi field (*G*). (a) ×9,000, (b) ×11,000 and a few polyribosomes. Mitochondria are sometimes very numerous. The Golgi field is medium-sized. There are a few lysosome-like granules nearby.

The follicles regularly contain another type of cell, although in smaller numbers, namely, blast cells (Fig. 253) with a large nucleus, sparse chromatin, abundant polyribosomes, and prominent marginal nucleoli. These cells find their equivalent in the centroblasts of germinal centers. As first described by KOJIMA[67] and LENNERT and NIEDORF,[68] there are also dendritic reticulum cells in the follicles. These cells can be clearly identified on electron microscopy by the presence of desmosomes.

The interfollicular area usually contains only a small number of centrocytes and centroblasts and no dendritic reticulum cells at all. On the other hand, it abounds with lymphocytes and epithelioid venules. The lymphocytes have an oval or indented nucleus, a ring-shaped nucleolus, and a cytoplasm containing monoribosomes. The epithelioid venules show the same structure as those in the paracortical area of normal lymph nodes. Sometimes they are surrounded by a thick basement membrane and collagenous fibers. Among the cylindrical endothelial cells there are sometimes numerous small lymphocytes that are cytologically identical with those predominating in the interfollicular area. We have never seen centrocytes or centroblasts within the venular wall. In some of our cases we found interdigitating reticulum cells in the interfollicular area. They showed the characteristically branched cytoplasmic projections and narrow invaginations of the cell membrane, a well-developed so-called tubulovesicular system, and a bizarrely shaped nucleus. Sometimes the interfollicular area also contains T-associated plasma cells and occasionally typical plasma cells. The interfollicular area therefore has numerous features of a T-dependent area, which is also characterized by epithelioid venules, interdigitating reticulum cells, and T-associated plasma cells.[69] As the studies of JAFFE *et al.*[70] and our own findings suggest, the small lymphocytes in this area are probably T-lymphocytes.

Based on ultrastructural findings, there is no fundamental difference between the cytologic spectrum of follicular and that of diffuse or partly diffuse, partly follicular centroblastic/centrocytic lymphoma.

Centroblastic/centrocytic lymphomas composed of typical centroblasts and centrocytes predominate heavily in our collection. We found a group of four out of 30 cases, however, in which the tumor cells had a somewhat larger diameter than typical centrocytes, an oval or only slightly indented nucleus, and abundant monoribosomes as well as polyribosomes. According to light-microscopic findings, these cells correspond to centrocytes, but cannot be clearly distinguished by electron microscopy from the small centroblasts of germinal centers described by LENNERT *et al.*[71] and MÜLLER-HERMELINK and CAESAR.[72]

There is another special form of centroblastic/centrocytic lymphoma (seven out of 30 cases) characterized by a few, in rare cases numerous tumor cells containing ergastoplasm, in addition to centrocytes and centroblasts.[73] The

[67] 1969.
[68] 1969.
[69] KAISERLING, 1976.
[70] JAFFE, SHEVACH, FRANK, BERARD *et al.*, 1974.
[71] LENNERT, CAESAR and MÜLLER, 1967.
[72] 1969.
[73] KAISERLING, 1976.

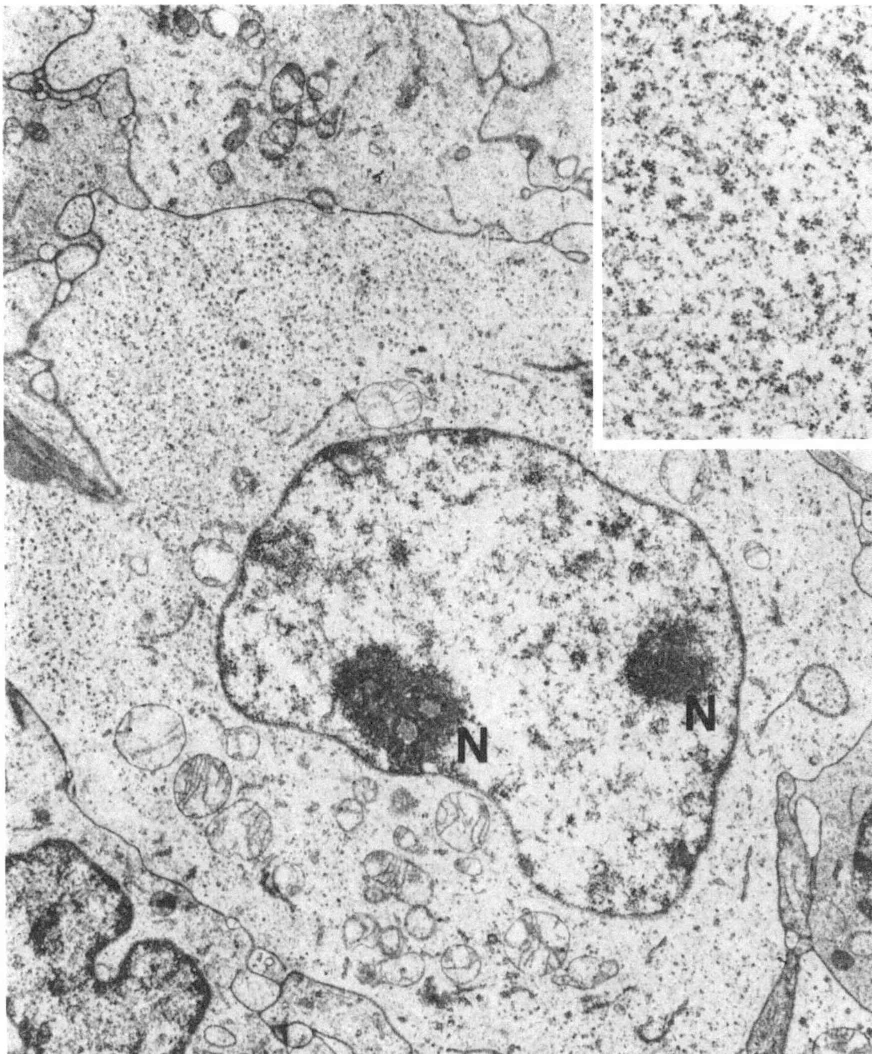


Fig. 253. Malignant lymphoma, centroblastic/centrocytic. Typical centroblast with a broad rim of cytoplasm and marginal nucleoli (*N*). The cytoplasm contains abundant polyribosomes (inset). × 9,200, inset: × 25,000

cells containing ergastoplasm are reminiscent of typical centrocytes owing to their size and nuclear shape, but differ from them by a large amount of rough endoplasmic reticulum. We interpret these cells as a special type of centrocyte or as immature plasma cells. The strands of rough endoplasmic reticulum are sometimes narrow, sometimes widened. When they are widened, they occasionally contain amorphous or crystalline inclusions. As already mentioned (p. 245ff.),

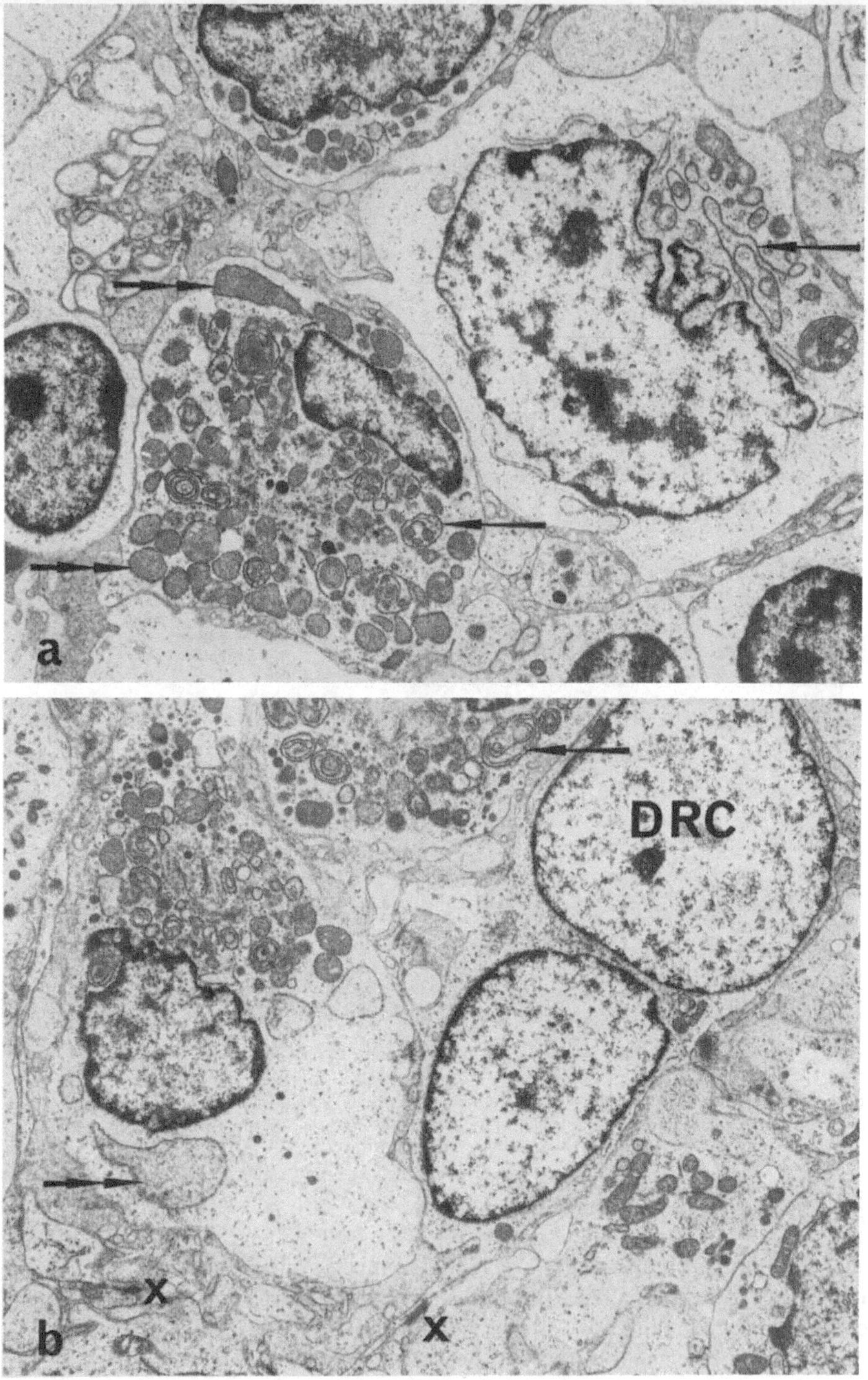
a
DRC
x
x
b

the amount of rough endoplasmic reticulum may be so large that in some cases it may be very difficult to draw a sharp border between centroblastic/centrocytic lymphoma and LP immunocytoma. Such a case is illustrated in Figure 117: on light microscopy, there were extremely large follicles, in which dendritic reticulum cells (Fig. 254) as well as typical centrocytes and centroblasts were evident on electron microscopy. In addition, there were numerous cells with signs of plasmacytic differentiation; some of them were still reminiscent of centrocytes, whereas others showed features of immature plasma cells. Some of the tumor cells contained widened cisterns, others contained narrow profiles of endoplasmic reticulum; some of the profiles looked like *Nebenkerne*. Immunochemical analysis revealed another special feature of this case, namely, a great increase in tissue Ig (IgM), with no increase in the serum-Ig level. This finding indicates that Ig secretion was completely blocked.

Enzyme cytochemically, centrocytes and centroblasts reveal a positive ATPase reaction in some cases;[74] in others they are enzyme-negative. There is no, or only an extremely weak reaction for 5-nucleotidase. The few lysosomes show a weakly positive acid phosphatase reaction. In only one of our cases, which revealed a great increase in lysosome-like granules, did we observe a strongly positive acid phosphatase reaction on light microscopy.

# II. High-Grade Malignant Lymphomas

## A. Malignant Lymphoma, Centroblastic

We distinguish a primary and a secondary centroblastic lymphoma. The primary type is directly derived from germinal-center cells. The secondary type develops from a centroblastic/centrocytic lymphoma.

*Primary centroblastic lymphoma*—four cases in our collection—consists chiefly of blast cells with large nuclei and a moderate (Fig. 255) or large number of polyribosomes. Cytologically, these cells correspond to centroblasts of germinal centers. The nucleus is usually oval, but occasionally indented, and contains sparse heterochromatin. Frequently, there are two or more large marginal nucleoli. The cytoplasm also contains a few rough ergastoplasmic profiles, a medium-sized Golgi field sometimes with abundant vesicles, and large mitochondria, which are often swollen and show rarefaction of cristae. Furthermore,

[74] KAISERLING, 1975.

◁ Fig. 254a and b. Malignant lymphoma, centroblastic/centrocytic, follicular. Borderline case to polymorphic immunocytoma. Tumor cells with numerous narrow strands (arrows) and cisterns (double arrows) of rough endoplasmic reticulum. Dendritic reticulum cells (*DRC*). Desmosomes (*x*). Same case as Figs. 117 and 118. (a) ×6,600, (b) ×7,000

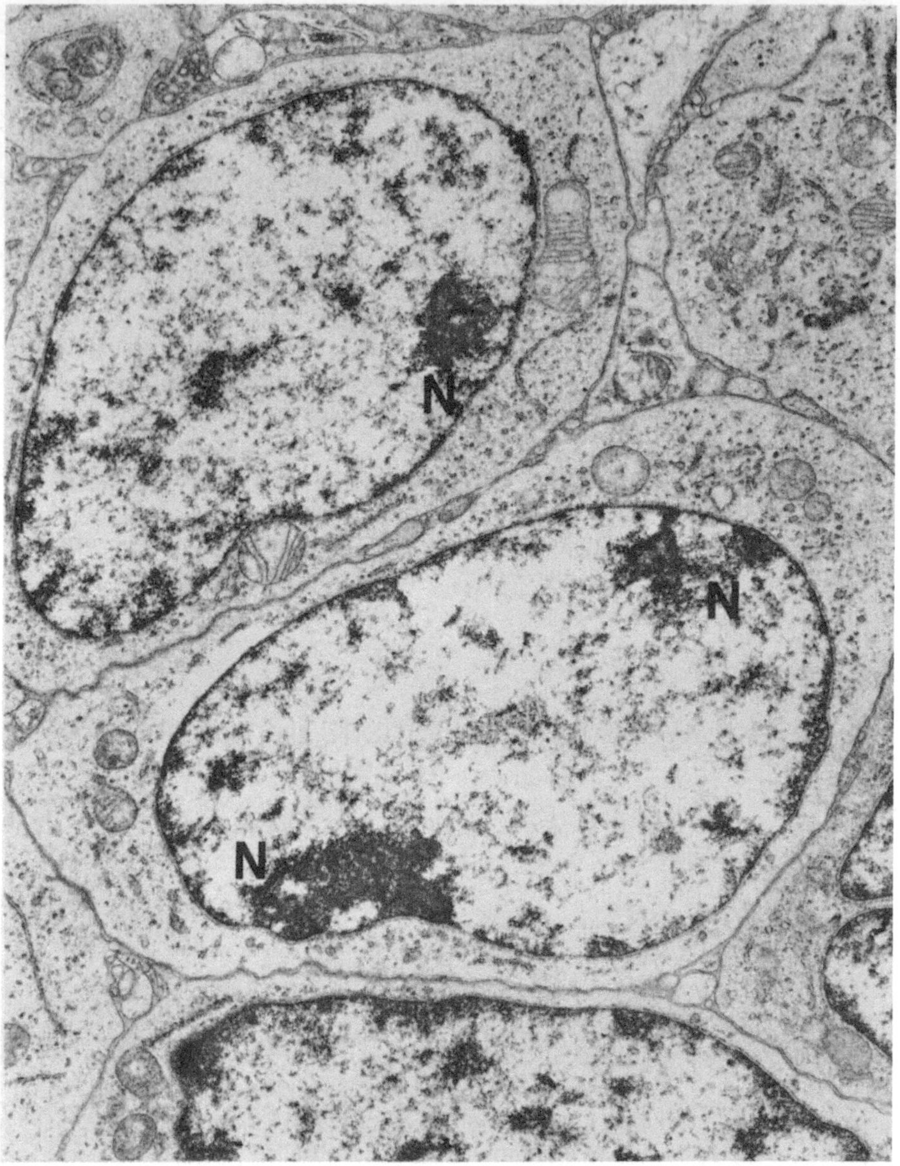


Fig. 255. Malignant lymphoma, centroblastic (primary). Tumor cells have an oval nucleus with little heterochromatin and marginal nucleoli (*N*). Cytoplasm contains chiefly polyribosomes. ×15,000

one finds a few smaller lymphoid cells with an irregularly shaped nucleus, which occasionally reveals nuclear pockets, and a cytoplasm containing monoribosomes. These cells are therefore reminiscent of centrocytes.

One of our primary centroblastic lymphomas was characterized by a large number of dendritic reticulum cells that sometimes revealed desmosomes. All of the tumors contained small lymphocytes, which varied in number from case to case. Three tumors showed typical epithelioid venules.

We have examined two cases of *secondary centroblastic lymphoma*. The ultrastructure of these two tumors was very different. In one case large tumor cells, in the other small tumor cells predominated. In the large-cell tumor we found almost the same picture as in primary centroblastic lymphoma: the predominating cells were blast cells with abundant polyribosomes and an oval, occasionally indented nucleus containing one or two nucleoli and little heterochromatin.

The small-cell secondary centroblastic lymphoma revealed cells that were reminiscent of typical centrocytes of germinal centers owing to the shape of the nucleus and organization of the cytoplasm. On the other hand, there were also tumor cells that were similar to centrocytes, but were somewhat larger (anaplastic centrocytes). The nucleus of these cells was bizarrely shaped, sometimes divided into segments by deep nuclear invaginations, and contained one or more prominent nucleoli. Now and then we also found nuclear pockets. The cytoplasm showed abundant short rough membrane profiles, mitochondria, and mono- and polyribosomes. Tumor cells with large nuclei and abundant polyribosomes, like the cells described in the previous case, were rarely found. Dendritic reticulum cells were seen occasionally. There were also a few small lymphocytes and some interdigitating reticulum cells.

Primary centroblastic lymphomas are therefore characterized by large tumor cells with abundant polyribosomes. These cells have the features of centroblasts. The presence of dendritic reticulum cells may be considered an indication of the germinal-center nature of this lymphoma. As in the primary type, centroblasts may predominate in secondary centroblastic lymphoma. Centrocytes, however, may also be very numerous and dominate the picture. The presence of dendritic and interdigitating reticulum cells is again an indication that this type of lymphoma develops from M.L. centroblastic/centrocytic.

## B. Malignant Lymphoma, Lymphoblastic

### *1. Burkitt Type*

Typical Burkitt's tumor, which is distinguished from other malignant lymphomas by special clinical features and its morphology, occurs almost exclusively in the equatorial regions of Africa and New Guinea. We call lymphomas with an essentially similar histology that are observed in temperate zones "lymphoblastic lymphomas of the Burkitt type" for two reasons. First, they show a different clinical picture. Second, the increased Epstein-Barr-virus (EBV) titer regularly demonstrated in Burkitt's tumor is usually not found in European and American lymphomas of the Burkitt type.

*Burkitt's tumor* is a lymphoma with quite constant cytologic and histologic features.[75] The ultrastructural characteristics of Burkitt's tumor, which apply in all important respects to lymphoblastic lymphoma of the Burkitt type, were summarized at a workshop in Bethesda in 1969 as follows:[76]

At low magnification the monomorphism of the dominant cells is striking. They are round or oval and have a relatively high nucleocytoplasmic ratio. Scattered macrophages are seen and usually contain phagocytosed cell debris. The ultrastructural features of the typical cells are as follows: ... The nucleus is round or oval, and shallow irregular indentations are frequently found. Rarely, these indentations are deep and significantly distort the nuclear shape. Projections of the nuclear envelope may appear as satellites or as invaginations of the nucleus. Such changes of the nuclear membrane are not, however, specific for these tumor cells. ... Chromatin is abundant and clumped at the nuclear envelope and around the nucleoli. The interchromatinic substance is relatively clear, an important characteristic of undifferentiated cells. ... Nucleoli are quite large and the nucleolonemas are usually visible.

... The cytoplasm is moderate but variable in amount and relatively dense. ... The most characteristic feature is the large number of polyribosomes. ... Ergastoplasmic lamellae are rare. ... Mitochondria are few, large, and have a tendency to polarize. ... Large inclusions consistent with lipid vacuoles are found in some cells.

As a rule, EBV or virus-like structures are missing in the primary tumor. As far as we know, they were detected only by GRIFFIN *et al.*[77] They are frequently demonstrated in cell cultures, however, as first shown by EPSTEIN *et al.*[78] The so-called undulating tubuli[79] occasionally described in Burkitt's lymphoma, which have also been called virus-like structures, are not a specific feature of this lymphoma, since one does find them in other lymphomas[80] and especially in lupus erythematosus. Furthermore, there is probably no relationship between them and EBV.[81]

In lymphomas of the *Burkitt type* the tumor cells had a round or oval nucleus, coarse heterochromatin condensations, and prominent nucleoli (Fig. 256a). The cytoplasm contained abundant polyribosomes. There was almost no rough endoplasmic reticulum. The same is true in African Burkitt's lymphoma in all but a few cases.[82] In contrast to African Burkitt's lymphoma, our cases rarely showed intracytoplasmic lipid droplets.

In one of our cases the tumor cells had an irregularly shaped nucleus (Fig. 256b); some had nuclear pockets. The chromatin was condensed at the nuclear membrane. The cytoplasm contained chiefly monoribosomes and only a few polyribosomes. Cases of Burkitt's lymphoma of similar morphol-

[75] EPSTEIN and ACHONG, 1965, 1970; STEWART, LOVELACE, WHANG and NGU, 1965; EPSTEIN, ACHONG, BARR, ZAJAC *et al.*, 1966; RABSON, O'CONOR, BARON, WHANG *et al.*, 1966; EPSTEIN, 1967; POPE, ACHONG, EPSTEIN and BIDDULPH, 1967; TOSHIMA, TAKAGI, MINOWADA and MOORE *et al.*, 1967; DORFMAN, 1968; POPE, ACHONG and EPSTEIN, 1968; BERNHARD, 1970; KATAYAMA, UEHARA, GLESER and WEINTRAUB, 1974.

[76] BERARD, O'CONOR, THOMAS and TORLONI, 1969.

[77] GRIFFIN, WRIGHT, BELL and ROSS, 1966.

[78] EPSTEIN, ACHONG and BARR, 1964.

[79] POPE, ACHONG, EPSTEIN and BIDDULPH, 1967; CHANDRA, 1968; BEDOYA, GRIMLEY and RABSON, 1969.

[80] CHANDRA, 1968; UZMAN, SAITO and KASAC, 1971; KAISERLING, 1972.

[81] EPSTEIN and ACHONG, 1970; KLIPPEL, DECKER, GRIMLEY, EVANS *et al.*, 1973; SPLINTER, HELDER, LUCAS and FELTKAMP-VROOM, 1975.

[82] EPSTEIN, ACHONG, BARR, ZAJAC *et al.*, 1966; RABSON, O'CONOR, BARON, WHANG *et al.*, 1966; DOUGLAS, BORJESON and CHESSIN, 1967.

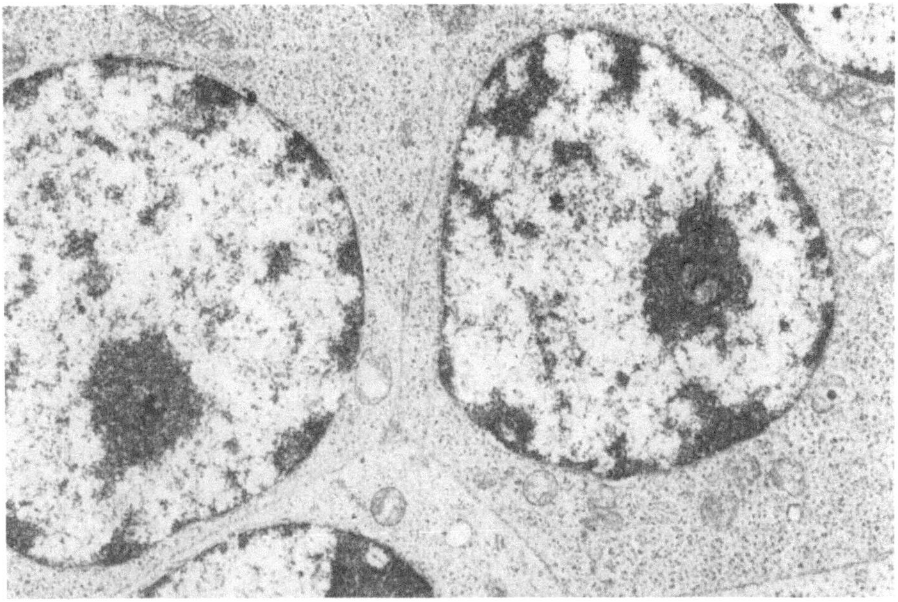
(a)

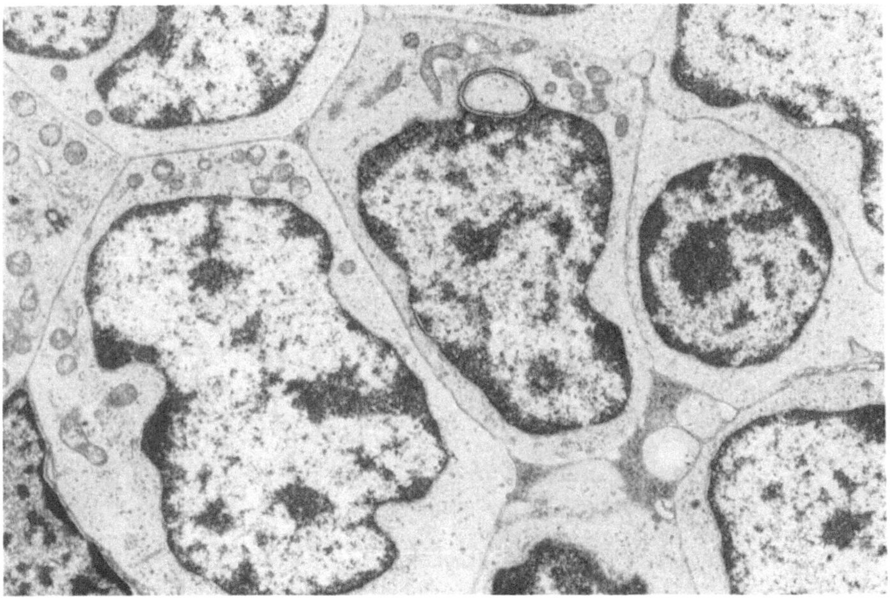
(b)

Fig. 256a and b. Malignant lymphoma, lymphoblastic, Burkitt type. (a) Tumor cells containing numerous polyribosomes and an oval nucleus. (b) Tumor cells from another case with a smaller, irregularly shaped nucleus and chiefly monoribosomes. × 11,000

ogy were also described by EPSTEIN and ACHONG[83] and BERNHARD.[83a] The tumor cells of this type of Burkitt's lymphoma, which is also said to be undifferentiated or "atypical," show certain cytologic similarities to centrocytes of germi-

[83] 1970. [83a] 1970.

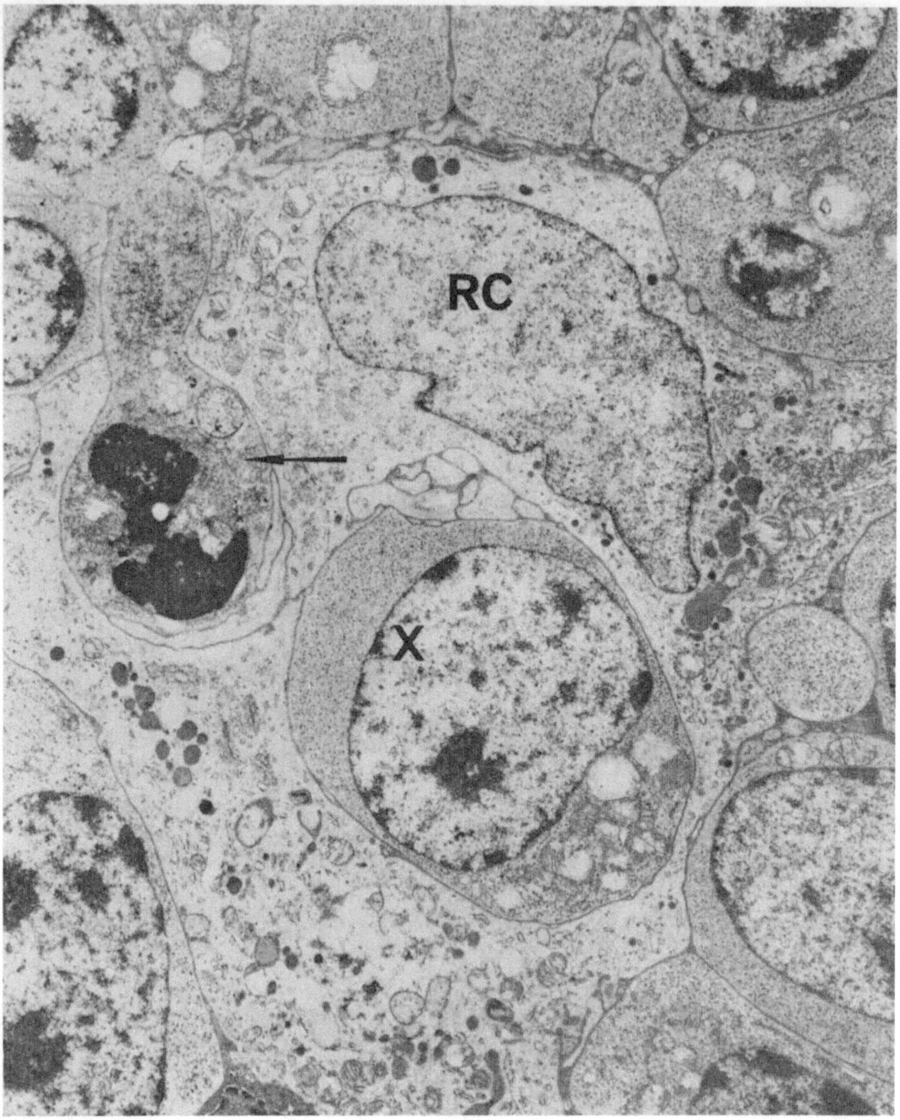


Fig. 257. Histiocytic reticulum cell (*RC*) in lymph node in lymphoblastic lymphoma of the Burkitt type. Cytoplasm contains numerous residual bodies (arrow) and an evidently phagocytosed tumor cell (*X*), whose cytology shows that it is probably vital. ×7,200

nal centers. According to various authors,[84] the cells of other ("differentiated") Burkitt's lymphomas are reminiscent of centroblasts or immunoblasts. In some cases we found a cytologic relationship to the small germinal-center blast cells that contain abundant polyribosomes; these cells have so far been called small centroblasts.

[84] BERNHARD, 1970; KRÜGER and O'CONOR, 1972; LUKES and COLLINS, 1975.

As in African Burkitt's lymphoma, we found numerous starry-sky cells (histiocytic reticulum cells) in all lymphomas of the Burkitt type that we studied. Like the cytologically similar starry-sky cells of germinal centers, these cells phagocytose lymphoid cells. The phagocytosed tumor cells are sometimes greatly degenerated. At times, however, one sees tumor cells that lack any sign of decay (Fig. 257). The studies of BEDOYA *et al.*[85] on cell cultures of Burkitt's lymphoma also showed that the reticulum cells phagocytose nondegenerated tumor cells, or not only degenerated tumor cells, but also cells that would be called "vital" because of their morphology.

## 2. *Convoluted-Cell Type (Acid Phosphatase Type)*

There have been only a few publications on the ultrastructure of lymphoblastic lymphoma of the convoluted-cell type.[86] According to our findings, this tumor is characterized by three types of cells: medium-sized lymphoid cells (Fig. 258), which dominate in number and are characterized by an irregularly shaped or greatly indented nucleus, sometimes divided into segments; considerably larger cells with a likewise greatly indented or segmented nucleus; and a few small lymphocytes with a nucleus containing abundant chromatin and a narrow rim of cytoplasm containing monoribosomes. The large and medium-sized cells have a relatively uniformly distributed, only partly condensed heterochromatin and one or more medium-sized nucleoli. The cytoplasm contains mono- and polyribosomes, almost no rough endoplasmic reticulum, and a well-developed Golgi field. Near the Golgi field there are a few small smooth or coated vesicles, in some of the cells numerous electron-dense lysosome-like granules[87] of variable size, and sometimes multivesicular bodies. The Golgi field and the lysosomes sometimes lie within a nuclear indentation. In two cases we found abundant intracytoplasmic glycogen. In all but a few cases, the cell surface is free of invaginations or cytoplasmic projections. Between the tumor cells there are wide intercellular clefts. Enzyme cytochemically, it has so far not been possible to achieve a positive acid phosphatase reaction using a modified Gomori method[88] with Na-$\beta$-glycerophosphate as substrate. In contrast to the cells of most other lymphomas, the tumor cells of this lymphoma react negatively for ATPase.[89]

Lymphoblastic lymphomas of the convoluted-cell type cannot always be clearly identified by ultrastructural parameters alone. Above all, it is not possible to make a definite distinction between this type of lymphoma and T-CLL or unclassified lymphoblastic lymphomas. Neither the presence nor the number of lysosomes is a reliable diagnostic criterion for lymphoblastic lymphoma of the convoluted-cell type, since some cases reveal hardly any lysosomes at all. In such cases the acid phosphatase activity seen on light microscopy probably represents an enzyme reaction of the Golgi field.

---

85 BEDOYA, GRIMLEY and RABSON, 1969.
86 BARCOS and LUKES, 1975; CATOVSKY, 1975; CATOVSKY, FRISCH and VAN NOORDEN, 1975; KAISERLING, 1975, 1976, 1977.
87 CATOVSKY, 1975.
88 BARKA and ANDERSON, 1963.
89 MÜLLER-HERMELINK and KAISERLING, 1975.

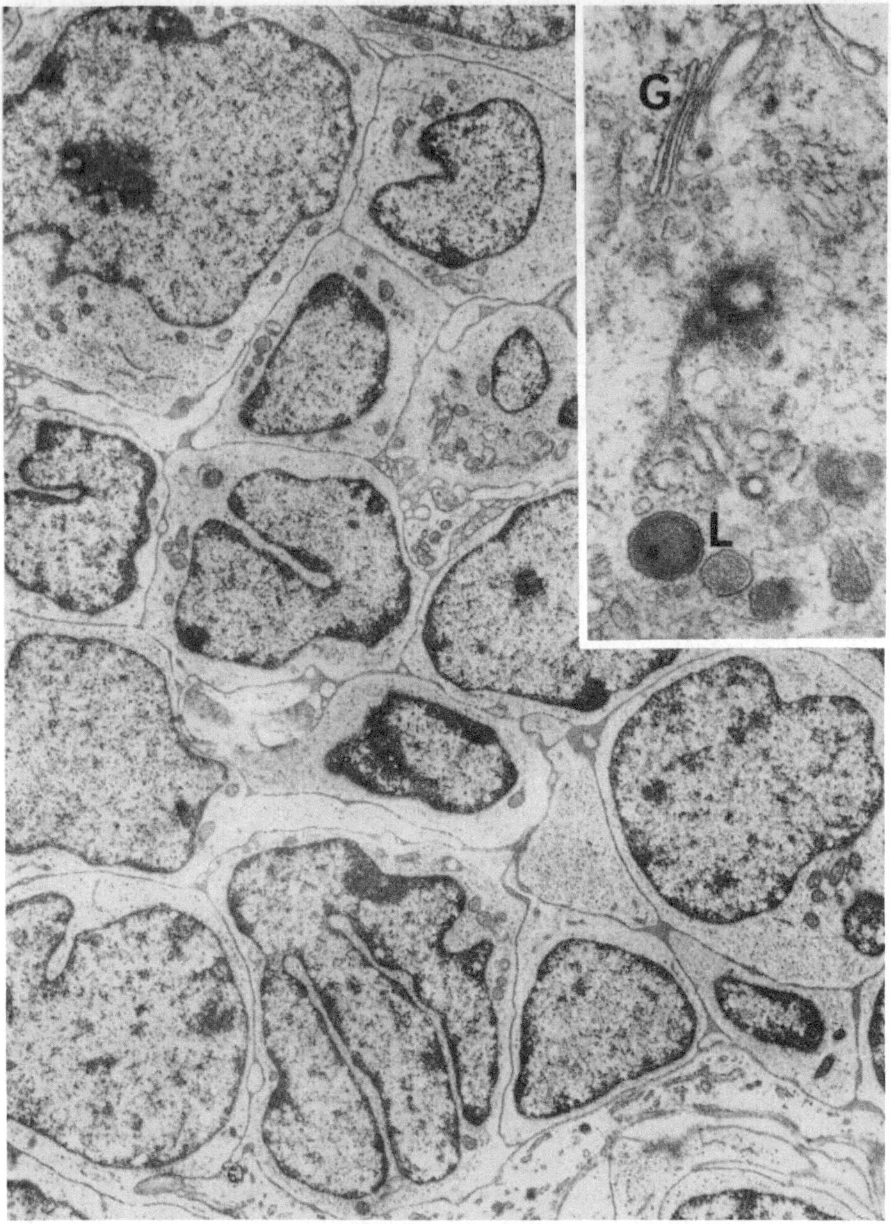


Fig. 258. Malignant lymphoma, lymphoblastic, convoluted-cell type. Lymphatic tissue consists of variable-sized tumor cells with sometimes oval, sometimes bizarrely shaped nuclei. Some of the tumor cells have a large Golgi field (*G*) surrounded by smooth and coated vesicles and lysosome-like granules (*L*). ×7,200, inset: ×44,000

### *3. A Case of T-Lymphoblastic Lymphoma without Convoluted Nuclei (Malignant Lymphoma of T-Associated Plasma Cells)*

Our electron-microscopic investigation of lymphoblastic lymphomas with a focal paranuclear acid phosphatase reaction in enzyme-cytochemical preparations turned up one tumor[89a] that contained no cells with convoluted nuclei. In contrast to all other lymphoblastic lymphomas of the acid phosphatase type (convoluted-cell type), the cells in this case had oval nuclei (Fig. 259). The clinical and light-microscopic findings (the patient had ataxia telangiectasia) are presented on page 399.

On electron microscopy, there were chiefly medium-sized tumor cells with a diameter of about 8 μm. The cells had an oval nucleus with a small ring-shaped nucleolus and relatively uniformly distributed chromatin. The cytoplasm usually contained numerous polyribosomes and only a few rough membrane profiles. Among these cells, however, there were a few cells with moderately or well-developed, lamellate or vesicular rough endoplasmic reticulum. The strands of ergastoplasm were usually short and filled with electron-dense material. There were also many transitional forms among the cells containing numerous polyribosomes or abundant ergastoplasm. The Golgi field consisted of a few parallel lamellae; there were often variable-sized lysosome-like granules nearby.

Small lymphocytes with marginally condensed heterochromatin were occasionally found among the tumor cells, especially near blood vessels. Furthermore, there were so-called dark reticulum cells with large cytoplasmic lacunae. Besides a few phagocytic reticulum cells, we found occasional interdigitating reticulum cells that showed characteristic, bizarrely shaped nuclei. Interdigitation and invaginations of the outer cell membrane had not developed to any great degree in the interdigitating reticulum cells. Near these cells there were both small lymphocytes and tumor cells containing numerous polyribosomes. The tissue contained a large number of epithelioid venules, which had no abnormal ultrastructural features.

Our ultrastructural findings in this lymphoma indicate that it is probably a tumor in which the cells showing the highest degree of differentiation may be interpreted as T-associated plasma cells. Since numerous transitional forms between the tumor cells containing numerous polyribosomes and the T-associated plasma cells could be demonstrated, we consider the cells containing numerous polyribosomes to be precursors of T-associated plasma cells. For these reasons, we have also interpreted this lymphoma as a "malignant lymphoma of T-associated plasma cells."

This case is significant, especially because it is the first lymphoma we have seen in which interdigitating reticulum cells and epithelioid venules, i.e., structural elements of thymus-dependent regions, proved to be important elements of the neoplasm. There is still no answer to the question about the significance of the T-associated plasma cells. Their ultrastructure is reminiscent of plasma cells; but we are still not sure whether we are justified in calling them plasma cells, especially since it has not been determined whether these cells also produce

---

[89a] KAISERLING 1975, 1977.

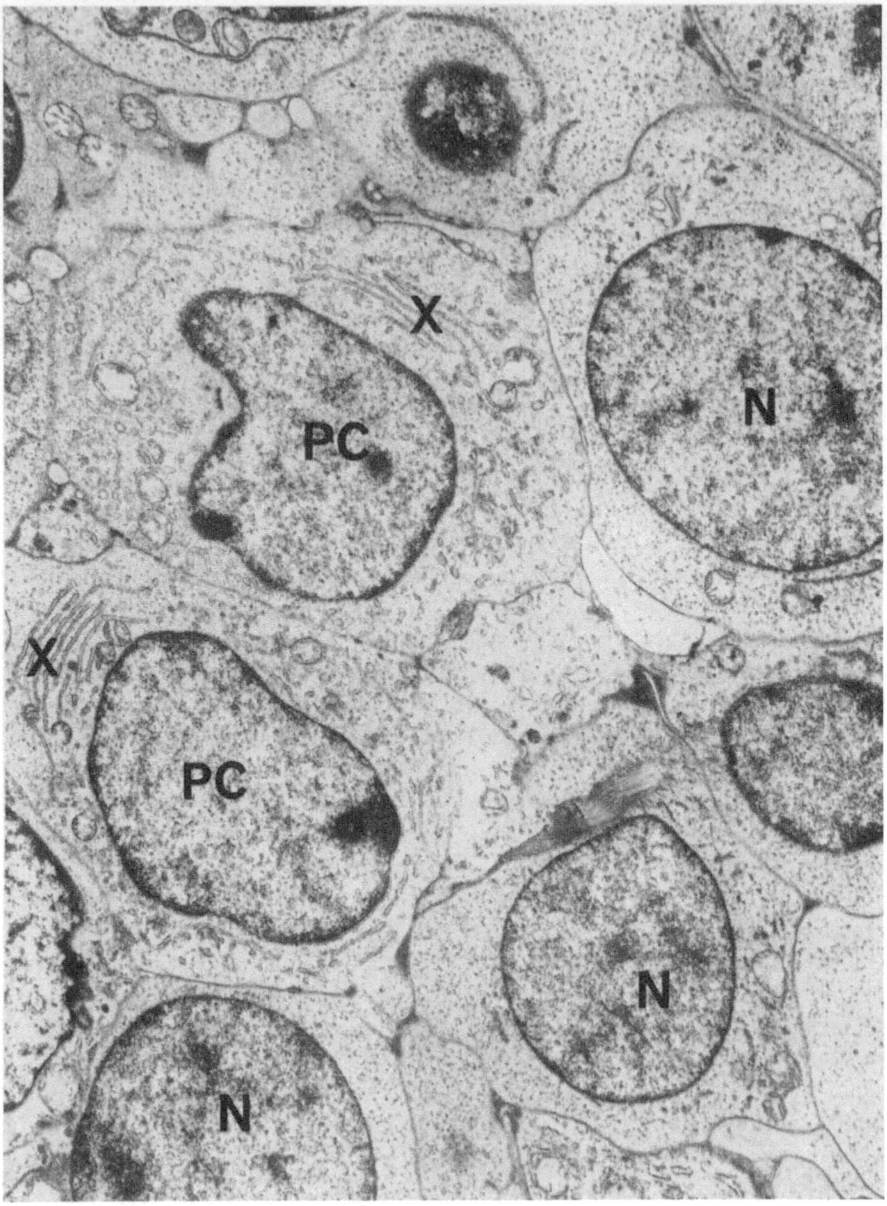


Fig. 259. Malignant lymphoma of T-associated plasma cells. Tumor cells with an oval (nonconvoluted) nucleus (*N*) and polyribosomes predominate. Two tumor cells (*PC*) with a moderate amount of rough endoplasmic reticulum (*X*) are reminiscent of T-associated plasma cells. ×8,800

secretory Ig. T-associated plasma cells are found almost regularly in nonspecific lymphadenitis. They are seen in or at the edge of T-nodules, often in the direct vicinity of interdigitating reticulum cells, which indicates interaction between these two types of cells. We have also observed T-associated plasma cells in various non-Hodgkin's lymphomas (centroblastic/centrocytic lymphoma, T-zone lymphoma, M.F., Sézary's syndrome) and occasionally in Hodgkin's disease. In contrast to the cells in the special case discussed in this section, however, the T-associated plasma cells seen in other lymphomas are not to be interpreted as tumor cells, but instead as passive participants in the neoplastic process.

### 4. *Unclassified*

In this tumor group we include all those lymphomas composed of blast cells that cannot be characterized as T- or B-cells, either because immunologic marker analyses could not be performed for technical reasons, or because the tumor cells expressed no, or no unequivocal immunologic markers. Most of the tumors belong to the group of acute lymphoblastic leukemias (ALL).

Ultrastructurally, these lymphoblastic lymphomas are divided into two cytologically different classes. We distinguish small-cell and large-cell lymphomas. The large-cell lymphomas consist of tumor cells with abundant polyribosomes and a high nuclear/cytoplasmic ratio. They have a small Golgi field with only a few lysosome-like granules and vesicles nearby, and an oval, sometimes indented nucleus with little chromatin and prominent nucleoli. They are reminiscent of the cells described as macrolymphoblasts by PAINTRAND *et al.*[90] Cells of similar morphology were also described by SCHUMACHER *et al.*[91] ALL of the small-cell type consists of tumor cells with an irregularly shaped nucleus and cytoplasm containing mostly monoribosomes. Neither the large-cell nor the small-cell form has a significant amount of rough endoplasmic reticulum. The nonlymphoid cells occasionally found in the lymphomas include histiocytic reticulum cells. Dendritic reticulum cells and interdigitating reticulum cells are absent.

Morphologically, it is not possible in either the large- or the small-cell lymphomas to discover a cytologic relationship between the tumor cells and cells of normal lymphatic tissue.

## C. Malignant Lymphoma, Immunoblastic (Immunoblastic Sarcoma)

Three forms of immunoblastic lymphoma, which used to be known as reticulosarcoma, can be distinguished by electron microscopy: tumors without and those with plasmablastic differentiation, and a rarer form described by MORI and LENNERT[92] in which the tumor cells are reminiscent of plasma cells, but contain exclusively smooth endoplasmic reticulum.

In the first type of immunoblastic lymphoma the tumor cells (Fig. 260) are most reminiscent of immunoblasts of germinal centers in size, chromatin

---

[90] PAINTRAND, DANTCHEV and MATHÉ, 1973.

[91] SCHUMACHER, SZEKELY, PARK and FISHER, 1973.

[92] 1969.

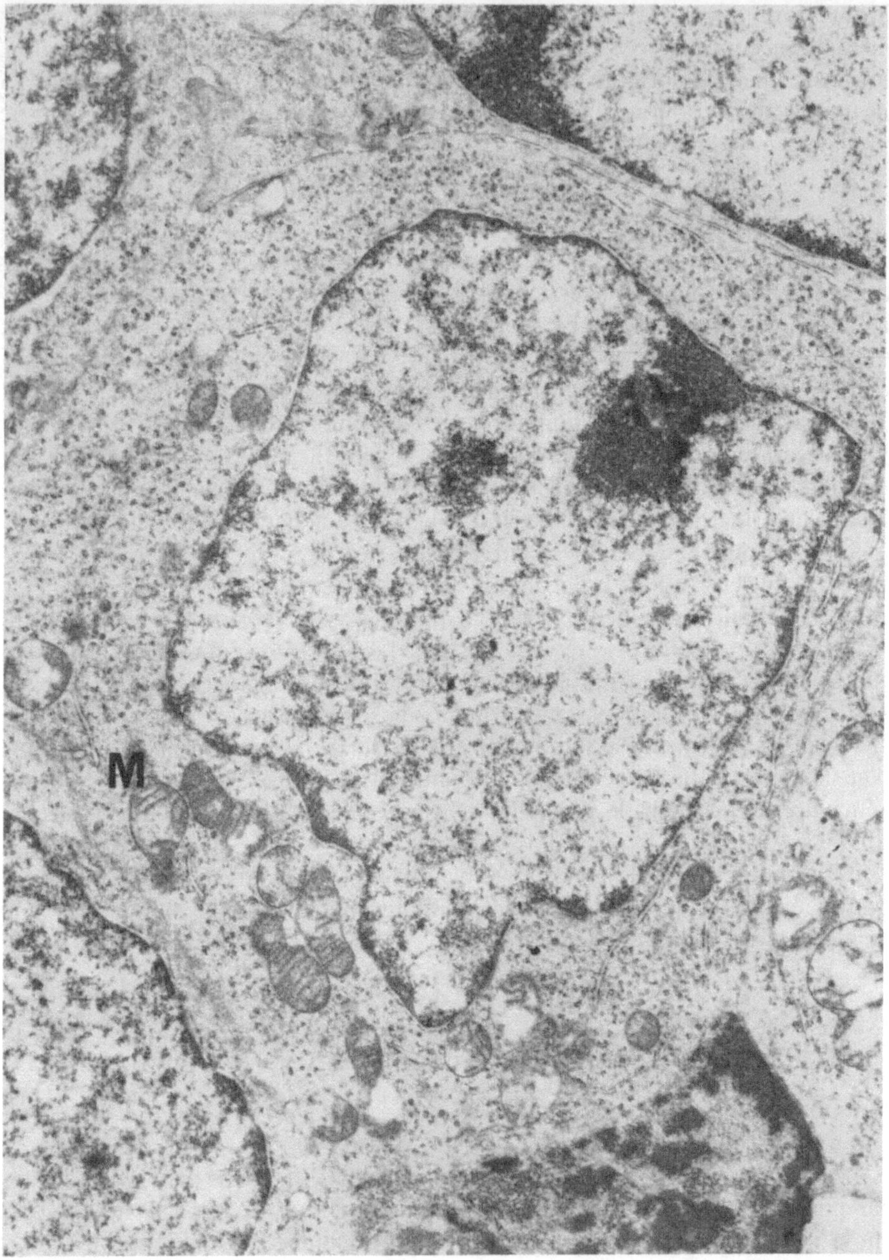


Fig. 260. Immunoblastic lymphoma. Tumor cell contains abundant polyribosomes, only a few strands of ergastoplasm, and several swollen mitochrondria (*M*). Nucleus is irregular in shape, like that of immunoblasts of germinal centers. × 19,000

distribution, and number of polyribosomes in the cytoplasm. It should be mentioned, however, that the tumor cells cannot be clearly differentiated from immunoblasts of other regions (marginal zone, T-nodules). The nucleus of the tumor cells is oval or indented. Occasionally, one finds nuclear pockets or narrow invaginations that penetrate deep into the nucleus. In some cases there are a few tumor cells with a cerebriform nucleus, as also described by LUTZNER *et al.*[93] in a so-called reticulosarcoma. Multinucleate tumor cells are found in large numbers in some cases. The nucleolus is large and sometimes marginal, sometimes central. Its morphology varies from case to case: it may be compact and then lies chiefly in the middle of the nucleus; or it is loosely joined, consists of nucleolonemata, and is chiefly marginal. Two or more nucleoli are not a rarity. The number of polyribosomes in the cytoplasm varies from case to case. The Golgi field is chiefly medium-sized and consists of parallel lamellae and a few vesicles. The number of lysosome-like granules is small. The mitochondria are electron-transparent and usually show rarefaction of cristae. They may be markedly hydropic and sometimes contain electron-dense material. There are abundant lipid droplets in some cases. In one case we found so-called ribosome-lamella complexes, as described in hairy-cell leukemia (see p. 483). Whereas in some cases no, or only a few, cytoplasmic projections are seen, in other cases they are found in large numbers in close connection with the projections of neighboring tumor cells.

In the second group—the lymphomas with plasmablastic differentiation—some of the tumor cells have a variably well-developed rough endoplasmic reticulum. Corresponding to the amount of ergastoplasm, the tumor cells are reminiscent of plasmablasts or proplasmacytes; the latter are predominant in number. Mature plasma cells are extremely rare. Occasionally, there are globular inclusions in the ergastoplasm. In contrast to the tumors with plasmablastic differentiation, those containing only immunoblastic tumor cells as a rule lack (Ig) inclusions. We found amorphous electron-dense precipitates in the perinuclear space in only one case (Fig. 261).[94] Immunochemical analysis proved that these precipitates represented IgM. They were electron-dense in periodic-acid silver-methenamine staining. The special feature of this case was that the Ig synthesis occurred at the membrane-bound ribosomes of the perinuclear space, as also shown in immunoblasts of rats.[95]

The third type of immunoblastic lymphoma is characterized by tumor cells that contain almost exclusively smooth endoplasmic reticulum. This type is probably very rare. Two such tumors were described by MORI and LENNERT.[95a] The tumor cells contain chiefly smooth vesicular membrane profiles as well as monoribosomes and free polyribosomes. Later, we found numerous *annulatae lamellae* in one of these cases. This feature was also described by FOA *et al.*[96] in reticulosarcoma. *Annulatae lamellae* have no diagnostic significance, however, since they occasionally occur in lymphoid cells in nonspecific lymphadenitis. It is possible that the third type of immunoblastic lymphoma is a neoplasm

[93] LUTZNER, HOBBS and HORVATH, 1971.
[94] KAISERLING, STEIN and LENNERT, 1973.
[95] AVRAMEAS and LEDUC, 1970.
[95a] 1969.
[96] FOA, FOA and MURATORE, 1970.

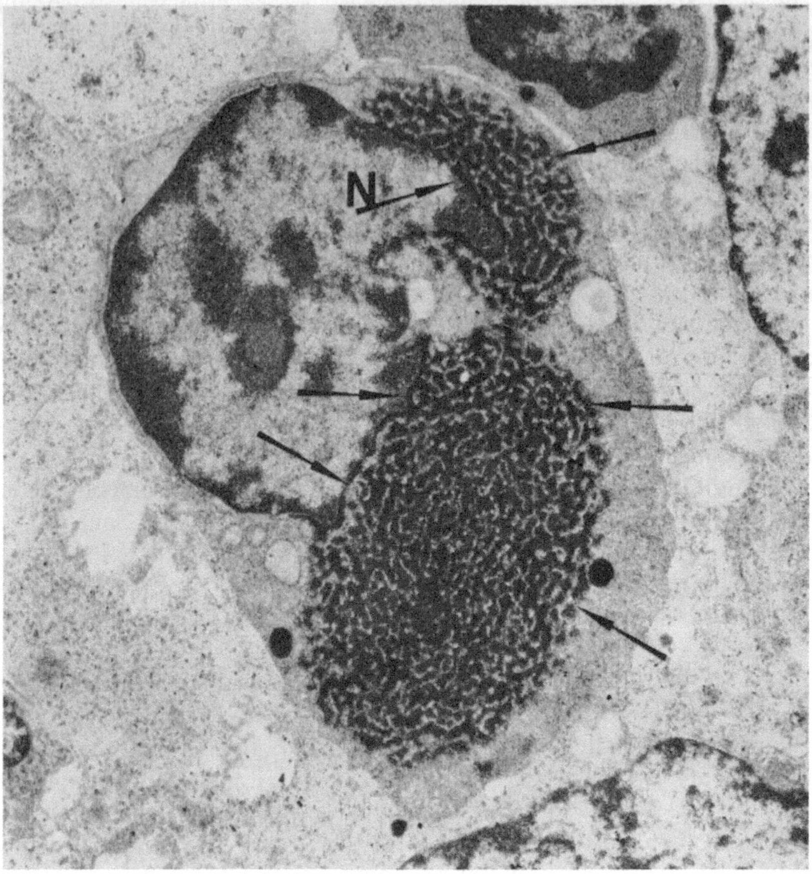


Fig. 261. Immunoblastic lymphoma. Widespread Ig precipitates in the perinuclear space (arrows). With silver methenamine staining they are electron-dense. Nucleus (*N*). × 14,000

in which the switch from the synthesis of cell-bound Ig to that of secretory Ig is disturbed.

In contrast to most other lymphomas, immunoblastic lymphoma is characterized by a large number of reticulum cells. A majority prove to be histiocytic reticulum cells with a variable number of phagosomes, but some prove to be so-called dark reticulum cells. Dendritic reticulum cells and interdigitating reticulum cells were not evident in any of our cases, with one exception. As shown in ultrastructural studies by SUCHI *et al.*,[97] epithelioid cells are seen in immunoblastic lymphoma. We found them in more than one third of our cases. These cells contain numerous lysosome-like granules and show typical deep cleavage of the cytoplasmic surface and parallel finger-shaped invaginations. Occasionally, one finds intracytoplasmic residual bodies. On electron microscopy, the histiocytic reticulum cells prove to be strongly acid phosphatase-positive. The tumor cells, on the other hand, show an extremely weak, lysosomal acid phosphatase reaction. In addition, they reveal a positive reaction for ATPase,

[97] SUCHI, SATO, KOBAYASHI, AKATSUKA *et al.*, 1973.

as already shown in light-microscopic studies of so-called reticulosarcoma by RINNEBERG,[98] WILLIGHAGEN,[98a] and JEFFREE.[99] According to our findings, however, some of the nonneoplastic cells (reticulum cells) also give a positive ATPase reaction.

Immunoblastic lymphomas can be classified as B-cell neoplasms by means of electron microscopy only when some of the tumor cells reveal plasmablastic differentiation or when Ig inclusions can be demonstrated morphologically. Tumors with purely immunoblastic differentiation may be either B- or T-cell neoplasms. Only one of the tumors we have observed so far could be clearly identified as a T-immunoblastic lymphoma. Light microscopy revealed numerous follicles with chiefly regressively transformed germinal centers. Around the follicles and in the broad interfollicular zone there were polymorphic tumor cells, sometimes with strongly basophilic cytoplasm, and numerous mitotic figures. On electron microscopy, the lymph-node regions containing tumor cells proved to be T-regions: they also contained numerous interdigitating reticulum cells, epithelioid venules, and T-associated plasma cells. The tumor cells proved to be blast cells with polyribosomes, a very high nuclear/cytoplasmic ratio, and prominent nucleoli. Mitotic figures and tumor cells were often seen in the direct vicinity of interdigitating reticulum cells; sometimes the tumor cells were surrounded on all sides by cytoplasmic projections of the interdigitating reticulum cells. Since all essential components of a T-area could be demonstrated in this tumor and since some of the tumor cells were in the immediate neighborhood of interdigitating reticulum cells, it may be assumed that this was a T-immunoblastic lymphoma. In contrast to all other immunoblastic lymphomas we have investigated, it showed an organoid structure.

## *Addendum*

### *Reticulosarcoma*

As far as we know, there are no ultrastructural descriptions of definitely proved cases of reticulosarcoma in the literature. We also have no such cases in our collection that have been definitely proved by receptor analyses. Nevertheless, we have seen a few tumors that, similar to cases described by HENRY,[100] probably arose primarily in lymph nodes and that might be derived from histiocytic reticulum cells.

The tumor cells had a wide rim of cytoplasm and large, oval or irregularly shaped nuclei. In two cases the tumor cells revealed numerous microvilli, but presented a quite uncharacteristic cytologic picture. The cytoplasm contained abundant mono- and polyribosomes and mostly short rough membrane profiles (Fig. 262). These were found chiefly near the Golgi field, which consisted of closely or loosely packed lamellae and smooth and coated vesicles. We have not clearly identified phagosomes in any of our cases, with one exception (Fig. 263). In some cases the tumor cells revealed intracytoplasmic cilia. Although so far we have found cilia in lymphatic tissue exclusively in reticulum

[98] 1961.
[98a] 1961.
[99] 1974.
[100] 1975.

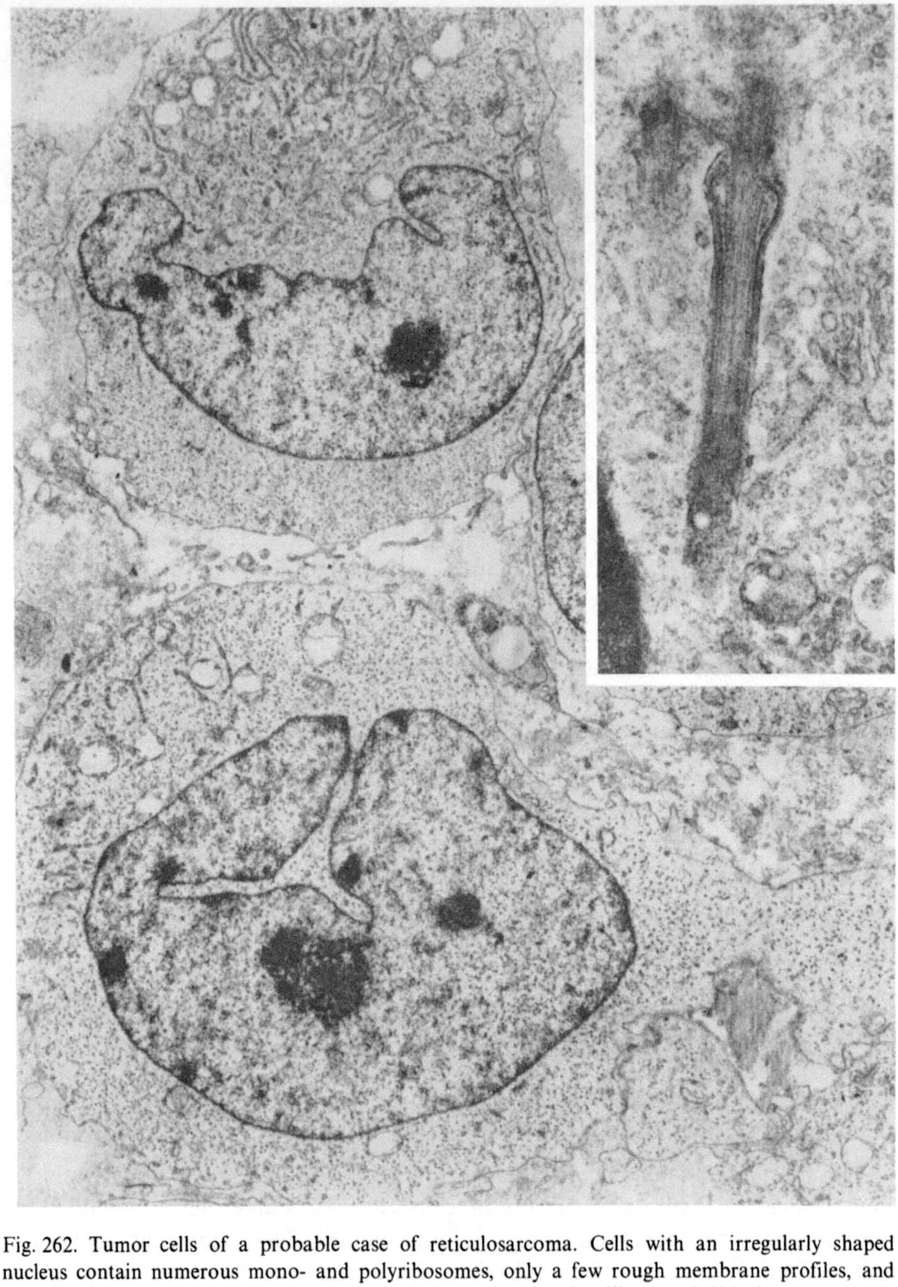

Fig. 262. Tumor cells of a probable case of reticulosarcoma. Cells with an irregularly shaped nucleus contain numerous mono- and polyribosomes, only a few rough membrane profiles, and a well-developed Golgi field. Inset shows an intracytoplasmic cilium. ×9,600, inset: ×30,000

cells (histiocytic, dendritic, interdigitating, and dark reticulum cells), this finding does not prove the reticulum-cell nature of the tumor cells, since cilia have also been demonstrated in numerous other (nonlymphatic) tumors and cells.

On the whole, there are only a few, relatively worthless ultrastructural criteria

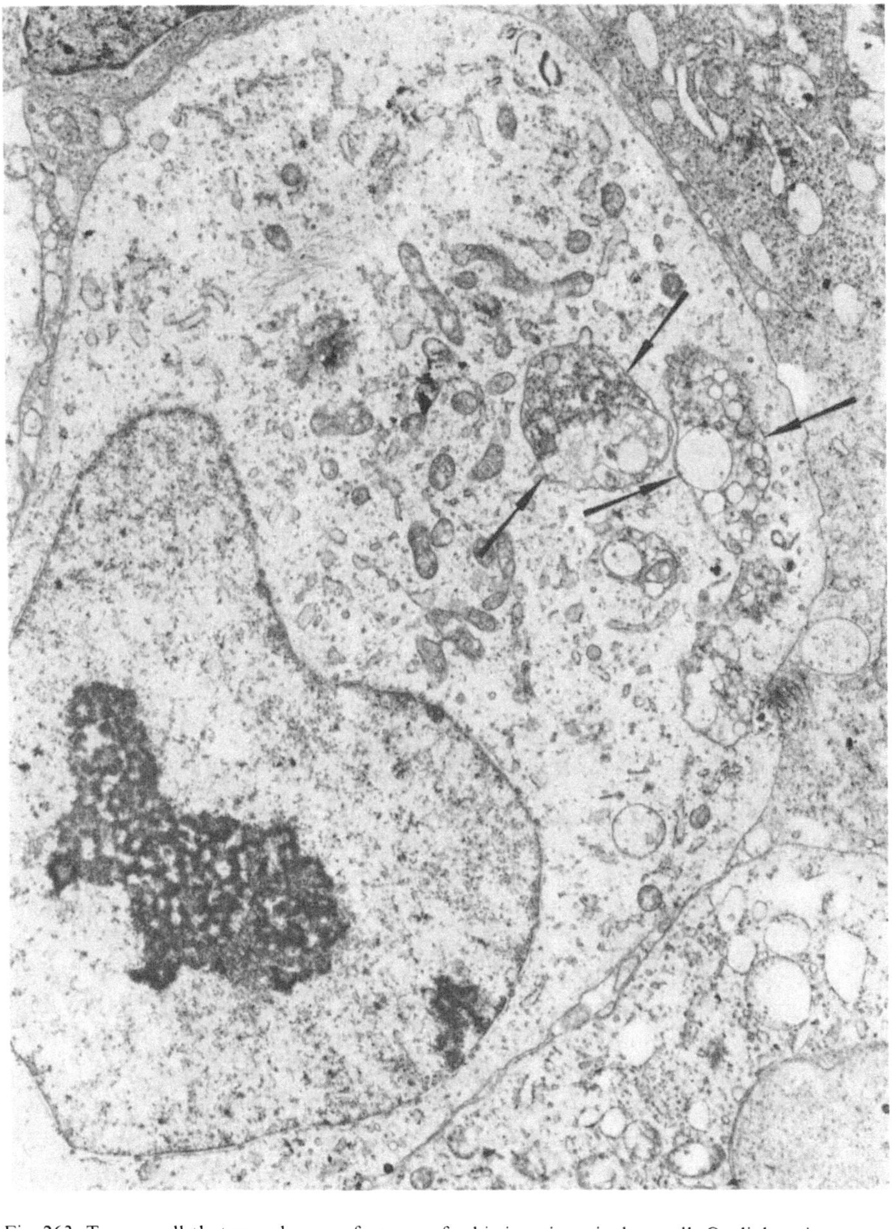

Fig. 263. Tumor cell that reveals some features of a histiocytic reticulum cell. On light microscopy, the tumor showed hemophagocytosis. This electron micrograph demonstrates residual bodies (probably heterophagosomes) surrounded by a unit membrane (arrows) in the tumor cell. × 12,000

for clearly characterizing a malignant lymphoma as a tumor of reticulum cells. The most important feature is probably phagocytosis (heterophagocytosis). One must remember, however, that phagocytosis is not a characteristic of all reticulum cells of lymphatic tissue and also that neoplastic reticulum cells may lose the ability to phagocytose. Another parameter would be the occurrence of desmosomes if the neoplasm is composed of dendritic reticulum cells. One would have to distinguish such neoplasms, however, from tumors of other cells with desmosomal junctions. The classification of tumor cells as dendritic reticulum cells is probably particularly difficult because dendritic reticulum cells are characterized by only a few morphologic features (above all by their nuclear shape, chromatin distribution, and branched cytoplasmic projections), which are not necessarily preserved when the cells become neoplastic.

Neoplasms of interdigitating reticulum cells are probably also difficult to identify. We have observed two tumors in which the tumor cells were reminiscent of interdigitating reticulum cells, mainly because of their nuclear shape. A definite classification was not possible, since significant interdigitation of the cytoplasmic projections was not found, circumscribed cytoplasmic invaginations were rarely observed, and a tubulovesicular system was only barely visible. Finally, one should bear in mind the fact that in many lymphomas reticulum cells often appear to have an abnormal ultrastructure, without necessarily having to be considered neoplastic. In Hodgkin's disease, the reticulum cells look particularly abnormal.[101] Our own studies have shown that this is also true for interdigitating reticulum cells in Hodgkin's disease of the mixed type and in nodular sclerosing Hodgkin's disease.

# Conclusions

Almost all cases of malignant non-Hodgkin's lymphoma can be clearly differentiated and classified on the basis of constant ultrastructural features. The ultrastructural findings agree with the results of light-microscopic, immunochemical, and immunocytochemical studies.

In the classification of non-Hodgkin's lymphomas, there are basically four electron-microscopic parameters for differentiation: (1) the cytology of the tumor cells and their relationships to cells of normal lymphatic tissue, (2) the spectrum of cellular differentiation, (3) morphologic parameters indicating a special function of the tumor cells, e.g., synthesis of exocrine antibodies, and (4) the presence of nonneoplastic elements, in particular of interdigitating reticulum cells, dendritic reticulum cells, epithelioid venules, and T-associated plasma cells, which are all components of the special microenvironment of normal lymphatic tissue.

Taking these four parameters into consideration, it is possible not only to differentiate the non-Hodgkin's lymphomas from one another, but also often to classify them with respect to their T- or B-cell nature or even with regard to their histogenetic nature.

In some cases cytologic parameters alone are sufficient to characterize the tumors and to reveal relationships to cells of normal lymphatic tissue. That is especially true for the germinal-center tumors, namely, M.L. centroblastic/cen-

[101] Carr, 1975.

trocytic, M.L. centrocytic, and M.L. centroblastic. In other lymphomas the tumors are characterized above all by the cytologic spectrum of the tumor cells. For example, in LP immunocytoma nearly the whole spectrum of a B-cell reaction, as found in normal lymphatic tissue, is repeated. In immunoblastic lymphoma the relationship to normal lymphatic tissue becomes clear, particularly when plasmablastic differentiation is evident.

In some lymphomas the ultrastructural findings are still of a descriptive nature. For instance, in hairy-cell leukemia, in most lymphoblastic lymphomas, and also in CLL, clear cytologic relationships to cells of normal lymphatic tissue cannot be drawn from the ultrastructural findings.

The occurrence of nonneoplastic elements in malignant lymphomas has hardly been taken into consideration in light- and electron-microscopic studies in the past. The consideration of such elements, particularly of those that belong to the specific microenvironment of normal lymphatic tissue, greatly facilitates the differentiation as well as the cytogenetic and histogenetic classification of lymphomas. For example, one can distinguish tumors with features of a thymus-dependent area from those with characteristics of a bone marrow-dependent area, in particular with those of germinal centers. The most important representative of the first group is T-zone lymphoma, in which all components of a thymus-dependent area can be found: interdigitating reticulum cells, T-associated plasma cells, and epithelioid venules. There are also components of thymus-dependent regions in Sézary's syndrome and mycosis fungoides, which have been clearly proved to be T-cell neoplasms. Some of the cases of T-CLL observed by LENNERT also revealed interdigitating reticulum cells and epithelioid venules (see p. 137ff.). In addition to these T-cell neoplasms, in which the components of a thymus-dependent area simulate an organoid structure, there are also "nonorganoid" T-cell neoplasms. Features of a thymus-dependent area are not found in these tumors, namely, lymphoblastic lymphomas of the convoluted-cell type.

The group of organoid B-cell neoplasms includes M.L. centroblastic/centrocytic, M.L. centrocytic, and some of the cases of M.L. centroblastic. At least in some cases, these tumors contain dendritic reticulum cells, i.e., cells that are found in germinal centers. On the whole, dendritic reticulum cells are seen only rarely in B-cell lymphomas. In CLL (B-type), immunoblastic lymphoma, and Burkitt's lymphoma they are completely absent. Only exceptional cases of immunocytoma reveal dendritic reticulum cells. Whereas dendritic reticulum cells are not found in Hodgkin's disease of the mixed type or in nodular sclerosing Hodgkin's disease, they were evident in a nodular Hodgkin's lymphoma with lymphocytic predominance (nodular paragranuloma). Thus, we may assume that this tumor took place in germinal centers.

It seems remarkable to us that interdigitating reticulum cells and T-associated plasma cells are occasionally found in some cases of M.L. centroblastic/centrocytic, which is definitely a B-cell lymphoma, as clearly proved by numerous findings.

There is still no answer to the question about the significance of the nonneoplastic components of malignant non-Hodgkin's lymphomas, in particular of the interdigitating and dendritic reticulum cells. From the ultrastructural picture, especially from the close topographic relationship between reticulum cells and tumor cells, one gets the impression that there is not only a topographic, but also a functional relationship between these two types of cells. It has not yet been determined just what this functional relationship is. It seems interesting in this context, however, that SWARTZENDRUBER *et al.*[102] found endogenous virus particles in close contact with dendritic reticulum cells in mice with a high rate of spontaneous leukemia, and that other authors[103] have reported the accumulation of oncogenic viruses (Rauscher leukemia virus) at the projections of dendritic reticulum cells.

One could compare the occurrence of interdigitating reticulum cells, dendritic reticulum cells, and epithelioid venules to a nonspecific stroma reaction. We consider this to be an unsatisfactory interpretation, however, since these elements have quite specific functions in normal lymphatic tissue.

---

[102] SWARTZENDRUBER, IL MA and MURPHY, 1967.

[103] SZAKAL and HANNA, 1968; HANNA, SZAKAL and TYNDALL, 1970.

Part Six

# The Immunologic and Immunochemical Basis for the Kiel Classification

H. STEIN

## Introduction

As can be seen from the history of the classification of lymphomas (see p. 83ff.), the morphologic analysis of lymphoproliferative diseases did not advance beyond a certain state of knowledge. The main reason is that characteristic morphologic features, such as certain organelles (granules, etc.), are not found in most lymphoid cells. Since the morphologic description and evaluation of normal and neoplastic lymphoid cells is highly subjective, very different concepts of classification were developed, and, as we now know, numerous misinterpretations appeared. For example, the large cells of lymphatic tissue were usually mistaken for reticulum cells or "thrown into one pot" with real reticulum cells. It is now known that these large cells represent definite functional forms of the lymphoid cell series that appear after antigenic stimulation. For decades, morphologists also misinterpreted the derivation of plasma cells. It was said that plasma cells are derived from reticulum cells,[1] since it was previously believed that there are transitional morphologic forms between them.

A relatively long time passed before pathologists and hematologists adopted immunologic methods and knowledge and applied them to their problems. Practically speaking, that did not occur until 1970 and later, when RAFF,[2] BIANCO *et al.*,[3] BACH and DORMONT,[4] JONDAL *et al.*,[5] and BASTEN *et al.*[6] discovered structural features on the surfaces of T- and B-cells of the lymphatic system. The B/T dichotomy of the lymphatic system was already known from functional studies.[6a] The demonstration of surface structures made it possible, however, to determine whether a particular lymphoid cell belongs to the B-cell or to the T-cell series. The first analyses of B- and T-cell characteristics in lymphoid tumor cells revealed that these features can also be found in neoplastic

[1] E.g., STOECKENIUS and NAUMANN, 1958; ROHR, 1960; RAPPAPORT, 1966.

[2] 1970.

[3] BIANCO, PATRICK and NUSSENZWEIG, 1970.

[4] 1971.

[5] JONDAL, HOLM and WIGZELL, 1972.

[6] BASTEN, MILLER, SPRENT and PYE, 1972.

[6a] WARNER, SZENBERG and BURNET, 1962; COOPER, PETERSON, SOUTH and GOOD, 1966; PARROTT, DE SOUSA and EAST, 1966; MILLER, BASTEN, SPRENT and CHEERS, 1971.

Table 93. Markers of "mature" B- and T-cells

| Marker | B-cell | T-cell |
|---|---|---|
| Surface immunoglobulin (SIg) | + | – |
| Tissue Ig in the saline extract | ↑ | ↓ or normal |
| Tissue Ig in the detergent 2nd extract | ↑ | ↓ |
| Cytoplasmic immunoglobulin (CIg) | +[a] | – |
| IgG-Fc receptor | + | – (activated T-cells are +) |
| Receptor for complement component | | |
| C3b (C4) | + | – (sometimes +) |
| C3d | + | – |
| Receptor for Epstein-Barr virus | + | – |
| Mouse-E receptor | + | – |
| Sheep-E receptor | – | + |
| Receptor for measles virus | – | + |
| Human T-lymphocyte antigen (HTLA) | – | + |
| Ia-like antigen (B-associated antigen or HL-B) | + | – |

↑ = increased; ↓ = decreased.
[a] Only secretory B-cells.

lymphoid cells, which would enable characterization of lymphoproliferative diseases with previously unknown reliability.

The immunologic features of mature B- and T-cells are listed in Table 93. Before discussing the immunologic findings that played a substantial role in the conception of the so-called Kiel Classification, we shall present the principle and the significance of the most important immunologic methods and markers used in our laboratory and by other researchers.

# I. Immunochemical and Immunologic Methods and Markers and Their Significance for the Characterization of Lymphoid-Cell Populations

## A. Immunoglobulin Content of Tissue Extracts

B-cells produce significant amounts of immunoglobulin (Ig), whereas T-cells synthesize only small amounts of Ig or none at all.[7] Considering this fact, one would expect significantly more Ig to be demonstrated in extracts of B-cell tumors than in extracts of T-cell tumors.

[7] Vitetta, Bianco, Nussenzweig and Uhr, 1972.

We decided to analyze Ig in tissue extracts, because this method is not restricted to the use of living lymphoid cells, in contrast to most of the other methods for demonstrating B- and T-cell features discussed below. Since deep-frozen or lyophilized lymphoma material can be used for the analysis of Ig in tissue extracts, it was possible for us to receive frozen biopsy material from hospitals all over Germany and even from hospitals in other countries. That allowed the investigation of a relatively large number of malignant lymphomas in a relatively short time.

As far as we know, McMaster and Hudack[8] were the first to study the antibody content of saline extracts from lymph-node tissue. They found specific antibodies earlier in saline extracts from regional lymph nodes after immunization than in serum, indicating that lymph nodes are probably the primary site of antibody production. In 1946, White and Dougherty separated saline extracts of lymph nodes from mice and rabbits by means of electrophoresis into four fractions. Two of these fractions revealed the mobility of $\beta$- and $\gamma$-globulins.

To our knowledge, the first analysis of $\gamma$-globulin in a saline extract from a malignant lymphoma was performed by Abrams *et al.*[9] In the extract of a lymphosarcoma, these authors found a cryoglobulin whose electrophoretic and biologic properties agreed with those of the serum cryoglobulin. It was another 15 years before the identification of the five Ig classes, the production of monospecific antisera against these Ig classes, and the development of radial immunodiffusion facilitated a reliable identification of the immunoglobulin classes and their quantitative measurement.

In 1970, we tested the significance of quantitative determination of Ig in tissue extracts and sera from malignant lymphomas. At the very beginning we found a greatly increased concentration of IgM in the autopsy-tissue extract from two so-called reticulosarcomas, although there was no measurable change in the serum-Ig value compared with the norm.[10] In 1971, we therefore began a systematic quantitative analysis of Ig in biopsy-tissue extracts from malignant lymphomas.

### *1. Results and Disadvantages of Extraction with Saline Alone*

In the first series of investigations, we performed the tissue extraction with saline. The procedure is outlined in Figure 264. Analysis of the first 30 malignant lymphomas revealed an increased Ig content in the tissue extracts from a large majority of the tumors, including so-called reticulosarcoma.[10] It was evident from these results that the previously used concepts of classification would have to be revised. The results also showed, however, that saline extraction solubilizes only very incompletely the Ig present in the tissue. That was particularly clear in lymphomas in which some of the cells contained PAS-positive cytoplasmic inclusions that could be labeled with anti-IgM antibodies, whereas increased amounts of IgM could not be demonstrated in the saline extracts. Furthermore, the saline-extraction procedure proved to be a relatively insignificant method for demonstrating Ig produced by tumor cells, since the serum Ig of the whole extracellular space is also included in the results of the analysis. That was clearly shown by comparing the results

---

[8] 1935.

[9] Abrams, Cohen and Meyer, 1949.

[10] Stein, Lennert and Parwaresch, 1972; Stein, Kaiserling and Lennert, 1973.

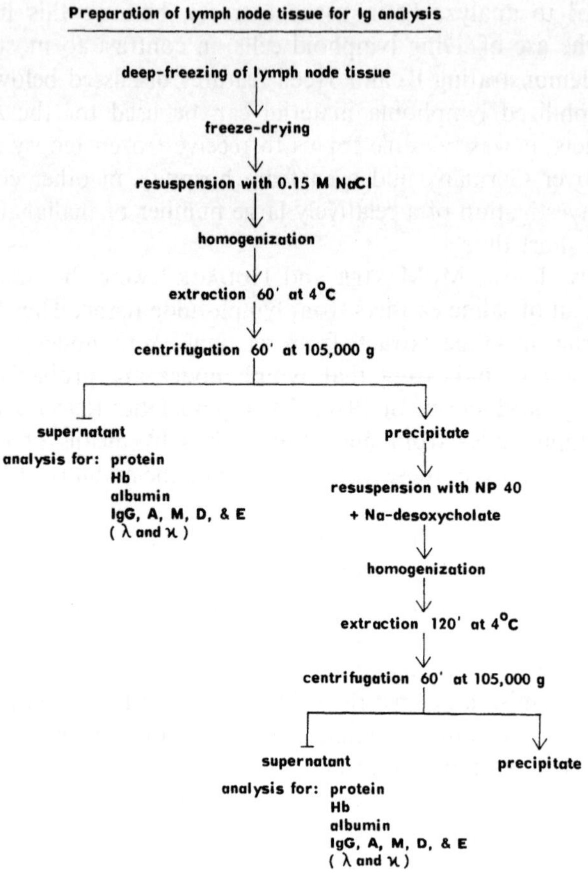


Fig. 264. Scheme of preparation of lymph-node tissue for immunoglobulin analysis

of extraction of tissue and washed cells from the same lymphatic organs.[10a] The Ig values for the saline tissue extracts from tonsils more or less reflected the proportionate Ig concentration of the corresponding sera. In contrast, the Ig values for the extracts of washed cells revealed a fundamentally different relationship of the Ig classes to one another, demonstrating that the Ig values for saline tissue extracts are considerably influenced by the serum Ig of the extracellular space (Fig. 265).

This interference could be reduced by using albumin instead of the dry substance or total protein for the reference value for the Ig concentration. In our opinion, using albumin as a reference has the following advantages. (1) The serum-albumin level is relatively constant; the serum albumin saturates the extracellular space quite uniformly owing to its relatively low molecular weight (65,000). (2) Albumin is not produced in lymphoid cells, only in the liver. An increase in the Ig/albumin quotient of lymphatic tissue therefore means a serum-independent accumulation of Ig in this tissue. A serum-dependent increase in Ig in the tissue can be proved or excluded by comparing the Ig/albumin quotient of the serum with that of the tissue. (3) Albumin is measured with the same method (radial immunodiffusion) as the Ig.

On the whole, however, it must be mentioned that the demonstration of tissue-derived Ig in saline tissue extracts is combined with much background owing to the inclusion of serum Ig. That is also evident from the relatively small differences between the Ig values for saline extracts of lymph nodes and thymus tissue. The Ig assay of saline extracts therefore allows only the distinction of lymphomas with highly active Ig synthesis from those with no Ig synthesis.

[10a] STEIN, 1975a.

## 2. *Results of a Second Extraction with Detergents*

To improve the significance of the method and to capture the insoluble, membrane-bound Ig, we expanded the tissue-extraction procedure by extracting the centrifugal precipitate of the saline extraction (saline 1st extraction) a second time with a detergent mixture of NP40 (Shell, U.S.A.) and sodium desoxycholate (DOC; detergent 2nd extraction). Details are provided in Figure 264. In numerous preliminary trials, the use of detergents instead of saline for the preparation of the first extract did not prove to be advantageous. The mixture NP40 and DOC turned out to be the most effective combination for the second extraction. For example, the IgM concentration measured in the extract of a malignant lymphoma obtained with NP40 and DOC was about six times higher than that of the extract prepared with NP40 alone. There was no IgM at all in the second extract prepared with saline alone.

To test the practical utility of Ig analysis of the second extract for distinguishing pure T-cell tissue from tissue containing B-cells, we studied extracts from thymuses, lymph nodes, and tonsils. We also analyzed extracts of washed cells from thymuses and tonsils to determine the influence of serum Ig of the extracellular space on the values for the detergent 2nd extract. The results are presented in Figure 265. The graph clearly shows that, although the saline extracts from thymuses and lymph nodes revealed differences in Ig concentration, these differences were not significant, particularly for IgA and IgM. The differences in Ig content between the various organs were much clearer when the values for the detergent 2nd extracts were compared with each other.

## 3. *Origin of the Extracted Immunoglobulin*

Fundamentally, two known compartments must be distinguished in the tissue: (1) the extracellular space and (2) the cellular space. As mentioned previously, the distribution of the Ig classes in saline tissue extracts from thymuses, tonsils, and lymph nodes is similar to that of the serum. Ig analysis of the saline 1st extracts of washed tonsil cells provides fundamentally different results (Fig. 265). Here, the IgM concentration is the highest, followed by IgG and IgA. This shows that serum Ig from the extracellular space considerably influences the total concentration of Ig in the saline 1st extract. The Ig from the cells practically gets lost in the large amount of extracellular Ig.

Detergent 2nd extraction, on the other hand, provided Ig values that were similar to those for the extracts of washed cells. This indicates that when extraction is performed with saline, the serum proteins of the extracellular space are present in the supernatant together with the soluble and loosely bound cell proteins. After centrifugation, the membrane structures with well-bound proteins are pelleted, and most of the serum proteins and particularly albumin are washed off these structures. The bound proteins are released through renewed extraction of the pellet with membrane-dissolving detergents. The Ig values for the detergent 2nd extracts are therefore influenced relatively little by serum Ig of the extracellular space (see Fig. 265).

## 4. *Correlation between the Tissue-Immunoglobulin Concentration and the B-Cell Content of the Tissue*

The low Ig content of extracts from thymuses is consistent with data reported in the literature showing that thymus lymphocytes do not produce[11] or bear

[11] Vitetta, Bianco, Nussenzweig and Uhr, 1972.

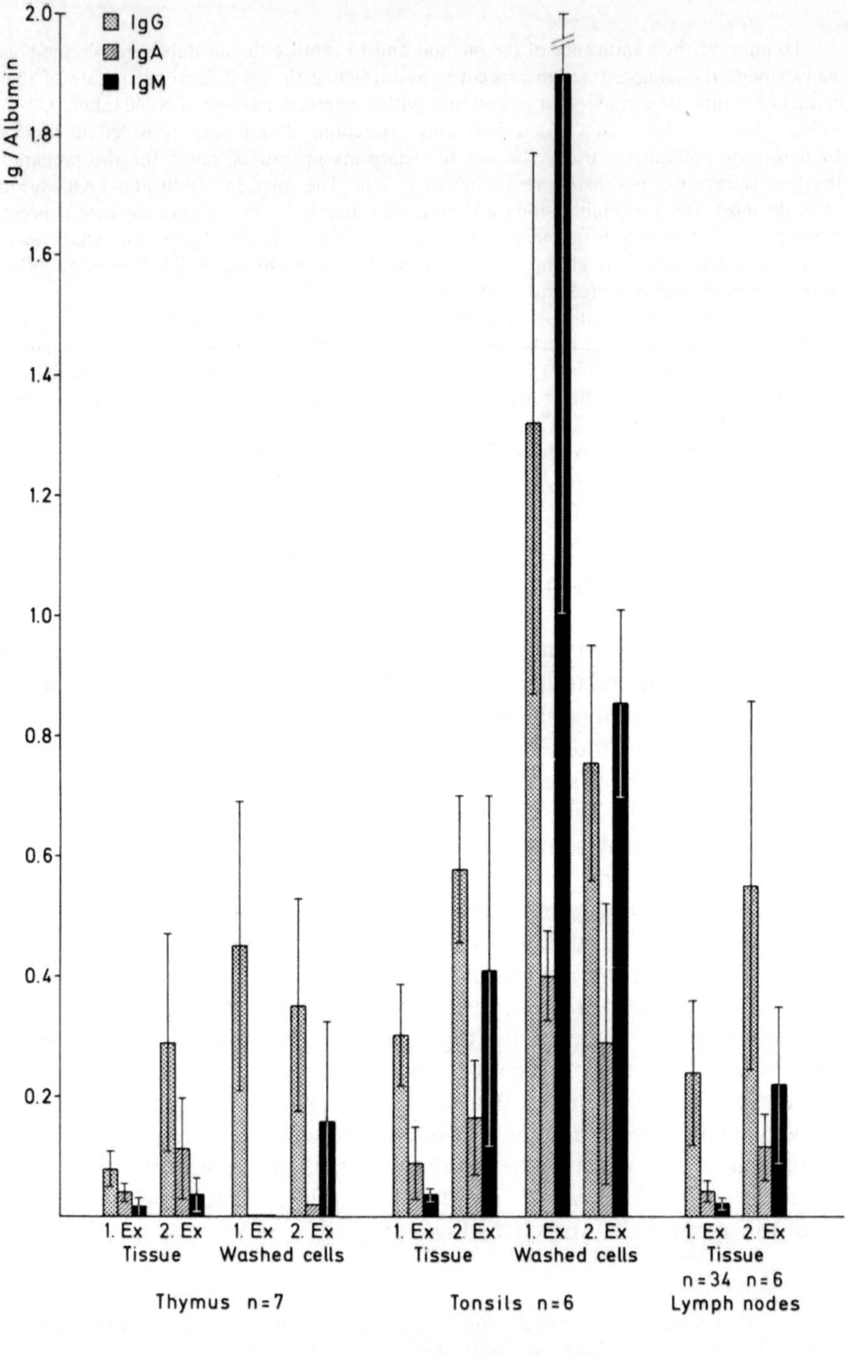


Fig. 265. Comparison of the immunoglobulin (*Ig*) concentrations of saline (*1. Ex.*) and detergent second extracts (*2. Ex.*) of thymus tissue, washed thymocytes, tonsil tissue, washed tonsil cells, and lymph-node tissue. The Ig values are referred to the albumin concentrations measured in the same extracts. The height of each column is the mean value. Vertical lines in the columns indicate standard deviation

significant amounts of Ig.[12] In addition, the thymus contains only a very small number of B-cells (less than 3%). It is remarkable that, like SMITH *et al.*,[13] we found a relatively large amount of IgG in the extracts of thymus tissue and thymus cells. The meaning of this finding has not yet been clarified.

More than 90% of the B-cells in lymph nodes and tonsils retain the produced Ig and fix it to their surface.[14] This Ig essentially serves the recognition of antigens. In the tonsils more than 56% of the nonsecreting B-cells produce IgM, only about 38% produce IgG, and less than 6% produce IgA.[15] In contrast to these nonsecreting B-cells, secreting B-cells reveal only small amounts of Ig on their surface.[16] Their cytoplasm contains large amounts of Ig (CIg), which is usually continually secreted into the extracellular space. As a rule, these secreting B-cells, commonly called plasma cells, amount to less than 10% of the cells in tonsils and lymph nodes. Nevertheless, this percentage is subject to great variation. Most of the plasma cells produce secretory Ig of class G (45%); class A is second (37%), and the lowest percentage is that of IgM-producing plasma cells (18%).[17] These data suggest that the Ig demonstrated in saline extracts is essentially locally produced secretory Ig as well as Ig derived from the serum.

The Ig demonstrated in detergent 2nd extracts, on the other hand, probably comes chiefly from the membranes. One would expect the IgM content of a detergent 2nd extract to be higher than the IgG content, since most of the membrane-bound Ig is of type M. During homogenization with saline, however, a large number of the IgG molecules produced by the ergastoplasm of secretory B-cells (plasma cells) and destined for secretion are enclosed in ergastoplasmic vesicles, as shown by the studies of POTTER.[18] These molecules are not released until the second extraction with detergents breaks up the membrane vesicles. That explains why the IgG class prevails in the detergent 2nd extract, in spite of the numerical predominance of surface IgM-bearing B-cells in the extracted tissue.

A comparison of the B-cell contents of tonsils and lymph nodes shows that tonsils contain about 26–51% surface Ig-positive cells,[15] whereas only 20–30% Ig-positive cells are found in lymph nodes.[19] Our analysis of eight tonsils revealed an average B-cell content of 60–70% when surface Ig (SIg) and the complement receptor were used as B-cell markers.[20] Thus, the B-cell content of the tonsil is about 2–4 times higher than that of the lymph node. A relationship similar to that between the B-cell contents of tonsils and of lymph nodes was shown by the IgM values for the detergent 2nd extracts of these organs. The amount of extracted IgM in the detergent 2nd extracts is therefore approximately proportional to the B-cell content of the examined tissue.

---

[12] PERNIS, FORNI and AMANTE, 1970; RAFF, 1970; RAFF, STERNBERG and TAYLOR, 1970; RABELLINO, COLON, GREY and UNANUE, 1971; NOSSAL, WARNER, LEWIS and SPRENT, 1972.

[13] SMITH, LADOULIS, MISRA, GILL *et al.*, 1975.

[14] BOSMAN and FELDMAN, 1970.

[15] FROLAND and NATVIG, 1973.

[16] PARASKEVAS, LEE and ISRAELS, 1970; PERNIS, FORNI and AMANTE, 1971.

[17] HIJMANS, 1974; VOSSEN, 1975.

[18] 1955.

[19] PAPAMICHAIL, BROWN and HOLBOROW, 1971; STEIN, 1975, unpublished data.

[20] PETERSEN and STEIN, 1976, unpublished data.

Application of the double-extraction procedure to normal lymphatic tissue clearly showed that the Ig assay of tissue extracts with the method used in our laboratory allows a distinction between pure T-cell tissue and tissue containing B-cells. A disadvantage of this method is that slight differences in the B-cell content cannot be determined because of the high serum contamination. Compared to the direct identification of B-cells in lymphatic tissue by means of labeled antibodies, however, this method has the advantage that it does not require living tissue or cells. In addition, it is considerably more sensitive than the immunofluorescence-microscopic demonstration of Ig on frozen sections or fixed cell smears, because SIg is usually not demonstrable on frozen sections by means of fluorescein-labeled antibodies. Ig assay of tissue extracts is therefore a suitable method of screening for both SIg- and CIg-producing lymphomas. Of course, this method should only be used for lymphomas that show homogeneous tumor-cell proliferation.

## B. Demonstration of Monoclonality

Immunoglobulin or antibodies produced in response to antigenic stimulation are as heterogeneous as the number of plasma-cell clones induced by the antigen to produce antibodies. In general, the number of clones stimulated by one antigen is very large. Since an organism continuously comes in contact with numerous antigens, the number of antibody-producing cell clones and therefore of antibodies of various specificities is immense. The heterogeneity of the antibodies lies only in the antigen-binding fraction, called the Fab fragment. The heterogeneity is based on different amino-acid sequences in the variable part of the Fab fragment. The cells of a plasmacytoma, on the other hand, all produce Ig of the same specificity, i.e., with an identical amino-acid sequence, not only in the constant region, but also in the variable region. Since a cell clone produces antibodies with identical amino-acid sequences, one may assume that the cells of a plasmacytoma are derived from a single cell clone. The Ig produced by plasmacytoma cells is therefore called monoclonal Ig, and the Ig produced by plasma cells in response to reactive antigenic stimuli is called polyclonal Ig.

The following methods have proved to be effective to varying degrees in the analysis of polyclonality or monoclonality of antibodies.

### *1. Discontinuous Polyacrylamide Electrophoresis*

When the buffer system described by ORNSTEIN[21] and DAVIS[22] is used, polyclonal IgG and IgA fractions show a wide migration zone in this electrophoretic system[23] (Fig. 266a–c). Monoclonal IgG or IgA fractions are demonstrated after electrophoretic separation as highly distinct, narrow bands[23] (Fig. 266e, f). Even without immunologic identification, monoclonal IgG can be distinguished from monoclonal IgA in this electrophoretic system in most instances. Monoclonal

[21] 1964.

[22] 1964.

[23] STEIN and PARWARESCH, 1971; STEIN, PARWARESCH, KAPER and MÄDER, 1973.

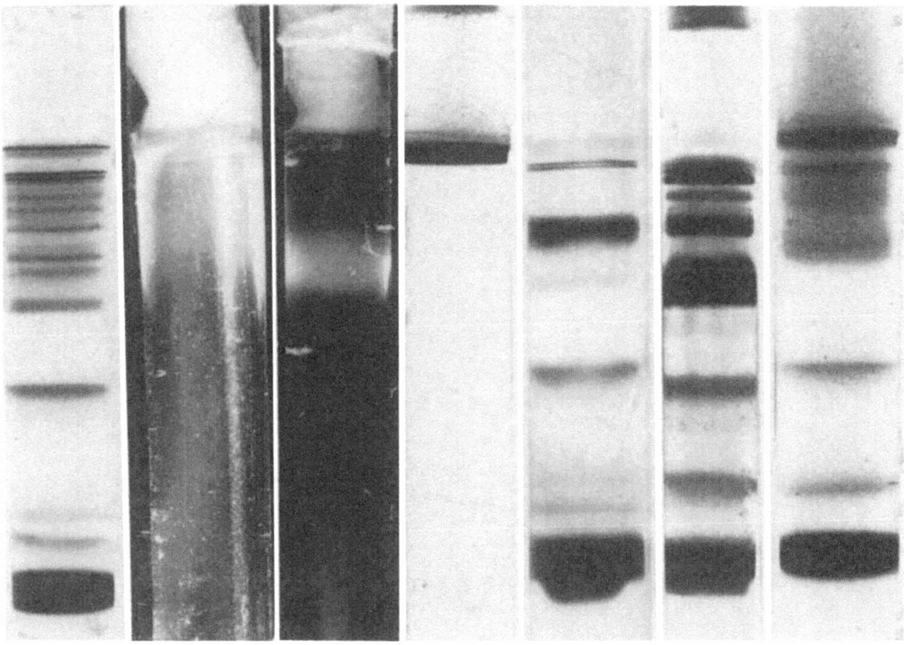


Fig. 266a–g. Discontinuous polyacrylamide-gel electrophoresis. (a) Normal serum. The gel was stained with amido black after the run. (b) Normal serum. After the run, the IgG fraction was precipitated by incubating the gel in monovalent anti-IgG serum. (c) Normal serum. After the run, the IgA fraction was precipitated by incubating the gel in monovalent anti-IgA serum. (d) Purified 19S IgM. (e) Serum from a patient with IgG-secreting plasmacytoma. (f) Serum from a patient with IgA-secreting plasmacytoma. (g) Serum from a patient with IgM-secreting LP immunocytoma (macroglobulinemia of Waldenström). (d–g) The gels were stained as in (a)

IgG is always demonstrated in the form of an isolated narrow distinct band, whereas monoclonal IgA usually shows not only the narrow band of the monomeric IgA molecules, but also further bands of polymerized IgA molecules in the gel (Fig. 266f). IgM can also be clearly distinguished from IgG and IgA in this electrophoretic system. Unfortunately, however, monoclonal IgM cannot be differentiated from polyclonal IgM with this method, since IgM is demonstrated in every case as a narrow distinct band (Fig. 266d, g) because of its slight migration into the separating gel.[23a]

## 2. *Immunoelectrophoresis*

With the help of immunoelectrophoresis, one can infer the monoclonality of an Ig fraction with a certain degree of probability after development with a polyvalent antiserum or a monovalent anti-heavy chain serum. Polyclonal Ig fractions are demonstrated in the form of elongate and repeatedly curved lines (Fig. 267a, b). Monoclonal Ig fractions show uniformly semicircular precipitation lines after electrophoretic separation and development with antibodies (Fig. 267c). The interpretation of such different precipitation lines is often extremely problematic and is frequently unclear when the concentration of the monoclonal Ig fraction is not high enough. With immunoelectrophoresis, the characterization of IgM again presents the greatest problem. One reason is that IgM has a strong tendency to aggregate and often remains at the site of application. Furthermore, it shows only slight electrophoretic mobility.

[23a] Stein and Parwaresch, 1971; Stein, Parwaresch, Kaper and Mäder, 1973.

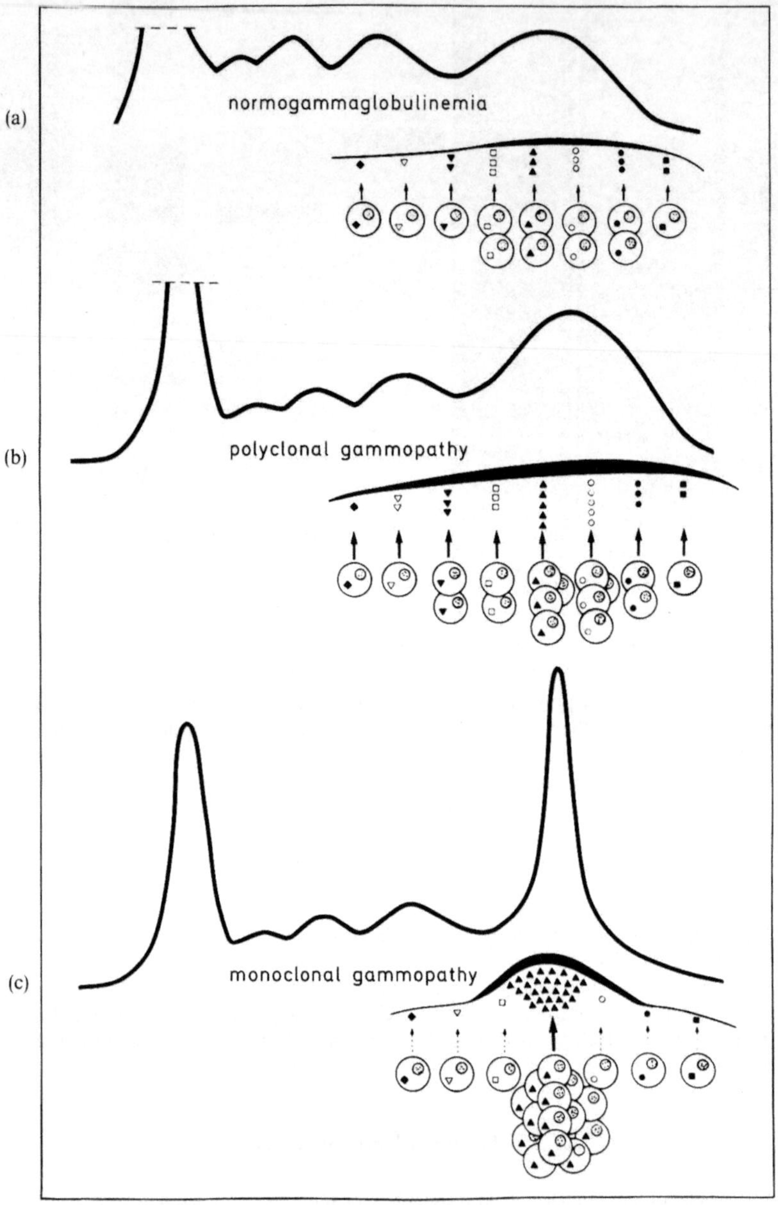


Fig. 267a–c. Schematic drawing of electrophoretograms of sera from healthy individuals (a) and patients with polyclonal (b) and monoclonal (c) gammopathy. In polyclonal gammopathy, various plasma-cell clones are increased in number. These produce antibodies of different specificity and electrophoretic mobility, resulting in a broad-based $\gamma$-globulin peak and an elongate, multiply curved precipitation line (b). Uncontrolled increase in one plasma-cell clone leads to an excessive increase in antigenically and electrophoretically homogeneous (monoclonal) immunoglobulins; this results in a small-based $\gamma$-globulin peak and a uniformly semicircular precipitation line (c). (From Fateh-Moghadam, 1976, with his kind permission)

The diagnosis of monoclonality of an Ig class can be made with a certain degree of probability when the immunoelectrophoresis plates are developed with an anti-light chain serum. If the suspected monoclonal Ig fraction is demonstrated with only one of the two anti-light chain sera, then there is practically no doubt as to the monoclonality of this fraction. A disadvantage is that the differentiation with anti-light chain sera is successful only when the monoclonal Ig fraction exceeds a certain quantity in the sample. Furthermore, one must bear in mind that not all anti-light chain sera are capable of recognizing and clearly precipitating all monoclonal light chains that are bound to the heavy chains of various classes.

## 3. *Isoelectric Focusing*

At present, the most sensitive method for demonstrating microheterogeneity or homogeneity of proteins is separation of the proteins according to their isoelectric point. In analytic use, this method is capable of separating proteins or immunoglobulins that differ in only one amino acid. The method is based on the following principle. A continuous pH gradient (through ampholines) is built up in a supporting medium, e.g., polyacrylamide gel. An electric potential is applied to the plate after application of the proteins to be analyzed. The proteins then migrate in the pH gradient until each one reaches the area of the plate where its charge concurs with the charge of the plate. The protein stops migrating and stays at this site. The method has been described in detail by KARLSSON *et al.*[24]

Until recently, only the isoelectric focusing of IgG, IgA, IgD, and IgE was possible. IgM could not be analyzed with this method because it cannot move freely in the polyacrylamide gel suitable for the analytic procedure, owing to its molecular size. In addition, IgM is not soluble in the electrolyte-free milieu necessary for this method. These problems have now been overcome by our research group[25] by reducing the dimension of IgM to that of the monomer, and increasing the solubility by introduction of carboxymethyl groups into the molecule.

The isoelectric-focusing method is of practical significance only when the Ig classes to be analyzed do not have to be applied to the isoelectric-focusing plates in a pure state. The reason is that isolation of the Ig before the isoelectric-focusing analysis would usually be impossible because of the small quantity of the samples; furthermore, it would also be exceedingly complicated. The necessity of isolation can be avoided by specifically precipitating the sought Ig class with $^{125}$I-labeled antibodies after the isoelectric-focusing separation. The unprecipitated proteins are washed from the plate. The precipitated Ig is then made visible by autoradiography (Fig. 268).

This method of demonstrating monoclonality proved to be extremely effective. In polyacrylamide electrophoresis, monoclonal Ig fractions migrated in a distinct band. In immunoelectrophoresis, they precipitated in semicircular lines. With isoelectric focusing, monoclonal Ig fractions are demonstrated in the form of several (2 – 14) bands. This means that the Ig, which appeared to be homogeneous in electrophoresis, clearly reveals heterogeneity in isoelectric focusing, demonstrating the extremely high resolving power of isoelectric focusing. AWDEH *et al.*[26] assumed that monoclonal Ig has a homogeneous primary structure in the protein moiety. Several causes for the microheterogeneity were considered by these authors. The most probable ones were postsynthetic deamidation of glutamine and asparagine, and removal or incomplete biosynthesis of carbohydrates attached to the Ig. The studies of BOUMAN *et al.*[27] revealed that the microheterogeneity of some monoclonal IgG and IgM fractions could be reduced by means of pretreatment with neuraminidase. Thus, the heterogeneity is due, to some extent, to the association of a variable number of sugar molecules to the Ig chains.[27] In spite of the microheterogeneity of monoclonal Ig fractions demonstrated in isoelectric focusing, they can be clearly distinguished from polyclonal Ig with this method. Polyclonal Ig is demonstrated as a diffuse zone, up to 5 cm wide (Fig. 268b), which is due to the almost infinite number of antibodies of various specificities of polyclonal Ig fractions. The bands of polyclonal Ig are so numerous and lie so close together that they "melt" into this

---

[24] KARLSSON, DAVIES, ÖHMAN and ANDERSSON, 1973.

[25] BOUMAN, LÜSEBRINK, HAVSTEEN and STEIN, 1976.

[26] AWDEH, ASKONAS and WILLIAMSON, 1967.

[27] BOUMAN, MEINCKE and HAVSTEEN, 1975; BOUMAN and STEIN, 1975, unpublished data.

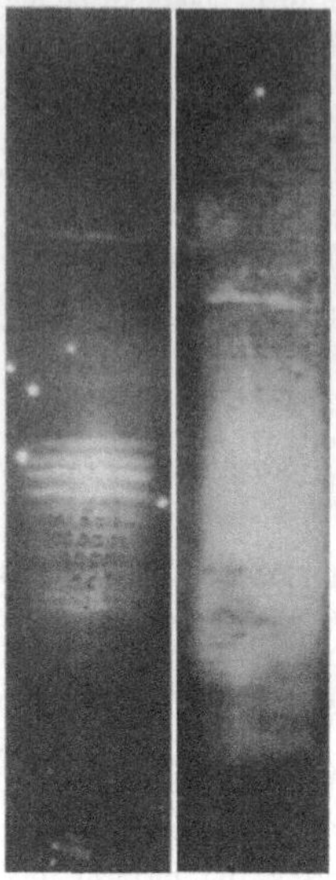


Fig. 268a and b. Autoradiographs of reduced and carboxymethylated isoelectrofocused IgM. (a) Serum from a patient with IgM-secreting LP immunocytoma (macroglobulinemia of Waldenström). (b) Normal serum

wide zone. In contrast, the monoclonal Ig fractions show only up to 15 bands, and the individual bands are clearly widened and easy to distinguish from one another (Fig. 268a). Through incubation of the isoelectric-focusing plates with $^{125}$I-labeled anti-light chain antibodies, one can demonstrate that the "monoclonal" Ig bands reveal only one light-chain type.

# C. Surface Immunoglobulin (SIg)

On the basis of indirect evidence, it had already been suspected for a long time that some lymphoid cells express Ig as antigen receptors on their cell membrane.[28] The direct demonstration of Ig localized on the cell membrane (SIg) was first successful in cells from an African Burkitt's lymphoma by incubating living tumor cells in fluorescein-labeled anti-IgM antibodies.[29]

In 1970, RAFF detected SIg on about one third of the peripheral blood lymphocytes and also of the lymph-node cells. These findings were confirmed in principle by various authors.[30]

## *1. Procedure*

A reliable demonstration of SIg is possible only with living cells. It can be performed with fluorochrome-labeled,[31] $^{125}$I-labeled,[32] or peroxidase-labeled anti-Ig sera[33] by means of the direct

[28] SELL and GELL, 1965; BERT, MASSARO and MAJA, 1968; ABDOU and RICHTER, 1969.

[29] KLEIN, KLEIN, NADKARNI, NADKARNI *et al.*, 1967.

[30] PERNIS, FORNI and AMANTE, 1970; RABELLINO, COLON, GREY and UNANUE, 1971.

[31] KLEIN, KLEIN, NADKARNI, NADKARNI *et al.*, 1967; PERNIS, FORNI and AMANTE, 1970; RABELLINO, COLON, GREY and UNANUE, 1971.

[32] RAFF, 1970; WILSON and NOSSAL, 1971.

[33] STEIN and DRESCHER, 1973.

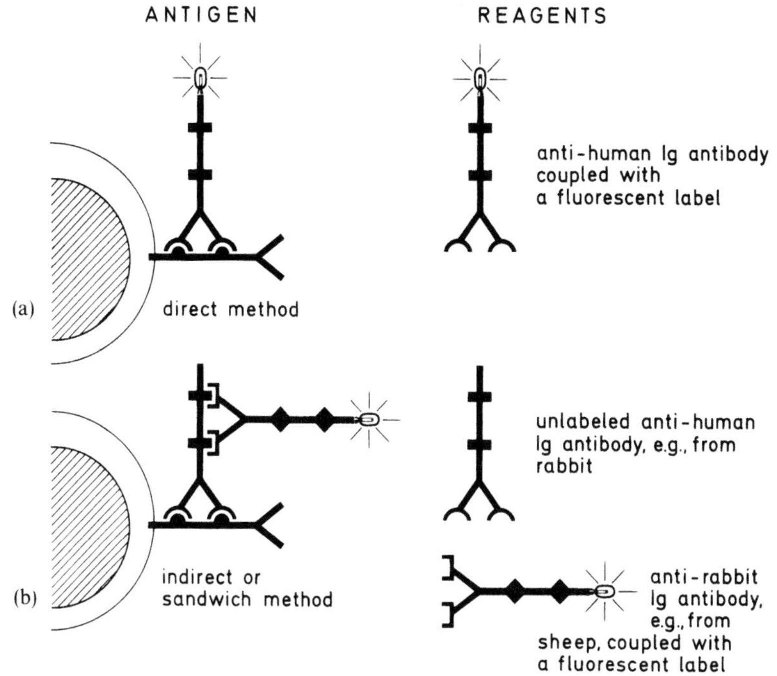


Fig. 269a and b. Symbolic representation of the immunofluorescence method for the microscopic localization of surface antigen. (a) Direct procedure. (b) Indirect procedure

or indirect procedure. In the direct procedure, cells that have been washed three times are incubated with the labeled IgG fraction of monospecific anti-Ig sera for 20–40 min. Then the unbound antibodies are removed by washing the cells three times. The cells labeled with fluorochrome-antibody conjugates are deposited in a mixture of glycerol and phosphate-buffered saline onto a microscopic slide and spread out with a cover glass. Evaluation is made within 4 hours with a fluorescence microscope. The immunofluorescence method is outlined in Figure 269. When cells are incubated with peroxidase-coupled antibodies, the cells are washed three times and centrifuged onto microscopic slides by means of a cytocentrifuge. The labeled antibodies are made visible with the peroxidase reaction according to GRAHAM and KARNOVSKY.[34] The use of living cells guarantees that the labeled antibodies react exclusively with the antigens on the cell membrane; the labeled antibodies cannot penetrate into the cell through the intact cell membrane. This procedure therefore leads to extremely selective SIg labeling with almost no background.

## *a) Immunofluorescence*

The demonstration of SIg with fluorochrome-coupled antibodies is less susceptible than that with peroxidase-coupled antibodies. The fluorochrome method as a rule provides good results when the IgG fraction of the antisera, isolated by DEAE-cellulose chromatography, is labeled with fluorochromes. Isolation of pure specific antibodies is not necessary with the fluorescence method. A disadvantage of this method is that the cytology of the cells labeled with fluorochrome conjugate can be evaluated only by phase microscopy.

Two fluorochromes are now used most often: (1) fluorescein and (2) rhodamine. The advantage of fluorescein is that it is relatively chemically stable. A disadvantage is that it is relatively quickly destroyed by the exciting radiation; thus, the labeling fades quickly during observation. In comparison, rhodamine is chemically less stable than fluorescein, but it reveals more intense fluorescence and is hardly affected by the exciting radiation. Our experience has shown that rhodamine conjugates

[34] 1966.

are preferable to fluorescein conjugates. Preparation of the conjugates, their final testing, and the labeling procedure have been described in detail by HIJMANS *et al.* and others.[35]

### *b) Two-Color Fluorescence*

Rhodamine and fluorescein conjugates can be used simultaneously, making it possible to simultaneously demonstrate two different antigen structures. When exciting light of the appropriate wavelength is used with the appropriate filters, either the structures labeled with rhodamine conjugate or only those in the same slide labeled with fluorescein are visible. Detailed information about light sources and filter combinations is provided by FAULK and HIJMANS.[36]

### *c) Immunoperoxidase Method*

The labeling of SIg with peroxidase conjugates has the advantage that the labeled cell can be morphologically differentiated much better (see Figs. 279 and 283a). Another very important advantage of the immunoperoxidase method is that the peroxidase-positive substance is electron-dense and can therefore be demonstrated by electron microscopy (see Figs. 237 and 240). A considerable disadvantage of this method is that the quality of the labeling is highly dependent on the peroxidase charge used. Furthermore, enrichment of the antibodies by isolating the IgG fraction has proved to be insufficient. Pure antibodies of the desired specificity must be isolated by affinity chromatography. That makes the immunoperoxidase method extremely complicated and expensive. Various methods for preparing horseradish-peroxidase-antibody conjugates have been described by AVRAMEAS and co-workers.[37] The labeling procedure has been outlined by us a number of times.[38]

## *2. Possibilities for Error*

Besides the specificity of monovalent antisera, the first major cause of interference with SIg on B-cells is the common occurrence of antibodies against lymphocytes in pathologic conditions[39] and even in some normal individuals.[40] These antibodies are autospecific and adhere to both T- and B-lymphocytes. They then mimic innate SIg on B-cells. A second main problem is that a number of lymphocytes bear IgG-Fc receptors and/or complement receptors that bind IgG, particularly when the IgG is aggregated or complexed with antigen and complement. As with autoantibodies, secondary fixation of complexed Ig to IgG-Fc receptors and/or to complement receptors simulates SIg and results in falsely high values for Ig-bearing cells. In peripheral blood there is apparently a third population[40] of lymphocytes that have avid IgG-Fc receptors, but lack true SIg. This population can frequently be assayed for B-cells by means of fluorescent anti-Ig analysis. Much of the interference can be eliminated, however, by incubation at 37° C for 2–24 hours, during which bound autoantibodies and immunocomplexes are shed from the lymphocyte surface, while the innate Ig is not affected or is resynthesized by the B-cells. Furthermore, it is advisable to utilize the fluorescent antigen-binding fragment

---

[35] HIJMANS, SCHUIT and KLEIN, 1969; VAN DALEN, KNAPP and PLOEM, 1973; KNAPP, HAAIJMAN, SCHUIT, RÁDL *et al.*, 1975.

[36] 1972.

[37] AVRAMEAS, 1969; AVRAMEAS and TERNYNCK, 1971.

[38] STEIN and DRESCHER, 1973; STEIN and KAISERLING, 1974b.

[39] WINCHESTER, WINFIELD, SIEGAL, WERNET *et al.*, 1974.

[40] WINCHESTER, FU, HOFFMAN and KUNKEL, 1975.

Table 94. Occurrence of surface markers on cells of the lymphatic and hemopoietic systems

| Type of cell | SIg | IgG-Fc receptor | Receptor for | | Mouse-E receptor | Sheep-E receptor | | HTLA |
|---|---|---|---|---|---|---|---|---|
| | | | C 3b | C 3d | | stable at 37° C | unstable at 37° C | |
| | % | % | % | % | % | % | % | % |
| Peripheral blood lymphocytes | 8–15[a] | 15–20 | 20 | 20 | 8,[b] 16[c] | low | 60–80 | 70–80 |
| Tonsil lymphocytes | 50–60 | 20–40 | 60–70 | 40–50 | n.d. | low | 20–40 | 20–40 |
| Lymphoid cells of the bone marrow | 20 | n.d. | n.d. | n.d. | n.d. | low | 70 | 80 |
| Thymocytes | 2–4 | 2–8 | 5 | 5 | 0 | 90 | 98 | 98–100 |
| Granulocytes | 0[a] | 80–100 | 100 | 0–20 | 0 | 0 | 0 | 0 |
| Monocytes | 0[a] | 80–100 | 100 | 100 | 0 | 0 | 0 | 0 |

n.d. = not determined.
[a] After overnight culture, fresh cells often stain for IgG.
[b] Without neuraminidase treatment.
[c] With neuraminidase treatment.

of the IgG molecule (Fab2) for detecting all surface antigens. The use of labeled Fab2 successfully prevents the labeled antibodies from adhering—*via* the Fc portion—to the IgG-Fc receptors on the lymphoid cells.

### *3. Occurrence and Significance*

The clearest difference between B- and T-cells is the occurrence of SIg on B-cells and its absence from T-cells, at least when the usual analytic methods are used. Numerous investigations have shown that SIg-positive cells originate from the bone marrow, mature without influence of the thymus, and transform under antigenic stimulation, usually with the help of T-helper cells, into Ig-secreting plasma cells.[41] According to findings of VOSSEN[42] and others,[42a] the expression of various Ig classes on the cell membranes changes during maturation of the cells and after transformation in response to antigenic stimulation.

GATIEN *et al.*[43] reported that cells flowing into the thymus anlage in the 9th–10th week of gestation bear SIg. The cells differ from normal B-cells in their behavior during gradient-density centrifugation. Upon maturation of these "T-precursor cells" into thymocytes, the SIg quickly disappears. Nevertheless, the findings show that SIg may be considered a reliable B-cell feature only after the 12th week of gestation, or even birth, and in normally developed individuals.

The percentage of SIg-bearing lymphoid cells from different sources is shown

[41] WARNER, SZENBERG and BURNET, 1962; COOPER, PETERSON and GOOD, 1965; CLAMAN, CHAPERON and TRIPLETT, 1966; DAVIES, LEUCHARS, WALLIS, MARCHANT *et al.*, 1967; MILLER and MITCHELL, 1969; RAFF, 1973.

[42] 1975.

[42a] PIERCE, ASOFSKY and SOLLIDAY, 1973; LITWIN, HÜTTEROTH, LIN, KENNARD *et al.*, 1974.

[43] GATIEN, SCHNEEBERGER and MERLER, 1975.

in Table 94. The main classes of SIg on all lymphoid cells are IgM and IgD.[44] As a rule, both Ig classes are simultaneously present on the surfaces of lymphoid cells. All other Ig classes, including IgG, are rarely expressed on blood B-cells. The difficulties in detecting surface IgG (possibility of falsely high values) have already been mentioned (see p. 542).

## D. Cytoplasmic Immunoglobulin (CIg)

In 1955, Ig was directly demonstrated for the first time in the cytoplasm of plasma cells on frozen sections or fixed smears by means of fluorochrome-labeled antisera.[45] In the 1950's and 1960's, this method still involved a high rate of error; the labeling results were frequently nonspecific. Progress in the purification of the IgG fraction, which is used for the staining conjugate, and the subsequent purification of the fluorochrome-labeled antibodies have finally eliminated almost all problems. Purification has greatly increased the efficiency of the fluorochrome method. Between 1965 and 1970, enzyme markers for the conjugation of antibodies were introduced.[46] The horseradish-peroxidase method has proved to be particularly useful.

Intracytoplasmic Ig, called cytoplasmic Ig (CIg) in this book, can only be demonstrated in fixed cells or in cells that have been killed through freezing, since fixing or freezing makes the cell membrane pervious to antibodies.

### *1. Procedure for Suspended Cells*

Conventional smears of blood cells, bone-marrow cells, etc., and imprints of lymphatic tissue are not very suitable for the demonstration of CIg with labeled antibodies. The reason is that the cells are surrounded by serum components, including all Ig classes. Staining of conventional smears or imprints therefore leads to much background staining, which often makes the evaluation of the labeling impossible. Such problems can be easily avoided if the cells to be studied are suspended and liberated from the serum Ig by washing two to three times. The washed cells are applied to microscopic slides by means of a cytocentrifuge and fixed in an ice-cold mixture of acetic acid and ethyl alcohol. These slides can be kept in a deep freeze for several years when wrapped in plastic film. For the demonstration of CIg the cells on the slides are coated with an anti-Ig-fluorochrome conjugate and incubated for 30 min. After repeated washing, the slides are evaluated with a fluorescence microscope. Positive demonstration of CIg is presented in Figure 282a. When two antibody fractions with different anti-Ig specificity, and different fluorescent stains (rhodamine and fluorescein) are used, heavy and light chains, or both light chains, for example, can be demonstrated simultaneously. This two-color labeling method considerably facilitates evaluation of whether a proliferation of antibody-producing cells is monoclonal or polyclonal. When plasma cells predominantly reveal only one heavy- and light-chain type, this is a strong indication of a monoclonal proliferation.

---

[44] Rowe, Hug, Faulk, McCormick *et al.*, 1973; Rowe, Hug, Forni and Pernis, 1973.

[45] Coons, Leduc and Connolly, 1955.

[46] Avrameas, 1969.

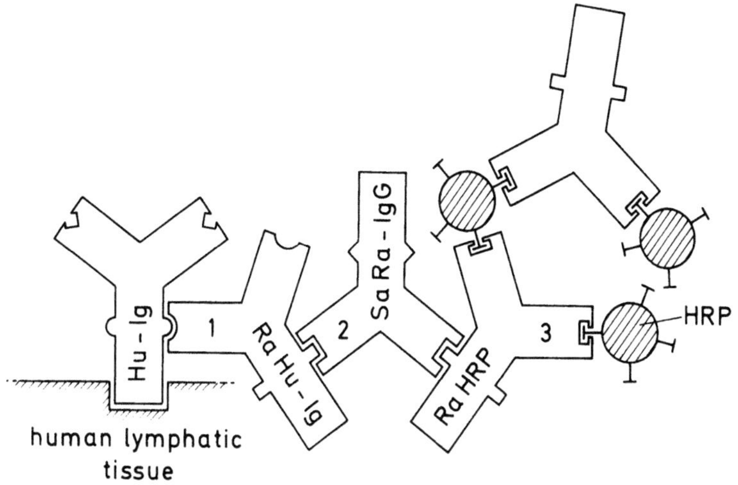


Fig. 270. Symbolic representation of horseradish peroxidase (*HRP*)-bridge method for detecting cellular antigens with the peroxidase-antiperoxidase (PAP) complex. *1* Rabbit anti-human immunoglobulin serum (*Ra Hu-Ig*). *2* Sheep anti-rabbit IgG serum (*Sa Ra-IgG*). *3* PAP complex consisting of two molecules of IgG antibody and three molecules of peroxidase

## 2. *Procedure for Tissue*

### *a) Frozen Sections*

Intracytoplasmic Ig can also be demonstrated on tissue sections. So far, that has usually been done on frozen sections. Previously, a nonspecific background was very frequently observed and deplored. As mentioned above, however, it could be eliminated through protein-chemical purification of the IgG fraction of the antisera before fluorochroming and through isolation of IgG labeled with a certain number of fluorochrome molecules. A great disadvantage of the demonstration of CIg with fluorochrome-labeled antibodies is that the cells cannot be evaluated cytologically.

### *b) Paraffin Sections and Enzyme-Bridge Method*

The enzyme-bridge method of STERNBERGER *et al.*[47] has proved to be a very promising method for the demonstration of CIg. The principle of it is presented in Figure 270. Tissue sections are incubated in a rabbit anti-Ig serum, for instance, and then washed. That is followed by incubation with a sheep anti-rabbit Ig serum. After careful washing, the slide is incubated in a solution containing a complex of horseradish peroxidase and rabbit anti-peroxidase antibodies (PAP). Then the bound PAP complex is made visible by means of the peroxidase reaction described by GRAHAM and KARNOVSKY.[48] The enzyme-bridge method is very sensitive and yields a specific reaction, even in paraffin sections.[49] Paraffin sections, however, must be pretreated in an appropriate manner. After being carefully deparaffinized, the sections are incubated in methanol containing 3% $H_2O_2$. Then the slides are incubated in sheep normal serum that has been absorbed with insolubilized human serum proteins. This method has two great advantages. (1) The demonstration of CIg is possible on conventionally prepared paraffin sections. Thus, old slides or sections from stored paraffin blocks can be analyzed for the presence of CIg. (2) The cytologic quality of the slides is nearly as good as that of conventional slides stained with hematoxylin and eosin. The labeling can also be easily recognized after counterstaining with hematoxylin (see Fig. 286).

---

[47] STERNBERGER, HARDY, CUCULIS and MEYER, 1970.

[48] 1966.

[49] TAYLOR and BURNS, 1974.

### 3. Occurrence and Significance

Intracytoplasmic Ig is demonstrable with labeled antibodies in the cells that produce Ig for secretion, i.e., plasma cells. Ig demonstrated in the cytoplasm is therefore "secretory Ig." CIg may be distributed in the cytoplasm in three different ways:

1. Diffusely distributed throughout the whole cytoplasm. It is then invisible with conventional stainings.
2. As amorphous globular homogeneous material, which is called Russell bodies when it occurs in plasma cells, and Russell body-like material when it occurs in lymphoid cells other than typical plasma cells. It shows a strong PAS-positive reaction.
3. As crystalline inclusions. They are usually not stainable with PAS.

Diffuse CIg is detectable only with labeled anti-Ig antibodies, whereas amorphous and crystalline inclusions are visible without specific labeling. Nevertheless, their Ig nature can be established only by labeling with antibodies.

The studies of MELCHERS and ANDERSSON[50] showed that the cells that produce exclusively SIg, i.e., Ig for their own use, reveal about 90% of it on the membrane and only about 10% in the cytoplasm. Thus, it is not surprising that CIg cannot be demonstrated with labeled antibodies in most SIg-bearing cells.

CIg can also be demonstrated in cells that are in the process of switching from the synthesis of nonsecretory Ig (SIg) to the synthesis of secretory Ig. These cells are immunoblasts and plasmablasts. In such cells, Ig is demonstrable with labeled antibodies both on the membrane and in the cytoplasm. The same is true for most IgM-producing plasma cells, but usually not for IgG- and IgA-producing plasma cells.

Finally, it should be mentioned that (ingested) IgG and trace amounts of IgM also occur in neutrophil granulocytes and monocytes of the peripheral blood. This can be demonstrated by applying the very sensitive immunoperoxidase-bridge technique to smears.[50a]

## E. IgG-Fc-Fragment Receptor (IgG-Fc Receptor)

The cytophilic antibodies discovered by BOYDEN and SORKIN in 1960 were bound by macrophages, as was later shown by BOYDEN.[51] BERKEN and BENACERRAF[52] proved that the binding site is localized on the Fc fragment of IgG molecules. The IgG-Fc fragment-binding membrane structure was accordingly called the Fc receptor or IgG-Fc receptor. The relatively weak binding of uncomplexed IgG antibodies could be considerably strengthened through reaction of the antibodies with antigens. Sheep erythrocytes (E) coated with anti-sheep erythrocyte antibodies (A) of the IgG type were usually used as antigen-antibody (IgGEA) complexes in the further characterization of the IgG-Fc receptor. Com-

[50] 1974.
[50a] MASON, LABAUME and PREUD'HOMME, 1977.
[51] 1964.
[52] 1966.

pared with molecular antigen-antibody complexes, the advantage of the IgG-sheepEA complexes is that they can be directly visualized by light microscopy.

It is generally reported in the literature[53] that IgG-sheepEA complexes are bound by a majority of monocytes and macrophages, but not by lymphocytes. We made the same observation.

Almost 10 years went by after the discovery of the IgG-Fc receptor on monocytes and macrophages before it was also demonstrated on lymphocytes. In 1972, BASTEN *et al.*[54] observed that antigen-antibody complexes were bound by some lymphocytes. They used radiolabeled molecular antigen-antibody complexes and made the binding to lymphocytes visible by autoradiography.

The same year, DICKLER and KUNKEL[55] discovered that heat-aggregated IgG was bound with a high affinity by some lymphocytes. Various research groups had previously shown that IgG molecules stick together over Fab fragments when heated.[56] Heat aggregation therefore causes development of IgG complexes, from which the Fc fragments project like quills of a hedgehog. Because of the Fab association of the IgG molecules, there is also activation of the Fc fragment, as is the case when the IgG molecules are complexed with an antigen. The Fc fragments of the aggregated IgG complexes bind complement, for example, to the same extent as do the Fc fragments of antibodies complexed with antigen. One may therefore assume that the determinants for the IgG-Fc receptor are also activated and become accessible through heat aggregation. The extremely stable binding of aggregated-IgG complexes to the IgG-Fc receptor on lymphocytes is probably based above all on the extreme density of the Fc fragments on these complexes.

## *1. Procedure*

The binding of aggregated IgG to lymphocytes can be easily and reliably visualized by labeling the IgG with fluorochromes or $^{125}I$ before heat aggregation. The IgG-Fc receptor on lymphocytes cannot be demonstrated as easily with erythrocyte-antibody complexes (IgGEA). Sheep erythrocytes that have been coated with rabbit anti-sheep erythrocyte antibodies of IgG type are practically not bound by lymphocytes. In contrast, SEILER *et al.*[57] and BRAIN and MARSTON[58] achieved binding of IgGEA to lymphocytes by sensitizing human erythrocytes with a high-titer anti-D serum. FERRARINI *et al.*[59] reported that the percentage of lymphocytes binding ox erythrocytes loaded with rabbit-IgG antibodies was similar to that of lymphocytes binding aggregated IgG.

In our studies, Rh-positive erythrocytes that had been thickly coated with antibodies by means of incubation in a high-titer incomplete anti-D serum consistently showed stable rosette formation with lymphocytes.

Several explanations can be given for the finding that IgG-sheepEA complexes are not bound by the IgG-Fc receptor on lymphocytes, whereas IgG-humanEA complexes are. (1) Stable binding of IgGEA requires a high concentration of antibodies on the erythrocyte membrane. Practically complete loading of the antigen structures on the erythrocytes is easily achieved through incubation in an undiluted or only slightly diluted, incomplete anti-D serum, since agglutination does not occur. Conditions are similar with ox erythrocytes, which are also not, or only incompletely, agglutinated by rabbit anti-ox erythrocyte sera. Agglutination is the limiting factor in the coating

---

[53] SHEVACH, JAFFE and GREEN, 1973.

[54] BASTEN, MILLER, SPRENT and PYE, 1972.

[55] 1972.

[56] AUGENER and GREY, 1970.

[57] SEILER, SEDLACEK, KANZY and LANG, 1972.

[58] 1973.

[59] FERRARINI, MORETTA, ABRILE and DURANTE, 1975.

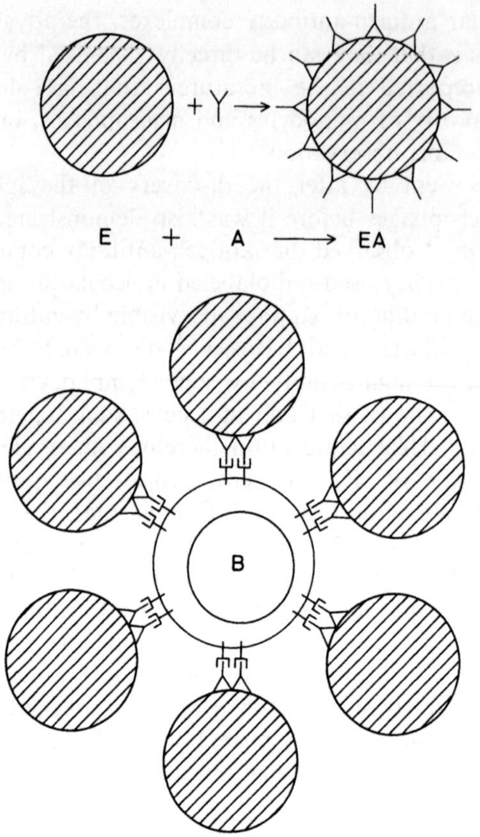


Fig. 271. Symbolic representation of the rosette assay for the detection of IgG-Fc receptors. At the top, how to prepare erythrocyte-antibody complexes (*EA*) by coating erythrocytes (*E*) with IgG antibodies (*A*). At the bottom, how these indicator cells form rosettes with IgG-Fc receptor-positive cells (*B*)

of sheep erythrocytes with rabbit anti-sheep erythrocyte antibodies. (2) The IgG-Fc receptor has a high affinity only to homologous IgG molecules.

Recently, we achieved binding of sheep erythrocytes coated with rabbit IgG to lymphocytes. The IgGEA was brought into close contact with the lymphocytes by pelleting the cell mixture and then incubating it for 30 min at room temperature. When applying this technique, it is essential to use trypsinized sheep erythrocytes in order to be sure that the binding of the IgGEA is specifically mediated only *via* the Fc portion of the membrane-bound IgG, and not *via* the sheep-erythrocyte determinants responsible for the spontaneous binding of sheep erythrocytes by T-cells.

The principle of demonstrating IgG-Fc receptors by means of IgG-humanEA complexes is presented in Figure 271. Compared with the demonstration of IgG-Fc receptors by means of aggregated IgG, the IgG-humanEA-rosette test has the advantage that the cells forming rosettes with IgGEA can be conventionally stained with Pappenheim and cytologically evaluated after centrifugation with a cytocentrifuge onto microscopic slides. That is especially important when tumor cells in cell suspensions are to be characterized according to receptor features.

## 2. *Occurrence and Significance*

Receptors for the Fc portion of the IgG molecule are expressed on various cells of the immune and phagocytic systems (see Table 94), on the cells of various organs, such as liver, kidney, breast, etc.,[60] and on various tumor cells.[61] Depleting studies[62] and double-labeling experiments[63] have revealed that IgG-Fc receptors predominantly occur on B-cells. The restriction of IgG-Fc receptors to the B-cell series was further substantiated by the demonstration of IgG-Fc receptors on CLL cells of the B-type, but not on those of the T-type.[64]

IgG-Fc receptors are also found on lymphocytes that are devoid of SIg and sheep-E receptors but bear receptors for complement (C3b).[65] These cells are capable of killing IgG-antibody-coated cells[65] and are therefore called killer cells.[66]

Various research groups have also shown, however, that IgG-Fc receptors are detectable on activated T-cells or develop on T-cells when the cells are activated by antigen.[67] The T-cells with IgG-Fc receptors also apparently function as killer cells. Recently, COOPER[68] reported that IgG-Fc receptor-positive T-cells exhibit suppressor-T-cell activity, in contrast to the T-cells that bear receptors for IgM (detectable with IgM-coated bovine erythrocytes [IgM-bovine-EA] after 20-hour incubation). The IgM receptor-positive cells were shown to be capable of inducing surface IgM-positive B-lymphocytes to transform into plasma cells. The IgMEA receptor-positive T-cells therefore appear to be T-helper cells. Surface IgM-positive B-cells revealed no signs of transformation into plasma cells in the presence of IgG-Fc receptor-positive T-cells.

Apart from antibody-mediated cytotoxicity and/or suppressor activity (lymphocytic series) and phagocytosis (phagocytic-cell series), the *in-vivo* function of the IgG-Fc receptor is unclear. Although the IgG-Fc receptor is predominantly expressed on B-cells, its significance as a marker of this lymphoid-cell subpopulation is limited, since the receptor is present on various subsets of cytogenetically and functionally different lymphoid cells, including T-cells.

## F. Complement Receptor

In 1968, HUBER *et al.*[69] discovered a receptor for antigen-antibody-complement complexes on human monocytes. It was called complement receptor. In 1970, BIANCO *et al.*[70] found that some lymphocytes also have complement receptors. Erythrocytes (E) coated with antibodies (A) and complement (C) were used for the demonstration of complement receptors. The same authors showed that the EAC was chiefly bound *via* the third component of complement (C 3), since EAC prepared in the presence of cobra-venom factor was not bound by complement receptor-bearing lymphocytes. EAC1243b produced with pure

[60] FRØLAND and NATVIG, 1973; SHEVACH, JAFFE and GREEN, 1973; TÖNDER, THUNOLD and SOLHAUG, 1976.
[61] KERBEL and DAVIES, 1974.
[62] FRØLAND and NATVIG, 1973; JONDAL, WIGZELL and AIUTI, 1973.
[63] DICKLER and KUNKEL, 1972.
[64] DICKLER, SIEGAL, BENTWICH and KUNKEL, 1973.
[65] FLAD, FINK and DIERICH, 1977.
[66] PERLMANN and PERLMANN, 1970; PERLMANN, PERLMANN and BIBERFELD, 1972.
[67] YOSHIDA and ANDERSSON, 1972; GREAVES, JANOSSY and DOENHOFF, 1974; VAN BOXEL and ROSENSTREICH, 1974; FERRARINI, MORETTA, ABRILE and DURANTE, 1975.
[68] 1976.
[69] HUBER, POLLEY, LINSCOTT, FUDENBERG *et al.*, 1968.
[70] BIANCO, PATRICK, and NUSSENZWEIG, 1970.

complement components was bound by complement receptor-bearing lymphocytes, whereas EAC14 did not show any binding. Furthermore, only the cleavage products of C 3 led to inhibition of the binding of EAC to complement receptor-bearing lymphocytes. In 1973, EDEN *et al.*[71] proved that the binding of EAC occurs *via* the C3b fragment. Later, ROSS and POLLEY[72] showed that the binding of EAC3b is mediated *via* C3c, a subfragment of C3b (see Fig. 272). Furthermore, both research groups[73] reported that, after removal of the C3c fragment by means of C3 inactivator, the EAC was still bound by lymphocytes *via* the remaining C3d fragment. The binding of EAC3b was inhibited only by C3b or C3c cleavage products and the binding of EAC3d only by C3d fragments. These findings indicated that there are two independent complement receptors on lymphocytes: the C3b and the C3d receptor. It was also evident that the C3d determinant is not accessible to the C3d receptor until the C3c fragment is separated from the C3b molecule. Moreover, ROSS and POLLEY[72] and BOKISCH and SOBEL[73a] observed that EAC can be bound not only *via* the C3b and C3d, but also *via* the C4 component, namely, when EAC1 is coated with a sufficiently thick layer of C4 molecules. Since the binding of EAC14 was inhibited by EAC3b but not by EAC3d, ROSS and POLLEY[72] suspected that the receptor for C3b is largely identical with that for C4.

THEOFILOPOULOS *et al.*[74] made the interesting observation that Raji cells, a cell line derived from Burkitt's lymphoma cells, can also bind uncleaved C 3, which peripheral blood lymphocytes cannot. Inhibition experiments suggested that the native C3 was bound only by the C3b receptor and not by the C3d receptor on Raji cells.

### *1. Procedure*

The simplest way of demonstrating complement receptors is with erythrocyte-antibody-complement complexes (EAC; Fig. 273). Erythrocytes are coated with anti-erythrocyte antibodies (EA). The use of anti-erythrocyte antibodies of the IgM type is recommended, since so far no receptor

[71] EDEN, BIANCO, NUSSENZWEIG and MAYER, 1973.
[72] 1975.
[73] EDEN, MILLER and NUSSENZWEIG, 1973; ROSS and POLLEY, 1975.
[73a] 1974.
[74] THEOFILOPOULOS, BOKISCH and DIXON, 1974.

Fig. 272a–h. Symbolic representation of sequence of binding of complement components to cell membrane *via* the classic pathway. When one IgM antibody or two IgG antibodies (shown here) are bound to adjacent sites of a cell membrane (e.g., of an erythrocyte, as shown here), the one IgM molecule or the two adjacent IgG antibodies can activate complement factor Cl, which is inactive until it binds to the antibodies. Cl consists of three subunits, Clq, Clr, and Cls, held together by a calcium ion ($Ca^{++}$). The Clq subunit is able to bind to the complement-binding sites on antibodies (a). When it is bound, the Cl complex becomes enzymatically active and will activate C4 that comes in contact with a Cls subunit (b, c). C4 breaks into two parts, C4a and C4b, and the latter binds to the cell surface nearby (d). When C2 comes in contact with the activated Cls (e), it too is split. In the presence of magnesium ions ($Mg^{++}$), the C2a fragment combines with C4b (f) to form an enzyme (C3 convertase), which splits C3 into C3a and C3b (g). The C3b fragment binds to the surface membrane. This EAC14b2a3b (abbreviated EAC3b)

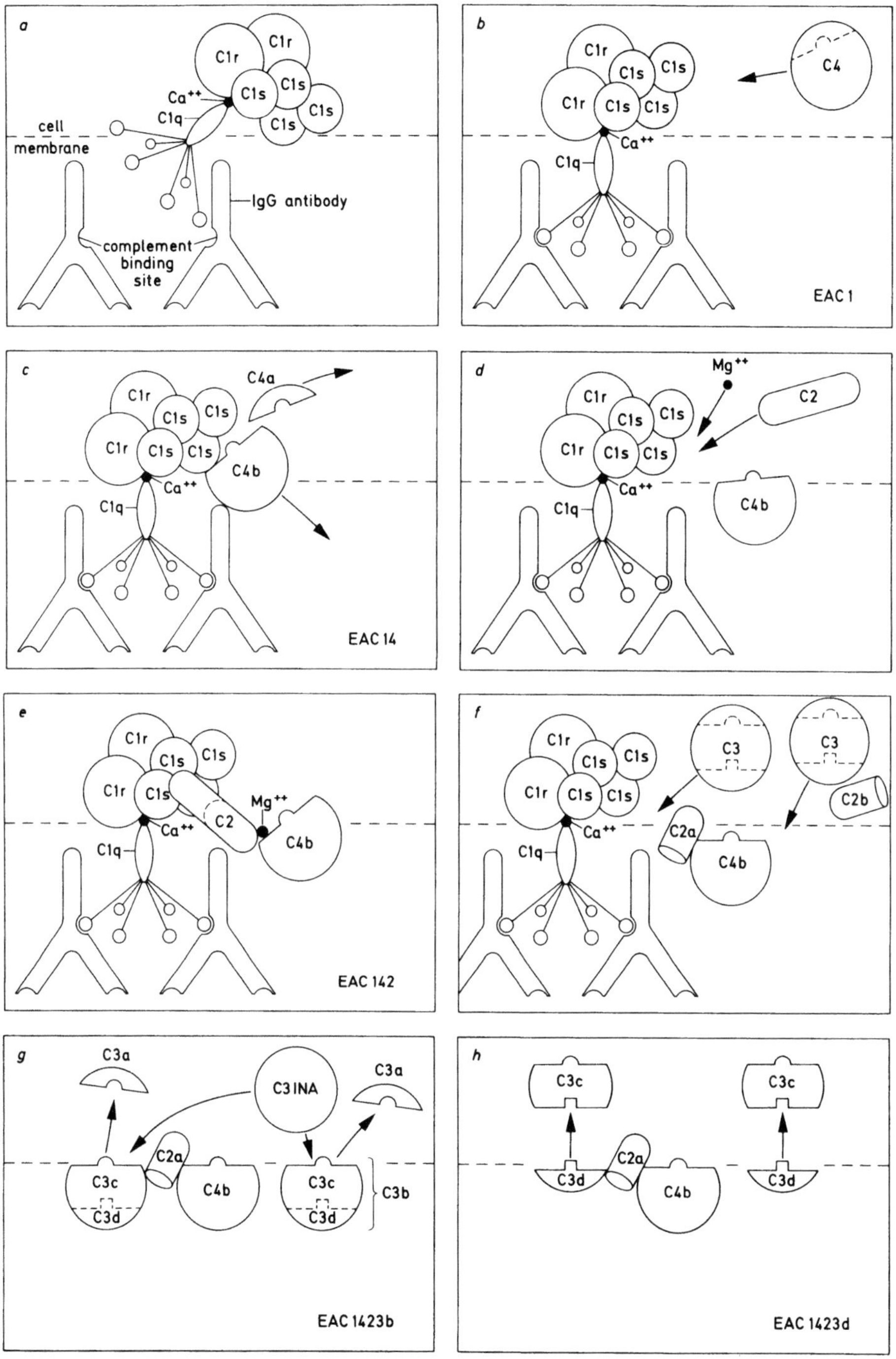


complex is used for the detection of C3b receptors. The EAC3b complex can be converted into an EAC3d complex by splitting the C3b into the subunits C3c and C3d with a C3b inactivator (*C3 INA*). The C3c fragment is released, whereas the C3d fragment remains membrane-bound. The C3d-specific binding site is uncovered by the cleavage of C3b (h). (Modification of diagram published by MAYER, 1973)

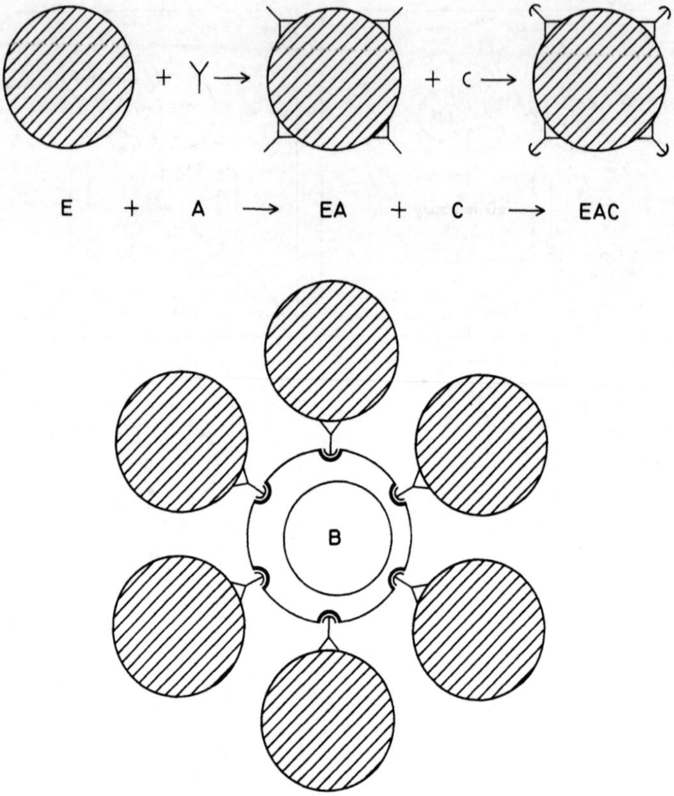


Fig. 273. Symbolic representation of the rosette assay for the detection of complement receptors. At the top, how to prepare erythrocyte-antibody-complement complexes (*EAC*) by coating erythrocytes (*E*) with antibodies (*A*) and complement (*C*). At the bottom, how these indicator cells form rosettes with complement receptor-bearing B-cell (*B*)

for IgM antibodies has been demonstrated on freshly drawn white blood cells. Erythrocytes that have been coated with IgG antibodies should not be used, because it is possible for them to be bound *via* the IgG-Fc receptor.

Sheep erythrocytes (E) are particularly suitable for the EAC assay, since they are much smaller than erythrocytes from other animals or humans. If one wants to use sheep EAC for the detection of complement receptors on T-cells or on cells of T-cell neoplasms, it is advisable to trypsinize the sheep erythrocytes before coating them with IgM and complement, since sheep erythrocytes can also be bound spontaneously by T-cells, particularly thymocytes and T-ALL cells, under non-sheep-E rosette-forming conditions (see p. 559). Pretreatment with trypsin destroys the surface determinants for sheep-E receptors without significantly affecting the surface antigenicity of the sheep erythrocytes. To achieve a sensitive assay for complement receptors, it is advisable to coat the sheep erythrocytes as thickly as possible with antibodies. We therefore incubate the sheep erythrocytes with the 19 S fraction of an anti-sheep-E antiserum at just the dilution at which the sheep erythrocytes do not agglutinate. The sheep EA thus prepared is then incubated in diluted (1:4) serum from NMRI or C5-deficient mice. That yields the EAC142356789 complex, usually abbreviated EACmouse; or, when serum from C5-deficient mice is used, the EAC1423 complex, called EAC (C5-deficient mouse). The IgMEA is not lysed when NMRI or C5-deficient-mouse serum is used as the source of complement, because the complement of the NMRI mouse strain has extremely low lytic activity, and that of the C5-deficient mice none at all. Coating of IgMEA with C 3 molecules is good in both cases.

Specific demonstration of complement-receptor subtypes on suspended cells is possible only when EAC is prepared with pure complement components. That is also true for the EAC prepared with C5-deficient-mouse serum. The latter type of EAC is thought to be specific for the C3d receptor.[75] In our tests, EAC (C5-deficient mouse) often clearly reacted with human erythrocytes, which are known to have receptors only for C3b. Nevertheless, EACmouse and EAC (C5-deficient mouse) appear to be bound mainly *via* the C3d fragment on tissue sections; this was suggested by the results of adherence tests on cryostat sections from tonsils using EAC3b and EAC3d prepared with purified complement components (Cordis, U.S.A.). The EAC3b was prepared according to the procedure of BORSOS and RAPP.[76] The EAC3d was converted into EAC3b by incubating the EAC3d with purified C3 inactivator for 2–4 hours. On tonsil sections the EAC3d exhibited a nodular adherence over germinal centers, similar to the adherence of EACmouse prepared with whole mouse serum or with C5-deficient-mouse serum and to the adherence of glutaraldehyde-fixed sheep erythrocytes thickly coated with human complement. In contrast, EAC3b adhered not only over germinal centers, but also over the interfollicular area between the germinal centers, resulting in a more diffuse adherence pattern (see Fig. 284a).[77]

DUKOR *et al.*[78] were the first investigators to demonstrate complement receptors on frozen sections. Frozen sections are layered with EAC and then washed thoroughly. EAC is extremely well bound by the complement receptors on frozen sections. After fixation and counterstaining with hematoxylin and eosin, the bound EAC is easy to recognize on dark-field microscopy as orange-red dots (see Figs. 283b and 285a). The sensitivity of the demonstration of complement receptors (probably C3d receptors) on frozen sections can be increased considerably when sheep erythrocytes are made resistent to hemolysis by means of glutaraldehyde fixation and are then coated to a maximum with antibodies and human complement. A further increase in sensitivity can be achieved by building a flat chamber over the frozen sections, filling it with EAC, and then centrifuging these slides at 200 g in a swinging rotor.

## 2. *Occurrence and Significance*

The complement receptor plays an important role in a variety of biologic processes: antibody- and antigen-triggering,[79] germinal center-cell formation,[80] antibody-mediated cytotoxicity *via* the C3b receptor,[81] phagocytosis,[82] clearance of large immunocomplexes by the phagocytic system and of small soluble immunocomplexes by the glomeruli apparatus,[83] and blood coagulation.[84] Nevertheless, the exact role of the complement receptor, and especially of its subtypes in the processes mentioned, is still unknown. In accordance with their different functions, complement receptors are expressed on a variety of cells, as documented in Table 94. In spite of the widespread occurrence of complement receptors, we regard them, particularly the subtypes, as important markers of lymphoid-cell subpopulations. Many studies have shown that a majority of complement receptor-bearing lymphocytes are SIg-positive and sheep-E receptor-negative.[85] DUKOR *et al.*[86] found that EACmouse on frozen sections of spleen and lymph node was bound exclusively to cells in

[75] DIERICH, PELLEGRINO, FERRONE and REISFELD, 1974.
[76] 1967.
[77] STEIN, SIEMSSEN and DIERICH, 1976, unpublished data.
[78] DUKOR, BIANCO and NUSSENZWEIG, 1970.
[79] PEPYS, 1972; MÖLLER and COUTINHO, 1975.
[80] DUKOR, BIANCO and NUSSENZWEIG, 1970; STEIN, 1976b; KLAUS and HUMPHREY, 1977.
[81] FLAD, FINK and DIERICH, 1977; PERLMANN, 1976.
[82] HUBER, POLLEY, LINSCOTT, FUDENBERG *et al.*, 1968; MANTOVANI, RABINOVITCH and NUSSENZWEIG, 1972.
[83] GELFAND, FRANK and GREEN, 1975.
[84] ROTHER and TILL, 1974.
[85] JONDAL, HOLM and WIGZELL, 1972; ROSS, RABELLINO, POLLEY and GREY, 1973.
[86] DUKOR, BIANCO and NUSSENZWEIG, 1970.

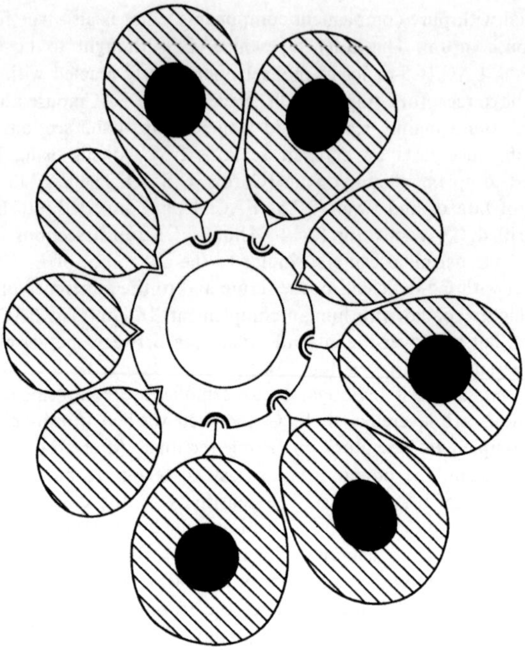

Fig. 274. Symbolic representation of the simultaneous demonstration of complement receptors and sheep-E receptors. Complement receptors are demonstrated with nucleated chicken erythrocytes coated with antibodies and complement. Sheep-E receptors are demonstrated with denucleated sheep erythrocytes

the follicles, whereas T-cell areas remained free. These and many other findings suggested that complement receptors are expressed exclusively on lymphoid cells of the B-cell system.

The situation recently became complicated after it was reported by SHEVACH *et al.*,[87] CHIAO *et al.*,[88] and our research group[89] that a small percentage (1–4%) of peripheral blood lymphocytes bear not only complement receptors, but also sheep-E receptors (see p. 559). The simultaneous presence of both receptors could be established in tests using IgM- and complement-coated nucleated erythrocytes (e.g., chicken EAC) and denucleated sheep erythrocytes. The principle of this technique is outlined in Figure 274. The simultaneous presence of complement receptors and sheep-E receptor on some peripheral blood lymphocytes became understandable after GATIEN *et al.*[90] detected complement receptors on thymocytes from human fetuses. They showed that fetal thymocytes of 9–10 weeks' gestation bore complement receptors, but no sheep-E receptors. With increasing fetal age, the thymocytes became complement receptor-negative and sheep-E receptor-positive. Our surface-marker studies[91] of fetal thymocytes confirmed the results of GATIEN *et al.*[90] Furthermore, we discovered that the switch in receptors on fetal thymocytes takes

[87] SHEVACH, EDELSON, FRANK, LUTZNER *et al.*, 1974.

[88] CHIAO, PANTIC and GOOD, 1974.

[89] STEIN, 1975a, b; STEIN, PETERSEN, GAEDICKE, LENNERT *et al.*, 1976.

[90] GATIEN, SCHNEEBERGER and MERLER, 1975.

[91] STEIN and MÜLLER-HERMELINK, 1977.

Table 95. Presence of the complement-receptor subtypes on cells of the two antigenic B-cell reactions and on T-cells in frozen sections

| Lymphatic subpopulation | Receptors for | |
|---|---|---|
| | C3b | C3d |
| B-cells of the plasma-cell reaction | + | − |
| B-cells of the germinal center-cell reaction | +++ | +++ |
| T-cells (postnatal) | − | − |

+++ = dense adherence of EAC reagent.

place *via* an intermediate cell type that simultaneously expresses complement receptors and sheep-E receptors. Recently, complement receptors were also detected on T-killer cells.[92] All of the mentioned findings demonstrate that the presence of complement receptors is not specific to B-cells. Thus, the complement receptor should not be used alone as a B-cell marker.

In our opinion, the analysis of complement-receptor subtypes may be of help in differentiating between B-cells of the plasma-cell reaction, first described by FAGRAEUS[93] and studied in detail by VELDMAN,[94] and B-cells of the germinal center-cell reaction. As mentioned previously, it was shown on frozen sections that C3d receptors are exclusively expressed by germinal-center cells, including the cells in the inner part of the follicular mantle zone.[95] C3b receptors are also expressed by germinal-center cells. In contrast to the C3d receptor, however, the C3b receptor is often present on cells in the outer part of the mantle zone and on cells in the interfollicular area between the follicles and germinal centers.[95] The interfollicular area contains not only T-cells, but also cells of the plasma-cell reaction.[96]

From these data we conclude that (1) the sole expression of the C3b receptor suggests cells related to the plasma-cell reaction, (2) the simultaneous expression of C3d and C3b receptors is indicative of cells related to germinal-center cells (Table 95), and (3) the adherence of EAC prepared with whole serum from NMRI mice, C5-deficient mice, or humans, on frozen sections suggests cells related to germinal-center cells. Nonadherence of such EAC reagents does not necessarily indicate a complete lack of complement receptors; it may mean only a lack of C3b receptors.

SHEVACH *et al.*[97] pointed out that the adherence of EAC on frozen sections can be used to demonstrate not only complement receptors on lymphoid cells, but also those on monocytes and macrophages. In contrast, through simultaneous detection of complement receptors by means of EACmouse and demonstration of nonspecific esterase and acid phosphatase in monocytes, macrophages, and reticulum cells, we showed that, as a rule, the complement receptors on lymphoid cells usually maintained their binding capacity on frozen sections, whereas most of the complement receptors on macrophages and monocytes often appeared to be inactivated.

[92] PERLMANN, 1976.
[93] 1948.
[94] 1970.
[95] STEIN, SIEMSSEN and LENNERT, 1978.
[96] VELDMAN, 1970.
[97] SHEVACH, JAFFE and GREEN, 1973.

# G. Mouse-Erythrocyte (E) Receptor

STATHOPOULOS and ELLIOT[98] reported that a subset (approximately 10%) of peripheral blood lymphocytes and chronic lymphocytic leukemia (CLL) cells were capable of spontaneously forming rosettes with mouse erythrocytes (E). Later, GUPTA *et al.*[99] observed enhanced binding of mouse erythrocytes when the lymphocytes were pretreated with neuraminidase.

### *1. Procedure*

Untreated lymphoid cells or lymphoid cells pretreated with neuraminidase are mixed with fetal calf serum (heat-inactivated and absorbed with mouse erythrocytes) and mouse erythrocytes. The mixture is centrifuged at 200 g for 5 min at room temperature, followed by incubation without agitation at 28° C for 1 hour. The pellet is gently resuspended by rotating the test tube around its long axis. Because the rosettes are very fragile, they have to be counted in a chamber.

### *2. Occurrence and Significance*

Using untreated lymphocytes, GUPTA *et al.*[99] recently showed that mouse-E receptors were chiefly detectable on cells that bore surface IgM. Mouse erythrocytes were not bound by thymocytes, peripheral T-cells, monocytes, or other myeloid cells (see Table 94). Treatment of peripheral blood lymphocytes with neuraminidase increased the percentage of mouse-E rosette-forming cells from 7.4 to 16.2%. T-cells pretreated with neuraminidase did not form rosettes with mouse erythrocytes. Thus, neuraminidase treatment presumably exposes hidden mouse E-binding sites on B-cells, but not on T-cells.

CATOVSKY *et al.*[100] reported that there was a significant difference between the cells of CLL and those of other non-Hodgkin's lymphomas in the capacity to bind mouse erythrocytes: the proportion of mouse-E receptor-positive cells was significantly higher in CLL. Intermediate results were observed in hairy-cell leukemia (see p. 585). GUPTA *et al.*[99] recently found large numbers of mouse-E rosette-forming cells in the blood of patients with CLL, even though SIg could not be detected on the lymphocytes.

# H. Sheep-Erythrocyte (E) Receptor

In 1969, BACH *et al.*[101] reported that some human lymphocytes form rosettes with sheep erythrocytes. In subsequent years, a large number of authors investigated this phenomenon.[102] The number of lymphocytes rosetting with sheep

---

[98] 1974.

[99] GUPTA, GOOD and SIEGAL, 1976a.

[100] CATOVSKY, CHERCHI, OKOS, HEGDE *et al.*, 1976.

[101] BACH, DORMONT, DARDENNE and BALNER, 1969.

[102] E.g., BRAIN, GORDON and WILLETTS, 1970; COOMBS, GURNER, WILSON, HOLM *et al.*, 1970; LAY, MENDES, BIANCO and NUSSENZWEIG, 1971; FRØLAND, 1972; JONDAL, HOLM and WIGZELL, 1972; ROSS, RABELLINO, POLLEY and GREY, 1973.

erythrocytes was steadily increased through improvement of the technical parameters. In 1970, the percentage of sheep-E rosette-forming blood lymphocytes was said to be 5–15%; in 1971, 15–40%; and in 1972 and 1973, 50–80%. These percentages illustrate that the amount of sheep-E rosette-forming lymphocytes is crucially dependent on the technical execution of the rosette test. The technical parameters that must be taken into consideration in the execution of the sheep E-rosette test will be discussed in the following section.

### *1. Technical Parameters*

1. Contamination of the lymphocyte population with autologous erythrocytes must not exceed a certain limit. Erythrocytes can be separated most effectively from the lymphocytes by means of the density-centrifugation method of BØYUM.[103] When this method is properly used to collect blood lymphocytes, they show practically no contamination with autologous erythrocytes.

2. LAY *et al.*[104] observed that the highest number of rosettes was achieved with incubation at 37° for a short time (15–60 min), followed by a longer period (1–2 hours) of incubation at 0–4°C. Several authors[105] reported on a further improvement in the results when the first incubation time was shortened to 5 min and the second incubation phase was prolonged to 10–12 hours.

3. In order to achieve high rosette values, close contact of the sheep erythrocytes with the lymphocytes is essential. Close contact is attained by centrifuging the lymphocyte-sheep-erythrocyte mixture at 200 g.

4. Resuspension of the centrifuged cells must be performed extremely carefully. We resuspend by slowly swinging the reaction mixture back and forth in the centrifuge tube, letting the mixture run up and down the sides of the tube until resuspension is complete.

5. The sheep E-rosette test did not become a truly reliable and reproducible method until pretreatment of the sheep erythrocytes with neuraminidase or AET was introduced. In 1972, SEILER *et al.*[106] discovered that incubation of the sheep erythrocytes in neuraminidase greatly increased the capacity of these cells to bind to lymphocytes. This observation was confirmed by WEINER *et al.*[107] In 1974, KAPLAN and CLARK reported that the sulfhydryl reagent 2-amino-ethylisothiouronium-bromide (AET) changed the erythrocyte membrane in such a manner that it developed a highly increased affinity to lymphocytes. Pretreatment of sheep erythrocytes with neuraminidase or AET reduces the differences caused by the use of cells obtained from different animals and of different ages. In addition, it increases the number of rosetting lymphocytes to a constantly high level. Figure 275 presents the way the treatment of sheep erythrocytes with neuraminidase or AET might work.

In our own experiments using sheep erythrocytes pretreated with neuraminidase or AET, we determined almost equally high percentages (70–80%) of sheep-E rosette-forming cells in peripheral blood. In comparison with neuraminidase treatment, the AET method has the advantage that AET-treated sheep erythrocytes can be kept for a week. In contrast, neuraminidase-treated erythrocytes must be made anew each day. A disadvantage of the AET method is sometimes that AET-treated sheep erythrocytes show more of a tendency to hemolyze.

### *2. Occurrence and Significance*

The postnatal thymus contains the most sheep-E rosette-forming cells (95–100%). After the thymus, the peripheral blood reveals the most sheep-E

[103] 1968.

[104] LAY, MENDES, BIANCO and NUSSENZWEIG, 1971.

[105] BACH and DORMONT, 1971; JONDAL, HOLM and WIGZELL, 1972; PAPAMICHAIL, HOLBOROW, KEITH and CURREY, 1972; ROSS, RABELLINO, POLLEY and GREY, 1973.

[106] SEILER, SEDLACEK, KANZY and LANG, 1972.

[107] WEINER, BIANCO and NUSSENZWEIG, 1973.

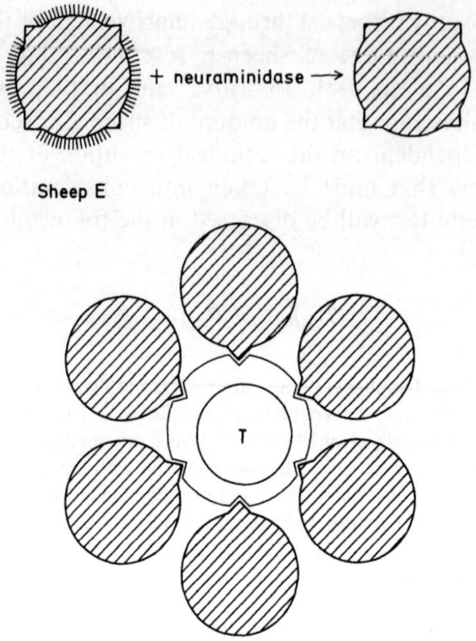


Fig. 275. Symbolic representation of the rosette assay for the detection of the T-cell-specific sheep-erythrocyte receptor. At the top, how neuraminidase might unmask sheep erythrocyte (*E*)-receptor determinants. At the bottom, how these indicator cells form rosettes with T-cells (*T*)

receptor-positive lymphocytes (see Table 94). The percentages reported by various authors varied between 50 and 80%.[108] In peripheral lymphatic organs, the number of sheep-E rosette-forming cells is clearly smaller: tonsils contain about 20–50%,[109] the spleen about 15–45%,[110] and lymph nodes about 20–70%.[111]

Inhibition experiments with antisera showed that anti-human Ig sera[112] do not lead to inhibition of sheep E-rosette formation. In contrast, inhibition of sheep E-rosette formation due to the presence of anti-lymphocyte sera[113] or anti-thymocyte serum[114] has been observed. Specific anti-B-cell sera did not inhibit rosette formation.[114] On the basis of these results, together with other data from cell-separation experiments and findings in immune-deficiency diseases, sheep-E rosette-forming cells may be considered to be T-cells.

---

[108] SEILER, SEDLACEK, KANZY and LANG, 1972; BENTWICH, DOUGLAS, SKUTELSKY and KUNKEL, 1973; FRØLAND and NATVIG, 1973; JONDAL, WIGZELL and AIUTI, 1973; ROSS, RABELLINO, POLLEY and GREY, 1973; WEINER, BIANCO and NUSSENZWEIG, 1973; STEIN, PETERSEN, GAEDICKE, LENNERT *et al.*, 1976.

[109] FRØLAND and NATVIG, 1973; SMITH and HAEGERT, 1974; KRÜGER, UHLMANN, HELLRIEGEL, SESTERHENN *et al.*, 1976.

[110] FRØLAND and NATVIG, 1973.

[111] ROSS, RABELLINO, POLLEY and GREY, 1973; AISENBERG and LONG, 1975; KRÜGER, UHLMANN, HELLRIEGEL, SESTERHENN *et al.*, 1976.

[112] BRAIN, GORDON and WILLETTS, 1970; COOMBS, GURNER, WILSON, HOLM *et al.*, 1970; FRØLAND, 1972; JONDAL, WIGZELL and AIUTI, 1973; WHITTINGHAM and MACKAY, 1973; DICKLER, ADKINSON and TERRY, 1974; KAPLAN and CLARK, 1974.

[113] BACH, DORMONT, DARDENNE and BALNER, 1969; KELLY, MEARS and SHELL, 1971; FRØLAND, 1972.

[114] WORTIS, COOPER and BROWN, 1973.

By using the sheep E-rosette test in combination with the demonstration of SIg, a number of authors[115] showed that SIg-positive lymphocytes do not form sheep-E rosettes. These results were corrected by DICKLER *et al.*[116] and KAPLAN and CLARK.[117] In their studies, a small percentage (2–6%) of peripheral blood lymphocytes proved to bear both SIg and sheep-E receptors.

The simultaneous demonstration of complement receptors and sheep-E receptors by means of EAC and sheep erythrocytes yielded contradictory results. The experimental data of the years 1972 and 1973 showed no overlapping of the mentioned receptors.[118] In contrast, more recent studies[119] revealed that a small percentage (1–2%) of peripheral blood lymphocytes do bear both types of surface receptors.

Early fetal thymocytes are apparently a special type of T-cell. As already mentioned in the discussion of the complement receptor, fetal thymocytes of the 10th–20th week of gestation chiefly reveal the complement receptors characteristic of B-cells, whereas the sheep-E receptors characteristic of T-cells are largely absent. The capacity of fetal thymocytes to form rosettes with sheep erythrocytes develops during the fetal period with increasing fetal age and is almost complete at the time of birth. As mentioned previously (see p. 554), complement receptors and sheep-E receptors are simultaneously present on fetal thymocytes of 12–22 weeks' gestation.[120]

MENDES *et al.*[120a] reported that, in contrast to T-lymphocytes, thymocytes reveal the capacity to form rosettes with sheep erythrocytes even after prolonged incubation at 37° C. SEN and BORELLA[121] confirmed this finding. Thus, testing of sheep-E rosettes that are stable or unstable at 37° C provides a simple procedure for distinguishing thymocytes and their neoplastic counterparts (e.g., some T-ALL cells) from peripheral T-cells and their neoplastic counterparts (e.g., cells from CLL, mycosis fungoides, or Sézary's syndrome). It should be mentioned, however, that blast cells of the T-type induced *in vitro* by mitogens also form sheep-E rosettes that are stable at 37° C.[121a]

## *Addendum*
## *Evaluation of Rosette Tests*

As already mentioned, complement receptors, IgG-Fc receptors, and mouse-E and sheep-E receptors can be demonstrated most easily and reliably by means of the rosette procedure. This procedure has therefore found widespread use in applied immunology. In the characterization of lymphoid tumor cells, the significance of the rosette test is crucially dependent on the evaluation of the results. Essentially, there are two parameters: (1) the number of cells in a suspension that form rosettes with the added indicator erythrocytes, and (2) the type of cell (myeloid or lymphoid, reactive or neoplastic cells) that binds the indicator cells.

---

[115] FRØLAND, 1972; PAPAMICHAIL, HOLBOROW, KEITH and CURREY, 1972; BRAIN and MARSTON, 1973; JONDAL, WIGZELL and AIUTI, 1973; ROSS, RABELLINO, POLLEY and GREY, 1973.

[116] DICKLER, ADKINSON and TERRY, 1974.

[117] 1974.

[118] JONDAL, HOLM and WIGZELL, 1972; BIANCO, WEINER and NUSSENZWEIG, 1973; GILBERTSEN and METZGAR, 1973.

[119] CHIAO, PANTIC and GOOD, 1974; SHEVACH, EDELSON, FRANK, LUTZNER *et al.*, 1974; STEIN, 1975a, b; STEIN, PETERSEN, GAEDICKE, LENNERT *et al.*, 1976.

[120] STEIN and MÜLLER-HERMELINK, 1977.

[120a] MENDES, TOLNAI, SILVEIRA, GILBERTSEN *et al.*, 1973.

[121] 1975.

[121a] SEN, MILLS and BORELLA, 1976.

In most laboratories, the number of rosetting cells is determined with a hemocytometer (counter chamber). The great disadvantage of this method is that one cannot distinguish between lymphoid cells and mononuclear cells of the myeloid cell series (especially monocytes and macrophages) in cell populations from the bone marrow, blood, or spleen. Subsequent correction, for example, of the lymphocyte-rosette values by subtracting the monocyte values according to the percentage of monocytes determined in a parallel centrifuge slide, is an uncertain procedure with a statistically high rate of error. Thus, we routinely prepare smears of resuspended reaction mixtures by adding a drop of 10% bovine albumin to each one before carefully applying it to a wide area on a microscopic slide. After being dried for a short time ($^1/_2$–1 min), the smears are centrifuged for 5 min at 200 g. During centrifugation, the cells are spread out on the slide without running off the slide or changing their position. The two-phase preparation of the slides (slight drying of the cell/albumin mixture on the slide and subsequent centrifugation) guarantees that the relationship between rosette-negative and rosette-forming cells does not change. Since the erythrocytes cannot change their position either, all rosettes remain intact. The centrifuge imprints are subsequently stained with May-Grünwald-Giemsa (Pappenheim) or with enzyme-cytochemical stains. The slides can be cytologically evaluated so well that most of the cells can be clearly differentiated. When difficulties arise, particularly with bone marrow-cell suspensions, additional cytochemical staining is recommended.

For the merely qualitative evaluation of rosette tests, equal amounts of the resuspended reaction mixture (about $5 \times 10^5$ white blood cells) mixed with 10% bovine albumin are centrifuged onto microscopic slides by means of a cytocentrifuge. Such "cyto"-slides are of excellent cytologic quality. Besides conventional hematologic stainings, such as May-Grünwald-Giemsa, the enzyme reactions for peroxidase and chloroacetate esterase can be performed on these slides without destruction of the rosettes. Partial destruction or leaching of the erythrocytes occurs with the enzyme reactions for acid phosphatase and acid and neutral nonspecific esterase, because these reactions must be performed on unfixed slides. When the slides are well dried before the enzyme reactions, however, the rosette-forming cells can still be evaluated, even after the enzyme-cytochemical reactions for acid phosphatase and acid and neutral nonspecific esterase.

The disadvantage of preparing slides by means of a cytocentrifuge is that selective accumulation of rosetting cells occurs on the cytoslides. Cytoslides are therefore not suitable for the quantification of rosette-forming cells.

## I. Human T-Associated Antigens

There are several different T-associated antigens that are more or less specific to T-cells. These antigens are listed in Table 96.

### *1. Human T-Lymphocyte Antigen (HTLA)*

Mouse T-lymphocytes bear a specific surface marker, called $\theta$-antigen or Thy-1 antigen, which is not present on other types of lymphocytes.[122] The first reports on specific anti-human T-cell antibodies were published in 1973.[123] The anti-T-cell sera were prepared by immunizing rabbits or other animals with human thymocytes. Multiple cross-reactions with other cells besides the T-cells in the xenogenic anti-T-cell sera were a great problem and, until recently, could be only partly eliminated by means of absorption. Thus, these anti-T-cell sera could be used only in cytotoxicity assays for human T-lymphocyte antigen (HTLA), but not in direct visualization of HTLA by labeling the antisera.

---

[122] Reif and Allen, 1964; Raff, 1970.

[123] Aiuti and Wigzell, 1973; Smith, Terry, Buell and Sell, 1973; Williams, DeBoard, Mellbye, Messner *et al.*, 1973.

Table 96. Occurrence and localization of T-associated antigens in various types of cells

| | HTLA[a] | THYSA[b] | HTHY-L[c] | CLL-THYA[d] | Brain-ass. TA[e] |
|---|---|---|---|---|---|
| Thymocytes | ++ | ++ | ++ | + | + |
| Peripheral T-lymphocytes | + | − | − | − | + |
| Peripheral B-lymphocytes | − | − | − | + | − |
| T-ALL cells | ++ | ++ | ++ | − | + |
| Null-ALL cells | − | − | + | + | − |
| Localization | Cell surface | Cell surface | Cytoplasm | Cell surface | Cell surface |

[a] Rodt, Thierfelder, Thiel, Götze *et al.*, 1975.
[b] Mills, Sen and Borella, 1975.
[c] Chechik, Pyke and Gelfand, 1976.
[d] Brouet, Valensi, Daniel, Flandrin *et al.*, 1976.
[e] Brain-associated T-cell antigen; Brown, Greaves, Lister, Rapson *et al.*, 1974.

The data on the occurrence of HTLA on malignant-lymphoma cells reported here were therefore chiefly gained from cytotoxicity assays.

Recently, Rodt *et al.*[124] succeeded in preparing a highly specific anti-T-cell serum by means of exhaustive absorptions with kidney homogenate and with a pool of CLL cells and of lymphoblastoid cell lines. This anti-T-cell serum showed a specific reaction with thymocytes, peripheral T-cells, and Molt-4-line cells, but not with cells from EBV-positive lymphoblastoid cell lines or with cells from CLL of the B-cell type. Since then, other research groups have prepared specific anti-T-cell sera suitable for immunofluorescence or other labeling procedures.[125]

It proved to be of considerable interest to determine not only the distribution, but also the amount of HTLA on normal and neoplastic lymphoid cells. Thiel and co-workers[126] developed an autoradiographic method for quantitating HTLA using the IgG fraction of an anti-T-cell serum labeled with $^{125}I$. When this method was used, the highest concentration of T-cell antigen was found on thymocytes. Peripheral blood and tonsil T-cells bore half the amount of HTLA. Similar differences between thymocytes and splenic T-cells were observed in mice.[127] Cells from malignant T-cell neoplasms also revealed different amounts of HTLA. Cells from acute lymphoblastic leukemia (ALL) of the T-cell type, for example, expressed HTLA in a density ranging from that of thymocytes to that of peripheral blood T-cells (see p. 636).[128] The number of HTLA sites on cells from three cases of CLL of the T-cell type was comparable to that on splenic or peripheral blood T-cells (see p. 575).

---

[124] Rodt, Thierfelder, Thiel, Götze *et al.*, 1975.
[125] E.g., Brouet, Flandrin, Sasportes, Preud'Homme *et al.*, 1975.
[126] Thiel, Rodt, Huhn and Thierfelder, 1976; Thiel, Dörmer, Rodt, Huhn *et al.*, 1977.
[127] Thiele and Stark, 1971.
[128] Thiel, Dörmer, Rodt, Huhn *et al.*, 1977.

## 2. *Thymocyte-Specific Antigen (THYSA)*

MILLS *et al.*[128a] demonstrated that an anti-thymocyte serum reacted with at least two distinct thymus-associated surface antigens. One of them was present on T-lymphocytes from peripheral blood and on thymocytes; it is probably identical with HTLA. The other antigen was present only on normal thymocytes and on a subset of T-ALL cells. The thymocyte-specific antiserum was obtained by absorption of the anti-thymocyte serum with peripheral blood T-lymphocytes. MILLS *et al.* called the antigen "TL-like antigen." In order to avoid confusion with terms for other T-associated antigens, however, we prefer the term "thymocyte-specific antigen" (THYSA).

## 3. *Human Thymus/Leukemia-Associated Antigen (HTHY-L)*

In 1968, CHECHIK detected a saline-extractable antigen in normal human thymic tissue and in leukemia cells. Unlike other T-cell-characteristic antigens, such as HTLA, this so-called human thymus/leukemia-associated antigen (HTHY-L) is not expressed on the surface of the cells—it occurs only in the cytoplasm. HTHY-L was found in extracts of normal human thymocytes, sheep-E rosette-positive T-cell lines, and cells from sheep-E rosette-positive ALL. HTHY-L was also present in sheep-E rosette-negative ALL and acute myeloid leukemia, whereas only trace amounts of this antigen were found in peripheral blood lymphocytes and in cells of B-cell lines.[128b] One explanation for these findings is that HTHY-L is clearly, but only temporarily expressed in all hemopoietic cells in the very early stages of differentiation, whereas it is expressed for a longer time in the T-cell axis up to mature thymocytes. During further differentiation of thymocytes into T-cells, the synthesis of HTHY-L appears to be suppressed. Thus, HTHY-L seems to be a differentiation antigen of the T-cell line until the development of mature thymocytes.

## 4. *CLL/Thymus Antigen (CLL-THYA)*

This antigen was detected with anti-CLL sera absorbed with peripheral T-cells from a patient with agammaglobulinemia.[128c] The antisera reacted with thymocytes, normal blood B-lymphocytes, B-ALL cells, and B-CLL cells. They showed negative reactions with T-derived ALL cells from 18 out of 19 cases and with acute myeloid leukemia cells, but positive reactions with cells from 30 out of 33 cases of null ALL. These findings indicate that CLL-THYA is different from HTLA and THYSA, which are both present on T-ALL cells, but absent from null-ALL, B-ALL, and B-CLL cells. The occurrence of CLL-THYA on both normal and leukemic cells suggests that it is not a leukemia-specific antigen, but rather a differentiation antigen that is present on hemopoietic cells of a very early stage of differentiation and retained in the B-cell line.

---

[128a] MILLS, SEN and BORELLA, 1975.
[128b] CHECHIK, PYKE and GELFAND, 1976.
[128c] BROUET, VALENSI, DANIEL, FLANDRIN *et al.*, 1976.

## J. Common-ALL Antigen

GREAVES *et al.*[128d] raised antisera in rabbits against cells of ALL lacking all known markers (null ALL). After exhaustive absorption with erythrocytes, tonsil cells, normal bone-marrow cells, and acute myeloid leukemia cells, these sera appeared to be leukemia-specific. They reacted with cells from 251 out of 348 (72%) cases of null ALL. GREAVES *et al.*[128d] called the null ALL with anti-ALL reactive cells "common ALL." We shall therefore use the term common-ALL antigen for the respective antigen. GREAVES *et al.* reported that the anti-common ALL sera also reacted with cells from other types of leukemia and lymphoma, namely, four out of 86 (5%) cases of acute myeloid leukemia, two out of 29 lymphomas, and, surprisingly, 26 out of 57 cases of $Ph^1$-positive chronic myeloid leukemia in blast crisis, but none out of 16 cases of chronic myeloid leukemia and none out of 16 cases of CLL. The blast-crisis cells in chronic myeloid leukemia cross-reacted completely with those of common ALL. All the common-ALL antigen-positive blast-crisis cells were lymphoid in appearance and lacked conventional myeloid markers.[128e]

Extensive screening studies showed that common-ALL antigen does not appear to cross-react with any of the known oncogenic viruses of murine, feline, or primate origin. Because of the non-cross-reactivity of anti-common ALL serum with oncogenic-virus antigen and because of the presence of common-ALL antigen on leukemic cells of different types, GREAVES *et al.*[128d] were of the opinion that common-ALL antigen might be a differentiation antigen that is exhibited only at a very early stage of differentiation and maturation, i.e., on pluripotent and oligopotent stem cells.

## K. Human B-Associated Antigens: Ia-Like Antigens

Recently, a surface glycoprotein complex was obtained from cell membranes of a human B-lymphoblast line.[129] The complex was solubilized with papain. It had a mass of 23,000 and 30,000 daltons. Rabbit antisera against this complex were specifically cytotoxic to B-lymphocytes of peripheral blood, to cells from B-lymphoblast lines, and to complement receptor-positive, SIg-negative (null) lymphocytes. The glycoprotein complex was not present on T-lymphocytes, complement receptor-negative null lymphocytes, or platelets.

There is strong evidence that the human glycoprotein complex under discussion resembles murine Ia-antigen in chemical structure, tissue distribution, linkage to the major histocompatibility complex, and biologic functions as judged by the effect of heteroantisera in various systems. Antibodies with similar specificity have been detected in pregnancy sera.[130] Other authors have also reported

[128d] GREAVES, JANOSSY, ROBERTS, RAPSON *et al.*, 1977.

[128e] JANOSSY, GREAVES, REVESZ, LISTER *et al.*, 1976.

[129] HUMPHREYS, MCCUNE, CHESS, HERRMAN *et al.*, 1976.

[130] WINCHESTER, FU, WERNET, KUNKEL *et al.*, 1975; KUNKEL, 1976.

on Ia-like human B-cell antigens.[131] These antigens have been given various names, e.g., HL-B, HuBLAA, Da-antigen, and Merrit B-cell alloantigen.

The Ia-like glycoprotein complex is immunochemically and functionally different from previously identified membrane antigens, including SIg, HL-A antigens, $\beta_2$-microglobulin, IgG-Fc receptors, and complement receptors. Because of the restriction of the Ia-like antigen to B-lymphocytes and to a subpopulation of null lymphocytes under normal conditions, it is of considerable interest to study the presence of this antigen on cells from malignant lymphomas, including ALL. Such studies have so far revealed that the Ia-like antigen is present not only on cells from B-derived chronic lymphocytic and acute lymphoblastic leukemias, but also on ALL cells that lack all other known surface markers except for common-ALL antigen,[132] and on the blast-crisis cells of chronic myeloid leukemia (see pp. 638 and 643).[133] The occurrence of Ia-like antigen on null-ALL cells and blast-crisis cells of chronic myeloid leukemia, and its absence from T-derived leukemias or lymphomas[134] suggest that it is expressed on stem cells, including myeloid progenitors, and is preserved in the B-cell axis only until full maturation. This hypothesis was substantiated by the recent finding that antisera directed against Ia-like antigen is cytotoxic to normal myeloid stem cells (colony-forming unit culture; CFU-C).[134a] There is recent evidence that Ia-like antigen may also be expressed by stimulated T-cells;[134b] but the meaning of these data is still unclear.

## L. Terminal Deoxynucleotidyl Transferase (Tdt)

In healthy persons, terminal deoxynucleotidyl transferase (Tdt), a unique type of DNA polymerase, had been found only in the thymus and was considered to be a specific property of thymocytes.[134c] In 1975, McCaffrey *et al.*[134d] reported that they found Tdt in a majority of patients with ALL and in patients with chronic myeloid leukemia in blast crisis. Similar findings were reported by Sarin and Gallo.[134e] Low levels of Tdt have also been found in normal bone marrow, probably in thymocyte precursor cells, of humans[134d] and mice.[134f]

These observations and the findings on the distribution of common-ALL antigen, Ia-like antigen, and HTLA on nonneoplastic and neoplastic hemopoietic cells lead to the assumption that Tdt is present in pluripotent stem cells, prethymic precursor cells, mature thymocytes, and early myeloid precursors, e.g., myeloblasts and probably promyelocytes.

[131] Arbeit, Sachs, Amos and Dickler, 1975; Naeim, Gossett and Walford, 1977.

[132] Fu, Winchester and Kunkel, 1975a; Wernet, Schunter, Wilms and Waller, 1977.

[133] Wernet, Schunter, Wilms and Waller, 1977.

[134] Fu, Winchester and Kunkel, 1975; Schlossman, Chess, Humphreys and Strominger, 1976; Wernet, Schunter, Wilms and Waller, 1977.

[134a] Cline and Billing, 1977.

[134b] Dickler, Arbeit, Henkart and Sachs, 1976; McKenzie and Parish, 1976; Vadas, Miller, McKenzie, Chism *et al.*, 1976.

[134c] Chang, 1971.

[134d] McCaffrey, Harrison, Kung, Parkman *et al.*, 1976.

[134e] 1974; Sarin, Anderson and Gallo, 1976.

[134f] Silverstone, Cantor, Goldstein and Baltimore, 1976.

### M. Receptor for Hemagglutinin A from the Snail *Helix Pomatia* (HP)

In normal peripheral blood, receptors for hemagglutinin A from the snail *Helix pomatia* (HP) are found on neuraminidase-treated T-cells, but not on most B-cells.[134g] Some B-cells in peripheral blood, however, may also have the HP receptor. Since the HP receptor is present on T-cells in adults and on a relatively large proportion of B-cells of cord blood, HELLSTRÖM *et al.*[134h] assumed that the HP receptor might be part of a fetal component present on immature lymphocytes of both the T- and B-types, but that it is preferentially preserved on T-cells during maturation. Our own experiments[134i] revealed that monocytes and granulocytes do not bind HP, suggesting that the HP receptor is a specific marker of the lymphoid-cell system.

# II. Immunologic Findings and Their Relevance to the Classification of Non-Hodgkin's Lymphomas

## A. Chronic Lymphocytic Leukemia (CLL)

**Surface Immunoglobulin (SIg).** SELIGMANN's group[135] demonstrated SIg in 165 out of 170 cases of CLL. AISENBERG *et al.*[136] found SIg in all 25 cases in their first series and in 46 out of the 48 cases in their second series. Thirty out of our 31 cases revealed SIg. In the series of GREY *et al.*[137] five out of 18 cases of CLL showed either no fluorescence for SIg or fluorescence only for light chains. In freeze-thaw extracts of cells from the SIg-negative cases of CLL, however, the total amount of immunoglobulin was very similar to that found in the SIg-positive cases.[137a] This finding suggested that the synthesized immunoglobulin could not be transported and/or fixed in the surface membrane.

PREUD'HOMME and SELIGMANN[138] and HIJMANS[139] regularly found both heavy and light chains on the surfaces of Ig-positive CLL lymphocytes. In contrast, GREY *et al.*[137] detected only light chains on lymphocyte surface membranes in 20% of their cases of CLL.

[134g] HAMMARSTRÖM, HELLSTRÖM, PERLMANN and DILLNER, 1973; HELLSTRÖM, MELLSTEDT, PERLMANN, HOLM *et al.*, 1976.
[134h] HELLSTRÖM, MELLSTEDT, PERLMANN, HOLM *et al.*, 1976.
[134i] STEIN and KAPPS, 1977, unpublished data.
[135] BROUET, PREUD'HOMME and SELIGMANN, 1975.
[136] AISENBERG and BLOCH, 1972; AISENBERG, BLOCH and LONG, 1973.
[137] GREY, RABELLINO and PIROFSKY, 1971.
[137a] KUBO, GREY and PIROFSKY, 1974.
[138] 1972a.
[139] 1974.

Table 97. Presence of $\mu$- and/or $\delta$-chains on the surfaces of cells from chronic lymphocytic leukemia

| Author | Ig class | | Incidence | Light-chain type |
|---|---|---|---|---|
| | $\mu$ | $\delta$ | | |
| PREUD'HOMME *et al.*[a] | + | + | 17/20 | κ (10), λ (5), κ and λ (2) |
| | + | − | 3/20 | κ (2), λ (1) |
| | − | + | 0/20 | |
| KUBO *et al.*[b] | + | + | 4/7 | κ (3), λ (1) |
| | + | − | 1/7 | κ |
| | − | + | 2/7 | κ (1; one case was not tested) |
| FU *et al.*[c] | + | + | 7/14 | |
| | + | − | 4/14 | |
| | − | + | 3/14 | |
| STEIN and BRUHN[d] | + | + | 10/12 | |
| | + | − | 0/12 | |
| | − | + | 2/12 | |

[a] PREUD'HOMME, BROUET, CLAUVEL and SELIGMANN, 1974.
[b] KUBO, GREY and PIROFSKY, 1974.
[c] FU, WINCHESTER and KUNKEL, 1974.
[d] Unpublished data.

In a majority of cases that were quantitatively measured, the amount of SIg was reduced four to 10 times compared with that on normal B-lymphocytes.[140] Immunofluorescence provided qualitative evidence of the same fact. The different percentages of SIg-negative cases of CLL described by various authors may have been due, however, to differences in sensitivity of their fluorescence methods.

The immunoglobulin found on the surfaces of CLL cells is usually restricted to a single light- and heavy-chain class, strongly suggesting monoclonality of the proliferating cells. According to the findings of several authors,[141] IgM was the predominant heavy-chain class on the surfaces of CLL cells. SELIGMANN *et al.*[142] reported the following distribution of heavy chains in CLL: the SIg was IgM in 71%, IgG in 26%, and IgA in 1.4% of the cases; two heavy chains (biclonal Ig pattern) were produced in 1.4%.

In 17% of the cases studied, SELIGMANN *et al.*[142] found a mixed staining pattern characterized by the simultaneous presence of $\mu$-, $\gamma$-, $\kappa$-, and $\lambda$-chain determinants on freshly drawn cells. Other investigators[143] observed a mixed staining pattern in a majority of cases of CLL. After overnight culture at 37° C or removal of the SIg by means of trypsin treatment followed by incubation

[140] GREY, KUBO, RABELLINO, POLLEY *et al.*, 1974; TERNYNCK, DIGHIERO, FOLLEZOU and BINET, 1974.

[141] E.g., GREY, RABELLINO and PIROFSKY, 1971; AISENBERG and BLOCH, 1972; PREUD'HOMME and SELIGMANN, 1972a.

[142] SELIGMANN, PREUD'HOMME and BROUET, 1973.

[143] PAPAMICHAIL, BROWN and HOLBOROW, 1971; PIESSENS, SCHUR, MOLONEY and CHURCHILL, 1973.

for 5–7 hours at 37° C in tissue-culture medium, however, only one heavy-chain type and one light-chain type were detected on the surface of the cells from all cases studied by SELIGMANN *et al.*[143a] NIES *et al.*[144] obtained similar results in short-term tissue-culture experiments using incorporation of radioactive amino acids. These findings clearly support the monoclonal nature of all cases of CLL. The mixed staining pattern that led to a false polyclonal appearance was shown to be either due to the attachment of autoantibodies directed against surface antigenic determinants on the CLL cells or of immune complexes *via* the IgG-Fc and/or complement receptor, or due in some cases to antibody activity of the monoclonal surface IgM directed against normal native human IgG (rheumatoid-factor activity of the monoclonal surface IgM).[145]

FRÖLAND and NATVIG[146] studied a case of CLL with IgG-bearing cells and showed that the IgG was restricted to one subclass and Gm allotype. The demonstration in several cases of defined antibody activity of the SIg – such as the anti-human IgG mentioned previously,[145] anti-sheep erythrocytes,[147] and anti-human blood group I[147a] – on all proliferating cells reflects identical variable regions of the SIg. That provides further substantiation of the monoclonal nature of CLL.

Recent studies have revealed that in most cases of CLL an additional heavy-chain class is present on the surfaces of lymphocytes, namely, IgD.[148] Table 97 summarizes the data obtained by various authors on the presence of $\mu$-chain and $\delta$-chain determinants on CLL cells. There is agreement on the finding that the cells from more than half of the cases of CLL bear both $\mu$-chain and $\delta$-chain determinants. The data on the expression of $\mu$- or $\delta$-chains alone, however, differed from author to author.

In contrast to the findings of AISENBERG and BLOCH,[149] who found predominantly $\mu$-chain-positive cells, equal numbers of $\delta$-chain- and $\mu$-chain-positive CLL cells were found by several authors[148] and by our research group in most cases. By using the two-color fluorescence technique in connection with cocapping experiments, we established that in the $\mu$-chain-positive and $\delta$-chain-positive cases more than 90% of the cells simultaneously bore both $\mu$- and $\delta$-chains. By quantitative analysis KUBO *et al.*[150] demonstrated that in five out of seven cases the amount of IgD was 1.5–5 times greater than the amount of IgM on the surfaces of CLL cells.

The simultaneous presence of heavy chains does not interfere with the concept of monoclonality, because other heavy-chain classes were not observed in the $\mu/\delta$-chain-positive cases of CLL and because the light chains were of a single type. It was recently demonstrated[151] that the $\mu$- and $\delta$-chains that were simultaneously expressed on the CLL cells shared the same variable regions.

---

[143a] SELIGMANN, PREUD'HOMME and BROUET, 1973.
[144] NIES, OBERLIN, BROWN and HALPEN, 1973.
[145] PREUD'HOMME and SELIGMANN, 1972b.
[146] 1972.
[147] BROUET and PRIEUR, 1974.
[147a] PREUD'HOMME and SELIGMANN, 1972a.
[148] FU, WINCHESTER and KUNKEL, 1974; KUBO, GREY and PIROFSKY, 1974; PREUD'HOMME, BROUET, CLAUVEL and SELIGMANN, 1974.
[149] 1972.
[150] KUBO, GREY and PIROFSKY, 1974.
[151] FU, WINCHESTER and KUNKEL, 1975b; SALSANO, FROLAND, NATVIG and MICHAELSEN, 1974.

**Tissue Immunoglobulin.** *Saline Extract.* In 10 out of 48 cases of CLL the Ig content was significantly higher than that of normal thymuses. There was an increase in IgM in nine cases, in IgG in two cases, and in IgA in one case. The results of the IgM assays are shown in Figure 276. It is evident that in most cases of CLL the IgM values lay in the range of normal thymuses and normal lymph nodes.

The mean IgM value for the saline extracts of CLL tissue was as high as that of lymphoblastic lymphoma of the Burkitt type, higher than that of centroblastic/centrocytic lymphoma and lymphoblastic lymphoma of the convoluted-cell and unclassified types, and lower than that of centrocytic lymphoma, LP immunocytoma, centroblastic lymphoma, and immunoblastic lymphoma. The difference between the mean values for CLL and LP immunocytoma was particularly clear.

*Detergent Second Extract.* The Ig content of the detergent 2nd extracts from 23 out of 38 cases of CLL was higher than that of the thymus. There was an increase in IgM in 23 cases, in IgG in five cases, and in IgA in two cases. That shows that in most cases the immunoglobulin produced by CLL cells was not effectively solubilized by saline alone. The detergent mixture of NP40 and Na-desoxycholate proved to be more effective.

The mean IgM value (Fig. 277) for the detergent 2nd extracts from CLL lay in about the same range as that of centroblastic lymphoma, was significantly higher than that of lymphoblastic lymphoma of the convoluted-cell and unclassified types, and was conspicuously lower than that of LP immunocytoma, centrocytic lymphoma, centroblastic/centrocytic lymphoma, lymphoblastic lymphoma of the Burkitt type, and immunoblastic lymphoma. The greatest difference was found again between the values for CLL and LP immunocytoma.

The results of Ig assays of tissue extracts are consistent with the thesis deduced from surface-labeling experiments that most cases of CLL are proliferations of B-cells and that IgM is the major Ig class produced by CLL cells.

In 20 cases of CLL we determined the amount of IgD and IgE in tissue extracts. The extracts from two cases contained a significant amount of IgD, and the extract from one case revealed IgE. Surface labeling with horseradish peroxidase-labeled anti-IgE serum showed that a high percentage of the cells from the CLL with a high IgE content bore surface IgE/κ.[152] The expression of only one heavy- and light-chain type suggested autosynthesis of IgE.

[152] Stein, Bartels, Wiemer and Kaiserling, 1975.

▷

Fig. 276. Concentration of IgM measured in saline extracts of biopsy material from normal lymph nodes (*LN*) and entities of the Kiel Classification: chronic lymphocytic leukemia (*CLL*), LP immunocytoma (*LPI*), centrocytic lymphoma (*CC*), centroblastic/centrocytic lymphoma (*CB/CC*), centroblastic lymphoma (*CB*), lymphoblastic lymphoma of the Burkitt type (*B*), of the convoluted-cell type (*C*), and of the unclassified type (*U*), and immunoblastic lymphoma (*IB*). Black dots indicate IgM concentrations of tissue extracts that were associated with normal or decreased levels of IgM in the corresponding sera; white dot stands for a value measured in an adult patient with lymphoblastic lymphoma of the unclassified type. Triangles indicate IgM concentrations of tissue extracts that were associated with a significant, monoclonal increase in the IgM level of the corresponding sera. Height of each column is the mean value

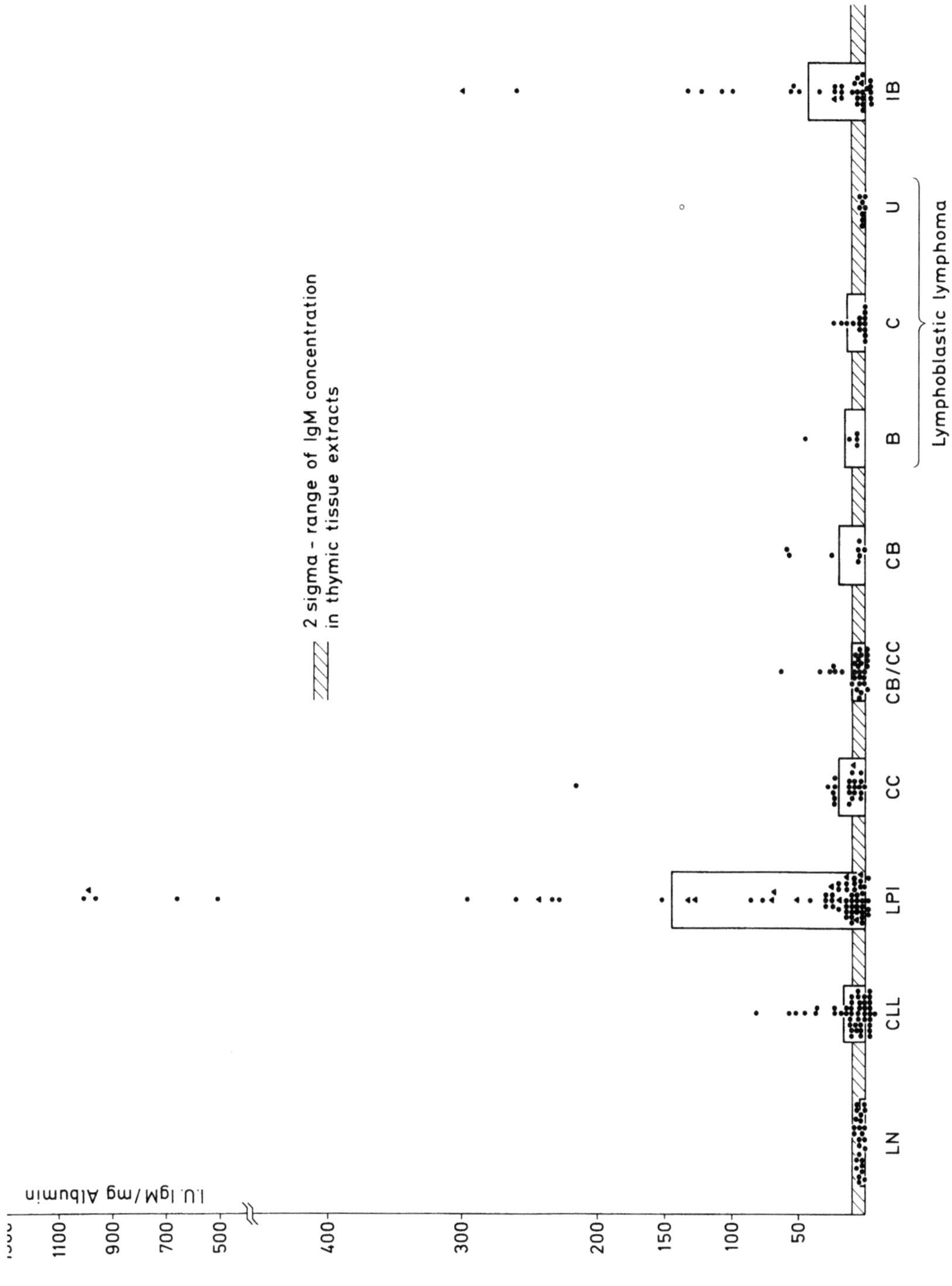
2 sigma - range of IgM concentration in thymic tissue extracts
I.U. IgM/mg Albumin
1100
900
700
500
400
300
200
150
100
50
LN
CLL
LPI
CC
CB/CC
CB
B
C
U
IB
Lymphoblastic lymphoma

The results of our IgD assays conflict with those of KUBO *et al.*[153] They found a significant amount of IgD in five out of seven freeze-thaw lysates of isolated, washed CLL cells. The IgD concentration, however, was never as high as the IgM values found in some cases. It is likely that we failed to detect IgD in most cases because we extracted whole tissue instead of washed cells or isolated surface membranes.

It may be of interest that the amount of IgM measured in freeze-thaw cell extracts from all cases was much greater (10–40 times) than that measured on the surface membranes of viable cells,[153] whereas the amount of IgD in the whole tissue extract was only two to five times greater. This finding indicates that IgD is much more concentrated at the cell membrane than IgM is in CLL.

In 10 cases we looked for the presence of free light chains in the tissue extracts. Free light chains can be distinguished from bound light chains by detecting determinants that are hidden when light chains are combined with heavy chains in whole proteins. Significant amounts of free $\kappa$-chains were measured in six cases and of free $\lambda$-chains in two cases. In one case no free light chains could be detected. These results are consistent with those of FU *et al.*,[154] who found readily detectable amounts of free light chains on cells from seven out of eight cases of CLL. The significance of free light chains on CLL cells is still unclear. In three out of 12 cases of CLL we found measurable amounts of free light chains in urine by means of the radial immunodiffusion assay.

**Serum Immunoglobulin.** In our 15 cases the serum-Ig levels were never above the $2\sigma$ range. They were usually in the lower normal range or even significantly reduced, which has also been reported by other authors.[155]

**Monoclonality of the Tissue and Serum Immunoglobulin.** The IgG fraction extracted from a surface IgG-positive CLL was monoclonal in polyacrylamide electrophoresis, whereas the serum IgG exhibited a polyclonal pattern (Fig. 278a, b).[156] The IgM extracted from the tissue from three patients with CLL was subjected to isoelectric focusing. A monoclonal IgM pattern was obtained in all three cases (Fig. 278c), whereas the serum IgM showed no restriction in heterogeneity (Fig. 278d).

[153] KUBO, GREY and PIROFSKY, 1974.
[154] FU, WINCHESTER and KUNKEL, 1974.
[155] DAMESHEK and GUNZ, 1964.
[156] STEIN, KAISERLING and LENNERT, 1974a.

Fig. 277. Concentration of IgM measured in detergent second extracts of biopsy material from normal lymph nodes (*LN*) and entities of the Kiel Classification: chronic lymphocytic leukemia (*CLL*), LP immunocytoma (*LPI*), centrocytic lymphoma (*CC*), centroblastic/centrocytic lymphoma (*CB/CC*), centroblastic lymphoma (*CB*), lymphoblastic lymphoma of the Burkitt type (*B*), of the convoluted-cell type (*C*), and of the unclassified type (*U*), and immunoblastic lymphoma (*IB*). Black dots indicate IgM concentrations of tissue extracts that were associated with normal or decreased levels of IgM in the corresponding sera; white dots stand for values measured in adult patients with lymphoblastic lymphoma of the unclassified type. Triangles indicate IgM concentrations of tissue extracts that were associated with a significant, monoclonal increase in the IgM level of the corresponding sera. Height of each column is the mean value

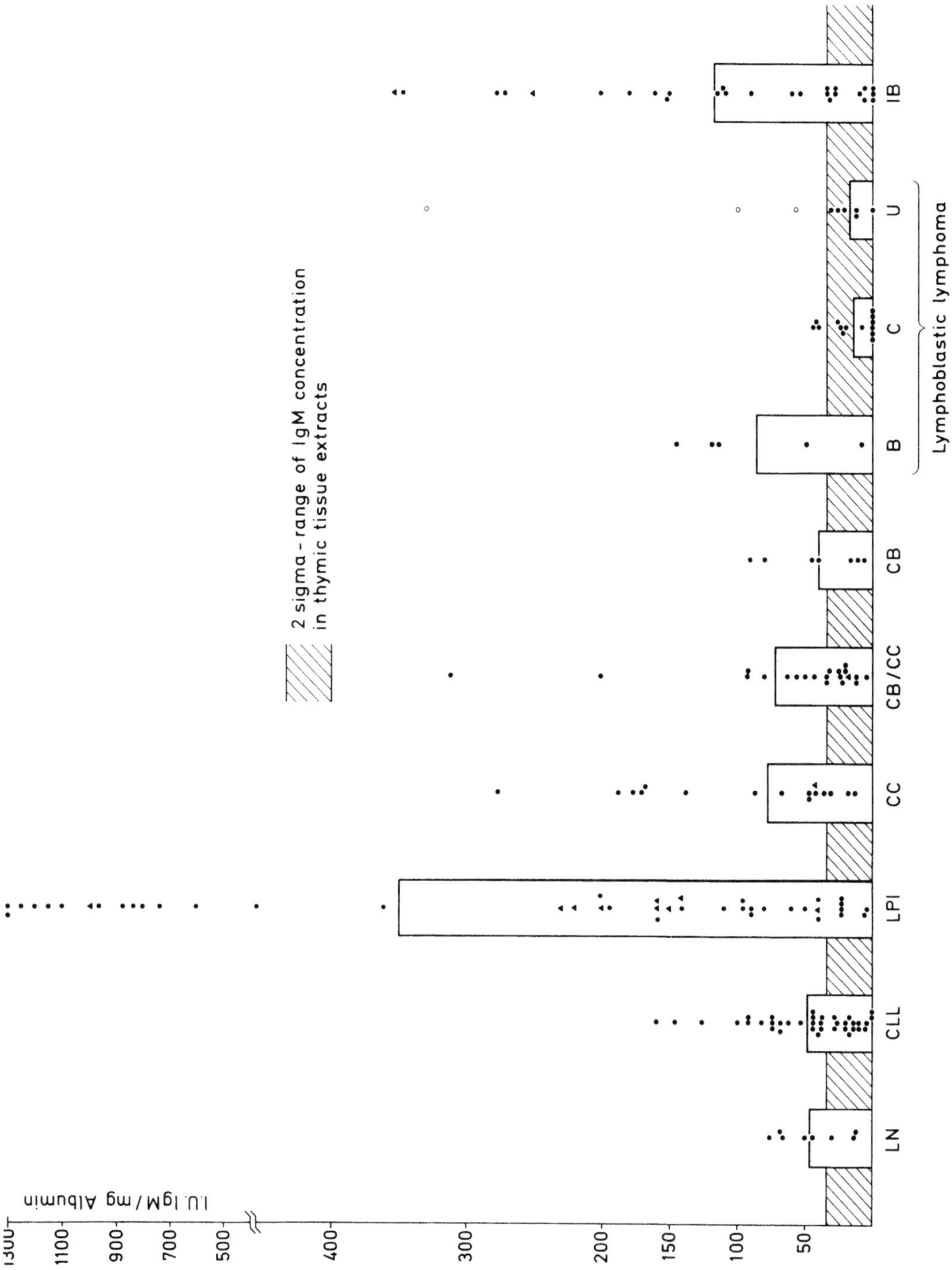
2 sigma - range of IgM concentration
in thymic tissue extracts
I.U. IgM / mg Albumin
1300
1100
900
700
500
400
300
200
150
100
50
LN
CLL
LPI
CC
CB/CC
CB
B
C
U
IB
Lymphoblastic lymphoma

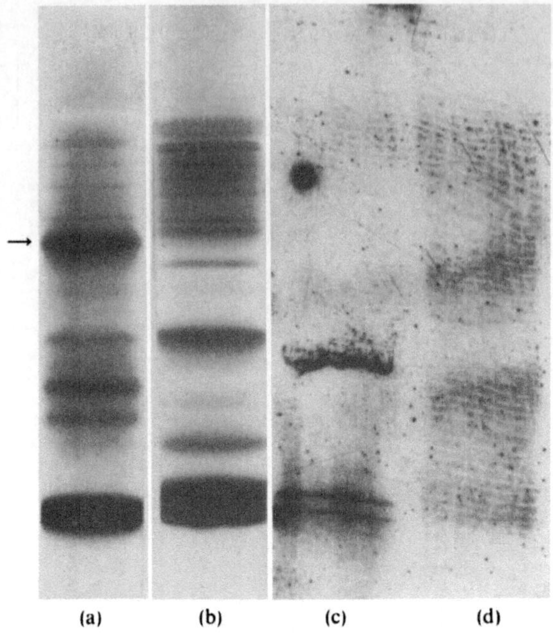


Fig. 278 (a–d). Chronic lymphocytic leukemia. (a, b) Polyacrylamide-gel electrophoresis of biopsy tissue extract (a) and serum (b). A monoclonal IgG fraction (arrow) is visible in (a), but not in (b). (c, d) Autoradiographs of reduced and carboxymethylated, isoelectrofocused IgM from biopsy tissue extract (c) and serum (d). The black band in the middle of (c) is the site of application

**Cytoplasmic Immunoglobulin (CIg).** CIg could not be demonstrated with fluorescein-labeled anti-Ig antibodies or by the very sensitive enzyme-bridge (PAP) method in the leukemic cells from any of the 15 cases of CLL we studied. PREUD'HOMME and SELIGMANN[157] observed CIg in only four out of 73 cases of CLL. It is likely, however, that these four cases were not representative of CLL as defined by the Kiel Classification, but were instead LP immunocytomas. KNAPP *et al.*[158] were also of the opinion that CLL cells do not contain CIg that can be easily detected.

**IgG-Fc Receptor.** The results of demonstration of IgG-Fc receptors on CLL cells vary greatly from investigator to investigator and depend on the marker substrate used (aggregated IgG, human IgGEA, IgG-sheepEA, IgG-oxEA, pelleting technique; see p. 547). SHEVACH *et al.*[159] found no binding of IgG-sheepEA by cells from seven cases, whereas BELPOMME *et al.*[160] achieved rosetting with 10–63% of the CLL cells from all 10 cases studied. We observed rosetting with IgG-humanEA in a percentage similar to that reported by BELPOMME *et al.*[160] FERRARINI *et al.*[161] reported a much higher percentage of CLL cells binding IgG-oxEA. The highest percentage of CLL cells with IgG-Fc

[157] 1972a.

[158] KNAPP, SCHUIT, BOLHUIS and HIJMANS, 1974.

[159] SHEVACH, JAFFE and GREEN, 1973.

[160] BELPOMME, DANTCHEV, DU RUSQUEC, GRANDJON *et al.*, 1974.

[161] FERRARINI, MORETTA, ABRILE and DURANTE, 1975.

receptors was detected by DICKLER *et al.*,[162] who used IgG aggregates. Almost all of the lymphocytes from all positive patients bound IgG aggregates (range: 88–100%, mean: 96%), as measured with the indirect labeling method. It may be of interest that DICKLER *et al.* noted a difference in some cases between the percentage of cells binding IgG aggregates measured with the more sensitive indirect method and that found with the direct method. That was not the case in normal subjects. This observation suggests that the quantity of IgG-Fc receptors expressed on CLL cells differs from patient to patient more than the amount of IgG-Fc receptors on normal lymphocytes. That would explain why the results on the frequency of IgG-Fc receptor-positive cells demonstrated with different marker substrates varied more in CLL than in normal subjects.

It may be concluded that nearly all cells from almost all cases of CLL bear IgG-Fc receptors. Under normal conditions, IgG-Fc receptors were expressed only on B-cells.[163] The presence of IgG-Fc receptors on lymphoid tumor cells was therefore used as a strong argument for the B-cell origin of the cells.

**Complement Receptor.** JONDAL *et al.*[164] detected complement receptors on none, or on only a very small proportion of CLL cells. That conflicts with other experimental results. The studies of various authors[165] and our own investigations showed that cells from nearly all cases of CLL bore complement receptors when EA complexes coated with mouse complement were used in the rosette assays. In contrast to the occurrence of SIg and of IgG-Fc receptors, however, the percentage of complement receptor-positive cells varied greatly from patient to patient (10–90%). We demonstrated complement receptors on frozen sections of CLL tissue in only 60% of our cases. The histologic distribution of the receptors was diffuse or nodular.

ROSS *et al.*[166] described a striking difference in the ability of EAC prepared with whole mouse serum and that prepared with purified human complement components to react with normal or leukemic lymphocytes. Whereas normal peripheral blood lymphocytes reacted similarly with mouse and human complement, CLL cells reacted preferentially (15/18) with mouse complement.

Later studies of ROSS and POLLEY[167] showed that the preferential binding of EACmouse was due to a C3b inactivator present in whole serum. The C3b inactivator cleaved cell-bound C3b into two fragments, namely, C3c and C3d, in such a way that the C3c fragment was liberated from the EAC, while the C3d fragment remained cell-bound (EAC3d).[168]

These studies demonstrated that the receptor for C3d is nearly always expressed on CLL cells, whereas the receptor for C3b is either absent or very much reduced in quantity in a majority of cases. This indicates that two

[162] DICKLER, SIEGAL, BENTWICH and KUNKEL, 1973.

[163] BASTEN, WARNER and MANDEL, 1972; DICKLER and KUNKEL, 1972; DICKLER and SACHS, 1974.

[164] JONDAL, WIGZELL and AIUTI, 1973.

[165] ROSS, RABELLINO, POLLEY and GREY, 1973; SHEVACH, JAFFE and GREEN, 1973; BELPOMME, DANTCHEV, DU RUSQUEC, GRANDJON *et al.*, 1974; BRAYLAN, JAFFE, BURBACH, FRANK *et al.*, 1976; STEIN, 1975a, 1976a, b.

[166] ROSS, POLLEY, RABELLINO and GREY, 1973.

[167] 1975.

[168] RUDDY and AUSTEN, 1971.

subgroups of CLL can be distinguished on the basis of complement-receptor subtypes:

1. CLL showing only, or preferentially, the C3d receptor (16/18, or 89% of the cases of ROSS and POLLEY[168a]).

2. CLL showing both the C3b and the C3d receptor (2/18, or 11% of the cases of ROSS and POLLEY[168a]).

In connection with the derivation of CLL cells, it may be of interest that nearly all peripheral blood lymphocytes bear both C3b and C3d receptors.[169]

**Mouse-Erythrocyte (E) Receptor.** STATHOPOULOS and ELLIOT[170] were the first to report that a high percentage of the cells from CLL form rosettes with mouse erythrocytes. GUPTA *et al.*[171] found a high percentage of mouse E-rosetting cells in all nine cases of CLL studied. We obtained similar results. CATOVSKY and co-workers[172] have reported on mouse-E rosette-forming capacity of cells of various malignant lymphomas. Their most recent finding was that all but one out of 25 cases of B-CLL showed spontaneous binding of mouse erythrocytes to neuraminidase-treated lymphocytes (median: 65%). No such constant pattern was seen in other B-cell neoplasms, such as prolymphocytic leukemia or lymphosarcoma-cell leukemia, especially the poorly differentiated cases. Intermediate results were observed in follicular lymphoma (see p. 619) and hairy-cell leukemia (see p. 585). Thus, mouse-E receptors appear to be characteristic, but not specific, markers of B-CLL.

**Sheep-Erythrocyte (E) Receptor.** In the largest CLL series (170 cases) investigated so far,[173] the cells from 3% of the cases formed rosettes with sheep erythrocytes. All of the sheep-E rosette-positive cases lacked B-characteristic SIg and IgG-Fc receptors, which confirmed the T-cell origin of the tumor cells. Findings on leukemic cells that reacted simultaneously with sheep erythrocytes and anti-Ig antibodies are discussed on page 638ff.

**Human T-Lymphocyte Antigen (HTLA) and Other T-Associated Antigens.** So far, only a few cases of CLL of the T-cell type have been investigated for their reactivity with anti-thymocyte serum. Recently, BROUET *et al.*[174] studied 11 cases of CLL (two of which morphologically resembled prolymphocytic leukemia) showing sheep E-rosette formation and reported on the reactivity of the cells with two different anti-thymocyte sera: (1) an antiserum to peripheral T-cells and (2) an antiserum to fetal thymocytes. Whereas normal peripheral blood lymphocytes were killed in equal proportions by both anti-T sera, the pattern of reactivity observed in CLL with the different anti-T sera varied from patient to patient. Three categories of T-CLL cells were apparent:

1. CLL cells killed in equal proportions by both antisera.

---

[168a] 1975.

[169] ROSS and POLLEY, 1975; STEIN, 1976, unpublished data.

[170] 1974.

[171] GUPTA, GOOD and SIEGAL, 1976b.

[172] CATOVSKY, CHERCHI, OKOS, HEGDE *et al.*, 1976; CATOVSKY and GALTON, 1977.

[173] BROUET, PREUD'HOMME and SELIGMANN, 1975.

[174] BROUET, FLANDRIN, SASPORTES, PREUD'HOMME *et al.*, 1975.

2. CLL cells reacting preferentially with anti-peripheral T-cell serum.
3. CLL cells more susceptible to anti-fetal T-cell serum.

An anti-human brain cell serum used in the same study labeled more than 80% of the cells from two out of five patients with CLL. Only occasional lymphocytes were positive in the other three cases.

It may be of interest that, in two out of 11 patients, surface IgG with a single light chain was present on most of the sheep-E receptor-positive and HTLA-positive leukemic cells. BROUET *et al.*[177] interpreted the surface-bound IgG, although it was of a single light-chain type, as autoantibodies to the leukemic cells. In our opinion, however, another possibility must be discussed. HSU *et al.*[175] reported on a case of CLL in which 50–90% of the cells formed sheep-E rosettes and 72% of the lymphocytes were labeled with a T-cell-specific antiserum. On initial examination, 15% of the lymphocytes were positively labeled for SIg. The percentage of Ig-bearing cells progressively increased to 92% over the ensuing four months. The SIg was found to consist of monoclonal IgM/$\lambda$. During the next four months, various percentages of cells developed SIg of other heavy-chain classes: 50–78% IgG, 23–30% IgA, 5–93% IgD, and 5–28% IgE. Incubation of the patient's serum with normal and leukemic lymphocytes did not increase the percentage of cells with SIg. GATIEN *et al.*[176] showed that fetal thymocytes of the 9th–10th week of gestation bear surface IgM. Taking this finding into consideration with the observations of HSU *et al.*,[175] it seems highly likely that there are some cases of CLL derived from T-cells, in which inert B-cell genes controlling synthesis of Ig are activated during malignant transformation or during the course of the disease. That might be the case for one CLL in the series of BROUET *et al.*,[177] since a high percentage of the cells from this T-CLL reacted with anti-fetal T-cell serum.

RODT *et al.*[178] quantitated the amount of HTLA on cells from two cases of CLL. In both cases the density of HTLA on the surface membrane was lower than on normal peripheral blood lymphocytes. That is analogous to CLL of the B-cell type, in which the cells usually bear a significantly lower quantity of SIg than do normal peripheral blood lymphocytes.

The same research group[179] also found that the density of HTLA varied less from cell to cell in patients with CLL than it did on normal T-cells. That suggested a clonal proliferation.

**Human B-Associated Antigens (Ia-Like Antigen).** Ia-like antigen, which is regarded as a primary B-cell antigen,[180] was demonstrated on the surfaces of cells from 27 out of 28 cases of CLL.[181] Cells from the 27 Ia-like antigen-positive cases were incapable of binding sheep erythrocytes, whereas a high percentage of the cells from the Ia-like antigen-negative case formed rosettes with sheep erythrocytes.

---

[175] HSU, MARTI, SCHREK and WILLIAMS, 1975.
[176] GATIEN, SCHNEEBERGER and MERLER, 1975.
[177] BROUET, FLANDRIN, SASPORTES, PREUD'HOMME *et al.*, 1975.
[178] RODT, THIERFELDER, THIEL, GÖTZE *et al.*, 1975.
[179] THIEL, RODT, HUHN and THIERFELDER, 1976.
[180] KUNKEL, 1976.
[181] WERNET, SCHUNTER, WILMS and WALLER, 1977.

**Terminal Deoxynucleotidyl Transferase (Tdt).** B-CLL cells were devoid of significant levels of Tdt in all cases.[181a] The same was true for the few cases of T-CLL that were analyzed for Tdt.[181b] Since Tdt is present in thymocytes, but not in peripheral T-cells, the absence of Tdt from T-CLL cells is further evidence that they resemble peripheral T-cells more than thymocytes.

**Receptor for *Helix-Pomatia* Hemagglutinin A (HP Receptor).** HELLSTRÖM *et al.*[181c] demonstrated binding of fluorescein-labeled HP to 90–100% of the leukemic cells from 11 cases of SIg-positive B-CLL.

**IgM-Fc Receptor.** PICHLER and KNAPP[181d] were recently able to demonstrate that 11–70% (mean: 42%) of the peripheral lymphocytes from 15 CLL patients bound IgMEA. In a mixed rosette assay using fluorescein-labeled IgGEA or fluorescein-labeled sheep erythrocytes and IgMEA, it was shown that not only residual T-cells, but also the leukemic (SIg-positive and sheep-E receptor-negative) B-CLL cells expressed receptors for IgM-Fc.

**Conclusions.** *Chronic Lymphocytic Leukemia of the B-Cell Type.* The cells from most cases (about 97%) of CLL have B-cell markers. Surface IgM, surface IgD, C3d receptors, IgG-Fc receptors, mouse-E receptors, and Ia-like antigens are most frequently present on CLL cells. Conventional methods do not allow the demonstration of CIg in CLL cells. The cytoplasm of CLL cells contains abundant ribosomes and little ergastoplasm (see p. 474). Thus, CLL of the B-cell type is a monoclonal proliferation of nonsecretory B-cells—in contrast to myeloma, which is a uniform proliferation of secretory B-cells (plasma cells). CLL cells appear to be arrested in the nonsecretory stage of differentation and therefore cannot transform into secretory B-cells (plasma cells). That is the main difference between CLL and LP immunocytoma, which is characterized by a proliferation of a clone of B-cells that mature from small, nonsecretory lymphocytoid cells into secretory cells (plasma cells).

The monoclonality of the proliferation in B-CLL was suggested by the finding of restricted heavy-chain classes and one light-chain type on the surface membranes. Monoclonality has been proved by the detection of the same idiotype of SIg on the cells from cases of CLL[182] and by the demonstration of a monoclonal electrophoretic[183] or isoelectric-focusing[184] pattern of the immunoglobulin extrated from CLL tissue.

The concept of monoclonality also holds true in those cases of CLL in which freshly drawn lymphocytes simultaneously bear $\mu$-, $\gamma$-, $\kappa$-, and $\lambda$-chains. This mixed staining could be converted into a monotypic staining pattern by means of overnight incubation of the CLL cells at 37° C. Furthermore, after stripping, the CLL lymphocytes of many cases synthesized monoclonal IgM.[185]

[181a] MCCAFFREY, HARRISON, KUNG, PARKMANN *et al.*, 1976; SARIN and GALLO, 1976.
[181b] SELIGMANN, BROUET and PREUD'HOMME, 1977.
[181c] HELLSTRÖM, MELLSTEDT, PERLMANN, HOLM *et al.*, 1976.
[181d] 1977.
[182] SALSANO, FRÖLAND, NATVIG and MICHAELSEN, 1974.
[183] STEIN, KAISERLING and LENNERT, 1974a.
[184] BOUMAN, LÜSEBRINK, HAVSTEEN and STEIN, 1976.
[185] SELIGMANN, PREUD'HOMME and BROUET, 1973.

An apparent exception to the rule is the simultaneous presence of $\delta$- and $\mu$-chains. The $\delta$- and $\mu$-chains, however, reveal the same light chains, idiotypic specificity,[186] and antibody activity,[187] suggesting that both molecules have the same variable regions and differ only in the constant part of the heavy chains.

Since the amount of SIg increases during the maturation of B-lymphocytes and since cells of most cases of B-CLL bear greatly reduced amounts of SIg, PREUD'HOMME and SELIGMANN[188] interpreted CLL as a proliferation of B-lymphocytes that are blocked at an early stage of the maturation process. CATOVSKY *et al.*[189] and STATHOPOULOS and ELLIOT[190] said that this hypothesis is supported by the presence of receptors for mouse erythrocytes on CLL cells. From the studies of these two groups of researchers, it seemed likely that mouse-E receptors occur only at an early stage in the immunologic maturation of B-lymphocytes. More recent findings showed, however, that the cells of LP immunocytoma and of follicular lymphoma are also capable of forming mouse-E rosettes,[191] indicating that the mouse-E receptor is also expressed on neoplastic cells that are derived from more mature B-cells.

KUBO *et al.*[191a] drew attention to the similarity between CLL cells and cord-blood lymphocytes: a large proportion of both types of cells bore IgM and IgD. In this respect, CLL cells resemble fetal lymphocytes more than blood lymphocytes of adults. LUKES and COLLINS[191b] speculated that CLL lymphocytes might be derived from lymphocytes of the mantle zone of follicular centers. That is consistent with the SIg pattern, since most lymphocytes from tonsils simultaneously express surface IgM and IgD,[191c] like CLL cells.

It should be stressed, however, that the cells of a majority of cases of B-CLL differ in several respects from normal B-cells of the blood and lymphatic tissue. In contrast to blood B-cells, B-CLL cells usually lack C3b receptors,[191d] bear less SIg in most instances,[191e] reveal a higher density of normal lymphoid-cell membrane antigens,[191f] and show an impaired proliferative response after antigenic or mitogenic stimulation.[191g] Furthermore, B-CLL cells bind HP[191h] and express a receptor for IgM-Fc.[191i] In normal peripheral blood, receptors for HP and IgM-Fc are found on T-cells, but not on most mature B-cells.[191j] B-cells of lymphatic tissue differ from cells of most cases of B-CLL in that the former lack receptors for mouse erythrocytes[191k] and express receptors for either both C3b and C3d or C3b alone.[191l] There is an especial distinction

[186] FU, WINCHESTER and KUNKEL, 1974; SALSANO, FRÖLAND, NATVIG and MICHAELSEN, 1974.
[187] PREUD'HOMME and SELIGMANN, 1972a, b; BROUET, PREUD'HOMME and SELIGMANN, 1975.
[188] 1972a.
[189] CATOVSKY, CHERCHI, OKOS, HEGDE *et al.*, 1976.
[190] 1974.
[191] CATOVSKY and GALTON, 1977; STEIN and TOLKSDORF, 1977, unpublished data.
[191a] KUBO, GREY and PIROFSKY, 1974.
[191b] 1973.
[191c] KRÜGER, UHLMANN, HELLRIEGEL, SESTERHENN *et al.*, 1976; STEIN, SIEMSSEN and LENNERT, 1978.
[191d] ROSS and POLLEY, 1975.
[191e] GREY, KUBO, RABELLINO, POLLEY *et al.*, 1974; TERNYNCK, DIGHIERO, FOLLEZOU and BINET, 1974.
[191f] HEKMAN and MELIS, 1975.
[191g] SMITH, COWLING and BARKER, 1972.
[191h] HELLSTRÖM, MELLSTEDT, PERLMANN, HOLM *et al.*, 1976.
[191i] PICHLER and KNAPP, 1977.
[191j] HAMMARSTRÖM, HELLSTRÖM, PERLMANN and DILLNER, 1973; MORETTA, FERRARINI, DURANTE and MINGARI, 1975; GMELIG-MEYLING, VAN DER HAM and BALLIEUX, 1976.
[191k] STEIN, 1977, unpublished data.
[191l] STEIN, SIEMSSEN and LENNERT, 1978.

between CLL cells and the morphologically similar cells of primary follicles or the mantle zone of germinal centers: CLL cells are consistently negative for alkaline phosphatase, whereas the cells of the follicular mantle zone are alkaline phosphatase-positive.[192]

In summary, the cells of most cases of B-CLL have mostly B-cell characteristics, but they also have some membrane properties that are not present on a majority of B-cells but are found on mature T-cells. There are various possibilities for interpreting this finding. One is that the expression of an atypical set of membrane markers (e.g., IgM-Fc receptors) is a virus-induced phenomenon analogous to the induction of IgG-Fc receptors in cytomegalovirus-infected fibroblasts. Another possibility is that the B-CLL cell originates from a precursor or immature lymphoid cell that occurs only in small numbers in normal adults and is a B-determined cell with some residual T-cell characteristics. Simultaneous presence of B- and T-markers is observed, for example, on bursal and thymic lymphoid cells in chickens before they hatch. At hatching, the structures specific to T-cells disappear from bursal cells and vice versa.[193] The B-determined cell fraction that proliferates in CLL and has some T-cell properties might still be unable to mature into plasma cells. That would explain why B-CLL cells do not show any maturation towards plasma cells and reveal an impaired proliferative response after mitogenic stimulation. It would also agree with laboratory findings that the serum of B-CLL patients does not show a monoclonal serum-Ig spike, but often reveals pronounced hypogammaglobulinemia.

It might be that the cells of the small group of cases of B-CLL that express receptors for both C3b and C3d and probably lack receptors for IgM-Fc are the malignant counterparts of normal peripheral blood B-lymphocytes or of lymphocytes of the follicular mantle zone. These two B-lymphocyte populations are apparently antigen-committed $B_2$-lymphocytes.

In order to clarify the exact nature of B-CLL cells, however, further work is needed. It will have to be determined whether and to what extent immature or activated normal B- and T-lymphocytes express membrane characteristics not usually found on mature or resting B- and T-lymphocytes.

*Chronic Lymphocytic Leukemia of the T-Cell Type*. Only 3% of the cases of CLL were found to be of the T-cell type. It was remarkable that the reactivity of the leukemic T-cells with different heteroantisera to T-cells differed from patient to patient, but was homogeneous in each case.[194] This finding suggests that the leukemic T-lymphocytes were derived from a single subset of T-cells or, in other words, that T-CLL is a monoclonal proliferation, as is CLL of the B-cell type.

T-CLL cells are probably derived from, or are more closely related to peripheral T-lymphocytes than to thymocytes. That was substantiated by the immunologic finding that T-CLL cells resembled peripheral T-cells and differed from thymocytes in their lower density of HTLA, in the inability to form sheep-E rosettes that were stable at 37° C, and in the absence, or low levels of Tdt.

---

[192] Nanba, Jaffe, Braylan, Soban *et al.*, 1977.
[193] Albini and Wick, 1975.
[194] Brouet, Flandrin, Sasportes, Preud'Homme *et al.*, 1975.

## B. Prolymphocytic Leukemia

**Surface Immunoglobulin (SIg).** BUSKARD *et al.*[195] studied nine cases of prolymphocytic leukemia. All cases were positive for SIg. Surface immunofluorescence was usually strong. IgM was the predominant immunoglobulin class. It was often associated with IgD. IgD was present alone in one case. One case showed a strongly positive reaction when tested with labeled anti-IgG antibodies. A similar reaction was obtained with labeled anti-IgG-Fab2 fragments, which ruled out attachment of the labeled antibodies to the IgG-Fc receptor. The cells from this case also showed a weak reaction with anti-IgM antibodies. The cells from the two cases we recently studied reacted strongly for $\mu$-, $\delta$-, and $\kappa$-chains on the surface membrane. CATOVSKY *et al.*[196] reported on one, BROUET *et al.*[194] on two, and LÖFFLER *et al.*[197] on one case of prolymphocytic leukemia in which the cells lacked SIg.

**Tissue Immunoglobulin.** No data are available.

**Serum Immunoglobulin.** No significant changes in serum-Ig levels have been reported in the literature.

**IgG-Fc Receptor.** There was a strong reaction for IgG-Fc receptors on a majority of cells from seven cases tested by BUSKARD *et al.*[195] They used fluorescein-labeled aggregated IgG as reagent. The cells from the two cases we studied also showed strong reactivity with IgG aggregates.

**Complement Receptor.** In the series of BUSKARD *et al.*[195] complement receptors were found on a variable number of cells—a low percentage in four cases and a high percentage in two cases. A high percentage (>50%) of cells from the two cases of prolymphocytic leukemia we tested bore complement receptors. Analysis of the complement-receptor subtypes revealed the presence of receptors for both C3d and C3b, with a predominance of C3b receptors, on a majority of the prolymphocytic leukemia cells. The cells from the case of prolymphocytic leukemia investigated by CATOVSKY *et al.*[196] lacked complement receptors as well as SIg.

**Mouse-Erythrocyte (E) Receptor.** BUSKARD *et al.*[195] investigated the affinity of mouse erythrocytes for prolymphocytic leukemia cells in seven cases. We tested two cases. A small number of mouse-E rosettes was observed in all nine cases. Recently, CATOVSKY and GALTON[198] detected among 11 prolymphocytic leukemias two cases with more than 40% cells that were capable of spontaneously binding mouse erythrocytes.

**Sheep-Erythrocyte (E) Receptor.** The SIg-positive prolymphocytic leukemia cells did not form rosettes with sheep erythrocytes. A large proportion of cells from the prolymphocytic leukemias without SIg described by CATOVSKY *et al.*[196]

---

[195] BUSKARD, CATOVSKY, OKOS, GOLDMAN *et al.*, 1976.

[196] CATOVSKY, GALETTO, OKOS, MILIANI *et al.*, 1974.

[197] LÖFFLER, GRAUBNER and DESAGA, 1977.

[198] 1977.

and BROUET *et al.*,[199] however, bound sheep erythrocytes. The cells from the case of prolymphocytic leukemia described by LÖFFLER *et al.*[200] formed only a few sheep-E rosettes (3%), but cytologic evaluation confirmed that the rosetted cells were indeed prolymphocytic leukemia cells.

**Human T-Lymphocyte Antigen (HTLA).** BROUET *et al.*[199] detected HTLA in two cases of prolymphocytic leukemia on cells that formed rosettes with sheep erythrocytes.

**Conclusions.** A majority of cases of prolymphocytic leukemia have B-cell characteristics (SIg). T-cell characteristics are rare in prolymphocytic leukemia, but more common than in CLL. Although initially recognized as a variant of CLL, prolymphocytic leukemia shows, besides morphologic and clinical differences (see p. 134ff.), three other main differences from CLL. (1) The staining for SIg on prolymphocytic leukemia cells is strong, whereas on CLL cells it is often weak or moderate. (2) The percentage of mouse-E rosette-forming cells is usually high in CLL and low in prolymphocytic leukemia. (3) In contrast to CLL cells, which always react weakly for acid phosphatase, prolymphocytic leukemia cells of both the B-[201] and the T-types[202] often seem to be positive for tartrate-resistant acid phosphatase.

## C. Hairy-Cell Leukemia (HCL)

Although hairy-cell leukemia (HCL) is a well-recognized clinicopathologic entity,[203] the origin of the neoplastic hairy cells is still a point of controversy. For some time, they were considered to be primitive reticulum cells,[204] but then they were said to be capable of synthesizing immunoglobulin[205] and to bear SIg.[206] More recently, IgG-Fc receptors were found on hairy cells in the absence of complement receptors.[207] That suggested a monocytic-histiocytic origin. Evidence has accumulated in recent years, however, favoring the concept that hairy cells are derived from lymphoid cells, in particular from B-lymphocytes.

**Surface Immunoglobulin (SIg).** A number of investigators have studied the presence of SIg on the tumor cells of hairy-cell leukemia.[208] All but two groups

---

[199] BROUET, FLANDRIN, SASPORTES, PREUD'HOMME *et al.*, 1975.
[200] LÖFFLER, GRAUBNER and DESAGA, 1977.
[201] CATOVSKY, GALETTO, OKOS, MILIANI *et al.*, 1974; STEIN, 1976, unpublished data.
[202] LÖFFLER, GRAUBNER and DESAGA, 1977.
[203] BOURONCLE, WISEMAN and DOAN, 1958.
[204] BOURONCLE, WISEMAN and DOAN, 1958; MITUS, MEDNICOFF, WITTELS and DAMESHEK, 1961; SCHREK and DONNELLY, 1966; YAM, CASTOLDI, GARVEY and MITUS, 1968.
[205] RUBIN, DOUGLAS, CHESSIN, GLADE *et al.*, 1969.
[206] PREUD'HOMME and SELIGMANN, 1972a.
[207] JAFFE, SHEVACH, FRANK and GREEN, 1974.
[208] PREUD'HOMME and SELIGMANN, 1972a; AISENBERG, BLOCH and LONG, 1973; CATOVSKY, PETTIT, GALETTO, OKOS *et al.*, 1974; HAAK, DE MAN, HIJMANS, KNAPP *et al.*, 1974; HAEGERT, CAWLEY, COLLINS, FLEMANS *et al.*, 1974; SILBERMAN and SCHREK, 1974; STEIN and KAISERLING, 1974b; DEBUSSCHER, BERNHEIM, COLLARD-RONGÉ, GOVAERTS *et al.*, 1975; HUBER, ASAMER, MICHLMAYR and BRAUNSTEINER, 1976; RIEBER, V. HEYDEN, LINKE, SAAL *et al.*, 1976; SCHEINBERG, BRENNER, SULLIVAN, CATHCART *et al.*, 1976.

Table 98. Presence of surface-immunoglobulin (SIg) chains on hairy cells after overnight culture[a, c] or after removal of SIg by capping with anti-Ig antibodies and short-term culture[b]

| Author | SIg class | Incidence | Light-chain type |
|---|---|---|---|
| Fu *et al.*[a] | IgM-D | 3/4 | $\kappa$ (3) |
| | IgD | 1/4 | $\kappa$ |
| Rieber *et al.*[b] | IgM-D | 2/4 | |
| | IgD-G | 1/4 | |
| | IgG | 1/4 | |
| Stein and Bruhn[c] | IgG | 2/2 | $\kappa$ (2) |

[a] Fu, Winchester, Rai and Kunkel, 1974.
[b] Rieber, Linke, Hadam, Saal *et al.*, 1977.
[c] 1977, unpublished data.

of authors found that cells from all cases of HCL bore SIg. Scheinberg *et al.*[209] could not demonstrate SIg on cells from two cases. Aisenberg *et al.*[210] reported a negative reaction for SIg on cells from one case and a positive reaction for IgD on some cells from a second case. Most other research groups, including our own, reported that HCL cells usually stained with more than one anti-heavy chain serum and more than one anti-light chain serum.[211] With $^{125}$I-labeled anti-Ig sera, Huber *et al.*[212] observed a marked difference in staining intensity between the various antisera. The hairy cells were labeled to the highest degree with anti-$\gamma$ and anti-$\kappa$ serum. In contrast to normal blood lymphocytes, a considerable proportion of the hairy cells were stained with rabbit antisera against albumin and transferrin. Haegert *et al.*,[213] on the other hand, detected only one light-chain type on hairy cells from three cases ($\kappa$ in two cases and $\lambda$ in one case). The predominant heavy chain proved in two cases to be $\delta$ alone and in one case $\delta$ combined with $\mu$. Fu *et al.*[214] analyzed the SIg pattern of four cases of HCL before and after overnight culture. They found $\gamma$-, $\lambda$-, and $\kappa$-chains and $\mu$- or $\delta$-chains on the surfaces of freshly drawn hairy cells. After overnight culture at 37° C, however, $\mu$- or $\delta$-chains, or both, and only one light chain persisted on the surfaces of the hairy cells (Table 98), whereas IgG was effectively removed under these conditions. We obtained similar results in two cases studied before and after overnight culture (Table 98).

Golde *et al.*[215] studied SIg on fresh hairy cells of two cases and on permanently growing HCL cell-line cells established from the two cases. In both cases the initial SIg chains were maintained in culture (IgM and IgD in the first case and IgG in the second case). Golde *et al.* did not mention the light-chain characteristics of their cases.

[209] Scheinberg, Brenner, Sullivan, Cathcart *et al.*, 1976.
[210] Aisenberg, Bloch and Long, 1973.
[211] Preud'Homme and Seligmann, 1972a; Haak, de Man, Hijmans, Knapp *et al.*, 1974; Stein and Kaiserling, 1974b; Huber, Asamer, Michlmayr and Braunsteiner, 1976.
[212] Huber, Asamer, Michlmayr and Braunsteiner, 1976.
[213] Haegert, Cawley, Collins, Flemans *et al.*, 1974.
[214] Fu, Winchester, Rai and Kunkel, 1974.
[215] Golde, Stevens, Quan and Saxon, 1977.

RIEBER *et al.*[216] studied the presence of SIg on cells from four cases of HCL by means of a combined cytochemical-autoradiographic method that allowed simultaneous demonstration of tartrate-resistant acid phosphatase and SIg on single cells. To be sure that the labeled anti-Ig antibodies were not bound by an IgG-Fc receptor, RIEBER *et al.* used the antigen-binding fragment (Fab2) of monospecific anti-Ig antibodies. Cells from two patients simultaneously expressed $\mu$- and $\delta$-chains. Cells from another patient bore only $\gamma$-chains. Both $\gamma$- and $\delta$-chains were found simultaneously on hairy cells from the fourth patient. Using anti-light chain antibodies, RIEBER *et al.* detected only one type of light chain on the tartrate-resistant acid phosphatase-positive hairy cells from all four patients. After removal of the SIg by capping with respective unlabeled bivalent anti-Ig antibodies, resynthesis of SIg was observed during cultivation of the hairy cells. Under the culture conditions used, however, the SIg reappeared much more slowly on hairy cells than on normal B-lymphocytes treated identically. Figure 279 shows hairy cells that are positively stained with peroxidase-coupled anti-IgG antibodies.

**Tissue Immunoglobulin.** *Saline Extract.* In one case we had the chance to compare the Ig content of splenic tissue that was massively infiltrated by hairy cells with that of a homogenate of pure washed hairy cells prepared from the same spleen. Significant amounts of IgG, IgA, IgM, and albumin were measured in the spleen homogenate. In the homogenate of pure hairy cells, on the other hand, only trace amounts of IgG, IgA, and albumin could be detected, whereas the IgM content was nearly the same as in the spleen homogenate. When the IgM value was referred to the albumin value, the ratio for the homogenate of pure hairy cells was more than 15 times greater than that for the whole spleen homogenate.[217]

*Detergent Second Extract.* In another case of HCL we studied the Ig content, including IgD, in both the saline extract and the detergent 2nd extract of the spleen. Whereas the saline extract contained normal amounts of the different Ig classes, the detergent 2nd extract revealed a large amount of IgD.[218]

**Serum Immunoglobulin.** No great changes in serum-Ig levels were reported in the literature, although an increase in one or all of the three major Ig classes is not uncommon.[219] Recently, however, GOLDE *et al.*[219a] described a case of HCL that was associated with macroglobulinemia. This finding is very unusual and makes the diagnosis somewhat questionable, although hairy-cell features and tartrate-resistant acid phosphatase activity were demonstrated. It should be stressed that the differential diagnosis between Waldenström's disease (LP immunocytoma) and HCL is sometimes very difficult and only possible when histologic and electron-microscopic investigation of splenic tissue is included in the diagnostic review. The demonstration of a tartrate-resistant acid

[216] RIEBER, LINKE, HADAM, SAAL *et al.*, 1977.
[217] STEIN and KAISERLING, 1974b; STEIN, 1975a, b.
[218] STEIN, 1975a, b.
[219] BOIRON, FLANDRIN, RIPAULT, LORTHOLARY *et al.*, 1968; DUHAMEL, 1971; GHADIALLY and SKINNIDER, 1972; STEIN, 1975a.
[219a] GOLDE, STEVENS, QUAN and SAXON, 1977.

(a)

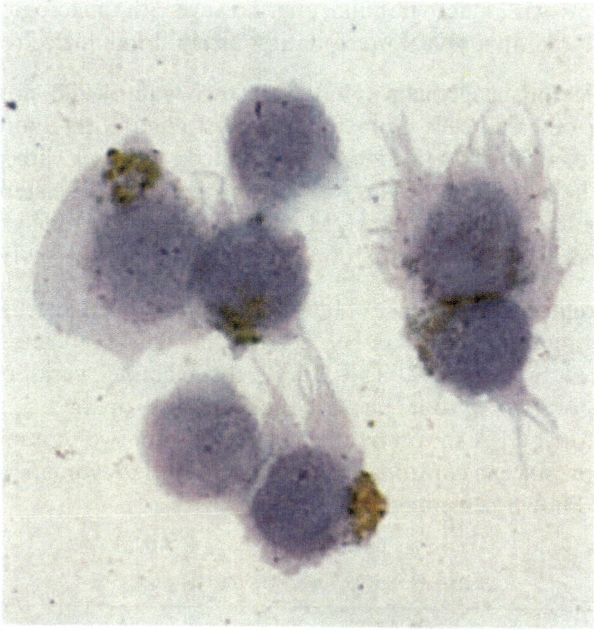

(b)

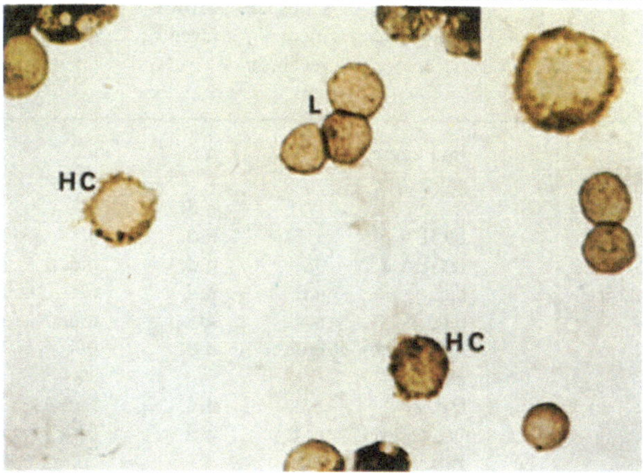


Fig. 279a and b. Hairy-cell leukemia. (a) Hairy cells labeled for surface IgG (brownish green spots) by means of horseradish peroxidase-coupled anti-IgG antibodies. Cytocentrifuge slide, counterstained with Pappenheim. ×2,000. (b) Hairy cells (*HC*) and lymphocytes (*L*) labeled for lymphocyte-specific surface antigen by means of horseradish peroxidase-coupled IgG obtained from a lymphocyte-specific antiserum. No counterstaining. ×400. Inset: labeled hairy cell. ×875

phosphatase reaction is not sufficient evidence, since this isoenzyme is occasionally found in other lymphomas[219b] of low-grade malignancy.

**Monoclonality of the Tissue and Serum Immunoglobulin.** Data from isoelectric-focusing studies of tissue Ig in HCL are not available. The increased serum-Ig

[219b] KATAYAMA, 1977.

fractions usually proved to be polyclonal in electrophoresis.[219c] In the case of GOLDE *et al.*[219d] with macroglobulinemia, however, the macroglobulin showed an M gradient and an atypical precipitation arc in immunoelectrophoresis.

**Cytoplasmic Immunoglobulin (CIg).** Our own studies did not reveal Ig in the cytoplasm of hairy cells from four cases studied with fluorescein-labeled antibodies. In contrast, GOLDE *et al.*[219d] presented two cases with positive staining for CIg. The cytoplasm of hairy cells from the case associated with macroglobulinemia and showing surface IgM and IgD stained strongly for IgM with fluorescein-labeled antibodies; the other case stained faintly for IgG.

**IgG-Fc Receptor.** The presence of IgG-Fc receptors on HCL cells was analyzed by several authors, who used either IgGEA or IgG aggregates. The results are summarized in Table 99. The hairy cells from all cases of HCL, with the exception of two of our cases, bound IgGEA or IgG aggregates. The nonreactivity for IgGEA shown by the hairy cells from two of our cases was not a technical error, since in control assays peripheral blood lymphocytes bound the IgGEA in the known percentage (15–20%).

Table 99. Surface markers on hairy cells

| Author | IgG-Fc receptor | Complement receptor | Mouse-E receptor | Sheep-E receptor | Ia, Da, or lymphocyte-specific antigen (LSA) |
|---|---|---|---|---|---|
| PREUD'HOMME and SELIGMANN[b] | IgG aggregates 2/2 | n.d.[a] | n.d. | n.d. | n.d. |
| CATOVSKY *et al.*[c] | + | 1/1 | n.d. | 0/3 | Ia+ |
| HAEGERT *et al.*[d] | IgGEA 5/5 | 3/5 | n.d. | 0/5 | n.d. |
| JAFFE *et al.*[e] | IgGEA 2/2 | 0/2 | n.d. | n.d. | n.d. |
| STEIN and KAISERLING[f] | n.d. | n.d. | n.d. | 0/1 | LSA 2/2 |
| CATOVSKY *et al.*[g] | n.d. | n.d. | 4/4 | n.d. | n.d. |
| HUBER *et al.*[h] | IgG aggregates 4/4 | n.d. | n.d. | 0/4 | n.d. |
| KUNKEL[i] | n.d. | n.d. | n.d. | n.d. | Da+ |
| RIEBER *et al.*[j] | IgG aggregates 4/4 | n.d. | n.d. | 0/4 | n.d. |
| SCHEINBERG *et al.*[k] | IgGEA 2/2 | 1/2 | n.d. | 0/2 | n.d. |
| CATOVSKY and GALTON[l] | n.d. | n.d. | 8/13 | n.d. | n.d. |
| STEIN[m] | IgGEA 3/5 | 3/5 | n.d. | 0/5 | LSA 4/4 |

[a] n.d. = not determined.
[b] 1972a.
[c] CATOVSKY, GALTON, OKOS, MILIANI *et al.*, 1974; CATOVSKY, PETTIT, GALETTO, OKOS *et al.*, 1974.
[d] HAEGERT, CAWLEY, COLLINS, FLEMANS *et al.*, 1974.
[e] JAFFE, SHEVACH, FRANK and GREEN, 1974.
[f] 1974b.
[g] CATOVSKY, PAPAMICHAIL, OKOS, MILIANI *et al.*, 1975.
[h] HUBER, ASAMER, MICHLMAYR and BRAUNSTEINER, 1976.
[i] 1976.
[j] RIEBER, LINKE, HADAM, SAAL *et al.*, 1977.
[k] SCHEINBERG, BRENNER, SULLIVAN, CATHCART *et al.*, 1976.
[l] 1977.
[m] 1977, unpublished data.

RIEBER *et al.*[220] investigated the amount of IgG aggregates bound by hairy cells from four cases. The hairy cells from all cases bound more IgG aggregates than did normal peripheral blood lymphocytes or monocytes, indicating a high density of IgG-Fc receptors on hairy cells.

**Complement Receptor.** Analysis of complement-receptor reactivity on hairy cells produced various results. They are shown in Table 99. JAFFE *et al.*[221] did not observe EAC-rosette formation by hairy cells. CATOVSKY *et al.*,[222] on the other hand, reported on one EAC-positive case. Three out of the five cases studied by HAEGERT *et al.*,[223] one out of the two cases analyzed by SCHEINBERG *et al.*,[224] and three out of five cases in our series revealed complement receptors.

In our three positive cases we specified the complement-receptor subtypes. In all three cases C3b receptors predominated; C3d receptors were also expressed, but on a smaller proportion of cells.

**Mouse-Erythrocyte (E) Receptor.** CATOVSKY and co-workers[225] reported on the capacity of HCL cells to form mouse-E rosettes. A significant proportion (25–45%) of the hairy cells from eight out of 13 cases showed spontaneous binding of mouse erythrocytes. Cytocentrifuge slides unequivocally revealed that almost all of the mouse-E rosette-forming cells were hairy cells.

**Sheep-Erythrocyte (E) Receptor.** As shown in Table 99, the sheep E-rosette assay of HCL cells consistently gave negative results.

**Human T-Associated Antigens.** No data are available.

**Lymphocyte-Specific Antigen and Human B-Associated Antigens (Ia-Like Antigen).** Using a specific anti-lymphocyte serum, we observed avid labeling of hairy cells from two cases (Fig. 279b).[226] CATOVSKY *et al.*[227] obtained positive labeling of hairy cells with two different anti-B-lymphocyte sera prepared by GREAVES and colleagues. These B-cell antisera were probably directed against the Ia-like antigen recently described.[228] KUNKEL[229] and NAEIM *et al.*[229a] reported similar findings. They found that hairy cells possess Da-antigens and Merrit B-cell alloantigens. Ia-like antigen, Da-antigen, and Merrit B-cell alloantigen were found to be primary B-cell antigens that are probably largely identical (see p. 564).[229] They are probably closely related to the lymphocyte-specific antigens that we detetcted.[226]

**Phagocytosis and Adherence.** There are several controversial findings on phagocytosis and adherence. Most investigators were not able to demonstrate signifi-

---

[219c] BOIRON, FLANDRIN, RIPAULT, LORTHOLARY *et al.*, 1968; DUAHMEL, 1971; GHADIALLY and SKINNIDER, 1972; STEIN, 1975a.

[219d] GOLDE, STEVENS, QUAN and SAXON, 1977.

[220] RIEBER, LINKE, HADAM, SAAL *et al.*, 1977.

[221] JAFFE, SHEVACH, FRANK, GREEN *et al.*, 1974.

[222] CATOVSKY, PETTIT, GALETTO, OKOS *et al.*, 1974.

[223] HAEGERT, CAWLEY, COLLINS, FLEMANS *et al.*, 1974.

[224] SCHEINBERG, BRENNER, SULLIVAN, CATHCART *et al.*, 1976.

[225] CATOVSKY, PAPAMICHAIL, OKOS, MILIANI *et al.*, 1975; CATOVSKY and GALTON, 1977.

[226] STEIN and KAISERLING, 1974b.

[227] CATOVSKY, GALTON, OKOS, MILIANI *et al.*, 1974.

[228] HUMPHREYS, MCCUNE, CHESS, HERRMAN *et al.*, 1976.

[229] KUNKEL, 1976.

[229a] NAEIM, GOSSETT and WALFORD, 1977.

cant phagocytosis by hairy cells. Furthermore, neither the cases described by CATOVSKY *et al.*[230] nor the three cases we tested revealed IgG- or C3-mediated phagocytosis (so-called immunophagocytosis), which is a common property of polymorphonuclear granulocytes, monocytes, and macrophages.[231] In contrast, FLANDRIN *et al.*[232] observed phagocytosis of latex particles of a certain size. This phenomenon was also reported by RIEBER *et al.*[233] and FU *et al.*[234]

While RUBIN *et al.*,[235] TRUBOWITZ *et al.*,[236] and our group[237] did not see retardation of hairy cells in nylon fiber columns, RIEBER *et al.*,[233] CATOVSKY *et al.*,[230] DEBUSSCHER *et al.*,[238] and KING *et al.*[239] recognized strong adherence of hairy cells to glass beads or nylon surfaces.

**Receptor for *Helix-Pomatia* Hemagglutinin A (HP Receptor).** After treatment with neuraminidase, hairy cells from three cases bound large amounts of fluorescein-conjugated HP.[240]

**Conclusions.** The data presented show that there are several controversial findings on the properties of hairy cells, particularly those on phagocytosis and SIg staining. Although SIg staining for all, or nearly all, Ig classes could be found on hairy cells by most authors, some reported a restriction of the SIg classes to one light-chain type and one or two heavy-chain classes. The cause of the mixed SIg staining now appears to have been clarified.[241] Comparison of the SIg-staining pattern of freshly drawn hairy cells with that of hairy cells after overnight culture showed that the mixed SIg staining was due to passively absorbed polytypic IgG. Whereas $\delta$- and/or $\mu$- or $\gamma$-chains persisted on the surfaces of the hairy cells after overnight culture, polytypic IgG and one light chain were effectively removed, which resulted in a light-chain staining restricted to one class. This finding is consistent with the results of tissue-Ig analysis in two cases. The tissue extract from one case contained considerable amounts of IgM;[237] the other revealed IgD.[242] The intrinsic nature of the "monoclonal" SIg on hairy cells was recently proved by the detection of *de-novo* SIg synthesis by the cells.[243] Further evidence for a lymphatic nature was provided by the observation that hairy cells are capable of forming rosettes with mouse erythrocytes.[244] Both Ig synthesis and the binding of mouse erythrocytes have so far been observed only as features of lymphoid cells of the B-type. The lymphatic nature of hairy cells has also been substantiated by the demonstration of lymphocyte-specific antigens[237] and primary

---

[230] CATOVSKY, PETTIT, GALETTO, OKOS *et al.*, 1974.
[231] HUBER, POLLEY, LINSCOTT, FUDENBERG *et al.*, 1968; MANTOVANI, RABINOVITCH and NUSSENZWEIG, 1972.
[232] FLANDRIN, DANIEL, FOURCADE and CHELLOUL, 1973.
[233] RIEBER, V. HEYDEN, LINKE, SAAL *et al.*, 1976.
[234] FU, WINCHESTER, RAI and KUNKEL, 1974.
[235] RUBIN, DOUGLAS, CHESSIN, GLADE *et al.*, 1969.
[236] TRUBOWITZ, MASEK and FRASCA, 1971.
[237] STEIN and KAISERLING, 1974b.
[238] DEBUSSCHER, BERNHEIM, COLLARD-RONGÉ, GOVAERTS *et al.*, 1975.
[239] KING, HURTUBISE, SAGONE, LOBUGLIO *et al.*, 1975.
[240] STEIN, 1977, unpublished data.
[241] FU, WINCHESTER, RAI and KUNKEL, 1974.
[242] STEIN, 1975a.
[243] RIEBER, LINKE, HADAM, SAAL *et al.*, 1977.
[244] CATOVSKY, PAPAMICHAIL, OKOS, MILIANI *et al.*, 1975.

B-cell antigens[245] on the cells. The binding of HP by hairy cells is further evidence of their lymphatic nature: HP receptors are found on lymphoid cells, but not on monocytes.[246]

These findings suggest that hairy-cell leukemia is a monoclonal proliferation of Ig-bearing cells like those of CLL. Another similarity between hairy-cell leukemia and CLL is the nearly regular expression of IgG-Fc receptors. Hairy cells differ, however, from CLL lymphocytes in the density of the IgG-Fc receptors on the surface membrane, in morphology, and in phagocytic potential. The ability of hairy cells to phagocytose seems to be limited to certain particles, e.g., latex beads. Candida and bacteria were not ingested by hairy cells. Attempts to induce hairy cells to ingest specific IgG- and complement-coated erythrocytes or bacteria also failed.[247] That is a marked difference between hairy cells and monocytes. Taking all of the known data into consideration, it appears that the hairy cell is derived from a subset of B-cells with limited phagocytic potential. It should be mentioned that relatively active phagocytosis of latex particles can also be observed in established B-cell neoplasms, e.g., prolymphocytic leukemia and some nonleukemic malignant lymphomas.[247a]

## D. Mycosis Fungoides

**Surface Immunoglobulin (SIg).** ZUCKER-FRANKLIN[248] analyzed the lymphoid-cell component for SIg in eight patients with mycosis fungoides. The number of SIg-positive cells was extremely low in all eight patients.

**Tissue Immunoglobulin.** *Saline Extract.* We studied the concentration of tissue Ig in an immunoblastic lymphoma that had arisen in a patient with mycosis fungoides. A greatly increased amount of IgE was measured in the saline tissue extract. There was also a significant, although merely slight, increase in IgM. Because there was not enough material, the IgE and IgM fractions could not be investigated for monoclonality. Thus, the significance of the increases in tissue Ig remains unclear.

*Detergent Second Extract.* No data are available.

**Serum Immunoglobulin.** The literature does not contain any reports of consistent, significant changes in serum-Ig levels in mycosis fungoides.

**IgG-Fc Receptor and Complement Receptor.** EDELSON *et al.*[249] found no adherence of IgMEAC or IgGEA on frozen sections from intradermic plaques (three patients), enlarged lymph nodes (three patients), or a lung nodule (one

[245] CATOVSKY, GALTON, OKOS, MILIANI *et al.*, 1974; KUNKEL, 1976; NAEIM, GOSSETT and WALFORD, 1977.
[246] STEIN and TOLKSDORF, 1977, unpublished data.
[247] CATOVSKY, PETTIT, GALETTO, OKOS *et al.*, 1974; FU, WINCHESTER, RAI and KUNKEL, 1974; STEIN, 1975a.
[247a] STEIN, 1977, unpublished data.
[248] 1974.
[249] EDELSON, KIRKPATRICK, SHEVACH, SCHEIN *et al.*, 1974; EDELSON, LUTZNER, KIRKPATRICK, SHEVACH *et al.*, 1974.

patient) of patients with mycosis fungoides. ZUCKER-FRANKLIN[249a] also did not detect binding of EAC by suspended mycosis-fungoides cells. These findings clearly indicate that there are no complement receptors on mycosis-fungoides cells. The data on IgG-Fc receptors are inconclusive.

**Mouse-Erythrocyte (E) Receptor.** GUPTA *et al.*[250] observed that cells from one case of mycosis fungoides did not bind mouse erythrocytes.

**Sheep-Erythrocyte (E) Receptor.** It has been shown by various authors that mycosis-fungoides cells isolated from the blood,[249a] from involved lymph nodes, and from skin lesions[251] bind sheep erythrocytes in a high percentage.

**Human T-Lymphocyte Antigen (HTLA).** EDELSON *et al.*[252] demonstrated the presence of HTLA on mycosis-fungoides cells from all of the cases they studied.

**Conclusions.** The absence of SIg, complement receptors, and mouse-E receptors and the presence of sheep-E receptors and HTLA on mycosis-fungoides cells prove their T-cell nature.

## E. Sézary's Syndrome

**Surface Immunoglobulin (SIg).** Several authors[253] showed that Sézary cells did not bear SIg.

**Tissue Immunoglobulin.** No data are available.

**Serum Immunoglobulin.** There are no reports of significant changes in serum-Ig levels in Sézary's syndrome.

**IgG-Fc Receptor.** Sézary cells from the series (6 cases) of BROUET *et al.*[254] did not bind IgG aggregates.

**IgM-Fc Receptor.** According to the findings of BROUET,[255] Sézary cells usually bear a receptor for IgM-Fc, as revealed by the IgMEA-rosette assay. That is consistent with the T-helper-cell activity revealed by cocultivation experiments (see p. 589).

**Complement Receptor.** ZUCKER-FRANKLIN *et al.*[256] investigated by electron microscopy EAC rosette-forming cells from patients with Sézary's syndrome. Sézary cells were not identified in the EAC rosettes.

---

249a ZUCKER-FRANKLIN, 1974.
250 GUPTA, GOOD and SIEGAL, 1976b.
251 EDELSON, KIRKPATRICK, SHEVACH, SCHEIN *et al.*, 1974; VAN LEEUWEN, MEIJER and DE MAN, 1975.
252 EDELSON, LUTZNER, KIRKPATRICK, SHEVACH *et al.*, 1974.
253 BROUET, FLANDRIN and SELIGMANN, 1973; FLANDRIN and BROUET, 1974; ZUCKER-FRANKLIN, MELTON III and QUAGLIATA, 1974.
254 BROUET, FLANDRIN and SELIGMANN, 1973.
255 1977.
256 ZUCKER-FRANKLIN, MELTON III and QUAGLIATA, 1974.

**Sheep-Erythrocyte (E) Receptor.** Normal or large numbers of sheep-E rosette-forming cells were measured in the blood of patients with Sézary's syndrome.[257] Morphologic and electron-microscopic examination established the presence of Sézary cells in most, but not all, sheep-E rosettes.[256]

**Human T-Lymphocyte Antigen (HTLA).** FLANDRIN and BROUET[258] studied cells from three cases and EDELSON *et al.*[259] analyzed cells from four cases of Sézary's syndrome for their reactivity with anti-T sera in the presence of complement. A high percentage (55–95%) of the cells were killed by the anti-T serum, indicating the presence of HTLA on the Sézary cells.

**Helper-Cell Function.** Like normal T-cells, leukemic cells from four out of five patients with Sézary's syndrome stimulated increased Ig synthesis by purified normal B-cells or even by B-cells from patients with antibody deficiency.[260] Unlike the situation observed when large numbers of normal T-cells were added to purified B-cells, however, there was no depression of Ig production at very high ratios of Sézary cells to B-cells. This finding indicates that Sézary cells are completely devoid of suppressor-cell activity.

**Terminal Deoxynucleotidyl Transferase (Tdt).** MCCAFFREY *et al.*[260a] found no Tdt activity in cells from two cases. The same was true in all but one of the cases studied by BROUET.[260b]

**Conclusions.** The data provided by the few studies of immunologic properties of Sézary cells clearly show that Sézary cells lack SIg, IgG-Fc receptors, and complement receptors, and that they have sheep-E receptors and HTLA. These findings are consistent with a T-cell origin. Sézary cells are distinguished from thymocytes by their weak capacity to bind sheep erythrocytes and their low levels of Tdt. Thus, it seems likely that Sézary cells are derived from a subset of peripheral T-lymphocytes having a low density of sheep-E receptors and cerebriform nuclei. The results of cocultivation of Sézary cells with normal B-cells or with B-cells from patients with agammaglobulinemia suggest that Sézary cells originate from a relatively mature subset of T-cells programmed exclusively for helper-like interaction with B-cells during their production of Ig molecules.

The similarities between Sézary cells and mycosis-fungoides cells in morphology and membrane-marker properties support the view that the two diseases are closely related or are variants of the same disorder.

---

[257] BRAYLAN, VARIAKOJIS and YACHNIN, 1973; BROUET, FLANDRIN and SELIGMANN, 1973; EDELSON, KIRKPATRICK, SHEVACH, SCHEIN *et al.*, 1974; FLANDRIN and BROUET, 1974; ZUCKER-FRANKLIN, MELTON III and QUAGLIATA, 1974.

[258] 1974.

[259] EDELSON, LUTZNER, KIRKPATRICK, SHEVACH *et al.*, 1974.

[260] BRODER, EDELSON, LUTZNER, NELSON *et al.*, 1976.

[260a] MCCAFFREY, HARRISON, KUNG, PARKMAN *et al.*, 1976.

[260b] 1977.

## F. Malignant Lymphoma, Lymphocytic, T-Zone Type (T-Zone Lymphoma)

**Surface Immunoglobulin (SIg).** SIg was found on nonneoplastic cells in two cases; the percentages ranged from 20–50%.

**Tissue Immunoglobulin.** *Saline and Detergent Second Extracts.* The amounts of Ig measured in the saline and detergent 2nd tissue extracts from the three cases studied varied from subnormal to slightly increased.

**Serum Immunoglobulin.** The serum-Ig levels of the one case studied were in the normal or subnormal range.

**Cytoplasmic Immunoglobulin (CIg).** No data are available.

**IgG-Fc Receptor.** No data are available.

**Complement Receptor.** The frozen sections of three cases showed a dense adherence of EAC to the follicles. The interfollicular regions infiltrated by neoplastic cells were spared. In suspension, the neoplastic cell fraction did not bind EAC. Labeling the cells of one case for SIg showed that the EAC-negative cells were devoid of SIg and the EAC-positive cells were positive for SIg in most instances.

**Mouse-Erythrocyte (E) Receptor.** No data are available.

**Sheep-Erythrocyte (E) Receptor.** A significant proportion (20–45%) of the cells from all three cases studied formed rosettes with sheep erythrocytes. Cytologic analysis of the cytocentrifuge slides clearly showed that the sheep-E rosette-forming cells were indeed neoplastic cells. That was particularly evident in one case in which the cytoplasm of neoplastic cells in interfollicular areas (see Fig. 90) contained vacuoles: the cells that formed sheep-E rosettes contained a similar amount of vacuoles of the same size (see Fig. 81).

**Human T-Associated Antigens.** No data are available.

**Conclusions.** Our immunologic data agree with the morphologic findings in T-zone lymphoma, which indicate that the tumor is usually composed of neoplastic T-cells and nonneoplastic B-cells. Both the nonneoplastic and the neoplastic cells are roughly situated in their normal lymph-node compartments. The B-cells are grouped in the form of follicles, often with germinal centers. The follicles – like those of normal or hyperplastic lymphatic tissue – bind EAC. At first glance, this type of tumor may thus resemble follicular lymphoma in morphology and in the distribution of complement receptor-positive cells in the tissue. In contrast to follicular lymphoma, however, the tumor cells of T-zone lymphoma are located between the follicles. The T-cell nature of the tumor cells was clearly demonstrated by the sheep E-rosette assay. Since the neoplastic T-cells varied in size and cytology like the stimulated cells of

T-regions and since T-characteristic interdigitating reticulum cells and T-associated plasma cells were usually found among the tumor cells, this neoplasm may be regarded as an organoid tumor of the T-region. The nonneoplastic follicular elements might be remnants of preexistent follicles; or they might be induced by the tumor cells, since it has been shown that T-cells are essential for reactive germinal-center formation.[260c]

## G. Malignant Lymphoma, Lymphoplasmacytic/Lymphoplasmacytoid (LP Immunocytoma)

A malignant lymphoma composed of lymphocytoid cells, blast cells, and plasmacytoid cells, and lacking macroglobulinemia was formerly not recognized as an entity. There are therefore no comprehensive reports on immunologic studies of lymphomas characterized by such a mixed cell proliferation. Lymphomas showing this type of morphology were called LP immunocytomas by our research group.[260d] Immunologic data are not lacking for all types of LP immunocytomas. They are not available for the lymphomas that do not reveal monoclonal changes in serum Ig. On the other hand, LP immunocytomas that exhibit active secretion of immunoglobulin, otherwise known as Waldenström's disease, have been subjected to immunologic study. The first group is much larger than the second. There are apparently no fundamental cytogenetic differences, however, between Waldenström's disease (LP immunocytoma with macroglobulinemia) and LP immunocytoma without macroglobulinemia. Thus, it would be worthwhile to compare the immunologic data collected on Waldenström's disease with the data on LP immunocytoma lacking a serum-Ig spike, in order to determine whether there is a close relationship between the two neoplasms.

**Surface Immunoglobulin (SIg).** *LP Immunocytoma with a Serum-Immunoglobulin Spike.* Seligmann and his colleagues[261] studied a relatively large series of LP immunocytomas for SIg. They classified the disease as a pleomorphic lymphoid proliferation. The results of the latest study[262] are given in Table 100. Most of the neoplastic cells from all 39 cases bore SIg. The cells from 36 cases (92%) reacted positively for surface IgM. All of these patients had macroglobulinemia. The neoplasm was therefore identical with Waldenström's disease. IgM was demonstrated alone in 31 cases. In two patients (5%) a serum-IgG spike was found in addition to monoclonal IgM. SIg analysis of these two cases revealed two distinct clones of cells: one bearing $\mu$- and the other $\gamma$-chains. The heavy-chain class and the light-chain type of the SIg were identical with those of the serum Ig in all cases. Two cases (5%) were positive for IgG, and one case (2.5%) was positive for IgA. In the IgM-positive cases nearly

[260c] Jacobson, Caporale and Thorbecke, 1974.
[260d] Lennert, Stein and Kaiserling, 1975; Stein, Kaiserling and Lennert, 1974c, 1975; Stein, 1975a, b, 1976a, b.
[261] Preud'Homme and Seligmann, 1972a, c; Seligmann, Preud'Homme and Brouet, 1973.
[262] Seligmann, Preud'Homme and Brouet, 1973.

Table 100. Surface immunoglobulin (SIg) on cells from LP immunocytoma with and without a serum-Ig spike

| Author | SIg class | Incidence | Light-chain type |
|---|---|---|---|
| *With serum-Ig spike:* | | | |
| SELIGMANN *et al.*[b] | Ig-PV[a] | 39/39 | |
| | IgM | 31/39 | |
| | IgG | 2/39 | κ (2) |
| | IgA | 1/39 | κ |
| | IgM + IgG | 2/39 | two populations |
| | mixed staining (μ, γ, κ, λ) | 3/39 | |
| PERNIS *et al.*[c] | IgM-D | 7/7 | |
| *Without serum-Ig spike:* | | | |
| SELIGMANN *et al.*[b] | IgM | 1/1 | κ |
| STEIN and LENNERT[d] | IgM | 11/12 | |
| | IgG | 1/12 | |
| | IgM-D | 4/4 | |

[a] Ig-PV = Ig demonstrated with a polyvalent anti-Ig serum.
[b] SELIGMANN, PREUD'HOMME and BROUET, 1973.
[c] PERNIS, BROUET and SELIGMANN, 1974.
[d] 1976, unpublished data.

all lymphoid cells, including plasmablasts and plasmacytes, bore surface IgM. In contrast, SIg was present only on the lymphocytoid cells from the cases with monoclonal IgG or IgA. SIg was not found on plasmacytes from such cases. A mixed SIg-staining pattern, characterized by the simultaneous presence of μ-, γ-, λ-, and κ-chain determinants, was observed in three of the patients with macroglobulinemia. In these cases, however, only one heavy- and one light-chain type were detected on the cells after removal of SIg by means of trypsin treatment, followed by 6–7 hours' incubation in a culture medium. In one case the mixed staining pattern was obviously due to anti-IgG activity of surface IgM. The surface IgM therefore had the same antibody activity as the patient's serum IgM, which led to the mixed cryoglobulinemia.

PERNIS *et al.*[263] (Table 100) studied seven cases of Waldenström's disease for surface IgM and surface IgD. In all cases they found bone-marrow lymphocytes bearing both Ig classes and also cells expressing only one class. The relative percentages of the three groups of lymphocytes varied from case to case. The group that expressed both Ig classes was predominant in all cases. The plasmablasts and/or plasmacytes that contained cytoplasmic IgM always exhibited surface IgM. IgD was not seen on the surfaces of true plasma cells, but it was present on some plasmablasts. Peripheral lymphocytes from the one case in which the macroglobulin and the surface IgM revealed anti-IgG reactivity also exhibited IgM and IgD on the membrane. By capping with anti-IgG sera or with IgG aggregates, PERNIS *et al.*[263] also showed that both classes of Ig receptors, i.e., IgM and IgD, were anti-IgG-reactive.

[263] PERNIS, BROUET and SELIGMANN, 1974.

*LP Immunocytoma without a Serum-Immunoglobulin Spike.* In their series of pleomorphic lymphoid proliferations, SELIGMANN and his colleagues[264] (Table 100) had one patient who lacked a serum-Ig spike in serum and urine. A majority of the cells from this patient were intensely stained by antisera against $\mu$- and $\kappa$-chains. The series of 12 LP immunocytomas we studied (Table 100) for SIg were all devoid of monoclonal serum Ig. In two cases small amounts of $\kappa$- or $\lambda$-chains were detected in the urine. SIg was found on most of the cells from the 12 cases: IgM in 11 cases and IgG in one case. Cells from four patients were additionally analyzed for $\delta$-chains and the light-chain type: $\delta$- and $\mu$-chains and a single light chain were demonstrated by two-color fluorescence on the surface membranes of the tumor cells.

In three cases cytologic evaluation of cells labeled with different horseradish peroxidase-coupled anti-Ig antibodies demonstrated that identical heavy and light chains were present on all three types of LP-immunocytoma cells, i.e., lymphocytoid cells, blast cells, and plasmablasts and/or plasma cells.

On the whole, the findings indicate that there is no fundamental difference in SIg labeling between LP immunocytoma with and that without a serum-Ig spike.

So-called CLL with crystalline inclusions is apparently an unusual lymphoma. In the Kiel Classification it is classified as LP immunocytoma of the lymphoplasmacytoid subtype. Cells from all such cases with crystalline inclusions that have been studied so far exhibited $\lambda$-chain determinants on the surface membrane (see Table 102). In contrast, the SIg in the one case of so-called CLL with amorphous globular cytoplasmic inclusions observed by HUREZ *et al.*[265] was not limited to $\lambda$-chains. The cells from their case revealed $\mu$- and $\kappa$-chain determinants on the surface membrane. We also observed some cases in which the light-chain type was not restricted to $\lambda$.

**Tissue Immunoglobulin.** *Saline Extract.* Figure 276 shows that in 39 (58%) out of 67 cases the IgM values were significantly and in 12 (18%) cases greatly above the thymic range. There was an increase in IgM together with IgG in one case (1.5%) and together with IgA in three cases (4.5%). In three cases (4.5%) the IgM, IgA, and IgG values were increased, and in one case (1.5%) the IgA value together with the IgE value. There was an increase in IgM alone in 31 cases (46%), in IgA alone in two cases (3%), and in IgG alone in one case (1.5%). IgD was not detectable in the 15 cases studied.

In three cases we had the opportunity of analyzing material at various stages of the disease. In one case the tissue-IgM values were almost identical, although the lymph-node biopsies were taken at two-month intervals. In the second case the tissue from the first biopsy showed only a small increase in the amount of IgM, whereas the second biopsy (12 months later) contained 30 times more IgM than the norm. In the third case the situation was reversed: in 1967 a monoclonal increase in IgM had been found in the serum, whereas five years later there was no increase in IgM in either the lymph-node tissue or the serum.

---

[264] SELIGMANN, PREUD'HOMME and BROUET, 1973.

[265] HUREZ, FLANDRIN, PREUD'HOMME and SELIGMANN, 1972.

*Detergent Second Extract* (Fig. 277). More distinctly than in the saline extracts, three groups of IgM values were measured in the detergent 2nd extracts: (1) IgM values within the thymic range (14%, n=6), (2) IgM values ranging from the upper limit of normal thymic values to 15 times the mean thymic value (51%, n=22), and (3) IgM values 40–200 times higher than the mean thymic value (35%, n=15). The third group included the cases that revealed abundant PAS-positive globules.

Of the six cases with IgM values within the thymic range, two showed a 15- to 18-fold increase in IgA in the tissue extract. In one case it was combined with an increase in IgE.

There was an increase in IgM together with IgA in two cases (4.6%) and together with IgG in one case (2.3%). In two cases (4.6%) the IgM, IgA, and IgG values were increased simultaneously. An increase in IgM alone was found in 34 cases (79%) and in IgA alone in two cases (4.6%), whereas an increase in IgG alone was not found in any case. Measurable amounts of IgD were not detected in any case.

Altogether, the results of tissue-Ig analysis provided evidence of Ig production in 95% (41/43) of the cases. IgM was by far the most predominant Ig class.

**Comparison of the Tissue-IgM Concentrations in the Morphologic Subtypes of LP Immunocytoma.** The tissue- and serum-Ig data on the lymphoplasmacytoid, lymphoplasmacytic, and polymorphic subtypes of immunocytoma are compared in Figure 280. It shows that the highest mean tissue-IgM value was found in the lymphoplasmacytic group. The next highest values were measured in the polymorphic group, and the lowest values in the lymphoplasmacytoid group. Cases with extremely high tissue-IgM values occurred in all three groups, but they were most common in the lymphoplasmacytic group. In the lymphoplasmacytoid group there was a relatively large number of cases with "slightly" increased tissue-IgM values. Our studies showed that the tissue IgM of the lymphoplasmacytic tumors could be efficiently solubilized with saline, whereas in many cases of the lymphoplasmacytoid and polymorphic types the tissue IgM could be solubilized only with detergents.

**Serum Immunoglobulin.** The amount of IgM in the serum was increased in 17% (12/67) of the cases in the saline-extracted group and in 21% (9/43) of the cases in the detergent-extracted group. The serum-IgG value was slightly increased above the norm in two cases. An increase in serum IgA was found in only one case together with an increase in serum IgM. The IgA and IgM values were also increased in the tissue extract of the same tumor.

When the data on the serum-Ig and tissue-Ig contents are compared, it is remarkable that there was no correlation between the IgM concentrations of the tissue and serum.[266] In the group with the highest tissue-IgM values, the serum-IgM level was increased only once (see Fig. 277). Nearly all of the increased serum-IgM values were found in the second group that exhibited

[266] Stein, Kaiserling and Lennert, 1974c, 1975; Stein, 1975a, b, 1976b; Stein, Bouman, Lennert, Fuchs *et al.*, 1977.

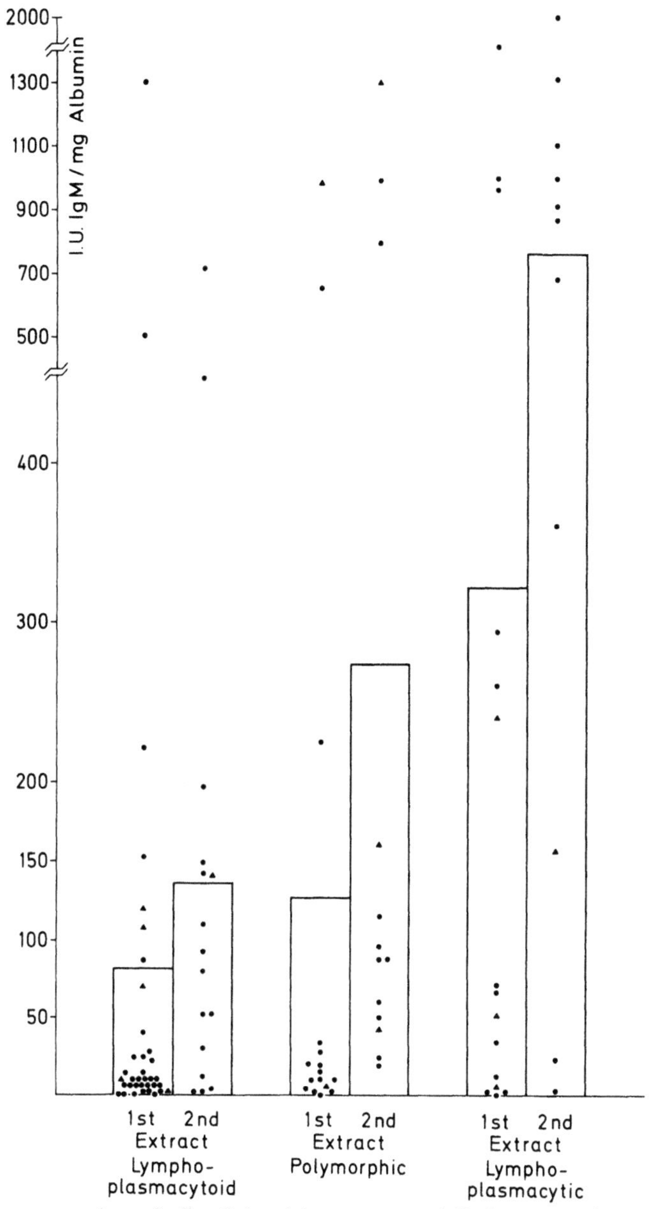


Fig. 280. IgM concentrations of saline (*1st*) and detergent second (*2nd*) extracts of the lymphoplasmacytoid, polymorphic, and lymphoplasmacytic subtypes of immunocytoma. Dots indicate IgM concentrations of tissue extracts that were associated with normal or decreased IgM levels in the corresponding sera. Triangles indicate IgM concentrations of tissue extracts that were associated with a significant, monoclonal increase in the IgM level of the corresponding sera. Height of each column is the mean value

significantly, but not markedly, increased tissue-IgM values. A similar relationship was found between the number of PAS-positive inclusions in the tumor cells and the serum-Ig levels. The largest number of inclusions was seen in the cases that lacked a monoclonal increase in serum Ig.

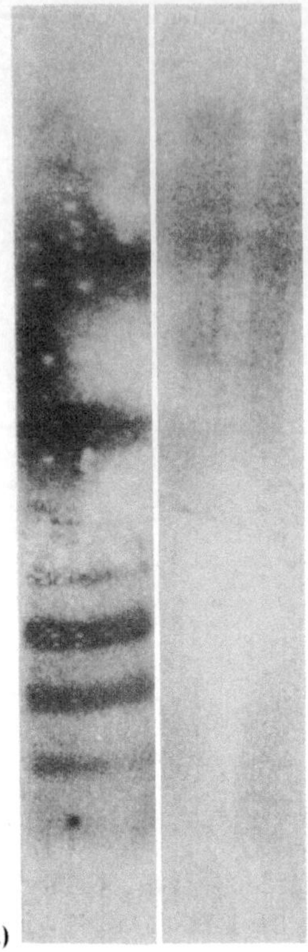


Fig. 281a and b. LP immunocytoma. Autoradiographs of reduced and carboxymethylated, isoelectrofocused IgM from biopsy tissue extract (a) and serum (b) of a patient with the lymphoplasmacytic subtype

**Monoclonality of the Tissue and Serum Immunoglobulin.** The previously mentioned increased serum-IgM fractions proved to be monoclonal in immunoelectrophoresis. Thus, those cases were equivalent with classic Waldenström's disease. The IgM and IgA fractions that were increased in the serum from one case were also monoclonal. In electrophoresis the tissue extract from this tumor showed an IgM and IgA band that could be developed only with an anti-$\kappa$ serum.

To obtain direct evidence for or against monoclonality of the increased tissue-IgM fractions in cases of LP immunocytoma without increased serum-IgM levels, the tissue extracts and sera from 18 cases were subjected to isoelectric focusing.[267] Then, the IgM fraction was made visible by means of $^{125}$I-labeled anti-IgM antibodies. The tissue IgM from all but one case revealed a monoclonal isoelectric-focusing pattern, whereas the serum-IgM pattern was of the polyclonal type in all cases (Fig. 281). In connection with the results of labeling for CIg, these findings strongly indicate (1) that the plasmacytoid cells were actually tumor cells, (2) that the IgM extracted from the biopsy material was

[267] BOUMAN, STEIN, HAVSTEEN and LENNERT, 1975, unpublished data; STEIN, BOUMAN, LENNERT, FUCHS *et al.*, 1977.

synthesized by the tumor cells themselves, and (3) that in most cases the IgM produced by the plasmacytoid cells was not released into the blood.

The tissue extracts that contained increased amounts of two or three Ig classes have not yet been subjected to isoelectric focusing. It is therefore unknown at this time whether all of the Ig classes found to be increased were produced by the LP-immunocytoma cells.

**Cytoplasmic Immunoglobulin (CIg).** *LP Immunocytoma with a Serum-Immunoglobulin Spike.* CIg was first observed in Waldenström's disease in the form of globular (PAS-positive) cytoplasmic or nuclear inclusions.[268] The CIg nature of these inclusions was confirmed in 1960 by DUTCHER and FAHEY, who showed that the inclusions could be stained with fluorescein-labeled anti-IgM antibodies. By means of labeled anti-Ig sera, it was found that the reaction for CIg was diffuse in a majority of cells from most cases (see Fig. 282a), but invisible when routine morphologic methods were used. CIg rarely occurred as crystalline inclusions (see p. 599). PREUD'HOMME *et al.*[269] investigated a large series of Waldenström's disease for CIg in the tumor cells. Only four out of 38 cases revealed a large number of cytoplasmic IgM-positive cells. In most other cases the incidence of cytoplasmic IgM-positive cells was strikingly low. The cells that did stain for cytoplasmic IgM exhibited, in most instances, features of lymphatic plasma cells and plasmablasts. Similar results had been reported by other authors.[270] These findings differ from the CIg-staining results in multiple myeloma, in which most, if not all, plasma cells were stained by monospecific, labeled anti-Ig sera. As shown in double-labeling experiments, in Waldenström's disease most lymphocytes bearing surface IgM and IgD did not contain detectable cytoplasmic IgM, whereas the cells with cytoplasmic IgM (identical with plasmacytoid cells) bore surface IgM with the same light-chain type as the cytoplasmic IgM, but were devoid of surface IgD.[270a]

In three cases with a lymphoplasmacytoid morphology the plasmacytoid cells and a small proportion of the lymphocytoid cells were positive for cytoplasmic IgG or IgA and negative for SIg. This indicates that lymphoplasmacytoid morphology is not limited to IgM-producing cells. In contrast to the IgM-producing cases, the IgG- or IgA-producing cases revealed SIg only on the surface of the lymphocytoid cells and not on the cytoplasmic IgG- or IgA-positive plasmacytoid cells.[271]

*LP Immunocytoma without a Serum-Immunoglobulin Spike.* SELIGMANN *et al.*[271] had in their series only one patient whose serum revealed no spike of monoclonal Ig. Thirteen percent of the proliferating cells from this patient contained IgM/$\kappa$ in the cytoplasm. Some of them revealed IgM/$\kappa$-positive intranuclear and morular cytoplasmic globules, i.e., Russell body-like material. SELIGMANN *et al.* called the lesion "nonsecreting macroglobulinemia." Thus, it was equivalent to the usual type of LP immunocytoma of the Kiel Classification.

[268] SCHAMAUN, 1954; LELBACH, 1957; ZOLLINGER, 1958; DUTCHER and FAHEY, 1959.

[269] PREUD'HOMME, HUREZ and SELIGMANN, 1970.

[270] SOLOMON, FAHEY and MALMGREN, 1963; MARMONT and DAMASIO, 1971.

[270a] PERNIS, BROUET and SELIGMANN, 1974.

[271] SELIGMANN, PREUD'HOMME and BROUET, 1973.

By means of two-color fluoresence, we studied three cases of LP immunocytoma without a serum-Ig spike for thc simultaneous occurrence of SIg and CIg. A majority of cells from all three cases bore surface IgM, whereas CIg was found in only 4–20% of the cells. Some, but not all, of the CIg-positive cells were also positive for SIg. The heavy- and light-chain types on the surface and in the cytoplasm were identical in all three cases.

In cases with a monoclonal serum-Ig spike, or in which identical Ig chains were immunologically demonstrated on the surface membrane and in the cytoplasm, it is easy to decide whether the plasmacytoid cells belong to the neoplastic cell population. When only routine sections and no immunologic data are available—as is the rule—classification of the lymphoplasmacytoid cells with or without PAS-positive globules as nonneoplastic or neoplastic may be difficult or even impossible.

To help clarify the significance of PAS-positive globules in the nucleus or cytoplasm, Kim *et al.*[272] studied the serum and urine from 18 patients for monoclonal increases in immunoglobulin. The lymphoid-cell proliferations in these cases had cytologic features that suggested Ig production: plasmablasts, plasmacytes, and/or PAS-positive globules. PAS-positive globules were found in the cells from only three out of 10 patients with a monoclonal increase in serum Ig. In contrast, abundant PAS-positive globules were present in four out of five lymphoid-cell proliferations without a monoclonal increase in serum Ig. Three of the five proliferations were interpreted by Kim *et al.*[272] as nonneoplastic. They therefore concluded that PAS-positive globules are more abundant and more consistent in lymphatic proliferations without monoclonal increases in serum Ig, and that abundant PAS-positive globules usually reflect synthesis of polyclonal Ig rather than of monoclonal Ig. Our data, on the other hand, indicate that abundant PAS-positive globules chiefly suggest highly active synthesis of monoclonal Ig and a block in the secretory mechanism. The block results in accumulation of the synthesized Ig in the cells.

In order to fully clarify the nature of cells of the plasma-cell series and of intranuclear or cytoplasmic PAS-positive inclusions in lymphoproliferative lesions, we consider it essential to specify the heavy- and light-chain types in the plasmacytoid cells from a large series of cases. Thus, we[273] attempted to demonstrate CIg on routine paraffin sections from a large number of LP immunocytomas without monoclonal increases in serum Ig by means of the enzyme-bridge method of Sternberger *et al.*[274] as modified by Taylor and Burns.[275] The LP immunocytomas were selected on the basis of morphologic criteria alone. The results are presented in Table 101. Of the 43 lymphomas with lymphoplasmacytoid morphology, five showed much background staining. Eighteen out of the other 38 cases clearly revealed a predominance of plasmacytoid cells and/or PAS-positive globules reacting for one light-chain type. This indicated that the plasmacytoid cells, including the cells containing PAS-positive globules, belonged to the tumor-cell population. The cytoplasm of the tumor cells and/or the PAS-

---

[272] Kim, Heller and Rappaport, 1973.

[273] Stein, Lennert and Fuchs, 1976, unpublished data.

[274] Sternberger, Hardy, Cuculis and Meyer, 1970.

[275] 1974.

Table 101. Results of labeling intracytoplasmic immunoglobulin (CIg) in LP immunocytoma by means of the peroxidase-bridge method

| CIg-labeling results | No. of observations |
|---|---|
| Predominance of one light-chain type | 18 ($\kappa$ [12], $\lambda$ [6]) |
| Equal amount of both light-chain types | 11 |
| No CIg-positive cells | 9 |
| Much background staining | 5 |
| Total | 43 |

positive globules often stained more weakly for CIg than did the cytoplasm of reactive plasma cells.

Nine cases were completely devoid of cells stainable for CIg. In two of the nine cases large amounts of protein deposits were visible among and within some of the cells with Giemsa staining. These deposits stained intensely with PAS but not with anti-Ig sera. Tissue extracts from the two cases, however, revealed a high concentration of IgM. It showed a monoclonal pattern in isoelectric focusing. This indicates that in some cases the antigenic sites of the Ig produced by the tumor cells are not accessible in paraffin sections or that they are destroyed during processing of the tissue. In such cases the enzyme-bridge method yields false negative results. It is noteworthy that, in contrast to the negative tumor cells, few reactive plasma cells, located mainly at the margins of the tumor, stained strongly for $\kappa$-, $\lambda$-, and $\gamma$-chains.

In 11 cases plasmacytoid cells that were positive for $\kappa$- or $\lambda$-chains were found in approximately equal amounts, suggesting their reactive nature. Apparently, however, not all of the plasmacytoid cells in all 11 cases were reactive in nature. In some cases transitional forms between plasmacytoid cells and blast cells, and between lymphocytoid cells and blast cells were visible. This indicated that some of the plasmacytoid cells belonged to the tumor-cell population. One such case was of special interest. Some of the cells from this case contained PAS-positive globular intranuclear and cytoplasmic inclusions. The inclusions stained strongly with antisera directed against IgM and $\kappa$- and $\lambda$-chains. It could not be decided whether an individual inclusion stained for both light-chain types or for only one. When the tissue extract from this case was subjected to isoelectric focusing, however, the fraction with $\mu$-chain antigenicity exhibited a monoclonal pattern. To clarify this phenomenon, we plan to subject tissue extracts from similar cases to isoelectric focusing and to label the Ig fractions with anti-$\lambda$ and anti-$\kappa$ sera as well as with anti-heavy chain sera.

In contrast to amorphous cytoplasmic globules, crystalline cytoplasmic inclusions are widely accepted as indications of the neoplastic nature of the cells containing them. Crystalline inclusions are very rare; but when they do occur, it is most often in cells that resemble CLL cells.[276] The occurrence of crystalline

[276] BERNARD, BESSIS, SOULIÉR and THIÉRY, 1959; DE MAN and MEINERS, 1962; HUREZ, FLANDRIN, PREUD'HOMME and SELIGMANN, 1972; NARDO and NORTON, 1972; CLARK, RYDELL and KAPLAN, 1973.

Table 102. Surface-immunoglobulin (SIg) and intracytoplasmic-immunoglobulin (CIg) labeling of cells from lymphoplasmacytoid subtype of LP immunocytoma with crystalline cytoplasmic inclusions

| Author | No. of cases studied | SIg | CIg | Serum-Ig spike | Bence-Jones proteinuria |
|---|---|---|---|---|---|
| HUREZ *et al.*[c] | 1 | $\mu$, $\lambda$ | $\mu$, $\lambda$ | n.p.[a] | n.p. |
| CAWLEY *et al.*[d] | 1 | $\mu$, ($\gamma$), $\lambda$ | $\alpha$, $\lambda$ | n.d.[b] | n.d. |
| CLARK *et al.*[e] | 4 | $\mu$, $\lambda$ | $\mu$, $\lambda$ | p. | n.p. |

[a] n.p. = not present.
[b] n.d. = not determined.
[c] HUREZ, FLANDRIN, PREUD'HOMME and SELIGMANN, 1972.
[d] CAWLEY, BARKER, BRITCHFORD and SMITH, 1973.
[e] CLARK, RYDELL and KAPLAN, 1973.

inclusions appears to be limited to lymphoplasmacytoid immunocytoma cells that produce $\lambda$-chains. In all cases studied so far, the inclusions gave a positive reaction for $\lambda$-chains (see Table 102). In the six cases described in the literature, the heavy chain was of the $\mu$-type in five[277] and of the $\alpha$-type in one case.[278]

**IgG-Fc Receptor.** As far as we know, no data are available.

**Complement Receptor.** The literature contains no reports on systematic studies of the presence of complement receptors on cells of LP immunocytoma or Waldenström's disease.

We demonstrated complement receptors on frozen sections of LP-immunocytoma tissue from 12 out of 25 cases by means of EACmouse or glutaraldehyde-fixed EAChuman. In all positive cases the histologic distribution of the complement receptors was more or less nodular. Cytologic analysis revealed that most of the lymphoid cells and some of the blast cells, but not the plasmablasts and plasmacytoid cells, formed rosettes with EAC (Fig. 282b).

ROSS and POLLEY[279] studied the expression of complement-receptor subtypes on cells from three cases of Waldenström's disease. The cells chiefly exhibited receptors for C3b (and C4), but not for C3d.

We specified the complement-receptor subtypes in frozen sections from 13 cases of LP immunocytoma. Cells from nine of the cases expressed receptors for both C3b and C3d; cells from one case bore receptors for C3b alone. Four cases did not reveal any complement-receptor activity.[279a] So far, we have not observed any cases of LP immunocytoma with cells having receptors for C3d alone. That receptor distribution is characteristic of B-CLL.

From the data from these complement-receptor studies, we conclude that there might be two immunologic subtypes of LP immunocytoma:

1. A subtype that expresses only receptors for C3b or no complement-receptor activity at all. The reaction of EACmouse and glutaraldehyde-fixed

[277] HUREZ, FLANDRIN, PREUD'HOMME and SELIGMANN, 1972; CLARK, RYDELL and KAPLAN, 1973.
[278] CAWLEY, BARKER, BRITCHFORD and SMITH, 1973.
[279] 1975.
[279a] STEIN, PAPADIMITRIOU, BOUMAN, LENNERT *et al.*, 1978, in press.

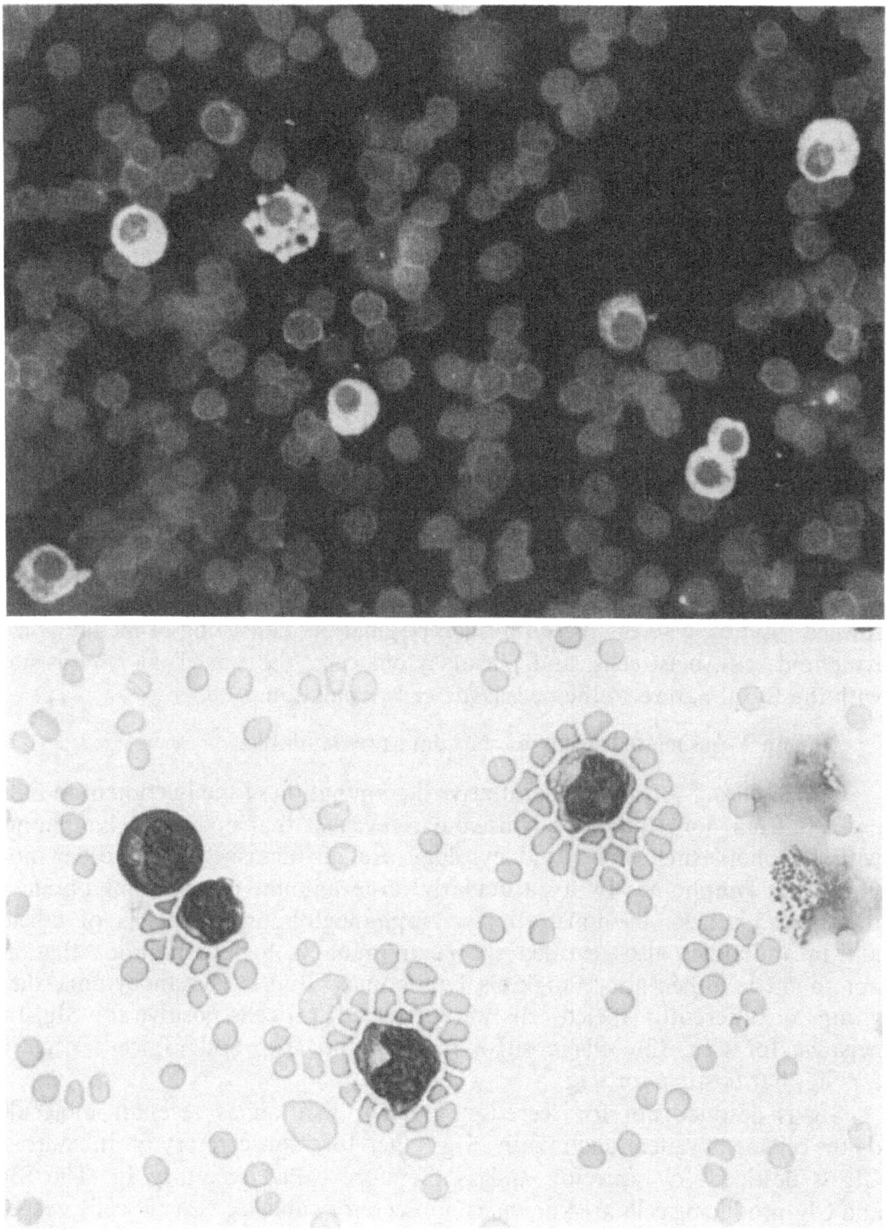

(a)

(b)

Fig. 282a and b. LP immunocytoma. (a) Suspended cells stained with monovalent rhodamine-conjugated anti-Ig antibodies. Plasmacytoid cells react positively for $\mu$- and $\kappa$-chains, whereas lymphocytes do not. In the serum of this patient, the levels of all three major Ig classes were decreased. $\times 440$. (b) Suspended cells from the same case as (a) subjected to the EAC-rosette assay. Lymphocytes form rosettes with EAC, whereas plasmacytoid cells do not. Double labeling with two-color fluorescence showed that the SIg of lymphocytes and the CIg of plasmacytoid cells shared the same heavy-chain class ($\mu$) and the same light-chain type ($\kappa$). Cytocentrifuge slide. Pappenheim. $\times 875$

EAChuman with C3d receptors, but not with C3b receptors, on frozen sections suggests that the EACmouse-negative or glutaraldehyde-fixed EAChuman-negative LP immunocytomas belong to this subtype.

2. A subtype that expresses both complement-receptor subtypes (C3b and C3d receptors). It includes our EACmouse-positive and glutaraldehyde-fixed EAChuman-positive cases of LP immunocytoma.

**Mouse-Erythrocyte (E) Receptor.** GUPTA *et al.*[280] found increased numbers of mouse-E rosette-forming cells (32%) in the peripheral blood of a patient with Waldenström's disease. The number of mouse-E rosette-forming cells from nine patients with CLL studied by the same authors, however, ranged from 45.5–96% with a mean value of 70%. CATOVSKY *et al.*[281] observed small numbers of mouse-E rosette-forming cells from one patient with Waldenström's disease. Further studies will have to show whether the mouse E-rosette assay is of help in distinguishing between CLL and LP immunocytoma. That would be of great interest, since the morphologic distinction between CLL and LP immunocytoma is often difficult (see p. 241 ff.).

**Sheep-Erythrocyte (E) Receptor.** Only a small percentage of the cells obtained from biopsies of five LP immunocytomas bound sheep erythrocytes. Cytologic evaluation of the rosette-forming cells revealed that only small lymphoid cells formed rosettes, whereas the tumor-cell population, consisting of medium-sized lymphoid cells, blast cells, and plasmacytoid cells, did not. That is consistent with the B-cell nature of the neoplastic cell population.

**Human T-Associated Antigens.** No data are available.

**Conclusions.** Systematic quantitative determination of the Ig content in tissue extracts from non-Hodgkin's lymphomas revealed that malignant lymphomas with lymphoplasmacytic/-cytoid cytology are distinguished from other non-Hodgkin's lymphomas by a particularly large amount of immunoglobulin in the tissue extracts. Demonstration of immunoglobulin by means of labeled anti-Ig antibodies also revealed special immunocytologic conditions that are not found in other non-Hodgkin's lymphomas. In LP immunocytoma three groups of differently labeled cells were detected: (1) cells positive for SIg, but negative for CIg, (2) cells positive for SIg and CIg, and (3) cells negative for SIg, but positive for CIg.

SIg is destined not for secretion, but for fixation as receptor molecules on the cell membrane. Functionally, SIg is therefore nonsecretory Ig. In contrast, CIg is destined for secretion and is therefore called secretory Ig. The SIg- and CIg-producing cells are known as nonsecretory and secretory B-cells, respectively.

Applying this functional terminology, LP immunocytoma is defined as a proliferation of functionally different B-cells, i.e., of both nonsecretory and secretory B-cells. In contrast, B-CLL, centrocytic lymphoma, centroblastic/centrocytic lymphoma, centroblastic lymphoma, and lymphoblastic lymphoma of the Burkitt type are proliferations of nonsecretory B-cells, and plasmacytoma is a proliferation of secretory B-cells (see Table 103).

---

[280] GUPTA, GOOD and SIEGAL, 1976a, b.

[281] CATOVSKY, CHERCHI, OKOS, HEGDE *et al.*, 1976.

Table 103. Immunoglobulin (Ig) staining pattern and serum-Ig levels in chronic lymphocytic leukemia (CLL), LP immunocytoma, B-type immunoblastic lymphoma, and plasmacytoma

| | Predominant heavy-chain class | SIg | CIg | Serum-Ig level |
|---|---|---|---|---|
| CLL | $\mu$ and $\delta$ | + | − | n or ↓ |
| LP immunocytoma | $\mu$ and $\delta$ on the surface, $\mu$ in the cytoplasm | + | + | 25% ↑ |
| Immunoblastic lymphoma | $\mu$ | + | + | rarely ↑ |
| Plasmacytoma | $\gamma$; $\alpha$ | − or + | +++ | 99% ↑ |

n = normal; ↓ = decreased; ↑ = increased.

LP immunocytoma resembles B-immunoblastic lymphoma in the simultaneous production of nonsecretory and secretory Ig, since SIg- and CIg-positive cells are also often demonstrable in B-immunoblastic lymphoma (see pp. 644f. and 647). In contrast to LP immunocytoma, however, B-immunoblastic lymphoma is a morphologically homogeneous proliferation of blast cells. They are apparently in the process of switching from the synthesis of nonsecretory Ig to the synthesis of secretory Ig. That explains why both SIg and CIg are often simultaneously demonstrable in B-immunoblastic lymphoma cells. LP immunocytoma, on the other hand, is a proliferation of the whole, or at least a part of, the B-cell transformation series, i.e., of lymphoid cells (nonsecretory cells), blast cells ("switching" cells), and plasmablasts and/or plasmacytes (secretory cells).

IgM is the predominant SIg and CIg class in LP immunocytoma. IgG and IgA are rarely found. The studies of PERNIS *et al.*[282] and of our own group suggest that most IgM-producing LP-immunocytoma cells bear both $\delta$- and $\mu$-chains on the surface membrane. $\delta$-Chains were never detected in the cytoplasm.

Because of the presence of secretory cells in LP immunocytoma, one would expect the serum—as in plasmacytoma—to reveal an increase in the same Ig class as that detected in the cytoplasm. Only a small number of cases, however, revealed a serum-Ig spike. When this serum Ig was of the IgM class, the neoplasm was identical with Waldenström's disease. The neoplastic nature of the plasmacytoid cells is generally accepted in such cases. In cases of LP immunocytoma without a serum-Ig spike, some hematologists doubt that the plasmacytoid cells belong to the malignant, proliferating cell clone. The data collected from our series indicate that in most instances the plasmacytoid cells definitely belonged to the tumor-cell population.

Since there was evidence of secretory-Ig synthesis, seen either as an increase in tissue Ig or as CIg, in nearly all of the cases of LP immunocytoma without a serum-Ig spike, we conclude that the secretory mechanism of the plasmacytoid cells, especially of those producing IgM, was often blocked. The tendency of the secretory mechanism of LP immunocytoma cells to fail may be related to the complexity of the mechanism for secretion of IgM. PARKHOUSE and ASKONAS[283] suggested that there is a link between the secretion and the pentamerization of monomeric IgM. This assumption was supported by our finding

[282] PERNIS, BROUET and SELIGMANN, 1974. [283] 1969.

that in four cases that revealed a high tissue- but a reduced serum-IgM content the tissue IgM consisted chiefly of monomeric 8 S IgM.[284]

The block in the mechanism for secretion of the produced Ig frequently led to accumulation of large amounts of Ig, seen as Russell body-like material or, less often, as crystalline inclusions in the plasmacytoid cells of LP immunocytoma. Thus, the blocked secretory mechanism would explain the large amount of Russell body-like material found in some malignant lymphomas without changes in serum-Ig levels.[285]

Even though complete absence of Ig synthesis appears to be rare in LP immunocytoma, partial disturbance of Ig synthesis sometimes occurs. Besides failures in carbohydrate incorporation, the failure of heavy and light chains to link must be mentioned. Such cases are well known as heavy-chain disease, in which free heavy chains are detectable in the serum. As far as we know, heavy-chain disease without secretion of heavy chains has not been described in the literature. Recently, we observed a case of nonsecreting heavy-chain disease. Morphologically, it proved to be a plasmacytoma (see p. 608).

The data presented here provide evidence that there are four phenotypic variants of LP immunocytoma:

1. Waldenström's syndrome = IgM-producing LP immunocytoma in which the cells are capable of releasing the IgM they have produced into the blood.
2. IgG or IgA paraproteinemia = IgG- or IgA-producing and -secreting LP immunocytoma.
3. Heavy-chain disease = LP immunocytoma in which the cells produce and secrete heavy chains that are not linked to light chains and/or are defective in structure.
4. LP immunocytoma with no changes in serum-Ig levels = Ig-producing LP immunocytoma in which the cells are incapable of releasing the Ig they have produced into the blood.

The nature of the proliferating cells is fundamentally the same in all variants. This means that functional properties alone are not always suitable for classifying tumor cells, particularly when the classification is based on only one functional property, such as production or secretion of immunoglobulin. As far as we know, a malignant proliferation of plasma cells is generally regarded as plasmacytoma, even when the malignant plasmacytoma cells have lost their capacity to produce and/or secrete immunoglobulin. Another example is malignant melanoma, which is always a malignant melanoma, even when it does not produce melanin.

Data on complement-receptor subtypes and the cytology of LP immunocytoma, in connection with findings in tonsillar tissue, suggest that there are two subtypes of LP immunocytoma of different cellular origin:

1. A subtype containing cells that are devoid of complement receptors or have receptors for C3b, but not for C3d, and thus resemble cells of the plasma-cell reaction. The nonsecretory cells are similar to CLL cells (small round lymphocytoid cells). Since cells of the plasma-cell reaction are apparently

[284] KAISERLING, STEIN and LENNERT, 1973; STEIN, KAISERLING, LENNERT and PARWARESCH, 1973; STEIN, 1974, unpublished data.

[285] KIM, HELLER and RAPPAPORT, 1973.

C3d receptor-negative and C3b receptor-positive or devoid of both complement-receptor subtypes (see p. 555), this subtype of LP immunocytoma may be the neoplastic equivalent of the plasma-cell reaction defined by FAGRAEUS[286] and described in detail by VELDMAN.[287]

2. A C3d receptor- and C3b receptor-positive form with nonsecretory cells resembling centrocytes and with blast cells resembling centroblasts. Since germinal-center cells are C3d and C3b receptor-positive (see p. 555), this subtype may be the neoplastic equivalent of a hyperimmune germinal-center reaction in which plasma cells usually develop.[288]

These two subtypes of LP immunocytoma do not fully correlate with the three subtypes (lymphoplasmacytoid, polymorphic, and lymphoplasmacytic; see p. 224ff.) distinguished by means of morphologic criteria alone.

The close relationship between germinal-center cells and some LP immunocytomas is substantiated by the observation of cytologically typical follicular centroblastic/centrocytic lymphomas in which some of the cells transformed into CIg-positive cells (i.e., cells with plasmacytoid appearance and/or cells containing intranuclear or intracytoplasmic Russell body-like material). Further study is necessary to determine whether such borderline cases should be classified as germinal center-cell lymphoma, LP immunocytoma, or a separate type of one of these entities.

## H. Malignant Lymphoma, Plasmacytic (Plasmacytoma), Including Multiple Myeloma

Most authors do not include all kinds of plasmacytoma among the non-Hodgkin's lymphomas, probably for historical reasons. Until recently, it was not generally accepted that the plasma cell is derived from a B-lymphocyte. Another reason is that most plasmacytomas appear to originate in the bone marrow and secondarily involve lymph nodes. Plasmacytomas that originate primarily in lymph nodes, however, are generally classified with the non-Hodgkin's lymphomas. Since there are no immunologic differences between plasmacytomas that primarily develop within (usually called multiple myeloma) and those that develop outside the bone marrow, we shall discuss the immunologic properties of both types of plasmacytoma together.

**Surface Immunoglobulin (SIg) and Cytoplasmic Immunoglobulin (CIg).** SELIGMANN *et al.*[288a] studied 40 cases of multiple myeloma for SIg and CIg. We have compiled their data in Table 104. Four main staining patterns were encountered. In the first and most common type the same monoclonal Ig chains were found on the surface and in the cytoplasm of plasmacytoma cells. In the second, next most common type the plasma-cell surface was stained with antisera to the two light-chain types and to more than one heavy-chain class. In the third type no SIg was detected on Ig-containing plasma cells. Four of these cases

[286] 1948.
[287] 1970.
[288] WHITE, 1960; STRAUS, 1970.
[288a] SELIGMANN, PREUD'HOMME and BROUET, 1973.

Table 104. Surface immunoglobulin (SIg) and cytoplasmic immunoglobulin (CIg) in multiple myeloma. Forty cases studied by SELIGMANN, PREUD'HOMME and BROUET (1973)

| Type | No. of cases | SIg | CIg |
|---|---|---|---|
| I | 14 | Same heavy and light chains as CIg | γ, α and/or only one light chain |
| II | 13 | Mixed staining (μ, γ, κ, λ) | γ, α and/or both light chains |
| III | 9 | None | γ, α and only one light chain |
| IV | 4 | μ and same light chain as CIg | γ, α and only one light chain |

secreted only light chains. The fourth type is of special interest because of the finding of IgM molecules on the surface of plasmacytoma cells, which contained Bence-Jones proteins or IgG or IgA myeloma protein. The SIg and CIg of these cases showed the same light chain.

The mixed SIg staining of the second type is probably a false polyclonal pattern, like the one in CLL and other lymphomas. This view is substantiated by our studies of one primary lymph-node plasmacytoma in an 11-year-old girl.[288b] The freshly drawn cells of this case exhibited μ-, δ-, γ-, α-, κ-, and λ-chains, but no ε-chains. After overnight culture, the mixed staining could be completely converted into a monoclonal staining for α- and κ-chains only (i.e., type I). Double-labeling assays for SIg and CIg revealed that most of the plasmacytoma cells containing α- and κ-chains in their cytoplasm also expressed α- and κ-chains on the cell surface membrane. These findings suggest that the mixed SIg staining was due only to passively absorbed Ig chains. Low-rate synthesis of SIg by the plasmacytoma cells, however, could not be ruled out by our studies.

In rare cases the plasmacytoma cells stain positively for CIg, although the serum lacks a monoclonal Ig component, indicating that Ig is produced but not secreted. Recently, we observed a multiple myeloma that resembled a case described by HUREZ *et al.*[288c] The cells from our case stained with fluorescein-conjugated antisera and only for α-chains, but not for light chains, with the highly sensitive enzyme-bridge method. The cell extracts also revealed only α- and no light chains.

SIg analysis of blood lymphocytes from plasmacytoma patients is of special interest. In the series of SELIGMANN *et al.*[288d] five out of 40 patients showed a monoclonal population of circulating B-lymphocytes bearing at their surfaces the same heavy and light chains as those found in the cytoplasm of plasmacytoma cells from the bone marrow. A large proportion of lymphocytes bearing μ- and λ-chains were present in the blood of one patient with λ-Bence-Jones myeloma showing μ- and λ-chains on the surface and in the cytoplasm of plasmacytoma cells. In extension of these studies, MELLSTEDT and colleagues[288e] investigated the SIg on blood lymphocytes of plasmacytoma patients by means of antiidiotypic antibodies that were specific for the unique hypervariable region

[288b] KRUSE, STEIN, HITZIG and LASSON, 1978.

[288c] HUREZ, PREUD'HOMME and SELIGMANN, 1970.

[288d] SELIGMANN, PREUD'HOMME and BROUET, 1973.

[288e] MELLSTEDT, HAMMARSTRÖM and HOLM, 1974.

of the heavy chain of each case of plasmacytoma and did not react with "normal" Ig components. These authors demonstrated that a proportion of circulating small lymphocytes bore SIg that was identical to the Ig secreted by the plasmacytoma cells. Trypsinization studies confirmed that the lymphocytes bearing the idiotypic monoclonal Ig were capable of synthesizing that Ig and had not simply absorbed it from the serum. These studies indicate that in plasmacytoma a proportion of the blood B-lymphocytes often belong to the same neoplastic cell clone as the plasmacytoma cells.

**Tissue Immunoglobulin.** *Saline Extract.* The Ig assay of the tissue extracts revealed a high concentration of IgG in all four cases of multiple myeloma studied.[288f] Whereas IgA was decreased in amount in all four tissue extracts, IgM was significantly increased in amount in one extract. In Sephadex G200 chromatography, most of the increased IgM fraction was monomeric 8S IgM. By means of affinity chromatography it could also be shown that the 8S-IgM fraction and the IgG fraction of that case shared the same light chain ($\kappa$).[288f]

**Serum Immunoglobulin.** Highly increased amounts of IgG were measured in the sera of all four cases studied. The IgM level was reduced in all four cases.[288f]

**Monoclonality of the Tissue and Serum Immunoglobulin.** In polyacrylamide-gel electrophoresis, both the tissue and the serum IgG of all cases proved to be monoclonal. The electrophoretic mobility of the tissue and serum IgG of each case was approximately equal, whereas the electrophoretic mobility of the monoclonal IgG varied markedly from case to case. For technical reasons, it was not possible to demonstrate monoclonality of the IgM fraction that was increased in the tissue extract of one plasmacytoma. As mentioned, however, we were able to show that the IgM fraction had the same light-chain type ($\kappa$) as the monoclonal IgG fraction.[288f]

**Membrane Markers Other than SIg.** Like reactive plasma cells, plasmacytoma cells were devoid of receptors for IgG-Fc, complement, mouse erythrocytes, sheep erythrocytes, and HP.[288g]

In one case of lymph-node plasmacytoma we studied the complement-receptor subtypes. The plasmacytoma cells were devoid of receptors for C3b and C3d. In contrast, the blood B-lymphocytes that bore SIg chains ($\alpha$ and $\kappa$) identical with those secreted by the plasmacytoma cells exhibited—unlike normal blood B-lymphocytes—only receptors for C3b and lacked those for C3d.[288h]

**Conclusions.** Plasmacytoma is a purebred proliferation of secretory Ig-producing B-cells, at least as far as the cells in the solid tumor nodules are concerned. In contrast to many former views, plasmacytoma cells frequently show a positive reaction for nonsecretory Ig, i.e., SIg. According to the SIg and CIg staining pattern, four types of plasmacytoma are discernible (Table 104). Most fre-

[288f] Stein and Kaiserling, 1974a.

[288g] Hellström, Mellstedt, Perlmann, Holm et al., 1976.

[288h] Kruse, Stein, Hitzig and Lasson, 1978.

quently, the SIg molecules appear to be produced by plasmacytoma cells (types I and III of Table 104), but in some instances they are passively absorbed (type II of Table 104). That is especially valid for plasmacytomas in which the cells exhibit a mixed SIg staining. In shedding experiments with overnight culture, we could convert the mixed SIg staining into a monotypic staining that was identical with the CIg staining pattern of that case, confirming the extrinsic nature of many of the surface-bound Ig molecules. The studies of ABDOU and ABDOU[288i] suggest that the extrinsic surface membrane-bound molecules are often anti-Ig antibodies. These authors and others[288j] found an increased incidence of anti-Ig antibodies in the sera of plasmacytoma patients.

Of the plasmacytomas with endogenous SIg, the cells of most cases have SIg and CIg (usually $\gamma$ or $\alpha$, seldom $\delta$ or $\varepsilon$) that are identical in heavy-chain class and light-chain type (type I of Table 104). These plasmacytomas might be derived from plasma cells that developed from surface IgG- or surface IgA-positive lymphocytes.

The surface IgM-positive plasmacytomas in which the surface IgM differed in heavy-chain class, but not in light-chain type, from the CIg, recall the findings of PERNIS *et al.*[288k] At the surface of IgG-containing plasma cells those authors demonstrated IgM molecules with the same light chains and the same allotypic markers of variable regions as those of the intracytoplasmic IgG. The surface IgM- and cytoplasmic IgG- or IgA-positive plasma cells might be secretory B-cells at a maturation stage relatively soon after the switch from synthesis of nonsecretory IgM to that of secretory IgG. The SIg-negative plasmacytoma cells might be the neoplastic equivalents of mature plasma cells that have completely ceased the production of surface-membrane Ig-receptor molecules.

In contrast to IgM-producing LP immunocytoma, the secretion mechanism of plasmacytoma cells is only rarely defect (less than 1% of cases).[288l] More common is the sole production and secretion of light chains in the absence of heavy chains (so-called light-chain myeloma). Synthesis and secretion only of heavy chains without light chains (heavy-chain disease) is rare. Recently, we observed a plasmacytoma that resembled the case previously described by HUREZ *et al.*[288m] In the cells of both cases only $\alpha$-chains and no light chains were detectable with fluorescein-labeled antibodies or by means of the sensitive enzyme-bridge method. In addition, extracts of plasmacytoma cells from our case revealed only $\alpha$-chains, but no light chains in measurable amounts. This case is apparently the first case of a nonsecretory type of heavy-chain disease to be reported.

Comparison of Ig classes on peripheral blood lymphocytes with those present on and within plasmacytoma cells and with secreted monoclonal Ig revealed a very remarkable finding. These studies showed that in many instances the SIg of a proportion of the small, morphologically typical blood lymphocytes and the CIg and secreted Ig of plasmacytoma cells shared the same light-chain type and the same idiotypic activity, indicating that both a proportion of the blood B-lymphocytes and the plasmacytoma cells are parts of the same neoplastic cell clone.

[288i] 1975.
[288j] LINDSTRÖM and WILLIAMS, 1975.
[288k] PERNIS, FORNI and AMANTE, 1971.
[288l] OSSERMAN and TAKATSUKI, 1963.
[288m] HUREZ, PREUD'HOMME and SELIGMANN, 1970.

# I. Malignant Lymphoma, Centrocytic

**Surface Immunoglobulin (SIg).** In our experiments, SIg was present on a large proportion of cells from all cases of centrocytic lymphoma. In contrast to CLL, which usually exhibits only faint SIg staining, the cells from centrocytic lymphoma showed dense labeling with peroxidase-coupled or fluorescein-coupled antibodies in most instances (Fig. 283a). Analysis of the heavy-chain class of the SIg revealed that it was of the $\mu$-chain type in all cases. In four cases $\gamma$-chains were also detected on the surfaces of centrocytic lymphoma cells. $\delta$-Chains were investigated in two cases and were found on 35% and 60% of the cells, respectively. Two-color fluorescent staining demonstrated that $\delta$-chains were present on the same cells that bore $\mu$-chains. Labeling for light chains

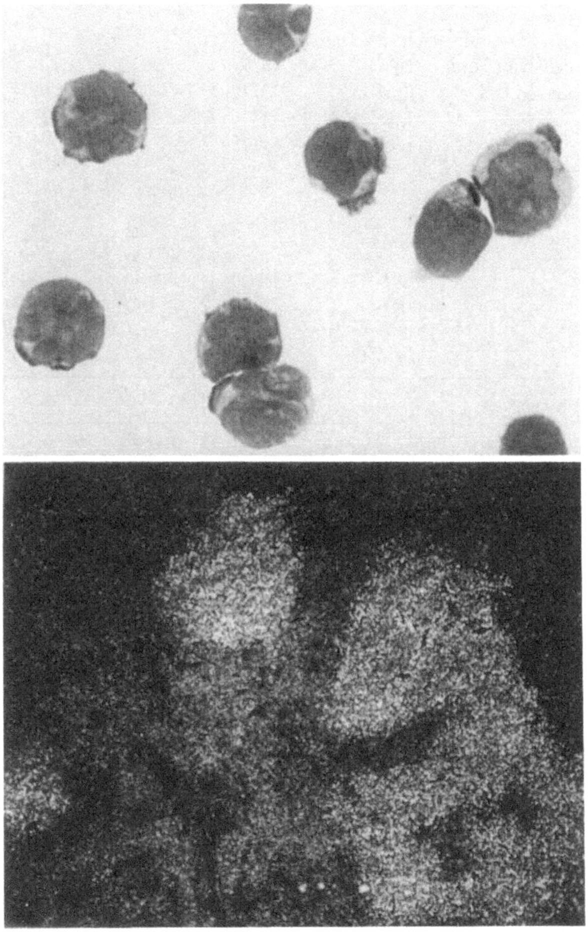

(a)

(b)

Fig. 283a and b. Centrocytic lymphoma. (a) Suspended cells stained for surface IgM by means of horseradish peroxidase-coupled antibodies. Surface IgM is represented by black staining on the surface membrane. Note the irregularly shaped, often cleaved nuclei of the labeled cells and the pronounced capping. Counterstaining with hemalum. ×1,500. (b) Frozen section treated with EAC. The reagent red cells (light spots) adhere to the section in a nodular pattern, although the tumor-cell proliferation is diffuse. Hematoxylin and eosin. Dark-field illumination. ×30

Table 105. Surface immunoglobulin (SIg) on cells from centrocytic lymphoma and apparently similar or equivalent entities of other lymphoma classifications

| Author/Term | SIg class | Incidence | Light-chain type |
|---|---|---|---|
| SILBERMAN and SCHREK:[b] | Ig-PV[a] | 7/7 | |
| Lymphosarcoma-cell leukemia | IgG | 1/7 | |
| | IgM-G | 5/7 | |
| | IgM-G-A | 1/7 | κ |
| BROUET et al.:[c] | Ig-PV | 12/13 | |
| Poorly differentiated | IgM | 8/12 | κ (3), λ (5) |
| lymphocytic lymphoma | IgG | 2/12 | κ (2) |
| (diffuse) | IgM-G | 1/12 | κ, λ |
| AISENBERG and LONG:[d] | Ig-PV | 12/12 | κ (6), λ (6) |
| M.L. lymphocytic, poorly | IgM | 11/12 | κ (5), λ (6) |
| differentiated, diffuse | IgM-G | 1/12 | κ |
| LEECH et al.:[e] | Ig-PV | 9/9 | |
| Follicular center cell lymphoma, | IgM | 4/9 | |
| small and large cleaved cell, | IgM-D | 3/7 | |
| diffuse | IgD | 1/7 | κ |
| | IgG | 1/7 | |
| PREUD'HOMME et al.:[f] | IgM-D | 8/9 | κ (3), λ (5) |
| Poorly differentiated | | | |
| lymphocytic lymphoma | | | |
| STEIN[g] | Ig-PV | 14/14 | κ (5), λ (4), κ and λ (5) |
| | IgM | 8/12 | κ (4), λ (1), κ and λ (3) |
| | IgM-G | 4/12 | λ (2), κ and λ (2) |
| | IgM-D | 2/2 | κ (1), λ (1) |
| Sum of SIg-positive cases | | 62/64 (97%) | |

[a] Ig-PV = Ig demonstrated with a polyvalent anti-Ig serum.
[b] 1974.
[c] BROUET, LABAUME and SELIGMANN, 1975.
[d] 1975.
[e] LEECH, GLICK, WALDRON, FLEXNER et al., 1975.
[f] PREUD'HOMME, BROUET, CLAUVEL and SELIGMANN, 1974.
[g] 1976, unpublished data.

did not provide clear-cut results, since the cells from five out of 14 cases stained for both light-chain types. In three out of the five cases, however, the labeling for one light-chain type was much more intense than that for the other. Capping was conspicuous on the stained cells in most cases (Fig. 283a).

The results of SIg-labeling experiments reported on in the literature and of our own are listed in Table 105. The cases studied by SILBERMAN and SCHREK[289] were originally classified as lymphosarcoma-cell leukemia. PREUD'HOMME et al.,[290] AISENBERG and LONG,[291] BROUET et al.,[292] and HOPPER[293] diagnosed their cases as diffuse lymphocytic poorly differentiated lymphoma,

[289] 1974.
[290] PREUD'HOMME, BROUET, CLAUVEL and SELIGMANN, 1974.
[291] 1975.
[292] BROUET, LABAUME and SELIGMANN, 1975.
[293] 1974.

and LEECH *et al.*[294] described malignant lymphoma, large cleaved, diffuse, and small cleaved, diffuse. Although we cannot be fully certain that all the cases described by those authors are equivalent to our centrocytic lymphoma, the following conclusions may be drawn from the data provided by their studies.

The cells from nearly all, if not all, centrocytic lymphomas bear SIg. The main heavy-chain class is IgM, followed by IgD, as revealed by the data of HOPPER,[295] PREUD'HOMME *et al.*,[296] and LEECH *et al.*[294] PREUD'HOMME *et al.*[296] found IgD simultaneously with IgM in all SIg-positive cases. HOPPER[295] confirmed the simultaneous presence of $\mu$- and $\delta$-chains by means of double labeling and showed that these separate Ig proteins cap independently. There is some controversy over the occurrence of $\gamma$- and $\alpha$-chains on cells bearing predominantly $\mu$-chains. The findings of PIESSENS *et al.*,[297] AUGENER *et al.*,[298] HOPPER,[295] and SILBERMAN and SCHREK[299] and our own results suggest the simultaneous expression of $\mu$- and $\gamma$-chains on the cells from some cases of centrocytic lymphoma. LEECH *et al.*[294] and BROUET *et al.*,[300] however, found no $\gamma$- or $\alpha$-chain labeling in cases with a large proportion of cells that were positive for $\mu$-chains. These controversial findings suggest that the surface IgG detected on centrocytic lymphoma cells by our group and others is an autoantibody, or that it is labile SIg, which was described by LOBO *et al.*[301] on normal blood lymphocytes.

**Tissue Immunoglobulin.** *Saline Extract.* The saline extracts from half of the cases of centrocytic lymphoma contained slightly increased amounts of immunoglobulin, compared with the Ig content of thymuses or normal lymph nodes. In all of the cases that revealed an increase in tissue Ig, the Ig was mainly of the IgM type. Figure 276 shows the IgM values measured in 23 saline extracts. A large amount of IgM was detected in only one case. In addition to IgM, an increase in IgG was found in two cases and IgA in one case.

*Detergent Second Extract.* The detergent 2nd extracts from 13 out of 15 cases revealed a significant increase in immunoglobulin. The predominant Ig class involved was IgM in all cases; in eight cases alone, in three with IgA, and in two with IgG. Two-color fluorescence demonstrated the presence of both $\mu$- and $\gamma$-chains and of only one light chain on the cells from the two cases with increased amounts of IgM and IgG in the tissue extract.

As shown in Figure 277, the IgM content was highly increased in six out of 14 cases. The mean IgM content was significantly higher than that found in CLL, centroblastic/centrocytic lymphoma, and lymphoblastic lymphoma of other than the Burkitt type, lower than that in LP immunocytoma and immunoblastic lymphoma, and as high as that in lymphoblastic lymphoma of the Burkitt type.

---

[294] LEECH, GLICK, WALDRON, FLEXNER *et al.*, 1975.
[295] 1974.
[296] PREUD'HOMME, BROUET, CLAUVEL and SELIGMANN, 1974.
[297] PIESSENS, SCHUR, MOLONEY and CHURCHILL, 1973.
[298] AUGENER, COHNEN and BRITTINGER, 1975.
[299] 1974.
[300] BROUET, LABAUME and SELIGMANN, 1975.
[301] LOBO, WESTERVELT and HORWITZ, 1975.

**Serum Immunoglobulin.** The serum-IgM level was in the normal ($2\sigma$) range in 67%, IgA in 61%, and IgG in 83% of the 23 cases studied. A reduction in the serum-IgM level was found in 29%, IgA in 26%, and IgG in 17% of the cases. The IgG level was never above normal. There was a slight increase in IgA in three out of 23 cases (13%), and in IgM in one out of 24 cases (4%).

**Monoclonality of the Tissue and Serum Immunoglobulin.** The tissue Ig extracted from centrocytic lymphomas has not yet been tested for monoclonality by means of isoelectric focusing. In one case the serum-IgM fraction, which revealed no increase, consisted of monoclonal IgM/$\kappa$.

**Cytoplasmic Immunoglobulin (CIg).** The cells from two representative cases of centrocytic lymphoma were completely negative for CIg, as demonstrated in our studies using fluorescein-labeled anti-Ig antibodies on cytocentrifuge slides of washed tumor cells and on frozen sections.

With the enzyme-bridge method, TAYLOR[302] observed CIg in cells from two out of 12 lymphomas, which he classified as lymphosarcoma (four cases) and lymphoblastic reticulosarcoma (eight cases). The latter group is considered by TAYLOR to be roughly equivalent to lymphocytic lymphoma, diffuse, well and poorly differentiated. Thus, the cases of TAYLOR might be equivalent to our centrocytic lymphoma, although we cannot be certain of it.

We observed one case of centrocytic lymphoma in which the cells were predominantly of the centrocytic lymphoma-cell type, but a considerable number of them demonstrated transformation into plasma cells. All types of intermediate cell forms between the centrocytic cell type and plasma cells were visible, whereas no blast cell-like forms were found. A large amount of IgM was measured in the extract from this special case. These observations are consistent with the view that centrocytes are capable of transforming directly into plasma cells without passing through a blast-cell stage.

**IgG-Fc Receptor.** In the four cases studied, the centrocytic lymphoma cells did not form rosettes with IgGEA. By applying the more sensitive method of detecting IgG-Fc receptors by means of IgG aggregates, BROUET *et al.*[303] found positively reacting cells in seven out of nine cases of poorly differentiated lymphoma. The difference between the results of the IgGEA and IgG-aggregate assays can be explained most easily by a low density of IgG-Fc receptors on the surface membranes of the centrocytic lymphoma cells, resulting in the capacity to bind only IgG aggregates, or to bind IgGEA only when the pelleting technique is used.

**Complement Receptor.** As far as we know, only a few studies on the occurrence of complement receptors on centrocytic lymphoma cells have been published. JAFFE *et al.*[304] found only a small percentage of EAC-reactive cells among those from lymphomas that they classified as poorly differentiated lymphoma, diffuse. A high percentage of the cells from their three cases bound neuraminidase-treated sheep erythrocytes instead of EAC, suggesting a T-cell origin. We

---

302 1974.

303 BROUET, LABAUME and SELIGMANN, 1975.

304 JAFFE, SHEVACH, SUSSMAN, FRANK *et al.*, 1975.

assume that the three cases were not equivalent to our centrocytic lymphoma, but more likely to lymphoblastic lymphoma of the convoluted-cell type.

We studied the cells from six cases of centrocytic lymphoma for the presence of complement receptors on frozen sections by means of the IgMEAC-adherence technique. The neoplastic cells from all cases bound IgMEAC either in a nodular or in a more diffuse pattern, although in histologic sections the growth pattern was always diffuse (Fig. 283b).

In five cases we had the opportunity to study the occurrence of complement receptors on suspended cells. In all cases 35–70% of the centrocytic lymphoma cells formed rosettes with IgMEACmouse. Cytologic examination of the Ig MEAC rosette-forming cells on cytocentrifuge slides revealed that they were indeed tumor cells. Analysis of the complement-receptor subtypes showed the presence of both C3b and C3d receptors in the three cases studied. Thus, the pattern of complement-receptor subtypes in centrocytic lymphoma is apparently different from that usually found in B-CLL.

**Mouse-Erythrocyte (E) Receptor.** CATOVSKY *et al.*[305] studied the mouse-E rosette-forming capacity of cells from six cases of lymphosarcoma-cell leukemia, poorly differentiated, which is probably identical with leukemic centrocytic lymphoma. None of the six neoplasms contained more than 20% rosetting cells, whereas all but one of the cases of CLL revealed a high percentage (30–80%) of mouse-E rosettes. That indicates a clear difference between centrocytic lymphoma and CLL.

**Sheep-Erythrocyte (E) Receptor.** The data reported by most authors on sheep E-rosette assays of cells from poorly differentiated lymphoma, diffuse, agree in that the percentage of sheep-E rosette-forming cells in tumor tissue was low,[306] ranging from 0–35%. The centrocytic lymphomas we studied also contained only a small proportion of sheep-E rosette-forming cells. LEECH *et al.*[307] and our group carried out cytologic studies of the sheep-E rosette-forming cells. The cells were usually small round lymphocytes, suggesting that they were merely nonneoplastic bystander cells. As mentioned previously, JAFFE *et al.*[308] reported on three cases of poorly differentiated lymphoma, diffuse, with a large proportion of sheep-E rosette-forming cells and a small proportion of EAC rosette-forming cells, indicating a T-cell origin of these neoplasms. We assume that the three cases described by JAFFE *et al.*[308] were equivalent to our lymphoblastic lymphoma of the convoluted-cell type, which sometimes cytologically resembles poorly differentiated lymphoma or centrocytic lymphoma.

**Human T-Lymphocyte Antigen (HTLA).** AISENBERG and LONG[309] evaluated the occurrence of HTLA in seven cases of poorly differentiated lymphoma, diffuse. They found only a slightly higher percentage of cells reacting with anti-thymocyte serum than with sheep erythrocytes. A majority of cells showed no staining with anti-thymocyte serum.

[305] CATOVSKY, CHERCHI, OKOS, HEGDE *et al.*, 1976.

[306] AISENBERG and LONG, 1975; BROUET, LABAUME and SELIGMANN, 1975; LEECH, GLICK, WALDRON, FLEXNER *et al.*, 1975.

[307] LEECH, GLICK, WALDRON, FLEXNER *et al.*, 1975.

[308] JAFFE, SHEVACH, SUSSMAN, FRANK *et al.*, 1975.

[309] 1975.

**Conclusions.** From the studies mentioned, including our own, it may be concluded that SIg is usually present on all centrocytic lymphoma cells. With few exceptions, Ig cannot be detected in the cytoplasm. Electron microscopy revealed that the tumor cells usually contain little ergastoplasm and abundant ribosomes, indicating that the cells are of a nonsecretory type (see p. 504). Correspondingly, the serum-Ig level in all cases was either decreased or within the normal range. Thus, centrocytic lymphoma is a proliferation of nonsecretory B-cells, as is CLL of the B-cell type. In contrast to B-CLL, however, centrocytic lymphoma displays the following immunologic characteristics:

1. The tumor cells usually bear large amounts of SIg, which tends to cap. In CLL the amount of SIg is small and capping of the labeled SIg seldom occurs.
2. Detergent tissue extracts from centrocytic lymphoma contain significantly larger amounts of Ig than do those from CLL.
3. Centrocytic lymphoma tends to express $\gamma$- and $\alpha$-chains as well as $\mu$- and $\delta$-chains.
4. Centrocytic lymphoma cells apparently do not bind mouse erythrocytes, whereas CLL cells do.
5. Centrocytic lymphoma cells appear to usually express receptors for both C3b and C3d, whereas in most cases of B-CLL the leukemic cells are devoid of receptors for C3b.

These characteristics indicate that centrocytic lymphoma cells are derived from a subset of B-cells that differs from the subset from which B-CLL cells originate.

Since we found that centrocytic lymphoma cells are very similar in morphology to small germinal-center cells (centrocytes), we suggested that these tumor cells are derived from centrocytes.[309a] The results of our marker studies are consistent with this hypothesis, because centrocytes bear a large amount of SIg, predominantly IgM and IgD, and they have complement receptors.

Hopper[310] and Hamburg *et al.*[311] pointed out the similarities between some cord-blood lymphocytes and cells of malignant lymphoma, poorly differentiated, diffuse, in morphology and SIg classes (IgM and IgD). They assumed that this neoplasm reflects an oncofetal arrest of maturation in the early lymphocytic development process. In our opinion, it is more likely that centrocytic lymphoma is derived from the noncirculating B-cell pool, i.e., small germinal-center cells, and not from circulating cord-blood lymphocytes. Our reasons are that most cases of centrocytic lymphoma do not show release of significant numbers of neoplastic cells into the blood and that centrocytic lymphoma cells do not form mouse-E rosettes, unlike blood B-lymphocytes, but like reactive centrocytes.

## J. Malignant Lymphoma, Centroblastic/Centrocytic

**Surface Immunoglobulin (SIg).** The results of SIg labeling by four different investigators are given in Table 106. Leech *et al.*[312] studied the greatest number

[309a] Lennert, Stein and Kaiserling, 1975; Stein, 1976b.
[310] 1974.
[311] Hamburg, Brynes, Reese and Golomb, 1976.
[312] Leech, Glick, Waldron, Flexner *et al.*, 1975.

Table 106. Surface immunoglobulin (SIg) on cells from centroblastic/centrocytic lymphoma and apparently equivalent entities of other lymphoma classifications

| Author/Term | SIg class | Incidence | Light-chain type |
|---|---|---|---|
| AISENBERG and LONG:[b] | Ig-PV[a] | 5/6 | |
| M.L. lymphocytic, poorly differentiated, | IgM | 3/6 | κ (3) |
| nodular | IgG | 2/6 | κ (2) |
| BROUET *et al.*:[c] | IgM | 1/1 | κ |
| Well differentiated lymphocytic lymphoma (nodular) | | | |
| LEECH *et al.*:[d] | Ig-PV | 14/15 | |
| Follicular center cell lymphoma, small | IgM | 7/11 | |
| and large cleaved cell, nodular | IgM-D | 2/5 | κ (2) |
| | IgM-G | 1/11 | κ |
| | IgD-A | 1/5 | κ |
| STEIN:[e] | Ig-PV | 6/6 | |
| Centroblastic/centrocytic lymphoma, | IgM | 6/6 | κ (4), λ (2) |
| nodular | IgM-D | 2/2 | κ (1), λ (1) |
| Sum of SIg-positive cases | | 26/28 (93%) | |

[a] Ig-PV = Ig demonstrated with a polyvalent anti-Ig serum.
[b] 1975.
[c] BROUET, LABAUME and SELIGMANN, 1975.
[d] LEECH, GLICK, WALDRON, FLEXNER *et al.*, 1975.
[e] 1976, unpublished data.

of cases. IgM was found to be the predominant Ig class (present in seven out of 11 cases). IgD was detectable in three out of five cases, combined twice with IgM and once with IgA. IgM and IgG were apparently expressed simultaneously on the cells from one patient. The only nodular lymphoma studied by BROUET *et al.*[313] revealed IgM/κ. IgD assays were not performed by the latter authors.

AISENBERG and LONG[314] detected IgM/κ on cells from three and IgG/κ on cells from two out of six cases of nodular lymphoma. They did not look for IgD. One case in the series of LEECH *et al.*[312] and one in that of AISENBERG and LONG[314] did not label for SIg.

In our own series, all cases of centroblastic/centrocytic lymphoma showed SIg on most of the cells. IgM was the dominant heavy chain. We recently investigated two cases for the presence of IgD by means of a strong anti-IgD-fluorescein conjugate combined with an anti-IgM-rhodamine conjugate. In these two cases IgD was demonstrated on 40% and 80%, respectively, of the cells bearing IgM.

**Tissue Immunoglobulin.** *Saline Extract.* In the saline extracts of tissue from 30 cases of centroblastic/centrocytic lymphoma, there was a great increase in IgM in five cases (see Fig. 276). The extracts from a majority of the other cases contained Ig in quantities slightly above or within the range of normal lymph nodes or thymuses. The mean IgM content was as high as that of CLL.

[313] BROUET, LABAUME and SELIGMANN, 1975. [314] 1975.

*Detergent Second Extract.* There was an increase in the Ig concentration of the detergent 2nd extracts from 11 out of 29 cases; in nine cases the predominant class was IgM (see Fig. 277), in one case IgG, and in one case IgA with IgE. The extracts from two out of the nine cases with an increase in IgM contained significant amounts of IgD. Two other cases attracted attention because the IgM concentration of the tissue extract was 20 times higher than that measured in thymus tissue. The cells from both patients contained PAS-positive Russell body-like inclusions, indicating synthesis of secretory IgM.

**Serum Immunoglobulin.** With the exception of three cases, the serum-Ig levels of centroblastic/centrocytic lymphoma lay within or below the normal range. That was also true of two cases in which the cells contained CIg in the form of PAS-positive Russell body-like material. Electron microscopy revealed that the cells from one of the two cases contained malformed ergastoplasm, which might have been the cause of the inability to secrete synthesized secretory IgM.[315]

The increased serum-Ig fractions found in three out of 30 cases appeared to be polyclonal in electrophoresis and were therefore not synthesized by the tumor cells.

**Monoclonality of the Tissue and Serum Immunoglobulin.** Data from isoelectric-focusing studies of tissue Ig are not available. The Ig fractions of classic cases usually proved to be polyclonal in electrophoresis. In borderline cases to LP immunocytoma, however, monoclonality of a serum-Ig class could be observed, especially when it was increased in amount.

**Cytoplasmic Immunoglobulin (CIg).** In rare cases (4/30)[315a] the centroblastic/centrocytic lymphoma cells produced such large amounts of CIg that the CIg was visible as intranuclear and/or cytoplasmic PAS-positive inclusions. The fluorescent-antibody technique that we applied to fixed centrifuge slides of suspended centroblastic/centrocytic lymphoma cells from four cases showed only occasional CIg-positive cells. The light-chain staining, however, was restricted to the same type as that found on the surface of these cells.

TAYLOR[316] demonstrated a much more common production of CIg. He investigated 20 cases of follicular lymphoma for the presence of CIg in paraffin sections by means of the enzyme-bridge method. The tumor cells from 14 of the cases were CIg-positive. Numerous CIg-positive cells were seen in the perifollicular tissue in many cases, whereas the neoplastic follicles, which consisted predominantly of small cells (centrocytes), revealed only a few cells with positive cytoplasmic staining. The CIg-positive cells appeared to contain only one light-chain type. In tumors with a greater number of larger cells (probably equivalent to our centroblasts), a positive reaction for CIg was observed in the cells with a more neoplastic appearance. In cases with sarcomatous transformation and with a loss of the follicular growth pattern, the large cells demonstrated a weak or negative reaction for CIg. Similar observations have been made by PAPADIMITRIOU.[316a]

[315] KAISERLING, 1975, unpublished data.
[315a] STEIN, 1975a, 1976b.
[316] 1976.
[316a] 1977, unpublished data.

**IgG-Fc Receptor.** There have been only a few studies on the presence of IgG-Fc receptors on cells from follicular lymphomas. JAFFE *et al.*[317] applied the IgGEA-rosette assay in six cases. They used sheep erythrocytes coated with rabbit anti-sheep-E antibodies (IgG-sheepEA). The neoplastic cells failed to bind this type of IgGEA. That is not surprising, because IgG-sheep EA has only a weak affinity for IgG-Fc receptors, as indicated by the binding to only a very small proportion of normal peripheral blood lymphocytes. In our tests, however, a small proportion of the centroblastic/centrocytic lymphoma cells formed rosettes with Rh-positive human erythrocytes that were thickly coated with human anti-D IgG. This type of IgGEA was bound by normal peripheral blood lymphocytes in the same percentage as IgG aggregates were.[318] BROUET *et al.*[319] found that IgG aggregates were capable of binding cells from the one case of follicular lymphoma they studied.

**Complement Receptor.** JAFFE *et al.*[320] studied cells from six cases of nodular (follicular) lymphoma for the presence of complement receptors. Three of the tumors revealed an abundance of centroblasts (mixed lymphocytic/histiocytic type), and in three cases centrocytes were predominant (poorly differentiated lymphoma). The neoplastic cells from all cases bound IgMEAC both in suspensions and on frozen sections. Our own studies provided similar results. Follicular adherence of IgMEAC was demonstrable on the frozen sections from 14 out of 15 centroblastic/centrocytic lymphomas. In four cases we also performed the EAC-rosette assay on suspended tumor cells. The rosette counts ranged from 18–74%. Cytologic evaluation of the EAC rosette-forming cells on cytocentrifuge slides confirmed that the rosetting cells were indeed tumor cells.

We specified the complement-receptor subtypes in seven cases. Most of the cells from all seven cases simultaneously had receptors for C3b and C3d on their surfaces. In frozen sections the neoplastic nodules bound both EAC3b and EAC3d, whereas the peripheral rim of the nodules and adjacent tissue bound only EAC3b (Fig. 284c, d).[321] Thus, centroblastic/centrocytic lymphoma not only expressed both complement-receptor subtypes, like normal germinal-center cells, but also showed a distribution of the complement-receptor subtypes similar to that of normal lymphatic tissue. This finding is another indication of the close relationship between the cells of centroblastic/centrocytic lymphoma and reactive germinal-center cells.

In 1969, BENNETT and MILLETT described a lymphoma that they referred to as nodular sclerosing lymphosarcoma. In a majority of cases the proliferating cells could be identified morphologically as centrocytes and centroblasts. On frozen sections from three such tumors, we observed a nodular adherence of EAC resembling that seen in typical centroblastic/centrocytic lymphoma. This finding supports the view that tumors with nodular fiber formation are variants of centroblastic/centrocytic lymphoma.

---

[317] JAFFE, SHEVACH, FRANK, BERARD *et al.*, 1974.
[318] STEIN and PETERSEN, 1975, unpublished data.
[319] BROUET, LABAUME and SELIGMANN, 1975.
[320] JAFFE, SHEVACH, FRANK, BERARD *et al.*, 1974.
[321] STEIN, SIEMSSEN and LENNERT, submitted for publication.

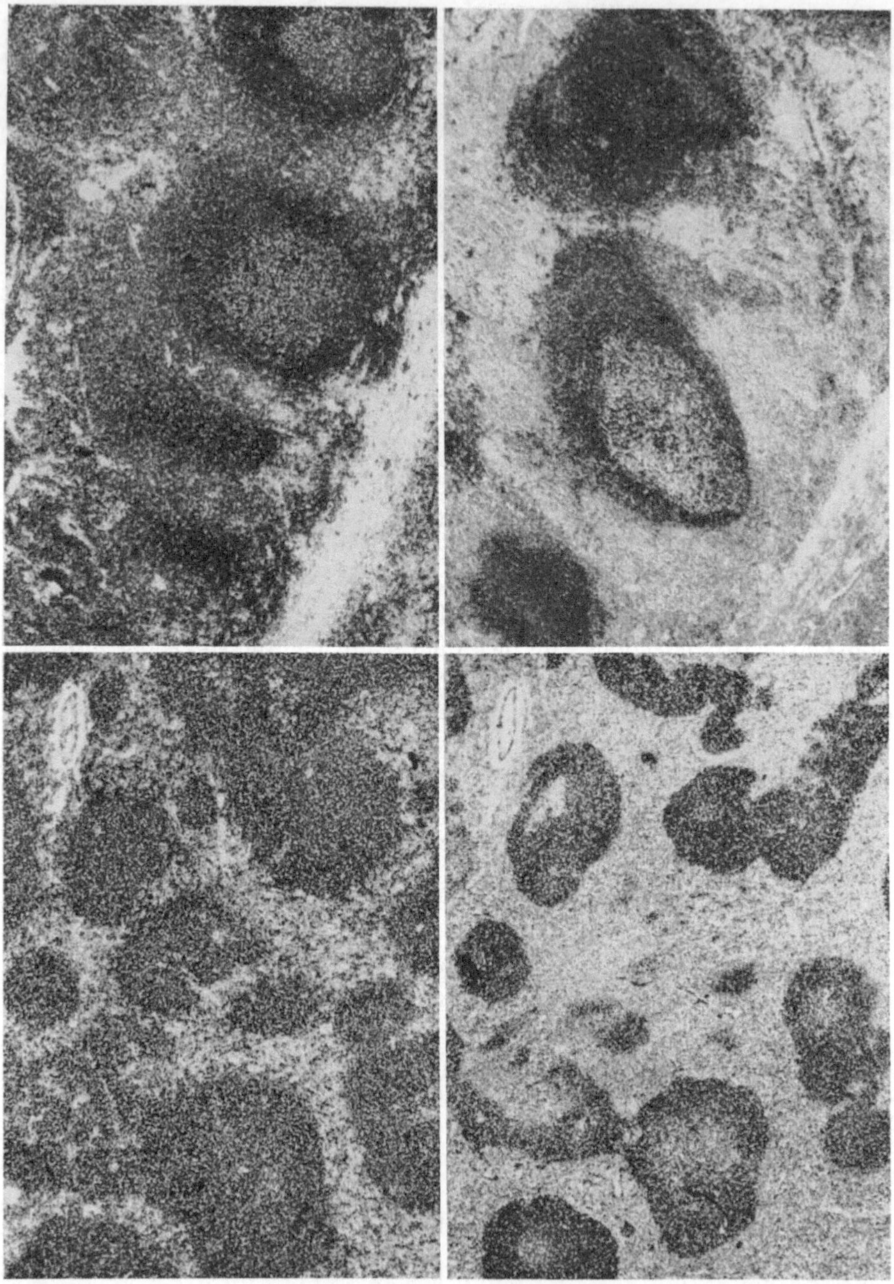

(a) (b) (c) (d)

Fig. 284a–d. Distribution of complement-receptor subtypes in normal tonsil and follicular lymphoma (centroblastic/centrocytic lymphoma). (a) Frozen section of a normal tonsil treated with IgM-EAC3b. The reagent red cells (dark spots) adhere to germinal centers, to the follicular mantle, and, less densely, to interfollicular regions. (b) Adjacent region of a serial frozen section of the same tonsil as (a), treated with IgM-EAC3d. The reagent red cells adhere exclusively to germinal centers and the follicular mantle, but completely spare interfollicular areas. (c) Frozen section from a follicular lymphoma treated with IgM-EAC3b. The reagent red cells adhere to all of the neoplastic nodules, including their outer rim, and, less densely, to the interfollicular cords. (d) The same region in a serial frozen section of the same case as (c), treated with IgM-EAC3d. The reagent red cells adhere to neoplastic nodules and spare the interfollicular cords and marginal parts of the neoplastic nodules. As in many reactive germinal centers, the reagent red cells frequently adhere less densely to central parts of the neoplastic nodules. (a–d) Hematoxylin and eosin. ×30

**Mouse-Erythrocyte (E) Receptor.** CATOVSKY and GALTON[321a] studied seven cases of follicular lymphoma. More than 20% of the cells from four out of the seven cases bound mouse erythrocytes. Unfortunately, however, the authors did not mention whether or not they had pretreated the cells with neuraminidase. In our own series (n = 10) we[321b] observed a nearly regular binding of mouse erythrocytes by centroblastic/centrocytic lymphoma cells when they had been pretreated with neuraminidase.

**Sheep-Erythrocyte (E) Receptor and Human T-Lymphocyte Antigen (HTLA).** According to the findings of AISENBERG and LONG,[322] BROUET *et al.*,[322a] JAFFE *et al.*,[323] and LEECH *et al.*,[324] and our own,[325] a relatively large proportion of centroblastic/centrocytic lymphoma cells form sheep-E rosettes. JAFFE *et al.*[323] and we observed the highest percentages (35% and 25%, respectively) of sheep-E rosette-positive cells, probably because sheep erythrocytes treated with neuraminidase were used – pretreatment with neuraminidase noticeably enhances the binding of sheep erythrocytes to T-cells.

Using anti-thymocyte serum, AISENBERG and LONG[322] studied five cases for the presence of HTLA on follicular lymphoma cells. Fourteen to 82% of the cells labeled with anti-thymocyte serum, the mean being $63.2 \pm 34.1\%$. In two of the cases in the series of AISENBERG and LONG, the sum of SIg-positive and anti-thymocyte serum-reactive cells greatly exceeded 100%. The authors did not interpret the overlapping of B- and T-marker labeling. Nevertheless, these findings confirm the results of the rosette assay with sheep erythrocytes treated with neuraminidase, indicating that there is a large proportion of T-cells in many follicular lymphomas. Since the neoplastic follicles chiefly consist of complement receptor-positive B-cells, as shown by the follicular adherence of EAC on frozen sections, the T-cells are probably located in perifollicular areas.

The electron-microscopic findings of KAISERLING[326] led to a similar conclusion. He found interdigitating reticulum cells in the perifollicular area. It has been shown that these cells occur only in the thymus and in thymus-dependent regions.[327] The presence of interdigitating reticulum cells therefore favors the T-cell nature of the interfollicular lymphocytes. These observations and assumptions are somewhat contrary to the findings of TAYLOR.[328] He described the occurrence of abundant plasma cells, which contained Ig with a single light-chain type, around the neoplastic follicles in 15 out of 17 cases. Further comprehensive study is necessary to resolve the contradictions.

In one case in the series of AISENBERG and LONG,[322] 82% of the cells reacted positively with anti-thymocyte serum and negatively for SIg. This suggests that, in rare instances, lymphomas originating from T-cells can display

[321a] 1977.

[321b] STEIN and TOLKSDORF, 1977, unpublished data.

[322] 1975.

[322a] BROUET, LABAUME and SELIGMANN, 1975.

[323] JAFFE, SHEVACH, SUSSMAN, FRANK *et al.*, 1975.

[324] LEECH, GLICK, WALDRON, FLEXNER *et al.*, 1975.

[325] STEIN, SIEMSSEN and LENNERT, 1978, in press.

[326] 1976.

[327] VELDMAN, 1970; HEUSERMANN, STUTTE and MÜLLER-HERMELINK, 1974; KAISERLING and LENNERT, 1974; KAISERLING, STEIN and MÜLLER-HERMELINK, 1974.

[328] 1974.

a follicular growth pattern. Our research group has also observed T-cell lymphomas that were associated with a follicular pattern. It could be shown, however, that the follicles were remnants of germinal centers and that the neoplastic cells were located between them. The tumor cells were identified as T-cells in the sheep E-rosette test (see p. 196).

**Conclusions.** Taken together, the data of AISENBERG and LONG,[328a] BROUET *et al.*,[329] LEECH *et al.*,[329a] and our own group show that a total of 26 out of 28 cases of centroblastic/centrocytic lymphoma (follicular lymphoma) were SIg-positive. The results of tissue-Ig analysis are in accordance with these findings. As a rule, monotypic CIg is easily demonstrated in only a few cells of centroblastic/centrocytic lymphoma.[330] That conforms with the usually high predominance of neoplastic cells with a nonsecretory-cell structure on electron microscopy.[331] The detection of cells with plasmacytoid features,[331a] ergastoplasm,[331b] and CIg[332] in centroblastic/centrocytic lymphoma showed, however, that the tumor cells may undergo transformation from nonsecretory- to secretory-cell (plasmacytic) differentiation. Such secretory-cell (plasmacytic) differentiation of neoplastic cells may be striking in some cases. Centroblastic/centrocytic lymphoma cells with plasmacytic differentiation are probably the neoplastic equivalent of a hyperimmune germinal-center reaction in which many cells become CIg-positive.[333] The centroblastic/centrocytic lymphomas with plasmacytic differentiation (presence of plasmacytoid cells, Russell body-like material, or CIg-positive cells) are borderline cases between centroblastic/centrocytic lymphoma and LP immunocytoma. It is therefore not always possible to make a clear distinction between these two entities (cf., p. 246).

RAPPAPORT and his school[334] maintained that there is no conclusive evidence supporting the contention that the so-called follicles of follicular lymphoma arise from or are related to reactive lymphoid nodules. Recently, however, it was found that the neoplastic follicles of nearly all follicular lymphomas studied[334a] consisted of complement receptor-positive cells resembling reactive germinal-center cells. This finding dispelled the skepticism of RAPPAPORT and his colleagues and led to general acceptance of the thesis that follicular lymphomas are indeed neoplastic equivalents of the germinal-center reaction. This thesis has been repeatedly proposed by LENNERT.[335]

Further strong evidence for the germinal center-cell origin of centroblastic/centrocytic lymphoma was provided by our recent studies of complement-receptor subtypes.[335a] We found that the expression and distribution of the complement-receptor subtypes on suspended cells and frozen sections were similar

---

[328a] 1975.
[329] BROUET, LABAUME and SELIGMANN, 1975.
[329a] LEECH, GLICK, WALDROW, FLEXNER *et al.*, 1975.
[330] TAYLOR, 1976; PAPADIMITRIOU, 1977, unpublished data.
[331] MORI and LENNERT, 1969; KAISERLING, 1976.
[331a] STEIN, 1975a.
[331b] KAISERLING, 1976.
[332] STEIN and PREUSSLER, 1976, unpublished data; TAYLOR, 1976; PAPADIMITRIOU, 1977, unpublished data.
[333] WHITE, 1960; STRAUS, 1970.
[334] RAPPAPORT, WINTER and HICKS, 1956; RAPPAPORT, 1966; DORFMAN, 1973; JONES, FUKS, BULL, KADIN *et al.*, 1973.
[334a] JAFFE, SHEVACH, FRANK, BERARD *et al.*, 1974; STEIN, 1975a, 1976b.
[335] 1964, 1967, 1971, 1973; LENNERT and STEIN, 1972.
[335a] STEIN, SIEMSSEN and LENNERT, 1978, in press.

to those of normal lymphatic tissue. The neoplastic nodules bound both EAC3b and EAC3d, whereas the peripheral rim of the nodules and the adjacent tissue bound only EAC3d. Thus, the follicular lymphoma cells not only expressed both complement-receptor subtypes, like normal germinal-center cells, but also showed a distribution of the complement-receptor subtypes similar to that of normal lymphatic tissue.

Studies of CIg also revealed similarities between follicular lymphoma and hyperplastic lymphatic tissue. The CIg-positive cells are usually scattered around the follicles in both reactive hyperplastic lymphatic tissue and centroblastic/centrocytic lymphoma.[336]

LEECH *et al.*[337] were the first to report IgD as a predominant SIg class besides IgM on follicular lymphoma cells. We recently confirmed this finding. HAMBURG *et al.*[338] noticed an analogy between the increased percentage of SIg-bearing cells with IgD in small and large cleaved follicular center-cell lymphomas or poorly differentiated lymphomas, and the increased percentage of SIg-bearing cells with IgD in cord blood. In spite of the parallel in SIg staining between cord-blood lymphocytes and follicular lymphoma cells, it appears unlikely that follicular lymphoma (centroblastic/centrocytic lymphoma) is derived from cord-blood lymphocytes, since all other morphologic and immunologic data tend to indicate concordance between germinal-center cells and centroblastic/centrocytic lymphoma cells. In addition, a large proportion of the lymphoid cells from infantile tonsils, which contain numerous germinal-center cells, also express IgM and IgD.[339] This finding shows that the presence of IgD on follicular lymphoma cells is not incompatible, but consistent with the germinal center-cell origin of the tumor cells.

It has recently been questioned[339a] whether the neoplastic cells in follicular lymphoma are present in the interfollicular tissue as well as in the neoplastic nodules, or whether the neoplastic cells are confined to the follicles and the interfollicular tissue is composed of normal lymphoid cells. The results of SIg and CIg analyses especially favor the first view. The SIg studies mentioned previously revealed a completely monotypic light-chain staining pattern of the suspended cells in all SIg-positive cases. Demonstration of CIg showed that the cytoplasmic staining of the intranodular and perinodular cells was consistently restricted to the same heavy- and light-chain types. Furthermore, in our cases, the CIg was of the same class as the Ig detected on the surface membrane. This indicates that most, or at least some, of the interfollicular cells and the cells of the nodules in centroblastic/centrocytic lymphoma are parts of the same neoplastic process.

Finally, it should be pointed out that all lymphomas exhibiting a follicular growth pattern are not necessarily of the B-type. In the rare cases that are

---

[336] TAYLOR, 1976; PAPADIMITRIOU, 1977, unpublished data; STEIN and FUCHS, 1977, unpublished data.

[337] LEECH, GLICK, WALDRON, FLEXNER *et al.*, 1975.

[338] HAMBURG, BRYNES, REESE and GOLOMB, 1976.

[339] KRÜGER, UHLMANN, HELLRIEGEL, SESTERHENN *et al.*, 1976; STEIN, 1976, unpublished data.

[339a] BUTLER, STRYKER and SHULLENBERGER, 1974; JAFFE, SHEVACH, FRANK, BERARD *et al.*, 1974.

not of the B-type, the SIg- and complement receptor-bearing cells in the follicles do not belong to the neoplastic cell population; the sheep-E receptor-positive T-cells in the interfollicular area (T-zone) are the actual tumor cells. LENNERT called this type of lymphatic neoplasm T-zone lymphoma (see pp. 196ff. and 590).

## K. Malignant Lymphoma, Centroblastic

**Surface Immunoglobulin (SIg).** LEECH *et al.*[340] studied four lymphomas classified as follicular center-cell lymphoma, large noncleaved. Two cases showed a diffuse, and two a nodular growth pattern. SIg was detectable on the cells from all four cases. The Ig classes were determined in three cases. It was remarkable that the cells from all three cases bore surface IgG, in two cases combined with λ-chains and in one case with κ-chains.

Most of the cells from the one case of centroblastic lymphoma that we had the opportunity to label for SIg also bore IgG. This labeling result was confirmed by immunoprecipitation of radioiodine-labeled surface membranes of the cells and subsequent SDS-gel electrophoresis. A significant amount of radioactivity was precipitated only with anti-IgG sera. The membrane fraction isolated with the anti-IgG serum migrated to the position of IgG in the SDS gel, confirming the IgG nature of the precipitated Ig molecules.

**Tissue Immunoglobulin.** *Saline Extract.* There was a significant increase in IgM in the saline extracts from three out of eight cases. The other Ig classes, IgG and IgA, were decreased in amount in all cases. The mean IgM concentration of the tissue extract was a high as that shown by centrocytic lymphoma and CLL, higher than that of centroblastic/centrocytic lymphoma, lymphoblastic lymphoma of the Burkitt type, and lymphoblastic lymphoma of other than the Burkitt type, and lower than that of LP immunocytoma and immunoblastic lymphoma (see Fig. 276).

*Detergent Second Extract.* Ig analysis of the detergent 2nd extracts revealed a significant increase in IgM in four out of seven cases (see Fig. 277). Only small amounts of IgG and IgA were detected in the tissue extracts. The mean IgM value for the 2nd extracts from centroblastic lymphoma was relatively low, but significantly higher than that of thymuses. It lay below that of LP immunocytoma, centroblastic/centrocytic lymphoma, centrocytic lymphoma, lymphoblastic lymphoma of the Burkitt type, and immunoblastic lymphoma. It was higher than that of lymphoblastic lymphoma of the convoluted-cell and unclassified types.

**Serum Immunoglobulin.** The serum-Ig levels of all cases studied were either within or below the normal range.

**Monoclonality of the Tissue and Serum Immunoglobulin.** Isoelectric-focusing studies of tissue Ig have not been performed.

---

[340] LEECH, GLICK, WALDRON, FLEXNER *et al.*, 1975.

**Cytoplasmic Immunoglobulin (CIg).** In two out of eight cases of centroblastic lymphoma, PAS-positive Russell body-like material was found in few, but definite, tumor cells. This indicates that direct transformation into the plasma-cell line is possible. With the enzyme-bridge method, the Russell body-like material proved to be IgM, a finding that agrees with the results of tissue-Ig determination. A systematic analysis of CIg in centroblastic lymphoma has yet to be carried out.

**IgG-Fc Receptor.** As far as we know, no data on the presence of IgG-Fc receptors are available.

**Complement Receptor.** In two out of the four cases investigated, EAC exhibited nodular adherence on frozen sections, indicating a nodular distribution of complement receptor-positive tumor cells.

**Mouse-Erythrocyte (E) Receptor.** No data are available.

**Sheep-Erythrocyte (E) Receptor.** LEECH *et al.*[341] determined the percentage of sheep-E rosette-forming cells in suspensions from two cases of follicular center-cell lymphoma, large noncleaved. The values were 5.8% and 23%. There was no overlapping of SIg-positive and sheep E-reactive cells.

**Human T-Associated Antigens.** No data are available.

**Conclusions.** Four out of seven cases of centroblastic lymphoma revealed increased amounts of IgM in the tissue extracts. In the other three cases there was no increase in Ig of any class. LEECH *et al.*[341] found SIg on the cells from four cases of large noncleaved-cell lymphoma, which is probably equivalent to centroblastic lymphoma. The predominant Ig class proved to be IgG. That was also true for the one case of centroblastic lymphoma from which we isolated the SIg by means of coprecipitation. The discrepancy between the results of tissue-Ig and SIg determination may well be due to the small number of cases studied, rather than to divergent morphologic criteria for follicular center-cell lymphoma, large noncleaved, and centroblastic lymphoma. The studies indicate, however, that centroblastic lymphoma usually reveals Ig synthesis and is therefore a lymphoma of the B-cell type.

It was observed that the produced Ig was not secreted. That is consistent with the electron-microscopic findings, which showed that centroblastic lymphoma cells are usually of the nonsecretory type: they contain abundant ribosomes and little ergastoplasm, similar to reactive centroblasts (see p. 509). A few cases demonstrated the production of secretory Ig in the form of Russell body-like material. There is still no answer to the question as to whether such a switch to synthesis of secretory Ig is possible under neoplastic conditions only, or whether it reflects a possible pathway of differentiation taken by reactive centroblasts.

---

[341] LEECH, GLICK, WALDRON, FLEXNER *et al.*, 1975.

Complement receptors were detectable on the centroblastic lymphoma cells from two representative cases. Reactive centroblasts also bear complement receptors.[342] These data support the close relationship between centroblastic lymphoma cells and reactive centroblasts. It is primarily based on the morphologic resemblance of centroblastic lymphoma cells to reactive centroblasts and on the observation of frequent transformation of centroblastic/centrocytic lymphoma into centroblastic lymphoma, a neoplasm in which centroblast-like cells are the predominant proliferating cells.

## L. Lymphoblastic Lymphoma, Burkitt Type

In 1958, BURKITT described a malignant lymphoma of the lymphoblastic type that occurred in Central Africa and New Guinea. Shortly thereafter, malignant lymphomas with identical morphology were observed outside Central Africa and New Guinea, namely, in America and Europe.[343] The immunologic data on the African and non-African cases with Burkitt-like morphology will be presented and compared in this section.

**Surface Immunoglobulin (SIg).** Reactivity for $\mu$- and $\kappa$-chains on the surface of African Burkitt's lymphoma cells was first detected by KLEIN *et al.*[344] In collaboration with KLEIN's group, FIALKOW *et al.*[345] studied 95 African Burkitt's lymphomas for the presence of SIg. In 58 cases they found surface IgM, associated with $\kappa$-chains in 40%. Only a few cases stained positively for IgG and none for IgA. The remaining cases did not show staining for SIg. $\lambda$-Chain determinants were not investigated.

Many assays for SIg were performed on lymphoblastoid cell lines established from various patients with African Burkitt's lymphoma. Most of these cell lines revealed SIg,[346] although some of them, e.g., the Raji cells, lacked SIg.[347] Raji cells appear to be derived from the SIg-negative Burkitt's lymphoma cells demonstrated by FIALKOW *et al.*[345] in 47 out of 95 cases.

There are only a few reports on SIg studies of lymphomas with Burkitt-like morphology that occurred outside Central Africa. The results of these studies are listed in Table 107 together with the data on African Burkitt's lymphoma.

In contrast to cells from African Burkitt's lymphomas, cells from all 17 cases of non-African lymphoma of the Burkitt type listed in Table 107 exhibited SIg. IgM was the predominant Ig class (16/17). IgG was detected on the cells from only one out of 17 cases (6%). The tumor cells from one case stained for $\alpha$- as well as $\mu$- and $\delta$-chains.[348]

There are no reliable data on the frequency of $\delta$-chains on cells from African Burkitt's lymphomas and from non-African lymphomas of the Burkitt type.

---

[342] STEIN, SIEMSSEN and LENNERT, 1978, in press.
[343] O'CONOR, 1963; DORFMAN, 1965, 1968; O'CONOR, RAPPAPORT and SMITH, 1965.
[344] KLEIN, KLEIN, NADKARNI, NADKARNI *et al.*, 1967.
[345] FIALKOW, KLEIN, KLEIN, CLIFFORD *et al.*, 1973.
[346] JONDAL and KLEIN, 1973.
[347] THEOFILOPOULOS, BOKISCH and DIXON, 1974.
[348] MANN, JAFFE, BRAYLAN, NANBA *et al.*, 1976.

Table 107. Surface immunoglobulin (SIg) on cells from Burkitt's lymphoma and lymphoma of Burkitt type

| Author/Term | SIg class | Incidence | Light-chain type |
|---|---|---|---|
| KLEIN *et al.*:[c] African Burkitt's lymphoma | IgM | 1/1 | κ |
| FIALKOW *et al.*:[d] African Burkitt's lymphoma | IgM | 55/95 | 40% κ, λ n.d.[a] |
| | IgG | a few cases | |
| FLANDRIN *et al.*:[e] Acute leukemia with Burkitt's tumor cells | Ig-PV[b] | 6/6 | κ (2), λ (4) |
| | IgM | 5/6 | |
| | IgG | 1/6 | |
| PREUD'HOMME *et al.*:[f] ALL of Burkitt type | IgM-D | 2/2 | κ (2) |
| GAJL-PECZALSKA *et al.*:[g] American Burkitt's lymphoma | IgM | 2/2 | κ (2) |
| BINDER *et al.*:[h] American Burkitt's lymphoma | IgM | 1/1 | |
| MANN *et al.*:[i] Non-endemic (American) Burkitt's lymphoma | Ig-PV | 7/7 | κ (6), λ (1) |
| | IgM | 6/7 | κ (5), λ (1) |
| | IgM-D-A | 1/7 | κ |

[a] n.d. = not determined.
[b] Ig-PV = Ig demonstrated with a polyvalent anti-Ig serum.
[c] KLEIN, KLEIN, NADKARNI, NADKARNI *et al.*, 1967.
[d] FIALKOW, KLEIN, KLEIN, CLIFFORD *et al.*, 1973.
[e] FLANDRIN, BROUET, DANIEL and PREUD'HOMME, 1975.
[f] PREUD'HOMME, BROUET, CLAUVEL and SELIGMANN, 1974.
[g] GAJL-PECZALSKA, BLOOMFIELD, COCCIA, SOSIN *et al.*, 1975.
[h] BINDER, JENCKS, CHUN and RATH, 1975.
[i] MANN, JAFFE, BRAYLAN, NANBA *et al.*, 1976.

The expression of δ-chains is probably common, however, since the two cases of non-African lymphoma of the Burkitt type studied by PREUD'HOMME *et al.*[349] were positive for δ-chains.

In two cases FLANDRIN *et al.*[350] showed in trypsinization experiments that SIg was actually synthesized by the lymphoma cells.

**Tissue Immunoglobulin.** *Saline Extract.* Of the five cases of European lymphoma of the Burkitt type we studied, two revealed slightly, but significantly increased amounts of IgM in the saline extract (see Fig. 276). Other Ig classes were not increased in amount.

*Detergent Second Extract.* Detergent 2nd extracts were analyzed in five European cases. A significant increase in IgM was detected in four cases; three of them showed a great increase (see Fig. 277). Other Ig classes could not be extracted in significant amounts. In the two cases analyzed, the light chain associated with the μ-chains proved to be of the κ-type.

[349] PREUD'HOMME, BROUET, CLAUVEL and SELIGMANN, 1974.

[350] FLANDRIN, BROUET, DANIEL and PREUD'HOMME, 1975.

These results agree with those of ESKELAND and KLEIN[351] and SHERR and UHR.[352] Both groups of authors extracted $\mu$- and $\kappa$-chain structures from the surfaces of Daudi cells, a Burkitt's lymphoma-derived cell line, by freezing and thawing or by solubilization with the detergent NP40.

**Serum Immunoglobulin.** As reported for African Burkitt's lymphoma, we found a decrease in the serum-Ig levels, especially of IgM, in all of the European cases studied.

**Monoclonality of the Tissue and Serum Immunoglobulin.** In immunoelectrophoresis the serum-Ig classes proved to be polyclonal. There are no data available on heterogeneity of Ig chains extracted from lymphoma cells of the Burkitt type and analyzed by isoelectric focusing.

**Cytoplasmic Immunoglobulin (CIg).** KLEIN *et al.*[353] reported that Daudi cells derived from an African Burkitt's lymphoma showed little or no cytoplasmic staining with fluorescein-conjugated anti-Ig sera. In cells of the Raji cell line, which is derived from cells of another Burkitt's lymphoma, CIg of the $\kappa$-type was detectable with the sensitive PAP enzyme-bridge method.[354]

**IgG-Fc Receptor.** As far as we know, the literature contains no data on IgG-Fc receptors on African Burkitt's lymphoma cells. On the other hand, there have been a number of studies of the expression and affinity of IgG-Fc receptors on cells from cell lines derived from African Burkitt's lymphomas. JONDAL and KLEIN[355] studied the presence of IgG-Fc receptors on cells of 10 such cell lines. Cells of five out of the 10 lines had receptors for IgG-Fc when measured with the IgGEA-rosette test (12–16%, mean 21%). When the more sensitive method of detecting IgG-Fc receptors by means of IgG aggregates was used, the number of IgG-Fc receptor-positive lines and cells within a line increased. For instance, Raji cells did not form IgGEA rosettes, but bound IgG aggregates. The IgG-aggregate assay also revealed a difference between the density of IgG-Fc receptors on cells of the Daudi cell line and that on cells of the Raji cell line. A much stronger staining was found on Daudi cells than on Raji cells.[356]

Like African Burkitt's lymphoma-derived cell lines, cells from European and American cases apparently bear IgG-Fc receptors with a variable frequency and density. With the sensitive test of IgG-aggregate binding, FLANDRIN *et al.*[357] detected IgG-Fc receptors on cells from all six cases they studied. MANN *et al.*[358] detected rosette formation in six out of eight American cases by means of the less sensitive IgGEA assay (Table 108).

---

[351] 1971.
[352] 1971.
[353] KLEIN, KLEIN, NADKARNI, NADKARNI *et al.*, 1967.
[354] PARKER, TAYLOR, PATTENGALE, ROYSTON *et al.*, 1977.
[355] 1973.
[356] THEOFILOPOULOS, BOKISCH and DIXON, 1974.
[357] FLANDRIN, BROUET, DANIEL and PREUD'HOMME, 1975.
[358] MANN, JAFFE, BRAYLAN, NANBA *et al.*, 1976.

Table 108. Surface markers on cells from Burkitt's lymphoma and lymphoma of Burkitt type

| Reference | Author's term | IgG-Fc receptors | EAC rosettes | Sheep-E rosettes |
|---|---|---|---|---|
| JONDAL *et al.*:[h] | Burkitt's lymphoma | n.d. | 0/3 | 0/3 |
| MAGRATH:[i] | Burkitt's lymphoma | n.d. | 6/6[a] | 5/6[b] |
| JONDAL *et al.*:[j] | Burkitt's lymphoma | n.d. | n.d. | 0/1 |
| FLANDRIN *et al.*:[k] | ALL, Burkitt type | 6/6[c] | n.d. | 0/6 |
| STEIN:[l] | Lymphoblastic lymphoma, Burkitt type | n.d. | 2/3[d] | n.d. |
| BINDER *et al.*:[m] | American Burkitt's lymphoma | n.d. | n.d. | 0/1 |
| MANN *et al.*:[n] | Non-endemic Burkitt's lymphoma | 6/8[e] | 3/8[f] | 0/8 |
| STEIN and TOLKSDORF:[o] | Lymphoblastic lymphoma, Burkitt type | n.d. | n.d. | 1/1[g] |

n.d. = not done.
[a] Range of positive cells: 2–33%.
[b] Range of positive cells: 3–18%.
[c] IgG aggregates were used.
[d] Detected on frozen sections.
[e] IgGEA were used; range of positive cells: 2–14%.
[f] Range of positive cells: 2–31%.
[g] Number of positive cells: 6%.
[h] JONDAL, HOLM and WIGZELL, 1972.
[i] 1974.
[j] JONDAL, SVEDMYR, KLEIN and SINGH, 1975.
[k] FLANDRIN, BROUET, DANIEL and PREUD'HOMME, 1975.
[l] 1975a, b; 1976b.
[m] BINDER, JENCKS, CHUN and RATH, 1975.
[n] MANN, JAFFE, BRAYLAN, NANBA *et al.*, 1976.
[o] 1977, unpublished data.

**Complement Receptor.** The literature contains little data on the presence of complement receptors on cells freshly obtained from African Burkitt's lymphomas. The available findings are summarized in Table 108. JONDAL *et al.*[359] reported that cells from three biopsies did not bind EACmouse. They also found that cells of 11 Burkitt's lymphoma-derived cell lines were not EAC-reactive. It is not clear whether these findings were valid, since, a year later, members of the same research group[360] stated that all Burkitt's lymphoma-derived cell lines tested (n=10) revealed the capacity to bind EAC. The percentage of EAC-positive cells varied from 2–100%, however, indicating a variable amount and affinity of complement receptors on the cells. SHEVACH *et al.*[361] found that cells from three out of five Burkitt's lymphoma-derived cell lines bound EACmouse.

In contrast to JONDAL *et al.*,[359] MAGRATH[362] found EACmouse-rosette formation by cells in fresh biopsies from six cases of African Burkitt's lymphoma (Table 108). As observed with the Burkitt's lymphoma-derived cell lines, the percentage of EAC-positive cells showed a wide range (2–33%).

359 JONDAL, HOLM and WIGZELL, 1972.
360 JONDAL and KLEIN, 1973.
361 SHEVACH, JAFFE and GREEN, 1973.
362 1974.

Complement-receptor subtypes have been studied on cells of only some of the Burkitt's lymphoma-derived cell lines, e.g., the Daudi and the Raji cell lines. Whereas Daudi cells formed rosettes only with EAC3d, Raji cells bound both EAC3b and EAC3d. These two Burkitt's lymphoma-derived cell lines also differed in the expression of SIg (see p. 624).

THEOFILOPOULOS *et al.*[363] reported that both Raji and Daudi cells can bind uncleaved C3. This feature distinguished complement receptors on Raji and Daudi cells from the complement receptors on human peripheral blood lymphocytes, which bind only cleaved C3, namely, C3b and C3d. The significance of the capacity to bind uncleaved C3 is not yet clear.

There are also few data on EAC rosette-forming capacity of cells from non-African lymphomas of the Burkitt type. The available data are presented in Table 108. Binding of EACmouse was observed by MANN *et al.*[364] in three out of eight American lymphomas of the Burkitt type. The range in the percentage of EAC-positive tumor cells was similar to that found by MAGRATH[365] for African Burkitt's lymphomas. Our own study revealed adherence of EAC-mouse on frozen sections from three out of five cases of European lymphoma of the Burkitt type.[366] In one of these cases EBV genomes were detected in the biopsy material by means of nuclear-acid hybridization.[367] Recently, we specified the complement-receptor subtypes in all complement receptor-positive cases of lymphoblastic lymphoma of the Burkitt type. Both the receptor for C3b and the receptor for C3d were present on some of the lymphoma cells from these three cases.[367a]

**Relationship between the Complement Receptor and the Receptor for Epstein-Barr Virus (EBV).** It has been established that EBV affects B-cells only.[368] An explanation for the B-cell tropism of EBV was given by JONDAL and KLEIN.[368] They succeeded in demonstrating that B-cells have a receptor that binds EBV. The specificity of this receptor was confirmed by blocking the binding of EBV by means of high-titer anti-viral-capsid antigen sera. T-cells did not bind EBV.[368a] GREAVES *et al.*[369] confirmed these findings and therefore regarded the EBV receptor as a reliable marker of B-lymphocytes.

JONDAL *et al.*[370] drew attention to the close relationship between EBV receptors and complement (C3d) receptors in a number of established human lymphoid cell lines. EBV receptor-positive lines proved to be positive for complement receptors, whereas not all EBV receptor-negative lines revealed complement receptors. EAC-rosette formation by cell lines was partially inhibited by concentrated EBV preparations. The inhibition could be neutralized by specific EBV antibody. Binding of EBV to virus receptor-positive cells was blocked by active mouse complement, but not by heat-inactivated complement. Furthermore, only

[363] THEOFILOPOULOS, BOKISCH and DIXON, 1974.
[364] MANN, JAFFE, BRAYLAN, NANBA *et al.*, 1976.
[365] 1974.
[366] STEIN, 1977, unpublished data.
[367] BORNKAMM, STEIN, LENNERT, RÜGGEBERG *et al.*, 1976.
[367a] STEIN and SIEMSSEN, 1977, unpublished data.
[368] JONDAL and KLEIN, 1973.
[368a] GREAVES, BROWN and RICKINSON, 1975; JONDAL, KLEIN, OLDSTONE, BOKISH *et al.*, 1976.
[369] GREAVES, BROWN and RICKINSON, 1975.
[370] JONDAL, KLEIN, OLDSTONE, BOKISH *et al.*, 1976.

complement receptor-positive lymphoid cell lines, including the T-ALL-derived, sheep-E receptor-positive and complement receptor-positive Molt 4 cell line, were susceptible to superinfection or primary infection with EBV, whereas complement receptor-negative cell lines were not susceptible.[370]

Two-color fluorescence combined with capping experiments showed complete overlapping of the labeling for EBV receptors and complement receptors. This indicated that EBV and complement (probably C3d) are probably bound to B-cells by the same receptor molecules, but not necessarily by the same binding site of these molecules.[371]

**Mouse-Erythrocyte (E) Receptor.** No data are available.

**Sheep-Erythrocyte (E) Receptor.** Whereas JONDAL *et al.*[372] found no binding of sheep erythrocytes by tumor cells from three African Burkitt's lymphomas, MAGRATH[373] observed sheep-E rosette-forming capacity in all six cases studied. She reported that the sheep E-rosetting cells could be clearly identified as tumor cells and that the percentage of contaminating lymphocytes was too low to explain the sheep E-rosette formation in the tumor-cell suspension. The percentage of sheep E-binding cells was low, however, ranging from 3–18% with a mean of 8% (Table 108). Recently, we[373a] confirmed the findings of MAGRATH. In one case we observed binding of sheep erythrocytes by the cells of a non-African lymphoma of the Burkitt type. Cytologic study of the rosette-forming cells clearly indicated that some of the sheep-E rosette-positive cells belonged to the neoplastic cell population.

JONDAL *et al.*[374] found 1% sheep E-binding cells in a suspension from an African Burkitt's lymphoma. The authors showed that these cells, or at least some of them, were cytotoxic to the tumor cells *in vitro*.

**Antigens Associated with Burkitt's Lymphoma Cells Containing Epstein-Barr Virus.** Several antigens have been demonstrated on Burkitt's lymphoma cells containing EBV genomes:

1. Membrane antigen (MA). It is detectable on Burkitt's lymphoma cells by means of direct immunofluorescence with the patient's serum.[375] MA has a macromolecular structure with different, probably three, antigenic determinants.

2. Viral-capsid antigen (VCA). It is present on the viral capsid of EBV.[376] VCA appeared only in MA- and early antigen-positive cells.[377]

3. Early antigen (EA). This antigen appeared after superinfection with EBV, but before VCA and DNA synthesis. It is therefore called early antigen.[378] EA has two components.[379] Demonstration of EA is a useful assay for successful EBV infection.

---

[371] YEFENOF, KLEIN, JONDAL and OLDSTONE, 1976.
[372] JONDAL, HOLM and WIGZELL, 1972.
[373] 1974.
[373a] STEIN and TOLKSDORF, 1977, unpublished data.
[374] JONDAL, SVEDMYR, KLEIN and SINGH, 1975.
[375] KLEIN, CLIFFORD, KLEIN and STJERNSWÄRD, 1966.
[376] BREMBERG, KLEIN and EPSTEIN, 1969.
[377] GERGELY, KLEIN and ERNBERG, 1971.
[378] HENLE, HENLE, ZAJAC, PEARSON *et al.*, 1970.
[379] HENLE, HENLE and KLEIN, 1971.

Table 109. Presence of Epstein-Barr-virus (EVB) genomes or Epstein-Barr nuclear antigen in lymphoblastic lymphoma with Burkitt-type morphology

| | African cases (endemic) % | Non-African cases (non-endemic) % |
|---|---|---|
| EBV-positive | 97–100 | 8–17 |
| EBV-negative | 0–3 | 83–92 |

4. Epstein-Barr nuclear antigen (EBNA). This antigen is localized at the nuclei of nearly all, if not all, cells that bear the EBV genome detected by nuclear-acid hybridization. EBNA can be demonstrated on methanol-fixed cells by means of anticomplementary immunofluorescence.[380] Thus, the EBNA test is a specific and sensitive tool for indirect detection of EBV genes at the cellular level.

**Epstein-Barr-Virus DNA (EBV-DNA) and Epstein-Barr Nuclear Antigen (EBNA).** Hybridization studies[381] have demonstrated that 97% of the cases of African Burkitt's lymphoma showed EBNA and/or EBV-DNA. In contrast, most American and European lymphoblastic lymphomas of the Burkitt type were devoid of EBV-DNA and EBV-associated antigens or antibodies.[382] More recent studies, however, have demonstrated EBV-DNA and/or EBNA in cases of non-African lymphoma of the Burkitt type.[383]

Taken together, these reports suggest a rate of 8–17% EBV-positive cases in the non-African group. This means that the non-African lymphomas should be divided into at least two subgroups (Table 109): one associated with EBV (8–17%) and one not associated with EBV (83–92%). The subdivision can easily be done with the EBNA test.[380] It also appears that African Burkitt's lymphomas should be separated into an EBNA-positive and an EBNA-negative subtype. Recent experimental findings have indicated, however, that the rate of EBV-negative African Burkitt's lymphomas is less than 3% (Table 109).

**Conclusions.** A majority of cases of African Burkitt's lymphoma and all cases of non-African lymphoblastic lymphoma of the Burkitt type exhibited SIg. IgM was most common, and IgG was rarely found. IgD was detected in only one out of seven cases in one study[385] and in both cases of non-African lymphoma of the Burkitt type in another study.[386] The SIg was restricted to a single light chain, usually κ. *De-novo* synthesis of surface IgM in African Burkitt's lymphoma has been established in a number of investigations.[387] Analysis of Ig in tissue extracts from non-African lymphoblastic lymphomas of

---

380 REEDMAN and KLEIN, 1973.
381 KLEIN, 1975a, b.
382 LEVINE, 1972; PAGANO, HUANG and LEVINE, 1973.
383 ANDERSSON, KLEIN, ZIEGLER and HENLE, 1976; BORNKAMM, STEIN, LENNERT, RÜGGEBERG *et al.*, 1976; EPSTEIN, HENLE, HENLE, HEWETSON *et al.*, 1976; GRAVELL, LEVINE, MCINTYRE, LAND *et al.*, 1976.
385 MANN, JAFFE, BRAYLAN, NANBA *et al.*, 1976.
386 PREUD'HOMME, BROUET, CLAUVEL and SELIGMANN, 1974.
387 SHERR and UHR, 1971; FLANDRIN, BROUET, DANIEL and PREUD'HOMME, 1975.

the B-type revealed a highly increased amount of IgM in four out of five cases.[388] That suggested synthesis of IgM by the tumor cells. ESKELAND and KLEIN[389] extracted IgM/$\kappa$ from the cells of an African Burkitt's lymphoma. Quantitative serum-Ig analysis showed that the Ig levels, especially those of IgM, were reduced in most cases of both African and non-African lymphoma. Thus, the functional (production but not secretion of Ig) and morphologic features (abundance of polyribosomes and paucity of ergastoplasm) indicate that lymphomas with Burkitt-like morphology belong to the group of B-cell lymphomas of the nonsecretory type.

The presence of IgG-Fc receptors on African Burkitt's lymphoma cells can be concluded only from studies of cell lines derived from Burkitt's lymphomas. By means of the IgGEA assay, the IgG-Fc receptor was found on cells in a majority of the cell lines. The sensitive assay for binding of IgG-aggregates revealed that nearly all the cell lines demonstrated this receptor. Similar results were obtained in non-African lymphoblastic lymphomas of the Burkitt type.

The percentage of complement receptor-positive tumor cells varied greatly from case to case in both the African and the non-African groups. It was also shown that, in many instances, complement receptors became detectable after cultivation. This finding provides evidence that the cells of nearly all, if not all, cases of lymphoblastic lymphoma of the Burkitt type bear complement receptors, but that the complement receptors are often blocked *in vivo* by a serum factor. It probably consists of complexes formed by antigens of the tumor cells and by host antibodies. In culture the blocking immunocomplexes are probably shed off the surface of the tumor cells. Consequently, the complement receptors become accessible to EAC. This hypothesis is substantiated by the following findings:

1. IgG-complement complexes were demonstrated in the glomeruli of two patients with African Burkitt's lymphoma (glomeruli have C3b receptors and are therefore able to specifically bind antigen-antibody-complement complexes).
2. The IgG fraction of the complexes found in the glomeruli revealed activity against viral-capsid antigen (VCA) and early antigen (EA).
3. Complexes with affinity to complement receptors on Raji cells were demonstrated in the sera of nine out of 15 (60%) patients with African Burkitt's lymphoma.[390]

The probable coating of Burkitt's and Burkitt-type lymphoma cells with immunocomplexes is interesting in connection with the starry-sky pattern seen in histologic sections from these tumors. The starry-sky pattern results from the presence of numerous light macrophages among the tumor cells. The macrophages actively phagocytose living tumor cells, even those in mitosis. It is therefore possible that the macrophages are captured within the tumor because they adhere *via* their complement receptors to the immunocomplexes that are bound to tumor cells. Because of the complement receptor-mediated binding and a possible additional binding *via* IgG-Fc receptors, the macrophages are induced to rapidly phagocytose living and even dividing tumor cells. In our opinion,

---

388 STEIN, 1975a.
389 1971.
390 OLDSTONE, THEOFILOPOULOS, GUNVEN and KLEIN, 1976.

avid phagocytosis of tumor cells is generally a reliable histologic indication of the presence of anti-tumor antibodies on the surfaces of tumor cells.

The collected data show that the neoplastic cells from African and non-African cases are similar not only in morphology and histochemistry, but also in immunologic markers. This suggests that in both groups of tumors, the same subset of nonsecretory lymphoid cells proliferates. LUKES and COLLINS[391] and the author (H.S.)[392] suggested that Burkitt-type lymphoma cells are derived from germinal-center cells. This hypothesis was based on morphologic findings (focal involvement of germinal centers),[393] cytologic similarity to a certain subtype of germinal-center cells (see Fig. 180), and immunologic data, i.e., abundant SIg and complement receptors, which are characteristic of germinal-center cells. The assumption of a close relationship between Burkitt-type lymphoma cells and germinal-center cells is substantiated above all by the findings on complement-receptor subtypes. The studies of JONDAL *et al.*[394] and our own[395] strongly suggest that cells of all Burkitt's and Burkitt-type lymphomas or of Burkitt's lymphoma-derived cell lines bear a receptor for C3d. We have shown that the receptor for C3d on noncirculating lymphoid cells is highly characteristic of germinal-center cells (see p. 354f.).[396] One problem with the hypothesis of germinal center-cell derivation is the large number of lymphomas with Burkitt-like morphology, chiefly African but also non-African, that are extralymphatic. For example, the mandible and ovary are sites that do not contain germinal centers under normal conditions. It may be, however, that germinal-center cells are present in the bone marrow under the conditions that favor the development of lymphomas with Burkitt-like morphology. Another problem with the hypothesis of a germinal center-cell, and thus B-cell, origin is the presence of sheep-E receptors on some tumor cells.[396a] At present, the only way to interpret this finding is to assume that EBV affects B-cells that activate genes controlling the derepression of sheep-E receptors during malignant transformation.

Although the nonsecretory B-cell subtypes proliferating in the African and non-African cases are apparently identical, there is overwhelming evidence that the African and most of the non-African tumors have different etiologies. Whereas the vast majority of cases of African Burkitt's lymphoma are associated with EBV, the non-African cases have to be subdivided into those associated with EBV (8–17%) and those not associated with EBV (83–92%).[397]

## M. Lymphoblastic Lymphomas Other than the Burkitt Type

Nearly all attempts at immunologic characterization of the tumor cells of lymphoblastic lymphoma have been made in cases of a type of leukemia that

---

[391] 1975.

[392] STEIN, 1975a, b, 1976b.

[393] MANN, JAFFE, BRAYLAN, NANBA *et al.*, 1976.

[394] JONDAL, KLEIN, OLDSTONE, BOKISH *et al.*, 1976.

[395] STEIN and SIEMSSEN, 1977, unpublished data.

[396] STEIN, SIEMSSEN and LENNERT, 1978, in press.

[396a] MAGRATH, 1974; STEIN and TOLKSDORF, 1977, unpublished data.

[397] KLEIN, 1975; ANDERSSON, KLEIN, ZIEGLER and HENLE, 1976; BORNKAMM, STEIN, LENNERT, RÜGGEBERG *et al.*, 1976; EPSTEIN, HENLE, HENLE, HEWETSON *et al.*, 1976; GRAVELL, LEVINE, MCINTYRE, LAND *et al.*, 1976.

is usually called acute lymphatic leukemia (ALL). It has not yet been determined whether the findings in ALL are also valid for nonleukemic lymphoblastic lymphoma. It appears to be likely that they are, however, since transitions from nonleukemic lymphoblastic lymphoma into the leukemic form (i.e., ALL) are common and there is no difference in cytology between the cells of the nonleukemic and leukemic forms of lymphoblastic lymphoma (see p. 416).

**Surface Immunoglobulin (SIg).** No cases of SIg-positive ALL were found in several relatively large series,[398] and SIg-positive cases were reported only occasionally.[399] SIg was found by BROUET *et al.*[400] in three out of 100, and by GAJL-PECZALSKA *et al.*[401] in one out of 34 cases of ALL. The SIg consisted of one heavy-chain and one light-chain type. The heavy chain was IgM in every case; the light chain was $\lambda$ in three cases and $\kappa$ in one case. Thus, the frequency of SIg in ALL is approximately 3%.

One case in our series was of particular interest. Thirty-three percent of the cells from this case of ALL reacted distinctly for $\mu$-, $\delta$-, and $\kappa$-chain determinants, 50% formed sheep-E rosettes, and 10% formed EAC rosettes. Ninety-eight percent of the cells revealed a strongly positive reaction for acid phosphatase in a localized region of the cytoplasm.

**Tissue Immunoglobulin.** *Saline Extract.* As illustrated in Figure 276, the mean IgM value for lymphoblastic lymphoma of the non-Burkitt type was within or only slightly above the normal thymic range, with one exception. When the lymphoblastic lymphomas were divided into morphologic subtypes, no great deviations in the tissue-IgM values above the thymic range were observed in the convoluted-cell type of lymphoblastic lymphoma. The tissue-IgM values of unclassified lymphoblastic lymphoma were also within or only slightly above the thymic range, with the one exception mentioned previously. The exceptional patient with a highly increased amount of IgM in the saline extract was a 50-year-old man.

*Detergent Second Extract.* As for the saline extract, the mean tissue-IgM value for the detergent 2nd extracts of the convoluted-cell type of lymphoblastic lymphoma was within the normal thymic range. That was also true for the unclassified type of lymphoblastic lymphoma of children and young adults. Two cases of the unclassified type of lymphoblastic lymphoma, however, showed a great increase in tissue IgM. Both patients were older than 30 years of age. One of them was the patient who also exhibited an increased amount of tissue IgM in the saline extract (see Fig. 277).

The results of the tissue-Ig assays suggest that there may be two subtypes

---

[398] BORELLA and SEN, 1973; BELPOMME, DANTCHEV, DU RUSQUEC, GRANDJON *et al.*, 1974; BROWN, GREAVES, LISTER, RAPSON *et al.*, 1974; KERSEY, NESBIT, LUCKASEN, HALLGREN *et al.*, 1974; SEN and BORELLA, 1975.

[399] BROUET, TOBEN, CHEVALIER and SELIGMANN, 1974; DAVEY and GOTTLIEB, 1974; GAJL-PECZALSKA, BLOOMFIELD, NESBIT and KERSEY, 1974; HAEGERT, CAWLEY, KARPAS and GOLDSTONE, 1974; BROUET, VALENSI, DANIEL, FLANDRIN *et al.*, 1976.

[400] BROUET, VALENSI, DANIEL, FLANDRIN *et al.*, 1976.

[401] GAJL-PECZALSKA, BLOOMFIELD, NESBIT and KERSEY, 1974.

of morphologically unclassifiable lymphoblastic lymphoma: one subtype without Ig synthesis and occurring predominantly in children and young adults, and one subtype with Ig synthesis and occurring in older patients.

**Serum Immunoglobulin.** In all but two cases of lymphoblastic lymphoma, the serum-Ig levels were within or below the normal range. The two exceptional cases were morphologically classified as lymphoblastic lymphoma of the convoluted-cell type. The serum Ig that was found to be increased belonged to the IgM class. It appeared to be polyclonal in immunoelectrophoresis.

**Monoclonality of the Tissue and Serum Immunoglobulin.** The IgM fraction of the tissue extracts and sera from all six cases of the non-Burkitt type of lymphoblastic lymphoma exhibited a polyclonal pattern in isoelectric focusing.

**Cytoplasmic Immunoglobulin (CIg).** Systematic studies of CIg have not been performed. We have studied five cases of ALL with a focal acid phosphatase reaction. Fixed cells on centrifuge slides of these cases did not stain with fluorescein-conjugated anti-Ig antibodies. With the very sensitive immunoperoxidase-bridge method, however, we observed a positive CIg staining in the case of lymphoblastic lymphoma whose cells showed strong focal acid phosphatase reactivity, SIg, complement receptors, and sheep-E receptors. It was remarkable that a positive staining of the cytoplasm was achieved with both anti-$\kappa$ and anti-$\lambda$ sera. Positive CIg staining of an HTLA-positive and complement receptor-positive cell line (RPMI-8402) was recently described by PARKER *et al.*[401a] The cells of their case also stained clearly for both $\kappa$- and $\lambda$-chains. CIg staining in apparently T-cell-derived ALL cells is puzzling, but might reflect the production of Ig-like molecules or a property of very early thymocyte precursor cells, which are said to produce Ig.[401b]

**IgG-Fc Receptor.** The percentage of cells from one case of ALL in the series of BELPOMME *et al.*[402] that bound IgGEA was higher than that of the non-ALL cells in the sample, suggesting the expression of IgG-Fc receptors by some of the blast cells. BELPOMME *et al.*, however, apparently did not systematically determine which cells formed the rosettes. We found lymphoblastic lymphoma cells that bound IgG-humanEA in two out of 20 cases. The cells from these cases also bound neuraminidase-treated sheep erythrocytes, but lacked SIg. BROUET *et al.*[403] found only two out of 74 cases of ALL that revealed the capacity to bind IgG aggregates. The blast cells from both cases were SIg-positive and were not killed by anti-thymocyte serum.

**IgM-Fc Receptor.** MORETTA *et al.*[403a] detected IgMEA-rosette formation by cells from two cases of T-ALL. Since COOPER[403b] demonstrated that T-cells

[401a] PARKER, TAYLOR, PATTENGALE, ROYSTON *et al.*, 1977.

[401b] DU PASQUIER, WEISS and LOOR, 1972; GATIEN, SCHNEEBERGER and MERLER, 1975.

[402] BELPOMME, DANTCHEV, DU RUSQUEC, GRANDJON *et al.*, 1974.

[403] BROUET, VALENSI, DANIEL, FLANDRIN *et al.*, 1976.

[403a] MORETTA, FERRARINI, DURANTE and MINGARI, 1975.

[403b] 1976.

bearing IgM-Fc receptors (detectable in the IgMEA-rosette test after 20-hour incubation) show T-helper functions, IgM-Fc receptor-positive ALL might be a clonal proliferation of a subset of (probably immature) T-helper cells, like the cells of Sézary's syndrome.

**Complement Receptor.** JONDAL *et al.*[404] found only a very small proportion of EAC-reactive cells in ALL. In our own study, we investigated the binding of EAC by lymphoblastic lymphoma cells on frozen sections and by suspended tumor cells. As previously reported,[405] we were surprised to find that the frozen sections from five out of 12 cases of lymphoblastic lymphoma exhibited adherence of EAC (see Fig. 285a) when glutaraldehyde-fixed sheep erythrocytes maximally coated with human complement were used. Sheep erythrocytes or sheep EA did not adhere to sections from any case of lymphoblastic lymphoma. Suspended cells from eight out of 21 cases of lymphoblastic lymphoma also formed EAC rosettes in a significant percentage. Cytologic evaluation confirmed that most of the EAC-binding cells were neoplastic blast cells.

Among our cases of lymphoblastic lymphoma there were some in which the cells had complement receptors, but completely lacked sheep-E receptors.[406] JAFFE *et al.*[407] and GAJL-PECZALSKA *et al.*[408] reported on similar findings. The cells of our complement receptor-positive and sheep-E receptor-negative cases always showed strong focal acid phosphatase reactivity. Recently, THIEL *et al.*[408a] studied the presence and amount of HTLA in three such cases. In two cases they found less HTLA than in thymocytes, but slightly more than in peripheral T-cells. THIEL *et al.*[408a] also observed two focally acid phosphatase-positive, complement receptor-positive, SIg-negative, and sheep-E receptor-negative cases of ALL whose cells expressed common-ALL antigen and HTLA simultaneously, suggesting the existence of hybrid types of ALL (null/T-ALL).

**Mouse-Erythrocyte (E) Receptor.** Cells from the few cases investigated so far did not form rosettes with mouse erythrocytes.[409]

**Sheep-Erythrocyte (E) Receptor.** Several authors have reported that cells from 30–40% of the cases of ALL formed sheep-E rosettes.[410] The spontaneous sheep-E rosette-forming capacity varied greatly from case to case. In half of the cases the percentage of sheep-E rosette-forming blast cells was higher than 60% and in the other half it was 10–16%. The number of sheep erythrocytes bound by ALL blast cells also differed from case to case. There were some cases in which the ALL blast cells constantly bound only two to four sheep erythrocytes. In many cases the percentage of sheep-E rosette-forming cells

[404] JONDAL, WIGZELL and AIUTI, 1973.
[405] STEIN, 1975a, b, 1976b.
[406] STEIN, BOUMAN, LENNERT, FUCHS *et al.*, 1977; STEIN and MÜLLER-HERMELINK, 1977.
[407] JAFFE, BRAYLAN, FRANK, GREEN *et al.*, 1976.
[408] GAJL-PECZALSKA, CHARTRAND, BLOOMFIELD, CORTE *et al.*, 1977.
[408a] THIEL, DÖRMER, RODT, HUHN *et al.*, 1977.
[409] CATOVSKY, CHERCHI, OKOS, HEGDE *et al.*, 1976.
[410] KERSEY, SABAD, GAJL-PECZALSKA, HALLGREN *et al.*, 1973; BROUET, TOBEN, CHEVALIER and SELIGMANN, 1974; GAJL-PECZALSKA, BLOOMFIELD, NESBIT and KERSEY, 1974; KAPLAN, MASTRANGELO and PETERSON, 1974; SCHWENK, 1974; KERSEY, NESBIT, HALLGREN, SABAD *et al.*, 1975; SEN and BORELLA, 1975.

and the number of sheep erythrocytes bound by the cells could be increased by using sheep erythrocytes treated with neuraminidase or AET. SEN and BORELLA[411] made the interesting observation that ALL blast cells with sheep-E receptors and thymocytes, but not peripheral blood lymphocytes, form sheep-E rosettes after prolonged incubation at 37°C. Our own studies revealed that in eight out of 21 cases the lymphoblastic lymphoma cells showed a significant binding of both EAC and sheep erythrocytes. If the percentages of EAC and sheep-E rosette-forming cells are added together, the sum exceeds 100% in all eight cases.

**Human T-Associated Antigens.** *1. Human T-Lymphocyte Antigen (HTLA).* CHIN *et al.*,[411a] KERSEY *et al.*,[412] and BROUET *et al.*[413] studied relatively large series of ALL for reactivity of the tumor cells with anti-thymocyte serum directed against thymocyte and peripheral T-cell antigens. They used either the cytotoxicity assay or indirect immunofluorescence. CHIN *et al.*[411a] found anti-thymocyte sera reactivity in 10 out of 15 (67%) cases; KERSEY *et al.*,[412] in 12 out of 20 (60%) cases; and BROUET *et al.*,[413] in 18 out of 54 (33%) cases of ALL. KERSEY *et al.*[412] reported that in all instances the ALL cells that bore sheep-E receptors also bore HTLA. In six out of 12 cases the cells revealed HTLA, but did not bear sheep-E receptors.

BROUET *et al.*[413] also observed contradictory results with anti-thymocyte serum and sheep-E reactivity. In three out of 19 cases the ALL cells did not form rosettes with sheep erythrocytes, but were killed by anti-thymocyte serum. In contrast to the findings of KERSEY *et al.*,[412] the cells from one case in the series studied by BROUET *et al.*[413] bound sheep erythrocytes but not anti-thymocyte antibodies.

A quantitative autoradiographic method has recently been developed for determining absolute amounts of surface antigen on individual cells.[414] Sixteen HTLA-positive cases selected from 42 cases of ALL were analyzed for the amount of HTLA on the cells and the capacity of the cells to form sheep-E rosettes with the following results. (1) In four cases a large amount of HTLA was found together with the capacity to form sheep-E rosettes that were stable at 37°C. Both features are comparable with those of thymocytes. All four patients presented with a mediastinal mass. In two cases the cells also showed complement receptors. (2) The cells from five cases expressed a large amount of HTLA, like thymocytes, but were capable of forming only dissociable (fragile at 37°C) sheep-E rosettes. All five cases were devoid of complement receptors. (3) In seven cases the density of HTLA on the cells was slightly higher than on blood T-lymphocytes, but there was no sheep-E rosette-forming capacity. The cells of two out of three cases simultaneously bore HTLA and complement receptors. In all 16 cases of ALL the cells showed strong focal acid phosphatase reactivity.

---

[411] 1975.

[411a] CHIN, SAIKI, TRUJILLO and WILLIAMS, 1973.

[412] KERSEY, NESBIT, HALLGREN, SABAD *et al.*, 1975.

[413] BROUET, VALENSI, DANIEL, FLANDRIN *et al.*, 1976.

[414] SHEVACH, EDELSON, FRANK, LUTZNER *et al.*, 1974.

*2. Thymocyte-Specific Antigen (THYSA).* In healthy persons THYSA is present only on thymocytes and not on peripheral T-cells (see p. 562).[414a] It was detected on the leukemic cells of all 12 sheep-E rosette-positive cases of ALL studied by MILLS *et al.*[414a] The cells of eight sheep-E rosette-negative cases of ALL were devoid of THYSA.

*3. Human Thymus/Leukemia-Associated Antigen (HTHY-L).* HTHY-L (see p. 562) is normally present only on thymocytes and not on peripheral T-cells or B-cells. This antigen has so far been found in three groups of leukemias: sheep-E rosette-positive ALL, sheep-E rosette-negative ALL, and acute myeloid leukemia (AML).[414b] The highest content of HTHY-L was measured in saline extracts of sheep-E rosette-positive ALL cells. Three to five times less HTHY-L was detected in extracts of cells from sheep-E rosette-negative cases of ALL and from AML. Cells of T-cell lines derived from sheep-E rosette-positive ALL, e.g., Molt cells, contained about the same amounts of HTHY-L as freshly obtained sheep-E rosette-positive ALL cells.

*4. CLL/Thymus Antigen (CLL-THYA).* The CLL-THYA shared by normal B-cells, B-CLL cells, and thymocytes (see p. 562) was detected on the cells of 30 out of 33 (91%) cases of non-B/non-T ALL, two cases of B-cell-derived ALL, and only one out of 19 (5%) cases of T-cell-derived ALL.[415]

**Common-ALL Antigen.** Common-ALL antigen has so far not been found on any type of normal cell (see p. 563). GREAVES *et al.*[416] detected common-ALL antigen on the cells of 251 out of 348 (72%) cases of ALL that lacked SIg, sheep-E receptors, and HTLA, but not in cases with B- or T-markers. The same research group found common-ALL antigen on cells with a lymphoid cytology in chronic myeloid leukemia in blast crisis, but not on cells with distinct myeloid characteristics.[417]

**Human B-Associated Antigens (Ia-Like Antigen).** In healthy persons Ia-like antigen is expressed on B-cells and on some special subsets of T-cells (see p. 563f.). FU *et al.*[418] and WERNET *et al.*[419] studied the occurrence of Ia-like antigen on leukemic cells by means of the complement-dependent cytotoxicity and/or the immunofluorescence technique. The results are summarized in Table 111. The primary association of Ia-like antigen with normal B-cells and its presence on B-CLL cells suggested that Ia-like antigen-positive leukemic cells are of B-cell lineage. This conclusion is consistent with the observation that all T-marker-positive ALL cells proved to be Ia-like antigen-negative.

[414a] MILLS, SEN and BORELLA, 1975.
[414b] CHECHIK, PYKE and GELFAND, 1976.
[415] BROUET, VALENSI, DANIEL, FLANDRIN *et al.*, 1976.
[416] GREAVES, JANOSSY, ROBERTS, RAPSON *et al.*, 1977.
[417] JANOSSY, GREAVES, REVESZ, LISTER *et al.*, 1976.
[418] FU, WINCHESTER and KUNKEL, 1975a.
[419] WERNET, SCHUNTER, WILMS and WALLER, 1977.

A striking observation was that Ia-like antigen was present in a vast majority of non-B and non-T ALL (19/24). Another interesting finding was provided by studies of myelogenous leukemia. They showed that Ia-like antigen was not expressed on chronic myeloid leukemia cells, whereas it was demonstrated on all acute myeloid leukemia cells and on cells from chronic myeloid leukemia in blast crisis. These findings support the view that common-ALL cells might be the neoplastic equivalents of precursor cells of the myeloid and B-lymphocyte series.

**Terminal Deoxynucleotidyl Transferase (Tdt) and α-N-Acetyl-Hexosaminidase Isoenzyme I (Hexosaminidase I).** Under nonneoplastic conditions, significant amounts of Tdt are found only in thymocytes (see p. 564). McCAFFREY *et al.*[420] reported on the occurrence of Tdt in leukemic cells. Tdt was found in a total of 32 out of 36 patients, both children and adults, with ALL, and in eight out of 22 patients with chronic myeloid leukemia in blast crisis. The enzyme was not present in cells from other types of leukemia such as CLL, acute myeloid leukemia, chronic myeloid leukemia, Sézary's syndrome, or lymphosarcoma-cell leukemia. In extension of these studies, JANOSSY *et al.*[421] correlated the presence of Tdt with the type of ALL. They found a large amount of Tdt in T-ALL and common-ALL antigen-positive non-B/non-T ALL, but not in B-ALL. GREAVES' group[421] and SARIN and GALLO[422] also measured large amounts of Tdt in cells from chronic myeloid leukemia in blast crisis. The largest amount of Tdt was measured in common ALL.[423]

The isoenzyme hexosaminidase I has been used by JANOSSY *et al.*[421] to further phenotype cells of ALL. So far, this enzyme has proved to be specific for common-ALL antigen-positive non-B/non-T ALL. Apparently, hexosaminidase I does not occur, or at least not in a significantly large population of cells, in healthy persons.

**Simultaneous Presence of Various Cell Markers.** There have been several reports of occasional leukemic human lymphocytes bearing both T- and B-cell surface markers (see Table 110). The lymphomas with such B- and T-markers were classified as lymphatic leukemia[424] or lymphosarcoma-cell leukemia.[425] In one case complement receptors and sheep-E receptors were demonstrated on the cells of an established cell line derived from a T-ALL.[426] It should be noted that simultaneous reactivity for SIg and sheep erythrocytes may be due to immunologic specificity of the SIg for sheep erythrocytes. Such a case was first described by BROUET *et al.*[427] and one was recently observed by FINK.[428] We also found such a case, in which the sheep-E rosette-forming capacity could be blocked only by anti-κ sera and not by anti-heavy chain

[420] McCAFFREY, HARRISON, PARKMAN and BALTIMORE, 1975.
[421] JANOSSY, ROBERTS and GREAVES, 1976; GREAVES, JANOSSY, ROBERTS, RAPSON *et al.*, 1977.
[422] 1976.
[423] BROUET, 1977; GREAVES, JANOSSY, ROBERTS, RAPSON *et al.*, 1977.
[424] SHEVACH, EDELSON, FRANK, LUTZNER *et al.*, 1974.
[425] LIN and HSU, 1976.
[426] WEST and HERBERMAN, 1974.
[427] BROUET and PRIEUR, 1974.
[428] 1976, personal communication.

Table 110. Simultaneous presence of surface markers on cells from lymphatic neoplasms

| Author/Term | n | SIg | IgG-Fc receptors | Complement receptors | Sheep-E receptors | HTLA | Common ALL antigen |
|---|---|---|---|---|---|---|---|
| SHEVACH *et al.*:[b] CLL | 1 | – | – | + | + | n.t. | n.t. |
| SANDILANDS *et al.*:[c] Lymphoproliferative disorder | 1 | – | + | n.t. | + | n.t. | n.t. |
| WEST and HERBERMAN:[d] T-ALL line (Molt 4) | 1 | n.t. | n.t. | + | + | n.t. | n.t. |
| LIN and HSU:[e] Lymphosarcoma-cell leukemia | 1 | + | n.t. | + | + | + | n.t. |
| HSU *et al.*:[f] Lymphosarcoma-cell leukemia | 1 | + | n.t. | n.t. | + | + | n.t. |
| STEIN *et al.*:[g] Lymphoblastic lymphoma, T-precursor type | 5[a] | – | n.t. | + | + | n.t. | n.t. |
| BRAYLAN *et al.*:[h] Lymphoblastic lymphoma | 3 | – | – | + | + | n.t. | n.t. |
| STEIN *et al.*:[i] Lymphoblastic lymphoma, T-precursor type | 1 | + | n.t. | + | + | n.t. | n.t. |
| THIEL *et al.*:[j] ALL | 2[a] | – | + | + | + | + | – |
| | 2[a] | – | + | + | – | + | + |
| | 2[a] | – | + | + | – | – | + |
| | 1 | – | + | – | – | – | + |
| MINOWADA *et al.*:[k] | | | | | | | |
| T-cell lines | 13 | – | n.t. | 4/13+ | 6/13+ | + | 11/13+ |
| Null-cell line | 1 | – | n.t. | – | – | + | + |

n = number of cases studied.
n.t. = not tested.
[a] Cases with a focal acid phosphatase reaction.
[b] SHEVACH, EDELSON, FRANK, LUTZNER *et al.*, 1974.
[c] SANDILANDS, GRAY, COONEY, BROWNING *et al.*, 1974.
[d] 1974.
[e] 1976.
[f] HSU, MARTI, SCHREK and WILLIAMS, 1975.
[g] STEIN, PETERSEN, GAEDICKE, LENNERT *et al.*, 1976
[h] BRAYLAN, JAFFE, MANN, FRANK *et al.*, 1977.
[i] STEIN, BOUMAN, LENNERT, FUCHS *et al.*, 1977.
[j] THIEL, DÖRMER, RODT, HUHN *et al.*, 1977.
[k] MINOWADA, TSUBOTA, NAKAZAWA, SRIVASTAVA *et al.*, 1977.

or anti-HTLA sera or by pretreatment of the sheep erythrocytes with trypsin. This indicates that the leukemic cells expressed SIg molecules with specific reactivity to sheep erythrocyte-membrane proteins that are resistant to trypsin.

The cases listed in Table 110, however, probably expressed both B- and T-markers for one of the following reasons: the leukemic cells lacked SIg;[428a] the SIg developed on the primarily sheep E-reactive leukemic cells in the course of the disease, and the neosynthesis of SIg was established in trypsinization experiments;[429] or both the complement receptors and sheep-E receptors were detectable on cultivated leukemic cells.[429a]

Our finding that a significant number of the cells from eight out of 20 cases of lymphoblastic lymphoma formed rosettes with EAC and with sheep erythrocytes suggests that the simultaneous presence of complement receptors and sheep-E receptors is a common property of lymphoblastic lymphoma cells. To establish the validity of this assumption, we decided to look for the simultaneous presence of complement receptors and sheep-E receptors on the same cells in a mixed rosette assay. In all eight cases that revealed EAC and sheep-E rosettes in the single assays, a considerable number of lymphoblastic lymphoma cells formed mixed rosettes, i.e., rosettes consisting of nucleated chicken EAC and sheep erythrocytes (Fig. 285b). The simultaneous presence of the two types of receptors could also be demonstrated with *Staphylococci aurei* coated with IgM antibodies and complement, and AET-treated sheep erythrocytes (Fig. 285c). The results of recent studies by various other authors[430] confirmed our findings.

THIEL *et al.*[431] analyzed the amount of HTLA on the surface of cells from four cases of ALL whose cells rosetted with both EAC and sheep erythrocytes. The amount of HTLA on these cells was about as large as that on thymocytes. The same authors reported on two further cases of ALL that were devoid of SIg and sheep-E receptors, but exhibited common-ALL antigen and HTLA simultaneously. MINOWADA *et al.*[432] also described the simultaneous presence of common-ALL antigen and HTLA on T-cell-line cells and cells from one null-cell line (Table 110).

**Conclusions.** The markers that helped to classify ALL cells are summarized in Table 111. On the basis of the presence of these markers, four main types of ALL can be distinguished:

*1. Common ALL.* Common ALL is characterized by the presence of the common-ALL antigen first described by GREAVES *et al.*[433] Classic B- and T-markers, such as SIg, sheep-E receptors, and HTLA, are lacking. In addition, common-ALL cells react positively for HTHY-L, CLL-THYA, Ia-like antigen, Tdt, and hexosaminidase I.

*2. T-ALL.* T-ALL cells are characterized by the presence of HTLA, THYSA, HTHY-L, Tdt, or sheep-E receptors, and sometimes by the simultaneous presence of sheep-E receptors and complement receptors. T-ALL cells are devoid of SIg, common-ALL antigen, CLL-THYA, Ia-like antigen, and hexosamini-

[428a] SHEVACH, EDELSON, FRANK, LUTZNER *et al.*, 1974.

[429] HSU, MARTI, SCHREK and WILLIAMS, 1975.

[429a] WEST and HERBERMAN, 1974.

[430] KERSEY, NESBIT, HALLGREN, SABAD *et al.*, 1975; BRAYLAN, JAFFE, MANN, FRANK *et al.*, 1977; CATOVSKY and GALTON, 1977; GAJL-PECZALSKA, CHARTRAND, BLOOMFIELD, CORTE *et al.*, 1977; KERSEY, COCCIA, BLOOMFIELD, NESBIT *et al.*, 1977.

[431] THIEL, DÖRMER, RODT, HUHN *et al.*, 1977.

[432] MINOWADA, TSUBOTA, NAKAZAWA, SRIVASTAVA *et al.*, 1977.

[433] GREAVES, BROWN, RAPSON and LISTER, 1975.

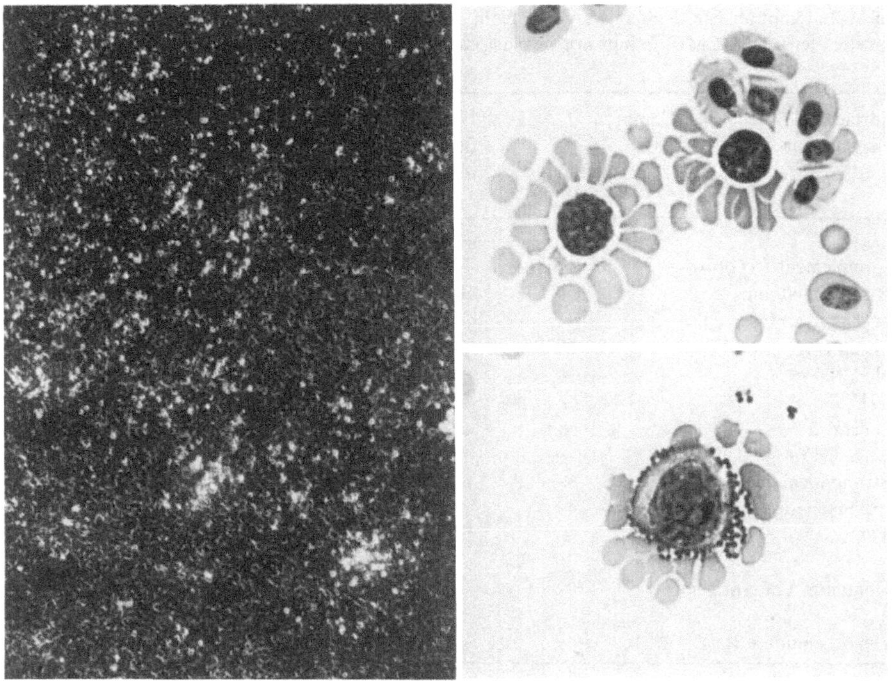

(a) (b) (c)

Fig. 285a–c. Lymphoblastic lymphoma, convoluted-cell type, with a strongly positive, focal acid phosphatase region. (a) Frozen section treated with EAC. Small number of reagent red cells (light spots) adhere diffusely to the section. Hematoxylin and eosin. Dark-field illumination. ×100. (b) Suspended tumor cells from the same case as (a) binding both sheep erythrocytes and nucleated chicken erythrocytes coated with IgM antibodies and mouse complement. Cytocentrifuge slide. Pappenheim. ×840. (c) Suspended tumor cells from the same case as (a) and (b) binding both sheep erythrocytes and glutaraldehyde-fixed *Staphylococci aurei* coated with IgM and human complement. Cytocentrifuge slide. Pappenheim. ×840

dase I. Most cases of T-ALL are also characterized by strong focal acid phosphatase reactivity. The cells from some cases with strong focal acid phosphatase reactivity bear only complement receptors. We also consider the cases with T-characteristic sheep-E receptors and B-characteristic complement receptors and those having complement receptors, but lacking sheep-E receptors, to be T-cell-derived. This view is supported by the following observations. (1) Fetal thymocytes of 9–10 weeks' gestation bear surface IgM and complement receptors, but no sheep-E receptors. With increasing fetal age, the thymocytes become complement receptor-negative and sheep-E receptor-positive.[434] This switch in receptors takes place *via* an intermediate cell type that simultaneously expressed complement and sheep-E receptors.[435] The fetal thymocytes that show only complement receptors, those with both complement and sheep-E receptors, and those having only sheep-E receptors all display strong focal acid phosphatase reactivity.[435] (2) A moderate amount of HTLA was demonstrated in two cases

[434] Gatien, Schneeberger and Merler, 1975. [435] Stein and Müller-Hermelink, 1977.

Table 111. Occurrence of surface and enzyme markers on cells from various immunologic subtypes of acute lymphoblastic leukemia (ALL), from acute myeloid leukemia (AML), and from chronic myeloid leukemia (CML) in and not in blast crisis. Summary of data from the literature and own studies

| Surface or enzyme marker | Common ALL | T-ALL | Unqualified ALL | B-ALL | AML | Blast-crisis cells in CML | CML |
|---|---|---|---|---|---|---|---|
| SIg | – | – | – | + | – | – | – |
| Complement receptor | –? | often + | ? | ? | + | –? | + |
| B-associated antigens (e.g., Ia) | + | – | 50% + | + | 80% + | 50% + | – |
| Sheep-E receptor | – | 60% + | – | – | – | – | – |
| HTLA | – | + | – | – | – | – | – |
| THYSA | – | + | – | – | – | – | – |
| HTHY-L | + | + | n.t. | – | + | n.t. | n.t. |
| CLL-THYA | + | – | n.t. | + | – | n.t. | n.t. |
| Strong focal acid phosphatase | – | + | – | – | – | sometimes + | – |
| Tdt | ++ | + | 50% + | – | sometimes + | 50% + | – |
| Common-ALL antigen | + | – | – | – | sometimes + | lymphoid cells + | – |
| Hexosaminidase I | + | – | – | – | – | – | – |

n.t. = not tested.

of ALL that showed strong focal acid phosphatase reactivity and complement receptors, but lacked sheep-E receptors.

Taking all of these findings, together with the results of quantitation of HTLA and the fragility of sheep-E rosettes at 37° C, into consideration, there is strong evidence that T-ALL can be subtyped into four groups:

(a) T-ALL that is probably derived from thymocyte precursor cells (*thymocyte-precursor subtype*). This subtype is based on the similar marker constellations of the tumor cells and thymocyte precursor cells. Both types of cells are characterized by focal acid phosphatase reactivity, complement receptors, and moderate amounts of HTLA; they are devoid of sheep-E receptors. This interpretation might explain why HTLA-positive cases of ALL were found more often than sheep-E rosette-positive cases, or, in other words, why HTLA-positive cases of ALL often lack sheep-E receptors.

(b) T-ALL that is probably derived from fetal prothymocytes, as suggested by the presence of complement receptors and HTLA and by the capacity to form sheep-E rosettes that are stable at 37° C (*prothymocytic subtype*).

(c) T-ALL that is probably derived from postnatal thymocytes (*postnatal or mature thymocytic subtype*). The close relationship between some T-ALL cells and mature thymocytes is confirmed by the common properties of forming sheep-E rosettes that are stable at 37° C and having large amounts of HTLA on the cell surface, but no complement receptors.

(d) T-ALL that is probably derived from peripheral T-cells (*peripheral T-cell subtype*). The ALL cells of this subtype are different from thymocytes and are similar to peripheral T-cells in their low density of HTLA and in the capacity to form sheep-E rosettes only at 4°C. This ALL subtype is probably closely related to T-CLL. It would be Tdt-negative.

As can be seen from the different marker constellations, not all cases of T-ALL clearly fit into these subtypes. The difficult cases have to be placed between the subtypes. This suggests that T-ALL cells are derived from T-cells of different stages of maturation and differentiation that fall between T-determined stem cells and peripheral T-cells.

*3. B-ALL.* B-ALL is rare. B-ALL cells are characterized by the presence of SIg, CLL-THYA, and Ia-like antigen. Common-ALL antigen, sheep-E receptors, HTLA, Tdt, and hexosaminidase I are lacking. Two subtypes can be recognized: (a) B-ALL of the Burkitt type, in which the cells have features resembling those of nonleukemic lymphoblastic lymphoma of the Burkitt type, and (b) B-ALL in which the cells resemble those of common ALL. B-ALL cells of the non-Burkitt type tend, however, to be more pleomorphic in morphology than those of common ALL.

*4. Unqualified ALL.* This type of ALL is characterized by the lack of classic B- and T-markers. It differs from common ALL in the lack of common-ALL antigen. Interestingly, unqualified ALL cells are positive for Ia-like antigen and Tdt in 50% of cases.

*Probable Derivation of the Common-ALL Antigen-Positive ALL Cell.* The partial overlapping of immunologic and enzyme markers, such as Ia-like antigen, complement receptors, HTHY-L, HTLA, CLL-THYA, and Tdt, in the different types of ALL speaks for a close relationship between the types. The data suggest that the common-ALL cell is derived from a pluripotent stem cell that has the capacity to develop (1) into thymocytes, as indicated by the usual presence of Tdt and HTHY-L in common-ALL cells and T-ALL cells, and by the occurrence of hybrid common-ALL antigen- and HTLA-positive ALL cells, and (2) into B-cells, as indicated by the presence of Ia-like antigen and CLL-THYA on common ALL cells and B-ALL cells. The stem-cell character of common-ALL cells is substantiated further by the demonstration of common-ALL antigen, Ia-like antigen, HTHY-L, and Tdt on acute myeloid leukemia cells and on cells from chronic myeloid leukemia in blast crisis (see Table 111). One may conclude from these findings that common-ALL cells are the precursor cells not only for the B- and T-lymphoid cell series, but also for the myeloid cell series.

**Relationship between the Immunologic and the Morphologic Subtypes of Lymphoblastic Lymphoma Other than the Burkitt Type.** At present, it is not possible to make a distinct correlation between the morphologic and the immunologic subtypes of lymphoblastic lymphoma of other than the Burkitt type. The reason is that there has been no systematic combined analysis of the relevant immunologic markers and histologic and cytologic features of lymphoblastic lymphomas, including ALL. Data from other studies and from our own investigations suggest, however, that the convoluted-cell type of lymphoblastic lymphoma is usually identical with the immunologic T-type. That is valid for both the imma-

Table 112. Assumed correlation between the histologic and immunologic subtypes of lymphoblastic lymphoma and ALL of non-Burkitt type

| Immunologic type | Histologic type | |
|---|---|---|
| | Convoluted-cell type | Unclassified type |
| Common ALL-antigen type | − | + |
| T-type | + | some + |
| Thymocyte-precursor subtype | + | − ? |
| Prothymocytic subtype | + | − ? |
| Mature thymocytic subtype | + | some + ? |
| Peripheral T-cell subtype | ? | some + ? |
| B-type | − | + |
| Unqualified type | − | + |

ture and mature thymocytic subtypes. The morphologically unclassified type seems to be highly heterogeneous. It probably includes the immunologically unqualified cases and some cases of the T-type, as well as all common-ALL antigen-positive cases and all B-types other than the Burkitt type (see Table 112).

## N. Malignant Lymphoma, Immunoblastic

A vast majority of the large-cell lymphomas, formerly classified as reticulum-cell sarcoma or malignant lymphoma, histiocytic, are equivalent to immunoblastic lymphoma in the Kiel Classification.

**Surface Immunoglobulin (SIg).** Only small series of reticulosarcomas or immunoblastic sarcomas have been studied for SIg (see Table 113). That is remarkable, since reticulum-cell sarcoma, or histiocytic lymphoma, was one of the most frequently described lymphoma classes in the statistics of various European authors[436] and of American and British pathologists.[437] In 1974, we reported on the presence of surface IgM on neoplastic cells from two reticulum-cell sarcomas or immunoblastic lymphomas.[438] AISENBERG and LONG[439] studied three lymphomas designated as diffuse histiocytic lymphoma, one well differentiated, one poorly differentiated, and one not qualified. They found the cells from these cases to be devoid of SIg. BROUET *et al.*[440] detected SIg with only one light-chain type on cells from two out of six reticulum-cell sarcomas. The SIg-positive reticulum-cell sarcomas had developed from other B-cell neoplasms (CLL in one case and macroglobulinemia of Waldenström in the other). The blast cell-like cells from these cases produced the same types of Ig chains as the neoplastic cells from the primary proliferations. In another case a small percentage (10−15%) of the large tumor cells reacted with antisera against

[436] LUMB, 1954; LENNERT, 1964.

[437] RAPPAPORT, WINTER and HICKS, 1956; DORFMAN, 1964; RAPPAPORT, 1966; FARRER-BROWN, BENNETT and HENRY, 1973; JONES, FUKS, BULL, KADIN *et al.*, 1973.

[438] STEIN, KAISERLING and LENNERT, 1974b.

[439] 1975.

[440] BROUET, LABAUME and SELIGMANN, 1975.

Table 113. Surface immunoglobulin (SIg) on cells from immunoblastic lymphoma and apparently equivalent entities of other lymphoma classifications

| Author/Term | SIg class | Incidence | Light-chain type |
|---|---|---|---|
| STEIN *et al.*:[b] | Ig-PV | 2/2 | |
| Reticulum-cell sarcoma or immunoblastic lymphoma | IgM | 2/2 | |
| AISENBERG and LONG:[c] | Ig-PV | 0/3 | |
| M.L. histiocytic, diffuse | | | |
| BROUET *et al.*:[d] | Ig-PV | 3/6[a] | |
| Poorly differentiated reticulum-cell sarcoma, diffuse | | | |
| MORRIS and DAVEY:[e] | Ig-PV | 5/6 | |
| Histiocytic and mixed histiocytic-lymphocytic lymphomas | IgM | 2/6 | κ (1), λ (1) |
| | IgG | 1/6 | κ |
| | IgM-G | 1/6 | κ |
| | IgM-D-G | 1/6 | κ |
| KRÜGER *et al.*:[f] | IgM | 1/6 | |
| M.L. histiocytic type | | | |
| SELIGMANN *et al.*:[g] | Ig-PV | 5/14 | |
| Large-cell lymphoma (reticulum-cell sarcoma or "histiocytic" lymphoma) | | | |
| BRAYLAN *et al.*:[h] | Ig-PV | 11/17 | |
| Large-cell malignant lymphoma | IgM | 6/7 | κ (6) |
| | κ | 1/7 | |
| STEIN:[i] | Ig-PV | 5/6 | |
| | IgM | 4/6 | κ (2), λ (1), κ and λ (1) |
| | IgG | 1/6 | κ |

Ig-PV = Ig demonstrated with a polyvalent anti-Ig serum.
[a] Two cases showed restricted light-chain staining, and one case was positive for μ, γ, α, λ, and κ.
[b] STEIN, KAISERLING and LENNERT, 1974b.
[c] 1975.
[d] BROUET, LABAUME and SELIGMANN, 1975.
[e] 1975.
[f] KRÜGER, UHLMANN, HELLRIEGEL, SESTERHENN *et al.*, 1976.
[g] SELIGMANN, BROUET and PREUD'HOMME, 1977.
[h] BRAYLAN, JAFFE, MANN, FRANK *et al.*, 1977.
[i] 1976, unpublished data.

μ-, γ-, α-, λ-, and κ-chains. HUBER *et al.*[441] detected IgM/κ on more than 80% of the cells from a reticulum-cell sarcoma.

KRÜGER *et al.*[442] reported on SIg-labeling results in six cases of histiocytic lymphoma. The tumor cells from all but one case were SIg-negative. MORRIS and DAVEY[443] studied a series of seven diffuse histiocytic lymphomas for the presence of SIg and found only one case devoid of SIg. In one case it was not clear whether the SIg-positive cells were actually tumor cells. In the SIg-

[441] HUBER, DWORZAK, FINK, MICHLMAYR *et al.*, 1974.

[442] KRÜGER, UHLMANN, HELLRIEGEL, SESTERHENN *et al.*, 1976.

[443] 1975.

positive group IgM proved to be the predominant Ig class, in two cases alone, in one case combined with IgG, and in one case combined with IgG and IgD. IgG was present alone on the lymphoma cells from one case. In all five SIg-positive cases only one light-chain type was expressed: κ in four and λ in one case.

SELIGMANN *et al.*[444] reported on the presence of SIg in five out of 14 large-cell lymphomas, including reticulum-cell sarcomas or "histiocytic" lymphomas of earlier nomenclatures. BRAYLAN *et al.*[445] studied 17 cases of large-cell malignant lymphoma, including neoplasms that had formerly been designated diffuse "histiocytic" lymphomas or undifferentiated pleomorphic lymphomas. Six of the patients had a previous history of follicular lymphoma. The predominant Ig class was IgM, which was restricted to one light chain. We assume that these six cases resembled centroblastic lymphoma rather than immunoblastic lymphoma. Of the 11 other cases of large-cell lymphoma described by BRAYLAN *et al.*[445] five showed a high percentage of neoplastic cells bearing SIg, which was restricted to one light chain in the four cases studied.

We investigated SIg in six cases of immunoblastic lymphoma. Cells from all but one of them were SIg-positive. IgM was predominant in four cases, and IgG was the main Ig class in one. The SIg was clearly restricted to one light-chain type in four cases. We did not look for the presence of surface IgD.

**Tissue Immunoglobulin.** *Saline Extract.* In 1972, we[446] reported on increased amounts of IgM in the saline extracts from all four cases studied. Twelve out of the 15 cases of so-called reticulum-cell sarcoma analyzed in 1974[447] also revealed an increase in tissue IgM. Since then, we have studied the Ig concentration of saline extracts from a total of 34 cases. In 18 of them significantly increased amounts of Ig could be extracted from biopsy tissue. There was an increase in IgM alone in 12 cases and in IgA in one. An increase in IgM and IgG above the normal level was observed in two cases. Another two cases revealed a combination of IgM and IgA above the normal range. The mean IgM content of the saline tissue extracts was higher than that of all other lymphoma classes, with the exception of LP immunocytoma (see Fig. 276).

*Detergent Second Extract.* Significantly increased amounts of Ig were detected in the detergent 2nd extracts from 11 out of 19 cases (see Fig. 277). The predominant Ig class was IgM. The IgM content was increased in eight cases alone, in two cases together with IgG, and in one case with IgA. Of the four extracts studied for the presence of IgD, one contained significant amounts of IgD together with IgM. Eight cases in this series of immunoblastic lymphoma showed no increase in tissue Ig.

**Serum Immunoglobulin.** Of 34 cases of immunoblastic lymphoma, three exhibited significantly increased serum-IgM concentrations. Tissue extracts from the three cases also revealed increased amounts of IgM. The serum-Ig values of

---

[444] SELIGMANN, BROUET and PREUD'HOMME, 1977.

[445] BRAYLAN, JAFFE, MANN, FRANK *et al.*, 1977.

[446] STEIN, LENNERT and PARWARESCH, 1972; STEIN, KAISERLING and LENNERT, 1973.

[447] STEIN, KAISERLING and LENNERT, 1974b.

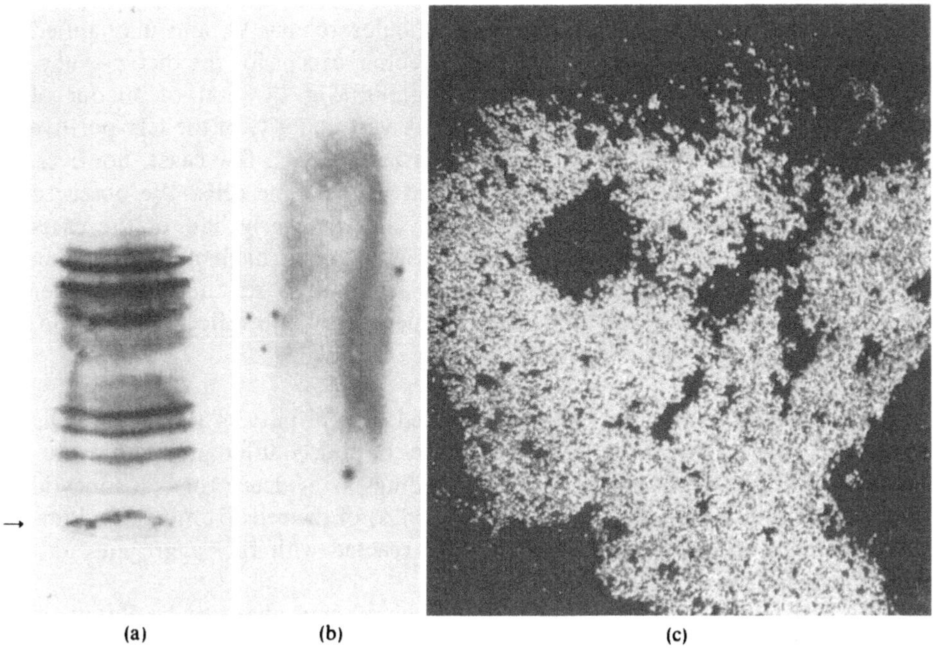

Fig. 286a–c. Immunoblastic lymphoma. (a, b) Autoradiographs of reduced and carboxymethylated, isoelectrofocused IgM from tumor tissue extract (a) and serum (b) of the same patient. Site of application is indicated by an arrow. (c) Frozen section treated with EAC. A dense layer of reagent red cells (light spots) adhere to the section in a nodular pattern, although the tumor-cell proliferation is diffuse. Hematoxylin and eosin. Dark-field illumination. ×60

the other cases were chiefly in the subnormal range. A comparison of the serum- and tissue-Ig concentrations of each case showed that there was no correlation between these values.

**Monoclonality of the Tissue and Serum Immunoglobulin.** The tissue extracts from five cases of immunoblastic lymphoma with increased levels of tissue IgM, but not of serum IgM, were subjected to isoelectric focusing. The IgM fractions of all five cases proved to be of highly restricted heterogeneity, similar to serum-IgM fractions of macroglobulinemia of Waldenström (Fig. 286a). In contrast, the IgM fractions of the sera from the five cases revealed a polyclonal isoelectric-focusing pattern (Fig. 286b).[447a] The serum-IgM fractions that were increased in three out of 34 cases of immunoblastic lymphoma appeared to be monoclonal in immunoelectrophoresis.

**Cytoplasmic Immunoglobulin (CIg).** CIg in the form of Russell body-like material could be demonstrated in tumor cells from eight out of 25 cases. The number of cells showing this material ranged from 0.1–10%. In most cases such material could be detected only after prolonged search.

With the enzyme-bridge method, Taylor[447b] studied a series of 55 large-cell lymphomas that were classified as syncytial reticulosarcoma (16 cases), dictyo-

[447a] Bouman, Stein, Havsteen and Lennert, in preparation.

[447b] 1974.

syncytial reticulosarcoma (5), dictyocytic/histiocytic reticulosarcoma (7), polymorphic reticulosarcoma (11), plasma-cell reticulosarcoma (9), and unqualified reticulosarcoma (7). In all types of reticulosarcoma, except for the dictyo-syncytial, he found cases with tumor cells containing CIg. A total of 40 out of the 55 cases (73%) proved to be CIg-positive. A vast majority of the CIg-positive cases showed restricted light-chain staining, usually $\kappa$. In a few cases, however, both $\kappa$- and $\lambda$-chains were apparently present in the same cells. We observed positive CIg staining of the blast-like tumor cells in nearly half of the cases we studied (Fig. 287).[448] In one case we also obtained distinct CIg staining of the tumor cells with both anti-$\kappa$ and anti-$\lambda$ sera. It is still unclear whether the occurrence of both $\kappa$- and $\lambda$-chains in the neoplastic cells reflects absorption, phagocytosis, or synthesis.

**IgG-Fc Receptor.** BROUET *et al.*[449] observed high affinity of the tumor cells for IgG aggregates in only one out of four cases of poorly differentiated reticulosarcoma (diffuse). They interpreted these findings as evidence for a histiocytic origin of the tumor cells. A high percentage (95%) of the cells from a reticulum-cell sarcoma investigated by HUBER *et al.*[450] reacted with IgG aggregates and with anti-$\mu$ and anti-$\kappa$ antibodies.

Only one out of the 17 cases of large-cell lymphoma observed by BRAYLAN *et al.*[451] revealed IgGEA-rosette formation by more than 25% of the cells. In three other cases less than 25% of the neoplastic cells bound IgGEA. Three of the IgGEA-positive neoplasms had developed from follicular lymphomas (centroblastic/centrocytic lymphoma). Cells from the fourth case were devoid of SIg and sheep-E receptors, but bore complement receptors. EAC was rapidly engulfed at 37°C by the cytoplasm of the cells, indicating that this tumor was a neoplasm either of monocytes or, less probably, of phagocytic reticulum cells.

We studied the presence of IgG-Fc receptors on cells from three immunoblastic lymphomas by means of the IgGEA-rosette test. The cells from all three cases formed rosettes only in very small percentages (2–4%) or not at all.

**Complement Receptor.** We investigated a series of 10 immunoblastic lymphomas for the presence of complement receptors on frozen sections. Nodular adherence of IgGEAC was observed in three out of the 10 cases (Fig. 286c).[452] By diluting the EAC reagent to reduce the thickness of the EAC layer on the section and by simultaneously demonstrating acid phosphatase and nonspecific esterase, it was ascertained that the EAC adhered to neoplastic enzyme-negative cells. Large amounts of both enzymes are characteristic of phagocytic reticulum cells or histiocytes.

In five cases we had the opportunity to study the binding of EAC to suspended cells. A significant proportion of EAC rosette-forming immunoblast-like cells were found in two cases. Cytologic evaluation confirmed that the

---

[448] STEIN, BOUMAN, LENNERT, FUCHS *et al.*, 1977; STEIN, PAPADIMITRIOU, BOUMAN, LENNERT *et al.*, 1978.

[449] BROUET, LABAUME and SELIGMANN, 1975.

[450] HUBER, DWORZAK, FINK, MICHLMAYR *et al.*, 1974.

[451] BRAYLAN, JAFFE, MANN, FRANK *et al.*, 1977.

[452] STEIN, 1975a, 1976a, b.

(a)

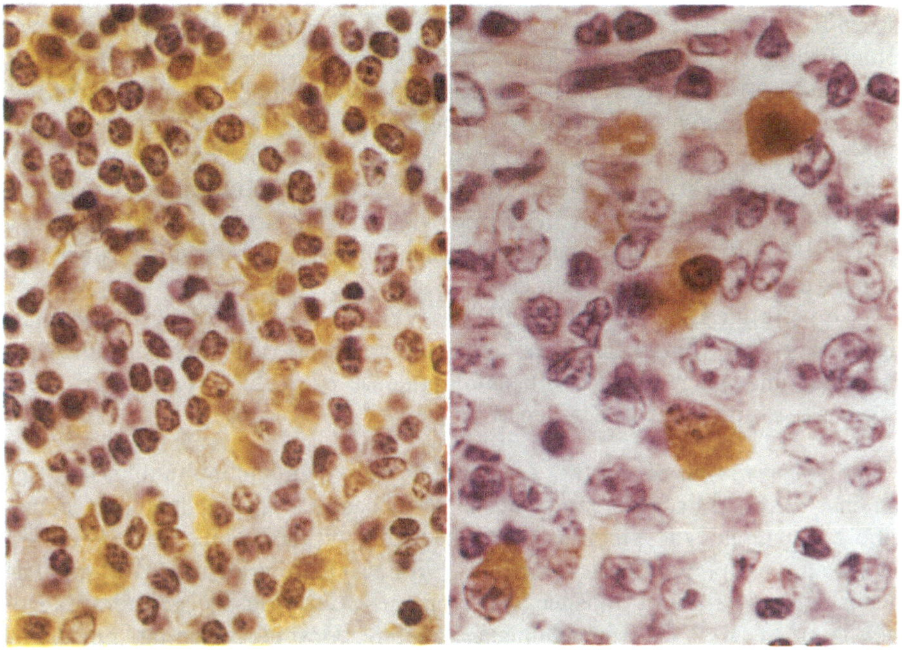

(b)

Fig. 287. (a) LP immunocytoma. Paraffin section stained for λ-chains by means of the immunoperoxidase technique. The staining for κ-chains was almost negative. (b) Immunoblastic lymphoma. Paraffin section stained for λ-chains by means of the immunoperoxidase technique. The staining for κ-chains was completely negative. (a, b) Counterstaining with hematoxylin and eosin. ×800

rosetting cells were tumor cells. In three complement receptor-positive cases we specified the complement-receptor subtypes on frozen sections. In all three cases EAC3b adhered to the frozen sections in an ill-defined nodular pattern. Only one case showed adherence of EAC3d. Thus, the cells of this case resembled reactive centroblasts in bearing both complement-receptor subtypes. The other two cases exhibited receptors for C3b and were devoid of receptors for C3d, like many immunoblasts of the plasma-cell reaction.

Complement receptors were detectable on cells from 12 out of the 16 cases of large-cell malignant lymphoma in the series of BRAYLAN *et al.*[453] All six cases with a previous history of follicular lymphoma and five of the other 10 "primary" large-cell lymphomas were complement receptor-positive. All but one of the "primary" complement receptor-positive cases were SIg-positive. Cells from the one case that exhibited complement receptors and lacked SIg bore IgG-Fc receptors and were capable of immunophagocytosis (cf., p. 648).

**Mouse-Erythrocyte (E) Receptor.** The literature does not contain any data.

**Sheep-Erythrocyte (E) Receptor and Human T-Lymphocyte Antigen (HTLA).** There have been only a few reports on sheep E-rosette and HTLA analyses of reticulosarcoma or immunoblastic lymphoma. LUKES[454] reported on one case

[453] BRAYLAN, JAFFE, MANN, FRANK *et al.*, 1977. [454] LUKES and LENNERT, 1974.

of immunoblastic lymphoma in which the cells were devoid of SIg and formed sheep-E rosettes. He made a cytologic analysis of the cells that spontaneously bound sheep erythrocytes and found that they were indeed tumor cells. AISENBERG and LONG[455] detected 51% sheep-E rosette-forming cells in a suspension from a well-differentiated histiocytic lymphoma; HTLA was present on only 20% of the cells from the same tumor. In another case they determined sheep E-rosette formation by 34% of the cells. AISENBERG and LONG did not mention, however, whether the tumor cells or bystander cells were the reactive cells. Of the 10 "primary" large-cell lymphomas of BRAYLAN *et al.*,[455a] only one displayed sheep-E receptors and lacked SIg.

We performed the sheep E-rosette assay on six immunoblastic lymphomas. The tumor cells from all six cases failed to bind sheep erythrocytes, both when untreated and when treated with neuraminidase or AET. Five of them were SIg-positive, and one was SIg-negative.

**Lymphocyte-Specific Surface Antigen.** The cells from two immunoblastic lymphomas were incubated in horseradish peroxidase-conjugated lymphocyte-specific anti-lymphocytic globulin. The specificity of the conjugate was judged by labeling peripheral blood leukocytes. Monocytes were identified by simultaneous demonstration of nonspecific esterase: the blue nonspecific esterase reaction contrasts well with the conjugate labeling. Granulocytes and monocytes did not react with the conjugate, whereas some of the lymphocytes exhibited a thick rim of surface labeling. The vast majority of the tumor cells from both cases of immunoblastic lymphoma revealed dense surface labeling with the conjugate, similar to that seen on peripheral blood lymphocytes. That confirms the lymphoid-cell origin of the tumor cells.

**Lysozyme (Muramidase).** TAYLOR[455b] examined a large number of cases of non-Hodgkin's lymphoma for the presence of lysozyme by means of the enzyme-bridge technique. Nearly all cases showed no trace of a positive reaction with anti-lysozyme in tumor cells, although varying numbers of reactive histiocytes and neutrophil leukocytes were seen in the sections. There were two cases, however, in which TAYLOR found that the neoplastic cells definitely contained lysozyme. One of these cases had been classified as syncytial reticulosarcoma and the other as unqualified reticulosarcoma. RALPH *et al.*[456] demonstrated synthesis of lysozyme by cells of a histiocytic lymphoma cell line.

**Conclusions.** In contrast to the results of SIg studies by AISENBERG and LONG[455] and to some of the findings of BROUET *et al.*[457] and KRÜGER *et al.*,[458] the SIg data reported by MORRIS and DAVEY,[459] BRAYLAN *et al.*, [455a] and our group[460] revealed that cells from most so-called reticulosarcomas bore SIg with one predominant light chain. BROUET *et al.*[457] observed SIg with a single

---

[455] 1975.
[455a] BRAYLAN, JAFFE, MANN, FRANK *et al.*, 1977.
[455b] 1976.
[456] RALPH, MOORE and NILSSON, 1976.
[457] BROUET, LABAUME and SELIGMANN, 1975.
[458] KRÜGER, UHLMANN, HELLRIEGEL, SESTERHENN *et al.*, 1976.
[459] 1975.
[460] STEIN, KAISERLING and LENNERT, 1974b.

light chain only in reticulosarcomas that developed from B-cell neoplasms, e.g., CLL or macroglobulinemia of Waldenström. It should be mentioned that all of the immunoblastic lymphomas or reticulosarcomas from our series studied for SIg were primary immunoblastic lymphomas, i.e., the diagnosis was made on the first biopsy after onset of the disease.

The results of tissue-Ig determination agreed with the data from SIg analyses by MORRIS and DAVEY[461] and with our own. The Ig content of the saline extracts from more than half of the cases of so-called reticulosarcoma were significantly, sometimes greatly, increased. A slightly higher percentage of increases in IgM was found in the detergent 2nd extracts. The predominant Ig class was IgM. On the basis of the tissue-Ig data, we concluded in 1972[462] that so-called reticulosarcomas are not reticulocytic, but lymphatic in origin.

The objection that the increased amounts of Ig measured in the tissue extracts were not produced by tumor cells, but might have been passively absorbed Ig (autoantibodies or immunocomplexes), was refuted by the results of CIg assays and isoelectric-focusing analyses. TAYLOR[463] demonstrated CIg with a single light chain in 73% of his cases of reticulum-cell sarcoma. We made similar observations.[464] It was generally accepted that CIg is produced by the cell in which it is detected.[465] Recently, however, MASON *et al.*[466] showed that IgG and trace amounts of IgM can be demonstrated in the cytoplasm of neutrophil granulocytes and monocytes on smears by means of the immunoperoxidase-bridge method. Therefore, CIg demonstrated by this technique on smears may be indicative not only of *de-novo* synthesis of CIg, but also of ingestion of Ig that has been bound to the cell membrane. In contrast to this finding in smears, we were not able to detect any Ig class in the cytoplasm of neutrophils or monocytes when paraffin-embedded tissue was used for the immunoperoxidase labeling. On the other hand, the neutrophils and monocytes on paraffin sections showed strong immunostaining for lysozyme. We conclude that the CIg detected in paraffin sections from large-cell malignant lymphomas is actually autosynthesized Ig. The CIg-positive lymphoma cells did not stain for lysozyme, whereas many reactive, strongly lysozyme-positive histiocytic reticulum cells were scattered among the tumor cells.

The IgM fraction of five so-called reticulosarcomas proved to be monoclonal in isoelectric focusing.[464] Monoclonal Ig is highly characteristic of malignant proliferation, as demonstrated by analysis of multiple myelomas and macroglobulinemia of Waldenström, and is therefore a strong argument in favor of production of the Ig by tumor cells.

The available experimental data indicate that most so-called reticulosarcomas or histiocytic lymphomas produce Ig and are thus actually lymphomas of the B-cell series. This view is supported by electron-microscopic, enzyme-cytochemical, and other immunologic findings. The cells from all "reticulosarcomas" showing a high tissue-Ig content were not similar to any type of reticulum

---

[461] 1975.
[462] STEIN, LENNERT and PARWARESCH, 1972; STEIN, KAISERLING and LENNERT, 1973, 1974a, b.
[463] 1974.
[464] STEIN, BOUMAN, LENNERT, FUCHS *et al.*, 1977.
[465] SELIGMANN, PREUD'HOMME and BROUET, 1973.
[466] MASON, LABAUME and PREUD'HOMME, 1977.

cell found in reactive lymphatic tissue.[467] The cells from the "reticulosarcomas" in our series lacked large amounts of acid phosphatase and nonspecific esterase,[467] which are characteristic of phagocytic reticulum cells or histiocytes. In the two cases analyzed, the "reticulosarcoma" cells bore lymphocyte-specific surface antigen in a density similar to that found on normal peripheral blood lymphocytes.[468]

The B-cell-derived so-called reticulosarcomas or histiocytic lymphomas are apparently not homogeneous in origin. In our opinion, it is highly probable that most of them are derived either from immunoblasts of the plasma-cell reaction or from particularly large centroblasts of the germinal center-cell reaction.

The first possibility is substantiated by the observation that the cells from many so-called reticulosarcomas are morphologically very similar to the blast cells of the plasma-cell reaction described in 1948 by FAGRAEUS and later in detail by VELDMAN.[469]

The plasma-cell reaction takes place in the interfollicular area of lymphatic tissue. The following events occur. Under antigenic stimulation, small to medium-sized lymphoid cells, called marginal-zone cells,[469] undergo transformation into large blast cells, called immunoblasts according to DAMESHEK.[470] The immunoblasts transform by mitotic division *via* plasmablasts (cells that develop ergastoplasm) into plasma cells. AVRAMEAS and LEDUC[471] and PANIJEL *et al.*[472] have shown that the reactive immunoblasts are the cells in the transformation series that switch from the synthesis of nonsecretory Ig to the synthesis of secretory Ig. Accordingly, immunoblasts and plasmablasts have nonsecretory Ig on their surface membranes and secretory Ig within the cytoplasm.[473]

Besides morphologic similarity, most B-cell-derived so-called reticulosarcoma cells and the described immunoblasts of the plasma-cell reaction show a resemblance in functional properties. Like immunoblasts of the plasma-cell reaction, the cells from many B-cell-derived "reticulosarcomas" have Ig both on the surface membrane and in the cytoplasm. In one case it could be demonstrated that the tumor cells resembled reactive immunoblasts with respect to the site of Ig production.[467] The cells from this case contained abundant polyribosomes and were almost completely devoid of ergastoplasm. Large amounts of IgM, however, were detectable in the distended perinuclear space. AVRAMEAS and LEDUC[471] and PANIJEL *et al.*[472] showed that the perinuclear space is the first site of secretory-Ig production in immunoblasts. Moreover, like reactive immunoblasts, the cells on frozen sections from most B-cell-derived "reticulosarcomas" did not bind EAC prepared with whole serum as the source of complement, or they bound only EAC3b.

Because of the great morphologic and functional similarities between immunoblasts of the plasma-cell reaction and reticulosarcoma cells, we assume that most so-called reticulosarcomas are actually proliferations of B-immunoblast-like cells. These cells either are arrested in the immunoblastic differential stage or have a capacity for transformation into plasmablasts, but not into plasma cells. That may also be valid for the so-called reticulosarcomas that develop

[467] STEIN, KAISERLING and LENNERT, 1974b.
[468] STEIN, 1975a, 1976b.
[469] VELDMAN, 1970.
[470] 1963.
[471] 1970.
[472] PANIJEL, DELAMETTE and LENEVEN, 1971.
[473] PERNIS, FORNI and AMANTE, 1971.

from CLL or macroglobulinemia of Waldenström. Immunoblast-like cells are found in both disorders, although in small numbers. In our opinion, it is likely that, in some instances, the immunoblast-like cells acquire a kinetic advantage and overgrow the other tumor-cell populations, resulting in a transformation of the original neoplasm into a B-immunoblastic lymphoma.

In some cases of so-called reticulosarcoma, however, there was morphologic similarity between the blast-like "reticulosarcoma" cells and centroblasts of the germinal center-cell reaction.[474] Furthermore, complement receptors could be demonstrated with EACmouse or EAChuman and with both EAC3b and EAC3d on frozen sections from such reticulosarcomas. The presence of complement receptors that react with EACmouse or EAChuman and especially of both complement-receptor subtypes on cells in frozen sections from solid lymphatic tissue is highly characteristic of germinal-center cells (see p. 555). These tumors were actually centroblastic lymphomas. "Large-cell lymphomas" that develop in cases of follicular centroblastic/centrocytic lymphoma are classified by the Kiel Classification as (secondary) centroblastic lymphomas. In analogy, it would be better to group the primary "reticulosarcomas" that appear to be derived from centroblasts under centroblastic lymphoma, as LENNERT has already done in Part Four (see pp. 348 and 424). It should be mentioned, however, that both immunoblast-like and centroblast-like cells are simultaneously present in many cases of so-called reticulum-cell sarcoma. Such cases cannot be clearly classified as either centroblastic or immunoblastic lymphoma.

Surface-marker studies by LUKES,[475] BROUET *et al.*,[476] and BRAYLAN *et al.*[477] revealed that cells from a minority of so-called reticulum-cell sarcomas were capable of forming rosettes with sheep erythrocytes and/or stained positively for HTLA, indicating the T-cell nature of these tumors. Furthermore, the cells with T-cell properties resembled PHA-stimulated blast cells. It is likely that such reticulosarcomas were derived from immunoblasts of the T-cell line.

The nature of the "reticulosarcomas" that lack all known markers (so-called unqualified or null-immunoblastic lymphoma) has not yet been clarified. The absence of markers, however, does not exclude the lymphoid origin of the large malignant cells. It is known from studies by various authors and by our own group that neoplastic cells can lose normal T- or B-markers, or undergo surface changes that prevent their identification by the known markers.

Since it is difficult, and often impossible, to reliably classify some cases from this group of lymphomas according to their cellular origin, it has been proposed[478] that all malignant lymphomas consisting of large cells be grouped under the heading "large-cell malignant lymphomas."

## *Addendum*
## *Reticulosarcoma*

BROUET *et al.*[476] and BRAYLAN *et al.*[477] each reported on a case of malignant lymphoma previously classified as reticulum-cell sarcoma or histiocytic lym-

[474] STEIN, 1976b.

[475] LUKES and LENNERT, 1974.

[476] BROUET, PREUD'HOMME, FLANDRIN, CHELLOUL *et al.*, 1976.

[477] BRAYLAN, JAFFE, MANN, FRANK *et al.*, 1977.

[478] BROUET, PREUD'HOMME, FLANDRIN, CHELLOUL *et al.*, 1976; BRAYLAN, JAFFE, MANN, FRANK *et al.*, 1977.

Table 114. A comparison of the most important immunochemical, immunologic, and cytochemical properties of non-Hodgkin's lymphomas. Tissue Ig = immunoglobulin content of biopsy tissue homogenate. SIg = surface-membrane immunoglobulin. CIg = intracytoplasmic immunoglobulin. Serum Ig = immunoglobulin content of blood serum. IgG-FcR = receptor for Fc fragment of IgG. EAC-mouse = erythrocytes coated with IgM antibodies and with complement obtained from mouse serum. EAC3b = erythrocytes coated with IgM antibodies and purified C 3b. EAC3d = EAC3b cleaved by C 3 inactivator and after liberation of C 3c. Mouse-E = mouse-erythrocyte receptor. Sheep-E 37° C = sheep-erythrocyte receptor that is stable at 37° C. Sheep-E 37→4° C = sheep-erythrocyte receptor that is labile at 37° C, but stable at 4° C. HTLA = human T-lymphocyte antigen. HTHY-

| | Tissue Ig | SIg | CIg | Serum Ig | IgG-FcR | Complement receptors | | |
|---|---|---|---|---|---|---|---|---|
| | | | | | | EAC mouse | EAC3b | EAC3c |
| Chronic lymphocytic leukemia | | | | | | | | |
| $B_1$-type | ↑ or n | + | − | ↓ | + | + | − | + |
| $B_2$-type | ↑ or n | ++ | − | ↓ | + | + | + | + |
| T-type | ↑ or n | − | − | n | − | − | − | − |
| Prolymphocytic leukemia | | | | | | | | |
| B-type | n.t. | +++ | − | n | + | + | + | + |
| T-type | n.t. | − | − | n | − | − | − | − |
| Hairy-cell leukemia | ↑ | ++ | − | ↑ or n | +++ | −/+ | −/+ | −/+ |
| Mycosis fungoides and Sézary's syndrome | ↓ | − | − | n | − | − | − | − |
| T-zone lymphoma | ↓ | − | n.t. | n | n.t. | n.t. | n.t. | n.t. |
| LP immunocytoma | ↑↑↑ | + | + | 25%↑ | (+) | 50%+ | >70%+ | >40%+ |
| Centrocytic lymphoma | ↑↑ | ++ | −/(+) | ↓ or n | (+) | ++ | ++ | ++ |
| Centroblastic/centrocytic lymphoma | ↑ | ++ | −/(+) | ↓ or n | (+) | +++ | ++ | ++ |
| Centroblastic lymphoma | ↑ | ++ | −/(+) | ↓ or n | n.t. | −/+ | n.t. | n.t. |
| Lymphoblastic lymphoma and/or ALL | | | | | | | | |
| B-lymphoblastic | | | | | | | | |
| Burkitt type | | | | | | | | |
| African (Burkitt's tumor) | n.t. | ++ | − | ↓ or n | −/+ | −/+ | n.t. | n.t. |
| Non-African | ↑↑ | ++ | − | ↓ or n | −/+ | −/+ | −/+ | −/+ |
| Other than Burkitt type | ↑ | + | − | n | −/+ | −/+ | n.t. | n.t. |
| T-lymphoblastic | | | | | | | | |
| Thymocyte precursor | ↓ or n | − | − | n | −/+ | ++ | n.t. | n.t. |
| Prothymocytic (convoluted-cell type) | ↓ or n | − | − | n | −/+ | ++ | ++ | ++ |
| Mature thymocytic (with and without convoluted nuclei) | ↓ or n | − | − | n | − | − | n.t. | n.t. |
| Peripheral T-cell (without convoluted nuclei) | ↓ | − | − | n | − | − | n.t. | n.t. |
| Common ALL (0-lymphoblastic) | ↓ | − | − | n | −/(+) | −/(+) | n.t. | n.t. |
| Unqualified | n.t. | − | − | n | n.t. | n.t. | n.t. | n.t. |
| Immunoblastic lymphoma | | | | | | | | |
| B-type | ↑↑ | ++ | + | n (or ↓) | (+) | ~30%+ | ~30%+ | <10%+ |
| T-type | ↓ | − | − | n | − | n.t. | n.t. | n.t. |
| Unqualified (null) | ↓ or n | − | − | n | −/+ | −/+ | n.t. | n.t. |
| Reticulum-cell sarcoma, phagocytic reticulum-cell type (histiocytic type) | n.t. | − | − | n | ++ | ++ | n.t. | n.t. |

L = human thymus/leukemia-associated antigen. cALL antigen = antigen on the surface membrane of acute lymphoblastic leukemia cells that lack B- and T-cell markers (common ALL). Ia-like antigen = glycoprotein complex that is present chiefly on B-lymphocytes of healthy individuals. Tdt = terminal deoxynucleotidyl transferase. EBV-DNA = deoxyribonucleic acid of the Epstein-Barr-virus genome. EBNA = Epstein-Barr virus-specific nuclear antigen. IP = immunophagocytosis. ↑ = increased. ↑↑ = markedly increased. ↑↑↑ = greatly increased. n = within normal 2 $\sigma$ range. ↓ = decreased. n.t. = not tested. + = positive. ++ = strongly positive. +++ = very strongly positive. (+) = weakly positive. – = negative. –/(+) = negative in some cases, but weakly positive in others. –/+ = negative in some cases, but positive in others. Percentages refer to number of cases

| ouse-E | Sheep-E 37° C | Sheep-E 37→4° C | HTLA | HTHY-L | cALL antigen | Ia-like antigen | Tdt | EBV-DNA or EBNA | Non-specific esterase | Lyso-zyme | IP |
|---|---|---|---|---|---|---|---|---|---|---|---|
| ++ | – | – | – | n.t. | – | + | n.t. | – | – | – | – |
| ++ | – | – | – | n.t. | – | + | n.t. | – | – | – | – |
| | – | + | + | n.t. | – | – | – | n.t. | – | – | – |
| | n.t. | – | – | n.t. | – | n.t. | n.t. | n.t. | – | n.t. | – |
| | n.t. | + | + | n.t. | – | n.t. | n.t. | n.t. | – | n.t. | – |
| | n.t. | – | n.t. | n.t. | n.t. | + | n.t. | – | –/+ | – | – |
| | – | + | + | n.t. | – | – | – | – | – | n.t. | – |
| . | n.t. | + | n.t. | n.t. | n.t. | n.t. | n.t. | n.t. | – | n.t. | – |
| /+ | – | – | n.t. | n.t. | n.t. | n.t. | n.t. | – | –/+[a] | n.t. | – |
| | – | – | – | n.t. | n.t. | n.t. | n.t. | – | – | n.t. | – |
| | – | – | – | n.t. | n.t. | n.t. | n.t. | – | – | n.t. | – |
| . | n.t. | – | n.t. | n.t. | n.t. | n.t. | n.t. | – | – | n.t. | – |
| . | – | –/(+) | – | n.t. | n.t. | n.t. | n.t. | 97% + | – | n.t. | – |
| . | – | –/(+) | – | n.t. | n.t. | n.t. | n.t. | 8–17% + | – | n.t. | – |
| . | – | – | – | n.t. | – | + | – | n.t. | – | n.t. | – |
| | – | – | + | + | – | – | – | – | – | n.t. | – |
| | + | + | ++ | ++ | – | – | + | – | – | n.t. | – |
| | + | + | ++ | ++ | – | – | + | – | – | n.t. | – |
| | – | + | + | n.t. | – | – | – | n.t. | – | n.t. | – |
| | – | – | – | + | + | + | + | – | – | n.t. | – |
| . | – | – | – | n.t. | – | 50% + | 50% + | n.t. | – | n.t. | – |
| | – | – | – | n.t. | n.t. | + | n.t. | – | – | – | – |
| . | n.t. | + | + | n.t. | n.t. | n.t. | n.t. | n.t. | – | – | – |
| . | n.t. | – | – | n.t. | n.t. | n.t. | n.t. | n.t. | – | – | – |
| . | n.t. | – | – | n.t. | n.t. | n.t. | n.t. | n.t. | +++[b] | + | + |

[a] Moderately positive in the plasmacytoid cells in some instances
[b] Diffuse, strongly positive reaction in most, if not all, tumor cells

phoma and now called large-cell lymphoma. Neoplastic cells from the two cases rapidly phagocytosed EAC. Complement- and IgG-mediated phagocytosis (immunophagocytosis) is specific to the phagocytic-cell series. Thus, these two cases were actually neoplasms of macrophages (histiocytic reticulum cells). In this context, it should be mentioned that phagocytosis of uncoated erythrocytes or particles such as latex beads is not a specific marker of phagocytic cells, since uncoated erythrocytes and latex beads can also be phagocytosed by stimulated T-cells and some neoplastic T- and B-lymphoma cells. The histiocytic nature of the case of BRAYLAN *et al.*[479] was also suggested by the presence of nonspecific esterase. One must remember, however, that even a large amount of nonspecific esterase is not an absolute specific marker of histiocytes, since large amounts of this enzyme may be found in immature plasmacytoma cells.[480]

TAYLOR's[481] series of so-called reticulosarcoma contained two cases in which the cells definitely showed staining for lysozyme. In one case of histiocytic lymphoma RALPH *et al.*[482] demonstrated that the tumor cells were able to synthesize lysozyme. So far, lysozyme has been detected only in myeloid cells and cells derived from myeloid cells, including monocytes and macrophages.[483] Therefore, such lysozyme-positive cases must be interpreted as true reticulum-cell sarcomas or histiocytic lymphomas, if it can be proved that they are not myeloid neoplasms. Myeloid neoplasms may resemble so-called reticulosarcoma or immunoblastic lymphoma in morphology, but are distinguishable by means of appropriate enzyme-cytochemical analyses (i.e., for endogenous peroxidase or chloroacetate esterase).

We have detected two leukemic neoplasms in our collection whose cells had abundant basophilic cytoplasm and were somewhat reminiscent of immature plasma cells; but the nuclei of the leukemic cells were larger and their chromatin was less dense. The leukemic cells were capable of immunophagocytosis (phagocytosis of IgGEA and EAC) and contained large amounts of nonspecific esterase and acid phosphatase that were diffusely distributed in the cytoplasm. The cells were devoid of SIg, CIg, peroxidase, and chloroacetate esterase. We therefore interpret these two leukemic neoplasms as proliferations of cells derived from histiocytic reticulum cells (macrophages).

# Summary and Final Remarks

The marker properties of the entites of the Kiel Classification and their immunologic subtypes are summarized in Table 114. Since most of these entities, and especially their subtypes, appear to be clonal proliferations of lymphoid cells, often arrested at some stage in their development or differentiation, marker studies of such neoplasms might also be of help in the definition of subsets of normal hemopoietic and lymphoid cells.

[479] BRAYLAN, JAFFE, MANN, FRANK *et al.*, 1977.
[480] LEDER, personal communication; STEIN, unpublished data.
[481] 1976.
[482] RALPH, MOORE and NILSSON, 1976.
[483] MASON, FARRELL and TAYLOR, 1975; MASON and TAYLOR, 1975; GREENBERGER, CAMPOS-NETO, PARKMAN, MOLONEY *et al.*, 1977.

Phenotypic identification of normal and neoplastic hemopoietic cells by means of current immunologic and enzyme-cytochemical markers has been performed in recent years as a prerequisite for an exact classification of the respective neoplasms; but that was merely a first step. Now, the search for leukemia-specific and leukemia-associated antigens has moved more and more into the center of interest. A number of leukemia-associated antigens have been detected in various cytologic types of leukemia. Some of them have been mentioned in this chapter. Many of the leukemia-associated antigens are shared by the cells of various leukemias. One such antigen, for example, is shared by acute myeloid leukemia and chronic myeloid leukemia cells,[484] one by CLL and ALL cells,[485] and one by CLL and acute myelomonocytic leukemia cells.[485] In addition, the common-ALL antigen present on most non-B/non-T-ALL cells is also detectable on the lymphoid cells of chronic myeloid leukemia in blast crisis (cf., Table 111).[486] The expression of such antigens in various neoplasms might reflect a common etiologic agent (e.g., oncogenic RNA virus[487]) that is responsible for the antigenic relationship. It might also be a reflection of derepression of similar neoantigens or of the fact that the neoplasms arise from the same, or closely related, target cells, irrespective of the exact etiologic agent.[486] Whatever their nature, extensive study of the properties and the actual incidence and distribution of neoplasm-associated antigens will surely lead to further advances in the diagnosis and classification of neoplasms, the evaluation of complete remission, and the monitoring of patients with malignant lymphoma or leukemia. It is hoped that antisera directed against leukemia- and lymphoma-associated antigens can be applied in the future not only in the classification of neoplastic disorders, but also in the search for etiologic agents and in therapy, perhaps as passive or active immunotherapeutic agents.

---

[484] Mohanakumar, Metzgar and Miller, 1974.

[485] Mohanakumar, Miller and Metzgar, 1976.

[486] Janossy, Greaves, Revesz, Lister *et al.*, 1976.

[487] Metzgar, Mohanakumar and Bolognesi, 1976.

# References

## *Part One*


ABDOU, N.L., ALAVI, J.B., ABDOU, N.I.: Human bone marrow lymphocytes: B and T cell precursors and subpopulations. Blood **47**, 423–430 (1976)

ABNEY, E.R., KEELER, K.D., PARKHOUSE, R.M.E., WILLCOX, H.N.A.: Immunoglobulin M receptors on memory cells of immunoglobulin G antibody-forming cell clones. Europ. J. Immunol. **6**, 443–450 (1976)

ACKERMAN, G.A.: Structural studies of the lymphocyte and lymphocyte development. In: Regulation of Hematopoiesis, Vol. 2, pp. 1297–1337. GORDON, A.S., Ed. New York: Appleton-Century-Crofts 1970

ADA, G.L., NOSSAL, G.J.V., AUSTIN, C.M.: Antigens in immunity. V. The ability of cells in lymphoid follicles to recognize foreignness. Aust. J. exp. Biol. med. Sci. **42**, 331–346 (1964)

AGNARSDOTTIR, G., VALDIMARSSON, H.: Measles virus receptors on human lymphocytes. Abstr. 6th Workshop on Leucocyte Cultures, p. 11, Basel 1975

AIUTI, F., SCHIRRMACHER, V., AMMIRATI, P., FIORILLI, M.: Effect of thymus factor on human precursor T lymphocytes. Clin. exp. Immunol. **20**, 499–503 (1975)

AIUTI, F., WIGZELL, H.: Function and distribution pattern of human T lymphocytes. I. Production of anti-T lymphocyte specific sera as estimated by cytotoxicity and elimination of function of lymphocytes. Clin. exp. Immunol. **13**, 171–181 (1973)

ALEXANDER, E., SANDERS, S., BRAYLAN, R.: Purported difference between human T- and B-cell surface morphology is an artifact. Nature **261**, 239–241 (1976)

ALEXANDER, E.L., WETZEL, B.: Human lymphocytes: Similarity of B and T cell surface morphology. Science **185**, 732–734 (1975)

AMANO, S.: Plasma cells and antibody—morphology, cytophysiology and immunochemistry. Jap. J. Allergy **6**, 409–433 (1958)

ARCHER, O., PIERCE, J.C.: Role of thymus in development of the immune response. Fed. Proc. **20**, 26 (1961)

ARCHER, O.K., SUTHERLAND, D.E.R., GOOD, R.A.: The developmental biology of lymphoid tissue in the rabbit. Consideration of the role of thymus and appendix. Lab. Invest. **13**, 259–271 (1964)

ARMERDING, D., KATZ, D.H.: Activation of T and B lymphocytes in vitro. I. Regulatory influence of bacterial lipopolysaccharide (LPS) on specific T-cell helper function. J. exp. Med. **139**, 24–43 (1974)

ARMSTRONG, J.A., D'ARCY HART, P.: Response of cultured macrophages to Mycobacterium tuberculosis, with observations on fusion of lysosomes with phagosomes. J. exp. Med. **134**, 713–740 (1971)

ARNASON, B.G., JANKOVIĆ, B.D., WAKSMAN, B.H., WENNERSTEN, C.: Role of the thymus in immune reactions in rats. II. Suppressive effect of thymectomy at birth on reactions of delayed (cellular) hypersensitivity and the circulating small lymphocyte. J. exp. Med. **116**, 177–186 (1962)

ASKONAS, B.A., ROELANTS, G.E., MAYOR-WITHEY, K.S., WELSTEAD, J.L.: Dual pathway of B lymphocyte differentiation in vitro. Europ. J. Immunol. **6**, 250–256 (1976)

BALFOUR, B.M., HUMPHREY, J.H.: Localization of γ-globulin and labeled antigen in germinal centers in relation to the immune response. In: Germinal Centers in Immune Responses, pp. 80–85. COTTIER, H., ODARTCHENKO, N., SCHINDLER, R., CONGDON, C.C., Eds. Berlin-Heidelberg-New York: Springer 1967

BARR, R.D., PERRY, S.: Lysosomal acid hydrolases in human lymphocyte subpopulations. Brit. J. Haemat. **32**, 565–572 (1976)

BARR, R.D., SARIN, P.S., PERRY, S.M.: Terminal transferase in human bone-marrow lymphocytes. Lancet 1976, I, pp. 508–509

BARR, R.D., WHANG-PENG, J.: Hemopoietic stem cells in human peripheral blood. Science **190**, 284–285 (1975)

BAST, JR., R.C., CLEVELAND, R.P., LITTMAN, B.H., ZBAR, B., RAPP, H.J.: Acquired cellular immunity: Extracellular killing of listeria monocytogenes by a product of immunologically activated macrophages. Cell. Immunol. **10**, 248–259 (1974)

BASTEN, A., MILLER, J.F.A.P., SPRENT, J., PYE, J.: A receptor for antibody on B lymphocytes. I. Method of detection and functional significance. J. exp. Med. **135**, 610–626 (1972)

BASTEN, A., WARNER, N.L., MANDEL, T.: A receptor for antibody on B lymphocytes. II. Immunochemical and electron microscopy characteristics. J. exp. Med. **135**, 627–642 (1972)

VAN BEKKUM, D.W., VAN NOORD, M.J., MAAT, B., DICKE, K.A.: Attempts at identification of hemopoietic stem cell in mouse. Blood **38**, 547–558 (1971)

BENNER, R., MEIMA, F., VAN DER MEULEN, G.M., VAN EWIJK, W.: Antibody formation in mouse bone marrow. III. Effects of route of priming and antigen dose. Immunology **27**, 747–760 (1974)

BENNER, R., MEIMA, F., VAN DER MEULEN, G.M., VAN MUISWINKEL, W.B.: Antibody formation in mouse bone marrow. I. Evidence for the development of plaque-forming cells in situ. Immunology **26**, 247–255 (1974)

BENNETT, M., CUDKOWICZ, G.: Functional and morphological characterization of stem cells: The unipotential role of 'lymphocytes' of mouse marrow. In: The Lymphocyte in Immunology and Haemopoiesis, pp. 183–194. YOFFEY, J.M., Ed. London: Edward Arnold Ltd. 1967

BENNETT, M., CUDKOWICZ, G.: Hemopoietic progenitor cells with limited potential for differentiation: Erythropoietic function of mouse marrow 'lymphocytes'. J. cell. Physiol. **72**, 129–139 (1968)

BENTWICH, Z., DOUGLAS, S.D., SKUTELSKY, E., KUNKEL, H.G.: Sheep red cell binding to human lymphocytes treated with neuraminidase; enhancement of T cell binding and identification of a subpopulation of B cells. J. exp. Med. **137**, 1532–1537 (1973)

BESSIS, M.: Traité de cytologie sanguine. Paris: Masson & Cie. 1954

BIANCO, C., PATRICK, R., NUSSENZWEIG, V.: A population of lymphocytes bearing a membrane receptor for antigen-antibody-complement complexes. I. Separation and characterization. J. exp. Med. **132**, 702–720 (1970)

BIBERFELD, P., PERLMANN, P.: Morphological observations on the cytotoxicity of human blood lymphocytes for antibody-coated chicken erythrocytes. Exp. Cell Res. **62**, 433–440 (1970)

BJÖRKHOLM, M., HOLM, G., JOHANSSON, B., MELLSTEDT, H.: T-lymphocyte deficiency following adult thymectomy in man. Scand. J. Haemat. **14**, 210–215 (1975)

BORELLA, L., SEN, L.: The distribution of lymphocytes with T- and B-cell surface markers in human bone marrow. J. Immunol. **112**, 836–843 (1974)

VAN BOXEL, J.A., ROSENSTREICH, D.L.: Binding of aggregated γ-globulin to activated T lymphocytes in the guinea pig. J. exp. Med. **139**, 1002–1012 (1974)

VAN BOXEL, J.A., STOBO, J.D., PAUL, W.E., GREEN, I.: Antibody-dependent lymphoid cell-mediated cytotoxicity: No requirement for thymus-derived lymphocytes. Science **175**, 194–196 (1972)

BRAIN, P., GORDON, J., WILLETTS, W.A.: Rosette formation by peripheral lymphocytes. Clin. exp. Immunol. **6**, 681–688 (1970)

VAN DEN BROEK, A.A.: Immune suppression and histophysiology of the immune response. Mode of action of 6-mercaptopurine, nitrogen mustard, cyclophosphamide and cortisone acetate. Thesis, Groningen: 1971. Groningen: Drukkerij van Denderen 1971a

VAN DEN BROEK, A.A.: Immunological effects of cortisone caused by interference with lymphoid cell traffic. In: Morphological and Functional Aspects of Immunity. Advances in Experimental Medicine and Biology, Vol. 12, pp. 667–672. LINDAHL-KIESSLING, G., ALM, G., HANNA, JR., M.G., Eds. New York-London: Plenum Press 1971b

VAN BUCHEM, F.L.: Histologisch onderzoek van de plasmacellulaire reactie en zijn plaats in de histophysiologie van de lymphklier. Doctoral thesis, Groningen 1962

BUCKTON, K.E., COURT BROWN, W.M., SMITH, P.G.: Lymphocyte survival in men treated with X-rays for ankylosing spondylitis. Nature **214**, 470–473 (1967)

BÜTTNER, D.W., HORSTMANN, E.: Haben die Sphaeridien in den Zellkernen kranker Gewebe eine pathognomonische Bedeutung? Virchows Arch. A. **343**, 142–163 (1967)

BURLESON, R., LEVEY, R.H.: Studies on the isolation of lymphocytes active in cell-mediated immune responses. I. Demonstration of an active population of thymus-derived cells in mouse bone marrow. Cell. Immunol. **4**, 305–315 (1972)

CAFFREY TYLER, R.W., EVERETT, N.B.: A radioautographic study of hemopoietic repopulation using irradiated parabiotic rats. Relation to the stem cell problem. Blood **28**, 873–890 (1966)

CANTOR, H., ASOFSKY, R.: Synergy among lymphoid cells mediating the graft-versus-host response. J. exp. Med. **135**, 764–779 (1972)

CARR, I.: The Macrophage. A Review of Ultrastructure and Function. London-New York: Academic Press 1973

CATOVSKY, D., CHERCHI, M., OKOS, A., HEGDE, U., GALTON, D.A.G.: Mouse red-cell rosettes in B-lymphoproliferative disorders. Brit. J. Haemat. **33**, 173–177 (1976)

CEROTTINI, J.-C., BRUNNER, K.T.: Cell-mediated cytotoxicity, allograft rejection, and tumor immunity. Advanc. Immunol. **18**, 67–132 (1974)

CHAPERON, E.A., SELNER, J.C., CLAMAN, H.N.: Migration of antibody-forming cells and antigen-sensitive precursors between spleen, thymus and bone marrow. Immunology **14**, 553–561 (1968)

CHESSIN, L.N., BÖRJESON, J., WELSH, P.D., DOUGLAS, S.D., COOPER, H.L.: Studies on human peripheral blood lymphocytes in vitro. II. Morphological and biochemical studies on the transformation of lymphocytes by pokeweed mitogen. J. exp. Med. **124**, 873–884 (1966)

CHIAO, J.W., PANTIC, V.S., GOOD, R.A.: Human peripheral lymphocytes bearing both B-cell complement receptors and T-cell characteristics for sheep erythrocytes detected by a mixed rosette method. Clin. exp. Immunol. **18**, 483–490 (1974)

CLEVELAND, W.W., FOGEL, B.J., BROWN, W.T., KAY, H.E.M.: Foetal thymic transplant in a case of DiGeorge's syndrome. Lancet 1968, II, pp. 1211–1214

COHEN, L., HOWE, M.L.: Synergism between subpopulations of thymus-derived cells mediating the proliferative and effector phases of the mixed lymphocyte reaction. Proc. nat. Acad. Sci. (Wash.) **70**, 2707–2710 (1973)

CONWAY, E.A.: Cyclic changes in lymphatic nodules. Anat. Rec. **69**, 487–513 (1937)

COOMBS, R.R.A., GURNER, B.W., WILSON, A.B., HOLM, G., LINDGREN, B.: Rosette-formation between human lymphocytes and sheep red cells not involving immunoglobulin receptors. Int. Arch. Allergy **39**, 658–663 (1970)

COOPER, E.H., BARKHAN, P., HALE, A.J.: Observations on the proliferation of human leucocytes cultured with phytohaemagglutinin. Brit. J. Haemat. **9**, 101–111 (1963)

COOPER, M.D., PEREY, D.Y., MCKNEALLY, M.F., GABRIELSEN, A.E., SUTHERLAND, D.E.R., GOOD, R.A.: A mammalian equivalent of the avian bursa of Fabricius. Lancet 1966, I, 1388–1391

COOPER, M.D., PETERSON, R.D.A., GOOD, R.A.: Delineation of the thymic and bursal lymphoid systems in the chicken. Nature (Lond.) **205**, 143–146 (1965)

COOPER, M.D., WELLER, E.M.: Developmental suppression of germinal center and IgG production by prednisolone and 6-mercaptopurine. In: Lymphatic Tissue and Germinal Centers in Immune Response. Advances in Esperimental Medicine and Biology, Vol. 5, pp. 277–284. FIORE-DONATI, L., HANNA, JR., M.G., Eds. New York: Plenum Press 1969

COTTIER, H., HESS, M.W., SCHÄDELI, J., BÜRKI, H.: Lymphocytenform: Herkunft und Entwicklungsmöglichkeiten. Verh. dtsch. Ges. inn. Med. **79**, 99–105 (1973)

COTTIER, H., SORDAT, B.: Lymphatic tissue and germinal centers in relation to antibody production. In: Morphological and Functional Aspects of Immunity. Advances in Experimental Medicine and Biology, Vol. 12, pp. 203–212. LINDAHL-KIESSLING, G., ALM, G., HANNA, JR., M.G., Eds. New York-London: Plenum Press 1971

COUTINHO, A., GRONOWICZ, E., BULLOCK, W.W., MÖLLER, G.: Mechanism of thymus-independent immunocyte triggering. Mitogenic activation of B cells results in specific immune responses. J. exp. Med. **139**, 74–92 (1974)

CRADDOCK, C.G.: Bone marrow lymphocytes of the rat as studied by autoradiography. Acta haemat. (Basel) **33**, 19–27 (1965)

CROSS, A.M., LEUCHARS, E., MILLER, J.F.A.P.: Studies on the recovery of the immune response in irradiated mice thymectomized in adult life. J. exp. Med. **119**, 837–850 (1964)

CUDKOWICZ, G., UPTON, A.C., SMITH, L.H., GOSSLEE, D.G., HUGHES, W.L.: An approach to the characterization of stem cells in mouse bone marrow. Ann. N.Y. Acad. Sci. **114**, 571–582 (1964)

DAEMS, W.T., BREDEROO, P.: The fine structure and peroxidase activity of resident and exudate peritoneal macrophages in the guinea pig. In: The Reticuloendothelial System and Immune Phenomena. Advances in Experimental Medicine and Biology, Vol. 15, pp. 19–31. DI LUZIO, N.R., FLEMMING, K., Eds. New York-London: Plenum Press 1971

DAEMS, W.T., KOERTEN, H.K., SORANZO, M.R.: Differences between monocyte-derived and tissue macrophages. In: The Reticuloendothelial System in Health and Disease: Functions and Characteristics. Advances in Experimental Medicine and Biology, Vol. 73A, pp. 27–40. REICHARD, S.M., ESCOBAR, M.R., FRIEDMAN, H., Eds. New York-London: Plenum Press 1976

DAMASHEK, W.: In: Case records of the Massachusetts General Hospital No. 26-1964. New Engl. J. Med. **270**, 1190–1197 (1964)

DEKRUYFF, R.H., DURKIN, H.G., GILMOUR, D.G., THORBECKE, G.J.: Migratory patterns of B lymphocytes. II. Fate of cells from central lymphoid organs in the chicken. Cell. Immunol. **16**, 301–314 (1975)

DENNERT, G., LENNOX, E.S.: Phagocytic cells as effectors in a cell-mediated immunity system. J. Immunol. **111**, 1844–1854 (1973)

DESAGA, J.F., PARWARESCH, M.R., MÜLLER-HERMELINK, H.K.: Die zytochemische Identifikation der Mastzellvorstufen bei der Ratte. Z. Zellforsch. **121**, 292–300 (1971)

DICKE, K.A., VAN NOORD, M.J., VAN BEKKUM, D.W.: Attempts at morphological identification of the hemopoietic stem cell in rodents and primates. Exp. Hemat. **1**, 36–45 (1973)

DICKLER, H.B., ADKINSON, JR., N.F., TERRY, W.D.: Evidence for individual human peripheral blood lymphocytes bearing both B and T cell markers. Nature **247**, 213–215 (1974)

DICKLER, H.B., KUNKEL, H.G.: Interaction of aggregated $\gamma$-globulin with B lymphocytes. J. exp. Med. **136**, 191–196 (1972)

DIENER, E., NOSSAL, G.J.V.: Phylogenetic studies on the immune response. I. Localization of antigens and immune response in the toad, Bufo marinus. Immunology **10**, 535–542 (1966)

DOBOZY, A., HUSZ, S., HUNYADI, J., SIMON, N.: Formation of mouse erythrocyte rosettes by human lymphocytes. A B-cell marker. Clin. exp. Immunol. **23**, 382–384 (1976)

DOUGLAS, S.D., HOFFMAN, P.F., BÖRJESON, J., CHESSIN, L.N.: Studies on human peripheral blood lymphocytes in vitro: III. Fine structural features of lymphocyte transformation by pokeweed mitogen. J. Immunol. **98**, 17–30 (1967)

DRESCHER, J., RÜSSLER, P.: Morphologische, zytochemische und autoradiographische Untersuchungen der Zellen in Lymphozytenkulturversuchen unter Zusatz von Phytohämagglutinin oder Tuberkulin. Folia haemat. (Lpz.) **101**, 196–212 (1974)

DUKOR, P., BIANCO, C., NUSSENZWEIG, V.: Tissue localization of lymphocytes bearing a membrane receptor for antigen-antibody-complement complexes. Proc. nat. Acad. Sci. (Wash.) **67**, 991–997 (1970)

DURKIN, H.G., CAPORALE, L., THORBECKE, G.J.: Migratory patterns of B lymphocytes. I. Fate of cells from central and peripheral lymphoid organs in the rabbit and its selective alteration by anti-immunoglobulin. Cell. Immunol. **16**, 285–300 (1975)

DURKIN, H.G., THORBECKE, G.J.: Homing of B-lymphocytes to follicles: Specific retention of immunologically committed cells. In: Microenvironmental Aspects of Immunity. Advances in Experimental Medicine and Biology, Vol. 29, pp. 63–70. JANKOVIĆ, B.D., ISAKOVIĆ, K., Eds. New York-London: Plenum Press 1973

EHRICH, W.: Studies of the lymphatic tissue. I. The anatomy of the secondary nodules and some remarks on the lymphatic and lymphoid tissue. Amer. J. Anat. **43**, 347–383 (1929)

EHRICH, W.E.: The role of the lymphocyte in the circulation of the lymph. Ann. N.Y. Acad. Sci. **46**, 823–857 (1946)

EVERETT, N.B., CAFFREY, R.W.: Radioautographic studies of bone marrow small lymphocytes. In: The Lymphocyte in Immunology and Haemopoieses, pp. 108–119. YOFFEY, J.M., Ed. London: E. Arnold 1967

EVERETT, N.B., CAFFREY, R.W., RIEKE, W.O.: Recirculation of lymphocytes. Ann. N.Y. Acad. Sci. **113**, 887–897 (1964) van Ewijk, W., Brons, N.H.C., Rozing, J.: Scanning electron microscopy of homing and recirculating lymphocyte populations. Cell. Immunol. **19**, 245–261 (1975)

Fagraeus, A.: Antibody production in relation to the development of plasma cells. In vivo and in vitro experiments. Acta med. scand. Suppl. **204**, 1–122 (1948)

Farnes, P., Barker, B.E., Brownhill, L.E., Fanger, H.: Mitogenic activity in Phytolacca americana (pokeweed). Lancet 1964, II, pp. 1100–1101

Ferrarini, M., Moretta, L., Abrile, R., Durante, M.L.: Receptors for IgG molecules on human lymphocytes forming spontaneous rosettes with sheep red cells. Eur. J. Immunol. **5**, 70–72 (1975)

Fichtelius, K.E.: The gut epithelium – a first level lymphoid organ? Exp. Cell Res. **49**, 87–104 (1968)

Fichtelius, K.E., Groth, O., Lidén, S.: The skin, a first level lymphoid organ? Int. Arch. Allergy **37**, 607–620 (1970)

Flemming, W.: Studien über Regeneration der Gewebe. Arch. mikr. Anat. **24**, 50–91 (1885)

Fliedner, T.M.: On the origin of tingible bodies in germinal centers. In: Germinal Centers in Immune Responses, pp. 218–224. Cottier, H., Odartchenko, N., Schindler, R., Congdon, C.C., Eds. Berlin-Heidelberg-New York: Springer 1967

Fliedner, T.M., Kesse, M., Cronkite, E.P., Robertson, J.S.: Cell proliferation in germinal centers of the rat spleen. Ann. N.Y. Acad. Sci. **113**, 578–594 (1964)

Ford, W.L., Gowans, J.L.: The traffic of lymphocytes. Semin. Hemat. **6**, 67–83 (1969)

Ford, W.L., Marchesi, V.T.: Lymphocyte recirculation and its immunological significance. In: Progress in Immunology, pp. 1159–1164. Amos, B., Ed. New York-London: Academic Press 1971

Freitas, A.A., de Sousa, M.: The role of cell interactions in the control of lymphocyte traffic. Cell. Immunol. **22**, 345–350 (1976)

Frey-Wettstein, M., Craddock, C.G.: Testosterone-induced depletion of thymus and marrow lymphocytes as related to lymphopoiesis and hematopoieses. Blood **35**, 257–271 (1970)

Fröland, S., Natvig, J.B., Berdal, P.: Surface-bound immunoglobulin as a marker of B lymphocytes in man. Nature [New Biol.] **234**, 251–252 (1971)

Fudenberg, H.H., Wybran, J., Robbins, D.: T-rosette-forming cells, cellular immunity and cancer. New Engl. J. Med. **292**, 475–476 (1975)

van Furth, R., Cohn, Z.A., Hirsch, J.G., Humphrey, J.H., Spector, W.G., Langevoort, H.L.: The mononuclear phagocyte system: A new classification of macrophages, monocytes, and their precursor cells. Bull. Wld Hlth Org. **46**, 845–852 (1972)

van Furth, R., Langevoort, H.L., Schaberg, A.: Mononuclear phagocytes in human pathology – prosposal for an approach to improved classification. In: Mononuclear Phagocytes in Immunity, Infection, and Pathology, pp. 1–15. van Furth, R., Ed. Oxford-London-Edinburgh-Melbourne: Blackwell 1975

Gatien, J.G., Schneeberger, E.E., Merler, E.: Analysis of human thymocyte subpopulations using discontinuous gradients of albumin: Precursor lymphocytes in human thymus. Eur. J. Immunol. **5**, 312–317 (1975)

Gatien, J.G., Schneeberger, E.E., Parkman, R., Merler, E.: Isolation on discontinuous gradients of bovine albumin of a subpopulation of human lymphocytes exhibiting precursor characteristics. Eur. J. Immunol. **5**, 306–312 (1975)

von Gaudecker, B., Hinrichsen, K.: Elektronenmikroskopische Untersuchungen zur Cytologie von Thymusrinde und Keimzentrum. Z. Zellforsch. **65**, 139–162 (1965)

Gengozian, N., Urso, I.S., Congdon, C.C., Conger, A.D., Makinodan, T.: Thymus specificity in lethally irradiated mice treated with rat bone marrow. Proc. Soc. exp. Biol. (N.Y.) **96**, 714–720 (1957)

Giacomelli, F., Wiener, J., Kruskal, J.B., Pomeranz, J.V., Loud, A.V.: Subpopulations of blood lymphocytes demonstrated by quantitative cytochemistry. J. Histochem. Cytochem. **19**, 426–433 (1971)

Glick, B., Chang, T.S., Jaap, R.G.: The bursa of Fabricius and antibody production. Poultry Sci. **35**, 224–225 (1956)

Globerson, A., Kirov, S.M., Parish, C.R.: Involvement of cells with 'B' properties in development of T helpers. In: Immune Reactivity of Lymphocytes. Advances in Experimental Medicine and Biology, Vol. 66, pp. 51–75. Feldman, M., Globerson, A., Eds. New York-London: Plenum Press 1976

GOLDSTEIN, A.L., GUHA, A., ZATZ, M.M., HARDY, M.A., WHITE, A.: Purification and biological activity of thymosin, a hormone of the thymus gland. Proc. nat. Acad. Sci. (Wash.) **69**, 1800–1803 (1972)

GOOD, R.A., DALMASSO, A.P., MARTINEZ, C., ARCHER, O.K., PIERCE, J.C., PAPERMASTER, B.W.: The role of the thymus in development of immunologic capacity in rabbits and mice. J. exp. Med. **116**, 773–795 (1962)

GORDON, S.: The secretion of lysozyme and a plasminogen activator by mononuclear phagocytes. In: Mononuclear Phagocytes in Immunity, Infection, and Pathology, pp. 463–470. VAN FURTH, R., Ed. Oxford-London-Edinburgh-Melbourne: Blackwell 1975

GOWANS, J.L., KNIGHT, E.J.: The route of re-circulation of lymphocytes in the rat. Proc. roy. Soc. Lond. B **159**, 257–282 (1964)

GREAVES, M.F., BAUMINGER, S., JANOSSY, G.: Lymphocyte activation. III. Binding sites for phytomitogens on lymphocyte subpopulations. Clin. exp. Immunol. **10**, 537–554 (1972)

GREAVES, M.F., HOGG, N.M.: Immunoglobulin determinants on the surface of antigen binding T- and B-lymphocytes in mice. In: Progress in Immunology, pp. 111–126, AMOS, B., Ed. New York-London: Academic Press 1971

GREAVES, M., JANOSSY, G.: Elicitation of selective T and B lymphocyte responses by cell surface binding ligands. Transplant. Rev. **11**, 87–130 (1972)

GREAVES, M., JANOSSY, G., DOENHOFF, M.: Selective triggering of human T and B lymphocytes in vitro by polyclonal mitogens. J. exp. Med. **140**, 1–18 (1974)

GREAVES, M.F., OWEN, J.J.T., RAFF, M.C.: T and B Lymphocytes: Origins, Properties and Roles in Immune Responses. Amsterdam: Excerpta Medica 1973

GREENBERG, A.H., HUDSON, L., SHEN, L., ROITT, I.M.: Antibody-dependent cell-mediated cytotoxicity due to a 'null' lymphoid cell. Nature [New Biol.] **242**, 111–113 (1973)

GREY, H.M., KUBO, R.T., CEROTTINI, J.-C.: Thymus-derived (T) cell immunoglobulins. Presence of a receptor site for IgG and absence of large amounts of 'buried' Ig determinants on T cells. J. exp. Med. **136**, 1323–1328 (1972)

GROBLER, P., BUERKI, H., COTTIER, H., HESS, M.W., STONER, R.D.: Cellular bases for relative radioresistance of the antibody-forming system at advanced stages of the secondary response to tetanus toxoid in mice. J. Immunol. **112**, 2154–2165 (1974)

GRUNDMANN, E.: Über die Unterscheidung von zwei Lymphocytentypen im Phasenkontrastmikroskop. Virchows Arch. path. Anat. **332**, 17–24 (1959)

GUDAT, F.G., HARRIS, T.N., HARRIS, S., HUMMELER, K.: Studies on antibody-producing cells. I. Ultrastructure of 19S and 7S antibody-producing cells. J. exp. Med. **132**, 448–474 (1970)

GUPTA, S., GRIECO, M.H.: Rosette formation with mouse erythrocytes: Probable marker for human B lymphocytes. Int. Arch. Allergy **49**, 734–742 (1975)

GUPTA, S., PAHWA, R., O'REILLY, R., GOOD, R.A., SIEGAL, F.P.: Ontogeny of lymphocyte subpopulations in human fetal liver. Proc. nat. Acad. Sci. (Wash.) **73**, 919–922 (1976)

HAAS, R.J., BOHNE, F., FLIEDNER, T.M.: On the development of slowly-turning-over cell types in neonatal rat bone marrow. (Studies utilizing the complete tritiated thymidine labeling method complemented by C-14 thymidine administration) Blood **34**, 791–805 (1969)

HAAS, R.J., FLAD, H.-D., FLIEDNER, T.M., FACHE, I.: Correlation between cytokinetically resting lymphocytes and bone marrow restoration: Experiments using a discontinuous albumin gradient. Blood **42**, 209–218 (1973)

HÄMMERLING, U., POLLIACK, A., LAMPEN, N., SABETY, M., DE HARVEN, E.: Scanning electron microscopy of tobacco mosaic virus-labeled lymphocyte surface antigens. J. exp. Med. **141**, 518–523 (1975)

HAMMARSTRÖM, S., HELLSTRÖM, U., PERLMANN, P., DILLNER, M.-L.: A new surface marker on T lymphocytes of human peripheral blood. J. exp. Med. **138**, 1270–1275 (1973)

HANNA, JR., M.G.: An autoradiographic study of the germinal center in spleen white pulp during early intervals of the immune response. Lab. Invest. **13**, 95–104 (1964)

HANNA, JR., M.G., SZAKAL, A.K., WALBURG, JR., H.E.: The relation of antigen and virus localization to the development and growth of lymphoid germinal centers. In: Lymphatic Tissue and Germinal Centers in Immune Response. Advances in Experimental Medicine and Biology, Vol. 5, pp. 149–165. FIORE-DONATI, L., HANNA, JR., M.G., Eds. New York: Plenum Press 1969

HANNIG, K., ZEILLER, K.: Zur Auftrennung und Charakterisierung immunkompetenter Zellen mit Hilfe der trägerfreien Ablenkungselektrophorese. Hoppe-Seylers Z. physiol. Chem. **350**, 467–472 (1969)

HARRIS, T.N., HUMMELER, K., HARRIS, S.: Electron microscopic observations on antibody-producing lymph node cells. J. exp. Med. **123**, 161–172 (1966)

HEUSERMANN, U., STUTTE, H.J., MÜLLER-HERMELINK, H.K.: Interdigitating cells in the white pulp of the human spleen. Cell Tiss. Res. **153**, 415–417 (1974)

HIJMANS, W., SCHUIT, H.R.E.: Immunofluorescence studies on immunoglobulins in the lymphoid cells of human peripheral blood. Clin. exp. Immunol. **11**, 483–494 (1972)

HIJMANS, W., SCHUIT, H.R.E., HULSING-HESSELINK, E.: An immunofluorescence study on intracellular immunoglobulins in human bone marrow cells. Ann. N.Y. Acad. Sci. **177**, 290–305 (1971)

HIRSCH, B.B., BROWN, M.B., NAGAREDA, C.S., KAPLAN, H.S.: Comparative activity of isologous versus homologous or heterologous mouse bone marrow in promoting regeneration of the irradiated mouse thymus. Radiat. Res. **5**, 52–57 (1956)

HOEFSMIT, E.C.M.: Mononuclear phagocytes, reticulum cells, and dendritic cells in lymphoid tissues. In: Mononuclear Phagocytes in Immunity, Infection, and Pathology, pp. 129–146. VAN FURTH, R., Ed. Oxford-London-Edinburgh-Melbourne: Blackwell 1975

HOWARD, J.C.: The life-span and recirculation of marrow-derived small lymphocytes from the rat thoracic duct. J. exp. Med. **135**, 185–199 (1972)

HOWARD, J.C., SCOTT, D.W.: The role of recirculating lymphocytes in the immunological competence of rat bone marrow cells. Cell. Immunol. **3**, 421–429 (1972)

HUMMELER, K., HARRIS, T.N., HARRIS, S., FARBER, M.B.: Studies on antibody-producing cells. IV. Ultrastructure of plaque-forming cells of rabbit lymph. J. exp. Med. **135**, 491–502 (1972)

INMAN, D.R., COOPER, E.H.: Electron microscopy of human lymphocytes stimulated by phytohaemagglutinin. J. Cell Biol. **19**, 441–445 (1963)

INMAN, D.R., COOPER, E.H.: The relation of ultrastructure to DNA synthesis in human leucocytes. I. Atypical lymphocytes in phytohaemagglutinin cultures and infectious mononucleosis. Acta haemat. (Basel) **33**, 257–278 (1965)

IVANYI, L., LEHNER, T.: Stimulation of human lymphocytes by B-cell mitogens. Clin. exp. Immunol. **18**, 347–356 (1974)

IVERSEN, J.-G., BENESTAD, H.B.: The presence of non-recirculating long-lived lymphocytes in rat blood. Scand. J. Haemat. **7**, 368–373 (1970)

IZARD, J., DEHARVEN, E.: Increased numbers of characteristic type of reticular cell in the thymus and lymph nodes of leukemic mice: An electron microscope study. Cancer Res. **28**, 421–433 (1968)

JACOBSON, E.B., CAPORALE, L.H., THORBECKE, G.J.: Effect of thymus cell injections on germinal center formation in lymphoid tissues of nude (thymusless) mice. Cell. Immunol. **13**, 416–430 (1974)

JANKOVIĆ, B.D., WAKSMAN, B.H., ARNASON, B.G.: Role of the thymus in immune reactions in rats. I. The immunologic response to bovine serum albumin (antibody formation, Arthus reactivity, and delayed hypersensitivity) in rats thymectomized or splenectomized at various times after birth. J. exp. Med. **116**, 159–176 (1962)

JERNE, N.K.: The immune system. A web of V-domains. In: The Harvey Lectures, New York 1975

JOEL, D.D., HESS, M.W., COTTIER, H.: Magnitude and pattern of thymic lymphocyte migration in neonatal mice. J. exp. Med. **135**, 907–923 (1972)

JØNSSON, V.: Technical aspects of the rosette technique for detecting human circulating B and T lymphocytes. Normal values and some remarks on null lymphocytes. Scand. J. Haemat. **13**, 361–369 (1974)

JONDAL, M., HOLM, G., WIGZELL, H.: Surface markers on human T and B lymphocytes. I. A large population of lymphocytes forming nonimmune rosettes with sheep red blood cells. J. exp. Med. **136**, 207–215 (1972)

JONDAL, M., KLEIN, G.: Surface markers on human B and T lymphocytes. II. Presence of Epstein-Barr virus (EBV) receptors on B lymphocytes. Cited by JONDAL, M., WIGZELL, H., AIUTI, F.: Human lymphocyte subpopulations: Classification according to surface markers and/or functional characteristics. Transplant. Rev. **16**, 163–195 (1973)

JONES, T.C., HIRSCH, J.G.: The interaction between Toxoplasma gondii and mammalian cells. II. The absence of lysosomal fusion with phagocytic vacuoles containing living parasites. J. exp. Med. **136**, 1173–1194 (1972)

JURÁŠKOVÁ, V., TKADLEČEK, L.: Character of primary and secondary colonies of haematopoiesis in the spleen of irradiated mice. Nature (Lond.) **206**, 951–952 (1965)

KAISERLING, E., LENNERT, K.: Die interdigitierende Reticulumzelle im menschlichen Lymphknoten. Eine spezifische Zelle der thymusabhängigen Region. Virchows Arch. B. **16**, 51–61 (1974)

KAISERLING, E., LENNERT, K., NITSCH, K., DRESCHER, J.: Ultrastruktur und Pathogenese der BCG-Histiocytose (sog. BCG-Granulomatose). Virchows Arch. A **355**, 333–353 (1972)

KAISERLING, E., STEIN, H., MÜLLER-HERMELINK, H.K.: Interdigitating reticulum cells in the human thymus. Cell Tiss. Res. **155**, 47–55 (1974)

KALINA, M., KLETTER, Y., SHAHAR, A., ARONSON, M.: Acid phosphatase release from intact phagocytic cells surrounding a large-sized parasite. Proc. Soc. exp. Biol. (N.Y.) **136**, 407–410 (1971)

KAPLAN, H.S., BROWN, M.B., PAULL, J.: Influence of bone marrow injections on involution and neoplasia of mouse thymus after systemic irradiation. J. nat. Cancer Inst. **14**, 303–316 (1953)

KAPLAN, M.E., CLARK, C.: An improved rosetting assay for detection of human T lymphocytes. J. immunol. Methods **5**, 131–135 (1974)

KEUNING, F.J.: Dynamics of immunoglobulin forming cells and their precursors. In: Immunoglobulins, pp. 1–14. Amsterdam: North-Holland Publ. 1972

KEUNING, F.J., BOS, W.H.: Regeneration patterns of lymphoid follicles in the rabbit spleen after sublethal X-irradiation. In: Germinal Centers in Immune Responses. Proc. of a Symp. held at the Univ. of Bern, June 22–24, 1966, pp. 250–257. COTTIER, H., ODARTCHENKO, N., SCHINDLER, R., CONGDON, C.C., Eds. Berlin-Heidelberg-New York: Springer 1967

KEUNING, F.J., VAN DER MEER, J., NIEUWENHUIS, P., OUDENDIJK, P.: The histophysiology of the antibody response. II. Antibody responses and splenic plasma cell reactions in sublethally X-irradiated rabbits. Lab. Invest. **12**, 156–170 (1963)

KINCADE, P.W., LAWTON, A.R., BOCKMAN, D.E., COOPER, M.D.: Suppression of immunoglobulin G synthesis as a result of antibody-mediated suppression of immunoglobulin M synthesis in chickens. Proc. nat. Acad. Sci. (Wash.) **67**, 1918–1925 (1970)

KIYONO, K.: Zur Frage der histiozytären Blutzellen. Folia haemat. (Lpz.) **18**, 149–170 (1914)

KLEBANOFF, S.J., HAMON, C.B.: Antimicrobial systems of mononuclear phagocytes. In: Mononuclear Phagocytes in Immunity, Infection, and Pathology, pp. 507–529. VAN FURTH, R., Ed. Oxford-London-Edinburgh-Melbourne: Blackwell 1975

KOJIMA, M., IMAI, Y.: Genesis and function of germinal centers. In: Malignant Diseases of the Hematopoietic System. GANN Monograph on Cancer Research, No. 15, pp. 1–24. AKAZAKI, K., RAPPAPORT, H., BERARD, C.W., BENNETT, J.M., ISHIKAWA, E., Eds. Baltimore-London-Tokyo: University of Tokyo Press 1973

KOLB, C., DI PAULI, R., WEILER, E.: Induction of IgG by lipid A in the newborn mouse. J. exp. Med. **139**, 467–478 (1974)

KOOK, A.I., YAKIR, Y., TRAININ, N.: Isolation and partial chemical characterization of THF, a thymus hormone involved in immune maturation of lymphoid cells. Cell. Immunol. **19**, 151–157 (1975)

KOTANI, M., NAWA, Y., FUJII, H., FUKUMOTO, T., MIYAMOTO, M., YAMASHITA, A.: Post-capillary venules as the pathway for migrating B lymphocytes. Cell Tiss. Res. **152**, 299–303 (1974)

KUHLMANN, W.D., AVRAMEAS, S.: Cellular differentiation and antibody localization during the primary immune response in peroxidase stimulated lymph nodes of rat. Cell. Immunol. **4**, 425–441 (1972)

LAFLEUR, L., MILLER, R.G., PHILLIPS, R.A.: A quantitative assay for the progenitors of bone marrow-associated lymphocytes. J. exp. Med. **135**, 1363–1374 (1972)

LAFLEUR, L., MILLER, R.G., PHILLIPS, R.A.: Restriction of specificity in the precursors of bone marrow-associated lymphocytes. J. exp. Med. **137**, 954–966 (1973)

LANDSTEINER, K., CHASE, M.W.: Experiments on transfer of cutaneous sensitivity to simple compounds. Proc. Soc. exp. Biol. (N.Y.) **49**, 688–690 (1942)

LANE, F.C., UNANUE, E.R.: Requirement of thymus (T) lymphocytes for resistance to listeriosis. J. exp. Med. **135**, 1104–1112 (1972)

LAWTON, A.R., SELF, K.S., ROYAL, S.A., COOPER, M.D.: Ontogeny of B-lymphocytes in the human fetus. Clin. Immunol. Immunopath. **1**, 84–93 (1972)

LAY, W.H., NUSSENZWEIG, V.: Receptors for complement on leukocytes. J. exp. Med. **128**, 991–1007 (1968)

LE BOUTEILLER, P., VUJANOVIC, N., DUC, H.T., KINSKY, R., VOISIN, G.A.: Ultrastructure des lymphocytes d'aspect thymique et d'aspect médullaire chez la souris: Identification par marquage immunoenzymatique. Ann. Immunol. **125** C, 445–450 (1974)

LEDER, L.D.: Der Nachweis der Naphthol-AS-D-Chloracetat-Esterase und seine Bedeutung für die histologische Diagnostik. Verh. dtsch. Ges. Path. **48**, 317–320 (1964)

LEDER, L.-D.: Der Blutmonocyt. (Experimentelle Medizin, Pathologie und Klinik, Bd 23) Berlin-Heidelberg-New York: Springer 1967

LEDUC, E.H., AVRAMEAS, S., BOUTEILLE, M.: Ultrastructural localization of antibody in differentiating plasma cells. J. exp. Med. **127**, 109–118 (1968)

LENNERT, K.: Über die Erkennung von Keimzentrumszellen im Lymphknotenausstrich. Klin. Wschr. **35**, 1130–1132 (1957)

LENNERT, K.: Lymphknoten. Diagnostik in Schnitt und Ausstrich. Bandteil A: Cytologie und Lymphadenitis. Handbuch der speziellen pathologischen Anatomie und Histologie 1,3 A. LUBARSCH, O., HENKE, F., RÖSSLE, R., UEHLINGER, E. (Hrsg.). Berlin-Göttingen-Heidelberg: Springer 1961

LENNERT, K.: Pathologie der Halslymphknoten. Ein Abriß für Pathologen, Kliniker und praktizierende Ärzte. Berlin-Göttingen-Heidelberg-New York: Springer 1964

LENNERT, K., CAESAR, R., MÜLLER, H.K.: Electron microscopic studies of germinal centers in man. In: Germinal Centers in Immune Responses, pp. 49–59. COTTIER, H., ODARTCHENKO, N., SCHINDLER, R., CONGDON, C.C., Eds. Berlin-Heidelberg-New York: Springer 1967

LENNERT, K., KAISERLING, E., MÜLLER-HERMELINK, H.K.: T-associated plasma-cells. [Letter to the Editor.] Lancet 1975, I, pp. 1031–1032

LENNERT, K., MITROU, P., MÜLLER-HERMELINK, H.K.: Cytophotometric and autoradiographic investigations on germinal center cells in man. In: Lymphatic Tissue and Germinal Centers in Immune Response. Advances in Experimental Medicine and Biology, Vol. 5, pp. 65–71. FIORE-DONATI, L., HANNA, JR., M.G., Eds. New York: Plenum Press 1969

LENNERT, K., MÜLLER-HERMELINK, H.K.: Lymphocyten und ihre Funktionsformen – Morphologie, Organisation und immunologische Bedeutung. (Vortrag) Verh. Anat. Ges. (Jena) **69**, 19–62 (1975)

LENNERT, K., NIEDORF, H.R.: Nachweis von desmosomal verknüpften Reticulumzellen im follikulären Lymphom (Brill Symmers). Virchows Arch. B **4**, 148–150 (1969)

LENNERT, K., REMMELE, W.: Karyometrische Untersuchungen an Lymphknotenzellen des Menschen. I. Mitt. Germinoblasten, Lymphoblasten und Lymphozyten. Acta haemat. (Basel) **19**, 99–113 (1958)

LENNERT, K., RINNEBERG, H.: Fermenthistochemische Untersuchungen des Lymphknotens. II. Adenosintriphosphatase und 5-Nucleotidase im Lymphknotenschnitt. Klin. Wschr. **39**, 923–924 (1961)

LIN, P.S., COOPER, A.G., WORTIS, H.H.: Scanning electron microscopy of human T-cell and B-cell rosettes. New Engl. J. Med. **289**, 548–551 (1973)

LIN, P.S., WALLACH, D.F.H., TSAI, S.: Temperature-induced variations in the surface topology of cultured lymphocytes are revealed by scanning electron microscopy. Proc. nat. Acad. Sci. (Wash.) **70**, 2492–2496 (1973)

MACKANESS, G.B.: The influence of immunologically committed lymphoid cells on macrophage activity in vivo. J. exp. Med. **129**, 973–992 (1969)

MACKANESS, G.B.: Cellular immunity. In: Mononuclear Phagocytes, pp. 461–475. VAN FURTH, R., Ed. Oxford-Edinburgh: Blackwell 1970

MACKANESS, G.B.: Delayed hypersensitivity and the mechanism of cellular resistance to infection. In: Progress in Immunology, pp. 413–424. AMOS, B., Ed. New York-London: Academic Press 1971

MACLENNAN, I.C.M.: Antibody in the induction and inhibition of lymphocyte cytotoxicity. Transplant. Rev. **13**, 67–90 (1972)

MACLENNAN, I.C.M., LOEWI, G.: Effect of specific antibody to target cells on their specific and non-specific interactions with lymphocytes. Nature **219**, 1069–1070 (1968)

MARCHESI, V.T., GOWANS, J.L.: The migration of lymphocytes through the endothelium of venules in lymph nodes: An electron microscope study. Proc. roy. Soc. Lond. B. **159**, 283–290 (1964)

MARSHALL, W.H., ROBERTS, K.B.: The growth and mitosis of human small lymphocytes after incubation with a phytohaemagglutinin. Quart. J. exp. Physiol. **48**, 146–155 (1963)

MATTER, A., LISOWSKA-BERNSTEIN, B., RYSER, J.E., LAMELIN, J.-P., VASSALLI, P.: Mouse thymus-independent and thymus-derived lymphoid cells. II. Ultrastructural studies. J. exp. Med. **136**, 1008–1030 (1972)

MATTHES, M.-L., AX, W., FISCHER, H.: Mikrokinematographische Studien über die Zellkooperation von Lymphocyten und Makrophagen nach primärem und sekundärem Stimulus mit löslichem Antigen. Z. ges. exp. Med. **154**, 253–264 (1971)

MAXIMOW, A.: Untersuchungen über Blut und Bindegewebe. II. Über die Histogenese des Thymus bei Säugetieren. Arch. mikr. Anat. **74**, 525–621 (1909)

MCCAFFREY, R., HARRISON, T.A., PARKMAN, R., BALTIMORE, D.: Terminal deoxynucleotidyl transferase activity in human leukemic cells and in normal human thymocytes. New Engl. J. Med. **292**, 775–780 (1975)

MCMILLAN, R., LONGMIRE, R.L., YELENOSKY, R.J., CRADDOCK, C.G.: Bone marrow as a major site of human IgG production. [Abstract] Blood **40**, 926 (1972)

MERK, K.F: Morphologische, zytochemische, autoradiographische und quantitative Untersuchungen der lymphatischen Reaktionsformen in Lymphozytenkulturen unter Zusatz von Tuberkulin und Anwendung einer neuen Ausstrichtechnik. Inaug.-Diss. Kiel 1976

METCALF, D.: The Thymus. Its Role in Immune Responses, Leukaemia Development and Carcinogenesis. (Recent Results in Cancer Research, Vol. 5) Berlin-Heidelberg-New York: Springer 1966

METCALF, D., MOORE, M.A.S.: Haemopoietic Cells. (Frontiers of Biology, Vol. 24) Amsterdam-London: North-Holland 1971

MICHALKE, W.D., HESS, M.W., RIEDWYL, H., STONER, R.D., COTTIER, H.: Thymic lymphopoiesis and cell loss in newborn mice. Blood **33**, 541–554 (1969)

MICKLEM, H.S., FORD, C.E.: Proliferation of injected lymph node and thymus cells in lethally irradiated mice. Transplant. Bull. **26**, 436–441 (1960)

MICKLEM, H.S., OGDEN, D.A., PAYNE, A.C.: Ageing, haemopoietic stem cells and immunity. In: Haemopoietic Stem Cells. Ciba Found. Symp. **13** N.S., 285–301. Amsterdam-London-New York: Elsevier, Excerpta Medical, North-Holland 1973

MILANESI, S.: Sulla presenza di dispositivi di giunzione tra le cellule dendritiche dei follicoli linfatici del linfonodo. Boll. Soc. ital. Biol. Sper. **41**, 1223–1225 (1965)

MILLER, J.F.A.P.: Immunological function of the thymus. Lancet 1961, II, pp. 748–749

MITCHELL, J.: Antigens in immunity. XVII. The migration of antigen-binding, bone-marrow-derived and thymus-derived spleen cells in mice. Immunology **22**, 231–245 (1972)

MITCHELL, J., ABBOT, A.: Ultrastructure of the antigen-retaining reticulum of lymph node follicles as shown by high-resolution autoradiography. Nature (Lond.) **208**, 500–502 (1965)

MITROU, P.S., QUEISSER, W., LENNERT, K., SANDRITTER, W.: Kombinierte autoradiographisch-cytophotometrische Untersuchungen von Keimzentrumszellen der menschlichen Tonsille. Virchows Arch. B **3**, 156–170 (1969)

MIYAKAWA, M.: The lymphatic system of germfree guinea pigs. Ann. N.Y. Acad. Sci. **78**, 221–236 (1959)

MODABBER, F., COONS, A.H.: Antibody cytophilic for lymphocytes. J. Immunol. **108**, 1447–1452 (1972)

MÖLLER, E.: Contact-induced cytotoxicity by lymphoid cells containing foreign isoantigens. Science **147**, 873–879 (1965)

MÖLLER, E., RUBIN, B.: New methods for the identification of T, B, and K cells. Workshop report. Transplant. Proc. **7**, Suppl. 1, 891–892 (1975)

MÖLLER, G.: Effect of B-cell mitogens on lymphocyte subpopulations possessing C'3 and Fc receptors. J. exp. Med. **139**, 969–982 (1974)

MÖLLER, G., SVEHAG, S.-E.: Specificity of lymphocyte-mediated cytotoxicity induced by in vitro antibody-coated target cells. Cell. Immunol. **4**, 1–19 (1972)

MOFFAT, D.J., ROSSE, C., YOFFEY, J.M.: Identity of the haemopoietic stem cell. Lancet 1967, II, pp. 547–548

MOLLO, F., MONGA, G., STRAMIGNONI, A.: Dark reticular cells in human lymphadenitis and lymphomas. Virchows Arch. B **3**, 117–126 (1969)

MORI, Y., LENNERT, K.: Electron microscopic atlas of lymph node cytology and pathology. Berlin-Heidelberg-New York: Springer 1969

MORSE, S.I.: Studies on the lymphocytosis induced in mice by Bordetella pertussis. J. exp. Med. **121**, 49–68 (1965)

MORSE, S.I., BARRON, B.A.: Studies on the leukocytosis and lymphocytosis induced by Bordetella pertussis. III. The distribution of transfused lymphocytes in pertussis-treated and normal mice. J. exp. Med. **132**, 663–672 (1970)

Movat, H.Z., Fernando, N.V.P.: The fine structure of the lymphoid tissue during antibody formation. Exp. mol. Path. **4**, 155–188 (1965)

Mueller, J., Brun del Re, G., Buerki, H., Keller, H.-U., Hess, M.W., Cottier, H.: Nonspecific esterase activity: A criterion for differentiation of T and B lymphocytes in mouse lymph nodes. Europ. J. Immunol. **5**, 270–274 (1975)

Müller-Hermelink, H.K.: Characterization of the B-cell and T-cell regions of human lymphatic tissue through enzyme histochemical demonstration of ATPase and 5'-nucleotidase activities. Virchows Arch. B **16**, 371–378 (1974)

Müller-Hermelink, H.K.: Herkunft der Lymphocyten und Mikroökologie der lymphatischen Gewebe. Habil. Schrift Kiel 1975

Müller-Hermelink, H.K., Caesar, R.: Elektronenmikroskopische Untersuchung der Keimzentren in menschlichen Tonsillen. Z. Zellforsch. **96**, 521–547 (1969)

Müller-Hermelink, H.K., Heusermann, U., Kaiserling, E., Stutte, H.-J.: Human lymphatic microecology — specificity, characterization and ontogeny of different reticulum cells in the B cell and T cell regions. In: Immune Reactivity of Lymphocytes. Advances in Experimental Medicine and Biology, Vol. 66, pp. 177–182. Feldman, M., Globerson, A., Eds. New York-London: Plenum Press 1976

Müller-Hermelink, H.K., Heusermann, U., Stutte, H.J.: Enzyme histochemical observations on the localization and structure of the T cell and B cell regions in the human spleen. Cell Tiss. Res. **154**, 167–179 (1974)

Müller-Hermelink, H.K., Kaiserling, E.: Seminar für elektronenmikroskopisch-histochemische Techniken. Verh. dtsch. Ges. Path. **59**, 522–527 (1975)

Müller-Hermelink, H.K., Kaiserling, E., Lennert, K.: Pseudofollikuläre Nester von Plasmazellen (eines besonderen Typs?) in der paracorticalen Pulpa menschlicher Lymphknoten. Virchows Arch. B **14**, 47–56 (1973)

Müller-Hermelink, H.K., Thiede, A., Sonntag, H.G., Müller-Ruchholtz, W., Leder, L.-D.: Elektronenmikroskopische Untersuchungen zur Herkunft von Gewebsmastzellen bei Ratten. Beitr. Path. **144**, 307–318 (1971)

Müller-Hermelink, H.K., Wottge, U., Müller-Ruchholtz, W.: Selective cytotoxicity of antisera on lymphoid cells in bone marrow. 2. Ann. Conf. Int. Soc. for Exp. Hemat., Paris 1973. [Abstract] Exp. Hemat. **1**, 294 (1973)

Müller-Ruchholtz, W., Müller-Hermelink, H.-K., Sonntag, H.-G.: Specific inactivation of lymphoid cells in bone marrow grafts. Transplant. Proc. **5**, 877–880 (1973)

Müller-Ruchholtz, W., Wottge, H.-U., Müller-Hermelink, H.K.: Selective grafting of hemopoietic cells. Transplant. Proc. **7**, Suppl. 1, 859–862 (1975)

Munro, A.J., Taussig, M.J.: Two genes in the major histocompatibility complex control immune response. Nature **256**, 103–106 (1975)

Nath, I., Poulter, L.W., Turk, J.L.: Effect of lymphocyte mediators on macrophages in vitro. A correlation of morphological and cytochemical changes. Clin. exp. Immunol. **13**, 455–466 (1973)

Newell, D.G., Roath, S., Smith, J.L.: The scanning electron microscopy of normal human peripheral blood lymphocytes. Brit. J. Haemat. **32**, 309–316 (1976)

Nieuwenhuis, P.: Germinal centers: A microenvironment for the production of antibody forming cell precursors? In: Microenvironmental Aspects of Immunity. Advances in Experimental Medicine and Biology, Vol. 29, pp. 95–100. Janković, B.D., Isaković, K., Eds. New York-London: Plenum Press 1973

Nieuwenhuis, P., Keuning, F.J.: Germinal centres and the origin of the B-cell system. II. Germinal centres in the rabbit spleen and popliteal lymph nodes. Immunology **26**, 509–519 (1974)

Nieuwenhuis, P., van Nouhuijs, C.E., Eggens, J.H., Keuning, F.J.: Germinal centres and the origin of the B-cell system. I. Germinal centres in the rabbit appendix. Immunology **26**, 497–507 (1974)

Niewisch, H., Vogel, H., Matioli, G.: Concentration, quantitation, and identification of hemopoietic stem cells. Proc. nat. Acad. Sci. (Wash.) **58**, 2261–2267 (1967)

Nopajaroonsri, C., Simon, G.T.: Phagocytosis of colloidal carbon in a lymph node. Amer. J. Path. **65**, 25–42 (1971)

Nossal, G.J.V.: Cellular genetics of immune responses. Advanc. Immunol. **2**, 163–204 (1962)

Nossal, G.J.V., Abbot, A., Mitchell, J., Lummus, Z.: Antigens in immunity. XV. Ultrastructural features of antigen capture in primary and secondary lymphoid follicles. J. exp. Med. **127**, 277–290 (1968)

NOSSAL, G.J.V., PIKE, B.L.: Studies on the differentiation of B lymphocytes in the mouse. Immunology **25**, 33–45 (1973)

NOSSAL, G.J.V., SZENBERG, A., ADA, G.L., AUSTIN, C.M.: Single cell studies on 19S antibody production. J. exp. Med. **119**, 485–502 (1964)

NOSSAL, G.J.V., WARNER, N.L., LEWIS, H., SPRENT, J.: Quantitative features of a sandwich radioimmunolabeling technique for lymphocyte surface receptors. J. exp. Med. **135**, 405–428 (1972)

NOWELL, P.C.: Phytohemagglutinin: An initiator of mitosis in cultures of normal human leukocytes. Cancer Res. **20**, 462–466 (1960)

NOWELL, P.C., HIRSCH, B.E., FOX, D.H., WILSON, D.B.: Evidence for the existence of multipotential lympho-hematopoietic stem cells in the adult rat. J. cell. Physiol. **75**, 151–158 (1970)

NUSSENZWEIG, V.: Receptors for immune complexes on lymphocytes. Advanc. Immunol. **19**, 217–258 (1974)

ODARTCHENKO, N., LEWERENZ, M., SORDAT, B., ROOS, B., COTTIER, H.: Kinetics of cellular death in germinal centers of mouse spleen. In: Germinal Centers in Immune Responses, pp. 212–217. COTTIER, H., ODARTCHENKO, N., SCHINDLER, R., CONGDON, C.C., Eds. Berlin-Heidelberg-New York: Springer 1967

ORDER, S.E., WAKSMAN, B.H.: Cellular differentiation in the thymus. Transplant. **8**, 783–800 (1969)

ORTEGA, L.G., MELLORS, R.C.: Cellular sites of formation of gamma globulin. J. exp. Med. **106**, 627–640 (1957)

OSMOND, D.G.: Formation and maturation of bone marrow lymphocytes. J. reticuloendothel. Soc. **17**, 99–114 (1975)

OSMOND, D.G., EVERETT, N.B.: Radioautographic studies of bone marrow lymphocytes in vivo and in diffusion chamber cultures. Blood **23**, 1–17 (1964)

OSMOND, D.G., NOSSAL, G.J.V.: Differentiation of lymphocytes in mouse bone marrow. I. Quantitative radioautographic studies of antiglobulin binding by lymphocytes in bone marrow and lymphoid tissues. Cell. Immunol. **13**, 117–131 (1974a)

OSMOND, D.G., NOSSAL, G.J.V.: Differentiation of lymphocytes in mouse bone marrow. II. Kinetics of maturation and renewal of antiglobulin-binding cells studied by double labeling. Cell. Immunol. **13**, 132–145 (1974b)

OWEN, J.J.T., COOPER, M.D., RAFF, M.C.: In vitro generation of B lymphocytes in mouse foetal liver, a mammalian 'bursa equivalent'. Nature **249**, 361–363 (1974)

OWEN, J.J.T., RITTER, M.A.: Tissue interaction in the development of thymus lymphocytes. J. exp. Med. **129**, 431–442 (1969)

PALVA, T., DAMMERT, K., PALVA, A.: On enzyme histochemistry of sarcoidosis. Acta path. microbiol. scand. Sect. A **81**, 189–194 (1973)

PARASKEVAS, F., LEE, S.-T., ORR, K.B., ISRAELS, L.G.: A receptor for Fc on mouse B-lymphocytes. J. Immunol. **108**, 1319–1327 (1972)

PARKHOUSE, R.M.E., JANOSSY, G., GREAVES, M.F.: Selective stimulation of IgM synthesis in mouse B lymphocytes by pokeweed mitogen. Nature **235**, 21–23 (1972)

PARROTT, D.M.V., DE SOUSA, M.A.B.: Changes in the thymus-dependent areas of lymph nodes after immunological stimulation. Nature (Lond.) **212**, 1316–1317 (1966)

PARROTT, D.M.V., DE SOUSA, M.A.B.: The persistence of donor-derived cells in thymus grafts, lymph nodes and spleens of recipient mice. Immunology **13**, 193–200 (1967)

PARROTT, D.M.V., DE SOUSA, M.A.B.: The source of cells within different areas of lymph nodes draining the site of primary stimulation with a contact sensitizing agent. In: Lymphatic Tissue and Germinal Centers in Immune Response. Advances in Experimental Medicine and Biology, Vol. 5, pp. 293–307. FIORE-DONATI, L., HANNA, JR., M.G., Eds. New York: Plenum Press 1969

PARROTT, D.M.V., DE SOUSA, M.: Thymus-dependent and thymus-independent populations: Origin, migratory patterns and lifespan. Clin. exp. Immunol. **8**, 663–684 (1971)

PARROTT, D.M.V., DE SOUSA, M.A.B., EAST, J.: Thymus-dependent areas in the lymphoid organs of neonatally thymectomized mice. J. exp. Med. **123**, 191–204 (1966)

PARWARESCH, M.R., MÜLLER-HERMELINK, H.K., DESAGA, J.F., ZAKARI, V., LENNERT, K.: Die Herkunft der Gewebsmastzellen bei der Ratte, zugleich ein Beitrag zur quantitativen Cytologie der sterilen Peritonitis. Virchows Arch. B **8**, 20–35 (1971)

PENFOLD, P.L., GREENBERG, A.H., ROITT, I.M.: Characteristics of the effector cells mediating cytotoxicity against antibody-coated target cells. III. Ultrastructural studies. Clin. exp. Immunol. **23**, 91–97 (1976)

PEREY, D.Y.E., FINSTAD, J., POLLARA, B., GOOD, R.A.: Evolution of the immune response. VI. First and second set skin homograft rejections in primitive fishes. Lab. Invest. **19**, 591–597 (1968)

PERLMANN, P., HOLM, G.: Cytotoxic effects of lymphoid cells in vitro. Advanc. Immunol. **11**, 117–193 (1969)

PERLMANN, P., PERLMANN, H.: Contactual lysis of antibody-coated chicken erythrocytes by purified lymphocytes. Cell. Immunol. **1**, 300–315 (1970)

PERLMANN, P., PERLMANN, H., WIGZELL, H.: Lymphocyte mediated cytotoxicity in vitro. Induction and inhibition by humoral antibody and nature of effector cells. Transplant. Rev. **13**, 91–114 (1972)

PERNIS, B.: The immunoglobulins present in the germinal centers. In: Germinal Centers in Immune Responses, pp. 112–119. COTTIER, H., ODARTCHENKO, N., SCHINDLER, R., CONGDON, C.C., Eds. Berlin-Heidelberg-New York: Springer 1967

PERNIS, B., FORNI, L., AMANTE, L.: Immunoglobulin spots on the surface of rabbit lymphocytes. J. exp. Med. **132**, 1001–1018 (1970)

PETERSON, R.D.A., COOPER, M.D., GOOD, R.A.: The pathogenesis of immunologic deficiency diseases. Amer. J. Med. **38**, 579–604 (1965)

DE PETRIS, S., KARLSBAD, G., PERNIS, B.: Localization of antibodies in plasma cells by electron microscopy. J. exp. Med. **117**, 849–862 (1963)

PLAYFAIR, J.H.L.: Cell cooperation in the immune response. Clin. exp. Immunol. **8**, 839–856 (1971)

POLLARD, M.: Immunologic activation of Peyer's patches in germfree mice. [Abstract] Fed. Proc. **29**, 811 (1970)

POLLIACK, A., LAMPEN, N., CLARKSON, B.D., DE HARVEN, E., BENTWICH, Z., SIEGAL, F.P., KUNKEL, H.G.: Identification of human B and T lymphocytes by scanning electron microscopy. J. exp. Med. **138**, 607–624 (1973)

POPP, R.A.: Repopulation of thymus by immunologically competent cells derived from donor marrow. Proc. Soc. exp. Biol. (N.Y.) **108**, 561–564 (1961)

POTWOROWSKI, E.F., LEFEBVRE, D., LUSSIER, G., TEODORCZYK, J.A.: Inhibition of T-cell differentiation by an antibody to a soluble thymic factor. Immunology **28**, 1115–1121 (1975)

QUEISSER, W., NOESKE, K., SANDRITTER, W., LENNERT, K.: Cytophotometrische Untersuchungen des DNS-, Histon- und Gesamtproteingehalts von Epitheloidzellen, Gewebsmastzellen und von Zellen der Plasmocytopoiese bei käsiger Lymphknotentuberkulose. Klin. Wschr. **45**, 1135–1142 (1967)

RABELLINO, E., COLON, S., GREY, H.M., UNANUE, E.R.: Immunoglobulins on the surface of lymphocytes. I. Distribution and quantitation. J. exp. Med. **133**, 156–167 (1971)

RABENHORST, G.: Fermentzytochemische Untersuchungen zur Herkunft und Entwicklung von Makrophagen und Fremdkörperriesenzellen bei Ratten. Inaug.-Diss. Kiel 1972

RACZ, P., KAISERLING, E., TENNER, K., WUTHE, H.H.: Experimental Listeria monocytogenes-lymphadenitis. Pathohistological observations. Virchows Arch. A **363**, 135–148 (1974)

RESCH, K., GELFAND, E.W., PRESTER, M.: Antibody-mediated target cell lysis by nonimmune cells: The use of anti-immunoglobulin to distinguish effector cell populations. J. Immunol. **112**, 792–803 (1974)

REYES, F., LEJONC, J.L., GOURDIN, M.F., MANNONI, P., DREYFUS, B.: The surface morphology of human B lymphocytes as revealed by immunoelectron microscopy. J. exp. Med. **141**, 392–410 (1975)

RIETHMÜLLER, G., RIEBER, E.P., RIETHMÜLLER, D.: Untersuchungen zur Heterogenität humaner Lymphocyten: Trennung peripherer Lymphocyten im Albumindichtegradienten und Untersuchung der einzelnen Zellpopulationen auf ihre proliferative Reaktion in vitro. Klin. Wschr. **48**, 1343–1349 (1970)

RIND, H.: Histochemie der Lymphocytenglanzkörner. Klin. Wschr. **33**, 731–732 (1955)

RINNEBERG, H.: Adenosintriphosphatase, 5-Nukleotidase und Glycerophosphatase im Schnitt und Ausstrich menschlicher Lymphknoten. Diss. med., Frankfurt 1961

RÖHLICH, K.: Beitrag zur Cytologie der Keimzentren der Lymphknoten. Z. mikr.-anat. Forsch. **20**, 287–297 (1930)

ROELANTS, G.E., MAYOR, K.S., HÄGG, L.-B., LOOR, F.: Ontogeny of T lymphocytes studied in athymic and foetal mice. In: Immune Reactivity of Lymphocytes. Advances in Experimental Medicine and Biology, Vol. 66, pp. 59–62. FELDMAN, M., GLOBERSON, A., Eds. New York-London: Plenum Press 1976

ROHR, K.: Das menschliche Knochenmark. 3. Ed. Stuttgart: G. Thieme 1960

ROSSE, C.: Lymphocyte production and life-span in the bone marrow of the guinea pig. Blood **38**, 372–377 (1971)

ROWE, D.S., HUG, K., FORNI, L., PERNIS, B.: Immunoglobulin D as a lymphocyte receptor. J. exp. Med. **138**, 965–972 (1973)

RUBINSTEIN, A.S., TROBAUGH, JR, F.E.: Ultrastructure of presumptive hematopoietic stem cells. Blood **42**, 61–80 (1973)

RUHENSTROTH-BAUER, G., LÜCKE-HUHLE, C.: Two populations of small lymphocytes. J. Cell Biol. **37**, 196–199 (1968)

SANDERSON, C.J., TAYLOR, G.A.: Antibody-dependent cell-mediated cytotoxicity in the rat. The role of macrophages. Immunology **30**, 117–121 (1976)

SANDILANDS, G.P., GRAY, K., COONEY, A., BROWNING, J.D., GRANT, R.M., ANDERSON, J.R.: Lymphocytes with T and B cell properties in a lymphoproliferative disorder. Lancet 1974, I, pp. 903–904

SARIN, P.S., GALLO, R.C.: Terminal deoxynucleotidyltransferase in chronic myelogenous leukemia. J. biol. Chem. **249**, 8051–8053 (1974)

SCHICK, P.: Lymphocytenkinetik bei lymphatischen Systemerkrankungen (chronische lymphatische Leukämie, Lymphogranulomatose). Verh. dtsch. Ges. inn. Med. **79**, 154–158 (1973)

SCHMIDT, M.E., DOUGLAS, S.D., RUBIN, A.D.: Human monocyte activation by supernatants from Concanavalin A (Con A) stimulated lymphocytes. Cell. Immunol. **9**, 45–59 (1973)

SCHULZE, W.: Untersuchungen über die Capillaren und postcapillären Venen lymphatischer Organe. Z. Anat. Entwickl.-Gesch. **76**, 421–462 (1925)

SCOTHORNE, R.J., MCGREGOR, I.A.: Cellular changes in lymph nodes and spleen following skin homografting in the rabbit. J. Anat. (Lond.) **89**, 283–292 (1955)

SEILER, F.R., SEDLACEK, H.H., KANZY, E.J., LANG, W.: Über die Brauchbarkeit immunologischer Nachweismethoden zur Differenzierung funktionell verschiedener Lymphozyten: Spontanrosetten, Komplementrezeptor-Rosetten und Immunglobulinrezeptoren. Behring Inst. Mitt. **52**, 26–72 (1972)

SERCARZ, E.E., WILLIAMSON, A.R., FOX, C.F. (Eds.): The Immune System – Genes, Receptors, Signals. New York: Academic Press 1974

SHARP, J.G., THOMAS, D.B., BRISCOE, C.V.: An approach to the morphological characterisation of the haematopoietic stem cell. J. Anat. (Lond.) **108**, 597–598 (1971)

SHELDON, P.J., HOLBOROW, E.J.: H-rosette formation in T-cell-proliferative diseases. Brit. med. J. 1975, IV, pp. 381–383

SHEVACH, E., EDELSON, R., FRANK, M., LUTZNER, M., GREEN, I.: A human leukemia cell with both B and T cell surface receptors. Proc. nat. Acad. Sci. (Wash.) **71**, 863–866 (1974)

SHEVACH, E.M., JAFFE, E.S., GREEN, I.: Receptors for complement and immunoglobulin on human and animal lymphoid cells. Transplant. Rev. **16**, 3–28 (1973)

SILVEIRA, N.P.A., MENDES, N.F., TOLNAI, M.E.A.: Tissue localization of two populations of human lymphocytes distinguished by membrane receptors. J. Immunol. **108**, 1456–1460 (1972)

SILVERSTEIN, A.M., PRENDERGAST, R.A.: The maturation of lymphoid tissue structure and function in ontogeny. In: Morphological and Functional Aspects of Immunity. Advances in Experimental Medicine and Biology, Vol. 12, pp. 37–42. LINDAHL-KIESSLING, G., ALM, G., HANNA, JR., M.G., Eds. New York-London: Plenum Press 1971

SORDAT, B., HESS, M.W., COTTIER, H.: IgG immunoglobulin in the wall of post-capillary venules: Possible relationship to lymphocyte recirculation. Immunology **20**, 115–118 (1971)

DE SOUSA, M.: Kinetics of the distribution of thymus and marrow cells in the peripheral lymphoid organs of the mouse: Ecotaxis. Clin. exp. Immunol. **9**, 371–380 (1971)

DE SOUSA, M.A.B.: Ecology of thymus dependency. In: Contemporary Topics in Immunobiology, Vol. 2, pp. 119–136. DAVIES, A.J.S., CARTER, R.L., Eds. New York-London: Plenum Press 1973

SPECTOR, W.G., MARIANO, M.: Macrophage behaviour in experimental granulomas. In: Mononuclear Phagocytes in Immunity, Infection, and Pathology, pp. 927–938. VAN FURTH, R., Ed. Oxford-London-Edinburgh-Melbourne: Blackwell 1975

STEIN, G., FLAD, H.D., PABST, R., TREPEL, F.: Separation of human lymphocytes according to their surface charge. Exp. Hemat. **1**, 266 (1973)

STEIN, H., MÜLLER-HERMELINK, H.K.: Simultaneous presence of receptors for complement and sheep red blood cells on human fetal thymocytes. Brit. J. Haemat. **36**, 227–233 (1977)

STEIN, H., PETERSEN, N.: Demonstration of three groups of human blood lymphocytes with double markers using the mixed rosette technique and a critical evaluation of the method. 1975, unpublished data.

STEPHAN, R., BLÜMCKE, S.: Elektronenhistochemischer Nachweis der sauren Phosphatase in Keimzentren menschlicher Tonsillen. Z. Zellforsch. **115**, 114–136 (1971)

STUART, A.E.: The Reticulo-Endothelial System. Edinburgh-London: Livingstone 1970

STUART, A.: Perspectives on the reticulum cell and fibre networks. In: Mononuclear Phagocytes in Immunity, Infection, and Pathology, pp. 111–118. VAN FURTH, R., Ed. Oxford-London-Edinburgh-Melbourne: Blackwell 1975

STUTMAN, O., YUNIS, E.J., GOOD, R.A.: Studies on thymus function. III. Duration of thymic function. J. exp. Med. **135**, 339–356 (1972)

SULLIVAN, A.K., ADAMS, L.S., SILKE, I., JERRY, L.M.: 'Hairy' B cell and 'smooth' T cells. New Engl. J. Med. **290**, 689–690 (1974)

SUTHERLAND, D.E.R., ARCHER, O.K., GOOD, R.A.: Role of the appendix in development of immunologic capacity. Proc. Soc. exp. Biol. (N.Y.) **115**, 673–676 (1964)

SWARTZENDRUBER, D.C.: Desmosomes in germinal centers of mouse spleen. Exp. Cell Res. **40**, 429–432 (1965)

SWARTZENDRUBER, D.C.: Observations on the ultrastructure of lymphatic tissue germinal centers. In: Germinal Centers in Immune Responses, pp. 71–76. COTTIER, H., ODARTCHENKO, N., SCHINDLER, R., CONGDON, C.C., Eds. Berlin-Heidelberg-New York: Springer 1967

TAMAOKI, N., ESSNER, E.: Distribution of acid phosphatase, β-glucuronidase and N-acetyl-β-glucosaminidase activities in lymphocytes of lymphatic tissues of man and rodents. J. Histochem. Cytochem. **17**, 238–243 (1969)

TANAKA, Y., EPSTEIN, L.B., BRECHER, G., STOHLMAN, JR., F.: Transformation of lymphocytes in cultures of human peripheral blood. Blood **22**, 614–629 (1963)

TAUSSIG, M.J.: A model for genetic control of the immune response. In: Immune Reactivity of Lymphocytes. Advances in Experimental Medicine and Biology, Vol. 66, pp. 551–553. FELDMAN, M., GLOBERSON, A., Eds. New York-London: Plenum Press 1976

THIEDE, A., MÜLLER-HERMELINK, H.K., SONNTAG, H.G., MÜLLER-RUCHHOLTZ, W., LEDER, L.-D.: Zur Entstehung von Gewebsmastzellen. Beitr. Path. **143**, 172–182 (1971)

THOMAS, D.B.: The radiation chimera as an experimental model for the study of haemopoietic stem cell populations. In: Haemopoietic Stem Cells. Ciba Foundation Symposium 13 (new series), pp. 71–99. Amsterdam-London-New York: Elsevier, Excerpta Medical, North-Holland 1973

THOMAS, E.D., FLIEDNER, T.M., THOMAS, D., CRONKITE, E.P.: The problem of the stem cell: Observations in dogs following nitrogen mustard. J. Lab. clin. Med. **65**, 794–803 (1965)

TITTOR, W., WALFORD, R.L.: Synergistic response between thymus and lymph node cells in the mixed lymphocyte culture. Nature **247**, 371–373 (1974)

TRENTIN, J.J., FAHLBERG, W.J.: An experimental model for studies of immunologic competence in irradiated mice repopulated with 'clones' of spleen cells. In: Conceptual Advances in Immunology and Oncology. CUMLEY, R.W., ALDRIDGE, D.M., HAROZ, J., MCCAY, J., Eds. New York: Hoeber Medical Books 1963 cited by TRENTIN, J.J.: Influence of hematopoietic organ stroma (hematopoietic inductive microenvironments) on stem cell differentiation. In: Regulation of Hematopoieses, Vol. 1: Red Cell Production, pp. 161–186. GORDON, A.S., Ed. New York: Appleton-Century-Crofts 1970

TREPEL, F.: Kinetik der Lymphocyten. Verh. dtsch. Ges. inn. Med. **79**, 105–111 (1973)

TREPEL, F.: Number and distribution of lymphocytes in man. A critical analysis. Klin. Wschr. **52**, 511–515 (1974)

TURK, J.L.: Delayed Hypersensitivity. Frontiers of Biology, Vol. 4. Amsterdam: North-Holland 1967

TURK, J.L., WATERS, M.F.R.: Immunological significance of changes in lymph nodes across the leprosy spectrum. Clin. exp. Immunol. **8**, 363–376 (1971)

UHLENBRUCK, G., WERNET, P., SCHUMACHER, K.: Specific T-cell marking by Helix pomatia agglutinin after neuraminidase treatment. Klin. Wschr. **51**, 1210–1211 (1973)

UNANUE, E.R.: Secretory function of mononuclear phagocytes. Amer. J. Path. **83**, 396–417 (1976)

URSO, P., CONGDON, C.C.: The effect of the amount of isologous bone marrow injected on the recovery of hematopoietic organs, survival and body weight after lethal irradiation injury in mice. Blood **12**, 251–260 (1957)

VALDIMARSSON, H., AGNARSDOTTIR, G., LACHMANN, P.J.: Measles virus receptor on human T lymphocytes. Nature **255**, 554–556 (1975)

VASSAR, P.S., LEVY, E.M., BROOKS, D.E.: Studies on the electrophoretic separability of B and T human lymphocytes. Cell. Immunol. **21**, 257–271 (1976)

VEERMAN, A.J.P.: On the interdigitating cells in the thymus dependent area of the rat spleen: A relation between the mononuclear phagocyte system and T-lymphocytes. Cell Tiss. Res. **148**, 247–257 (1974)

VELDMAN, J.E.: Histophysiology and Electron Microscopy of the Immune Response. Thesis, Groningen 1970. Groningen: N.V. Boekdrukkerij Dijkstra Niemeyer 1970

WAKEFIELD, J.D., THORBECKE, G.J.: Relationship of germinal centers in lymphoid tissue to immunological memory. I. Evidence for the formation of small lymphocytes upon transfer of primed splenic white pulp to syngeneic mice. J. exp. Med. **128**, 153–169 (1968a)

WAKEFIELD, J.D., THORBECKE, G.J.: Relationship of germinal centers in lymphoid tissue to immunological memory. II. The detection of primed cells and their proliferation upon cell transfer to lethally irradiated syngeneic mice. J. exp. Med. **128**, 171–187 (1968b)

WAKSMAN, B.H., ARNASON, B.G., JANKOVIĆ, B.D.: Role of the thymus in immune reactions in rats. III. Changes in the lymphoid organs of thymectomized rats. J. exp. Med. **116**, 187–206 (1962)

WALDMANN, H., MUNRO, A.: The inter-relationship of antigenic structure, thymus-independence and adjuvanticity. IV. A general model for B-cell induction. Immunology **28**, 509–522 (1975)

WALLIS, V.J., LEUCHARS, E., CHWALINSKI, S., DAVIES, A.J.S.: On the sparse seeding of bone marrow and thymus in radiation chimaeras. Transplant. **19**, 2–11 (1975)

WARNER, N.L.: Membrane immunoglobulins and antigen receptors on B and T lymphocytes. Advanc. Immunol. **19**, 67–216 (1974)

WARNER, N.L., SZENBERG, A., BURNET, F.M.: The immunological role of different lymphoid organs in the chicken. I. Dissociation of immunological responsiveness. Aust. J. exp. Biol. med. Sci. **40**, 373–388 (1962)

WATANABE, Y., TAMAOKI, N., HABU, S., TASHIRO, Y., AKATSUKA, S., ENOMOTO, Y.: Fine structural study on human T- and B-lymphocytes. Acta haemat. jap. **37**, 655–666 (1974)

WEINER, M.S., BIANCO, C., NUSSENZWEIG, V.: Enhanced binding of neuraminidase-treated sheep erythrocytes to human T lymphocytes. Blood **42**, 939–946 (1973)

WEISSMAN, I.L., GUTMAN, G.A., FRIEDBERG, S.H., JERABEK, L.: Lymphoid tissue architecture. III. Germinal centers, T cells, and thymus-dependent vs thymus-independent antigens. In: Immune Reactivity of Lymphocytes. Advances in Experimental Medicine and Biology, Vol. 66, pp. 229–237. FELDMAN, M., GLOBERSON, A., Eds. New York-London: Plenum Press 1976

WERB, Z., GORDON, S.: Secretion of a specific collagenase by stimulated macrophages. J. exp. Med. **142**, 346–360 (1975a)

WERB, Z., GORDON, S.: Elastase secretion by stimulated macrophages. J. exp. Med. **142**, 361–377 (1975b)

WHITE, R.G.: The relation of the cellular responses in germinal or lymphocytopoietic centres of lymph nodes to the production of antibody. In: Mechanisms of Antibody Formation, pp. 25–29. HOLUB, M., JAROŠKOVÁ, L. Eds. Prague: Publishing House Czech. Acad. Sci. 1960 (Distrib., New York: Academic Press)

WHITTINGHAM, S., MACKAY, I.R.: Rosette formation by human thymocytes. Cell. Immunol. **6**, 362–367 (1973)

WIIG, J.N.: Electrophoresis of lymphoid cells. Differences in the cell membrane structure of murine thymocytes, T and B cells revealed by enzyme and formalin treatment. Clin. exp. Immunol. **22**, 91–101 (1975)

WIIG, J.N., THUNOLD, S.: Electrophoresis of lymphoid cells. Characterization of human B and T cells in peripheral lymphoid tissues. Clin. exp. Immunol. **15**, 497–506 (1973)

WILLIAMS, JR., R.C., DEBOARD, J.R., MELLBYE, O.J., MESSNER, R.P., LINDSTRÖM, F.D.: Studies of T- and B-lymphocytes in patients with connective tissue diseases. J. clin. Invest. **52**, 283–295 (1973)

WILLIAMS, D., WILLIAMS, W.J., WILLIAMS, J.E.: Enzyme histochemistry of epithelioid cells in sarcoidosis and sarcoid-like granulomas. J. Path. **97**, 705–709 (1969)

WILSON, J.D., NOSSAL, G.J.V.: Identification of human T and B lymphocytes in normal peripheral blood and in chronic lymphocytic leukaemia. Lancet 1971, II, pp. 788–791

WOODRUFF, J., GESNER, B.M.: Lymphocytes: Circulation altered by trypsin. Science **161**, 176–178 (1968)

WOODRUFF, J.J., GESNER, B.M.: The effect of neurminidase on the fate of transfused lymphocytes. J. exp. Med. **129**, 551–567 (1969)

WU, A.M., TILL, J.E., SIMINOVITCH, L., MCCULLOCH, E.A.: A cytological study of the capacity for differentiation of normal hemopoietic colony-forming cells. J. cell. Physiol. **69**, 177–184 (1967)

WU, A.M., TILL, J.E., SIMINOVITCH, L., MCCULLOCH, E.A.: Cytological evidence for a relationship between normal hematopoietic colony-forming cells and cells of the lymphoid system. J. exp. Med. **127**, 455–464 (1968)

WYBRAN, J., FUDENBERG, H.H.: Thymus-derived rosette forming cells. New Engl. J. Med. **288**, 1072–1073 (1973)

YAMORI, T.: On phagocytes: Their structures and participation in inflammation. Acta path. jap. **14**, 1–43 (1964)

YATA, J., TSUKIMOTO, I., TACHIBANA, T.: Human lymphocyte subpopulations. Human thymus-lymphoid tissue (HTL) antigen-positive lymphocytes forming rosettes with sheep erythrocytes and HTL antigen-negative lymphocytes interacting with antigen-antibody-complement complexes. Clin. exp. Immunol. **14**, 319–326 (1973)

YOFFEY, J.M.: Stem cell role of the lymphocyte-transitional cell (LT) compartment. In: Haemopoietic Stem Cells. Ciba Foundation Symposium 13 (new series), pp. 5–39. Amsterdam-London-New York: Elsevier, Excerpta Medica, North-Holland 1973

YOFFEY, J.M., HUDSON, G., OSMOND, D.G.: The lymphocyte in guinea-pig bone marrow. J. Anat. (Lond.) **99**, 841–860 (1965)

YOFFEY, J.M., WINTER, G.C.B., OSMOND, D.G., MEEK, E.S.: Morphological studies in the culture of human leucocytes with phytohaemagglutinin. Brit. J. Haemat. **11**, 488–497 (1965)

YOSHIDA, T.O., ANDERSSON, B.: Evidence for a receptor recognizing antigen complexed immunoglobulin on the surface of activated mouse thymus lymphocytes. Scand. J. Immunol. **1**, 401–408 (1972)

YOSHIDA, Y., OSMOND, D.G.: Identity and proliferation of small lymphocyte precursors in cultures of lymphocyte-rich fractions of guinea pig bone marrow. Blood **37**, 73–86 (1971)

ZIGHELBOIM, J., BONAVIDA, B., FAHEY, J.L.: Evidence for several cell populations active in antibody dependent cellular cytotoxicity. J. Immunol. **111**, 1737–1742 (1973)

ZUCKER-FRANKLIN, D., GRUSKY, G., L'ESPERANCE, P.: Granulocyte colonies derived from lymphocyte fractions of normal human peripheral blood. Blood **42**, 1010 (1973)

# References

## *Parts Two, Three and Four*


ABLASHI, D.V., DE THÉ, G.B., EASTON, J.M., LIABEUF, A., LEVINE, P.H., ARMSTRONG, G.R.: Antibodies to Epstein-Barr virus (EBV) antigens in sera of American Burkitt lymphoma patients. Biomedicine **20**, 288–293 (1974)

AHLSTRÖM, C.G.: Gleichzeitiges Vorkommen eines Retikelzellsarkoms und einer lymphatischen Leukämie. Virchows Arch. path. Anat. **301**, 49–61 (1938)

AISENBERG, A.C.: Malignant lymphoma. New Engl. J. Med. **288**, 883–890, 935–941 (1973)

AISENBERG, A.C., BLOCH, K.J.: Immunoglobulins on the surface of neoplastic lymphocytes. New Engl. J. Med. **287**, 272–276 (1972)

AISENBERG, A.C., BLOCH, K.J., LONG, J.C.: Cell-surface immunoglobulins in chronic lymphocytic leukemia and allied disorders. Amer. J. Med. **55**, 184–191 (1973)

AISENBERG, A.C., LONG, J.C.: Lymphocyte surface characteristics in malignant lymphoma. Amer. J. Med. **58**, 300–306 (1975)

AKAZAKI, K.: Reticulosarcoma. (Japanese) Byorigaku Zasshi **2**, 483–515 (1943), cit. of AKAZAKI, 1953

AKAZAKI, K.: Tumors of the reticulo-endothelial system. Acta path. jap. **3**, 24–43 (1953)

AKAZAKI, K.: Reticulosarcoma in Japan. In: Malignant Diseases of the Hematopoietic System. GANN Monograph on Cancer Research, Vol. 15, pp. 71–82. AKAZAKI, K., RAPPAPORT, H., BERARD, C.W., BENNETT, J.M., ISHIKAWA, E., Eds. Tokyo: University of Tokyo Press 1973

AKAZAKI, K., WAKASA, H.: Pathological studies of tumors of RES in Japan. Tohoku J. exp. Med. **82**, 21–41 (1964)

AKAZAKI, K., WAKASA, H.: Frequency of lymphoreticular tumors and leukemias in Japan. J. nat. Cancer Inst. **52**, 339–343 (1974)

VON ALBERTINI, A., RÜTTNER, J.R.: Über das Wesen des großfollikulären Lymphoblastoms (Brill-Symmers-Disease). Dtsch. med. Wschr. **75**, 27–29 (1950)

ALY, F.W., BRAUN, H.J., MISSMAHL, H.P.: Amyloid involvement and monoclonal immunoglobulins. Curr. Probl. Immunol., Bayer-Symp. I, 295–301 (1969)

ANDAY, G.J., GOODMAN, J.R., TISHKOFF, G.H.: An unusual cytoplasmic ribosomal structure in pathologic lymphocytes. Blood **41**, 439–449 (1973)

ANDAY, G.J., SCHMITZ, H.L.: Follicular lymphoma with transient leukemic phase. Brief review of literature and report of a case. Arch. intern. Med. **89**, 621–634 (1952)

ANDERSEN, P.E.: Extramedullary plasmocytomas. Acta radiol. (Stockh.) **32**, 365–374 (1949)

ANDERSON, R.E., WALFORD, R.L.: Fibroblastic type of leukemic reticuloendotheliosis. Cancer (Philad.) **16**, 993–997 (1963)

ANDRÉ, R., DREYFUS, B.: La ponction ganglionnaire. Atlas de cytologie ganglionnaire pathologique. Expansion scientifique française 1955

APITZ, K.: Die Leukämien als Neubildungen. Virchows Arch. path. Anat. **299**, 1–69 (1937a)

APITZ, K: Über die Bildung Russellscher Körperchen in den Plasmazellen multipler Myelome. (2. Beitrag zur Pathologie des Zellkernes.) Virchows Arch. path. Anat. **300**, 113–129 (1937b)

APITZ, K.: Allgemeine Pathologie der menschlichen Leukämien. Ergebn. allg. Path. path. Anat. **35**, 1–104 (1940)

ARESU, M., SCALABRINO, R.: Iperplasie e sarcomatosi delle ghiandole linfatiche. Tumori **1**, 307–345 u. 403–571 (1927)

ARSENAU, J.C., CANELLOS, G.P., BANKS, P.M., BERARD, C.W., GRALNICK, H.R., DEVITA, JR., V.T.: American Burkitt's lymphoma: A clinicopathologic study of 30 cases. I. Clinical factors relating to prolonged survival. Amer. J. Med. **58**, 314–321 (1975)

ASTALDI, G., BERNARDELLI, E., RONDANELLI, E.G.: Ricerche sul contenuto in glicogeno delle cellule del sangue e del midollo osseo. Haematologica **36**, 749–771 (1952)

ASTALDI, G., VERGA, L.: The glycogen content of the cells of lymphatic leukaemia. Acta haemat. (Basel) **17**, 129–135 (1957)

AUR, R.J.A., PINKEL, D.: Total therapy of acute lymphocytic leukemia. Progr. clin. Cancer **5**, 155–170 (1973)

AZAR, H.A.: Pathology of multiple myeloma and related growths. In: Multiple Myeloma and Related Disorders, Vol. 1, pp. 1–85. AZAR, H.A., POTTER, M., Eds. New York: Harper & Row 1973

AZAR, H.A., HILL, W.T., OSSERMAN, E.F.: Malignant lymphoma and lymphatic leukemia associated with myeloma-type serum proteins. Amer. J. Med. **23**, 239–249 (1957)

BACCAREDDA, A.: Reticulohistiocytosis cutanea hyperplastica benigna cum melanodermia. Arch. Derm. Syph. (Berl.) **179**, 209–256 (1939)

BALLARD, H.S., HAMILTON, L.M., MARCUS, A.J., ILLES, C.H.: A new variant of heavy-chain disease ($\mu$-chain disease). New Engl. J. Med. **282**, 1060–1062 (1970)

BARANDUN, S., SORDAT, B., SPENGLER, G.A.: The giant follicular lymphoma (Brill-Symmers' disease). In: Germinal Centers in Immune Responses, pp. 447–449. COTTIER, H., ODARTCHENKO, N., SCHINDLER, R., KONGDON, C.C., Eds. Berlin-Heidelberg-New York: Springer 1967

BARCOS, M.P., LUKES, R.J.: Malignant lymphoma of convoluted lymphocytes: A new entity of possible T-cell type. In: Conflicts in Childhood Cancer. An Evaluation of Current Management, Vol. 4, pp. 147–178. SINKS, L.F., GODDEN, J.O., Eds. New York: Liss 1975

BASSET, A., SCAPIER, J.: Sur un cas d'un plasmocytome cervical. Monde méd. **47**, 7–8 (1937)

BAUER-SIC, P., LAMBERS, K.: Zur Glykogenverteilung in Blutzellen. In: Zyto- und Histochemie in der Hämatologie, pp. 426–431. MERKER, H., Ed. Berlin-Göttingen-Heidelberg: Springer 1963

BEARD, M.E.J.: A tentative classification of the non-Hodgkin's tumors of the lymphoid system to enable inclusion of the lymphoid leukaemias. Brit. J. Cancer **31**, Suppl. II, 94–95 (1975)

BECKER, E. Ein Beitrag zur Lehre von den Lymphomen. Dtsch. med. Wschr. **27**, 726–728 (1901)

BECKMANN, H., LANDBECK, G., NETH, R., SCHMIDTKE, H.: Akute Leukämien mit erythropoetischen Differenzierungsmerkmalen. Ein Beitrag zur Differenzierung der Leukämien des Kindesalters. Mschr. Kinderheilk. **119**, 8–13 (1971)

BELPOMME, D., DANTCHEV, D., DU RUSQUEC, E., GRANDJON, D., HUCHET, R., PINON, F., POUILLART, P., SCHWARZENBERG, L., AMIEL, J.-L., MATHÉ, G.: La nature T ou B des cellules néoplasiques des leucémies lymphoides. Bull. Cancer **61**, 387–402 (1974)

BEN-BASSAT, H., GOLDBLUM, N., MITRANI, S., GOLDBLUM, T., YOFFEY, J.M., COHEN, M.M., BENTWICH, Z., RAMOT, B., KLEIN, E., KLEIN, G.: Establishment in continuous culture of a new type of lymphocyte from a "Burkitt-like" malignant lymphoma (Line D.G.-75). Int. J. Cancer **19**, 27–33 (1977)

BENNETT, J.M.: Discussion for: CATOVSKY, D., FRISCH, B., VAN NOORDEN, S.: B, T and 'null' cell leukaemias. Electron cytochemistry and surface morphology. Blood Cells **1**, 125 (1975)

BENNETT, J.M., REED, C.E.: Acute leukemia cytochemical profile: Diagnostic and clinical implications. Blood Cells **1**, 101–108 (1975)

BENNETT, M.H.: Discussion. Workshop on Non-Hodgkin's Lymphomas, Chicago, June 1973

BENNETT, M.H.: Sclerosis in non-Hodgkin's lymphomata. Brit. J. Cancer **31**, Suppl. II, 44–52 (1975a)

BENNETT, M.H.: Sclerosis in non-Hodgkin's lymphomas. 5th Congr. Europ. Soc. Path., Vienna 1975b

BENNETT, M.H., FARRER-BROWN, G., HENRY, K., JELLIFFE, A.M.: Classification of non-Hodgkin's lymphomas. [Letter to the Editor.] Lancet 1974, II, pp. 405–406

BENNETT, M.H., MILLETT, Y.L.: Nodular sclerotic lymphosarcoma. A possible new clinico-pathological entity. Clin. Radiol. **20**, 339–343 (1969)

BENTWICH, Z., KUNKEL, H.G.: Specific properties of human B and T lymphocytes and alterations in disease. Transplant. Rev. **16**, 29–50 (1973)

BERARD, C.W.: Histopathology of the lymphomas. In: Hematology, pp. 901–912. WILLIAMS, W.J., BEUTLER, E., ERSLEV, A.J., RUNDLES, R.W., Eds. New York-Düsseldorf: McGraw-Hill 1972

BERARD, C.W.: Reticuloendothelial system: an overview of neoplasia. In: The Reticuloendothelial

System. Monographs in Pathology, No. 16, pp. 301–317. REBUCK, J.W., BERARD, C.W., ABELL, M.R., Eds. Baltimore: Williams & Wilkins 1975

BERARD, C.W., DORFMAN, R.F.: Histopathology of malignant lymphomas. In: Hodgkin's Disease and Other Lymphomas. Clinics in Haematology, Vol. 3,1, pp. 39–76. ROSENBERG, S.A., Ed. London-Philadelphia-Toronto: W.B.Saunders 1974

BERARD, C., O'CONOR, G.T., THOMAS, L.B., TORLONI, H.: Histopathological definition of Burkitt's tumour. Bull. Wld Hlth Org. **40**, 601–607 (1969)

BERG, B., BRANDT, L.: The cytology, distribution and function of the neoplastic cells in leukaemic reticuloendotheliosis. Scand. J. Haemat. **7**, 428–434 (1970)

BERMAN, L.: Malignant lymphomas. Their classification and relation to leukemia. Blood **8**, 195–210 (1953)

BERNARD, J.: Les sarcomes africains. Nouv. Rev. franç. Hémat. **3**, 101–104 (1963)

BERNARD, J.: La tumeur de Burkitt en 1966. Nouv. Rev. franç. Hémat. **6**, 183–186 (1966)

BERNHARD, W.: Fine structure of Burkitt's lymphoma. In: Burkitt's Lymphoma, pp. 103–117. BURKITT, D.P., WRIGHT, D.H., Eds. Edinburgh-London: Livingstone 1970

BERNHARD, W., LAMBERT, D.: Ultrastructure des tumeurs de Burkitt de l'enfant africain. In: Symposium on Lymphoreticular Tumours in Africa, Paris 1963, pp. 270–284. ROULET, F.C., Ed. Basel-New York: Karger 1964

BESSIS, M.: Contribution à l'étude cytologiques des réticulo-sarcomes. Sang **18**, 7–33 (1946)

BESSIS, M.: Études au microscope électronique des leucocytes normaux et leucémiques. Acta Un. int. Cancr. **7**, 646–659 (1951)

BESSIS, M.: Traité de cytologie sanguine. Paris: Masson & Cie. 1954

BICHEL, J., BING, J., HARBOE, N.: Another case of hyperglobulinemia and affection of the central nervous system. Acta med. scand. **138**, 1–14 (1950)

BICHEL, J., EFFERSØE, P., GORMSEN, H., HARBOE, N.: Leukemic myelomatosis (plasma cell leukemia). A review with report of four cases. Acta radiol. (Stockh.) **37**, 196–207 (1952)

BILGER, R.: Das großfollikuläre Lymphoblastom (die Brill-Symmerssche Krankheit). Ergebn. inn. Med. Kinderheilk. N.F. **5**, 642–706 (1954)

BILLINGTON, R.W., ITZHAKI, R.F.: Ribosomal RNA synthesis in chronic lymphocytic leukaemia. Brit. J. Cancer **29**, 318–323 (1974)

BINDER, R.A., JENCKS, J.A., CHUN, B., RATH, C.E.: 'B' cell origin of malignant cells in a case of American Burkitt's lymphoma. Characterization of cells from a pleural effusion. Cancer (Philad.) **36**, 161–168 (1975)

BLATRIX, C., FINE, J.-M., YEME, D., LAMBIN, P.: Les formes tumorales de la macroglobulinémie de Waldenström. À propos d'un cas comportant deux localisations, orbitaire et hépatique. Sem. Hôp. Paris **49**, 2847–2851 (1973)

BLOCK, J.B., EDGCOMB, J., EISEN, A., VAN SCOTT, E.J.: Mycosis fungoides. Natural history and aspects of its relationship to other malignant lymphomas. Amer. J. Med. **34**, 228–235 (1963)

BLOOMFIELD, C.D., GOLDMAN, A., DICK, F., BRUNNING, R.D., KENNEDY, B.J.: Multivariate analysis of prognostic factors in the non-Hodgkin's malignant lymphomas. Cancer (Philad.) **33**, 870–879 (1974)

BLUMENBERG, R.M., OLSON, K.B., STEIN, A.A., HAWKINS, T.L.: Giant follicle lymphoma. A clinicopathologic review of forty-six cases, with special emphasis on prognosis. Amer. J. Med. **35**, 832–841 (1963)

BÖSKEN, W., NOLTENIUS, H.: Großzelliges Retikulumzellsarkom als Spätzustand einer endoxanbehandelten Makroglobulinämie Waldenström. Zbl. allg. Path. **111**, 407–413 (1968)

BOGNEL, J.C., RAMBAUD, J.C., MODIGLIANI, R., MATUCHANSKY, C., BOGNEL, C., BERNIER, J.J., SCOTTO, J., HAUTEFEUILLE, P., MIHAESCO, E., HUREZ, D., PREUD'HOMME, J.L., SELIGMANN, M.: Étude clinique, anatomo-pathologique et immunochimique d'un nouveau cas de maladie des chaînes alpha suivi pendant cinq ans. Rev. europ. Étud. clin. biol. **17**, 362–374 (1972)

BOIRON, M., JACQUILLAT, C., LÉVY, D.: Bilan de l'asparaginase. In: Actualités hématol. IV, 79–86. Paris: Masson & Cie., 1970

BONHOMME, J., SELIGMANN, M., MIHAESCO, C., CLAUVEL, J.P., DANON, F., BROUET, J.C., BOUVRY, P., MARTINE, J., CLERC, M.: MU-chain disease in an African patient. Blood **43**, 485–492 (1974)

BOOTH, K., BURKITT, D.P., BASSETT, D.J., COOKE, R.A., BIDDULPH, J.: Burkitt lymphoma in Papua, New Guinea. Brit. J. Cancer **21**, 657–664 (1967)

BORELLA, L., SEN, L.: T cell surface markers on lymphoblasts from acute lymphocytic leukemia. J. Immunol. **111**, 1257–1260 (1973)

BORELLA, L., SEN, L.: T- and B-lymphocytes and lymphoblasts in untreated acute lymphocytic leukemia. Cancer (Philad.) **34**, 646–654 (1974)

BORNKAMM, G.W., STEIN, H., LENNERT, K., RÜGGEBERG, F., BARTELS, H., ZUR HAUSEN, H.: Attempts to demonstrate virus-specific sequences in human tumors. IV. EB viral DNA in European Burkitt lymphoma and immunoblastic lymphadenopathy with excessive plasmacytosis. Int. J. Cancer **17**, 177–181 (1976)

BOSMAN, F.T., VAN VLOTEN, W.A.: Sézary's syndrome: A cytogenetic, cytophotometric and autoradiographic study. J. Path. **118**, 49–57 (1975)

BOURONCLE, B.A., WISEMAN, B.K., DOAN, C.A.: Leukemic reticuloendotheliosis. Blood **13**, 609–630 (1958)

BOUSSER, J., DELARUE, J., BILSKI-PASQUIER, G., DIEBOLD, J., ZITTOUN, R., DAO, C.: Lymphome nodulaire de la rate. Nouv. Rev. franç. Hémat. **10**, 289–297 (1970)

BOUTIS, L., OBRECHT, P., MUSSHOFF, K., JOCHMANN, P.: Zur Prognose der chronischen lymphatischen Leukämie. Freiburger Ergebnisse 1946–1966. Dtsch. med. Wschr. **93**, 2111–2114 (1968)

BRABAND, H.: Der Burkitt-Tumor. Dtsch. med. J. **18**, 573–578 (1967)

BRABAND, H.: Burkitt-Tumor. Stuttgart Thieme 1968

BRADFIELD, J.W.B.: Classification of non-Hodgkin's lymphomas. [Letter to the Editor.] Lancet 1974, II, pp. 652–653

BRASS, K.: Die Eiweißstoffwechselstörungen des Plasmocytomkranken. Frankfurt. Z. Path. **57**, 367–480 (1943a)

BRASS, K.: Zur Cytologie und Funktion der Plasma- und Plasmocytomzellen. Frankfurt. Z. Path. **57**, 481–491 (1943b)

BRASS, K.: Die Eiweißstoffwechselstörungen des Plasmocytomkranken. III. Mitteilung. Frankfurt. Z. Path. **59**, 413–433 (1947/48)

BRAUN, H.J.: Beziehungen zwischen monoklonalen Gammopathien und Amyloidosen. In: Maligne Lymphome und monoklonale Gammopathien. Hämatologie und Bluttransfusion, Bd. 18, pp. 419–432. LÖFFLER, H., Ed. München: Lehmanns 1976

BRAUN, H.J., BRUCHHAUS, K.-F., ALY, F.W.: Monoklonale Makroglobulinämien. Dtsch. med. Wschr. **98**, 1835–1842 (1973)

BRAUNSTEIN, H., FREIMAN, D.G., THOMAS, JR., W., GALL, E.A.: A histochemical study of the enzymatic activity of lymph nodes. II. Further investigation of normal and hyperplastic lymph nodes. Cancer (Philad.) **15**, 130–138 (1962a)

BRAUNSTEIN, H., FREIMAN, D.G., THOMAS, JR., W., GALL, E.A.: A histochemical study of the enzymatic activity of lymph nodes. III. Granulomatous and primary neoplastic conditions of lymphoid tissue. Cancer (Philad.) **15**, 139–152 (1962b)

BRAUNSTEINER, H., SAILER, S.: Lymphatische Leukämie mit Makroglobulinämie Waldenström. Acta haemat. (Basel) **23**, 306–308 (1960)

BRAYLAN, R.C., RAPPAPORT, H.: Tissue immunoglobulins in nodular lymphomas as compared with reactive follicular hyperplasias. Blood **42**, 579–589 (1973)

BRAYLAN, R., VARIAKOJIS, D., YACHNIN, S.: The Sézary syndrome lymphoid cell: Abnormal surface properties and mitogen responsiveness. Brit. J. Haemat. **31**, 553–564 (1975)

BRECHER, G., TANAKA, Y., MALMGREN, R.A., FAHEY, J.L.: Morphology and protein synthesis in multiple myeloma and macroglobulinemia. Ann. N.Y. Acad. Sci. **113**, 642–653 (1963)

BREMER, K.: Chronische lymphatische Leukämie: Störungen der Kinetik der Lymphozyten. Pathophysiologische Aspekte und therapeutische Überlegungen. Dtsch. med. Wschr. **100**, 1250–1255 (1975)

BREMER, K., COHNEN, G., AUGENER, W., BRITTINGER, G.: Normal recirculation of T lymphocytes in chronic lymphocytic leukaemia. [Letter to the Editor.] Lancet 1975, I, p. 1247

BRILL, N.E., BAEHR, G., ROSENTHAL, N.: Generalized giant lymph follicle hyperplasia of lymph nodes and spleen. A hitherto undescribed type. Amer. J. Med. **13**, 570–574 (1952). Republished from J. Amer. med. Ass. **84**, 668–671 (1925)

BRITTIN, G.M., TANAKA, Y., BRECHER, G.: Intranuclear inclusions in multiple myeloma and macroglobulinemia. Blood **21**, 335–351 (1963)

BRITTINGER, G., BARTELS, H., BREMER, K., DÜHMKE, E., GUNZER, U., KÖNIG, E., STEIN, H. (Kieler Lymphomgruppe): Klinik der malignen Non-Hodgkin-Lymphome entsprechend der Kiel-

Klassifikation: Centrocytisches Lymphom, centroblastisch-centrocytisches Lymphom, lymphoblastisches Lymphom, immunoblastisches Lymphom. In: Maligne Lymphome und monoklonale Gammopathien. Hämatologie und Bluttransfusion, Bd. 18, pp. 211–223. LÖFFLER, H., Ed. München: Lehmanns 1976

BRITTINGER, G., KÖNIG, E., ABERLE, H.G., ZIMMERSCHITT, E.: Lysosomale Enzyme in Blutlymphozyten von Gesunden und Patienten mit chronischer Lymphadenose bei kurzdauernder unspezifischer Stimulierung in vitro. Schweiz. med. Wschr. **100**, 341–344 (1970)

BRITTINGER, G., KÖNIG, E., COHNEN, G., ABERLE, H.G.: Lysosomale Enzyme in Lymphozyten. I. Lymphoretikuläre Erkrankungen: Vergleich des Enzymgehaltes (saure Phosphatase, β-Glucuronidase) unstimulierter Blutlymphozyten mit der Blastentransformation nach Phytohämagglutinin-Stimulierung in vitro. Acta haemat. (Basel) **44**, 205–221 (1970)

BRODER, S., EDELSON, R.L., LUTZNER, M.A., NELSON, D.L., MACDERMOTT, R.P., DURM, M.E., GOLDMAN, C.K., MEADE, B.D., WALDMANN, T.A.: The Sézary syndrome. A malignant proliferation of helper T cells. J. clin. Invest. **58**, 1297–1306 (1976)

BRODY, J.I., OSKI, F.A., SINGER, D.E.: Impaired pentose phosphate shunt and decreased glycolytic activity in lymphocytes of chronic lymphocytic leukemia. Metabolic pathway ...? Blood **34**, 421–429 (1969)

BROOME, J.D., ZUCKER-FRANKLIN, D., WEINER, M.S., BIANCO, C., NUSSENZWEIG, V.: Leukemic cells with membrane properties of thymus-derived (T) lymphocytes in a case of Sézary's syndrome: Morphologic and immunologic studies. Clin. Immunol. Immunopath. **1**, 319–329 (1973)

BROUET, J.-C., FLANDRIN, G., SASPORTES, M., PREUD'HOMME, J.-L., SELIGMANN, M.: Chronic lymphocytic leukaemia of T-cell origin. Immunological and clinical evaluation in eleven patients. Lancet 1975, II, pp. 890–893

BROUET, J.-C., FLANDRIN, G., SELIGMANN, M.: Indications of the thymus-derived nature of the proliferating cells in six patients with Sézary's syndrome. New Engl. J. Med. **289**, 341–344 (1973)

BROUET, J.C., LABAUME, S., SELIGMANN, M.: Evaluation of T and B lymphocyte membrane markers in human non-Hodgkin malignant lymphomata. Brit. J. Cancer **31**, Suppl. II, 121–127 (1975)

BROUET, J.C., PREUD'HOMME, J.L., FLANDRIN, G., CHELLOUL, N., SELIGMANN, M.: Membrane markers in 'histiocytic' lymphomas (reticulum cell sarcomas). J. nat. Cancer Inst. **56**, 631–633 (1976)

BROUET, J.-C., PREUD'HOMME, J.-L., SELIGMANN, M.: The use of B and T membrane markers in the classification of human leukemias, with special reference to acute lymphoblastic leukemia. Blood Cells **1**, 81–90 (1975)

BROUET, J.-C., PREUD'HOMME, J.-L., SELIGMANN, M., BERNARD, J.: Blast cells with monoclonal surface immunoglobulin in two cases of acute blast crisis supervening on chronic lymphocytic leukaemia. Brit. med. J. 1973, IV, pp. 23–24

BROUET, J.C., PRIEUR, A.-M.: Membrane markers on chronic lymphocytic leukemia cells: A B cell leukemia with rosettes due to anti-sheep erythrocyte antibody activity of the membrane bound IgM and a T cell leukemia with surface Ig. Clin. Immunol. Immunopath. **2**, 481–487 (1974)

BROUET, J.C., TOBEN, H.R., CHEVALIER, A., SELIGMANN, M.: T and B membrane markers on blast cells in 69 patients with acute lymphoblastic leukemia. Ann. Immunol. **125C**, 691–696 (1974)

BROWN, R.S., SCHIFF, M., MITCHELL, M.S.: Reticulum-cell sarcoma of host origin arising in a transplanted kidney. Ann. intern. Med. **80**, 459–463 (1974)

BROWN, T.C., PETERS, M.V., BERGSAGEL, D.E., REID, J.: A retrospective analysis of the clinical results in relation to the Rappaport histological classification. Brit. J. Cancer **31**, Suppl. II, 174–186 (1975)

BRUCE, R.M., BLAESE, R.M.: Monoclonal gammopathy in the Wiskott-Aldrich syndrome. J. Pediat. **85**, 204–207 (1974)

BUFFA, F., RAPPAPORT, H.: Chronic lymphocytic leukemia associated with dysproteinemia and acquired hemolytic anemia. Amer. J. Med. **22**, 504–510 (1957)

BURCHENAL, J.H.: Summary of conference and implications for acute leukemia. In: Treatment of Burkitt's Tumour. UICC Monograph Series, Vol. 8, pp. 258–262. BURCHENAL, J.H., BURKITT, D.P., Eds. Berlin-Heidelberg-New York: Springer 1967

BURCHENAL, J.H., BURKITT, D.P. (Eds.): Treatment of Burkitt's Tumour. Proceedings of a Conference organized by the Chemotherapy Panel of the International Union Against Cancer. (UICC Monograph Series, Vol. 8.) Berlin-Heidelberg-New York: Springer 1967

BURCHENAL, J.H., WOLLNER, N.: Present status of research on Burkitt's tumor. In: Neoplasia in Childhood, pp. 293–303. Chicago: Year Book Medical Publ. 1969

BURKE, J.S., BYRNE, JR., G.E., RAPPAPORT, H.: Hairy cell leukemia (leukemic reticuloendotheliosis). I. A clinical pathologic study of 21 patients. Cancer (Philad.) **33**, 1399–1410 (1974)

BURKE, J.S., MACKAY, B., RAPPAPORT, H.: Hairy cell leukemia (leukemic reticuloendotheliosis). II. Ultrastructure of the spleen. Cancer (Philad.) **37**, 2267–2274 (1976)

BURKITT, D.P.: A sarcoma involving the jaws in African children. Brit. J. Surg. **46**, 218–223 (1958/59)

BURKITT, D.P.: A lymphoma syndrome in tropical Africa. With a note on histology, cytology, and histochemistry by D.H. WRIGHT. In: International Review of Experimental Pathology, Vol. 2, pp. 67–138. RICHTER, G.W., EPSTEIN, M.A., Eds. New York-London: Academic Press 1963

BURKITT, D.P.: A lymphoma syndrome dependent on environment. Part I. Clinical aspects. In: Symposium on Lymphoreticular Tumours in Africa, Paris 1963, pp. 80–93. ROULET, F.C., Ed. Basel-New York: Karger 1964a

BURKITT, D.P.: A lymphoma syndrome dependent on environment. Part II. Epidemiological features. In: Symposium on Lymphoreticular Tumours in Africa, Paris 1963, pp. 119–136. ROULET, F.C., Ed. Basel-New York: Karger 1964b

BURKITT, D.P.: Possible Relationships between the African Lymphoma and Acute Leukemia. Third guest lecture. Leukaemia Research Fund. London: Queen Anne Press 1967a

BURKITT, D.P.: African lymphoma. Epidemiological evidence suggesting a viral aetiology. In: Racial and Geographical Factors in Tumour Incidence, pp. 19–23. SHIVAS, A.A., Ed. Edinburgh: University Press 1967b

BURKITT, D.P.: Recent developments in geographical distribution. In: Treatment of Burkitt's Tumour. UICC Monograph Series, Vol. 8, pp. 36–41. BURCHENAL, J.H., BURKITT, D.P., Eds. Berlin-Heidelberg-New York: Springer 1967c

BURKITT, D.P.: Clinical demonstration of long-term survivors. In: Treatment of Burkitt's Tumour. UICC Monograph Series, Vol. 8, pp. 102–104. BURCHENAL, J.H., BURKITT, D.P., Eds. Berlin-Heidelberg-New York: Springer 1967d

BURKITT, D.P.: General features and facial tumours. In: Burkitt's Lymphoma, pp. 6–15. BURKITT, D.P., WRIGHT, D.H., Eds. Edinburgh-London: Livingstone 1970a

BURKITT, D.P.: Lesions outside the jaws. In: Burkitt's Lymphoma, pp. 16–22. BURKITT, D.P., WRIGHT, D.H., Eds. Edinburgh-London: Livingstone 1970b

BURKITT, D.P.: Treatment. General features. In: Burkitt's Lymphoma, pp. 43–51. BURKITT, D.P., WRIGHT, D.H., Eds. Edinburgh-London: Livingstone 1970c

BURKITT, D.P.: Geographical distribution. In: Burkitt's Lymphoma, pp. 186–197. BURKITT, D.P., WRIGHT, D.H., Eds. Edinburgh-London: Livingstone 1970d

BURKITT, D.P.: An alternative hypothesis to a vectored virus. In: Burkitt's Lymphoma, pp. 210–214. BURKITT, D.P., WRIGHT, D.H., Eds. Edinburgh-London: Livingstone 1970e

BURKITT, D.P., HUTT, M.S.R., WRIGHT, D.H.: The African lymphoma. Preliminary observations on response to therapy. Cancer (Philad.) **18**, 399–410 (1965)

BURKITT, D.P., O'CONOR, G.T.: Malignant lymphoma in African children. I. A clinical syndrome. Cancer (Philad.) **14**, 258–269 (1961)

BURKITT, D.P., WRIGHT, D.: Geographical and tribal distribution of the African lymphoma in Uganda. Brit. med. J. 1966, I, pp. 569–573

BURKITT, D.P., WRIGHT, D.H. (Eds.): Burkitt's lymphoma. Edinburgh-London: Livingstone 1970

BUSKARD, N.A., CATOVSKY, D., OKOS, A., GOLDMAN, J.M., GALTON, D.A.G.: Prolymphocytic leukaemia: Cell studies and treatment by leucapheresis. In: Maligne Lymphome und monoklonale Gammopathien. Hämatologie und Bluttransfusion, Bd. 18, pp. 237–253. LÖFFLER, H., Ed. München: Lehmanns 1976

BUTLER, J.J., STRYKER, J.A., SHULLENBERGER, C.C.: A clinicopathological study of Stages I and II non-Hodgkin's lymphomata using the Lukes-Collins classification. Brit. J. Cancer **31**, Suppl. II, 208–216 (1975)

BYRNE, JR., E., RAPPAPORT, H.: Malignant histiocytosis. In: Malignant Diseases of the Hematopoietic System. GANN Monograph on Cancer Research, Vol. 15, pp. 145–162. AKAZAKI, K.,

RAPPAPORT, H., BERARD, C.W., BENNETT, J.M., ISHIKAWA, E., Eds. Tokyo: University of Tokyo Press 1973

CAMAIN, R., BAYLET, R., BRES, P., LAMBERT, D.: Les hématosarcomes de la face chez l'enfant en Afrique Occidentale et Centrale francophone. III. Histopathologie, tentatives de culture et autres examens biologiques. In: Symposium on Lymphoreticular Tumours in Africa, Paris 1963, pp. 265–269. ROULET, F.C., Ed. Basel-New York: Karger 1964

CAMAIN, R., LAMBERT, D.: Les hématosarcomes de la face chez l'enfant en Afrique Occidentale et Centrale francophone. I. Considérations générales, répartition géographique, incidence de l'âge et du sexe. In: Symposium on Lymphoreticular Tumours in Africa, Paris 1963, pp. 94–100. ROULET, F.C., Ed. Basel-New York: Karger 1964

CARBONE, P.P., KAPLAN, H.S., MUSSHOFF, K., SMITHERS, D.W., TUBIANA, M.: Report of the committee on Hodgkin's disease staging classification. Cancer Res. **31**, 1860–1861 (1971)

CATOVSKY, D.: T-cell origin of acid-phosphatase-positive lymphoblasts. Lancet 1975, II, pp. 327–328

CATOVSKY, D., FRISCH, B., VAN NOORDEN, S.: B, T and 'null' cell leukaemias. Electron cytochemistry and surface morphology. Blood Cells **1**, 115–124 (1975)

CATOVSKY, D., FRISCH, B., OKOS, A., VAN NOORDEN, S.: Scanning electron microscopy and the nature of the hairy cell. [Letter to the Editor.] Lancet 1975, I, p. 462

CATOVSKY, D., GALETTO, J., OKOS, A., GALTON, D.A.G., WILTSHAW, E., STATHOPOULOS, G.: Prolymphocytic leukaemia of B and T cell type. Lancet 1973, II, pp. 232–234

CATOVSKY, D., GALETTO, J., OKOS, A., MILIANI, E., GALTON, D.A.G.: Cytochemical profile of B and T leukaemic lymphocytes with special reference to acute lymphoblastic leukaemia. J. clin. Path. **27**, 767–771 (1974)

CATOVSKY, D., GALTON, D.A.G.: Lysozyme activity and nitroblue-tetrazolium reduction in leukaemic cells. J. clin. Path. **26**, 60–69 (1973)

CATOVSKY, D., GOLDMAN, J.M., OKOS, A., FRISCH, B., GALTON, D.A.G.: T-lymphoblastic leukaemia: A distinct variant of acute leukaemia. Brit. med. J. 1974, II, pp. 643–646

CATOVSKY, D., PAPAMICHAIL, M., OKOS, A., MILIANI, E., HOLBOROW, E.J.: Formation of mouse red cell rosettes by "hairy" cells. Biomedicine **23**, 81–84 (1975)

CATOVSKY, D., PETTIT, J.E., GALETTO, J., OKOS, A., GALTON, D.A.G.: The B-lymphocyte nature of the hairy cell of leukaemic reticuloendotheliosis. Brit. J. Haemat. **26**, 29–37 (1974)

CATOVSKY, D., PETTIT, J.E., GALTON, D.A.G., SPIERS, A.S.D., HARRISON, C.V.: Leukaemic reticuloendotheliosis ('hairy' cell leukaemia): A distinct clinico-pathological entity. Brit. J. Haemat. **26**, 9–27 (1974)

ČEJKA, J., BOLLINGER, R.O., SCHUIT, H.R.E., LUSHER, J.M., CHANG, C.-H., ZUELZER, W.W.: Macroglobulinemia in a child with acute leukemia. Blood **43**, 191–199 (1974)

CHANTAR, C., ESCARTÍN, P., PLAZA, A.G., CORUGEDO, A.F., ARENAS, J.I., SANZ, E., ANAYA, A., BOOTELLO, A., SEGOVIA, J.M.: Diffuse plasma cell infiltration of the small intestine with malabsorption associated to IgA monoclonal gammapathy. Cancer (Philad.) **34**, 1620–1630 (1974)

CHELLOUL, N.: Moyens d'approche d'une classification nosologique des sarcomes ganglionnaires. Bull. Cancer **61**, 35–36 (1974)

CHELLOUL, N., DANIEL, M.T., FLANDRIN, G.: Histiolymphocytose de l'adulte ou leucémie à tricholeucocytes. Étude histologique, cytologique et ultrastructurale. Path. Europ. **8**, 235–251 (1973)

CHELLOUL, N., DIEBOLD, J., FLANDRIN, G., GÉRARD-MARCHANT, R., NEZELOF, C.: Commentaires sur la classification du centre de références de l'O.M.S. Les hématosarcomes non hodgkiniens. Ann. Anat. path. **21**, 301–304 (1976)

CHIARI, H.: Über eigentümliche Verlaufsformen von Haemoblastosen. Beitr. path. Anat. **130**, 51–68 (1964)

CHIN, A.H., SAIKI, J.H., TRUJILLO, J.M., WILLIAMS, JR., R.C.: Peripheral blood T- and B-lymphocytes in patients with lymphoma and acute leukemia. Clin. Immunol. Immunopath. **1**, 499–510 (1973)

CHURG, J., GORDON, A.J.: Multiple myeloma. Lesions of the extra-osseous hematopoietic system. Amer. J. clin. Path. **20**, 934–945 (1950)

CLAUDY, A.L.: The immunological identification of the Sézary cell. Brit. J. Derm. **91**, 597–600 (1974)

CLENDENNING, W.E., BRECHER, G., VAN SCOTT, E.J.: Mycosis fungoides. Relationship to malignant cutaneous reticulosis and the Sézary syndrome. Arch. Derm. **89**, 785–792 (1964)

CLIFFORD, P.: Malignant disease of the nose, paranasal sinuses and post-nasal space in East Africa. J. Laryng. **75**, 707–733 (1961)
CLIFFORD, P.: Treatment of Burkitt's lymphoma. Lancet 1968, I, p. 599
CLIFFORD, P.: Treatment. Response in particular chemotherapeutic and other agents and treatment of CNS involvement. In: Burkitt's Lymphoma, pp. 52–63. BURKITT, D.P., WRIGHT, D.H., Eds. Edinburgh-London: Livingstone 1970
COCCHI, U., MEIER, E.: Zur Frage der Therapie des großfollikulären Lymphoblastoms. Oncologia (Basel) **3**, 1–26 (1950)
COHEN, M.H., BENNETT, J.M., BERARD, C.W., ZIEGLER, J.L., VOGEL, C.L., SHEAGREN, J.N., CARBONE, P.P.: Burkitt's tumor in the United States. Cancer (Philad.) **23**, 1259–1272 (1969)
COHNEN, G.: Klinisch-diagnostische Bedeutung der Oberflächenmarker menschlicher T- und B-Lymphozyten. Dtsch. med. Wschr. **99**, 2302–2307 (1974)
COHNEN, G.: T- and B-Lymphozyten bei chronischer lymphatischer Leukämie und Lymphogranulomatose. Elektronenmikroskopische und immunologische Untersuchungen. Veröff. Path. H. 97. Stuttgart: G. Fischer 1975
COHNHEIM, J.: Ein Fall von Pseudoleukämie. Virchows Arch. A **33**, 451–454 (1865)
COOKE, J.V.: Mediastinal tumor in acute leukemia. A clinical and roentgenologic study. Amer. J. Dis. Child. **44**, 1153–1177 (1932)
COOPER, E.H., FRANK, G.L., WRIGHT, D.H.: Cell proliferation in Burkitt tumours. Europ. J. Cancer **2**, 377–384 (1966)
COOPER, J.H., HAQ, B.M., BAGNELL, H.: Intrafollicular hyalinosis and arterial hyalinosis of the spleen: Histochemical and immunofluorescence studies. J. Path. **98**, 193–199 (1969)
COOPER, M.D., PETERSON, R.D.A., GABRIELSEN, A.E., GOOD, R.A.: Lymphoid malignancy and development, differentiation, and function of the lymphoreticular system. Cancer Res. **26**, 1165–1169 (1966)
COTTIER, H., HESS, M.W., KELLER, H.U., LUSCIETI, P., SORDAT, B.: Immunological deficiency states and malignancy. Sympos. on "Interaction of Radiation and Host Immune Defense Mechanisms in Malignancy," Greenbrier, W.Va., March 1974
COX, J.N., WIDGREN, S.: Tumeur de Burkitt. A propos de sept cas au Libéria. Schweiz. med. Wschr. **95**, 355–360 (1965)
CRACIUN, E.C., URSU, A.: Le réticulo-sarcome des ganglions lymphatiques. Bull. Ass. franç. Cancer **22**, 711–756 (1933)
CRONKITE, E.P., SCHIFFER, L.M.: Kinetics of normal lymphopoiesis and chronic lymphocytic leukemia. In: Regulation of Hematopoiesis, Vol. 2, pp. 1455–1476. GORDON, A.S., Ed. New York: Appleton-Century-Crofts 1970
CROSSEN, P.E., MELLOR, J.E.L., FINLEY, A.G., RAVICH, R.B.M., VINCENT, P.C., GUNZ, F.W.: The Sézary syndrome. Cytogenetic studies and identification of the Sézary cell as an abnormal lymphocyte. Amer. J. Med. **50**, 24–34 (1971)
CUSTER, R.P., BERNHARD, W.G.: The interrelationship of Hodgkin's disease and other lymphatic tumors. Amer. J. med. Sci. **216**, 625–642 (1948)
CUTLER, S.J., AXTELL, L., HEISE, H.: Ten thousand cases of leukemia: 1940–1962. J. Nat. Cancer Inst. **39**, 993–1026 (1967)
CYR, D.P., GEOKAS, M.C.G., WORSLEY, G.H.: Mycosis fungoides. Hematologic findings and terminal course. Arch. Derm. (Chic.) **94**, 558–573 (1966)
DA GRADI, A., DE AMICIS, M.: Ein Fall von primärem Endotheliom der Lymphdrüsen. Virchows Arch. path. Anat. **207**, 323–330 (1912)
DAMESHEK, W.: In: Case records of the Massachusetts General Hospital No. 26-1964. New Engl. J. Med. **270**, 1190–1197 (1964)
DAMMACCO, F., BONOMO, L., FRANKLIN, E.C.: A new case of mu heavy chain disease: Clinical and immunochemical studies. Blood **43**, 713–719 (1974)
DANIEL, M.T., FLANDRIN, G.: Fine structure of abnormal cells in hairy cell (tricholeukocytic) leukemia, with special reference to their in vitro phagocytic capacity. Lab. Invest. **30**, 1–8 (1974)
DANON, F., CLAUVEL, J.P., SELIGMANN, M.: Les "paraprotéines" de type IgG et IgA en dehors de la maladie de Kahler. Rev. franç, Étud. clin. biol. **12**, 681–701 (1967)
DA SILVA PARREIRA, F., SALVIDIO, E.: Osservazioni sul sangue periferico nei reticolosarcomi. Haematologica (Pavia) **36**, 705–715 (1952)

DAVIES, J.N.P.: Lymphomas and leukaemias in Uganda Africans. In: Symposium on Lymphoreticular Tumours in Africa, Paris 1963, pp. 67–79. ROULET, F.C., Ed. Basel-New York: Karger 1964

DAVIS, B.J., ORNSTEIN, L.: High resolution enzyme localization with a new diazo reagent, 'Hexazonium' pararose aniline. J. Histochem. Cytochem. **7**, 297–298 (1959)

DAWSON, E.K., INNES, J.R.M., HARVEY, W.F.: Debatable tumours. II. Lymphosarcoma. Edinb. med. J. **44**, 645–657 (1937)

DEBUSSCHER, L., BERNHEIM, J.L., COLLARD-RONGÉ, E., GOVAERTS, A., HOOGHE, R., LEJEUNE, F.J., ZEICHER, M., STRYCKMANS, P.A.: Hairy cell leukemia: Functional, immunologic, kinetic, and ultrastructural characterization. Blood **46**, 495–507 (1975)

DEGOS, R., OSSIPOVSKI, B., CIVATTE, J., TOURAINE, R.: Réticuloses cutanées. (Réticuloses histiomonocytaires). Ann. Derm. Syph. (Paris) **84**, 125–152 (1957)

DELMAS-MARSALET, Y., VOISIN, D., HENNACHE, G., BAUTERS, F., GOUDEMAND, M.: Étude clinique et biologique de la maladie des chaînes lourdes gamma. À propos d'une nouvelle observation. Nouv. Rev. franç. Hémat. **11**, 717–734 (1971)

DESAGA, J.F., SCHMIDT, D.M.R., SCHMIDT-MENARD, A., LÜCK, R., LÖFFLER, H.: Die proliferative Aktivität der Blastenpopulationen bei Leukämien vom PAS-Typ. Verh. Dtsch. Ges. inn. Med. **80**, 1490–1492 (1974)

DESAI, P.B., MEHER-HOMJI, D.R., PAYMASTER, J.C.: Malignant lymphomas. A clinical study of 800 Indian patients. Cancer (Philad.) **18**, 25–33 (1965)

DEVITA, JR., V.T., CANELLOS, G.P., CHABNER, B., SCHEIN, P., HUBBARD, S.P., YOUNG, R.C.: Advanced diffuse histiocytic lymphoma, a potentially curable disease. Results with combination chemotherapy. Lancet 1975, I, p. 248

DEWAR, A.E., HABESHAW, J.A., YOUNG, G.A., STUART, A.E., PARKER, A.C., WILSON, C.D.: Mixed receptors. [Letter to the Editor.] Lancet 1974, II, p. 216

DICKLER, H.B., SIEGAL, F.P., BENTWICH, Z.H., KUNKEL, H.G.: Lymphocyte binding of aggregated IgG and surface Ig staining in chronic lymphocytic leukaemia. Clin. exp. Immunol. **14**, 97–106 (1973)

DIEBOLD, J.: Classification morphologique des hématosarcomes lymphoïdes non hodgkiniens. Nouv. Presse méd. **3**, 1818 (1974a)

DIEBOLD, J.: Réflexions sur les classifications morphologiques des hématosarcomes lymphoides. Bull. Cancer **61**, 37–38 (1974b)

DIEBOLD, J., REYNES, M., KALIFAT, R., TRICOT, G.: Les inclusions intranucléaires de la maladie de Waldenström. Nouv. Presse méd. **3**, 1067–1070 (1974)

DIEBOLD, J., REYNES, M., KALIFAT, R., TRICOT, G.: Les expressions morphologiques de la maladie de Waldenström. Sem. Hôp. Paris **51**, 2927–2934 (1975)

DIEBOLD, J., ZITTOUN, R., FINE, J.M., TRICOT, G., CAMILLERI, J.P., SIMON, F., ALCALAY, M., BOUSSER, J.: Syndrome lymphoprolifératif avec production de macroglobuline IgM purement intracellulaire. Nouv. Rev. franç. Hémat. **11**, 429–433 (1971)

DOE, W.F.: Alpha chain disease. Clinicopathological features and relationship to so-called Mediterranean lymphoma. Brit. J. Cancer **31**, Supp. II, 350–355 (1975)

DOE, W.F., HENRY, K., HOBBS, J.R., AVERY JONES, F., DENT, C.E., BOOTH, C.C.: Five cases of alpha chain disease. Gut **13**, 947–957 (1972)

DÖRING, G.: Beiträge zur Kenntnis des Retothelsarkoms. Beitr. path. Anat. **101**, 348–374 (1938)

DOMENICI, A.: Considerazioni sui processi iperplastici e neoplastici dei linfonodi. (Rilievi citologici sulle iperplasie secondarie, iperplasie primitive, granuloma maligno e tumori del reticolo.) Arch. De Vecchi Anat. pat. **24**, 187–233 (1956)

DORFMAN, R.F.: Enzyme histochemistry of the cells in Hodgkin's disease and allied disorders. Nature (Lond.) **190**, 925–926 (1961)

DORFMAN, R.F.: Enzyme histochemistry of normal, hyperplastic and neoplastic lymphoreticular tissues. In: Symposium on Lymphoreticular Tumours in Africa, Paris 1963, pp. 304–326. ROULET, F.C., Ed. Basel-New York: Karger 1964a

DORFMAN, R.F.: Follicular (nodular) lymphoma in South Africa. A study of 94 cases. In: Symposium on Lymphoreticular Tumours in Africa, Paris 1963, pp. 211–228. ROULET, F.C., Ed. Basel-New York: Karger 1964b

DORFMAN, R.F.: Childhood lymphosarcoma in St. Louis, Missouri, clinically and histologically resembling Burkitt's tumor. Cancer (Philad.) **18**, 418–430 (1965)

DORFMAN, R.F.: Classical concepts of nodular (follicular) lymphomas. In: Malignant Diseases of the Hematopoietic System. GANN Monograph on Cancer Research, Vol. 15, pp. 177–194. AKAZAKI, K., RAPPAPORT, H., BERARD, C.W., BENNETT, J.M., ISHIKAWA, E., Eds. Tokyo: University of Tokyo Press 1973

DORFMAN, R.F.: Classification of non-Hodgkin's lymphomas. [Letter to the Editor.] Lancet 1974a, I, pp. 1295–1296

DORFMAN, R.F.: Classification of non-Hodgkin's lymphomas. [Letter to the Editor.] Lancet 1974b, II, pp. 961–962

DORFMAN, R.F.: The non-Hodgkin's lymphomas. In: The Reticuloendothelial System. Monographs in Pathology, No. 16, pp. 262–281. REBUCK, J.W., BERARD, C.W., ABELL, M.R., Eds. Baltimore: Williams & Wilkins 1975

DOUGLAS, S.D., COHNEN, G., KÖNIG, E., BRITTINGER, G.: Lymphocyte lysosomes and lysosomal enzymes in chronic lymphocytic leukemia. Blood **41**, 511–518 (1973)

DRESCHER, J., HANSEN, H.G., ALTHOFF, H., GRAUCOB, E.: Das Di-Guglielmo-Syndrom im Kindesalter. Dtsch. med. Wschr. **94**, 2415–2421 (1969)

DRESCHER, J., LEDER, L.-D.: Zur Frage der akuten, extrem unreifzelligen Erythrämie. Z. Kinderheilk. **108**, 117–137 (1970)

DRESCHFELD, J.: Clinical lecture on acute Hodgkin's disease. Brit. med. J. 1892, I, pp. 893–896

DREYFUS, B., ANDRÉ, R.: Le diagnostic précoce des sarcomes des organes lymphoïdes. Rev. Hémat. **5**, 57–77 (1950)

DÜLLMANN, J., WULFHEKEL, U., DRESCHER, S., HAUSMANN, K.: Die Haarzellenhämoblastose ("hairy cell leukemia"). Klinische, licht- und elektronenmikroskopische Befunde. Dtsch. med. Wschr. **99**, 859–863 (1974)

DUHAMEL, G.: Histopathologie du ganglion lymphatique. Paris: Masson 1969

DUHAMEL, G.: Histopathologie clinique de la moelle osseuse. Paris: Masson 1974

DUHAMEL, G., GUERRA, L.: Un syndrome hématologique difficile à définir: La myélofibrose lymphoide. Étude nosologique de 6 observations. Presse méd. **74**, 585–596 (1966)

DUMONT, J., DUFFILLOT, C., FLANDRIN, G., CHELLOUL, N., TRISTANT, H., BERNARD, J.: Non-Hodgkin's lymphomata: Clinical and immunological data in relation to histology. Brit. J. Cancer **31**, Suppl. II, 187–200 (1975)

DUMONT, J., DUFFILLOT, C., THIEBAUT, F., CHELLOUL, N., BERNARD, J.: Étude de la durée de vie des lympho- et réticulosarcomes en fonction de différents facteurs cliniques et histologiques. Bull. Cancer **61**, 51–60 (1974)

DUMONT, J., FLANDRIN, G., BASCH, A., RIPAULT, J., LORTHOLARY, P., BERNARD, J.: Le syndrome de Richter. Nouv. Rev. franç. Hémat. **11**, 496–502 (1971)

DUTCHER, T.F., FAHEY, J.L.: The histopathology of the macroglobulinemia of Waldenström. J. nat. Cancer Inst. **22**, 887–918 (1959)

DUTZ, W., ASVADI, S., SADRI, S., KOHOUT, E.: Intestinal lymphoma and sprue: A systematic approach. Gut **12**, 804–810 (1971)

EDELSON, R.L.: Cutaneous T-cell lymphomas: Clues of a skin-thymus interaction. J. invest. Derm. **67**, 419–424 (1976)

EDELSON, R.L., KIRKPATRICK, C.H., SHEVACH, E.M., SCHEIN, P.S., SMITH, R.W., GREEN, I., LUTZNER, M.: Preferential cutaneous infiltration by neoplastic thymus-derived lymphocytes. Morphologic and functional studies. Ann. intern. Med. **80**, 685–692 (1974)

EDELSON, R.L., LUTZNER, M.A., KIRKPATRICK, C.H., SHEVACH, E.M., GREEN, I.: Morphologic and functional properties of the atypical T lymphocytes of the Sezary syndrome. Mayo Clin. Proc. **49**, 558–566 (1974)

EDINGTON, G.M., MACLEAN, C.M.U.: The relative incidence of tumours of the reticulo-endothelial system in Ibadan, Nigeria. In: Symposium on Lymphoreticular Tumours in Africa, Paris 1963, pp. 54–66. ROULET, F.C., Ed. Basel-New York: Karger 1964

EDINGTON, G.M., MACLEAN, C.M.U., OKUBADEJO, O.A.: 101 necropsies on tumours of the reticulo-endothelial system in Ibadan, Nigeria, with special reference to childhood lymphoma. In: Symposium on Lymphoreticular Tumours in Africa, Paris 1963, pp. 236–252. ROULET, F.C., Ed. Basel-New York: Karger 1964

[Editorial:] Follicular lymphomas. Lancet 1974, I, pp. 1088–1089

EICHENBERGER-DE BEER, H., STORCK, H.: Zur Klinik und Therapie der Mycosis fungoides. Hautarzt **21**, 458–464 (1970)

EIDELMANN, S., PARKINS, R., RUBIN, C.E.: Abdominal lymphoma presenting as malabsorption. A clinico-pathological study of nine cases in Israel and review of the literature. Medicine (Balt.) **45**, 111–137 (1966)

EL CASTRO, B., LEWIS, J.S., STRONG, E.W.: Plasmacytoma of paranasal sinuses and nasal cavity. Arch. Otolaryng. **97**, 326–329 (1973)

EMBERGER, J.M., NAVARRO, M., RIZKALLA, N., IZARN, P.: Étude histologique et cytologique de la moelle osseuse et de la rate au cours de l'histiolymphocytose primitive médullaire et splénique. Nouv. Rev. franç. Hémat. **13**, 365–375 (1973)

ENGESET, A., FRØLAND, S.S., BREMER, K.: Studies of human peripheral lymph. II. Low lymphocyte count and few B-lymphocytes in peripheral lymph of patients with chronic lymphocytic leukaemia. Scand. J. Haemat. **13**, 93–100 (1974)

EPSTEIN, JR., E.H., LEVIN, D.L., CROFT, JR., J.D., LUTZNER, M.A.: Mycosis fungoides. Survival, prognostic features, response to therapy and autopsy findings. Medicine (Baltimore) **51**, 61–72 (1972)

EPSTEIN, M.A., ACHONG, B.G., BARR, Y.M.: Virus particles in cultured lymphoblasts from Burkitt's lymphoma. Lancet 1964, I, pp. 702–703

EPSTEIN, M.A., HUNT, R.D., RABIN, H.: Pilot experiments with EB virus in owl monkeys (aotus trivirgatus). I. Reticuloproliferative disease in an inoculated animal. Int. J. Cancer **12**, 309–318 (1973)

ERKMAN-BALIS, B., RAPPAPORT, H.: Cytogenetic studies of lymph nodes in patients with mycosis fungoides. [Abstr.] Amer. J. Path. **59**, 54a (1970)

ERKMAN-BALIS, B., RAPPAPORT, H.: Cytogenetic studies in mycosis fungoides. Cancer (Philad.) **34**, 626–633 (1974)

EVANS, R.W.: Histological Appearances of Tumours. With a consideration of their histogenesis and certain aspects of their clinical features and behaviour. Edinburgh-London: Livingstone 1966

EWALD, O.: Die leukämische Reticuloendotheliose. Dtsch. Arch. klin. Med. **142**, 222–228 (1923)

EWING, J.: Neoplastic Diseases. A Treatise on Tumors. 3. Ed., pp. 368–373. Philadelphia-London: Saunders 1928

EWING, J.: Neoplastic Diseases. 4. Ed. Philadelphia-London: Saunders 1940

EWING, M.R., FOOTE, JR., F.W.: Plasma-cell tumors of the mouth and upper air passages. Cancer (Philad.) **5**, 499–513 (1952)

FABER, V.: Mycosis fungoides in den inneren Organen ohne Hautveränderungen. Zbl. allg. Path. **72**, 152–153 (1939)

FARRER-BROWN, G.: Discussion. Workshop on Non-Hodgkin's Lymphomas, Chicago, June 1973

FATEH-MOGHADAM, A.: Paraproteinämische Hämoblastosen. In: Handbuch der inneren Medizin, Bd. 2,5: Krankheiten des lymphocytären Systems. pp. 245–452. BEGEMANN, H., Ed. Berlin-Heidelberg-New York: Springer 1974

FATEH-MOGHADAM, A., PRECHTEL, K., WOLF-HORNUNG, B., LAMERZ, R., EHRHART, H.: Pulmonale Verlaufsform der Makroglobulinämie Waldenström. Dtsch. med. Wschr. **99**, 87–90 (1974)

FAUX, J.A., CRAIN, J.D., ROSEN, F.S., MERLER, E.: An alpha heavy chain abnormality in a child with hypogammaglobulinemia. Clin. Immunol. Immunopath. **1**, 282–290 (1973)

FAYOLLE, J., CŒUR, P., BRYON, P.A., GENTILHOMME, O., MOREL, P.: Valeur pronostique de l'atteinte de la peau au cours de la leucémie lymphoïde chronique. Nouv. Rev. franç. Hémat. **11**, 462–468 (1971)

FELDGES, A.J., AUR, R.J.A., VERZOSA, M.S., DANIELS, S.: Periodic acid-Schiff reaction, a useful index of duration of complete remission in acute childhood lymphocytic leukemia. Acta haemat. (Basel) **52**, 8–13 (1974)

FERGUSON, D.J., ALLEN, L.W., GRIEM, M.L., MORAN, M.E., RAPPAPORT, H., ULTMANN, J.E.: Surgical experience with staging laparotomy in 125 patients with lymphoma. Arch. intern. Med. **131**, 356–361 (1973)

FIRAT, D., STUTZMAN, L., STUDENSKI, E.R., PICKREN, J.: Giant follicular lymph node disease. Clinical and pathological review of sixty-four cases. Amer. J. Med. **39**, 252–259 (1965)

FISCHER, R., LORBACHER, P., KÄUFER, C.: Untersuchungen zur enzymhistochemischen Differenzierung von leukämischen Erkrankungen am Schnittpräparat. Virchows Arch. path. Anat. **337**, 525–534 (1964)

FITZGERALD, P.H., RASTRICK, J.M., HAMER, J.W.: Acute plasma cell leukaemia following chronic

lymphatic leukaemia: Transformation or two separate diseases? Brit. J. Haemat. **25**, 171–177 (1973)
FLAD, H.-D., HUBER, C., BREMER, K., MENNE, H.-D., HUBER, H.: Impaired recirculation of B lymphocytes in chronic lymphocytic leukemia. Europ. J. Immunol. **3**, 688–693 (1973)
FLANDRIN, G.: Discussion for: CATOVSKY, D., FRISCH, B., VAN NOORDEN, S.: B, T and 'null' cell leukaemias. Electron cytochemistry and surface morphology. Blood Cells **1**, 125 (1975)
FLANDRIN, G., BERNARD, J.: Cytological classification of acute leukemias. A survey of 1400 cases. Blood Cells **1**, 7–15 (1975)
FLANDRIN, G., BROUET, J.-C.: The Sézary cell: Cytologic, cytochemical and immunologic studies. Mayo Clin. Proc. **49**, 575–583 (1974)
FLANDRIN, G., BROUET, J.C., DANIEL, M.T., PREUD'HOMME, J.L.: Acute leukemia with Burkitt's tumor cells: A study of six cases with special reference to lymphocyte surface markers. Blood **45**, 183–188 (1975)
FLANDRIN, G., DANIEL, M.-T., BLANCHET, P., BRIÈRE, J., BERNARD, J.: La leucémie aiguë monocytaire. Situation clinique et pronostique actuelle à la lumière des techniques de détermination des estérases spécifiques. Nouv. Rev. franç. Hémat. **11**, 241–254 (1971)
FLANDRIN, G., DANIEL, M.T., EL YAFI, G., CHELLOUL, N.: Sarcomatoses ganglionnaires diffuses à différenciation plasmocytaire avec anémie hémolytique auto-immune. Actualités Hémat. **6**, 25–41 (1972)
FLANDRIN, G., DANIEL, M.T., FOURCADE, M., CHELLOUL, N.: Leucémie à "tricholeucocyte" (hairy cell leukemia), étude clinique et cytologique de 55 observations. Nouv. Rev. franç. Hémat. **13**, 609–640 (1973)
FLASHMAN, D.H., LEOPOLD, S.S.: Leukosarcoma. With report of a case beginning with a primary retroperitoneal lymphosarcoma and terminating with leukemia. Amer. J. med. Sci. **177**, 651–663 (1929)
FLAXMAN, B.A., ZELAZNY, G., VAN SCOTT, E.J.: Nonspecificity of characteristic cells in mycosis fungoides. Arch. Derm. **104**, 141–147 (1971)
FLEISCHMAJER, R., EISENBERG, S.: Sézary's reticulosis. Its relationship with neoplasias of the lymphoreticular system. Arch. Derm. **89**, 69–79 (1964)
FOOT, N.C.: Report of a case of malignant endothelioma with necropsy. J. med. Res. **44**, 417–430 (1924)
FORKNER, C.E.: Material from lymph nodes of man. I. Method to obtain material by puncture of lymph nodes for study with supravital and fixed stains. Arch. intern. Med. **40**, 532–537 (1927a)
FORKNER, C.F.: Material from lymph nodes of man. II. Studies on living and fixed cells withdrawn from lymph nodes of man. Arch. intern. Med. **40**, 647–660 (1927b)
FORSTER, G., MOESCHLIN, S.: Extramedulläres, leukämisches Plasmocytom mit Dysproteinämie und erworbener hämolytischer Anämie. Schweiz. med. Wschr. **84**, 1106–1110 (1954)
FORTE, F.A., PRELLI, F., YOUNT, W.J., JERRY, L.M., KOCHWA, S., FRANKLIN, E.C., KUNKEL, H.G.: Heavy chain disease of the μ (γM) type: Report of the first case. Blood **36**, 137–144 (1970)
FOULIS, A.K., COCHRAN, A.J., ANDERSON, J.R.: Surface immunoglobulins of leukaemic cells. Clin. exp. Immunol. **14**, 481–490 (1973)
FRANGIONE, B., FRANKLIN, E.C.: Heavy chain diseases: Clinical features and molecular significance of the disordered immunoglobulin structure. Semin. Hemat. **10**, 53–64 (1973)
FRANKLIN, E.C., LOWENSTEIN, J., BIGELOW, B., MELTZER, M.: Heavy chain disease—A new disorder of serum γ-globulins. Report of the first case. Amer. J. Med. **37**, 332–350 (1964)
FRAUMENI, JR., J.F.: Clinical epidemiology of leukemia. Semin. Hemat. **6**, 250–260 (1969)
FRESEN, O.: Untersuchungen zur Struktur und Genese des Tuberkels als Beitrag zur tuberkulösen Entzündung. I. Mitteilung. Die Epitheloidzelle. Virchows Arch. path. Anat. **317**, 491–516 (1949/50)
FRESEN, O.: Die retothelialen Hämoblastosen. Virchows Arch. path. Anat. **323**, 312–350 (1953)
FRESEN, O.: Über Örtlichkeit und Wertigkeit des Morbus Brill-Symmers. Zbl. allg. Path. path. Anat. **95**, 284–306 (1956)
FRITZE, E., VAN DE LOO, J.: Makroglobulinämie Waldenström mit plasmazellulärer Leukämie. Med. Klin. **60**, 173–176 (1965)

FRIZZERA, G., MORAN, E.M., RAPPAPORT, H.: Angio-immunoblastic lymphadenopathy with dysproteinaemia. Lancet 1974, I, pp. 1070–1073

FRUHLING, L., CHADLI, A.: Le sarcome plasmocytaire extrasquelettique. Ann. Anat. path. **8**, 317–376 (1963)

FÜLLE, H.H., ALBRECHT, M.: Plasmazellenleukämie. In: Leukämie, pp. 365–368. GROSS, R., VAN DE LOO, J., Eds. Berlin-Heidelberg-New York: Springer 1972

FÜLLE, H.H., PRIBILLA, W.: Diagnose und Therapie der Plasmazellenleukämie. Dtsch. med. Wschr. **98**, 874–881 (1973)

FUKS, Z.Y., BAGSHAW, M.A., FARBER, E.M.: Prognostic signs and the management of the mycosis fungoides. Cancer (Philad.) **32**, 1385–1395 (1973)

FUKS, Z.Y., CASTELLINO, R.A., CARMEL, J.A., FARBER, E.M., BAGSHAW, M.A.: Lymphography in mycosis fungoides. Cancer (Philad.) **34**, 106–112 (1974)

VAN FURTH, R., COHN, Z.A., HIRSCH, J.G., HUMPHREY, J.H., SPECTOR, W.G., LANGEVOORT, H.L.: The mononuclear phagocyte system: A new classification of macrophages, monocytes, and their precursor cells. Bull. Wld Hlth Org. **46**, 845–852 (1972)

VAN FURTH, R., GORTER, H., NADKARNI, J.S., NADKARNI, J.J., KLEIN, E., CLIFFORD, P.: Synthesis of immunoglobulins by biopsied tissues and cell lines from Burkitt's lymphoma. Immunology **22**, 847–857 (1972)

GAJL-PECZALSKA, K.J., BLOOMFIELD, C.D., COCCIA, P.F., SOSIN, H., BRUNNING, R.D., KERSEY, J.H.: B and T cell lymphomas. Analysis of blood and lymph nodes in 87 patients. Amer. J. Med. **59**, 674–685 (1975)

GAJL-PECZALSKA, K.J., BLOOMFIELD, C.D., NESBIT, M.E., KERSEY, J.H.: B-cell markers on lymphoblasts in acute lymphoblastic leukaemia. Clin. exp. Immunol. **17**, 561–569 (1974)

GALL, E.A., MALLORY, T.B.: Malignant lymphoma. A clinico-pathologic survey of 618 cases. Amer. J. Path. **18**, 381–429 (1942)

GALL, E.A., MORRISON, H.R., SCOTT, A.T.: The follicular type of malignant lymphoma; a survey of 63 cases. Ann. intern. Med. **14**, 2073–2090 (1941)

GALLMEIER, W.M., GÖBEL, F.W., HARTUNG, W., SCHMIDT, C.G.: Studien an einem Burkitt-Lymphom. Klin. Wschr. **48**, 537–542 (1970)

GALTON, D.A.G.: Chronic lymphocytic leukaemia: Its pathogenesis and relationship to lymphosarcoma. In: Symposium on Lymphoreticular Tumours in Africa, Paris 1963, pp. 163–172. ROULET, F.C., Ed. Basel-New York: Karger 1964

GALTON, D.A.G.: The pathogenesis of chronic lymphocytic leukemia. Canad. med. Ass. J. **94**, 1005–1010 (1967)

GALTON, D.A.G., GOLDMAN, J.M., WILTSHAW, E., CATOVSKY, D., HENRY, K., GOLDENBERG, G.J.: Prolymphocytic leukaemia. Brit. J. Haemat. **27**, 7–23 (1974)

GANS, O., STEIGLEDER, G.K.: Histologie der Hautkrankheiten. Bd. 1 u. 2. 2. Aufl. Berlin-Göttingen-Heidelberg: Springer 1955, 1957

GARNER, A.: Pathology of "pseudotumours" of the orbit: A review. J. clin. Path. **26**, 639–648 (1973)

GARWICZ, S., LANDBERG, T., ÅKERMAN, M.: Malignant lymphomas in children. A clinico-pathologic retrospective study. II. Non-Hodgkin's lymphomas. Acta paediat. scand. **63**, 679–686 (1974)

GASTON, E.A., DOLLINGER, M.R., STRONG, E.W., HAJDU, S.I.: Primary plasmacytoma of lymph nodes. Lymphology **2**, 7–15 (1969)

GATIEN, J.G., SCHNEEBERGER, E.E., MERLER, E.: Analysis of human thymocyte subpopulations using discontinuous gradients of albumin: Precursor lymphocytes in human thymus. Eur. J. Immunol. **5**, 312–317 (1975)

GATIEN, J.G., SCHNEEBERGER, E.E., PARKMAN, R., MERLER, E.: Isolation on discontinuous gradients of bovine albumin of a subpopulation of human lymphocytes exhibiting precursor characteristics. Eur. J. Immunol. **5**, 306–312 (1975)

GEE, T.S., HAGHBIN, M., DOWLING, JR., M.D., CUNNINGHAM, I., MIDDLEMAN, M.P., CLARKSON, B.D.: Acute lymphoblastic leukemia in adults and children. Differences in response with similar therapeutic regimens. Cancer (Philad.) **37**, 1256–1264 (1976)

GÉRARD-MARCHANT, R.: Une nouvelle approche physio-morphologique des lymphomes malins non hodgkiniens. Bull. Cancer **61**, 1–10 (1974a)

GÉRARD-MARCHANT, R.: Conceptions nosologiques actuelles des lymphomes malins non hodgkiniens. Ann. Anat. path. **19**, 149–162 (1974b)

GÉRARD-MARCHANT, R., HAMLIN, I., LENNERT, K., RILKE, F., STANSFELD, A.G., VAN UNNIK, J.A.M.: Classification of non-Hodgkin's lymphomas. [Letter to the Editor.] Lancet 1974, II, pp. 406–408

GERMANN, H.-J., WESTERHAUSEN, M., KICKHÖFEN, B.: μ-Kettenkrankheit. Dtsch. med. Wschr. **97**, 1902–1905 (1972)

GHON, A., ROMAN, B.: Über das Lymphosarkom. Frankfurt. Z. Path. **19**, 1–138 (1916)

GINGOLD, N., STOICA, G.: Protéines pathologiques du type gamma G et gamma M au cours de la leucémie lymphatique chronique. In: Proc. 10. Congr. europ. Soc. Haemat., Strasbourg 1965; part II, pp. 756–760. Basel-New York: Karger 1967

GIVLER, R.L.: Lymphocytic leukemia with coexistent localized reticulum cell sarcoma. Cancer (Philad.) **21**, 1184–1192 (1968)

GLATSTEIN, E., KIM, H., DONALDSON, S.S., DORFMAN, R.F., GRIBBLE, T.J., WILBUR, J.R., ROSENBERG, S.A., KAPLAN, H.S.: Non-Hodgkin's lymphomas. VI. Results of treatment in childhood. Cancer (Philad.) **34**, 204–211 (1974)

GLEICHMANN, E., GLEICHMANN, H., SCHWARTZ, R.S.: Immunologic induction of malignant lymphoma: Genetic factors in the graft-versus-host model. J. nat. Cancer Inst. **49**, 793–804 (1972)

GLEICHMANN, H., GLEICHMANN, E., ANDRÉ-SCHWARTZ, J., SCHWARTZ, R.S.: Chronic allogeneic disease. III. Genetic requirements for the induction of glomerulonephritis. J. exp. Med. **135**, 516–532 (1972)

GLENNER, G.G., EIN, D., TERRY, W.D.: The immunoglobulin origin of amyloid. Amer. J. Med. **52**, 141–147 (1972)

GLENNER, G.G., TERRY, W.D., ISERSKY, C.: Amyloidosis: its nature and pathogenesis. Semin. Hemat. **10**, 65–86 (1973)

GLICK, A.D., LEECH, J.H., WALDRON, J.A., FLEXNER, J.M., HORN, R.G., COLLINS, R.D.: Malignant lymphomas of follicular center cell origin in man. II. Ultrastructural and cytochemical studies. J. nat. Cancer Inst. **54**, 23–36 (1975)

GODEAU, P., SICARD, D., HERREMAN, G., SLAMA, G.: Macroglobulinémie de Waldenström de localisation pleuro-pulmonaire, orbitaire et sous-cutanée. Effet favorable du chlorambucil. Sem. Hôp. Paris **48**, 3111–3116 (1972)

GOETZ, O., LAMPERT, F., PELLER, P., PRECHTEL, K.: Histologisch und virologisch gesicherter Burkitt-Tumor bei einem 10jährigen Knaben. Münch. med. Wschr. **112**, 1373–1376 (1970)

GOLDBERG, A.F., BARKA, T.: Acid phosphatase activity in human blood cells. Nature (Lond.) **195**, 297 (1962)

GOLDNER, J.: A modification of the Masson trichrome technique for routine laboratory purposes. Amer. J. Path. **14**, 237–243 (1938)

GOLDSTONE, A.H., CAWLEY, J.C., ROBERTS, S.O., LEVENTINE, A., BARKER, C.R.: A case of small-cell Sézary's syndrome with null-cell features. J. clin. Path. **29**, 848–851 (1976)

GOLOMB, H.M., BRAYLAN, R., POLLIACK, A.: "Hairy" cell leukaemia (leukaemic reticuloendotheliosis): A scanning electron microscopic study of eight cases. Brit. J. Haemat. **29**, 455–460 (1975)

GOMEZ ORBANEJA, J., SANCHEZ YUS, E., DIAZ-FLORES, L., SIMON HUARTE, P.: Cytology of the mycosis fungoides and the Sézary syndrome. Correlation between light and electron microscopy. Brit. J. Derm. **87**, 96–105 (1972)

GOOD, R.A.: Congenital and acquired abnormalities of the immune system in relation to the aetiology of the lymphomas. Symposium on Non-Hodgkin's Lymphomata, London, Oct. 1973

GOORMAGHTIGH, N.: Sur la prolifération maligne du tissu réticulo-endothélial des ganglions lymphatiques. C.R. Soc. Biol. (Paris) **92**, 457–458 (1925)

GOOS, M., KAISERLING, E., LENNERT, K.: Mycosis fungoides: Model for T-lymphocyte homing to the skin. Brit. J. Derm. **94**, 221–222 (1976)

GORDON, S.: Problems in the laboratory diagnosis of acute leukaemias. Med. J. Aust. 1974, I, pp. 989–991

DE GRACIANSKY, P., TIMSIT, E., DANIEL, F., REVUZ, J., LARRÈGUE, M.: Les manifestations ganglionnaires du mycosis fongoïde. Étude anatomo-pathologique et essai d'interprétation. Sem. Hôp. Paris **43**, 3412–3419 (1967)

GRAVELL, M., LEVINE, P.H., MCINTYRE, R.F., LAND, V.J., PAGANO, J.S.: Epstein-Barr virus in an American patient with Burkitt's lymphoma: detection of viral genome in tumor tissue and establishment of a tumor-derived cell line (NAB). J. nat. Cancer Inst. **56**, 701–704 (1976)

GRAY, J.L., JACOBS, A., BLOCK, M.: Bone marrow and peripheral blood lymphocytosis in the prognosis of chronic lymphocytic leukemia. Cancer (Philad.) **33**, 1169–1178 (1974)

GREAVES, M.F.: Leukaemia-associated membrane antigens. 7th Workshop on Leucocyte Cultures, Ulm, 31.3.–2.4.1976

GREAVES, M., CAPELLARO, D., BROWN, G., REVESZ, T., JANOSSY, G., LISTER, T.A., BEARD, M., RAPSON, N., CATOVSKY, D.: Analysis of human leukaemic cells using cell surface binding probes and the fluorescence activated cell sorter. In: Modern Trends in Human Leukemia II. Hämatologie und Bluttransfusion, Bd. 19, pp. 243–260. NETH, R., GALLO, R.C., MANNWEILER, K., MOLONEY, W.C., Eds. München: Lehmanns 1976

GREEN, I., JAFFE, E.S., SHEVACH, E.M., EDELSON, R.L., FRANK, M.M., BERARD, C.W.: Determination of the origin of malignant reticular cells by the use of surface membrane markers. In: The Reticuloendothelial System. Monographs in Pathology, No. 16, pp. 282–300. REBUCK, J.W., BERARD, C.W., ABELL, M.R., Eds. Baltimore: Williams & Wilkins 1975

GREENWOOD, M.F., HOLLAND, P.: Plasma membrane characteristics in acute leukemia. J. reticuloendothel. Soc. **16**, Abstr. Suppl., p. 1a (1974)

GROSS, R.L., STEEL, C.M., LEVIN, A.G., SINGH, S., BRUBAKER, G.: In vitro immunological studies on East African cancer patients. III. Spontaneous rosette formation by cells from Burkitt lymphoma biopsies. Int. J. Cancer **15**, 139–143 (1975)

GRUNDMANN, E., HOBIK, H.P.: Graft-Versus-Host-Reaktion – Allogen-Krankheiten – Lymphome. Beitr. Path. **150**, 323–329 (1973)

GUNVÉN, P., KLEIN, G., HENLE, G., HENLE, W., CLIFFORD, P.: Antibodies to EBV-associated membrane and viral capsid antigens in Burkitt lymphoma patients. Nature (Lond.) **228**, 1053–1056 (1970)

GUNZ, F.W., ANGUS, H.B.: Leukemia and cancer in the same patient. Cancer (Philad.) **18**, 145–152 (1965)

GUNZ, F.W., HOUGH, R.F.: Acute leukemia over the age of fifty: A study of its incidence and natural history. Blood **11**, 882–901 (1956)

GUNZER, U., NÜRNBERGER, R., THIEMANN, R.: Nachweis von Epstein-Barr-Virus-Capsidantigen, IgG-Antikörpern und Early Antigen bei malignen Non-Hodgkin-Lmphomen. Paper presented at Meeting of the German-Austrian Society of Hematology, Bad Nauheim, Sept. 29–Oct. 10, 1975

GUTHRIE, C.G.: Gland puncture as a diagnostic measure. Bull. Johns Hopk. Hosp. **32**, 266–269 (1921)

GUTTERMAN, J., RODRIGUEZ, V., MCMULLAN, G.: Remission induction of acute leukemia developing in Burkitt's lymphoma. Cancer (Philad.) **29**, 626–629 (1972)

HAAK, H.L., DE MAN, J.C.H., HIJMANS, W., KNAPP, W., SPECK, B.: Further evidence for the lymphocytic nature of leukaemic reticuloendotheliosis (hairy-cell leukaemia). Brit. J. Haemat. **27**, 31–38 (1974)

HAAS, W., KNORRE, D.: Über eine ungewöhnliche Kombination einer malignen Retikulose mit kavernösen Lymphangiomen der peripheren Lymphknoten. Dtsch. Arch. klin. Med. **203**, 335–350 (1956)

HABESHAW, J.A., STUART, A.E.: Cell receptor studies on seven cases of diffuse histiocytic malignant lymphoma (reticulum cell sarcoma). J. clin. Path. **28**, 289–297 (1975)

HADDOW, A.J.: Epidemiological evidence suggesting an infective element in the aetiology. In: Burkitt's Lymphoma, pp. 198–209. BURKITT, D.P., WRIGHT, D.H., Eds. Edinburgh-London: Livingstone 1970

HAEGERT, D.G., CAWLEY, J.C., COLLINS, R.D., FLEMANS, R.J., SMITH, J.L.: Leukaemic reticuloendotheliosis: A morphological and immunological study of four cases. J. clin. Path. **27**, 967–972 (1974)

HAEGERT, D.G., CAWLEY, J.C., KARPAS, A., GOLDSTONE, A.H.: Combined T and B cell acute lymphoblastic leukaemia. Brit. med. J. 1974, IV, pp. 79–82

HAFERKAMP, O., ROSENAU, W., LENNERT, K.: Vascular transformation of lymph node sinuses due to venous obstruction. Arch. Path. **92**, 81–83 (1971)

HAMBURG, A., BRYNES, R.K., REESE, C., GOLOMB, H.M.: Human cord blood lymphocytes. Ultrastructural and immunologic surface marker characteristics; a comparison with B- and T-cell lymphomas. Lab. Invest. **34**, 207–215 (1976)

HAMILTON-FAIRLEY, G., FREEMAN, J.E.: Blood and neoplastic diseases. Treatment of the lymphomas. Brit. med. J. 1974, IV, pp. 761–765

HANSEN, J.A., GOOD, R.A.: Malignant disease of the lymphoid system in immunological perspective. Hum. Path. **5**, 567–599 (1974)

HARMS, D.: Milz und Blutgerinnung. In: Die Milz, pp. 306–316. LENNERT, K., HARMS, D., Eds. Berlin-Heidelberg-New York: Springer 1970

HARRIS, J., BAGAI, R.C.: Immune deficiency states associated with malignant disease in man. Med. Clin. N. Amer. **56**, 501–514 (1972)

HARRIS, O.D., COOKE, W.T., THOMPSON, H., WATERHOUSE, J.A.H.: Malignancy in adult coeliac disease and idiopathic steatorrhoea. Amer. J. Med. **42**, 899–912 (1967)

HARRIS, R.J.C.: Aetiology of central African lymphomata. Brit. med. Bull. **20**, 149–153 (1964)

HARRISON, C.V.: The morphology of the lymph node in the macroglobulinaemia of Waldenström. J. clin. Path. **25**, 12–16 (1972)

HAYES, D.W., BENNETT, W.A., HECK, F.J.: Extramedullary lesions in multiple myeloma. Review of literature and pathologic studies. Arch. Path. **53**, 262–272 (1952)

HAYHOE, F.G.J.: Leukaemia. Research and Clinical Practice. London: J. & A. Churchill Ltd. 1960

HAYHOE, F.G.J.: Cytochemical aspects of leukemia and lymphoma. In: Leukemia and Lymphoma, pp. 37–46. HOLLAND, J.F., MIESCHER, P.A., JAFFÉ, E.R., Eds. New York-London: Grune & Stratton 1969

HAYHOE, F.G.J., QUAGLINO, D., DOLL, R.: The Cytology and Cytochemistry of Acute Leukemias. London: Her Majesty's Stationary Office 1964

HECKNER, F.: Extramedulläres lymphatisches Plasmocytom. Acta haemat. (Basel) **5**, 158–168 (1951)

HECKNER, F.: Polysaccharide in Blut- und Knochenmarkszellen. In: Zyto- und Histochemie in der Hämatologie, pp. 408–425. MERKER, H., Ed. Berlin-Göttingen-Heidelberg: Springer 1963

HECKNER, F., VOTH, H.: Cytologische Begriffsbestimmung der Reticulumzellen. II. Mitteilung. Untersuchungen am Lymphknoten. Dtsch. Arch. klin. Med. **201**, 582–595 (1954)

HEENAN, P.J., MASON, D.Y., SKINNER, J.M., TAYLOR, C.R.: Waldenström's disease of the jejunum. Beitr. Path. **157**, 76–83 (1976)

VAN HEERDE, P., HIJMANS, W., WAGENAAR, S.S., SCHUIT, H.R.E., BLEEKER, G.M.: Twee gevallen van lymforeticulaire orbitatumoren. Ned. T. Geneesk. **118**, p. 488 (1974)

HEIDELBERGER, K.P., LEGOLVAN, D.P.: Wiskott-Aldrich syndrome and cerebral neoplasia: Report of a case with localized reticulum cell sarcoma. Cancer (Philad.) **33**, 280–284 (1974)

HEILMEYER, L., BEGEMANN, H.: Atlas der klinischen Hämatologie und Cytologie. Berlin-Göttingen-Heidelberg: Springer 1955

HEINE, J.: Lymphozytom der Lunge und generalisierte Plasmozytose. Zbl. allg. Path. path. Anat. **96**, 16–20 (1957)

HELLER, A.: Cytochemische Befunde bei M. Waldenström. In: Leukämie, pp. 429–432. GROSS, R., VAN DE LOO, J., Eds. Berlin-Heidelberg-New York: Springer 1972

HELLWIG, C.A.: Extramedullary plasma cell tumors as observed in various locations. Arch. Path. **36**, 95–111 (1943)

HENDERSON, E.S.: Treatment of acute leukemia. Sem. Hemat. **6**, 271–319 (1969)

HENLE, G., HENLE, W.: Immunofluorescence in cells derived from Burkitt's lymphoma. J. Bact. **91**, 1248–1256 (1966)

HENLE, G., HENLE, W., DIEHL, V.: Relation of Burkitt's tumor-associated herpes-type virus to infectious mononucleosis. Proc. nat. Acad. Sci. (Wash.) **59**, 94–101 (1968)

HENLE, W.: Evidence for viruses in acute leukemia and Burkitt's tumor. Cancer (Philad.) **21**, 580–586 (1968)

HENLE, W., DIEHL, V., KOHN, G., ZUR HAUSEN, H., HENLE, G.: Herpes-type virus and chromosome marker in normal leukocytes after growth with irradiated Burkitt cells. Science **157**, 1064–1065 (1967)

HENLE, W., HENLE, G.: Epstein-Barr virus and infectious mononucleosis. New Engl. J. Med. **288**, 263–264 (1973)

HENLE, W., HENLE, G.E., HORWITZ, C.A.: Epstein-Barr virus specific diagnostic tests in infectious mononucleosis. Hum. Path. **5**, 551–565 (1974)

HENLE, W., HENLE, G., ZAJAC, B.A., PEARSON, G., WAUBKE, R., SCRIBA, M.: Differential reactivity of human serums with early antigens induced by Epstein-Barr virus. Science **169**, 188–190 (1970)

HENNEMANN, H.H., RATHENOW, H.W.: Leukämiestudien (III). Das elektrophoretische Serumeiweißbild bei Leukämien. Z. ges. inn. Med. **10**, 616–621 (1955)

HENRY, K.: Electron microscopy in the non-Hodgkin's lymphomata. Brit. J. Cancer **31**, Suppl. II, 73–93 (1975)

HENRY, K., HOWARTH, C., FARRER-BROWN, G.: New concepts of primary gastrointestinal lymphomas. XI Congress Intern. Acad. Path., Washington, Oct. 1976

HERTL, M.: Zytochemie der Zellen der akuten Leukose. In: Zyto- und Histochemie in der Hämatologie, pp. 5–19. MERKER, H., Ed. Berlin-Göttingen-Heidelberg: Springer 1963

HERTL, M.: Zytochemie der Zellen der akuten Leukose. (Theoretische und klinische Medizin in Einzeldarstellungen, Bd. 30) Heidelberg: Hüthig 1966

HERTL, M., LANDBECK, G. [Eds.]: Leukämie bei Kindern. Stuttgart: Thieme 1969

HESS, M.W.: Discussion for: CATOVSKY, D., FRISCH, B., VAN NOORDEN, S.: B, T and 'null' cell leukaemias. Electron cytochemistry and surface morphology. Blood Cells **1**, 126 (1975)

HEUCHEL, G., EITNER, H.: Über besondere Bluteiweißbefunde bei Retothelsarkomatose. Acta haemat. (Basel) **12**, 27–34 (1954)

VON HEYDEN, H.W., WALLER, H.D., PAPE, G.R., BENÖHR, H.C., BRAUN, H.J., WILMS, K., RIEBER, E.P., RIETHMÜLLER, G.: Haarzell-Leukämie. I. Klinik, Zytochemie, Phagozytosefähigkeit von Haarzellen, Etablierung permanent wachsender Zellinien. Dtsch. med. Wschr. **101**, 3–8 (1976)

HIRSCHER, H.: Über extramedulläres lympho-retikuläres diffuses Plasmocytom. Folia haemat. (Lpz.) **72**, 74–86 (1953/54)

HITTMAIR, A.: Zur Ätiologie lymphatischer Hyperplasien bzw. lymphatischer Leukämien. Schweiz. med. Wschr. **82**, 1130–1131 (1952)

HOAGLAND, H.C.: Atypical lymphocytes. Morphologic features. Mayo Clin. Proc. **49**, 526–530 (1974)

HOBBS, J.R.: Growth rates and responses to treatment in human myelomatosis. Brit. J. Haemat. **16**, 607–617 (1969)

HOBBS, J.R.: Immunocytoma o' mice an' men. Brit. med. J. 1971, II, pp. 67–72

HOBBS, J.R., JACOBS, A.: A half-molecule GK plasmacytoma. Clin. exp. Immunol. **5**, 199–207 (1969)

HODGKIN, T.: On some morbid appearances of the absorbent glands and spleen. Med.-Chir. Trans. **17**, 68–114 (1832)

HOERNI, B., LAPORTE, G.: Immunological disorders in the aetiology of lymphoreticular neoplasms. Europ. J. clin. biol. Res. **15**, 841–850 (1970)

HOHL, K., GRETENER, A.: Das Reticulosarkom. Zürcher Material von 1936–1951 (39 Fälle). Oncologia (Basel) **9**, 338–352 (1956)

HOLDAWAY, D.R., WINKELMANN, R.K.: Histopathology of Sezary syndrome. Mayo Clin. Proc. **49**, 541–547 (1974)

HOLTON, C.P., VIETTI, T.J., NORA, A.H., DONALDSON, M.H., STUCKEY, JR., W.J., WATKINS, W.L., LANE, D.M.: Clinical study of Daunomycin and prednisone for induction of remission in children with advanced leukemia. New Engl. J. Med. **280**, 171–174 (1969)

HOPPER, J.E.: Immunoglobulin D: A predominant surface Ig in poorly differentiated lymphocytic (PDL) lymphoma. [Abstr.] Clin. Res. **22**, 394A (1974)

HORSTER, J.A.: Über das großfollikuläre Lymphoblastom. Dtsch. Arch. klin. Med. **198**, 295–304 (1951)

HUANG, C.C., HOU, Y., WOODS, L.K., MOORE, G.E., MINOWADA, J.: Cytogenetic study of human lymphoid T-cell lines derived from lymphocytic leukemia. J. nat. Cancer Inst. **53**, 655–660 (1974)

HUBER, C., MICHLMAYR, G., HUBER, H.: Immunologische Marker in der Differentialdiagnose lymphatischer Systemerkrankungen. Dtsch. med. Wschr. **99**, 2262–2268 (1974)

HUBER, H., BRAUNSTEINER, H.: Pathophysiologie und Differentialdiagnose der chronischen lymphatischen Leukämie. In: Leukämie, pp. 415–421. GROSS, R., VAN DE LOO, J., Eds. Berlin-Heidelberg-New York: Springer 1972

HUHN, D., DOBBELSTEIN, H., ENGELHARDT, D.: Sézary-Syndrom. Blut **25**, 352–363 (1972)

HUHN, D., STICH, W.: Fine Structure of Blood and Bone Marrow. An Introduction in Electron Microscopic Hematology. München: J.F. Lehmanns 1969

HUREZ, D., FLANDRIN, G., PREUD'HOMME, J.L., SELIGMANN, M.: Unreleased intracellular monoclonal macroglobulin in chronic lymphocytic leukaemia. Clin. exp. Immunol. **10**, 223–234 (1972)

HURST, D.W., MEYER, O.O.: Giant follicular lymphoblastoma. Cancer (Philad.) **14**, 753–778 (1961)

HUTT, M.S.R.: The pathology of Burkitt's tumour in the context of lymphomas and leukaemias. In: Treatment of Burkitt's Tumour. UICC Monograph Series, Vol. 8, pp. 11–13. BURCHENAL, J.H., BURKITT, D.P., Eds. Berlin-Heidelberg-New York: Springer 1967

Hutt, M.S.R.: Introduction and historical background. In: Burkitt's Lymphoma, pp. 1–5. Burkitt, D.P., Wright, D.H., Eds. Edinburgh-London: Livingstone 1970

Hutter, Jr., J.J., Favara, B.E., Nelson, M., Holton, C.P.: Non-Hodgkin's lymphoma in children. Correlation of CNS disease with initial presentation. Cancer (Philad.) **36**, 2132–2137 (1975)

Iijima, S.: Leukemic reticuloendotheliosis. Tohoku J. exp. Med. **89**, 35–44 (1966)

Iijima, S.: Leukemic reticuloendotheliosis. In: Malignant Diseases of the Hematopoietic System. GANN Monograph on Cancer Research, Vol. 15, pp. 163–176. Akazaki, K., Rappaport, H., Berard, C.W., Bennett, J.M., Ishikawa, E., Eds. Tokyo: University of Tokyo Press 1973

Insel, R.A., Melewicz, F.M., La Via, M.F., Balch, C.M.: Morphology, surface markers, and in vitro responses of a human leukemic T cell. Clin. Immunol. Immunopath. **4**, 382–391 (1975)

Isaacs, R.: 'Notched nucleus cell' leukemia. Proc. Cent. Soc. clin. Res. **12**, 37 (1939)

Isobe, T., Osserman, E.F.: Patterns of amyloidosis and their association with plasma-cell dyscrasia, monoclonal immunoglobulins and Bence-Jones proteins. New Engl. J. Med. **290**, 473–477 (1974)

Iversen, O.H., Harket, R.: Burkitt's tumour in Norway. A survey of possible cases occurring in the period 1953–1962. Europ. J. Cancer **4**, 383–389 (1968)

Iversen, O.H., Iversen, U., Ziegler, J.L., Bluming, A.Z.: Cell kinetics in Burkitt lymphoma. Europ. J. Cancer **10**, 155–163 (1974)

Iversen, U., Iversen, O.H., Bluming, A.Z., Ziegler, J.L., Kyalwasi, S.: Cell kinetics of African cases of Burkitt lymphoma. A preliminary report. Europ. J. Cancer **8**, 305–308 (1972)

Jackson, Jr., H., Parker, Jr., F.: Hodgkin's Disease and Allied Disorders. New York: Oxford University Press 1947

Jackson, Jr., H., Parker, Jr., F., Bethea, J.M.: Studies of diseases of the lymphoid and myeloid tissues. II. Plasmatocytomata and their relation to multiple myelomata. Amer. J. med. Sci. **181**, 169–180 (1931)

Jacobs, M.L.: Malignant lymphomas and their management. (Recent Results in Cancer Research, Vol. 16.) Berlin-Heidelberg-New York: Springer 1968

Jacquillat, C., Weil, M., Gemon, M.-F., Auclerc, G., Loisel, J.-P., Delobel, J., Flandrin, G., Schaison, G., Izrael, V., Bussel, A., Dresch, C., Weisgerber, C., Rain, D., Tanzer, J., Najean, Y., Seligmann, M., Boiron, M., Bernard, J.: Combination therapy in 130 patients with acute lymphoblastic leukemia (Protocol 06 LA 66-Paris). Cancer Res. **33**, 3278–3284 (1973)

Jaeger, E.: Das extramedulläre Plasmocytom. Z. Krebsforsch. **52**, 349–383 (1942)

Jaffe, E.S., Shevach, E.M., Frank, M.M., Berard, C.W., Green, I.: Nodular lymphoma – evidence for origin from follicular B lymphocytes. New Engl. J. Med. **290**, 813–819 (1974)

Jaffe, E.S., Shevach, E.M., Sussman, E.H., Frank, M., Green, I., Berard, C.W.: Membrane receptor sites for the identification of lymphoreticular cells in benign and malignant conditions. Brit. J. Cancer **31**, Suppl. II, 107–120 (1975)

Jaiyesimi, F., Oluboyede, O., Taylor, D., Familusi, J.B.: Burkitt's lymphoma presenting as acute leukaemia. Acta haemat. (Basel) **54**, 115–119 (1975)

Jarvis, J.E., Ball, G., Rickinson, A.B., Epstein, M.A.: Cytogenetic studies on human lymphoblastoid cell lines from Burkitt's lymphomas and other sources. Int. J. Cancer **14**, 716–721 (1974)

Jellinger, K., Radaszkiewicz, T., Slowik, F.: Primary malignant lymphomas of the central nervous system in man. Acta neuropath. (Berl.) Suppl. **6**, 95–102 (1975)

Jenkin, R.D.T.: Report on patterns of disease in lymphosarcoma and reticulum cell sarcoma. Meeting Internat. Soc. Paediat. Oncology, Oct. 1972, Manchester

Jéquier-Doge, E., Nicod, J.-L., Chapuis, J.-P.: Un cas de plasmocytome à localisation ganglionnaire observé cliniquement pendant plus de 6 ans et contrôlé anatomiquement. Schweiz. med. Wschr. **77**, 186–190 (1947)

Jønsson, V., Videbaek, A., Axelsen, N.H., Harboe, M.: μ-Chain disease in a case of chronic lymphocytic leukaemia and malignant histiocytoma. I. Clinical aspects. Scand. J. Haemat. **16**, 209–217 (1976)

Jondal, M., Wigzell, H., Aiuti, F.: Human lymphocyte subpopulations: Classification according to surface markers and/or functional characteristics. Transplant. Rev. **16**, 163–195 (1973)

Jones, S.E.: Autoimmune disorders and malignant lymphoma. Cancer (Philad.) **31**, 1092–1098 (1973)

Jones, S.E., Fuks, Z., Bull, M., Kadin, M.E., Dorfman, R.F., Kaplan, H.S., Rosenberg, S.A.,

KIM, H.: Non-Hodgkin's lymphomas. IV. Clinicopathologic correlation in 405 cases. Cancer (Philad.) **31**, 806–823 (1973)

JONES, S.E., KAPLAN, H.S., ROSENBERG, S.A.: Non-Hodgkin's lymphomas. III. Preliminary results of radiotherapy and a proposal for new clinical trials. Radiology **103**, 657–662 (1972)

JOSEPH, R.R., ZARAFONETIS, C.J.D., DURANT, J.R.: 'Lymphoma' in chronic granulocytic leukemia. Amer. J. med. Sci. **251**, 417–427 (1966)

KAHN, L.B.: Pathology of the lymphomas. S. Afr. med. J. **46**, 1153–1159 (1972)

KAISERLING, E.: Feinstrukturelle Befunde bei Non-Hodgkin-Lymphomen. Habil. Schrift, Kiel 1975

KAISERLING, E.: Elektronenmikroskopische Befunde bei Non-Hodgkin-Lymphomen. In: Maligne Lymphome und monoklonale Gammopathien. Hämatologie und Bluttransfusion, Bd. 18, pp. 185–198. LÖFFLER, H., Ed. München: Lehmanns 1976

KAPLAN, H.S.: Hodgkin's Disease. Cambridge, Mass.: Harvard University Press 1972

KAPLAN, J., MASTRANGELO, R., PETERSON, JR., W.D.: Childhood lymphoblastic lymphoma, a cancer of thymus-derived lymphocytes. Cancer Res. **34**, 521–525 (1974)

KAPPELER, R., KREBS, A., RIVA, G.: Klinik der Makroglobulinämie Waldenström. Beschreibung von 21 Fällen und Übersicht der Literatur. Helv. med. Acta **25**, 54–152 (1958)

KARITZKY, D., JACOBI, H.: IgM-Paraproteinämie bei lymphoblastischem Lymphosarkom im Kindesalter. Dtsch. med. Wschr. **99**, 954–957 (1974)

KATAYAMA, I., FINKEL, H.E.: Leukemic reticuloendotheliosis. A clinicopathologic study with review of the literature. Amer. J. Med. **57**, 115–126 (1974)

KATAYAMA, I., LI, C.Y., YAM, L.T.: Histochemical study of acid phosphatase isoenzyme in leukemic reticuloendotheliosis. Cancer (Philad.) **29**, 157–164 (1972a)

KATAYAMA, I., LI, C.Y., YAM, L.T.: Ultrastructural characteristics of the "hairy cells" of leukemic reticuloendotheliosis. Amer. J. Path. **67**, 361–370 (1972b)

KATAYAMA, I., NAGY, G.K.: Hairy-cell leukemia versus leukemic reticuloendotheliosis. [Letter to the Editor.] Amer. J. clin. Path. **62**, 442 (1974)

KATAYAMA, I., NAGY, G.K., BALOGH, JR., K.: Light microscopic identification of the ribosome-lamella complex in "hairy cells" of leukemic reticuloendotheliosis. Cancer (Philad.) **32**, 843–846 (1973)

KATAYAMA, I., PECHET, L.: Classification of non-Hodgkin's lymphomas. [Letter to the Editor.] Lancet 1974, II, p. 1211

KAUFMANN, E.: Lehrbuch der speziellen pathologischen Anatomie für Studierende und Ärzte. Bd. 1, S. 207 u. Bd. 2. 7. u. 8. Aufl. Berlin-Leipzig: de Gruyter 1928/29

KAY, H.E.M.: Classification of non-Hodgkin's lymphomas. [Letter to the Editor.] Lancet 1974, II, p. 586

KEISER, G., UEHLINGER, E., VIRIEUX, C.: Zwei Fälle von chronisch-lymphatischer Leukämie und Morbus Hodgkin. Acta haemat. (Basel) **26**, 29–43 (1961)

KELLER, H., SPENGLER, G.A., SKVAŘIL, F., FLURY, W., NOSEDA, G., RIVA, G.: Zur Frage der Heavy chain disease. Ein Fall von IgG-heavy-chain-Fragment- und IgM-Typ K-Paraproteinämie mit Plasmazellenleukämie. Schweiz. med. Wschr. **100**, 1012–1022 (1970)

KELLNER, B., LAPIS, K., ECKHARDT, S.: Lymphknotengeschwülste. Budapest: Akadémiai Kiadó 1966

KERSEY, J.H., GAJL-PECZALSKA, K.J., NESBIT, M.E.: The lymphoid system: Abnormalities in immunodeficiency and malignancy. J. Pediat. **84**, 789–796 (1974)

KERSEY, J.H., NESBIT, M., HALLGREN, H., SABAD, A., YUNIS, E., GAJL-PECZALSKA, K.: Evidence for origin of certain childhood acute lymphoblastic leukemias and lymphomas in thymus-derived lymphocytes. Cancer (Philad.) **36**, 1348–1352 (1975)

KERSEY, J.H., NESBIT, M.E., LUCKASEN, J.R., HALLGREN, H.M., SABAD, A., YUNIS, E.J., GAJL-PECZALSKA, K.J.: Acute lymphoblastic leukemic and lymphoma cells with thymus-derived (T) markers. Mayo Clin. Proc. **49**, 584–587 (1974)

KEUNING, F.J.: Dynamics of immunoglobulin forming cells and their precursors. In: Immunoglobulins, pp. 1–14. Amsterdam: North Holland Publ. 1972

KEUNING, F.J., BOS, W.H.: Regeneration patterns of lymphoid follicles in the rabbit spleen after sublethal X-irradiation. In: Germinal Centers in Immune Responses. Proc. of a Symp. held at the Univ. of Bern, June 22–24, 1966, pp. 250–257. COTTIER, H., ODARTCHENKO, N., SCHINDLER, R., CONGDON, C.C., Eds. Berlin-Heidelberg-New York: Springer 1967

KHAN, A.G.: The multifocal lymphoma syndrome in African children in Kenya. J. Laryng. **78**, 480–498 (1964)

KHARAZMI, A., HAGHIGHI, P., HAGHSHENAS, M., NASR, K., ABADI, P., REZAI, H.R.: Alpha-chain disease and its association with intestinal lymphoma. Clin. exp. Immunol. **26**, 124–128 (1976)

KIM, H., DORFMAN, R.F.: Morphological studies of 84 untreated patients subjected to laparotomy for the staging of non-Hodgkin's lymphomas. Cancer (Philad.) **33**, 657–674 (1974)

KIM, H., HELLER, P., RAPPAPORT, H.: Monoclonal gammopathies associated with lymphoproliferative disorders: A morphologic study. Amer. J. clin. Path. **59**, 282–294 (1973)

KIMURA, K.: Clinical and statistical studies of tumors of the reticuloendothelial system in Japan. Tohoku J. exp. Med. **82**, 1–20 (1964)

KING, G.W., HURTUBISE, P.E., SAGONE, JR., A.L., LOBUGLIO, A.F., METZ, E.N.: Leukemic reticuloendotheliosis. A study of the origin of the malignant cell. Amer. J. Med. **59**, 411–416 (1975)

KLAJMAN, A., YARETZKY, A., MANOR, J., STEINER, Z.: Acute lymphoblastic crisis in a patient with chronic lymphatic leukemia. Acta haemat. (Basel) **54**, 306–311 (1975)

KLEIN, G.: Some immunological studies. In: Burkitt's Lymphoma, pp. 172–185. BURKITT, D.P., WRIGHT, D.H., Eds. Edinburgh-London: Livingstone 1970

KLEIN, G., GEERING, G., OLD, L.J., HENLE, G., HENLE, W., CLIFFORD, P.: Comparison of the anti-EBV titer and the EBV-associated membrane reactive and precipitating antibody levels in the sera of Burkitt lymphoma and nasopharyngeal carcinoma patients and controls. Int. J. Cancer **5**, 185–194 (1970)

KLIMA, R., HERZOG, E.: Beziehungen der lymphatischen Leukämie zu Entzündung und Karzinom. Zehnjährige klinische Beobachtungen. Wien. med. Wschr. **106**, 6–10 (1956)

KNAPP, W., SCHUIT, H.R.E., BOLHUIS, R.L.H., HIJMANS, W.: Surface immunoglobulins in chronic lymphatic leukaemia, macroglobulinaemia and myelomatosis. Clin. exp. Immunol. **16**, 541–552 (1974)

KNOSPE, W.H., LOEB, JR., V., HUGULEY, JR., C.M.: Bi-weekly chlorambucil treatment of chronic lymphocytic leukemia. Cancer (Philad.) **33**, 555–562 (1974)

KNOTH, W.: Zur Cyto- und Histogenese und zur klinischen Einteilung der reticulo-histiocytären Erkrankungen der Haut. Arch. klin. exp. Derm. **209**, 130–170 (1959)

KÖNIG, E., BRITTINGER, G., COHNEN, G.: Relation of lysosomal fragility in CLL lymphocytes to PHA reactivity. Nature (Lond.) **244**, 247–248 (1973)

KOJIMA, M., IMAI, Y., MORI, N.: A concept of follicular lymphoma. A proposal for the existence of a neoplasm originating from the germinal center. In: Malignant Diseases of the Hematopoietic System. GANN Monograph on Cancer Research, No. 15, pp. 195–207. AKAZAKI, K., RAPPAPORT, H., BERARD, C.W., BENNETT, J.M., ISHIKAWA, E., Eds. Tokyo: University of Tokyo Press 1973

KOMOCKI, W.: Über eine Geschwulst von eigenartigem Bau (Reticuloma s. Adenoidoma). Virchows Arch. path. Anat. **250**, 517–521 (1924)

KRÄMER, F.: PAS-positive Zelleinschlüsse beim Plasmozytom und bei der Makroglobulinämie Waldenström. Diss. med., Kiel 1971

KRAUSS, S., SOKAL, J.E.: Paraproteinemia in the lymphomas. Amer. J. Med. **40**, 400–413 (1966)

KRÜGER, G.: Chronic immunosuppression and lymphomagenesis in man and mice. Nat. Cancer Inst. Monogr. **35**, 183–190 (1972)

KRÜGER, G., HARRIS, D., SUSSMAN, E.: Effect of dilantin in mice. II. Lymphoreticular tissue atypia and neoplasia after chronic exposure. Z. Krebsforsch. **78**, 290–302 (1972)

KRÜGER, G., O'CONOR, G.T.: Epidemiologic and immunologic considerations on the pathogenesis of Burkitt's tumor. In: Recent Results in Cancer Research, Vol. 39, pp. 211–224. GRUNDMANN, E., TULINIUS, H., Eds. Berlin-Heidelberg-New York: Springer 1972

KUNDRAT, H.: Ueber Lympho-Sarkomatosis. Wien. klin. Wschr. **6**, 211–213 u. 234–239 (1893)

KURZ, R., HAAS, H.: Value of the combined cytological and cytochemical classification in the management of acute childhood leukemia. Acta haemat. (Basel) **52**, 1–7 (1974)

KYLE, R.A., BAYRD, E.D., MCKENZIE, B.F., HECK, F.J.: Diagnostic criteria for electrophoretic patterns of serum and urinary proteins in multiple myeloma. Study of one hundred and sixty-five multiple myeloma patients and of seventy-seven nonmyeloma patients with similar electrophoretic patterns. J. Amer. med. Ass. **174**, 245–251 (1960)

LADEWIG, P.: Über eine einfache und vielseitige Bindegewebsfärbung (Modifikation der Mallory-Heidenhainschen Methode). Z. wiss. Mikr. **55**, 215–217 (1938)

LAMPERT, F.: Diagnose, Ätiologie und Therapie des Burkitt-Lymphoms. In: Leukämien und maligne Lymphome, pp. 483–486. STACHER, A., Ed. München-Berlin-Wien: Urban & Schwarzenberg 1973

LANDBECK, G.: Besonderheiten maligner Lymphome im Kindesalter. In: Leukämien und maligne Lymphome, pp. 487–493. STACHER, A., Ed. München-Berlin-Wien: Urban & Schwarzenberg 1973

LANDBECK, G., GAEDICKE, G., WINKLER, K., STEIN, H.: Besonderheiten der malignen Lymphome im Kindesalter. In: Maligne Lymphome und monoklonale Gammopathien. Hämatologie und Bluttransfusion, Bd. 18, pp. 225–235. LÖFFLER, H., Ed. München: Lehmanns 1976

LANDBERG, T., GARWICZ, S., ÅKERMAN, M.: A clinico-pathological study of non-Hodgkin's lymphomata in childhood. Brit. J. Cancer **31**, Suppl. II, 332–336 (1975)

LANE, C.G., GREENWOOD, A.M.: Lymphoblastoma (mycosis fungoides) and hemorrhagic sarcoma of Kaposi in the same person. Arch. Derm. Syph. (Chic.) **27**, 643–657 (1933)

LASZLO, J., GERBER, H.J., SOMMER, J.R.: Composition and structure of cytoplasmic globules in leukemic lymphocytes. Blood **29**, 77–86 (1967)

LE BEUX, Y., GANTER, P.: Étude histopathologique et cytologique de la maladie de Waldenström. (À propos de 8 cas de macroglobulinémie.) Ann. Anat. path. **8**, 377–416 (1963)

LEDER, L.-D.: Über die selektive fermentcytochemische Darstellung von neutrophilen myeloischen Zellen und Gewebsmastzellen im Paraffinschnitt. Klin. Wschr. **42**, 553 (1964)

LEDER, L.-D.: Fermenthistochemische Befunde bei chronischer Erythroblastose und akuter Erythrämie. Klin. Wschr. **43**, 795–796 (1965)

LEDER, L.-D.: Der Blutmonocyt. (Experimentelle Medizin, Pathologie und Klinik, Bd. 23.) Berlin-Heidelberg-New York: Springer 1967a

LEDER, L.-D.: Die fermentcytochemische Erkennung normaler und neoplastischer Erythropoesezellen in Schnitt und Ausstrich. Blut **15**, 289–293 (1967b)

LEDER, L.-D.: Die Herkunft der Blutmonozyten und ihre Beziehungen zu den sog. Histiozyten. In: Der Monozyt. Hämatologie und Bluttransfusion, Bd. 7, pp. 19–26. BRÜCHER, H., Ed. München: Lehmanns 1969a

LEDER, L.-D.: On the PAS reaction in acute paraerythroblastic hemoblastoses. Acta haemat. (Basel) **41**, 328–330 (1969b)

LEDER, L.-D.: Zur Praxis der bioptischen Hämoblastosediagnostik mit zytochemischen Methoden. Beitr. Path. **141**, 396–401 (1970)

LEDER, L.-D.: Diagnostic application of cytochemistry in hematology. Proc. 8. Wld Congr. of Anat. Clin. Path., Munich, Sept. 1972. Int. Congr. Ser. No. 285: Anatomic and Clinical Pathology, pp. 105–109. Amsterdam: Excerpta Medica 1973

LEDER, L.-D., LENNERT, K.: Über iatrogene Lymphknotenveränderungen. Verh. dtsch. Ges. Path. **56**, 310–320 (1972)

LEDER, L.-D., STUTTE, H.J.: Seminar für hämatologisch-zytochemische Techniken. Verh. dtsch. Ges. Path. **59**, 503–509 (1975)

LEE, S.L., ROSNER, F., RUBERMAN, W., GLASBERG, S.: Mu-chain disease. Ann. intern. Med. **75**, 407–414 (1971)

LEECH, J.H., GLICK, A.D., WALDRON, J.A., FLEXNER, J.M., HORN, R.G., COLLINS, R.D.: Malignant lymphomas of follicular center cell origin in man. I. Immunologic studies. J. nat. Cancer Inst. **54**, 11–21 (1975)

VAN LEEUWEN, A.W.F.M., MEIJER, C.J.L.M., DE MAN, J.C.H.: T-cell membrane characteristics of 'mycosis cells' in the skin and lymph node. J. invest. Derm. **65**, 367–369 (1975)

LEIBETSEDER, F.: Lymphdrüsenpunktion beim großfollikulären Lymphoblastom. Klin. Med. (Wien) **4**, 131–135 (1949)

LEIBETSEDER, F., TUBA, J.: Splenektomie bei Lymphomen. Folia haemat. (Frankfurt) N.F. **1**, 116–131 (1956)

LEJEUNE, F., TURPIN, F., LECOUTURIER, J.-P., BOUVIER, J.-B., LORTHOLARY, P.: Plasmocytome ganglionnaire. Association à une anémie hémolytique à auto-anticorps avec agglutinines froides. Nouv. Presse méd. **1**, 1065–1068 (1972)

LELBACH, W.K.: Ein Beitrag zur Morphologie der Makroglobulinämie Waldenström. Frankfurt. Z. Path. **68**, 440–464 (1957)

LEMERLE, M., GÉRARD-MARCHANT, R., SANCHO, H., SCHWEISGUTH, O.: Natural history of non-Hodgkin's malignant lymphomata in children. A retrospective study of 190 cases. Brit. J. Cancer **31**, Suppl. II, 324–331 (1975)

LENNERT, K.: Über Morphologie und Mechanismus der Urethanwirkung. Klin. Wschr. **26**, 735–736 (1948)

LENNERT, K.: Zur Praxis der pathologisch-anatomischen Knochenmarksuntersuchung. Frankfurt. Z. Path. **63**, 267–299 (1952a)

LENNERT, K.: Zur histologischen Diagnose der Lymphogranulomatose. Habil. Schrift Frankfurt/M. 1952b

LENNERT, K.: Die pathologische Anatomie der Makroglobulinämie Waldenström. Frankfurt. Z. Path. **66**, 201–226 (1955)

LENNERT, K.: Über die Erkennung von Keimzentrumszellen im Lymphknotenausstrich. Klin. Wschr. **35**, 1130–1132 (1957)

LENNERT, K.: Über Morphologie, Funktion und maligne Neoplasien der Lymphocyten. Z. Haut- u. Geschl.-Kr. **28**, 389–406 (1960)

LENNERT, K.: Lymphknoten. Diagnostik in Schnitt und Ausstrich. Bandteil A: Cytologie und Lymphadenitis. Handbuch der speziellen pathologischen Anatomie und Histologie **1**, 3 A. LUBARSCH, O., HENKE, F., RÖSSLE, R., UEHLINGER, E., (Eds.). Berlin-Göttingen-Heidelberg: Springer 1961

LENNERT, K.: Pathologie der Halslymphknoten. Ein Abriß für Pathologen, Kliniker und praktizierende Ärzte. Berlin-Göttingen-Heidelberg-New York: Springer 1964a

LENNERT, K.: Zur normalen und pathologischen Histologie hautnaher Lymphknoten. In: Handbuch der Haut- und Geschlechtskrankheiten. Ergänzungswerk **1**, 2: Normale und pathologische Anatomie der Haut II, pp. 830–896. Berlin-Göttingen-Heidelberg-New York: Springer 1964b

LENNERT, K.: Classification of malignant lymphomas (European concept). In: Progress in Lymphology, pp. 103–109. RÜTTIMANN, A., Ed. Stuttgart: G. Thieme 1967

LENNERT, K.: Pathologisch-anatomische Klassifikation der malignen Lymphome. Strahlentherapie, Sonderbd. **69**, 1–7 (1969a)

LENNERT, K.: Die derzeitige Häufigkeit der einzelnen Lymphknotenerkrankungen in Schleswig-Holstein. Dtsch. med. Wschr. **94**, 2194–2202 (1969b)

LENNERT, K.: Germinal centers and germinal center neoplasms. Acta haemat. jap. **32**, 495–500 (1969c)

LENNERT, K.: Pathologie und Klassifikation der malignen Lymphome. Paper presented at the Congr. of Jap. Soc. Path., Fukuoka 1969d

LENNERT, K.: Follicular lymphoma: A special entity of malignant lymphomas. In: Plenary Session Papers. 1. Meeting Europ. Div. of Int. Soc. of Haemat., Milano 1971, pp. 109–122. Milano: Arti Grafiche Fratelli Ferrari 1971

LENNERT, K.: Follicular lymphoma and other malignant lymphomas as neoplasias of the B cell system. Symposium at the 9. Int. Congr. of the Int. Academy of Path., Helsinki/Finland, Sept. 1972

LENNERT, K.: Follicular lymphoma. A tumor of the germinal centers. In: Malignant Diseases of the Hematopoietic System. GANN Monograph on Cancer Research, Vol. 15, pp. 217–231. AKAZAKI, K., RAPPAPORT, H., BERARD, C.W., BENNETT, J.M., ISHIKAWA, E., Eds. Tokyo: University of Tokyo Press 1973a

LENNERT, K.: Ancillary approaches to the cellular identification and classification of non-Hodgkin's lymphomas. A) Histochemistry and immunochemistry. Paper presented at a workshop on non-Hodgkin's-lymphomas, Chicago 1973b

LENNERT, K.: Pathologisch-histologische Klassifizierung der malignen Lymphome. In: Leukämien und maligne Lymphome, pp. 181–194. STACHER, A., Ed. München-Berlin-Wien: Urban & Schwarzenberg 1973c

LENNERT, K.: Origin of malignant lymphomas. [Letter to the Editor.] Lancet 1974a, II, p. 586

LENNERT, K.: The germinal centers and their tumors. [Span.] Patologia **7**, 81–88 (1974b)

LENNERT, K.: Reticuloses and Reticulosarcoma. [Span.] Patologia **7**, 35–38 (1974c)

LENNERT, K.: Morphology and classification of malignant lymphomas and so-called reticuloses. In: Malignant Lymphomas of the Nervous System. JELLINGER, K., SEITELBERGER, F., Eds. Acta neuropath. (Berlin) Suppl. **6**, 1–16 (1975)

LENNERT, K.: Klassifikation und Morphologie der Non-Hodgkin-Lymphome. In: Maligne Lymphome und monoklonale Gammopathien. Hämatologie und Bluttransfusion, Bd. 18, pp. 145–166. LÖFFLER, H., Ed. München: Lehmanns 1976

LENNERT, K., ELSCHNER, H.: Zur Kenntnis der lipomelanotischen Reticulo(cyto)se. Frankfurt. Z. Path. **65**, 559–577 (1954)

LENNERT, K., ILLERT, E.: Die Häufigkeit der Gewebsmastzellen im Lymphknoten bei verschiedenen Erkrankungen. Frankfurt. Z. Path. **70**, 121–131 (1959)

LENNERT, K., KAISERLING, E., MÜLLER-HERMELINK, H.K.: T-associated plasma-cells. [Letter to the Editor.] Lancet 1975, I, pp. 1031–1032

LENNERT, K., LEDER, L.-D., LÖFFLER, H.: Fermenthistochemische Untersuchungen des Lymphknotens. V. Mitt. Saure Phosphatase in Schnitt und Ausstrich. Virchows Arch. path. Anat. **338**, 285–304 (1965)

LENNERT, K., LÖFFLER, H., GRABNER, F.: Fermenthistochemische Untersuchungen des Lymphknotens. IV. Mitt. Esterase in Schnitt und Ausstrich. Virchows Arch. path. Anat. **335**, 491–512 (1962)

LENNERT, K., LÖFFLER, H., LEDER, L.-D.: Fermenthistochemische Untersuchungen des Lymphknotens. I. Mitt. Alkalische Phosphatase in Schnitt und Ausstrich. Virchows Arch. path. Anat. **334**, 399–418 (1961)

LENNERT, K., LÖFFLER, H., LEDER, L.-D.: Fermenthistochemische Untersuchungen am lymphoretikulären Gewebe. In: Zyto- und Histochemie in der Hämatologie, pp. 363–383. MERKER, H., Ed. Berlin-Göttingen-Heidelberg: Springer 1963

LENNERT, K., MESTDAGH, J.: Lymphogranulomatosen mit konstant hohem Epitheloidzellgehalt. Virchows Arch. A **344**, 1–20 (1968)

LENNERT, K., MOHRI, N.: Zur Pathologie der Leukämien und malignen Lymphome im Kindesalter. (Referat) Verh. dtsch. Ges. Path. **55**, 216–269 (1971)

LENNERT, K., MOHRI, N.: Histologische Klassifizierung und Vorkommen des M. Hodgkin. Internist **15**, 57–65 (1974)

LENNERT, K., MOHRI, N., STEIN, H., KAISERLING, E.: The histopathology of malignant lymphoma. Brit. J. Haemat. **31** (Suppl.), 193–203 (1975)

LENNERT, K., NAGAI, K., SCHWARZE, E.-W.: Patho-anatomical features of the bone marrow. Clin. Haemat. **4**, 331–351 (1975)

LENNERT, K., STEIN, H., KAISERLING, E.: New criteria for the classification of malignant lymphomas. In: Present Problems in Haematology, pp. 113–119. LÍBANSKÝ, J., DONNER, L., Eds. Amsterdam: Excerpta Medica 1974

LENNERT, K., STEIN, H., KAISERLING, E.: Cytological and functional criteria for the classification of malignant lymphomata. Brit. J. Cancer **31**, Suppl. II, 29–43 (1975)

LEVINE, P.H., CHO, B.R., CONNELLY, R.R., BERARD, C.W., O'CONOR, G.T., DORFMAN, R.F., EASTON, J.M., DEVITA, V.T.: The American Burkitt lymphoma registry: A progress report. Ann. intern. Med. **83**, 31–36 (1975)

LI, F.P., WILLARD, D.R., GOODMAN, R., VAWTER, G.: Malignant lymphoma after diphenylhydantoin (Dilantin) therapy. Cancer (Philad.) **36**, 1359–1362 (1975)

LIEBOW, A.A., CARRINGTON, C.B.: Diffuse pulmonary lymphoreticular infiltrations associated with dysproteinemia. Med. Clin. N.Amer. **57**, 809–843 (1973)

LILLE, I., DESPLACES, A., MEEUS, L., SARACINO, R.T., BROUET, J.C.: Thymus-derived proliferating lymphocytes in chronic lymphocytic leukaemia. Lancet 1973, II, pp. 263–264

LINDQVIST, K.J., RAGAB, A.H., OSTERLAND, C.K.: Paraproteinemia in a child with leukemia. Blood **35**, 213–221 (1970)

LINKE, A., FREUDENBERGER, B.: Über die Chemotherapie der Hämoblastosen und malignen Tumoren. In: Symposien aktueller therapeutischer Probleme, H. 3, pp. 38–134. Stuttgart: F. Enke 1960

LITOVITZ, T.L., LUTZNER, M.A.: Quantitative measurements of blood lymphocytes from patients with chronic lymphocytic leukemia and the Sézary syndrome. J. nat. Cancer Inst. **53**, 75–77 (1974)

LÖFFLER, H.: Zur Differenzierung unreifzelliger (akuter) Leukosen mit cytochemischen Methoden. Folia haemat. (Frankfurt) N.F. **8**, 112–117 (1963)

LÖFFLER, H.: Eine Klassifizierung als Grundlage der Behandlung unreifzelliger Leukosen. In: Hämatologie u. Bluttransfusion **8**, 105–107. München: J.F. Lehmanns 1969a

LÖFFLER, H.: Zytochemische Klassifizierung der akuten Leukosen. In: Chemo- und Immuntherapie der Leukosen und malignen Lymphome, pp. 120–127. STACHER, A., Ed. Wien: Bohmann 1969b

LÖFFLER, H.: Cytologische Befunde beim Sézary-Syndrom. Verh. dtsch. Ges. inn. Med. **78**, 285–287 (1972a)

LÖFFLER, H.: Cytochemie bei Leukosen: Einleitung und Übersicht. In: Leukämie, pp. 119–126. GROSS, R., VAN DE LOO, J., Eds. Berlin-Heidelberg-New York: Springer 1972b

LÖFFLER, H.: Indications and limits of cytochemistry in acute leukemia. In: Recent Results in Cancer Res. **43**, 57–62. Berlin-Heidelberg-New York: Springer 1973

LÖFFLER, H., GRAUBNER, M., DESAGA, J.F., JUNG, M.: Prolymphocytic leukemia with T cell properties and tartrate resistant acid phosphatase. In: Immunological Diagnosis of Leukemias and Lymphomas. Haematology and Blood Transfusion, Vol. 20, pp. 175–178. THIERFELDER, S., RODT, H., THIEL, E., Eds. Berlin-Heidelberg-New York: Springer 1977

LÖFFLER, H., KALTENBACH, T.: Koexistenz von chronischer lymphatischer Leukämie und Lymphogranulomatose bei zwei Patienten. Verh. dtsch. Ges. inn. Med. **75**, 513–515 (1969)

LÖFFLER, H., MEYHÖFER, W., LANGE, R.H., EHLERS, G., REMMELE, W.: Sézary-Syndrom – eine leukämische Variante der Mykosis fungoides. Dtsch. med. Wschr. **99**, 429–434 (1974)

LÖFFLER, H., PRÄLLE, H., LÜCK, R., FISCHER, J., ROUX, A.: Behandlungsergebnisse bei cytochemisch klassifizierten unreifzelligen Leukosen. Verh. dtsch. Ges. inn. Med. **79**, 357–360 (1973)

LÖFFLER, H., PRALLE, H., LÜCK, R., FISCHER, J., ROUX, A.: Der cytochemisch ermittelte Leukosetyp als prognostischer Parameter bei unreifzelligen Leukosen. Klin. Wschr. **52**, 134–137 (1974)

LOESCH, J.: Systematische reticulo-endotheliale Hyperplasien mit tumorähnlichen Bildungen in einem Falle von chronischer lymphatischer Leukämie. Frankfurt. Z. Path. **44**, 351–359 (1933)

LONG, J.C., AISENBERG, A.C.: Richter's syndrome. A terminal complication of chronic lymphocytic leukemia with distinct clinicopathologic features. Amer. J. clin. Path. **63**, 786–795 (1975)

LONG, J.C., MIHM, M.C.: Mycosis fungoides with extracutaneous dissemination: A distinct clinicopathologic entity. Cancer (Philad.) **34**, 1745–1755 (1974)

LORBACHER, P., YAM, L.T., MITUS, W.J.: Cytochemical demonstration of β-glucuronidase activity in blood and bone marrow cells. J. Histochem. Cytochem. **15**, 680–687 (1967)

LORENZ, W.: Über die Bedeutung der Lymphknotenpunktion für die Strahlenheilkunde. Strahlentherapie **79**, 435–464 (1949)

LORTHOLARY, P., BOIRON, M., RIPAULT, J., LEVACHER, A., MIELOT, F., BERNARD, J.: Trois observations de transformation aiguë d'hémopathies lymphocytaires chroniques. Nouv. Rev. franç, Hémat. **6**, 637–656 (1966)

LORTHOLARY, P., BOIRON, M., RIPAULT, P., LEVY, J.P., MANUS, A., BERNARD, J.: Leucémie lymphoide chronique secondairement associée à une réticulopathie maligne, syndrome de Richter. Nouv. Rev. franç. Hémat. **4**, 621–644 (1964)

LOUWAGIE, A.C., DESMET, V.J., VAN DEN BERGHE, H.: Coexistence of a myelo- and lymphoproliferative disorder. Scand. J. Haemat. **11**, 350–355 (1973)

LOWENBRAUN, S., SUTHERLAND, J.C., FELDMAN, M.J., SERPICK, A.A.: Transformation of reticulum cell sarcoma to acute leukemia. Cancer (Philad.) **27**, 579–585 (1971)

LOYAU, G., BARRÉ, J.P., L'HIRONDEL, J.L., LANIÈCE, M., PREUD'HOMME, J.L.: Maladie des chaînes lourdes gamma. À propos d'une nouvelle observation. Nouv. Presse méd. **4**, 957–959 (1975)

LUCAS, P.F.: Lymph node smears in the diagnosis of lymphadenopathy: a review. Blood **10**, 1030–1054 (1955)

LÜDIN, H.: Die Organpunktion in der klinischen Diagnostik. Basel: S. Karger 1955

LUKES, R.J.: The American concept of malignant lymphoma. Saishin Igaku **19**, 1630–1648 (1964)

LUKES, R.J.: A review of the American concept of malignant lymphoma. The evolution of a modern classification. In: Progress in Lymphology. Proc. of Int. Symp. on Lymphology, Zurich, July 1966, pp. 109–119. RÜTTIMANN, A., Ed. Stuttgart: G. Thieme 1967

LUKES, R.J.: The pathologic picture of the malignant lymphomas. In: Proceedings of the International Conference on Leukemia-Lymphoma, pp. 333–356. ZARAFONETIS, C.J.D., Ed. Philadelphia: Lea & Febiger 1968

LUKES, R.J.: Discussion. Workshop on Non-Hodgkin's Lymphomas, Chicago, June 1973

LUKES, R.J., COLLINS, R.D.: New observations on follicular lymphoma. In: Malignant Diseases of the Hematopoietic System. GANN Monograph on Cancer Research, Vol. 15, pp. 209–215. AKAZAKI, K., RAPPAPORT, H., BERARD, C.W., BENNETT, J.M., ISHIKAWA, E., Eds. Tokyo: University of Tokyo Press 1973

LUKES, R.J., COLLINS, R.D.: A functional approach to the classification of malignant lymphoma. In: Recent Results in Cancer Res. **46**, 18–30. Berlin-Heidelberg-New York: Springer 1974a

LUKES, R.J., COLLINS, R.D.: Immunologic characterization of human malignant lymphomas. Cancer (Philad.) **34**, 1488–1503 (1974b)

LUKES, R.J., COLLINS, R.D.: New approaches to the classification of the lymphomata. Brit. J. Cancer **31**, Suppl. II, 1–28 (1975a)

LUKES, R.J., COLLINS, R.D.: A functional classification of malignant lymphomas. In: The Reticuloendothelial System. Monographs in Pathology, No. 16, pp. 213–242. REBUCK, J.W., BERARD, C.W., ABELL, M.R., Eds. Baltimore: Williams & Wilkins 1975b

LUKES, R.J., LENNERT, K.: Malignant lymphoma, Slide Seminar. 10. Int. Congr. Int. Acad. Path., Hamburg 1974
LUKES, R.J., TINDLE, B.H.: Workshop on Classification of Non-Hodgkin's Lymphomas, Chicago, June 1973
LUKES, R.J., TINDLE, B.H.: Immunoblastic lymphadenopathy. A hyperimmune entity resembling Hodgkin's disease. New Engl. J. Med. **292**, 1–12 (1975)
LUMB, G.: Tumours of Lymphoid Tissue. Edinburgh-London: Livingstone 1954
LUMB, G., NEWTON, K.A.: Prognosis in tumors of lymphoid tissue. An analysis of 602 cases. Cancer (Philad.) **10**, 976–993 (1957)
LUTZNER, M.A., EMERIT, I., DUREPAIRE, R., FLANDRIN, G., GRUPPER, C., PRUNIERAS, M.: Cytogenetic, cytophotometric, and ultrastructural study of large cerebriform cells of the Sézary syndrome and description of a small-cell variant. J. nat. Cancer Inst. **50**, 1145–1162 (1973)
LUTZNER, M.A., HOBBS, J.W., HORVATH, P.: Ultrastructure of abnormal cells. In Sezary syndrome, mycosis fungoides, and parapsoriasis en plaque. Arch. Derm. **103**, 375–386 (1971)
LUTZNER, M.A., JORDAN, H.W.: The ultrastructure of an abnormal cell in Sézary's syndrome. Blood **31**, 719–726 (1968)
MACHADO, J.C., JAMRA, M., OKUYAMA, M.H., MARIGO, C.: Lymphoreticular tumors in Sao Paulo, Brazil. J. nat. Cancer Inst. **50**, 1651–1655 (1973)
MACKENZIE, M.R., FUDENBERG, H.H.: Macroglobulinemia: An analysis for forty patients. Blood **39**, 874–889 (1972)
MÄRKI, H.H., SIEGENTHALER, R.: Über eine unter dem Bilde einer Paraleukoblastenleukämie verlaufende Form der Makroglobulinämie. Schweiz. med. Wschr. **94**, 1557–1561 (1964)
MAGRATH, I.T.: Burkitt's lymphoma: A B or T cell tumour? Europ. J. Cancer **10**, 83–88 (1974)
MALDONADO, J.E., WILLIAMS, JR., R.C., SILVERSTEIN, M.N., HARRISON, JR., E.G.: Lymphosarcoma with Bence-Jones proteinuria (type K) and IgG serum M-component (type L): A bitypic gammopathy. Mayo Clin. Proc. **45**, 413–425 (1970)
MALLARMÉ, J.: L'adénogramme des sarcomes ganglionnaires. Sang **26**, 553–568 (1955)
DE MAN, J.C.H., MEINERS, W.B.H.: Crystals of protein nature in the cytoplasm of lymphatic cells in a case of lymphoreticular malignancy. Blood **20**, 492–500 (1962)
MANN, R.B., JAFFE, E.S., BRAYLAN, R.C., EGGLESTON, J.C., RANSOM, L., KAIZER, H., BERARD, C.W.: Immunologic and morphologic studies of T cell lymphoma. Amer. J. Med. **58**, 307–313 (1975)
MANN, R.B., JAFFE, E.S., BRAYLAN, R.C., NANBA, K., FRANK, M.M., ZIEGLER, J.L., BERARD, C.W.: Non-endemic Burkitt's lymphoma. A B-cell tumor related to germinal centers. New Engl. J. Med. **295**, 685–691 (1976)
MANN, H.B., WHITNEY, D.R.: On a test of whether one of two random variables is stochastically larger than the other. Ann. math. Statist. **18**, 50–60 (1947)
MANOLOV, G., MANOLOVA, Y.: Marker band in one chromosome 14 from Burkitt lymphomas. Nature (Lond.) **237**, 33–34 (1972)
MARCHAL, G., FINE, J.-M., BILSKI-PASQUIER, G.: Macroglobulinémie dans un cas de leucose plasmocytaire. Presse méd. **70**, 425–428 (1962)
MARESCH, R.: Über ein plasmazelluläres Lymphogranulom. Verh. dtsch. Ges. Path. **13**, 257–263 (1909)
MARIN-PADILLA, M., FAHIMI, H.D., MOLONEY, W.C.: Leukemic reticulum-cell sarcoma (reticulum-cell sarcoma terminating in acute leukemia). Report of two cases and review of the literature. Amer. J. clin. Path. **41**, 402–410 (1964)
MARSDEN, H.B., STEWARD, J.K.: Non-leukaemic reticuloendothelial tumours and leucosarcomas. In: Tumours in Children. Recent Results in Cancer Research, Vol. 13, pp. 63–85. MARSDEN, H.B., STEWARD, J.K., Eds. Berlin-Heidelberg-New York: Springer 1968
MARSHALL, A.H.E.: An Outline of the Cytology and Pathology of the Reticular Tissue, p. 129ff. Edinburgh-London: Oliver & Boyd 1956.
MARTINI, G.A., WENDEROTH, H.: Zur Klinik und Pathologie des follikulären Lymphoblastoms (Brill-Symmers). Z. klin. Med. **147**, 235–260 (1950)
MATHÉ, G., BELPOMME, D., DANTCHEV, D., KHALIL, A., AFIFI, A.M., TALEB, N., POUILLART, P., SCHWARZENBERG, L., HAYAT, M., DE VASSAL, F., JASMIN, C., MISSET, J.L., MUSSET, M.: Immunoblastic lymphosarcoma, a cytological and clinical entity? Biomedicine **22**, 473–488 (1975)
MATHÉ, G., BELPOMME, D., DANTCHEV, D., POUILLART, P., JASMIN, C., MISSET, J.L., MUSSET,

M., Amiel, J.L., Schlumberger, J.R., Schwarzenberg, L., Hayat, M., de Vassal, F., Lafleur, M.: Immunoblastic acute lymphoid leukaemia: An undescribed type. Biomedicine **20**, 333–340 (1974)

Mathé, G., Belpomme, D., Dantchev, D., Pouillart, P., Navares, L., Hauss, G., Schlumberger, J.R., Lafleur, M.: Search for correlations between cytological types and therapeutic sensitivity of acute leukaemias. Blood Cells **1**, 37–52 (1975)

Mathé, G., Gérard-Marchant, R., Texier, J.L., Schlumberger, J.R., Berumen, L., Paintrand, M.: The two varieties of lymphoid tissue "reticulosarcomas", histiocytic and histioblastic types. Brit. J. Cancer **24**, 687–695 (1970)

Mathé, G., Pouillart, P., Sterescu, M., Amiel, J.L., Schwarzenberg, L., Schneider, M., Hayat, M., de Vassal, F., Jasmin, C., Lafleur, M.: Subdivision of classical varieties of acute leukemia. Correlation with prognosis and cure expectancy. Europ. J. clin. biol. Res. **16**, 554–560 (1971)

Mathé, G., Pouillart, P., Weiner, R., Hayat, M., Steresco, M., Lafleur, M.: Classification and subclassification of acute leukemias correlated with clinical expression, therapeutic sensitivity and prognosis. In: Nomenclature, Methodology and Results of Clinical Trials in Acute Leukemias. Recent Results in Cancer Research, Vol. 43, pp. 6–20. Mathé, G., Pouillart, P., Schwarzenberg, L., Eds. Berlin-Heidelberg-New York: Springer 1973

Mathé, G., Rappaport, H., O'Conor, G.T., Torloni, H.: Histological and cytological typing of neoplastic diseases of haematopoietic and lymphoid tissues. (International Histological Classification of Tumors, No. 14.) Geneva: World Health Organization 1976

Mayer, Jr., S., Thomas, H.M.: Follicular lymphoblastoma and a related form of lymphosarcoma. Bull. Johns Hopkins Hosp. **64**, 315–338 (1939)

McKenna, R.W., Bloomfield, C.D., Brunning, R.D.: Nodular lymphoma: Bone marrow and blood manifestations. Cancer (Philad.) **36**, 428–440 (1975)

McNutt, D.R., Fudenberg, H.H.: IgG myeloma and Waldenström macroglobulinemia. Arch. intern. Med. **131**, 731–734 (1973)

Meister, H., Fuchs, R.: Zytochemie der malignen Erythroblastose. Folia haemat. (Lpz.) **98**, 71–80 (1972)

Michaux, J.-L., Heremans, J.F.: Thirty cases of monoclonal immunoglobulin disorders other than myeloma or macroglobulinemia. A classification of diseases associated with the production of monoclonal-type immunoglobulins. Amer. J. Med. **46**, 562–579 (1969)

Michlmayr, G., Huber, C., Fink, U., Falkensammer, M., Huber, H.: T-Lymphozyten in peripherem Blut und Lymphknoten bei lymphatischen Systemerkrankungen. Schweiz. med. Wschr. **104**, 815–820 (1974)

Michlmayr, G., Pathouli, C., Falkensammer, M., Huber, C., Huber, H., Braunsteiner, H.: Rosettentests bei lymphoproliferativen Erkrankungen. Schweiz. med. Wschr. **106**, 794–799 (1976)

Mielke, H.-G.: Serumeiweiß-Befunde beim Retothel- und Lympho-Sarkom. Ärztl. Wschr. **11**, 1086–1089 (1956)

Miller, D.G.: Immunological deficiency and malignant lymphoma. Cancer (Philad.) **20**, 579–588 (1967a)

Miller, D.G.: The association of immune disease and malignant lymphoma. Ann. intern. Med. **66**, 507–521 (1967b)

Millett, Y.L., Bennett, M.H., Jelliffe, A.M., Farrer-Brown, G.: Nodular sclerotic lymphosarcoma. A further review. Brit. J. Cancer **23**, 683–692 (1969)

Minowada, J., Klein, G., Clifford, P., Klein, E., Moore, G.E.: Studies of Burkitt lymphoma cells. I. Establishment of a cell line (B35M) and its characteristics. Cancer (Philad.) **20**, 1430–1437 (1967)

Mintz, U., Sachs, L.: Changes in the surface membrane of lymphocytes from patients with chronic lymphocytic leukemia and Hodgkin's disease. Int. J. Cancer **15**, 253–259 (1975)

Missmahl, H.P.: Amyloidose. Klinik, Therapie, Prognose. Fortschr. Med. **85**, 621–626 (1967)

Missmahl, H.P.: Amyloidosen bei chronisch-rheumatischen Erkrankungen. Verh. dtsch. Ges. inn. Med. **74**, 1102–1116 (1968)

Missmahl, H.P., Gafni, J.: Peri-collagen and peri-reticular amyloidoses—their differentiation by polarization microscopy. Path. et Microbiol. (Basel) **27**, 826–832 (1964)

Mitchell, L.A.: Malignant monoblastoma. A variant of monocytic leukemia. Ann. intern. Med. **8**, 1387–1403 (1935)

MITROU, P., SCHUBERT, J.C.F., MARTIN, H.: Die Behandlung der Makroglobulinämie Waldenström mit Procarbazin. Dtsch. med. Wschr. **97**, 1864–1869 (1972)
MITUS, A.: Presentation at Meeting of the International Society of Paediatric Oncology, Manchester, October 1972.
MITUS, W.J., BERGNA, L.J., MEDNICOFF, I.B., DAMESHEK, W.: Cytochemical studies of glycogen content of lymphocytes in lymphocytic proliferations. Blood **13**, 748–756 (1958)
MITUS, W.J., MEDNICOFF, I.B., WITTELS, B., DAMESHEK, W.: Neoplastic lymphoid reticulum cells in the peripheral blood: A histochemical study. Blood **17**, 206–215 (1961)
MOESCHLIN, S.: Klinik der Reticulosen – mit speziellem Hinweis auf Sensibilisierungserscheinungen durch die gebildeten Paraproteine. Helv. med. Acta **28**, 306–338 (1961)
MOESCHLIN, S.: Macroglobulinemia Waldenström with miliary lung infiltrations and terminal plasmacell-leukemia. Acta med. scand. Suppl. **445**, 154–162 (1966)
MOHR, U., KINZEL, V.: Das Burkitt-Lymphom. Dtsch. med. Wschr. **93**, 2229–2231 (1968)
MOLLO, F., MONGA, G., CODA, R., PALESTRO, G.: Ultrastructural features of human lymphomas. Acta neuropath. (Berl.) Suppl. **6**, 17–20 (1975)
MOORE, D.F., MIGLIORE, P.J., SHULLENBERGER, C.C., ALEXANIAN, R.: Monoclonal macroglobulinemia in malignant lymphoma. Ann. intern. Med. **72**, 43–47 (1970)
MOORE, G.E., MINOWADA, J.: T or B lymphocytes in chronic lymphocytic leukemia. Lancet 1972, I, pp. 38–39
MORI, Y., LENNERT, K.: Electron microscopic atlas of lymph node cytology and pathology. Berlin-Heidelberg-New York: Springer 1969
MORRISON, M., SAMWICK, A.A., RUBINSTEIN, J., STICH, M., LOEWE, L.: Lymph node aspiration. Am. J. clin. Path. **22**, 255–262 (1952)
MORROW, R.H., PIKE, M.C., KISUULE, A.: Survival of Burkitt's lymphoma patients in Mulago Hospital, Uganda. Brit. med. J. 1967, IV, pp. 323–327
MORROW, R.H., PIKE, M.C., SMITH, P., ZIEGLER, J.L.: Preliminary epidemiological findings of Burkitt's lymphoma in the Mengo Districts, Uganda, 1959–1968. [Abstr.] Cancer Res. **34**, 1211–1212 (1974)
MOSS, W.T., ACKERMAN, L.V.: Plasma cell leukemia. Blood **1**, 396–406 (1946)
MUELLER, J., BRUN DEL RE, G., BUERKI, H., KELLER, H.-U., HESS, M.W., COTTIER, H.: Nonspecific esterase activity: A criterion for differentiation of T and B lymphocytes in mouse lymph nodes. Europ. J. Immunol. **5**, 270–274 (1975)
MÜLLER-HERMELINK, H.K., KAISERLING, E.: Seminar für elektronenmikroskopisch-histochemische Techniken. Verh. dtsch. Ges. Path. **59**, 522–527 (1975)
MÜLLER-HERMELINK, H.K., KAISERLING, E., LENNERT, K.: Pseudofollikuläre Nester von Plasmazellen (eines besonderen Typs?) in der paracorticalen Pulpa menschlicher Lymphknoten. Virchows Arch. B **14**, 47–56 (1973)
MUNDT, E.: Das Retothelsarkom und die Retothelsarkomatose. Ergebn. inn. Med. Kinderheilk. N.F. **3**, 365–374 (1952)
MUSGER, A.: Zur Kenntnis der Reticulohistiocytosen der Haut. Hautarzt **5**, 56–62 (1954)
MUSGER, A.: Erythrodermatische Retikulose der Haut mit analogen feingeweblichen Veränderungen der hautnahen Lymphknoten und subleukämischem Blutbild. Wien. klin. Wschr. **68**, 403–405 (1956)
MUSGER, A.: Erythrodermatische Hautretikulosen. (Vorkommen, Krankheitsbild, Pathogenese). Hautarzt **17**, 148–152 (1966)
MUSSHOFF, K.: Therapy and prognosis of two different forms of organ involvement in cases of malignant lymphoma (Hodgkin's disease, reticulum cell sarcoma, lymphosarcoma) as well as a report about stage division in these diseases. Klin. Wschr. **48**, 673–678 (1970)
MUSSHOFF, K.: Die Strahlenbehandlung der Hodgkinschen Erkrankung. In: Maligne Lymphome und monoklonale Gammopathien. Hämatologie und Bluttransfusion, Bd. 18, pp. 119–134. LÖFFLER, H., Ed. München: Lehmanns 1976
MUSSHOFF, K., SCHMIDT-VOLLMER, H., LENNERT, K., SANDRITTER, W.: Preliminary clinical findings on the Kiel classification of malignant lymphomas. Z. Krebsforsch. **87**, 229–238 (1976)
MUSSHOFF, K., SLANINA, J.: Stadieneinteilung der malignen Lymphome. Zugleich ein Beitrag über die Bedeutung der Laparotomie mit Splenektomie. Klin. Wschr. **52**, 109–117 (1974)
NAEIM, F., SMITH, G.S.: Leukemic reticuloendotheliosis. Cancer (Philad.) **34**, 1813–1821 (1974)
NAGAYO, M.: Reticulum cellular lymphosarcoma. Chiryo-oyobi-Shoho **10**, 1255–1259 (1929), cit. of AKAZAKI, 1973

NANBA, K., ITAGAKI, T., IIJIMA, S.: Enzyme histochemical investigations of human malignant lymphomas. Beitr. Path. **154**, 233–242 (1975)
NATHWANI, B.N., KIM, H., RAPPAPORT, H.: Malignant lymphoma, lymphoblastic. Cancer (Philad.) **38**, 964–983 (1976)
NEIDHARDT, M., FOLTIN, E. (Eds.): Maligne Tumoren im Kindesalter. Ergebnisse einer kooperativen Therapiestudie mit Operation, Bestrahlung und Polychemotherapie. Arbeitsgemeinschaft „Tumoren im Kindesalter". Dtsch. med. Wschr. **98**, 2267–2274 (1973)
NELSON, M.G., LYONS, A.R.: Plasmacytoma of lymph glands. Cancer (Philad.) **10**, 1275–1280 (1957)
NEUHOLD, R., WOLFRAM, S.: Über Reticulohistiocytosen der Haut. Beitr. path. Anat. **112**, 137–149 (1952)
NEWALL, J., FRIEDMAN, M.: Reticulum-cell sarcoma. Part III: Prognosis. Radiology **97**, 99–102 (1970)
NEZELOF, C., BASSET, F., ROUSSEAU, M.F.: Histiocytosis X. Histogenetic arguments for a Langerhans cell origin. Biomedicine **18**, 365–371 (1973)
NGU, V.A.: The African lymphoma (Burkitt tumour): Survivals exceeding two years. Brit. J. Cancer **19**, 101–107 (1965)
NGU, V.A., BURKITT, D.P., OSUNKOYA, B.O.: Clinical and related evidence of host defence mechanisms. In: Burkitt's Lymphoma, pp. 158–163. BURKITT, D.P., WRIGHT, D.H., Eds. Edinburgh-London: Livingstone 1970
NIES, K.M., MARSHALL, J., OBERLIN, M.A., HALPERN, M.S., BROWN, J.C.: Chronic lymphocytic leukemia with gamma chain cytoplasmic inclusions. Amer. J. clin. Path. **65**, 948–956 (1976)
NIEUWENHUIS, P., KEUNING, F.J.: Germinal centres and the origin of the B-cell system. II. Germinal centres in the rabbit spleen and popliteal lymph nodes. Immunology **26**, 509–519 (1974)
NKRUHMAH, F.K., PERKINS, I.V.: Burkitt's lymphoma. A clinical study of 110 patients. Cancer (Philad.) **37**, 671–676 (1976a)
NKRUMAH, F.K., PERKINS, I.V.: Relapse in Burkitt's lymphoma. Int. J. Cancer **17**, 455–460 (1976b)
OBERLING, C.: Les réticulosarcomes et les réticulo-endothélio-sarcomes de la moelle osseuse (sarcomes d'Ewing). Bull. Ass. franç. Cancer **17**, 259–296 (1928)
OBERLING, C., HAGUENAU, F.: Histogénèse des tumeurs du système lymphatique. Acta Un. int. Cancr. **10**, 177–187 (1954)
O'CONOR, G.T.: Malignant lymphoma in African children. II. A pathological entity. Cancer (Philad.) **14**, 270–283 (1961)
O'CONOR, G.T.: Significant aspects of childhood lymphoma in Africa. Cancer Res. **23**, 1514–1518 (1963)
O'CONOR, G.T.: Persistent immunologic stimulation as a factor in oncogenesis, with special reference to Burkitt's tumor. Amer. J. Med. **48**, 279–285 (1970)
O'CONOR, G.T., DAVIES, J.N.P.: Malignant tumors in African children. With special reference to malignant lymphoma. J. Pediat. **56**, 526–535 (1960)
O'CONOR, G.T., RAPPAPORT, H., SMITH, E.B.: Childhood lymphoma resembling "Burkitt tumor" in the United States. Cancer (Philad.) **18**, 411–417 (1965)
OEHME, J.: Akute Leukämie im Kindesalter. Häufigkeit, Disposition, Behandlung. Dtsch. med. Wschr. **82**, 110–113 (1957)
OEHME, J., JANSSEN, W., HAGITTE, C.: Leukämie im Kindesalter. Beiträge zur Morphologie, Klinik, Pathophysiologie und Therapie. (Abhandl. aus d. Gebiet d. prakt. Kinderheilk., Bd. 4.) Leipzig: Thieme 1958
OEHMICHEN, M., GÄRTNER, H.-V., KNITTEL-JUNG, U.: T cell type immunoblastic sarcoma diagnosed primarily by CSF cell membrane features. Klin. Wschr. **55**, 37–40 (1977)
OETTGEN, H.F., MURPHY, M.L.: Malignant lymphoma of childhood in the United States and Burkitt's tumour in Africa: Therapeutic results. In: Treatment of Burkitt's Tumour. UICC Monograph Series, Vol. 8, pp. 105–108. BURCHENAL, J.H., BURKITT, D.P., Eds. Berlin-Heidelberg-New York: Springer 1967a
OETTGEN, H.F., MURPHY, M.L.: Malignant lymphoma in the United States and Burkitt's tumour in Africa: Some aspects of their natural history. In: Treatment of Burkitt's Tumour. UICC Monograph Series, Vol. 8, pp. 7–10. BURCHENAL, J.H., BURKITT, D.P., Eds. Berlin-Heidelberg-New York: Springer 1967b
OETTGEN, H.F., QUITMANN, K.: Weitere Untersuchungen zur Morphologie der Makroglobulinämie Waldenström. Frankfurt. Z. Path. **67**, 599–621 (1956)

Oettlé, A.G.: Lymphoreticular malignant neoplasms in South African races, mortality and morbidity studies. In: Symposium on Lymphoreticular Tumours in Africa, Paris 1963, pp. 1–23. Roulet, F.C., Ed. Basel-New York: Karger 1964a

Oettlé, A.G.: Primary malignant neoplasms of the lymphoreticular tissues (200–203, 205): A histopathological series from White and Bantu races in the Transvaal, 1949–1953. In: Symposium on Lymphoreticular Tumours in Africa, Paris 1963, pp. 24–35. Roulet, F.C., Ed., Basel-New York: Karger 1964b

Ogata, T.: Über die Geschwülste des reticuloendothelialen Systems. GANN **33**, 455–478 (1939), cit. of Akazaki, 1973

O'Gorman Hughes, D.W.: The prognosis of acute leukaemia in childhood. Med. J. Aust. 1974, I, pp. 991–994

Okano, H., Azar, H.A., Osserman, E.F.: Plasmacytic reticulum cell sarcoma. Case report with electron microscopic studies. Amer. J. clin. Path. **46**, 546–555 (1966)

Old, L.J., Boyse, E.A., Oettgen, H.F., de Harven, E., Geering, G., Williamson, B., Clifford, P.: Precipitating antibody in human serum to an antigen present in cultured Burkitt's lymphoma cells. Proc. nat. Acad. Sci. (Wash.) **56**, 1699–1704 (1966)

de Oliveira, G.: Über die Stellung der Retothelsarkome im System der Lymphdrüsengeschwülste. Virchows Arch. path. Anat. **298**, 464–514 (1936)

Oliver, R.T.D.: Linking lymphomas with immunodeficiency. Nature (Lond.) **256**, 262–263 (1975)

Olmer, J., Mongin, M., Muratore, R., Denizet, D.: Myélomes. Macroglobulinémies et dysglobulinémies voisines. Paris: Masson et Cie. 1961

Orsós, F.: Das Bindegewebsgerüst der Lymphknoten im normalen und pathologischen Zustand. Beitr. path. Anat. **75**, 15–134 (1926)

Osserman, E.F., Takatsuki, K.: Clinical and immunochemical studies of four cases of heavy ($H^{\gamma^2}$) chain disease. Amer. J. Med. **37**, 351–373 (1964)

Osunkoya, B.O., McFarlane, H., Luzzatto, L., Udeozo, I.O.K., Mottram, F.C., Williams, A.I.O., Ngu, V.A.: Immunoglobulin synthesis by fresh biopsy cells and established cell lines from Burkitt's lymphoma. Immunology **14**, 851–860 (1968)

Otani, M., Maruya, K., Shibue, K.: On the correlation between the reticulumcell and the monocyte in lymphatic reticulosarcomatosis. Extr. No. 268. 43. Annual Meeting Jap. Path. Soc. 1954. Acta path. jap. **4**, 205 (1954)

Paltauf, R.: Lymphosarkom (Lymphosarkomatose, Pseudoleukämie, Myelom, Chlorom). Ergebn. allg. Path. path. Anat. **3**, 652–691 (1897)

Paltauf, R., von Zumbusch, L.: Mycosis fungoides der Haut und inneren Organe. Arch. Derm. Syph. (Berl.) **118**, 699–742 (1913)

Palutke, M., McDonald, J.M.: Monoclonal gammopathies associated with malignant lymphomas. Amer. J. clin. Path. **60**, 157–165 (1973)

Palutke, M., Tranchida, L.: T-cell lymphoma. Report of a case. Amer. J. clin. Path. **64**, 26–33 (1975)

Pascoe, H.R.: Tumors composed of immature granulocytes occurring in the breast in chronic granulocytic leukemia. Cancer (Philad.) **25**, 697–704 (1970)

Patchefsky, A.S., Brodovsky, H.S., Menduke, H., Southard, M., Brooks, J., Nicklas, D., Hoch, W.S.: Non-Hodgkin's lymphomas: A clinicopathologic study of 293 cases. Cancer (Philad.) **34**, 1173–1186 (1974)

Paufique, L., Girard, P., Schott, B., Creyssel, R., Trillet, M., Chazot, G.: Pseudolymphome de l'orbite macroglobulino-secrétant associé à une méningolymphomatose avec macroglobulinorachie. Ann. Oculist. (Paris) **202**, 1033–1045 (1969)

Pautrier, L.-M., Woringer, F.: Mycosis fongoïde généralisé, forme érythrodermique et tumorale. Le ganglion mycosique. Bull. Soc. franç. Derm. Syph. **49**, 498–505 (1939)

Pavlovsky, A.: La Puncion Ganglionar. Buenos Aires: Aniceto Lopez 1934

Pavlovsky, A.: Contribution of cytology to the study of lymphopathies. Acta haemat. (Basel) **36**, 296–312 (1966)

Payet, M., Camain, R., Pene, P., Sankale, M., Lambert, D.: Les hématosarcomes en Afrique Noire Occidentale et Centrale francophone. II. Considérations cliniques, biologiques et anatomopathologiques. In: Symposium on Lymphoreticular Tumours in Africa, Paris 1963, pp. 104–118. Roulet, F.C., Ed. Basel-New York: Karger 1964

Penn, I., Halgrimson, C.G., Starzl, T.E.: De novo malignant tumors in organ transplant recipients. Transplant. Proc. **3**, 773–778 (1971)

PENN, I., STARZL, T.E.: Malignant tumors arising de novo in immunosuppressed organ transplant recipients. Transplantation **14**, 407–417 (1972)
PERERA, D.J.B., PEGRUM, G.D.: The lymphocyte in chronic lymphatic leukaemia. Lancet 1974, I, pp. 1207–1209
PETERS, M.V.: The contribution of radiation therapy in the control of early lymphomas. Amer. J. Roentgenol. **90**, 956–967 (1963)
PETERSON, L.C., BLOOMFIELD, C.D., SUNDBERG, R.D., GAJL-PECZALSKA, K.J., BRUNNING, R.D.: Morphology of chronic lymphocytic leukemia and its relationship to survival. Amer. J. Med. **59**, 316–324 (1975)
PFISTERER, H., NENNHUBER, J., BOLLAND, H., STICH, W.: Lymphocytenabbau nach in-vitro-Markierung mit $Na_2{}^{51}CrO_4$. II. Untersuchungen bei chronischer lymphatischer Leukämie. Klin. Wschr. **45**, 1073–1076 (1967)
PIKE, M.C.: Chemotherapy in Burkitt's tumour. Lancet 1966, II, p. 856
PINKEL, D.: Five-year follow-up of "total therapy" of childhood lymphocytic leukemia. J. Amer. med. Ass. **216**, 648–652 (1971)
PINKEL, D., JOHNSON, W., AUR, R.J.A.: Non-Hodgkin's lymphoma in children. Brit. J. Cancer **31**, Suppl. II, 298–323 (1975)
PLENDERLEITH, I.H.: Hairy cell leukemia. Canad. med. Ass. J. **102**, 1056–1060 (1970)
POLLIACK, A., BRAYLAN, R., GOLOMB, H.: [Letter to the Editor] Scanning electron microscopy of hairy cells in hairy-cell leukaemia. Lancet 1974, II, pp. 1013–1014
POOLE, A.G., MARCHETTA, F.C.: Extramedullary plasmacytoma of the head and neck. Cancer (Philad.) **22**, 14–21 (1968)
POPE, J.H., HORNE, M.K., WETTERS, E.J.: Significance of a complement-fixing antigen associated with herpes-like virus and detected in the Raji cell line. Nature (Lond.) **222**, 186–187 (1969)
POPKES, B.: Über Größe und Polymorphie der Zellkerne bei Lymphadenose und Lymphosarkom. Frankfurt. Z. Path. **66**, 252–267 (1955)
POUJOL, G.: Un cas de tumeur primitive des ganglions lymphatiques d'origine réticulo-endothéliale. Bull. Ass. franç. Cancer **16**, 627–655 (1927)
PREUD'HOMME, J.L., SELIGMANN, M.: Surface bound immunoglobulins as a cell marker in human lymphoproliferative diseases. Blood **40**, 777–794 (1972)
PRIGOGINA, E.L., FLEISCHMAN, E.W.: Marker chromosome 14q+ in two non-Burkitt lymphomas. Humangenetik **30**, 109–112 (1975)
PRUNIERAS, M.: DNA content and cytogenetics of the Sezary cell. Mayo Clin. Proc. **49**, 548–552 (1974)
PRUZANSKI, W., PLATTS, M.E., OGRYZLO, M.A.: Leukemic form of immunocytic dyscrasia (plasma cell leukemia). A study of ten cases and a review of the literature. Amer. J. Med. **47**, 60–74 (1969)
PULVERTAFT, R.J.V.: The use of tissue culture in the diagnosis of Burkitt's tumour. In: Treatment of Burkitt's Tumour. UICC Monograph Series, Vol. 8, pp. 24–28. BURCHENAL, J.H., BURKITT, D.P., Eds. Berlin-Heidelberg-New York: Springer 1967
PULVERTAFT, R.J.V., PLATT, H.S.: Tissue culture of bone marrow and biopsy material in African childhood lymphoma. A preliminary report. In: Symposium on Lymphoreticular Tumours in Africa, Paris 1963, pp. 285–288. ROULET, F.C., Ed. Basel-New York: Karger 1964
QAZI, R., AISENBERG, A.C., LONG, J.C.: The natural history of nodular lymphoma. Cancer (Philad.) **37**, 1923–1927 (1976)
QUAGLINO, D., COWLING, D.C., HAYHOE, F.G.J.: Cytochemical and autoradiographic studies on normal and leukaemic cells in short-term tissue cultures. Brit. J. Haemat. **10**, 417–436 (1964)
QUAGLINO, D., HAYHOE, F.G.J.: Observations on the periodic acid-Schiff reaction in lymphoproliferative diseases. J. Path. **78**, 521–532 (1959)
RADASZKIEWICZ, T., LENNERT, K.: Lymphogranulomatosis X. Klinisches Bild, Therapie und Prognose. Dtsch. med. Wschr. **100**, 1157–1163 (1975)
RAI, K.R., SAWITZKY, A., CRONKITE, E.P., CHANANA, A.D., LEVY, R.N., PASTERNACK, B.S.: Clinical staging of chronic lymphocytic leukemia. Blood **46**, 219–234 (1975)
RAIN, J.D., FLANDRIN, G., BINET, J.L., BERNARD, J.: Formes ganglionnaires tumorales des leucémies lymphoïdes chroniques. Nouv. Rev. franç. Hémat. **11**, 447–452 (1971)
RAMOT, B.: Malabsorption due to lymphomatous disease. Ann. Rev. Med. **22**, 19–24 (1971)
RAMOT, B., HULU, N.: Primary intestinal lymphoma and its relation to alpha heavy chain disease. Brit. J. Cancer **31**, Suppl. II, 343–349 (1975)

RAMOT, B., MANY, A.: Primary intestinal lymphoma: Clinical manifestations and possible effect of environmental factors. In: Current Problems in the Epidemiology of Cancer and Lymphomas. Recent Results in Cancer Research, Vol. 39, pp. 193–199. GRUNDMANN, E., TULINIUS, H., Eds. Berlin-Heidelberg-New York: Springer 1972

RAMOT, B., SHAHIN, N., BUBIS, J.J.: Malabsorption syndrome in lymphoma of small intestine. A study of 13 cases. Israel J. med. Sci. **1**, 221–226 (1965)

RAPPAPORT, H.: The histologic aspects of malignant lymphoreticular neoplasms. In: Symposium on Lymphoreticular Tumours in Africa, Paris 1963, pp. 174–210. ROULET, F.C., Ed. Basel-New York: Karger 1964a

RAPPAPORT, H.: Classification of neoplastic diseases of the reticular system. In: Symposium on Lymphoreticular Tumours in Africa, Paris 1963, pp. 394–409. ROULET, F.C., Ed. Basel-New York: Karger 1964b

RAPPAPORT, H.: Tumors of the Hematopoietic System. Atlas of Tumor Pathology, Sect. 3, Fasc. 8. Washington, D.C.: Armed Forces Institute of Pathology 1966

RAPPAPORT, H.: Nouveaux concepts dans la classification des hémopathies malignes. Bull. Cancer **61**, 11–22 (1974)

RAPPAPORT, H.: The pathologic anatomy of α chain disease. In: Maligne Lymphome und monoklonale Gammopathien. Hämatologie und Bluttransfusion, Bd 18, pp. 377–382. LÖFFLER, H., Ed. München: Lehmanns 1976

RAPPAPORT, H., BRAYLAN, R.C.: Changing concepts in the classification of malignant neoplasms of the hematopoietic system. In: The Reticuloendothelial System. IAP Monograph No. 16, pp. 1–19. Baltimore, Md.: Williams & Wilkins 1975

RAPPAPORT, H., EDGCOMB, J., THOMAS, L.: Mycosis fungoides: A reevaluation of its position in the scheme of lymphoreticular neoplasms. [Abstr.] Amer. J. clin. Path. **50**, 625 (1968)

RAPPAPORT, H., JOHNSON, F.B.: Intracellular protein resembling Russell bodies in malignant lymphomas associated with acquired hemolytic anemia. Blood **10**, 132–144 (1955)

RAPPAPORT, H., MORAN, E.M.: Angio-immunoblastic (immunoblastic) lymphadenopathy. New Engl. J. Med. **292**, 42–43 (1975)

RAPPAPORT, H., RAMOT, B., HULU, N., PARK, J.K.: The pathology of so-called Mediterranean abdominal lymphoma with malabsorption. Cancer (Philad.) **29**, 1502–1511 (1972)

RAPPAPORT, H., THOMAS, L.B.: Mycosis fungoides: The pathology of extracutaneous involvement. Cancer (Philad.) **34**, 1198–1229 (1974)

RAPPAPORT, H., WINTER, W.J., HICKS, E.B.: Follicular lymphoma. A re-evaluation of its position in the scheme of malignant lymphoma, based on a survey of 253 cases. Cancer (Philad.) **9**, 792–821 (1956)

RAU, R., MUELLER-ECKHARDT, C., HUTH, K., LÖFFLER, H.: Paraproteinämie und Antikörpermangelsyndrom bei chronischer lymphatischer Leukämie. Med. Welt **19** (N.F.), 801–806 (1968)

REED, D.M.: On the pathological changes in Hodgkin's disease, with especial reference to its relation to tuberculosis. Johns Hopkins Hosp. Rep. **10**, 133–196 (1902)

REEDMAN, B.M., KLEIN, G.: Cellular localization of an Epstein-Barr virus (EBV)-associated complement-fixing antigen in producer and non-producer lymphoblastoid cell lines. Int. J. Cancer **11**, 499–520 (1973)

REHMAN, K.L., ROSNER, F., GRÜNWALD, H.W.: The leukemic phase of histiocytic lymphoma: Report of four cases. Amer. J. med. Sci. **268**, 353–359 (1974)

REIS, H.E.: Immunsuppression, Tumorentstehung und Tumorwachstum. Z. Krebsforsch. **78**, 42–50 (1972)

RENNKE, H., LENNERT, K.: Käsig-tuberkuloide Reaktion bei Lymphknotenmetastasen lymphoepithelialer Carcinome (Schmincke-Tumoren). Virchows Arch. A **358**, 241–247 (1973)

REYNAUD, J., QUÉRÉ, M.A., LAMBERT, D.: Les hématosarcomes de la face chez l'enfant en Afrique Occidentale et Centrale francophone. II. Aspects cliniques, radiologiques et biologiques. In: Symposium on Lymphoreticular Tumours in Africa, Paris 1963, pp. 137–149. ROULET, F.C., Ed. Basel-New York: Karger 1964

RICHTER, M.N.: Generalized reticular cell sarcoma of lymph nodes associated with lymphatic leukemia. Amer. J. Path. **4**, 285–299 (1928)

RICHTER, M.N.: Origin of leukemic cells in monocytic leukemia. Lab. Invest. **5**, 155–161 (1956)

RIEBER, E.P., v. HEYDEN, H.W., LINKE, R.P., SAAL, J.G., RIETHMÜLLER, G., WALLER, H.D.: Haarzell-Leukämie. Charakterisierung der leukämischen Zelle: Oberflächenimmunglobuline, Fc-Rezeptoren und Stimulation durch Mitogene. Klin. Wschr. **54**, 1011–1019 (1976)

RIEGEL, R.: Plasmazellenleukämie nach Behandlung mit Thorium X. Ärztl. Wschr. **11**, 1093–1096 (1956)

RIEHM, H., GADNER, H., WELTE, K.: Die West-Berliner Studie zur Behandlung der akuten lymphoblastischen Leukämie des Kindes – Erfahrungsbericht nach 6 Jahren. Klin. Pädiat. **189**, 89–102 (1977)

RILKE, F., CLEMENTE, C., PILOTTI, S., MUSUMECI, R.: Il linfoma linfoblastico a cellule convolute. Tumori **61**, 377–391 (1975)

RIND, H.: Zytomorphologie und Prognose der Leukämie des Kindes. In: Chemo- und Immunotherapie der Leukosen und malignen Lymphome, pp. 183–184. STACHER, A., Ed. Wien: Bohmann 1969

RINNEBERG, H., LENNERT, K.: Fermenthistochemische Untersuchungen des Lymphknotens. III. Adenosintriphosphatase und 5-Nucleotidase in den Zellen des Lymphknotentupfpräparates. Klin. Wschr. **39**, 971 (1961)

RITTER, J., GAEDICKE, G., WINKLER, K., BECKMANN, H., LANDBECK, G.: Possible T-cell origin of lymphoblasts in acid-phosphatase-positive acute lymphatic leukaemia. Lancet 1975, II, p. 75

RITTER, J., GAEDICKE, G., WINKLER, K., LANDBECK, G.: Immunologische Oberflächenmarker von Lymphoblasten bei der saure Phosphatase-positiven akuten Leukämie. Z. Kinderheilk. **120**, 211–215 (1975)

ROATH, S., ISRAËLS, M.C.G., WILKINSON, J.F.: The acute leukaemias: A study of 580 patients. Quart. J. Med. N.S. **33**, 257–283 (1964)

ROBB-SMITH, A.H.T.: Reticulosis and reticulosarcoma: A histological classification. J. Path. **47**, 457–480 (1938)

ROBB-SMITH, A.H.T.: The lymph-node biopsy. In: Recent Advances in Clinical Pathology, pp. 350–370. DYKE, S.C., Ed. London: J. & A. Churchill 1947

ROBB-SMITH, A.H.T.: Introduction: The classification and natural history of the lymphadenopathies. In: Lymphomas and Related Diseases. Treatment of Cancer and Allied Diseases, Vol. 9, pp. 1–27. PACK, G.T., ARIEL, I.M., Eds. New York: Hoeber Medical Division, Harper & Row 1964

ROBB-SMITH, A.H.T.: Immuno-topography of lymphoreticular disorders. Lancet 1974, I, pp. 513–514

RODT, H., THIEL, E., THIERFELDER, S., HUHN, D., GÖTZE, D., BREHM, G.: Spezifisches Anti-T-Lymphocyten-Globulin (sATG) für die Diagnostik lymphoproliferativer Erkrankungen. Klin. Wschr. **54**, 361–366 (1976)

RÖSSLE, R.: Das Retothelsarkom der Lymphdrüsen. Seine Formen und Verwandtschaften. Beitr. path. Anat. **103**, 385–415 (1939)

ROHR, K.: Das menschliche Knochenmark. 3. Ed. Stuttgart: G. Thieme 1960

ROSAS-URIBE, A., RAPPAPORT, H.: Malignant lymphoma, histiocytic type with sclerosis (sclerosing reticulum cell sarcoma). Cancer (Philad.) **29**, 946–953 (1972)

ROSAS-URIBE, A., VARIAKOJIS, D., MOLNAR, Z., RAPPAPORT, H.: Mycosis fungoides: An ultrastructural study. Cancer (Philad.) **34**, 634–645 (1974)

ROSAS-URIBE, A., VARIAKOJIS, D., RAPPAPORT, H.: Proteinaceous precipitate in nodular (follicular) lymphomas. Cancer (Philad.) **31**, 534–542 (1973)

ROSENBERG, S.A., DIAMOND, H.D., DARGEON, H.W., CRAVER, L.F.: Lymphosarcoma in childhood. New Engl. J. Med. **259**, 505–512 (1958)

ROSENBERG, S.A., DIAMOND, H.D., JASLOWITZ, B., CRAVER, L.F.: Lymphosarcoma: A review of 1269 cases. Medicine (Baltimore) **40**, 31–84 (1961)

ROSENBERG, S.A., DORFMAN, R.F., KAPLAN, H.S.: A summary of the results of a review of 405 patients with non-Hodgkin's lymphoma at Stanford University. Brit. J. Cancer **31**, Suppl. II, 168–173 (1975)

ROSENTHAL, N.: The lymphomas and leukemias. Bull. N.Y. Acad. Med. 2. Ser. **30**, 583–600 (1954)

ROSENTHAL, N., DRESKIN, O.H., VURAL, I.L., ZAK, F.G.: The significance of hematogones in blood, bone marrow and lymph node aspiration in giant follicular lymphoblastoma. Acta haemat. (Basel) **8**, 368–377 (1952)

ROSSIER, P.-H., SPÜHLER, O.: Beitrag zum großfollikulären Lymphoblastom, Brill-Symmers Krankheit. Schweiz. med. Wschr. **78**, 1246–1249 (1948)

ROULET, F.: Das primäre Retothelsarkom der Lymphknoten. Virchows Arch. path. Anat. **277**, 15–47 (1930)

ROULET, F.: Weitere Beiträge zur Kenntnis des Retothelsarkoms der Lymphknoten und anderer Lymphoiden-Organe. Virchows Arch. path. Anat. **286**, 702–732 (1932)

ROULET, F.: Das Verhalten der Milz beim Retothelsarkom der Lymphknoten. Schweiz. Z. Path. Suppl. **10**, 88–101 (1947)

ROULET, F.C.: Die ausgesprochen blastomatösen Retikulosen. Verh. dtsch. Ges. Path. **37**, 105–127 (1953)

ROULET, F.C. (Ed.): Symposion on Lymphoreticular Tumours in Africa. Basel-New York: Karger 1964

ROWLANDS, B., SHAW, N.: Extramedullary plasmocytoma. Brit. med. J. 1954, I, pp. 1302–1303

RUBIN, A.D., DOUGLAS, S.D., CHESSIN, L.N., GLADE, P.R., DAMESHEK, W.: Chronic reticulolymphocytic leukemia. Reclassification of "leukemic reticuloendotheliosis" through functional characterization of the circulating mononuclear cells. Amer. J. Med. **47**, 149–162 (1969)

RUBIN, A.D., HAVEMANN, K., DAMESHEK, W.: Studies in chronic lymphocytic leukemia: Further studies of the proliferative abnormality of the blood lymphocyte. Blood **33**, 313–328 (1969)

RUDDERS, R.A.: B lymphocyte subpopulations in chronic lymphocytic leukemia. Blood **47**, 229–235 (1976)

RÜTTNER, J.R., VON ALBERTINI, A.: Das großfollikuläre Lymphoblastom. Schweiz. Z. Path. Suppl. **10**, 119–124 (1947)

SALMON, S.E., MCINTYRE, O.R., OGAWA, M.: IgE myeloma: Total body tumor cell number and synthesis of IgE and DNA. Blood **37**, 696–705 (1971)

SALMON, S.E., SELIGMANN, M.: B-cell neoplasia in man. Lancet 1974, II, p. 1230

SANDILANDS, G.P., GRAY, K., COONEY, A., BROWNING, J.D., GRANT, R.M., ANDERSON, J.R.: Lymphocytes with T and B cell properties in a lymphoproliferative disorder. Lancet 1974, I, pp. 903–904

SATODATE, R., SCHWARZE, E.-W., LENNERT, K.: Gewebsmastzellenzahl bei Immunocytom und chronischer lymphatischer Leukämie. Virchows Arch. A **373**, 303–309 (1977)

SCHAMAUN, M.: Zur pathologischen Anatomie der sog. Macroglobulinaemie Waldenstroem. Schweiz. Z. allg. Path. **17**, 25–46 (1954)

SCHAUB, F.: Zum Krankheitsbild und zur Differentialdiagnose der Makroglobulinanämie Waldenström. Schweiz. med. Wschr. **82**, 890–895 (1952)

SCHAUB, F.: Gleichzeitiges Vorkommen von Makroglobulinämie Waldenström und von malignen Tumoren. Schweiz. med. Wschr. **83**, 1256–1257 (1953)

SCHEINBERG, M., BRENNER, A.I., SULLIVAN, A.L., CATHCART, E.S., KATAYAMA, I.: The heterogeneity of leukemic reticuloendotheliosis, "hairy cell leukemia". Evidence for its monocytic origin. Cancer (Philad.) **37**, 1302–1307 (1976)

SCHEURLEN, P.G., HAUN, W., MÄUSLE, E., WOLFF, G.: Generalisierte tumorförmige Lymphknotenamyloidose mit Polyneuropathie und Makroglobulinämie. Dtsch. med. Wschr. **98**, 1947–1951 (1973)

SCHEURLEN, P.G., SCHWARZ, J.A.: Immunglobulinmangel und Defekte der spezifischen immunologischen Abwehr. In: Innere Medizin in Praxis und Klinik, Bd. III, pp. 11-115–11-120. HORNBOSTEL, H., KAUFMANN, W., SIEGENTHALER, W., Eds. Stuttgart: Thieme 1973

SCHICK, P.: Lymphocytenkinetik bei lymphatischen Systemerkrankungen (chronische lymphatische Leukämie, Lymphogranulomatose). Verh. dtsch. Ges. inn. Med. **79**, 154–158 (1973)

SCHILD, C.-A.: Notions générales sur le réticulosarcome des ganglions lymphatiques et des formations lymphoïdes. Oncologia (Basel) **2**, 1–19 (1949)

SCHILLING, V.: Das Blutbild und seine klinische Verwertung. Jena: G. Fischer 1943

SCHLEICHER, E.M.: Giant Russell bodies in neoplastic cells in a case of leukemic lymphosarcomatosis. Minn. Med. **48**, 1125–1130 (1965)

SCHMALZL, F., HUHN, D., ASAMER, H., BRAUNSTEINER, H.: Hairy cell leukemia ('leukemic reticuloendotheliosis'), reticulosarcoma, and monocytic leukemia. Cytochemical and ultrastructural investigations. Acta haemat. (Basel) **53**, 257–276 (1975)

SCHNITZER, B.: Classification of non-Hodgkin lymphomas. [Letter to the Editor.] Brit. med. J. 1975, I, p. 680

SCHNITZER, B., HAMMACK, W.J.: B-lymphocyte nature of hairy cells in hairy-cell leukaemia. [Letter to the Editor.] Lancet 1974, II, p. 649

SCHNITZER, B., KASS, L.: Leukemic phase of reticulum cell sarcoma (histiocytic lymphoma). Cancer (Philad.) **31**, 547–559 (1973)

SCHNITZER, B., KASS, L.: Hairy-cell leukemia. A clinicopathologic and ultrastructural study. Amer. J. clin. Path. **61**, 176–187 (1974)

SCHNITZER, B., LOESEL, L.S., REED, R.E.: Lymphosarcoma cell leukemia. A clinicopathologic study. Cancer (Philad.) **26**, 1082–1096 (1970)

SCHOEN, R., HECKNER, F., MARSCH, A.: Das vielseitige Erscheinungsbild der lymphatischen Leukämie. Dtsch. med. Wschr. **78**, 515–518 (1953)

SCHREK, R., DONNELLY, W.J.: "Hairy" cells in blood in lymphoreticular neoplastic disease and "flagellated" cells of normal lymph nodes. Blood **27**, 199–211 (1966)

SCHREK, R., DONNELLY, W.J.: Cytology in lymphosarcoma cell leukemia. Amer. J. clin. Path. **55**, 646–654 (1971)

SCHREK, R., KNOSPE, W.H., TROBAUGH, JR., F.E.: Chromatin and other cytologic indices in chronic lymphocytic leukemia. J. Lab. clin. Med. **75**, 217–224 (1970)

SCHUBERT, J.C.F., MONDORF, W.: Doppelerkrankung an Makroglobulinämie Waldenström und multiplem Myelom. In: Fortschritte der Krebsforschung, pp. 419–422. SCHMIDT, C.G., WETTER, O., Eds. Stuttgart-New York: F.K. Schattauer 1969

SCHWARTZ, R.S., ANDRÉ-SCHWARTZ, J.: Malignant lymphoproliferative diseases: Interactions between immunological abnormalities and oncogenic viruses. Ann. Rev. Med. **19**, 269–282 (1968)

SCHWARZE, E.-W., RADASZKIEWICZ, T., PÜLHORN, G., GOOS, M., LENNERT, K.: Maligne und benigne Lymphome des Auges, der Lid- und Orbitalregion. Virchows Arch. A **370**, 85–96 (1976)

SCHWARZE, E.-W., UDE, P.: Immunoblastic sarcoma with leukemic blood picture in the terminal stage of mycosis fungoides. Virchows Arch. A **369**, 165–172 (1975)

SCHWENK, H.U.: Immunological cell markers on lymphoblasts of patients with acute lymphatic leukemia. Z. Kinderheilk. **118**, 87–95 (1974)

SCOTT, R.B., ROBB-SMITH, A.H.T.: Histiocytic medullary reticulosis. Lancet 1939, II, pp. 194–198

SEEBER, S., SCHMIDT, C.G.: Makromolekulare Besonderheiten des Lymphocyten der chronisch-lymphatischen Leukämie (CLL). Klin. Wschr. **52**, 1093–1102 (1974)

SELIGMANN, M.: Principaux caractères des maladies des chaines lourdes. Bull. Cancer **59**, 381–388 (1972a)

SELIGMANN, M.: Heavy chain diseases. Rev. europ. Étud. clin. biol. **17**, 349–355 (1972b)

SELIGMANN, M.: Immunochemical, clinical, and pathological features of α-chain disease. Arch. intern. Med. **135**, 78–82 (1975)

SELIGMANN, M., BROUET, J.-C., PREUD'HOMME, J.-L.: The immunological diagnosis of human leukemias and lymphomas: an overview. In: Immunological Diagnosis of Leukemias and Lymphomas. Haematology and Blood Transfusion, Vol. 20, pp. 1–15. THIERFELDER, S., RODT, H., THIEL, E., Eds. Berlin-Heidelberg-New York: Springer 1977

SELIGMANN, M., DANON, F., HUREZ, D., MIHAESCO, E., PREUD'HOMME, J.-L.: Alpha-chain disease: A new immunoglobulin abnormality. Science **162**, 1396–1397 (1968)

SELIGMANN, M., PREUD'HOMME, J.-L., BROUET, J.-C.: B and T cell markers in human proliferative blood diseases and primary immunodeficiencies, with special reference to membrane bound immunoglobulins. Transplant. Rev. **16**, 85–113 (1973)

SELIGMANN, M., PREUD'HOMME, J.L., BROUET, J.C.: Surface cell markers in human lymphoid malignancies. In: Lymphocytes, Macrophages, and Cancer. Recent Results in Cancer Research, Vol. 56, pp. 91–97. MATHÉ, G., FLORENTIN, I., SIMMLER, M.-C., Eds. Berlin-Heidelberg-New York: Springer 1976

SEN, L., BORELLA, L.: Clinical importance of lymphoblasts with T markers in childhood acute leukemia. New Engl. J. Med. **292**, 828–832 (1975)

SENO, S., MONDEN, H., SHIBATA, T., SEKI, S., ASAKURA, H., HAMADA, H., MATSUOKA, K., TOYAMA, Y., KATANO, T., HAYASHI, K., NAKATSUKA, A.: Leukemia autopsies in Japan. Acta Med. Okayama **18**, 45–52 (1964)

SERCK-HANSSEN, A., PUROHIT, G.P.: Histiocytic medullary reticulosis. Brit. J. Cancer **22**, 506–516 (1968)

SERCK-HANSSEN, A.: Histiocytic medullary reticulosis. In: Tumours in a Tropical Country. Recent Results in Cancer Research, Vol. 41, pp. 292–297. TEMPLETON, A.C., Ed. Berlin-Heidelberg-New York: Springer 1973

SÉZARY, A.: Une nouvelle réticulose cutanée. La réticulose maligne leucémique à histio-monocytes monstrueux et à forme d'érythrodermie œdémateuse et pigmentée. Ann. Derm. Syph. (Paris) Sér. 8, **9**, 5–22 (1949)

SÉZARY, A., BOUVRAIN, Y.: Erythrodermie avec présence de cellules monstrueuses dans le derme et le sang circulant. Bull. Soc. franç. Derm. Syph. **45**, 254–260 (1938)

SÉZARY, A., HOROWITZ, A., MASCHAS, H.: Erythrodermie avec présence de cellules monstrueuses dans le derme et dans le sang circulant (second cas). Bull. Soc. franç. Derm. Syph. **45**, 395–400 (1938)

SHAHID, M.J., ALAMI, S.Y., NASSAR, V.H., BALIKIAN, J.B., SALEM, A.A.: Primary intestinal lymphoma with paraproteinemia. Cancer (Philad.) **35**, 848–858 (1975)

SHAW, M.T., ISHMAEL, D.R.: Acute lymphocytic leukemia with atypical cytochemical features. Amer. J. clin. Path. **63**, 415–420 (1975)

SHELDON, P.J., HOLBOROW, E.J.: H-rosette formation in T-cell-proliferative diseases. Brit. med. J. 1975, IV, pp. 381–383

SHERR, C.J., UHR, J.W.: Immunoglobulin synthesis and secretion. VI. Synthesis and intracellular transport of immunoglobulin in nonsecretory lymphoma cells. J. exp. Med. **133**, 901–920 (1971)

SHEVACH, E., EDELSON, R., FRANK, M., LUTZNER, M., GREEN, I.: A human leukemia cell with both B and T cell surface receptors. Proc. nat. Acad. Sci. (Wash.) **71**, 863–866 (1974)

SHEVACH, E.M., HERBERMAN, R., FRANK, M.M., GREEN, I.: Receptors for complement and immunoglobulin on human leukemic cells and human lymphoblastoid cell lines. J. clin. Invest. **51**, 1933–1938 (1972)

SHEVACH, E.M., JAFFE, E.S., GREEN, I.: Receptors for complement and immunoglobulin on human and animal lymphoid cells. Transplant. Rev. **16**, 3–28 (1973)

SHIMKIN, M.B., LOVELAND, D.B.: A note on mortality from lymphatic leukemia in oriental populations of the United States. Blood **17**, 763–766 (19617

SHIMOYAMA, M., MIKUNI, M.: Some clinical characteristics of reticulum cell sarcoma and lymphoblastic lymphosarcoma with reference to leukemic transformation. Recent Advanc. RES Res. **12**, 166–182 (1973)

SHIRAKURA, T., KOBAYASHI, Y., MURAI, Y., INOUE, T., IMAMURA, Y.: A case of gamma heavy chain disease associated with autoimmune haemolytic anaemia: Clinical, haematological, immunological and pathological details. Scand. J. Haemat. **16**, 387–393 (1976)

SHOPE, T., DECHAIRO, D., MILLER, G.: Malignant lymphoma in cottontop marmosets after inoculation with Epstein-Barr virus. Proc. nat. Acad. Sci. (Wash.) **70**, 2487–2491 (1973)

SHTERN, R.D.: Topography of organic affections in reticuloblastomatosis. [Russisch.] Probl. Gemat. **13**, 17–23 (1968)

SHTERN, R.D.: Reticulosarcoma. [Russisch.] Arkh. Pat. **32**, 9–24 (1970)

SILBERMAN, S., SCHREK, R.: Surface immunoglobulins of lymphocytes in chronic lymphocytic leukemia and disseminated lymphosarcoma. Exp. mol. Path. **20**, 33–39 (1974)

SILHOL, J., ROUSLACROIX, A.: Sarcome d'origine ganglionnaire à disposition strictement périthéliale. (Tumeur de l'aisselle). Bull. Ass. franç. Cancer **13**, 739–744 (1924)

SILVESTRINI, R., PIAZZA, R., RICCARDI, A., RILKE, F.: Correlation of cell kinetic findings with morphology of non-Hodgkin's malignant lymphomas. J. nat. Cancer Inst. **58**, 499–504 (1977)

SIMON, M.A., EIDLOW, S.: Plasmacytoma of lymph node. Report of a case with multiple myeloma. New Engl. J. Med. **243**, 335–338 (1950)

SJOEVALL, E.: Die diagnostischen Kennzeichen des Retikelzellsarkoms in den Lymphdrüsen. [Abstr.] Verh. 6. skand. Path. Kongr., Oslo 1935. Zbl. allg. Path. path. Anat. **65**, 125 (1936)

SKINNER, J.M., MANOUSOS, O.N., ECONOMIDOU, J., NICOLAOU, A., MERIKAS, G.: Alpha-chain disease with localized plasmacytoma of the intestine. Immunoperoxidase study. Clin. exp. Immunol. **25**, 112–116 (1976)

SLUITER, J.T.F.: De histologie van de ziekte van Brill in haar verschillende phasen. Diss. med., Amsterdam 1956

SMITH, J.L., BARKER, C.R., CLEIN, G.P., COLLINS, R.D.: Characterisation of malignant mediastinal lymphoid neoplasm (Sternberg sarcoma) as thymic in origin. Lancet 1973, I, pp. 74–77

SNAPPER, I., KAHN, A.: Myelomatosis. Fundamentals and Clinical Features. Basel-München-Paris-London-New York-Sydney: Karger 1971

SÖDERSTRÖM, N.: Cytologie der Milz in Punktaten. In: Die Milz – The Spleen, pp. 1–10. LENNERT, K., HARMS, D., Eds. Berlin-Heidelberg-New York: Springer 1970

SÖDERSTRÖM, N., NORBERG, B.: Observations regarding the specific post-capillary venules of lymph nodes in malignant lymphomas. Acta path. microbiol. scand. A **82**, 71–79 (1974)

SOLNIK, C., GLEICHMANN, H., KAVANAH, M., SCHWARTZ, R.S.: Immunosuppression and malignant lymphomas in graft-versus-host reactions. Cancer Res. **33**, 2068–2077 (1973)

SPIRO, S., GALTON, D.A.G., WILTSHAW, E., LOHMANN, R.C.: Follicular lymphoma: A survey of 75 cases with special reference to the syndrome resembling chronic lymphocytic leukaemia. Brit. J. Cancer **31**, Suppl. II, 60–72 (1975)

STACHER, A., BÖHNEL, J.: Über die Relation von lymphatischen Leukämien bzw. Reaktionen zu Malignomen. Wien. klin. Wschr. **78**, 633–636 (1966)

STACHER, A., WALDNER, R., THEML, H. (Kieler Lymphomgruppe): Klinik der malignen Non-Hodgkin-Lymphome entsprechend der Kieler Klassifikation: Lymphoplasmozytoides Lymphom (LPL) und chronisch lymphatische Leukämie (CLL). In: Maligne Lymphome und monoklonale Gammopathien. Hämatologie und Bluttransfusion, Bd. 18, pp. 199–209. LÖFFLER, H., Ed. München: Lehmanns 1976

STAHEL, R.: Diagnostische Drüsenpunktion. Leipzig: Thieme 1939

STAHEL, R.: Über großfollikuläres Lymphoblastom (Brill Symmers disease). Helv. med. Acta Ser. A **15**, 448–456 (1948)

STEGAGNO, G.: L'adenocitogramma nella leucemia linfatica acuta dell'infanzia. Arch. ital. Pediat. **15**, 397–427 (1950)

STEIN, H.: Immunchemische und immunzytologische Befunde bei Non-Hodgkin-Lymphomen. In: Maligne Lymphome und monoklonale Gammopathien. Hämatologie und Bluttransfusion, Bd. 18, pp. 167–183. LÖFFLER, H., Ed. München: Lehmanns 1976

STEIN, H., KAISERLING, E.: Surface immunoglobulins and lymphocyte-specific surface antigens on leukaemic reticuloendotheliosis cells. Clin. exp. Immunol. **18**, 63–71 (1974)

STEIN, H., KAISERLING, E., LENNERT, K.: Neue Gesichtspunkte zur Systematik maligner Lymphome auf dem Boden immunchemischer Analysen. In: Leukämien und maligne Lymphome, pp. 195–201. STACHER, A., Ed. München-Berlin-Wien: Urban & Schwarzenberg 1973

STEIN, H., KAISERLING, E., LENNERT, K.: Evidence for B-cell origin of reticulum cell sarcoma. Virchows Arch. A **364**, 51–67 (1974a)

STEIN, H., KAISERLING, E., LENNERT, K.: Immunoglobulin-production and surface-bound immunoglobulins in chronic lymphocytic leukemia, lymphosarcoma, and so-called reticulum cell sarcoma. In: Modern Trends in Human Leukemia. Hämatologie und Bluttransfusion, Vol. 14, pp. 97–106. NETH, R., GALLO, R.C., SPIEGELMAN, S., STOHLMAN, JR., F., Eds. München: J.F. Lehmanns 1974b

STEIN, H., KAISERLING, E., LENNERT, K., PARWARESCH, M.R.: Makroglobulinbildende chronische lymphatische Leukämie ohne Makroglobulinämie. Klin. Wschr. **51**, 389–396 (1973)

STEIN, H., LENNERT, K., PARWARESCH, M.R.: Malignant lymphomas of B-cell type. Lancet 1972, II, pp. 855–857

STEIN, H., PETERSEN, N., GAEDICKE, G., LENNERT, K., LANDBECK, G.: Lymphoblastic lymphoma of convoluted or acid phosphatase type—a tumor of T precursor cells. Int. J. Cancer **17**, 292–295 (1976)

STERNBERG, C.: Über eine eigenartige unter dem Bilde der Pseudoleukämie verlaufende Tuberculose des lymphatischen Apparates. Ztschr. Heilk. **19**, 21–90 (1898)

STERNBERG, C.: Über Leukosarcomatose. Wien. klin. Wschr. **21**, 475–480 (1908)

STERNBERG, C.: Leukosarkomatose und Myeloblastenleukämie. Beitr. Path. **61**, 75–100 (1916)

STJERNSWÅRD, J., CLIFFORD, P., SVEDMYR, E.: General and tumor-distinctive cellular immunological reactivity. In: Burkitt's Lymphoma, pp. 164–171. BURKITT, D.P., WRIGHT, D.H., Eds. Edinburgh-London: Livingstone 1970

STOOP, J.W., BALLIEUX, R.E., HIJMANS, W., ZEGERS, B.J.M.: Alpha-chain disease with involvement of the respiratory tract in a Dutch child. Clin. exp. Immunol. **9**, 625–635 (1971)

STOOP, J.W., ZEGERS, B.J.M., VAN DER HEIDEN, C., BALLIEUX, R.E.: Monoclonal gammopathy in a child with leukemia. Blood **32**, 774–786 (1968)

STORTI, E.: L'istochimica applicata all'ematologia. C.R. 3. Congr. Soc. europ. Hémat., Rome 1951, pp. 79–112. Rome: Edizioni Mediche e Scientifiche 1952

STOUT, A.P., KENNEY, F.R.: Primary plasma-cell tumors of the upper air passages and oral cavity. Cancer (Philad.) **2**, 261–278 (1949)

STRUNGE, T.: La Ponction des ganglions lymphatiques. Kopenhagen: Munksgaard 1944

STUTTE, H.J., SCHLÜTER, E.: Zur Ätiologie von Fibrinpräcipitaten in den Lymphfollikeln der menschlichen Milz. Untersuchungen an autoptischem Material. Virchows Arch. A **356**, 32–41 (1972)

SUCHI, T., OTA, K.: Clinical, cytological, and histopathological studies of cases of reticulum cell sarcoma-like tumors developing during the terminal phase of chronic myelogenous leukemia. In: Malignant Diseases of the Hematopoietic System. GANN Monograph on Cancer Research, Vol. 15, pp. 97–110. AKAZAKI, K., RAPPAPORT, H., BERARD, C.W., BENNETT, J.M., ISHIKAWA, E., Eds. Tokyo: University of Tokyo Press 1973

SUCHI, T., SATO, T., KOBAYASHI, H., AKATSUKA, H., AKAZA, T., KURITA, S., HOSHINO, M.: Reticulum cell sarcoma. Some characteristics of reticulum-cell-sarcoma cells. [Japanese.] Jap. J. Cancer Clin. **19**, 419–425 (1973)

SUISSA, L., LAROSA, J., LINN, B.: Plasmacytoma of lymph nodes. A case report. J. Amer. med. Ass. **197**, 136–140 (1966)

SUMIYA, M., MIZOGUCHI, H., KOSAKA, K., MIURA, Y., TAKAKU, F., YATA, J.: Chronic lymphocytic leukaemia of T-cell origin? Lancet 1973, II, p. 910

SUNDBERG, R.D.: Lymphocytogenesis in human lymph nodes. J. Lab. clin. Med. **32**, 777–792 (1947)

ŠVEJDA, J., KOSTELNÍK, J., CHURÝ, Z.: Beitrag zu den pathologisch-anatomischen Befunden bei Waldenströms Makroglobulinämie. Zbl. allg. Path. path. Anat. **98**, 497–504 (1958)

SYMMERS, D.: Follicular lymphadenopathy with splenomegaly. A newly recognized disease of the lymphatic system. Arch. Path. **3**, 816–820 (1927)

SYMMERS, D.: Giant follicular lymphadenopathy with or without splenomegaly. Arch. Path. **26**, 603–647 (1938)

SYMMERS, D.: Lymphoid diseases. Arch. Path. **45**, 73–131 (1948)

SYMMERS, W.STC.: Primary malignant diseases of the lymphoreticular system. In: Cancer **2**, 2: Pathology of Malignant Tumours, pp. 448–483. RAVEN, R.W., Ed. London: Butterworth 1958

SYMMERS, W.STC.: Survey of the eventual diagnosis in 226 cases referred for a second histological opinion after an initial biopsy diagnosis of reticulum cell sarcoma. J. clin. Path. **21**, 654–655 (1968)

TAKATSUKI, K., UCHIYAMA, T., SAGAWA, K., YODOI, J.: Adult T-cell leukemia in Japan. Proc. 16th Int. Congr. Hematol., in press.

TALAL, N., BUNIM, J.J.: The development of malignant lymphoma in the course of Sjögren's syndrome. Amer. J. Med. **36**, 529–540 (1964)

TALAL, N., SOKOLOFF, L., BARTH, W.F.: Extrasalivary lymphoid abnormalities in Sjögren's syndrome (reticulum cell sarcoma, 'pseudolymphoma', macroglobulinemia). Amer. J. Med. **43**, 50–65 (1967)

TALERMAN, A.: Clinico-pathological study of malignant lymphoma in Jamaica. Brit. J. Cancer **24**, 37–47 (1970)

TALERMAN, A., PLATENBURG, H.P.J.M.: Follicular lymphoma with deposits of amorphous hyaline material. J. Path. **112**, 27–31 (1974)

TANAKA, N.: Malignant reticulohistiocytosis. Border-line lesion between reactive and neoplastic. In: Malignant Diseases of the Hematopoietic System. GANN Monograph on Cancer Research, Vol. 15, pp. 123–143. AKAZAKI, K., RAPPAPORT, H., BERARD, C.W., BENNETT, J.M., ISHIKAWA, E., Eds. Tokyo: University of Tokyo Press 1973

TASWELL, H.F., WINKELMANN, R.K.: Sézary syndrome—a malignant reticulemic erythroderma. J. Amer. med. Ass. **177**, 465–472 (1961)

TAYLOR, C.R.: The nature of Reed-Sternberg cells and other malignant "reticulum" cells. Lancet 1974, II, pp. 802–807

TEN SELDAM, R.E.J., COOKE, R., ATKINSON, L.: Childhood lymphoma in the Territories of Papua and New Guinea. Cancer (Philad.) **19**, 437–446 (1966)

THEML, H., TREPEL, F., SCHICK, P., KABOTH, W., BEGEMANN, H.: Kinetics of lymphocytes in chronic lymphocytic leukemia: Studies using continuous $^{3}$H-thymidine infusion in two patients. Blood **42**, 623–636 (1973)

THIEL, E., RODT, H., HUHN, D., THIERFELDER, S.: Decrease and altered distribution of human T antigen on chronic lymphatic leukemia cells of T type, suggesting a clonal origin. Blood **47**, 723–736 (1976)

THIERBACH, R., HUTH, J.: Ein speicherndes Lymphoreticulom der Lunge. Frankfurt. Z. Path. **73**, 127–137 (1963)

THOMAS, L.B., RAPPAPORT, H.: Mycosis fungoides and its relationship to other malignant lymphomas. In: The Reticuloendothelial System. Monographs in Pathology, No. 16, pp. 243–261. REBUCK, J.W., BERARD, C.W., ABELL, M.R., Eds. Baltimore: Williams & Wilkins 1975

TINDLE, B.H., PARKER, J.W., LUKES, R.J.: "Reed-Sternberg cells" in infectious mononucleosis? Amer. J. clin. Path. **58**, 607–617 (1972)

TISCHENDORF, W.: Diagnostische Lymphdrüsenpunktion. Münch. med. Wschr. **1938**, 853–854

TISCHENDORF, W.: Über die Verwertbarkeit von Lymphknotenpunktaten zur Differentialdiagnose der Lymphdrüsenerkrankungen. Dtsch. Arch. klin. Med. **183**, 448–466 (1939)

TISCHENDORF, W.: Lymphosarkomatose und Leukämiebegriff. Dtsch. med. Wschr. **71**, 220–224 (1946)

TISCHENDORF, W.: Cytodiagnostik des Lymphknotenpunktates. Erg. inn. Med. Kinderheilk., N.F. **2**, 183–263 (1951)

TISCHENDORF, W.: Lymphknoten. In: Handbuch der gesamten Hämatologie, 2. Aufl., Bd. I, pp. 453–488. München-Berlin-Wien: Urban & Schwarzenberg 1957

TISCHENDORF, W., HARTMANN, F.: Makroglobulinaemie (Waldenström) mit gleichzeitiger Hyperplasie der Gewebsmastzellen. Acta haemat. (Basel) **4**, 374–383 (1950)

TISCHENDORF, W., HECKNER, F.: Zur Zytologie und Klinik der großfollikulären Lymphadenopathie (Brill-Symmerssche Krankheit). Neue med. Welt 1950, 1013–1018

TORNYOS, K., MACOSSAY, C.R., GYORKEY, F.: Chronic lymphocytic leukemia and Hodgkin's disease in the same patient. Report of a case, giving immunological and diagnostic considerations. Cancer (Philad.) **20**, 552–557 (1967)

TREPEL, F., SCHICK, P.: Proliferation und Wachstum von lymphatischen Zellpopulationen bei Malignen Lymphomen. In: Maligne Lymphome und monoklonale Gammopathien. Hämatologie und Bluttransfusion, Bd. 18, pp. 33–47. LÖFFLER, H., Ed. München: Lehmanns 1976

TREPEL, F., THEML, H., SCHICK, P., SCHNEBLE, G., BREMER, K., FLIEDNER, T.M., BEGEMANN, H.: Kontinuierliche $^{3}$H-Thymidininfusion bei CLL: II. Proliferation der Lymphknotenzellen. In: Leukämie, pp. 187–191. GROSS, R., VAN DE LOO, J., Eds. Berlin-Heidelberg-New York: Springer 1972

TRUBOWITZ, S., MASEK, B., FRASCA, J.M.: Leukemic reticuloendotheliosis. Blood **38**, 288–298 (1971)

TRUJILLO, J.M., BUTLER, J.J., AHEARN, M.J., SHULLENBERGER, C.C., LIST-YOUNG, B., GOTT, C., ANSTALL, H.B., SHIVELY, J.A.: Long-term culture of lymph node tissue from a patient with lymphocytic lymphoma. II. Preliminary ultrastructural, immunofluorescence and cytogenetic studies. Cancer (Philad.) **20**, 215–224 (1967)

TUBIANA, M., LE BOURGEOIS, J.-P.: La classification et le bilan des hématosarcomes. Bull. Cancer **61**, 39–50 (1974)

UHLMANN, E.M.: The significance of giant follicular lymphadenopathy. (Brill-Symmers disease). Radiology **50**, 147–156 (1948)

UNDRITZ, E.: Hämatologische Tafeln. Sandoz 1952

VAN UNNIK, J.A.M., BREUR, K., BURGERS, J.M.V., CLETON, F., HART, A.A.M., STENFERT KROESE, W.F., SOMERS, R., VAN TURNHOUT, J.M.M.P.M.: Non-Hodgkin's lymphomata: Clinical features in relation to histology. Brit. J. Cancer **31**, Suppl. II, 201–207 (1975)

VARIAKOJIS, D., ROSAS-URIBE, A., RAPPAPORT, H.: Mycosis fungoides: Pathologic findings in staging laparotomies. Cancer (Philad.) **33**, 1589–1600 (1974)

VERONESI, U., MUSUMECI, R., PIZZETTI, F., GENNARI, L., BONADONNA, G.: The value of staging laparotomy in non-Hodgkin's lymphomas. Cancer (Philad.) **33**, 446–459 (1974)

VETTE, J.P.: De ziekte van Brill en de folliculaire reticulosen. Thesis, Amsterdam 1950

VIDEBAEK, A.: Unusual cases of myelomatosis. Brit. med. J. 1971, II, p. 326

VIDEBAEK, A.: Leukaemia and cancer in relation to immunosuppressive therapy. Scand. J. Haemat. **10**, 241–243 (1973)

VIDEBAEK, A., POULSEN, H.: Myelofibrosis complicated by lymphogenous leukaemia. Acta haemat. (Basel) **17**, 250–256 (1957)

VIRCHOW, R.: Weißes Blut. Neue Notizen aus dem Gebiet der Natur- und Heilkunde. Froriep's neue Notizen **36**. 151–156 (1845)

VIRCHOW, R.: Zur pathologischen Physiologie des Bluts. II. Weißes Blut (Leukämie). Virchows Arch. path. Anat. **1**, 563–572 (1847)

VIRCHOW, R.: Die krankhaften Geschwülste. Dreißig Vorlesungen, gehalten während des Wintersemesters 1862–1863 an der Universität zu Berlin. Vol. 2. Berlin: A. Hirschwald 1864–65

WAITZ, R., MAYER, S., BIGEL, P., FITZENKAM-SAITO, A.: Myéloscléroses chroniques à forme lymphoïde. Nouv. Rev. franç. Hémat. **3**, 490–496 (1963)

WAITZ, R., MAYER, G., MAYER, S.: Myélophtisies à réaction lymphoïde. Importance de l'étude histologique de la moelle osseuse pour le diagnostic différentiel des états lymphoïdes dits subleucémiques. Rev. belge Path. **24**, 399–409 (1955)

WAKASA, H.: Histopathological differential diagnosis of malignant lymphogranulomatosis (Hodgkin's disease) from lymphatic reticulosarcomatosis. Tohoku J. exp. Med. **68**, 325–335 (1958)

WALDENSTRÖM, J.G.: Incipient myelomatosis or "essential" hyperglobulinemia with fibrinogenopenia – a new syndrome? Acta med. scand. **117**, 216–247 (1944)

WALDENSTRÖM, J.G.: Die Makroglobulinämie. Ergebn. inn. Med. Kinderheilk. **9**, 586–621 (1958)

WALDENSTRÖM, J.G.: Monoclonal and Polyclonal Hypergammaglobulinemia. Clinical and Biological Significance. London: Cambridge University Press 1968

WALDENSTRÖM, J.G.: Diagnosis and Treatment of Multiple Myeloma. New York-London: Grune & Stratton 1970

WALDMANN, T.A., STROBER, W., BLAESE, R.M.: Immunodeficiency disease and malignancy. Various immunologic deficiencies of man and the role of immune processes in the control of malignant disease. Ann. intern. Med. **77**, 605–628 (1972)

WANNER, J., SIEBENMANN, R.: Über eine subakut verlaufende osteolytische Form der Makroglobulinämie Waldenström mit Plasmazellenleukämie. Schweiz. med. Wschr. **87**, 1243–1246 (1957)

WARNER, N.L., POTTER, M., METCALF, D. (Eds.): Multiple Myeloma and Related Immunoglobulin-Producing Neoplasms. (UICC Technical Report Series, Vol. 13.) Geneva: International Union Against Cancer 1974

WASASTJERNA, C., VUORINEN, E., LEHTINEN, M., IKKALA, E., HUHTALA, E.: The cytochemical β-glucuronidase reaction in the differential diagnosis of acute leukaemias. Acta haemat. (Basel) **53**, 277–284 (1975)

WAUBKE, R.: Epstein-Barr-Virus, infektiöse Mononukleose und Burkitt-Lymphom. Dtsch. med. Wschr. **95**, 1572–1578 (1970)

WEISZER, L.: Zur Frage der Ausscheidung des Bence-Jones'-Eiweißkörpers. Z. klin. Med. **140**, 30–44 (1942)

WERNER, J., WOLF, H., APODACA, J., ZUR HAUSEN, H.: Lymphoproliferative disease in a cotton-top marmoset after inoculation with infectious mononucleosis-derived Epstein-Barr virus. Int. J. Cancer **15**, 1000–1008 (1975)

WESTERHAUSEN, M.: Immunglobulinveränderungen bei chronischer Lymphadenose. In: Der Lymphozyt, pp. 171–175. PIETSCHMANN, H., Ed. Wien: Verlag der Wiener Medizinischen Akademie 1972

WESTERHAUSEN, M.: Immunglobulinveränderungen bei der chronischen Lymphadenose (CLL). In: Leukämien und maligne Lymphome, pp. 268–272. STACHER, A., Ed. München-Berlin-Wien: Urban & Schwarzenberg 1973

WETHERLEY-MEIN, G., SMITH, P., GEAKE, M.R., ANDERSON, H.J.: Follicular lymphoma. Quart. J. Med. N.S. **21**, 327–351 (1952)

WETTER, O.: μ-Kettenkrankheit und Hyper-γ-Globulinämie – eine ungewöhnliche Immunglobulinstörung mit allgemeiner Lymphadenopathie. Verh. dtsch. Ges. inn. Med. **79**, 350–352 (1973)

WIDMANN, H.: Akute subleukämische Plasmozytose – auf der Basis eines Retikulosarkoms mit erworbener hämolytischer Anämie. Dtsch. med. Wschr. **82**, 1298–1301 (1957)

WILCOXON, F.: Individual comparisons by ranking methods. Biomet. Bull. **1**, 80–83 (1945)

WILLEMIN-CLOG, L., CAVAROC, M., MENUT, G., RAYNAUD, J.-E.: La maladie de Burkitt hors d'Afrique. Nouv. Rev. franç. Hémat. **7**, 367–380 (1967)

WILLIAMS, M.C.: Implications of the geographical distribution of Burkitt's lymphoma. In: Treatment of Burkitt's Tumour. UICC Monograph Series, Vol. 8, pp. 42–51. BURCHENAL, J.H., BURKITT, D.P., Eds. Berlin-Heidelberg-New York: Springer 1967

WILLIS, R.A.: Pathology of Tumours. London: Butterworths 1960

WILMS, H.: Beitrag zum Germinoblastom (Noduläres Lymphom, Brill-Symmers). Zytophotometrische Untersuchungen. Diss. med., Kiel 1970

WILSON, J.D., NOSSAL, G.J.V.: Identification of human T and B lymphocytes in normal peripheral blood and in chronic lymphocytic leukaemia. Lancet 1971, II, pp. 788–791

WILTSHAW, E.: The natural history of extramedullary plasmacytoma and its relation to solitary myeloma of bone and myelomatosis. Thesis submitted for the Degree of Doctor of Medicine at the University of Wales, 1969

WILTSHAW, E.: Extramedullary plasmacytoma. Myeloma Workshop, London 1971. Brit. med. J. 1971, II, pp. 319–328

WINKELMANN, R.K.: Clinical studies of T-cell erythroderma in the Sezary syndrome. Mayo Clin. Proc. **49**, 519–525 (1974)

WINKELMANN, R.K., PERRY, H.O., MULLER, S.A., SCHROETER, A.L., JORDON, R.E., ROGERS, R.S.: The pre-Sezary erythroderma syndrome. Mayo Clin. Proc. **49**, 588–589 (1974)

WINKLER, K., GAEDICKE, G., GROSCH-WÖRNER, I., MARSMANN, G., LANDBECK, G.: Zur Behandlung der akuten lymphoblastischen Leukämie im Kindesalter – Erfahrungsbericht. Klin. Pädiat. **189**, 74–88 (1977)

WISLOCKI, G.B., RHEINGOLD, J.J., DEMPSEY, E.W.: The occurrence of the periodic acid-Schiff reaction in various normal cells of blood and connective tissue. Blood **4**, 562–568 (1949)

WÖCKEL, W., SCHREIBER, D.: Ein Beitrag zum Gestaltwandel der Brill-Symmersschen Krankheit. Frankfurt. Z. Path. **68**, 97–108 (1957)

WOLF, H., WERNER, J., ZUR HAUSEN, H.: EBV DNA in nonlymphoid cells of nasopharyngeal carcinomas and in a malignant lymphoma obtained after inoculation of EBV into cottontop marmosets. Cold Spr. Harb. Symp. quant. Biol. **39**, 791–796 (1975)

WOLF, H., ZUR HAUSEN, H., BECKER, V.: EB viral genomes in epithelial nasopharyngeal carcinoma cells. Nature [New Biol.] **244**, 245–247 (1973)

WOLFF, J.A., BRUBAKER, C.A., MURPHY, M.L., PIERCE, M.I., SEVERO, N.: Prednisone therapy of acute childhood leukemia: Prognosis and duration of response in 330 treated patients. J. Pediat. **70**, 626–631 (1967)

WOLLNER, N., BURCHENAL, J.H., LIEBERMAN, P.H., EXELBY, P., D'ANGIO, G., MURPHY, M.L.: Non-Hodgkin's lymphoma in children. A comparative study of two modalities of therapy. Cancer (Philad.) **37**, 123–134 (1976)

WOLTER, J., HAMANN, W., OSTENDORF, P.: Ein Fall von großfollikulärem Lymphoblastom (Brill-Symmers) mit finalem Lymphoma malignum Hodgkin. Med. Welt (Stuttg.) **21**, 1778–1784 (1970)

WRIGHT, C.J.E.: Macrofollicular lymphoma. Amer. J. Path. **32**, 201–233 (1956)

WRIGHT, D.H.: Cytology and histochemistry of the Burkitt lymphoma. Brit. J. Cancer **17**, 50–55 (1963)

WRIGHT, D.H.: Cytology and histochemistry of the malignant lymphomas seen in Uganda. In: Symposium on Lymphoreticular Tumours in Africa, Paris 1963, pp. 291–303. ROULET, F.C., Ed. Basel-New York: Karger 1964a

WRIGHT, D.H.: Burkitt's tumour. A post-mortem study of 50 cases. Brit. J. Surg. **51**, 245–251 (1964b)

WRIGHT, D.H.: The gross and microscopic pathology of Burkitt's tumour. In: Treatment of Burkitt's Tumour. UICC Monograph Series, Vol. 8, pp. 14–23. BURCHENAL, J.H., BURKITT, D.P., Eds. Berlin-Heidelberg-New York: Springer 1967

WRIGHT, D.H.: Gross distribution and haematology. In: Burkitt's Lymphoma, pp. 64–81. BURKITT, D.P., WRIGHT, D.H., Eds. Edinburgh-London: Livingstone 1970a

WRIGHT, D.H.: Microscopic features, histochemistry, histogenesis and diagnosis. In: Burkitt's Lymphoma, pp. 82–102. BURKITT, D.P., WRIGHT, D.H., Eds. Edinburgh-London: Livingstone 1970b

WRIGHT, D.H., MCALPINE, J.C.: Ribonucleic acid content of Burkitt tumour cells. J. clin. Path. **19**, 257–259 (1966)

WU, S.D.: Lymphoblastom mit Riesenfollikeln. [Engl.] Chin. med. J. Suppl. **3** (1940). Ref. Zbl. allg. Path. path. Anat. **78**, 311 (1942)

WUKETICH, S., SIEGMUND, G.: Zur Diagnose der Makroglobulinämie Waldenström. Wien. klin. Wschr. **69**, 977–980 (1957)

YAM, L. T., LI, C.-Y., FINKEL, H.E.: Leukemic reticuloendotheliosis. The role of tartrate-resistant acid phosphatase in diagnosis and splenectomy in treatment. Arch. intern. Med. **130**, 248–256 (1972)

YAM, L.T., LI, C.Y., LAM, K.W.: Tartrate-resistant acid phosphatase isoenzyme in the reticulum cells of leukemic retikuloendotheliosis. New Engl. J. Med. **284**, 357–360 (1971)

YODOI, J., TAKATSUKI, K., MASUDA, T.: Two cases of T-cell chronic lymphocytic leukemia in Japan. New Engl. J. Med. **290**, 572–573 (1974)

YOSHIDA, T., EDELSON, R., COHEN, S., GREEN, I.: Migration inhibitory activity in serum and cell supernatants in patients with Sezary syndrome. J. Immunol. **114**, 915–918 (1975)

ZAJICEK, J., BARTELS, P.H., BAHR, G.F., BIBBO, M., WIED, G.L.: Computer analysis of lymphocytes from cases with lymphadenitis and lymphocytic lymphoma. Acta cytol. (Philad.) **16**, 284–296 (1972)

ZECH, L., HAGLUND, U., NILSSON, K., KLEIN, G.: Characteristic chromosomal abnormalities in biopsies and lymphoid-cell lines from patients with Burkitt and non-Burkitt lymphomas. Int. J. Cancer **17**, 47–56 (1976)

ZEFFREN, J.L., ULTMANN, J.E.: Reticulum cell sarcoma terminating in acute leukemia. Blood **15**, 277–284 (1960)

ZIEGLER, J.L., ANDERSSON, M., KLEIN, G., HENLE, W.: Detection of Epstein-Barr virus DNA in American Burkitt's lymphoma. Int. J. Cancer **17**, 701–706 (1976)

ZIEGLER, J.L., MORROW, JR., R.H., FASS, L., KYALWAZI, S.K., CARBONE, P.P.: Treatment of Burkitt's tumor with cyclophosphamide. Cancer (Philad.) **26**, 474–484 (1970)

ZIPPIN, C., CUTLER, S.J., REEVES, JR., W.J., LUM, D.: Survival in chronic lymphocytic leukemia. Blood **42**, 367–376 (1973)

ZOLLINGER, H.U.: Die pathologische Anatomie der Makroglobulinämie Waldenström. Helv. med. Acta **25**, 153–183 (1958)

ZUCKER-FRANKLIN, D.: Virus-like particles in the lymphocytes of a patient with chronic lymphocytic leukemia. Blood **21**, 509–512 (1963)

ZUCKER-FRANKLIN, D.: Properties of the Sezary lymphoid cell. An ultrastructural analysis. Mayo Clin. Proc. **49**, 567–574 (1974)

ZUCKER-FRANKLIN, D., MELTON III, J.W., QUAGLIATA, F.: Ultrastructural, immunologic, and functional studies on Sézary cells: A neoplastic variant of thymus-derived (T) lymphocytes. Proc. nat. Acad. Sci. (Wash.) **71**, 1877–1881 (1974)

ZUR HAUSEN, H.: Oncogenic Herpes viruses. Biochim. biophys. Acta (Amst.) **417**, 25–53 (1975)

ZUR HAUSEN, H.: Biochemical approaches to detection of Epstein-Barr virus in human tumors. Cancer Res. **36**, 678–680 (1976)

ZUR HAUSEN, H., SCHULTE-HOLTHAUSEN, H.: Presence of EB virus nucleic acid homology in a "virus-free" line of Burkitt tumour cells. Nature (Lond.) **227**, 245–248 (1970)

ZUR HAUSEN, H., SCHULTE-HOLTHAUSEN, H., KLEIN, G., HENLE, W., HENLE, G., CLIFFORD, P., SANTESSON, L.: EBV DNA in biopsies of Burkitt tumours and anaplastic carcinomas of the nasopharynx. Nature (Lond.) **228**, 1056–1058 (1970)

# References

## *Part Five*


ADA, G.L., NOSSAL, G.J.V., AUSTIN, C.M.: Antigens in immunity. V. The ability of cells in lymphoid follicles to recognize foreignness. Aust. J. exp. Biol. med. Sci. **42**, 331–346 (1964).

AKASAKA, K.: Proliferative diseases of the RES presenting a leukemic blood picture: Phase-contrast and electron microscopic studies. Recent Adv. RES Res. **12**, 183–213 (1973).

ANDAY, G.J., GOODMAN, J.R., TISHKOFF, G.H.: An unusual cytoplasmic ribosomal structure in pathologic lymphocytes. Blood **41**, 439–449 (1973).

ANDERSON, D.R.: Ultrastructure of normal and leukemic leukocytes in human peripheral blood. J. Ultrastruct. Res. Suppl. **9** (1966).

ARGANI, I., KIPKIE, G.F.: The cellular origin of macroglobulins. A study of the protein-secreting cells in Waldenstrom's disease. Lab. Invest. **14**, 720–728 (1965).

AVRAMEAS, S., LEDUC, E.H.: Detection of simultaneous antibody synthesis in plasma cells and specialized lymphocytes in rabbit lymph nodes. J. exp. Med. **131**, 1137–1168 (1970).

BARCOS, M.P., LUKES, R.J.: Malignant lymphoma of convoluted lymphocytes: A new entity of possible T-cell type. In: Conflicts in Childhood Cancer. An Evaluation of Current Management, Vol. 4, pp. 147–178. SINKS, L.F., GODDEN, J.O., Eds. New York: Liss 1975.

BARKA, T., ANDERSON, P.J.: Histochemistry. Theory, Practice, and Bibliography. New York-Evanston-London: Harper & Row 1963.

BEACHEY, E.H., HASHIMOTO, K., BURKETT, L.L.: Histiocytic leukemia: ultrastructure and phagocytic capacity of hairy cells. [Abstr.] Clin. Res. **17**, 530 (1969).

BEDOYA, V., GRIMLEY, P.M., RABSON, A.S.: Ultrastructural evidence of in vitro interaction among Burkitt lymphoma cells: Possible relevance to the "phagocytic" activity of starry sky histiocytes in vivo. Cancer Res. **29**, 753–762 (1969).

BERARD, C., O'CONOR, G.T., THOMAS, L.B., TORLONI, H.: Histopathological definition of Burkitt's tumour. Bull. Wld Hlth Org. **40**, 601–607 (1969).

BERNARD, J., BESSIS, M., SOULIER, J.P., THIÉRY, J.P.: Étude au microscope électronique d'une leucémie lymphoide avec cristaux intra-cytoplasmiques. Rev. Hémat. **14**, 227–237 (1959).

BERNHARD, W.: Elektronenmikroskopischer Beitrag zum Studium der Kanzerisierung und der malignen Zustände der Zelle. Verh. dtsch. Ges. Path. **45**, 8–37 (1961).

BERNHARD, W.: Fine structure of Burkitt's lymphoma. In: Burkitt's Lymphoma, pp. 103–117. BURKITT, D.P., WRIGHT, D.H., Eds. Edinburgh-London: Livingstone 1970.

BERNHARD, W., LEPLUS, R.: Structure fine du ganglion humain normal et malin. Oxford: Pergamon Press [usw.] 1964.

BESSIS, M.: Études au microscope électronique des leucocytes normaux et leucémiques. Acta Un. int. Cancer **7**, 646–659 (1951).

BESSIS, M.C.: Ultrastructure of lymphoid and plasma cells in relation to globulin and antibody formation. Lab. Invest. **10**, 1040–1067 (1961).

BESSIS, M.: Living Blood Cells and Their Ultrastructure. Berlin-Heidelberg-New York: Springer 1973.

BONNEAU, H., CESARINI, J.-P.: Étude ultrastructurale d'un cas de mycosis fongoïde. Bull. Soc. franç. Derm. Syph. **74**, 612–617 (1967)

BOSMAN, F.T., VAN VLOTEN, W.A.: Sézary's syndrome: A cytogenetic, cytophotometric and autoradiographic study. J. Path. **118**, 49–57 (1976).

BRITTINGER, G., AUGENER, W., BREMER, K., COHNEN, G., DABAG, S., FISCHER, K., KÖNIG, E., MEUSERS, P.: Der Lymphozyt bei der chronischen lymphatischen Leukämie. Blut **30**, 293–308 (1975).

BROUET, J.-C., FLANDRIN, G., SASPORTES, M., PREUD'HOMME, J.-L., SELIGMANN, M.: Chronic lymphocytic leukaemia of T-cell origin. Immunological and clinical evaluation in eleven patients. Lancet 1975, II, pp. 890–893.

BROWNLEE, T.R., MURAD, T.M.: Ultrastructure of mycosis fungoides. Cancer (Philad.) **26**, 686–698 (1970).

BRUNNING, R.D., PARKIN, J.: Ultrastructural studies of parallel tubular arrays in human lymphocytes. Amer. J. Path. **78**, 59–70 (1975).

BURKE, J. S., MACKAY, B., RAPPAPORT, H.: Hairy cell leukemia (leukemic reticuloendotheliosis). II. Ultrastructure of the spleen. Cancer (Philad.) **37**, 2267–2274 (1976).

CARR, I.: The ultrastructure of the abnormal reticulum cells in Hodgkin's disease. J. Path. **115**, 45–50 (1975).

CATOVSKY, D.: T-cell origin of acid-phosphatase-positive lymphoblasts. Lancet 1975, II, pp. 327–328.

CATOVSKY, D., FRISCH, B., VAN NOORDEN, S.: B, T and 'null' cell leukaemias. Electron cytochemistry and surface morphology. Blood Cells **1**, 115–124 (1975).

CAWLEY, J.C., BARKER, C.R., BRITCHFORD, R.D., SMITH, J.L.: Intracellular IgA immunoglobulin crystals in chronic lymphocytic leukaemia. Clin. exp. Immunol. **13**, 407–416 (1973).

CAWLEY, J.C., EMMINES, J., GOLDSTONE, A.H., HAMBLIN, T., HOUGH, D., SMITH, J.L.: Distinctive cytoplasmic inclusions in chronic lymphocytic leukaemia. Europ. J. Cancer **11**, 91–92 (1975).

CAWLEY, J.C., SMITH, J., GOLDSTONE, A.H., EMMINES, J., HAMBLIN, J., HOUGH, L.: IgA and IgM cytoplastic inclusions in a series of cases of chronic lymphocytic leukaemia. Clin. exp. Immunol. **23**, 78–82 (1976).

CHANDRA, S.: Undulating tubules associated with endoplasmic reticulum in pathologic tissues. Lab. Invest. **18**, 422–428 (1968).

CHELLOUL, N., DAUMAS-DUPORT, C., BONVALLET, D., BRIERE, J., VORHAUER-ATLAN, W., BERNUAU, D.: Pathologie ganglionnaire au cours des dermatoses avec cellules de Sézary circulantes. Biomedicine **24**, 62–77 (1976).

CLARK, C., RYDELL, R.E., KAPLAN, M.E.: Frequent association of IgM$\lambda$ with crystalline inclusions in chronic lymphatic leukemic lymphocytes. New Engl. J. Med. **289**, 113–117 (1973).

COHNEN, G.: T- und B-Lymphozyten bei chronischer lymphatischer Leukämie und Lymphogranulomatose. Elektronenmikroskopische und immunologische Untersuchungen. Veröff. Path. H. 97. Stuttgart: G. Fischer 1975.

COHNEN, G., FISCHER, K., LUDWIG, H., BRITTINGER, G.: Rasterelektronenmikroskopische Beobachtungen an Blutlymphozyten von Normalpersonen und Patienten mit chronischer lymphatischer Leukämie (Vortrag). Blut **31**, 180 (1975).

DANIEL, M.T., FLANDRIN, G.: Fine structure of abnormal cells in hairy cell (tricholeukocytic) leukemia with special reference to their in vitro phagocytic capacity. Lab. Invest. **30**, 1–8 (1974).

DEBUSSCHER, L., BERNHEIM, J.L., COLLARD-RONGÉ, E., GOVAERTS, A., HOOGHE, R., LEJEUNE, F.J., ZEICHER, M., STRYCKMANS, P.A.: Hairy cell leukemia: Functional, immunologic, kinetic, and ultrastructural characterization. Blood **46**, 495–507 (1975).

DIEBOLD, J., REYNES, M., KALIFAT, R., TRICOT, G.: Les inclusions intranucléaires de la maladie de Waldenström. Signification biologique et valeur diagnostique. Nouv. Presse méd. **3**, 1067–1070 (1974).

DIEBOLD, J., REYNES, M., KALIFAT, R., TRICOT, G.: Les expressions morphologiques de la maladie de Waldenström. Sem. Hôp. Paris **51**, 2927–2934 (1975).

DJALDETTI, M., LANDAU, M., MANDEL, E.M., HAR-ZAAV, L., LEWINSKI, U.: Electron microscopic study of lymphosarcoma cell leukemia. Blut **29**, 210–215 (1974).

DORFMAN, R.F.: Diagnosis of Burkitt's tumor in the United States. Cancer **21**, 563–574 (1968).

DOUGLAS, S.D., BORJESON, J., CHESSIN, L.N.: Studies on human lymphocytes in vitro. IV. Comparative fine structural features of the established Burkitt lymphoma cell lines AL-1, EB-2 and phytomitogen-transformed lymphocytes. J. Immunol. **99**, 340–346 (1967).

DOUGLAS, S.D., COHNEN, G., BRITTINGER, G.: Ultrastructural comparison between phytomitogen transformed normal and chronic lymphocytic leukemia lymphocytes. J. Ultrastruct. Res. **44**, 11–26 (1973).

Douglas, S.D., Cohnen, G., König, E., Brittinger, G., Fischer, K., Bremer, K.: Electron microscopic and biochemical studies on lysosomes and lysosomal enzymes in "resting" and phytohemagglutinin (PHA) stimulated lymphocytes from patients with chronic lymphatic leukemia (CLL). In: Leukämie, pp. 29–35. Gross, R., van de Loo, J., Eds. Berlin-Heidelberg-New York: Springer 1972.

Edelson, R.L., Kirkpatrick, C.H., Shevach, E.M., Schein, P.S., Smith, R.W., Green, I., Lutzner, M.: Preferential cutaneous infiltration by neoplastic thymus-derived lymphocytes. Morphologic and functional studies. Ann. intern. Med. **80**, 685–692 (1974).

Edelson, R.L., Lutzner, M.A., Kirkpatrick, C.H., Shevach, E.M., Green, I.: Morphologic and functional properties of the atypical T lymphocytes of the Sezary syndrome. Mayo Clin. Proc. **49**, 558–566 (1974).

Epstein, M.A.: Histogenesis of the Burkitt lymphoma. In: Treatment of Burkitt's Tumour. UICC Monograph Series, Vol. 8, pp. 29–33. Burchenal, J.H., Burkitt, D.P., Eds. Berlin-Heidelberg-New York: Springer 1967.

Epstein, M.A., Achong, B.G.: Fine structural organization of human lymphoblasts of a tissue culture strain (EB1) from Burkitt's lymphoma. J. nat. Cancer Inst. **34**, 241–253 (1965).

Epstein, M.A., Achong, B.G.: The fine structure of cultured Burkitt lymphoblasts of established in vitro strains. In: Burkitt's Lymphoma, pp. 118–133. Burkitt, D.P., Wright, D.H., Eds. Edinburgh-London: Livingstone 1970.

Epstein, M.A., Achong, B.G., Barr, Y.M.: Virus particles in cultured lymphoblasts from Burkitt's lymphoma. Lancet 1964, I, pp. 702–703.

Epstein, M.A., Achong, B.G., Barr, Y.M., Zajac, B., Henle, G., Henle, W.: Morphological and virological investigations on cultured Burkitt tumor lymphoblasts (strain Raji). J. nat. Cancer Inst. **37**, 547–559 (1966).

Fagraeus, A.: Antibody production in relation to the development of plasma cells. In vivo and in vitro experiments. Acta med. scand. **130**, Suppl. 204 (1948).

Flad, H.-D., Huber, C., Bremer, K., Menne, H.-D., Huber, H.: Impaired recirculation of B lymphocytes in chronic lymphocytic leukemia. Europ. J. Immunol. **3**, 688–693 (1973).

Flandrin, G., Daniel, M.T.: La leucémia à tricholeucocytes (hairy cell leukemia). Une variété rare et mal connue d'hématopathie maligne. Nouv. Presse méd. **3**, 581–586 (1974).

Flaxman, B.A., Zelazny, G., van Scott, E.J.: Nonspecificity of characteristic cells in mycosis fungoides. Arch. Derm. **104**, 141–147 (1971).

Foa, R., Foa, C., Muratore, R.: Aspects particuliers du réticulum endoplasmique dans trois cas de leucose et un cas de réticulosarcome. C.R. Soc. Biol. (Paris) **164**, 1048–1054 (1970).

Ghadially, F.N., Skinnider, L.F.: Ultrastructure of hairy cell leukemia. Cancer (Philad.) **29**, 444–452 (1972).

Glick, A.D., Leech, J.H., Waldron, J.A., Flexner, J.M., Horn, R.G., Collins, R.D.: Malignant lymphomas of follicular center cell origin in man. II. Ultrastructural and cytochemical studies. J. nat. Cancer Inst. **54**, 23–36 (1975).

Golomb, H.M., Braylan, R., Polliack, A.: 'Hairy' cell leukaemia (Leukaemic reticuloendotheliosis): A scanning electron microscopic study of eight cases. Brit. J. Haemat. **29**, 455–460 (1975).

Gomez Orbaneja, J., Sanchez Yus, E., Diaz-Flores, L., Simon Huarte, P.: Cytology of the mycosis fungoides and the Sézary syndrome. Correlation between light and electron microscopy. Brit. J. Derm. **87**, 96–105 (1972).

Goos, M., Kaiserling, E., Lennert, K.: Mycosis fungoides: model for T-lymphocyte homing to the skin? Brit. J. Derm. **94**, 221–222 (1976).

Griffin, E.R., Wright, D.H., Bell, T.M., Ross, M.G.R.: Demonstration of virus particles in biopsy material from cases of Burkitt tumor. Europ. J. Cancer **2**, 235–358 (1966).

Haak, H.L., de Man, J.C.H., Hijmans, W., Knapp, W., Speck, B.: Further evidence for the lymphocytic nature of leukaemic reticuloendotheliosis (hairy-cell-leukaemia). Brit. J. Haemat. **27**, 31–38 (1974).

Haegert, D.G., Cawley, J.C., Collins, R.D., Flemans, R.J., Smith, J.L.: Leukaemic reticuloendotheliosis: A morphological and immunological study of four cases. J. clin. Path. **27**, 967–972 (1974).

HAMBURG, A., BRYNES, R.K., REESE, C., GOLOMB, H.M.: Human cord blood lymphocytes. Ultrastructural and immunologic surface marker characteristics; a comparison with B- and T-cell lymphomas. Lab. Invest. **34**, 207–215 (1976).

HANNA, JR., M.G., SZAKAL, A.K., TYNDALL, R.L.: Histoproliferative effect of Rauscher leukemia virus on lymphatic tissue: Histological and ultrastructural studies of germinal centers and their relation to leukemogenesis. Cancer Res. **30**, 1748–1763 (1970).

HENRY, K.: Electron microscopy in the non-Hodgkin's lymphomata. Brit. J. Cancer **31**, Suppl. II, 73–93 (1975).

HUHN, D.: Feinstruktur peripherer Lymphozyten bei chronischer lymphatischer Leukämie. Dtsch. med. Wschr. **95**, 897–901 (1970).

HUHN, D., DOBBELSTEIN, H., ENGELHARDT, D.: Sézary-Syndrom. Blut **25**, 352–363 (1972).

HUHN, D., RODT, H., THIEL, E., GROSSE-WILDE, H., FINK, U., THEML, H., JÄGER, G., STEIDLE, C., THIERFELDER, S.: T-Zell-Leukämien des Erwachsenen. Blut **33**, 141–160 (1976).

HUHN, D., THIEL, E., RODT, H.: Immunglobulin-Ablagerungen in Lymphadenose-Zellen. Klin. Wschr. **53**, 317–320 (1975).

HUREZ, D., FLANDRIN, G., PREUD'HOMME, J.L., SELIGMANN, M.: Unreleased intracellular monoclonal macroglobulin in chronic lymphocytic leukaemia. Clin. exp. Immunol. **10**, 223–234 (1972).

INSEL, R.A., MELEWICZ, F.M., LA VIA, M.F., BALCH, C.M.: Morphology, surface markers, and in vitro responses of a human leukemic T cell. Clin. Immunol. Immunopath. **4**, 382–391 (1975).

ITO, S.: Study on the in vitro Rieder cell. Scand. J. Haemat. **12**, 355–365 (1974).

JAFFE, E.S., SHEVACH, E.M., FRANK, M.M., BERARD, C.W., GREEN, I.: Nodular lymphoma—evidence for origin from follicular B lymphocytes. New Engl. J. Med. **290**, 813–819 (1974).

JEFFREE, G.M.: Enzymes of round cell tumours in bone and soft tissue: A histochemical survey. J. Path. **113**, 101–115 (1974).

KAISERLING, E.: Verzweigte tubuläre Cytoplasmaeinschlüsse im menschlichen Lymphknoten. Beitr. Path. **147**, 237–248 (1972).

KAISERLING, E.: Feinstrukturelle Befunde bei Non-Hodgkin-Lymphomen. Habil. Schrift, Kiel 1975.

KAISERLING, E.: Elektronenmikroskopische Befunde bei Non-Hodgkin-Lymphomen. In: Maligne Lymphome und monoklonale Gammopathien. Hämatologie und Bluttransfusion, Bd. 18, pp. 185–198. LÖFFLER, H., Ed. München: Lehmanns 1976.

KAISERLING, E.: Non-Hodgkin-Lymphome. Ultrastruktur und Cytogenese. Veröff. Path., Heft 105. Stuttgart: G. Fischer 1977

KAISERLING, E., LENNERT, K.: Die interdigitierende Reticulumzelle im menschlichen Lymphknoten. Eine spezifische Zelle der thymusabhängigen Region. Virchows Arch. B**16**, 51–61 (1974).

KAISERLING, E., STEIN, H., LENNERT, K.: IgM-producing malignant lymphomas without macroglobulinemia. Morphological and immunochemical findings. Virchows Arch. B **14**, 1–18 (1973).

KATAYAMA, I., LI, C.Y., YAM, L.T.: Ultrastructural characteristics of the "hairy cells" of leukemic reticuloendotheliosis. Amer. J. Path. **67**, 361–370 (1972a).

KATAYAMA, I., LI, C.Y., YAM, L.T.: Ultrastructural characteristics of the "hairy cells" of leukemic reticuloendotheliosis. Amer. J. Path. **67**, 361–370 (1972b).

KATAYAMA, I., NAGY, G.K., BALOGH, JR., K.: Light microscopic identification of the ribosome-lamella complex in "hairy cells" of leukemic reticuloendotheliosis. Cancer (Philad.) **32**, 843–846 (1973).

KATAYAMA, I., UEHARA, H., GLESER, R.A., WEINTRAUB, L.: The value of electron microscopy in the diagnosis of Burkitt's lymphoma. Amer. J. clin. Path. **61**, 540–548 (1974).

KIM, H., HELLER, P., RAPPAPORT, H.: Monoclonal gammopathies associated with lymphoproliferative disorders: A morphologic study. Amer. J. clin. Path. **59**, 282–294 (1973).

KING, G.W., HURTUBISE, P.E., SAGONE, JR., A.L., LOBUGLIO, A.F., METZ, E.N.: Leukemic reticuloendotheliosis. A study of the origin of the malignant cell. Amer. J. Med. **59**, 411–416 (1975).

KLIPPEL, J.H., DECKER, J.L., GRIMLEY, P.M., EVANS, A.S., ROTHFIELD, N.F.: Epstein-Barr virus antibody and lymphocyte tubuloreticular structures in systemic lupus erythematosus. Lancet 1973, II, pp. 1057–1058.

KNAPP, W., SCHUIT, H.R.E., BOLHUIS, R.L.H., HIJMANS, W.: Surface immunoglobulins in chronic lymphatic leukaemia, macroglobulinaemia and myelomatosis. Clin. exp. Immunol. **16**, 541–552 (1974).

KOJIMA, M.: Cytopathological study on lymph node, especially reference to germinal center. [Jap.] Nippon Byōri Gakkai Kaishi (Trans. Soc. Path. Jap.) **58**, 3–28 (1969).

KOJIMA, M., IMAI, Y., MORI, N.: A concept of follicular lymphoma. A proposal for the existence of a neoplasm originating from the germinal center. In: Malignant Diseases of the Hematopoietic System. GANN Monograph on Cancer Research, No. 15, pp. 195–207. AKAZAKI, K., RAPPAPORT, H., BERARD, C.W., BENNETT, J.M., ISHIKAWA, E., Eds. Baltimore-London-Tokyo: University of Tokyo Press 1973.

KRÜGER, G., O'CONOR, G.T.: Epidemiologic and immunologic considerations on the pathogenesis of Burkitt's tumor. In: Current Problems in the Epidemiology of Cancer and Lymphomas. Recent Results in Cancer Research, Vol. 39, pp. 211–224. GRUNDMANN, E., TULINIUS, H., Eds. Berlin-Heidelberg-New York: Springer 1972.

KUHN, C.: Nuclear bodies and intranuclear globulin inclusions in Waldenström's macroglobulinemia. Lab. Invest. **17**, 404–415 (1967).

LABAZE, J.J., MOSCOVIC, E.A., PHAM, T.D., AZAR, H.A.: Histological and ultrastructural findings in a case of the Sézary syndrome. J. clin. Path. **25**, 312–319 (1972).

LASZLO, J., GERBER, H.J., SOMMER, J.R.: Composition and structure of cytoplasmic globules in leukemic lymphocytes. Blood **29**, 77–86 (1967).

VAN LEEUWEN, A.W.F.M., MEIJER, C.J.L.M., DE MAN, J.C.H.: T-cell membrane characteristics of 'mycosis cells' in the skin and lymph node. J. invest. Derm. **65**, 367–369 (1975).

VAN LEEUWEN, A.W.F.M., MEIJER, C.J.L.M., VAN VLOTEN, W.A., SCHEFFER, E., DE MAN, J.C.H.: Further evidence for the T-cell nature of the atypical mononuclear cells in mycosis fungoides. Virchows Arch. B **21**, 179–187 (1976).

LENNERT, K.: Follicular lymphoma. A tumor of the germinal centers. In: Malignant Diseases of the Hematopoietic System. GANN Monograph on Cancer Research, Vol. 15, pp. 217–231. AKAZAKI, K., RAPPAPORT, H., BERARD, C.W., BENNETT, J.M., ISHIKAWA, E., Eds. Tokyo: University of Tokyo Press 1973.

LENNERT, K.: Klassifikation und Morphologie der Non-Hodgkin-Lymphome. In: Maligne Lymphome und monoklonale Gammopathien. Hämatologie und Bluttransfusion, Bd. 18, pp. 145–166. LÖFFLER, H., Ed. München: Lehmanns 1976.

LENNERT, K., CAESAR, R., MÜLLER, H.K.: Electron microscopic studies of germinal centers in man. In: Germinal Centers in Immune Responses, pp. 49–59. COTTIER, H., ODARTCHENKO, N., SCHINDLER, R., CONGDON, C.C., Eds. Berlin-Heidelberg-New York: Springer 1967.

LENNERT, K., KAISERLING, E., MÜLLER-HERMELINK, H.K.: T-associated plasma-cells. [Letter to the Editor.] Lancet 1975, I, pp. 1031–1032.

LENNERT, K., KAISERLING, E., MÜLLER-HERMELINK, H.K.: Malignant lymphomas: Models of differentiation and cooperation of lymphoreticular cells. Paper presented at Cold Spring Harbor Meeting on "Differentiation of Normal and Neoplastic Hematopoietic Cells" in Cold Spring Harbor, New York, USA, Sept. 6–11, 1977. In press.

LENNERT, K., NIEDORF, H.R.: Nachweis von desmosomal verknüpften Reticulumzellen im follikulären Lymphom (Brill Symmers). Virchows Arch. B **4**, 148–150 (1969).

LEVINE, G.D., DORFMAN, R.F.: Nodular lymphoma: An ultrastructural study of its relationship to germinal centers and a correlation of light and electron microscopic findings. Cancer (Philad.) **35**, 148–164 (1975).

LITOVITZ, T.L., LUTZNER, M.A.: Quantitative measurements of blood lymphocytes from patients with chronic lymphocytic leukemia and the Sézary syndrome. J. nat. Cancer Inst. **53**, 75–77 (1974).

LÖFFLER, H., MEYHÖFER, W., LANGE, R.H., EHLERS, G., REMMELE, W.: Sézary-Syndrom – eine leukämische Variante der Mykosis fungoides. Dtsch. med. Wschr. **99**, 429–434 (1974).

LÖFFLER, H., ROUX, A., FISCHER, J., DESAGA, J.F., PRALLE, H., GRAUBNER, M.: Hairy cell-Leukämie. In: Maligne Lymphome und monoklonale Gammopathien. Hämatologie und Bluttransfusion, Bd. 18, pp. 255–272. LÖFFLER, H., Ed. München: Lehmanns 1976.

LUKES, R.J., BUTLER, J.J., HICKS, E.B.: Natural history of Hodgkin's disease as related to its pathologic picture. Cancer (Philad.) **19**, 317–344 (1966).

LUKES, R.J., COLLINS, R.D.: New approaches to the classification of the lymphomata. Brit. J. Cancer **31**, Suppl. II, 1–28 (1975).

LUTZNER, M.A., EMERIT, I., DUREPAIRE, R., FLANDRIN, G., GRUPPER, C., PRUNIERAS, M.: Cytogenetic, cytophotometric, and ultrastructural study of large cerebriform cells of the Sézary syndrome and description of a small-cell variant. J. nat. Cancer Inst. **50**, 1145–1162 (1973).

LUTZNER, M.A., HOBBS, J.W., HORVATH, P.: Ultrastructure of abnormal cells. In Sezary syndrome, mycosis fungoides, and parapsoriasis en plaque. Arch. Derm. **103**, 375–386 (1971).

LUTZNER, M.A., JORDAN, H.W.: The ultrastructure of an abnormal cell in Sézary's syndrome. Blood **31**, 719–726 (1968).

DE MAN, J.C.H., MEINERS, W.B.H.: Crystals of protein nature in the cytoplasm of lymphatic cells in a case of lymphoreticular malignancy. Blood **20**, 492–500 (1962).

DE MARTINO, C., ZAMBONI, L.: Silver methenamine stain for electron microscopy. J. Ultrastruct. Res. **19**, 273–282 (1967).

MCLAUGHLIN, H., WETHERLY-MEIN, G., PITCHER, C., HOBBS, J.R.: Non-immunoglobulin-bearing 'B' lymphocytes in chronic lymphatic leukaemia? Brit. J. Haemat. **25**, 7–14 (1973).

MOLLO, F., MONGA, G., STRAMIGNONI, A.: Dark reticular cells in human lymphadenitis and lymphomas. Virchows Arch. B **3**, 117–126 (1969).

MOLLO, F., MONGA, G., STRAMIGNONI, A.: Electron microscopy in morphological classification of human lymphomas. J. submicroscop. Cytol. **3**, 105–120 (1971).

MORAGAS, A., GUARDIA, J., MARTINEZ-VAZQUEZ, J.M., VILASECA, J., FERRAGUT, A., BACARDI, R., TORNOS, J.: Lymphome nodulaire associé à une macroglobulinémie. Lyon méd. **230**, 691–694 (1973).

MORI, Y., LENNERT, K.: Electron microscopic atlas of lymph node cytology and pathology. Berlin-Heidelberg-New York: Springer 1969.

MÜLLER-HERMELINK, H.K., CAESAR, R.: Elektronenmikroskopische Untersuchung der Keimzentren in menschlichen Tonsillen. Z. Zellforsch. **96**, 521–547 (1969).

MÜLLER-HERMELINK, H.K., KAISERLING, E.: Seminar für elektronenmikroskopisch-histochemische Techniken. Verh. dtsch. Ges. Path. **59**, 522–527 (1975).

MÜLLER-HERMELINK, H.K., KAISERLING, E., LENNERT, K.: Pseudofollikuläre Nester von Plasmazellen (eines besonderen Typs?) in der paracorticalen Pulpa menschlicher Lymphknoten. Virchows Arch. B**14**, 47–56 (1973).

NIES, K.M., MARSHALL, J., OBERLIN, M.A., HALPERN, M.S., BROWN, J.C.: Chronic lymphocytic leukemia with gamma chain cytoplasmic inclusions. Amer. J. clin. Path. **65**, 948–956 (1976).

ORFANOS, C., STÜTTGEN, G.: Elektronenmikroskopische Beobachtungen bei der Mycosis fungoides. Nachweis von cytoplasmatischen „Zelleinschlüssen". Arch. klin. exp. Derm. **215**, 438–460 (1963).

OTTÓ, S., BALOGH, I., JÁKÓ, J.: Electron microscopic study of plasma cells in immunoproliferative diseases. Acta morph. Acad. Sci. hung. **22**, 331–336 (1974).

PADILLA, F., SOLOFF, B.L.: Electron microscopic observations on 'hairy' lymphoreticular cells. [Abstr.] Clin. Res. **17**, 32 (1969).

PADILLA, F., SOLOFF, B.L.: Leukemic reticuloendotheliosis. Electron microscopy of circulating lymphoid cells. Nouv. Rev. franç. Hémat. **11**, 547–554 (1971).

PAINTRAND, M., DANTCHEV, D., MATHÉ, G.: Electron microscopic aspects of cells in the four subvarieties of acute lymphoid leukemia. In: Recent Results Cancer Res. **43**, 71–75. Berlin-Heidelberg-New York: Springer 1973.

PEDIO, G., RÜTTNER, J.R., SPYCHER, M.A., GUT, D.: Virus-bearing plasma cells in peripheral blood of a patient with 'hairy cell' leukemia. Acta haemat. (Basel) **54**, 297–305 (1975).

POLLIACK, A., SIEGAL, F.P., CLARKSON, B.D., FU, S.M., WINCHESTER, R.J., LAMPEN, N., SIEGAL, M., DEHARVEN, E.: A scanning electron microscopy and immunological study of 84 cases of lymphocytic leukaemia and related lymphoproliferative disorders. Scand. J. Haemat. **15**, 359–376 (1975).

POPE, J.H., ACHONG, B.G., EPSTEIN, M.A.: Cultivation and fine structure of virus-bearing lymphoblasts from a second New Guinea Burkitt lymphoma: Establishment of sublines with unusual cultural properties. Int. J. Cancer **3**, 171–182 (1968).

POPE, J.H., ACHONG, B.G., EPSTEIN, M.A., BIDDULPH, J.: Burkitt lymphoma in New Guinea: Establishment of a line of lymphoblasts in vitro and description of their fine structure. J. nat. Cancer Inst. **39**, 933–945 (1967).

RABSON, A.S., O'CONOR, G.T., BARON, S., WHANG, J.J., LEGALLAIS, F.Y.: Morphologic, cytogenetic and virologic studies in vitro of a malignant lymphoma from an African child. Int. J. Cancer **1**, 89–106 (1966).

RINNEBERG, H.: Adenosintriphosphatase, 5-Nukleotidase und Glycerophosphatase im Schnitt und Ausstrich menschlicher Lymphknoten. Diss. med., Frankfurt 1961.

RIVAS, C., OLIVA, H.: El diagnóstico óptico de reticulosarcoma, revisado y corregido por la microscopia electrónica. Bol. Fund. Jiminez Diaz **7**, 71–80 (1975).

ROBINOWITZ, B.N., NOGUCHI, S., ROENIGK, JR., H.H.: Tumor cell characterization in mycosis fungoides. Cancer (Philad.) **57**, 1747–1753 (1976).

RODT, H., THIEL, E., THIERFELDER, S., HUHN, D., GÖTZE, D., BREHM, G.: Spezifisches Anti-T-Lymphocyten-Globulin (sATG) für die Diagnostik lymphoproliferativer Erkrankungen. Klin. Wschr. **54**, 361–366 (1976).

ROSAS-URIBE, A., VARIAKOJIS, D., MOLNAR, Z., RAPPAPORT, H.: Mycosis fungoides: An ultrastructural study. Cancer (Philad.) **34**, 634–645 (1974).

ROSENTHAL, A.S., DAVIE, J.M., ROSENSTREICH, D.L., CEHRS, K.U.: Antibody-mediated internalization of B lymphocyte surface membrane immunoglobulin. Exp. Cell Res. **81**, 317–329 (1973).

ROZENSZAJN, L.A., GUTMAN, A., RADNAY, J., BEN DAVID, E., SHOHAM, D.: A study of the nature of 'hairy' cells, with emphasis on enzymatic markers. Amer. J. clin. Path. **66**, 432–441 (1976).

RUBIN, A.D., DOUGLAS, S.D., CHESSIN, L.N., GLADE, P.R., DAMESHEK, W.: Chronic reticulolymphocytic leukemia. Reclassification of 'leukemic reticuloendotheliosis' through functional characterization of the circulating mononuclear cells. Amer. J. Med. **47**, 149–162 (1969).

RYAN, E.A., SANDERSON, K.V., BARTÁK, P., SAMMAN, P.D.: Can mycosis fungoides begin in the epidermis? A hypothesis. Brit. J. Derm. **88**, 419–429 (1973).

SANDBANK, M.: Mycosis fungoides. Ultrastructural study with demonstration of atypical cells and nuclear bodies. Arch. Derm. **103**, 206–214 (1971).

SANDBANK, M., BEN-BASSAT, M.: Mycosis fungoides and Sézary's syndrome. Israel J. med. Sci. **7**, 1262–1270 (1971).

SCHAEFER, H.-E.: Die Ultrastruktur maligner Lymphome. In: Maligne Lymphome und monoklonale Gammopathien. Hämatologie und Bluttransfusion, Bd. 18, pp. 49–61. LÖFFLER, H., Ed. München: Lehmanns 1976.

SCHAEFER, H.E., KRÜGER, G.R.F., FISCHER, R.: Morphological classification of malignant lymphomas: Ultrastructural, cytochemical and immunological results. Acta neuropath. (Berl.) Suppl. **6**, 21–29 (1975).

SCHMALZL, F., HUHN, D., ASAMER, H., BRAUNSTEINER, H.: Hairy cell leukemia ('leukemic reticuloendotheliosis'), reticulosarcoma, and monocytic leukemia. Cytochemical and ultrastructural investigations. Acta haemat. (Basel) **53**, 257–276 (1975).

SCHNITZER, B., HAMMACK, W.J.: B-lymphocyte nature of hairy cells in hairy-cell leukaemia. [Letter to the Editor.] Lancet 1974, II, p. 649.

SCHNITZER, B., HAMMACK, W.J.: The hairy cell. [Letter to the Editor.] Hum. Path. **6**, 262–263 (1975).

SCHNITZER, B., KASS, L.: Hairy-cell leukemia. A clinicopathologic and ultrastructural study. Amer. J. clin. Path. **61**, 176–187 (1974).

SCHREK, R.: Ultrastructure of blood lymphocytes from chronic lymphocytic and lymphosarcoma cell leukemia. J. nat. Cancer Inst. **48**, 51–64 (1972).

SCHREK, R., DONNELLY, W.J.: "Hairy" cells in blood in lymphoreticular neoplastic disease and "flagellated" cells of normal lymph nodes. Blood **27**, 199–211 (1966).

SCHUMACHER, H.R., MAUGEL, T.K., DAVIS, K.D.: The lymphocyte of chronic lymphatic leukemia. I. Electron microscopy–onset. Cancer (Philad.) **26**, 895–903 (1970).

SCHUMACHER, H.R., SZEKELY, I.E., PARK, S.A., FISHER, D.R.: Ultrastructural studies on the acute leukemic lymphoblast. Blut **27**, 396–406 (1973).

SCHWARZE, E.-W., RADASZKIEWICZ, T., PÜLHORN, G., GOOS, M., LENNERT, K.: Maligne und benigne Lymphome des Auges, der Lid- und Orbitalregion. Virchows Arch. A **370**, 85–96 (1976).

SHIGEMATSU, T., KOZURU, M., HATTORI, K.: The fine structure of human myeloma cells and macroglobulin-producing cells. Acta haemat. jap. **33**, 37–50 (1970).

SMETANA, K., GYORKEY, F., GYORKEY, P., BUSCH, H.: Comparative studies on the ultrastructure of nucleoli in human lymphosarcoma cells and leukemic lymphocytes. Cancer Res. **30**, 1149–1155 (1970).

SMETANA, K., HEŘMANSKY, F., JANELE, J., BUSCH, H.: A further note on the ultrastructure of leukemic lymphocytes. Folia haemat. (Lpz.) **89**, 1–14 (1968).

SMITH, J.L., CAWLEY, J.C., BARKER, C.R.: The response to plant mitogens of two subpopulations of lymphocytes in a case of chronic lymphocytic leukaemia. Clin. exp. Immunol. **14**, 397–408 (1973).

SÖDERSTRÖM, N., NORBERG, B.: Observations regarding the specific post-capillary venules of lymph nodes in malignant lymphomas. Acta path. microbiol. scand. A **82**, 71–79 (1974).

SPLINTER, T.A.W., HELDER, A.W., LUCAS, C.J., FELTKAMP-VROOM, T.M.: Tubuloreticular structures in human lymphoid cell lines. A cell biological study. Brit. J. exp. Path. **56**, 124–132 (1975).

STEIN, H., KAISERLING, E., LENNERT, K.: Immunoglobulin-production and surface-bound immunoglobulins in chronic lymphocytic leukemia, lymphosarcoma, and so-called reticulum cell sarcoma. In: Modern Trends in Human Leukemia. Hämatologie und Bluttransfusion, Bd. 14, pp. 97–106. NETH, R., GALLO, R.C., SPIEGELMAN, S., STOHLMAN, JR., F., Eds. München: Lehmanns 1974.

STEIN, H., KAISERLING, E., STEIN, G.: Surface markers on hairy cells. Boll. Ist. sieroter. milan. Suppl. **53**, 305 (1974).

STEMPAK, J.G., WARD, R.T.: An improved staining method for electron microscopy. J. Cell Biol. **22**, 697–701 (1964).

STEWART, S.E., LOVELACE, E., WHANG, J.J., NGU, V.A.: Burkitt tumor: Tissue culture, cytogenetic and virus studies. J. nat. Cancer Inst. **34**, 319–327 (1965).

STOCKINGER, L.: Elektronenoptische Darstellung einer Makroglobulinretention in Plasmazellen des menschlichen Knochenmarks. J. Cell Biol. **15**, 131–136 (1962).

SUCHI, T., SATO, T., KOBAYASHI, H., AKATSUKA, H., AKAZA, T., KURITA, S., HOSHINO, M.: Reticulum cell sarcoma. Some characteristics of reticulum-cell-sarcoma cells. [Jap.] Jap. J. Cancer Clin. **19**, 419–425 (1973).

SWARTZENDRUBER, D.C., IL MA, B., MURPHY, W.H.: Localization of C-type virus particles in lymphoid germinal centers of C58 mice. Proc. Soc. exp. Biol. (N.Y.) **126**, 731–734 (1967).

SZAKAL, A.K., HANNA, JR., M.G.: The ultrastructure of antigen localization and virus-like particles in mouse spleen germinal centers. Exp. mol. Path. **8**, 75–89 (1968).

THIEL, E., RODT, H., HUHN, D., THIERFELDER, S.: Decrease and altered distribution of human T antigen on chronic lymphatic leukemia cells of T type, suggesting a clonal origin. Blood **47**, 723–736 (1976).

TOSHIMA, S., TAKAGI, N., MINOWADA, J., MOORE, G.E., SANDBERG, A.A.: Electron microscopic and cytogenetic studies of cells derived from Burkitt's lymphoma. Cancer Res. **27**, 753–771 (1967).

TRUBOWITZ, S., MASEK, B., FRASCA, J.M.: Leukemic reticuloendotheliosis. Blood **38**, 288–298 (1971).

UZMAN, B.G., SAITO, H., KASAC, M.: Tubular arrays in the endoplasmic reticulum in human tumor cells. Lab. Invest. **24**, 492–498 (1971).

VARIAKOJIS, D., ROSAS-URIBE, A., RAPPAPORT, H.: Mycosis fungoides: Pathologic findings in staging laparotomies. Cancer (Philad.) **33**, 1589–1600 (1974).

VELDMAN, J.E.: Histophysiology and Electron Microscopy of the Immune Response. Thesis, Groningen 1970. Groningen: N.V. Boekdrukkerij Dijkstra Niemeyer 1970.

VENABLE, J.H., COGGESHALL, R.: A simplified lead citrate stain for use in electron microscopy. J. Cell Biol. **25**, 407–408 (1965).

VYKOUPIL, K.F., THIELE, J., GEORGII, A.: Hairy cell leukemia. Bone marrow findings in 24 patients. Virchows Arch. A **370**, 273–289 (1976).

WARD, A.M., SHORTLAND, J.R., DARKE, C.S.: Lymphosarcoma of the lung with monoclonal (IgM) gammopathy. A clinicopathologic, histochemical, immunologic, and ultrastructural study. Cancer (Philad.) **27**, 1009–1028 (1971).

WILLIGHAGEN, R.G.J.: Histochemistry of enzymes in tumours. Ned. T. Geneesk. **105**, 1356–1357 (1961).

WOESSNER, S., ROZMAN, C.: Ribosome-lamellae complex in chronic lymphatic leukaemia. Blut **33**, 23–28 (1976).

ZUCKER-FRANKLIN, D.: Virus-like particles in the lymphocytes of a patient with chronic lymphocytic leukemia. Blood **21**, 509–512 (1963).

ZUCKER-FRANKLIN, D.: Structural features of cells associated with the paraproteinemias. Semin. Hemat. **1**, 165–198 (1964).

ZUCKER-FRANKLIN, D.: Properties of the Sezary lymphoid cell. An ultrastructural analysis. Mayo Clin. Proc. **49**, 567–574 (1974).

ZUCKER-FRANKLIN, D., MELTON III, J.W., QUAGLIATA, F.: Ultrastructural, immunologic, and functional studies on Sézary cells: A neoplastic variant of thymus-derived (T) lymphocytes. Proc. nat. Acad. Sci. (Wash.) **71**, 1877–1881 (1974).

# References

## *Part Six*


ABDOU, N.I., ABDOU, N.L.: The monoclonal nature of lymphocytes in multiple myeloma. Ann. intern. Med. **83**, 42–45 (1975).

ABDOU, N.I., RICHTER, M.: Cells involved in the immune response. X. The transfer of antibody-forming capacity to irradiated rabbits by antigen-reactive cells isolated from normal allogeneic rabbit bone marrow after passage through antigen-sensitized glass bead columns. J. exp. Med. **130**, 141–163 (1969).

ABRAMS, A., COHEN, P.P., MEYER, O.O.: Physical properties of a cryoglobulin obtained from lymph nodes and serum of a case of lymphosarcoma. J. biol. Chem. **181**, 237–245 (1949).

AISENBERG, A.C., BLOCH, K.J.: Immunoglobulins on the surface of neoplastic lymphocytes. New Engl. J. Med. **287**, 272–276 (1972).

AISENBERG, A.C., BLOCH, K.J., LONG, J.C.: Cell-surface immunoglobulins in chronic lymphocytic leukemia and allied disorders. Amer. J. Med. **55**, 184–191 (1973).

AISENBERG, A.C., LONG, J.C.: Lymphocyte surface characteristics in malignant lymphoma. Amer. J. Med. **58**, 300–306 (1975).

AIUTI, F., WIGZELL, H.: Function and distribution pattern of human T lymphocytes. I. Production of anti-T lymphocyte specific sera as estimated by cytotoxicity and elimination of function of lymphocytes. Clin. exp. Immunol. **13**, 171–181 (1973).

ALBINI, B., WICK, G.: Ontogeny of lymphoid cell surface determinants in the chicken. Int. Arch. Allergy **48**, 513–529 (1975).

ANDERSSON, M., KLEIN, G., ZIEGLER, J.L., HENLE, W.: Association of Epstein-Barr viral genomes with American Burkitt lymphoma. Nature **260**, 357–359 (1976).

ARBEIT, R.D., SACHS, D.H., AMOS, D.B., DICKLER, H.B.: Human lymphocyte alloantigen(s) similar to murine Ir region-associated (Ia) antigens. J. Immunol. **115**, 1173–1175 (1975).

AUGENER, W., COHNEN, G., BRITTINGER, G.: Correlation of expression of surface membrane markers with different stages of B cell differentiation in malignant lymphomas in man. [Abstr.] Fed. Proc. **34**, 842 (1975).

AUGENER, W., GREY, H.M.: Studies on the mechanism of heat aggregation of human γG. J. Immunol. **105**, 1024–1030 (1970).

AVRAMEAS, S.: Coupling of enzymes to proteins with glutaraldehyde. Use of the conjugates for the detection of antigens and antibodies. Immunochemistry **6**, 43–52 (1969).

AVRAMEAS, S., LEDUC, E.H.: Detection of simultaneous antibody synthesis in plasma cells and specialized lymphocytes in rabbit lymph nodes. J. exp. Med. **131**, 1137–1168 (1970).

AVRAMEAS, S., TERNYNCK, T.: Communication to the editors. Peroxidase labeled antibodies. Fab-conjugates with enhanced intracellular penetration. Immunochemistry **8**, 1175–1179 (1971).

AWDEH, Z.L., ASKONAS, B.A., WILLIAMSON, A.R.: The homogeneous γG-immunoglobulin produced by mouse plasmacytoma 5563 and its subsequent heterogeneity on serum. Biochem. J. **102**, 548–553 (1967).

BACH, J.-F., DORMONT, J.: Further developments of the rosette inhibition test for the testing of antihuman lymphocyte serum. Transplantation **11**, 96–100 (1971).

BACH, J.F., DORMONT, J., DARDENNE, M., BALNER, H.: In vitro rosette inhibition by antihuman antilymphocyte serum. Correlation with skin graft prolongation in subhuman primates. Transplantation **8**, 265–280 (1969).

Basten, A., Miller, J.F.A.P., Sprent, J., Pye, J.: A receptor for antibody on B lymphocytes. I. Method of detection and functional significance. J. exp. Med. **135**, 610–626 (1972).

Basten, A., Warner, N.L., Mandel, T.: A receptor for antibody on B lymphocytes. II. Immunochemical and electron microscopy characteristics. J. exp. Med. **135**, 627–794 (1972).

Belpomme, D., Dantchev, D., Du Rusquec, E., Grandjon, D., Huchet, R., Pouillart, P., Schwarzenberg, L., Amiel, J.L., Mathé, G.: T and B lymphocyte markers on the neoplastic cell of 20 patients with acute and 10 patients with chronic lymphoid leukemia. Biomedicine **20**, 109–118 (1974).

Bennett, M.H., Millett, Y.L.: Nodular sclerotic lymphosarcoma. A possible new clinico-pathological entity. Clin. Radiol. **20**, 339–343 (1969).

Bentwich, Z., Douglas, S.D., Skutelsky, E., Kunkel, H.G.: Sheep red cell binding to human lymphocytes treated with neuraminidase; enhancement of T cell binding and identification of a subpopulation of B cells. J. exp. Med. **137**, 1532–1537 (1973).

Berken, A., Benacerraf, B.: Properties of antibodies cytophilic for macrophages. J. exp. Med. **123**, 119–144 (1966).

Bernard, J., Bessis, M., Souliér, J.P., Thiéry, J.P.: Étude au microscope électronique d'une leucémie lymphoide avec cristaux intracytoplasmique. Rev. Hémat. **14**, 227–237 (1959).

Bert, G., Massaro, A.L., Maja, M.: Electrophoretic study of immunoglobulin on the lymphocyte surface. Nature **218**, 1078–1079 (1968).

Bianco, C., Patrick, R., Nussenzweig, V.: A population of lymphocytes bearing a membrane receptor for antigen-antibody-complement complexes. J. exp. Med. **132**, 702–720 (1970).

Bianco, C., Weiner, M., Nussenzweig, V.: Neuraminidase enhancement of the binding of sheep erythrocytes (E) to human T lymphocytes. [Abstr.] Fed. Proc. **32**, 975 (1973).

Binder, R.A., Jencks, J.A., Chun, B., Rath, C.E.: "B" cell origin of malignant cells in a case of American Burkitt's lymphoma. Characterization of cells from a pleural effusion. Cancer (Philad.) **36**, 161–168 (1975).

Bøyum, A.: Isolation of mononuclear cells and granulocytes from human blood. Scand. J. clin. Lab. Invest. Suppl. **97**, 77–89 (1968).

Boiron, M., Flandrin, G., Ripault, J., Lortholary, P., Teillet, F., Jacquillat, C., Bernard, J.: Histio-lymphocytose médullaire et splénique d'apparence primitive. Nouv. Rev. franç. Hémat. **8**, 179–199 (1968).

Bokisch, V.A., Sobel, A.T.: Receptor for the fourth component of complement on human B lymphocytes and cultured human lymphoblastoid cells. J. exp. Med. **140**, 1336–1347 (1974).

Borella, L., Sen, L.: T cell surface markers on lymphoblasts from acute lymphocytic leukemia. J. Immunol. **111**, 1257–1260 (1973).

Bornkamm, G.W., Stein, H., Lennert, K., Rüggeberg, F., Bartels, H., zur Hausen, H.: Attempts to demonstrate virus-specific sequences in human tumors. IV. EB viral DNA in European Burkitt lymphoma and immunoblastic lymphadenopathy with excessive plasmocytosis. Int. J. Cancer **17**, 177–181 (1976).

Borsos, T., Rapp, H.J.: Immune hemolysis: A simplified method for the preparation of EAC 4 with guinea pig or human complement. J. Immunol. **99**, 263–268 (1967).

Bosman, C., Feldman, J.D.: The proportion and structure of cells forming antibody, γG and γM immunoglobulins, and γG and γM antibodies. Cell. Immunol. **1**, 31–50 (1970).

Bouman, H., Lüsebrink, W.D., Havsteen, B., Stein, H.: Discrimination between monoclonal and heterogeneous immunoglobulin M by isoelectric focusing and radioautography. Febs lett. **64**, 201–203 (1976).

Bouman, H., Meincke, G., Havsteen, B.: Microheterogeneity of immunoglobulin G from plasmacytomas. Identification of two types of IgG by isoelectric focusing. Z. Immun.-Forsch. **150**, 370–377 (1975).

Bouroncle, B.A., Wiseman, B.K., Doan, C.A.: Leukemic reticuloendotheliosis. Blood **13**, 609–630 (1958).

van Boxel, J.A., Rosenstreich, D.L.: Binding of aggregated γ-globulin to activated T lymphocytes in the guinea pig. J. exp. Med. **139**, 1002–1012 (1974).

Boyden, S.V.: Cytophilic antibody in guinea-pigs with delayed-type hypersensitivity. Immunology **7**, 474–483 (1964).

BOYDEN, S.V., SORKIN, E.: The adsorption of antigen by spleen cells previously treated with antiserum in vitro. Immunology **3**, 272–283 (1960).

BRAIN, P., GORDON, J., WILLETTS, W.A.: Rosette formation by peripheral lymphocytes. Clin. exp. Immunol. **6**, 681–688 (1970).

BRAIN, P., MARSTON, R.H.: Rosette formation by human T and B lymphocytes. Europ. J. Immunol. **3**, 6–9 (1973).

BRAYLAN, R.C., JAFFE, E.S., BURBACH, J.W., FRANK, M.M., JOHNSON, R.E., BERARD, C.W.: Similarities of surface characteristics of neoplastic well-differentiated lymphocytes from solid tissues and from peripheral blood. Cancer Res. **36**, 1619–1625 (1976).

BRAYLAN, R.C., JAFFE, E.S., MANN, R.B., FRANK, M.M., BERARD, C.W.: Surface receptors of human neoplastic lymphoreticular cells. In: Immunological Diagnosis of Leukemias and Lymphomas. Haematology and Blood Transfusion, Vol. 20, pp. 47–52. THIERFELDER, S., RODT, H., THIEL, E., Eds. Berlin-Heidelberg-New York: Springer 1977.

BRAYLAN, R.C., VARIAKOJIS, D., YACHNIN, S.: The Sézary syndrome lymphoid cell: Abnormal mitogenic responsiveness and surface properties. [Abstr.] Blood **42**, 1024 (1973).

BREMBERG, S., KLEIN, G., EPSTEIN, A.: Direct membrane fluorescence reaction of EBV-carrying human lymphoblastoid cells: blocking tests with xenogenetic antisera. Int. J. Cancer **4**, 761–766 (1969).

BRODER, S., EDELSON, R.L., LUTZNER, M.A., NELSON, D.L., MACDERMOTT, R.P., DURM, M.E., GOLDMAN, C.K., MEADE, B.D., WALDMANN, T.A.: The Sézary syndrome. A malignant proliferation of helper T cells. J. clin. Invest. **58**, 1297–1306 (1976).

BROUET, J.C.: T-cell neoplasia. Immuno-Oncology Week, Villejuif-Paris, June 1977.

BROUET, J.-C., FLANDRIN, G., SASPORTES, M., PREUD'HOMME, J.-L., SELIGMANN, M.: Chronic lymphocytic leukaemia of T-cell origin. Immunological and clinical evaluation in eleven patients. Lancet 1975, II, pp. 890–894.

BROUET, J.-C., FLANDRIN, G., SELIGMANN, M.: Indications of the thymus-derived nature of the proliferating cells in six patients with Sézary's syndrome. New Engl. J. Med. **289**, 341–344 (1973).

BROUET, J.C., LABAUME, S., SELIGMANN, M.: Evaluation of T and B lymphocyte membrane markers in human non-Hodgkin malignant lymphomata. Brit. J. Cancer **31**, Suppl. II, 121–127 (1975).

BROUET, J.C., PREUD'HOMME, J.L., FLANDRIN, G., CHELLOUL, N., SELIGMANN, M.: Membrane markers in 'histiocytic' lymphomas (reticulum cell sarcomas). J. nat. Cancer Inst. **56**, 631–633 (1976).

BROUET, J.-C., PREUD'HOMME, J.-L., SELIGMANN, M.: The use of B and T membrane markers in the classification of human leukemias, with special reference to acute lymphoblastic leukemia. Blood Cells **1**, 81–90 (1975).

BROUET, J.C., PRIEUR, A.-M.: Membrane markers on chronic lymphocytic leukemia cells: A B cell leukemia with rosettes due to anti-sheep erythrocytes antibody activity of the membrane bound IgM and a T cell leukemia with surface Ig. Clin. Immunol. Immunopath. **2**, 481–487 (1974).

BROUET, J.C., TOBEN, H.R., CHEVALIER, A., SELIGMANN, M.: T and B membrane markers on blast cells in 69 patients with acute lymphoblastic leukemia. Ann. Immunol. **125C**, 691–696 (1974).

BROUET, J.-C., VALENSI, F., DANIEL, M.-T., FLANDRIN, G., PREUD'HOMME, J.-L., SELIGMANN, M.: Immunological classification of acute lymphoblastic leukaemias: Evaluation of its clinical significance in a hundred patients. Brit. J. Haemat. **33**, 319–328 (1976).

BROWN, G., GREAVES, M.F., LISTER, T.A., RAPSON, N., PAPAMICHAEL, M.: Expression of human T and B lymphocyte cell-surface markers on leukaemic cells. Lancet 1974, II, pp. 753–755.

BURKITT, D.: A sarcoma involving the jaws in African children. Brit. J. Surg. **46**, 218–223 (1958/59).

BUSKARD, N.A., CATOVSKY, D., OKOS, A., GOLDMAN, J.M., GALTON, D.A.G.: Prolymphocytic leukaemia: Cell studies and treatment by leucapheresis. In: Maligne Lymphome und monoklonale Gammopathien. Hämatologie und Bluttransfusion, Bd. 18, pp. 237–253. LÖFFLER, H., Ed. München: Lehmanns 1976.

BUTLER, J.J., STRYKER, J.A., SHULLENBERGER, C.C.: A clinicopathological study of stages I and II non-Hodgkin's lymphomata using the Lukes-Collins classification. Brit. J. Cancer **31**, Suppl. II, 208–216 (1974).

CATOVSKY, D., CHERCHI, M., OKOS, A., HEGDE, U., GALTON, D.A.G.: Mouse red-cell rosettes in B-lymphoproliferative disorders. Brit. J. Haemat. **33**, 173–177 (1976).

CATOVSKY, D., GALETTO, J., OKOS, A., MILIANI, E., GALTON, D.A.: Cytochemical profile of B and T leukaemic lymphocytes with special reference to acute lymphoblastic leukaemia. J. clin. Path. **27**, 767–771 (1974).

CATOVSKY, D., GALTON, D.A.G.: Cell markers and the classification of acute leukaemia. In: Immunological Diagnosis of Leukemias and Lymphomas. Haematology and Blood Transfusion, Vol. 20, pp. 25–31. THIERFELDER, S., RODTH, H., THIEL, E., Eds. Berlin-Heidelberg-New York: Springer 1977.

CATOVSKY, D., GALTON, D.A.G., OKOS, A., MILIANI, E., GALETTO, J., PAPAMICHAIL, M.: The B-lymphocyte features of the "hairy" cell of LRE. Abstr., p. 57. XVth Congress of the Int. Soc. Haemat., Jerusalem 1974.

CATOVSKY, D., PAPAMICHAIL, M., OKOS, A., MILIANI, E., HOLBOROW, E.J.: Formation of mouse red cell rosettes by "hairy" cells. Biomedicine **23**, 81–84 (1975).

CATOVSKY, D., PETTIT, J.E., GALETTO, J., OKOS, A., GALTON, D.A.G.: The B-lymphocyte nature of the hairy cell of leukaemic reticuloendotheliosis. Brit. J. Haemat. **26**, 29–37 (1974).

CAWLEY, J.C., BARKER, C.R., BRITCHFORD, R.D., SMITH, J.L.: Intracellular IgA immunoglobulin crystals in chronic lymphocytic leukaemia. Clin. exp. Immunol. **13**, 407–416 (1973).

CHANG, L.M.S.: Development of terminal deoxynucleotidyl transferase activity in embryonic calf thymus gland. Biochem. biophys. Res. Commun. **44**, 124–131 (1971).

CHECHIK, B.E.: Serological similarity between blood hemocytoblasts of patients with acute leukemia and human fetal thymus tissue. [Russian] Byull. éksp. Biol. Med. **66**, 85–88 (1968).

CHECHIK, B.E., PYKE, K.W., GELFAND, E.W.: Human thymus/leukemia-associated antigen in normal and leukemic cells. Int. J. Cancer **18**, 551–556 (1976).

CHIAO, J.W., PANTIC, V.S., GOOD, R.A.: Human peripheral lymphocytes bearing both B-cell complement receptors and T-cell characteristics for sheep erythrocytes detected by a mixed rosette method. Clin. exp. Immunol. **18**, 483–490 (1974).

CHIN, A.H., SAIKI, J.H., TRUJILLO, J.M., WILLIAMS, JR., R.C.: Peripheral blood T- and B-lymphocytes in patients with lymphoma and acute leukemia. Clin. Immunol. Immunopath. **1**, 499–510 (1973).

CLAMAN, H.N., CHAPERON, E.A., TRIPLETT, R.F.: Thymus-marrow cell combinations. Synergism in antibody production. Proc. Soc. exp. Biol. (N.Y.) **122**, 1167–1171 (1966).

CLARK, C., RYDELL, R.E., KAPLAN, M.E.: Frequent association of IgMλ with crystalline inclusions in chronic lymphatic leukemic lymphocytes. New Engl. J. Med. **289**, 113–117 (1973).

CLINE, M.J., BILLING, R.: Antigens expressed by human B lymphocytes and myeloid stem cells. J. exp. Med. **146**, 1143–1145 (1977).

COOMBS, R.R.A., GURNER, B.W., WILSON, A.B., HOLM, G., LINDGREN, B.: Rosette-formation between human lymphocytes and sheep red cells not involving immunoglobulin receptors. Int. Arch. Allergy **39**, 658–663 (1970).

COONS, A.H., LEDUC, E.H., CONNOLLY, J.M.: Studies on antibody production. I. A method for the histochemical demonstration of specific antibody and its application to a study of the hyperimmune rabbit. J. exp. Med. **102**, 49–60 (1955).

COOPER, M.D.: Immunodeficiency with special reference to molecular defects. VIIth Immunopathology Symposium, Bad Schachen, Western Germany, June 1976.

COOPER, M.D., PETERSON, R.D.A., GOOD, R.A.: Delineation of the thymic and bursal lymphoid systems in the chicken. Nature (Lond.) **205**, 143–146 (1965).

COOPER, M.D., PETERSON, R.D.A., SOUTH, M.A., GOOD, R.A.: The functions of the thymus system and the bursa system in the chicken. J. exp. Med. **123**, 75–102 (1966).

VAN DALEN, J.P.R., KNAPP, W., PLOEM, J.S.: Microfluorometry on antigen-antibody interaction in immunofluorescence using antigens covalently bound to agarose beads. J. immunol. Methods **2**, 383–392 (1973).

DAMESHEK, W.: "Immunoblasts" and "immunocytes"—An attempt at a functional nomenclature. Blood **21**, 243–245 (1963).

DAMESHEK, W., GUNZ, F.: Leukemia. 2nd Ed., p. 243. New York-London: Grune&Stratton 1964.

DAVEY, F.R., GOTTLIEB, A.J.: Lymphocyte surface markers in acute lymphocytic leukemia. Amer. J. clin. Path. **62**, 818–822 (1974).

DAVIES, A.J.S., LEUCHARS, E., WALLIS, V., MARCHANT, R., ELLIOTT, E.V.: The failure of thymus-derived cells to produce antibody. Transplantation **5**, 222–231 (1967).

DAVIS, B.J.: Disc electrophoresis—II. Method and application to human serum proteins. Ann. N.Y. Acad. Sci. **121**, 404–427 (1964).

DEBUSSCHER, L., BERNHEIM, J.L., COLLARD-RONGÉ, E., GOVAERTS, A., HOOGHE, R., LEJEUNE, F.J., ZEICHER, M., STRYCKMANS, P.A.: Hairy cell leukemia: functional, immunologic, kinetic, and ultrastructural characterization. Blood **46**, 495—507 (1975).

DICKLER, H.B., ADKINSON, JR., N.F., TERRY, W.D.: Evidence for individual human peripheral blood lymphocytes bearing both B and T cell markers. Nature **247**, 213—215 (1974).

DICKLER, H.B., ARBEIT, R.D., HENKART, P.A., SACHS, D.H.: Association between Ia antigens and the Fc receptors of certain T lymphocytes. J. exp. Med. **144**, 282—287 (1976).

DICKLER, H.B., KUNKEL, H.G.: Interaction of aggregated γ-globulin with B lymphocytes. J. exp. Med. **136**, 191—196 (1972).

DICKLER, H.B., SACHS, D.H.: Evidence for identity or close association of the B Fc receptor of B lymphocytes and alloantigens determined by the Ir region of the H-2 complex. J. exp. Med. **140**, 779—796 (1974).

DICKLER, H.B., SIEGAL, F.P., BENTWICH, Z.H., KUNKEL, H.G.: Lymphocyte binding of aggregated IgG and surface Ig staining in chronic lymphocytic leukaemia. Clin. exp. Immunol. **14**, 97—106 (1973).

DIERICH, M.P., PELLEGRINO, M.A., FERRONE, S., REISFELD, R.A.: Evaluation of C3 receptors on lymphoid cells with different complement sources. J. Immunol. **122**, 1766—1773 (1974).

DORFMAN, R.F.: Enzyme histochemistry of normal, hyperplastic and neoplastic lymphoreticular tissues. In: Symp. Lymph. Tumours in Africa, Paris 1963, pp. 304—326, ROULET, F.C., Ed. Basel-New York: Karger 1964.

DORFMAN, R.F.: Childhood lymphosarcoma in St. Louis, Missouri, clinically and histologically resembling Burkitt's tumor. Cancer (Philad.) **18**, 418—430 (1965).

DORFMAN, R.F.: Diagnosis of Burkitt's tumor in the United States. Cancer (Philad.) **21**, 563—574 (1968).

DORFMAN, R.F.: Classical concepts of nodular (follicular) lymphomas. In: Malignant Diseases of the Hematopoietic System. GANN Monograph on Cancer Research, Vol. 15, pp. 177—194. AKAZAKI, K., RAPPAPORT, H., BERARD, C.W., BENNETT, J.M., ISHIKAWA, E., Eds. Tokyo: University Press 1973.

DUHAMEL, G.: Lymphoid myelofibrosis. About 10 further observations. Acta haemat. (Basel) **45**, 89—98 (1971).

DUKOR, P., BIANCO, C., NUSSENZWEIG, V.: Tissue localization of lymphocytes bearing a membrane receptor for antigen-antibody-complement complexes. Proc. nat. Acad. Sci. (Wash.) **67**, 991—997 (1970).

DUTCHER, T.F., FAHEY, J.L.: The histopathology of the macroglobulinemia of Waldenström. J. nat. Cancer Inst. **22**, 887—918 (1959).

DUTCHER, T.F., FAHEY, J.L.: Immunocytochemical demonstration of intranuclear localization of 18S gamma macroglobulin in macroglobulinemia of Waldenström. Proc. Soc. exp. Biol. (N.Y.) **103**, 452—455 (1960).

EDELSON, R.L., KIRKPATRICK, C.H., SHEVACH, E.M., SCHEIN, P.S., SMITH, R.W., GREEN, I., LUTZNER, M.: Preferential cutaneous infiltration by neoplastic thymus-derived lymphocytes. Morphologic and functional studies. Ann. intern. Med. **80**, 685—692 (1974).

EDELSON, R.L., LUTZNER, M.A., KIRKPATRICK, C.H., SHEVACH, E.M., GREEN, I.: Morphologic and functional properties of the atypical T lymphocyte of the Sezary syndrome. Mayo Clin. Proc. **49**, 558—566 (1974).

EDEN, A., BIANCO, C., NUSSENZWEIG, V., MAYER, M.M.: C3 split products inhibit the binding of antigen-antibody-complement complexes to B lymphocytes. J. Immunol. **110**, 1452—1453 (1973).

EDEN, A., MILLER, G.W., NUSSENZWEIG, V.: Human lymphocytes bear membrane receptors for C3b and C3d. J. clin. Invest. **52**, 3239—3242 (1973).

EPSTEIN, A.L., HENLE, W., HENLE, G., HEWETSON, J.F., KAPLAN, H.S.: Surface marker characteristics and Epstein-Barr virus studies of two established North American Burkitt's lymphoma cell lines. Proc. nat. Acad. Sci. (Wash.) **73**, 228—232 (1976).

ESKELAND, T., KLEIN, E.: Isolation of 7S IgM and kappa chains from the surface membrane of tissue culture cells derived from a Burkitt lymphoma. J. Immunol. **107**, 1368—1375 (1971).

FAGRAEUS, A.: Antibody production in relation to the development of plasma cells. In vivo and in vitro experiments. Acta med. scand. Suppl. **204**, 1—122 (1948).

FARRER-BROWN, G., BENNETT, M.H., HENRY, K.: (1973) In: BERARD, C.W., DORFMAN, R.F.: Histopathology of malignant lymphomas. Clin. Haemat. **3**, 39—76 (1974).

FATEH-MOGHADAM, A.: Zur Diagnostik paraproteinämischer Hämoblastosen. Fortschr. Med. **94**, 821–828 (1976).

FAULK, W.P., HIJMANS, W.: Recent developments in immunofluorescence. Progr. Allergy **16**, 9–39 (1972).

FERRARINI, M., MORETTA, L., ABRILE, R., DURANTE, M.L.: Receptors for IgG molecules on human lymphocytes forming spontaneous rosettes with sheep red cells. Eur. J. Immunol. **5**, 70–72 (1975).

FIALKOW, P.J., KLEIN, E., KLEIN, G., CLIFFORD, P., SINGH, S.: Immunoglobulin and glucose-6-phosphate dehydrogenase as markers of cellular origin in Burkitt lymphoma. J. exp. Med. **138**, 89–102 (1973).

FLAD, H.-D., FINK, U., DIERICH, M.P.: K cell activity of normal and chronic lymphocytic leukaemia lymphocytes: Association with lymphocytes bearing receptors for human C3b. In: Immunological Diagnosis of Leukemias and Lymphomas. Haematology and Blood Transfusion, Vol. 20, pp. 197–202. THIERFELDER, S., RODT, H., THIEL, E., Eds. Berlin-Heidelberg-New York: Springer 1977.

FLANDRIN, G., BROUET, J.-C.: The Sézary cell: Cytologic, cytochemical, and immunologic studies. Mayo Clin. Proc. **49**, 575–583 (1974).

FLANDRIN, G., BROUET, J.C., DANIEL, M.T., PREUD'HOMME, J.L.: Acute leukemia with Burkitt's tumor cells: A study of six cases with special reference to lymphocyte surface markers. Blood **45**, 183–188 (1975).

FLANDRIN, G., DANIEL, M.T., FOURCADE, M., CHELLOUL, N.: Leucémie à «tricholeucocyte» (hairy cell leukemia), étude clinique et cytologique de 55 observations. Nouv. Rev. franç. Hémat. **13**, 609–640 (1973).

FRØLAND, S.S.: Binding of sheep erythrocytes to human lymphocytes. A probable marker of T lymphocytes. Scand. J. Immunol. **1**, 269–280 (1972).

FRØLAND, S.S., NATVIG, J.B.: Class, subclass, and allelic exclusion of membrane-bound Ig of human B lymphocytes. J. exp. Med. **136**, 409–414 (1972).

FRØLAND, S.S., NATVIG, J.B.: Identification of three different human lymphocyte populations by surface markers. Transplant. Rev. **16**, 114–162 (1973).

FU, S.M., WINCHESTER, R.J., KUNKEL, H.G.: Occurrence of surface IgM, IgD, and free light chains on human lymphocytes. J. exp. Med. **139**, 451–456 (1974).

FU, S.M., WINCHESTER, R.J., KUNKEL, H.G.: The occurrence of the HL-B alloantigens on the cells of unclassified acute lymphoblastic leukemias. J. exp. Med. **142**, 1334–1338 (1975a).

FU, S.M., WINCHESTER, R.J., KUNKEL, H.G.: Similar idiotypic specificity for the membrane IgD and IgM of human B lymphocytes. J. Immunol. **114**, 250–252 (1975b).

FU, S.M., WINCHESTER, R.J., RAI, K.R., KUNKEL, H.G.: Hairy cell leucemia: Proliferation of a cell with phagocytic and B-lymphocyte properties. Scand. J. Immunol. **3**, 847–851 (1974).

GAJL-PECZALSKA, K.J., BLOOMFIELD, C.D., COCCIA, P.F., SOSIN, H., BRUNNING, R.D., KERSEY, J.H.: B and T cell lymphomas. Analysis of blood and lymph nodes in 87 patients. Amer. J. Med. **59**, 674–685 (1975).

GAJL-PECZALSKA, K.J., BLOOMFIELD, C.D., NESBIT, M.E., KERSEY, J.H.: B-cell markers on lymphoblasts in acute lymphoblastic leukaemia. Clin. exp. Immunol. **17**, 561–569 (1974).

GAJL-PECZALSKA, K.J., CHARTRAND, S., BLOOMFIELD, C.D., CORTE, J., COCCIA, P.F., NESBIT, M.E., KERSEY, J.H.: Lymphocytes bearing receptors for both sheep erythrocytes and complement in patients with neoplastic and non-neoplastic diseases. Clin. Immunol. Immunopath. **8**, 292–299 (1977).

GATIEN, J.G., SCHNEEBERGER, E.E., MERLER, E.: Analysis of human thymocyte subpopulations using discontinuous gradients of albumin: Precursor lymphocytes in human thymus. Eur. J. Immunol. **5**, 312–317 (1975).

GELFAND, M.C., FRANK, M.M., GREEN, I.: A receptor for the third component of complement in the human renal glomerulus. J. exp. Med. **142**, 1029–1034 (1975).

GERGELY, L., KLEIN, G., ERNBERG, I.: The action of DNA antagonists on Epstein-Barr virus (EBV)-associated early antigen (EA) in Burkitt lymphoma lines. Int. J. Cancer **7**, 293–302 (1971).

GHADIALLY, F.N., SKINNIDER, L.F.: Ultrastructure of hairy cell leukemia. Cancer (Philad.) **29**, 444–452 (1972).

GILBERTSEN, R.B., METZGAR, R.S.: Human T and B lymphocytes: Characterization of rosette-forming properties. [Abstr.] Fed. Proc. **32**, 975 (1973).

GMELIG-MEYLING, F., VAN DER HAM, M., BALLIEUX, R.E.: Binding of IgM by human T lymphocytes. Scand. J. Immunol. **5**, 487–495 (1976).

GOLDE, D.W., STEVENS, R.H., QUAN, S.G., SAXON, A.: Immunoglobulin synthesis in hairy cell leukaemia. Brit. J. Haemat. **35**, 359–365 (1977).

GRAHAM, JR., R.C., KARNOVSKY, M.J.: The early stages of absorption of injected horseraddish peroxidase in the proximal tubules of mouse kidney: Ultrastructural cytochemistry by a new technique. J. Histochem. Cytochem. **14**, 291–302 (1966).

GRAVELL, M., LEVINE, P.H., MCINTYRE, R.F., LAND, V.J., PAGANO, J.S.: Epstein-Barr virus in an American patient with Burkitt's lymphoma: Detection of viral genome in tumor tissue and establishment of a tumor-derived cell line (NAB). J. nat. Cancer Inst. **56**, 701–704 (1976).

GREAVES, M.F., BROWN, G., RAPSON, N.T., LISTER, T.A.: Antisera to acute lymphoblastic leukemia cells. Clin. Immunol. Immunopath. **4**, 67–84 (1975).

GREAVES, M.F., BROWN, G., RICKINSON, A.B.: Epstein-Barr virus binding sites on lymphocyte subpopulations and the origin of lymphoblasts in cultured lymphoid cell lines and in the blood of patients with infectious mononucleosis. Clin. Immunol. Immunopath. **3**, 514–524 (1975).

GREAVES, M., JANOSSY, G., DOENHOFF, M.: Selective triggering of human T and B lymphocytes in vitro by polyclonal mitogens. J. exp. Med. **140**, 1–18 (1974).

GREAVES, M.F., JANOSSY, G., ROBERTS, M., RAPSON, N.T., ELLIS, R.B., CHESSELS, J., LISTER, T.A., CATOVSKY, D.: Membrane phenotyping: Diagnosis, monitoring and classification of acute 'lymphoid' leukaemias. In: Immunological Diagnosis of Leukemias and Lymphomas. Haematology and Blood Transfusion, Vol. 20, pp. 61–74. THIERFELDER, S., RODT, H., THIEL, E., Eds. Berlin-Heidelberg-New York: Springer 1977.

GREENBERGER, J.S., CAMPOS-NETO, A., PARKMAN, R., MOLONEY, W.C., KARPAS, A., SCHLOSSMAN, S.F., ROSENTHAL, D.S.: Immunologic detection of intracellular and cell-surface lysosyme with human and experimental leukemic leukocytes. Clin. Immunol. Immunopath. **8**, 318–334 (1977).

GREY, H.M., KUBO, R.T., RABELLINO, E.M., POLLEY, M., ROSS, G.D.: Immunoglobulins and complement receptors on CLL cells. In: Schering Symp. Immunopath., Cavtat, June 1973. Advances in the Biosciences, Vol. 12, pp. 213–218. RASPÉ, G., Ed. Braunschweig: Pergamonn Press. Vieweg 1974.

GREY, H.M., RABELLINO, E., PIROFSKY, B.: Immunoglobulins on the surface of lymphocytes. IV. Distribution in hypogammaglobulinemia, cellular immune deficiency, and chronic lymphatic leukemia. J. clin. Invest. **50**, 2368–2375 (1971).

GUPTA, S., GOOD, R.A., SIEGAL, F.P.: Rosette-formation with mouse erythrocytes. II. A marker for human B and non-T lymphocytes. Clin. exp. Immunol. **25**, 319–327 (1976a).

GUPTA, S., GOOD, R.A., SIEGAL, F.P.: Rosette formation with mouse erythrocytes. III. Studies in patients with primary immunodeficiency and lymphoproliferative disorders. Clin. exp. Immunol. **26**, 204–213 (1976b).

HAAK, H.L., DE MAN, J.C.H., HIJMANS, W., KNAPP, W., SPECK, B.: Further evidence for the lymphocytic nature of leukaemic reticuloendotheliosis (hairy-cell leukaemia). Brit. J. Haemat. **27**, 31–38 (1974).

HAEGERT, D.G., CAWLEY, J.C., COLLINS, R.D., FLEMANS, R.J., SMITH, J.L.: Leukaemic reticuloendotheliosis: A morphological and immunological study of four cases. J. clin. Path. **27**, 967–972 (1974).

HAEGERT, D.G., CAWLEY, J.C., KARPAS, A., GOLDSTONE, A.H.: Combined T and B cell acute lymphoblastic leukaemia. Brit. med. J. 1974, IV, pp. 79–82.

HAMBURG, A., BRYNES, R.K., REESE, C., GOLOMB, H.M.: Human cord blood lymphocytes. Ultrastructural and immunologic surface marker characteristics; a comparison with B- and T-cell lymphomas. Lab. Invest. **34**, 207–215 (1976).

HAMMARSTRÖM, S., HELLSTRÖM, U., PERLMANN, P., DILLNER, M.-L.: A new surface marker on T lymphocytes of human peripheral blood. J. exp. Med. **138**, 1270–1275 (1973).

HEKMAN, A., MELIS, M.H.G.: Increased expression of a normal lymphocyte membrane antigen on chronic lymphatic leukemia cells. Cancer Res. **35**, 3656–3662 (1975).

HELLSTRÖM, U., MELLSTEDT, H., PERLMANN, P., HOLM, G., PETTERSSON, D.: Receptors for Helix pomatia A haemagglutinin on leukaemic lymphocytes from patients with chronic lymphocytic leukaemia (CLL). Clin. exp. Immunol. **26**, 196–203 (1976).

HENLE, G., HENLE, W., KLEIN, G.: Demonstration of two distinct components in the early antigen complex of Epstein-Barr virus-infected cells. Int. J. Cancer **8**, 272–282 (1971).

HENLE, W., HENLE, G., ZAJAC, B.A., PEARSON, G., WAUBKE, R., SCRIBA, M.: Differential reactivity of human serums with early antigens induced by Epstein-Barr virus. Science **169**, 188–190 (1970).

HEUSERMANN, U., STUTTE, H.J., MÜLLER-HERMELINK, H.K.: Interdigitating cells in the white pulp of the human spleen. Cell. Tiss. Res. **153**, 415–417 (1974).

HIJMANS, W.: Immunocytes in health and disease. Boll. Ist. sieroter. milan., Special Issue **53**, 174–175 (1974).

HIJMANS, W., SCHUIT, H.R.E., KLEIN, F.: An immunofluorescence procedure for the detection of intracellular immunoglobulins. Clin. exp. Immunol. **4**, 457–472 (1969).

HOPPER, J.E.: Immunoglobulin D: A predominant surface Ig in poorly differentiated lymphocytic (PDL) lymphoma. [Abstr.] Clin. Res. **22**, 394A (1974).

HSU, C.C.S., MARTI, G.E., SCHREK, R., WILLIAMS, JR., R.C.: Lymphocytes bearing B- and T-cell markers in patient with lymphosarcoma cell leukemia. Clin. Immunol. Immunopath. **3**, 385–395 (1975).

HUBER, C., ASAMER, H., MICHLMAYR, G., BRAUNSTEINER, H.: Surface immunoglobulins and receptor sites for aggregated IgG on leukemic reticuloendotheliosis cells. Blut **32**, 21–28 (1976).

HUBER, C., DWORZAK, E., FINK, U., MICHLMAYR, G., BRAUNSTEINER, H., HUBER, H.: Receptor sites for aggregated gammaglobulin (AGG) on lymphocytes in lymphoproliferative diseases. Brit. J. Haemat. **27**, 643–654 (1974).

HUBER, H., POLLEY, M.J., LINSCOTT, W.D., FUDENBERG, H.H., MÜLLER-EBERHARD, H.J.: Human monocytes: distinct receptor sites for the third component of complement and for immunoglobulin G. Science **162**, 1281–1283 (1968).

HUMPHREYS, R.E., MCCUNE, J.M., CHESS, L., HERRMAN, H.C., MALENKA, D.J., MANN, D.L., PARHAM, P., SCHLOSSMAN, S.F., STROMINGER, J.L.: Isolation and immunologic characterization of a human B-lymphocyte-specific, cell surface antigen. J. exp. Med. **144**, 98–112 (1976).

HUREZ, D., FLANDRIN, G., PREUD'HOMME, J.L., SELIGMANN, M.: Unreleased intracellular monoclonal macroglobulin in chronic lymphocytic leukaemia. Clin. exp. Immunol. **10**, 223–234 (1972).

HUREZ, D., PREUD'HOMME, J.-L., SELIGMANN, M.: Intracellular "monoclonal" immunoglobulin in non-secretory human myeloma. J. Immunol. **104**, 263–264 (1970).

JACOBSON, E.B., CAPORALE, L.H., THORBECKE, G.J.: Effect of thymus cell injections on germinal center formation in lymphoid tissues of nude (thymusless) mice. Cell. Immunol. **13**, 416–430 (1974).

JAFFE, E.S., BRAYLAN, R.C., FRANK, M.M., GREEN, I., BERARD, C.W.: Heterogeneity of immunologic markers and surface morphology in childhood lymphoblastic lymphoma. Blood **48**, 213–222 (1976).

JAFFE, E.S., SHEVACH, E.M., FRANK, M.M., BERARD, N.C., GREEN, I.: Nodular lymphoma–evidence for origin from follicular B lymphocytes. New Engl. J. Med. **290**, 813–819 (1974).

JAFFE, E.S., SHEVACH, E.M., FRANK, M.M., GREEN, I.: Leukemic reticuloendotheliosis: Presence of a receptor for cytophilic antibody. Amer. J. Med. **57**, 108–114 (1974).

JAFFE, E.S., SHEVACH, E.M., SUSSMAN, E.H., FRANK, M., GREEN, I., BERARD, C.W.: Membrane receptor sites for the identification of lymphoreticular cells in benign and malignant conditions. Brit. J. Cancer **31**, Suppl. II, 107–120 (1975).

JANOSSY, G., GREAVES, M.F., REVESZ, T., LISTER, T.A., ROBERTS, M., DURRANT, J., KIRK, B., CATOVSKY, D., BEARD, M.E.J.: Blast crisis of chronic myeloid leukaemia (CML). II. Cell surface marker analysis of "lymphoid" and myeloid cases. Brit. J. Haemat. **34**, 179–192 (1976).

JANOSSY, G., ROBERTS, M., GREAVES, M.F.: Target cell in chronic myeloid leukaemia and its relationship to acute lymphoid leukaemia. Lancet 1976, II, pp. 1058–1061.

JONDAL, M., HOLM, G., WIGZELL, H.: Surface markers on human T and B lymphocytes. I. A large population of lymphocytes forming nonimmune rosettes with sheep red blood cells. J. exp. Med. **136**, 207–215 (1972).

JONDAL, M., KLEIN, G.: Surface markers on human B and T lymphocytes. II. Presence of Epstein-Barr virus receptors on B lymphocytes. J. exp. Med. **138**, 1365–1378 (1973).

JONDAL, M., KLEIN, G., OLDSTONE, M.B.A., BOKISH, V., YEFENOF, E.: Surface markers on human B and T lymphocyts. III. Association between complement and Epstein-Barr virus receptors on human lymphoid cells. Scand. J. Immunol. **5**, 401–410 (1976).

JONDAL, M., SVEDMYR, E., KLEIN, E., SINGH, S.: Killer T cells in a Burkitt's lymphoma biopsy. Nature **255**, 405–407 (1975).

JONDAL, M., WIGZELL, H., AIUTI, F.: Human lymphocyte subpopulations: Classification according to surface markers and/or functional characteristics. Transplant. Rev. **16**, 163–195 (1973).

JONES, S.E., FUKS, Z., BULL, M., KADIN, M.E., DORFMAN, R.F., KAPLAN, H.S., ROSENBERG, S.A., KIM, H.: Non-Hodgkin's lymphomas. IV. Clinicopathologic correlation in 405 cases. Cancer (Philad.) **31**, 806–823 (1973).

KAISERLING, E.: Elektronenmikroskopische Befunde bei Non-Hodgkin-Lymphomen. In: Maligne Lymphome und monoklonale Gammopathien. Hämatologie und Bluttransfusion, Bd. 18, pp. 185–198. LÖFFLER, H., Ed. München: Lehmanns 1976.

KAISERLING, E., LENNERT, K.: Die interdigitierende Reticulumzelle im menschlichen Lymphknoten. Eine spezifische Zelle der thymusabhängigen Region. Virchows Arch. B **16**, 51–61 (1974).

KAISERLING, E., STEIN, H., LENNERT, K.: IgM-producing malignant lymphomas without macroglobulinemia. Morphological and immunochemical findings. Virchows Arch. B. **14**, 1–18 (1973).

KAISERLING, E., STEIN, H., MÜLLER-HERMELINK, H.K.: Interdigitating reticulum cells in the human thymus. Cell Tiss. Res. **155**, 47–55 (1974).

KAPLAN, M.E., CLARK, C.: An improved rosetting assay for detection of human T lymphocytes. J. immunol. Methods **5**, 131–135 (1974).

KAPLAN, J., MASTRANGELO, R., PETERSON, JR., W.D.: Childhood lymphoblastic lymphoma, a cancer of thymus-derived lymphocytes. Cancer Res. **34**, 521–525 (1974).

KARLSSON, C., DAVIES, H., ÖHMAN, J., ANDERSSON, U.-B.: LKB multiphor. I. Analytical thin layer gel electrofocusing in polyacrylamide gel. Application Note, March 1973, LKB Produkter AB, Bromma, Sweden.

KATAYAMA, I.: Hairy-cell leukemia. New Engl. J. Med. **296**, 881 (1977).

KELLY, G.E., MEARS, D.C., SHELL, A.G.R.: Relationship of the immunosuppressive potency of antilymphocyte globulin to three in vitro tests. Close correlation with rosette inhibition. Transplantation **12**, 443–447 (1971).

KERBEL, R.S., DAVIES, A.J.S.: The possible biological significance of Fc receptors on mammalian lymphocytes and tumor cells. Cell **3**, 105–112 (1974).

KERSEY, J., COCCIA, P., BLOOMFIELD, C., NESBIT, M., MCKENNA, R., BRUNNING, R., HALLGREN, H., GAJL-PECZALSKA, K.: Surface markers define human lymphoid malignancies with differing prognoses. In: Immunological Diagnosis of Leukemias and Lymphomas. Haematology and Blood Transfusion, Vol. 20, pp. 17–24. THIERFELDER, S., RODT, H., THIEL, E., Eds. Berlin-Heidelberg-New York: Springer 1977.

KERSEY, J.H., NESBIT, M., HALLGREN, H., SABAD, A., YUNIS, E., GAJL-PECZALSKA, K.: Evidence for origin of certain childhood acute lymphoblastic leukemias and lymphomas in thymus-derived lymphocytes. Cancer (Philad.) **36**, 1348–1352 (1975).

KERSEY, J.H., NESBIT, M.E., LUCKASEN, J.R., HALLGREN, H.M., SABAD, A., YUNIS, E.J., GAJL-PECZALSKA, K.J.: Acute lymphoblastic leukemic and lymphoma cells with thymus-derived (T) markers. Mayo Clin. Proc. **49**, 584–587 (1974).

KERSEY, J.H., SABAD, A., GAJL-PECZALSKA, K., HALLGREN, H.M., YUNIS, E.J., NESBIT, M.E.: Acute lymphoblastic leukemic cells with T (thymus-derived) lymphocyte markers. Science **182**, 1355–1356 (1973).

KIM, H., HELLER, P., RAPPAPORT, H.: Monoclonal gammopathies associated with lymphoproliferative disorders: A morphologic study. Amer. J. clin. Path. **59**, 282–294 (1973).

KING, G.W., HURTUBISE, P.E., SAGONE, JR., A.L., LOBUGLIO, A.F., METZ, E.N.: Leukemic reticuloendotheliosis. A study of the origin of the malignant cell. Amer. J. Med. **59**, 411–416 (1975).

KLAUS, G.G.B., HUMPHREY, J.H.: The generation of memory cells. I. The role of C3 in the generation of B memory cells. Immunology **33**, 31–40 (1977).

KLEIN, G.: Studies on Epstein-Barr virus genome and the EBV-determined nuclear antigen in human malignant disease. Cold Spr. Harb. Symp. quant. Biol. **39**, 783–790 (1975a).

KLEIN, G.: The Epstein-Barr virus and neoplasia. New Engl. J. Med. **293**, 1353–1357 (1975b).

KLEIN, G., CLIFFORD, P., KLEIN, E., STJERNSWÄRD, J.: Search for tumor-specific immune reactions in Burkitt lymphoma patients by the membrane immunofluorescence reaction. Proc. nat. Acad. Sci. (Wash.) **55**, 1628–1635 (1966).

KLEIN, E., KLEIN, G., NADKARNI, J.S., NADKARNI, J.J., WIGZELL, H., CLIFFORD, P.: Surface IgM specificity on cells derived from a Burkitt's lymphoma. Lancet 1967, II, 1068–1070.

KNAPP, W., HAAIJMAN, J.J., SCHUIT, H.R.E., RÁDL, J., VAN DEN BERG, P., PLOEM, J.S., HIJMANS,

W.: Microfluorometric evaluation of conjugate specificity with the defined antigen substrate spheres (DASS) system. Ann. N.Y. Acad. Sci. **254**, 94–107 (1975).

KNAPP, W., SCHUIT, H.R.E., BOLHUIS, R.L.H., HIJMANS, W.: Surface immunoglobulins in chronic lymphatic leukaemia, macroglobulinaemia and myelomatosis. Clin. exp. Immunol. **16**, 541–552 (1974).

KRÜGER, G., UHLMANN, C., HELLRIEGEL, K.P., SESTERHENN, K., SAMII, H., FISCHER, R., WUSTROW, F., GROSS, R.: Membranrezeptoren lymphoreticulärer Zellen bei hyperplastischen und neoplastischen Erkrankungen des lymphatischen Systems. In: Maligne Lymphome und monoklonale Gammopathien. Hämatologie und Bluttransfusion, Bd. 18, pp. 17–31. LÖFFLER, H., Ed. München: Lehmanns 1976.

KRUSE, K., STEIN, H., HITZIG, W.H., LASSON, U.: Lymph-node plasmacytoma in a child. Clinical and immunological findings. 1978, submitted for publication.

KUBO, R.T., GREY, H.M., PIROFSKY, B.: IgD: A major immunoglobulin on the surface of lymphocytes from patients with chronic lymphatic leukemia. J. Immunol. **112**, 1952–1954 (1974).

KUNKEL, H.G.: Surface markers of human lymphocytes. Behring Inst. Mitt. **59**, 1–10 (1976).

LAY, W.H., MENDES, N.F., BIANCO, C., NUSSENZWEIG, V.: Binding of sheep red blood cells to a large population of human lymphocytes. Nature **230**, 531–532 (1971).

LEECH, J.H., GLICK, A.D., WALDRON, J.A., FLEXNER, J.M., HORN, R.G., COLLINS, R.D.: Malignant lymphomas of follicular center cell origin in man. I. Immunologic studies. J. nat. Cancer Inst. **54**, 11–21 (1975).

VAN LEEUWEN, A.W.F.M., MEIJER, C.J.L.M., DE MAN, J.C.H.: T-cell membrane characteristics of "mycosis cells" in the skin and lymph node. J. invest. Derm. **65**, 367–369 (1975).

LELBACH, W.K.: Ein Beitrag zur Morphologie der Makroglobulinämie Waldenström. Frankfurt. Z. Path. **68**, 440–464 (1957).

LENNERT, K.: Pathologie der Halslymphknoten. Ein Abriß für Pathologen, Kliniker und praktizierende Ärzte. Berlin-Göttingen-Heidelberg-New York: Springer 1964.

LENNERT, K.: Classification of malignant lymphomas (European concept). In: Progress in Lymphology, pp. 103–109. RÜTTIMANN, A., Ed. Stuttgart: Thieme 1967.

LENNERT, K.: Follicular lymphoma: A special entity of malignant lymphomas. In: Plenary Session Papers. 1. Meeting Europ. Div. of Int. Soc. of Haemat., Milano 1971, pp. 109–122. Milano: Arti Grafiche Fratelli Ferrari 1971.

LENNERT, K.: Follicular lymphoma. A tumor of the germinal centers. In: Malignant Diseases of the Hematopoietic System. GANN Monograph on Cancer Research, Vol. 15, pp. 217–231. AKAZAKI, K., RAPPAPORT, H., BERARD, C.W., BENNETT, J.M., ISHIKAWA, E., Eds. Tokyo: University of Tokyo Press 1973.

LENNERT, K., STEIN, H.: Follicular lymphoma and other malignant lymphomas as neoplasias of the B cell system. Symposium at the 9. Int. Congr. of the Int. Academy of Path., Helsinki/Finland, Sept. 1972.

LENNERT, K., STEIN, H., KAISERLING, E.: Cytological and functional criteria for the classification of malignant lymphomata. Brit. J. Cancer **31**, Suppl. II, 29–43 (1975).

LEVINE, P.H.: Relationship of Epstein-Barr virus antibodies to disease state in Hodgkin's disease, chronic lymphocytic leukemia and American Burkitt's lymphoma. In: Oncogenesis and Herpesviruses, pp. 384–389. BIGGS, P.M., DE THÉ, G., PAYNE, L.N., Eds. Lyon: IARC Scientific Publications 1972.

LIN, P.S., HSU, C.C.S.: Human leukaemic T cells with complement receptors. Clin. exp. Immunol. **23**, 209–213 (1976).

LINDSTRÖM, F.D., WILLIAMS, JR., R.C.: Serum anti-immunoglobulins in multiple myeloma and benign monoclonal gammopathy. Clin. Immunol. Immunopath. **3**, 503–513 (1975).

LITWIN, S.D., HÜTTEROTH, T.H., LIN, P.K., KENNARD, J., CLEVE, H.: Immunoglobulin expression of cells from human lymphoblastoid lines. II. Interrelationship among surface, cellular, and secreted immunoglobulins. J. Immunol. **113**, 668–672 (1974).

LOBO, P.I., WESTERVELT, F.B., HORWITZ, D.A.: Identification of two populations of immunoglobulin-bearing lymphocytes in man. J. Immunol. **114**, 116–119 (1975).

LÖFFLER, H., GRAUBNER, M., DESAGA, J.F., JUNG, M.: Prolymphocytic leukemia with T cell properties and tartrate resistant acid phosphatase. In: Immunological Diagnosis of Leukemias and Lymphomas. Haematology and Blood Transfusion, Vol. 20, pp. 175–178. THIERFELDER, S., RODT, H., THIEL, E., Eds. Berlin-Heidelberg-New York: Springer 1977.

LUKES, R.J., COLLINS, R.D.: New observations on follicular lymphoma. In: Malignant Diseases of the Hematopoietic System. GANN Monograph on Cancer Research, Vol. 15, pp. 209–215. AKAZAKI, K., RAPPAPORT, H., BERARD, C.W., BENNETT, J.M., ISHIKAWA, E., Eds. Tokyo: University of Tokyo Press 1973.

LUKES, R.J., COLLINS, R.D.: New approaches to the classification of the lymphomata. Brit. J. Cancer **31**, Suppl. II, 1–28 (1975).

LUKES, R.J., LENNERT, K.: Malignant lymphoma. Slide Seminar. 10th Int. Congr. Int. Acad. Path., Hamburg 1974.

LUMB, G.: Tumours of Lymphoid Tissue. Edinburgh-London: Livingstone 1954.

MAGRATH, I.T.: Burkitt's lymphoma: A B or T cell tumour? Europ. J. Cancer **10**, 83–88 (1974).

DE MAN, J.C.H., MEINERS, W.B.H.: Crystals of protein nature in the cytoplasm of lymphatic cells in a case of lymphoreticular malignancy. Blood **20**, 492–500 (1962).

MANN, R.B., JAFFE, E.S., BRAYLAN, R.C., NANBA, K., FRANK, M.M., ZIEGLER, J.L., BERARD, C.W.: Non-endemic Burkitt's lymphoma. A B-cell tumor related to germinal centers. New Engl. J. Med. **295**, 685–691 (1976).

MANTOVANI, B., RABINOVITCH, M., NUSSENZWEIG, V.: Phagocytosis of immune complexes by macrophages. Different roles of the macrophage receptor sites for complement (C3) and for immunoglobulin (IgG). J. exp. Med. **135**, 780–792 (1972).

MARMONT, A.M., DAMASIO, E.E.: B lymphocytes in macroglobulinemia. Lancet II, p. 1326 (1971).

MASON, D.Y., FARRELL, C., TAYLOR, C.R.: The detection of intracellular antigens in human leucocytes by immunoperoxidase staining. Brit. J. Haemat. **31**, 361–370 (1975).

MASON, D.Y., LABAUME, S., PREUD'HOMME, J.-L.: The detection of membrane and cytoplasmic immunoglobulins in human leucocytes by immunoperoxidase staining. Clin. exp. Immunol. **29**, 413–421 (1977).

MASON, D.Y., TAYLOR, C.R.: The distribution of muramidase (lysozyme) in human tissues. J. clin. Path. **28**, 124–132 (1975).

MAYER, M.M.: The complement system. A foreign cell in the body is identified by antibody, but the cell is detroyed by other agents. Among them is "complement", an intricately linked set of enzymes. Sci. Am. **229**, 54–66 (1973).

MCCAFFREY, R., HARRISON, T.A., KUNG, P.C., PARKMAN, R., SILVERSTONE, A.E., BALTIMORE, D.: Terminal deoxynucleotidyl transferase in normal and neoplastic hematopoietic cells. In: Modern Trends in Human Leukemia II. Hämatologie und Bluttransfusion, Bd. 19, pp. 503–513. NETH, R., GALLO, R.C., MANNWEILER, K., MOLONEY, W.C., Eds. München: Lehmanns 1976.

MCCAFFREY, R., HARRISON, T.A., PARKMAN, R., BALTIMORE, D.: Terminal deoxynucleotidyl transferase activity in human leukemic cells and in normal human thymocytes. New Engl. J. Med. **292**, 775–780 (1975).

MCKENZIE, I.F.C., PARISH, C.R.: Secretion of Ia antigens by a subpopulation of T cells which are Ly-$1^+$, Ly-$2^-$, and $Ia^-$. J. exp. Med. **144**, 847–851 (1976).

MCMASTER, P.D., HUDACK, S.S.: The formation of agglutinins within lymph nodes. J. exp. Med. **61**, 783–805 (1935).

MELCHERS, F., ANDERSSON, J.: IgM in bone marrow-derived lymphocytes. Changes in synthesis, turnover and secretion, and in numbers of molecules on the surface of B cells after mitogenic stimulation. Eur. J. Immunol. **4**, 181–188 (1974).

MELLSTEDT, H., HAMMARSTRÖM, S., HOLM, G.: Monoclonal lymphocyte population in human plasma cell myeloma. Clin. exp. Immunol. **17**, 371–384 (1974).

MENDES, N.F., TOLNAI, M.E.A., SILVEIRA, N.P.A., GILBERTSEN, R.B., METZGAR, R.S.: Technical aspects of the rosette tests used to detect human complement receptor (B) and sheep erythrocyte-binding (T) lymphocytes. J. Immunol. **111**, 860–867 (1973).

METZGAR, R.S., MOHANAKUMAR, T., BOLOGNESI, D.P.: Relationship between membrane antigens of human leukemic cells and oncogenic RNA virus structural components. J. exp. Med. **143**, 47–63 (1976).

MILLER, J.F.A.P., BASTEN, A., SPRENT, J., CHEERS, C.: Interaction between lymphocytes in immune responses. Cell. Immunol. **2**, 469–495 (1971).

MILLER, J.F.A.P., MITCHELL, G.F.: Thymus and antigen-reactive cells. Antigen-sensitive cells, their source and differentiation. Transplant. Rev. **1**, 3–42 (1969).

MILLS, B., SEN, L., BORELLA, L.: Reactivity of antihuman thymocyte serum with acute leukemic blasts. J. Immunol. **115**, 1038–1044 (1975).

MINOWADA, J., TSUBOTA, T., NAKAZAWA, S., SRIVASTAVA, B.I.S., HUANG, C.C., OSHIMURA, M., SONTA, S., HAN, T., SINKS, L.F., SANDBERG, A.A.: Establishment and characterization of leukemic T-cell lines, B-cell lines, and null-cell line: a progress report on surface antigen study of fresh lymphatic leukemias in man. In: Immunological Diagnosis of Leukemias and Lymphomas. Haematology and Blood Transfusion, Vol. 20, pp. 241–250. THIERFELDER, S., RODT, H., THIEL, E., Eds. Berlin-Heidelberg-New York: Springer 1977.

MITUS, W.J., MEDNICOFF, I.B., WITTELS, B., DAMESHEK, W.: Neoplastic lymphoid reticulum cells in the peripheral blood: A histochemical study. Blood **17**, 206–215 (1961).

MÖLLER, G., COUTINHO, A.: Role of C3 and Fc receptors in B-lymphocyte activation. J. exp. Med. **141**, 647–663 (1975).

MOHANAKUMAR, T., METZGAR, R.S., MILLER, D.S.: Human leukemia cell antigens: Serologic characterization with xenoantisera. J. nat. Cancer Inst. **52**, 1435–1444 (1974).

MOHANAKUMAR, T., MILLER, D.S., METZGAR, R.S.: Human acute myelomonocytic leukemia: Serologic studies with simian antisera. Blood **48**, 339–350 (1976).

MORETTA, L., FERRARINI, M., DURANTE, M.L., MINGARI, M.C.: Expression of a receptor for IgM by human T cells in vitro. Europ. J. Immunol. **5**, 565–569 (1975).

MORI, Y., LENNERT, K.: Electron microscopic atlas of lymph node cytology and pathology. Berlin-Heidelberg-New York: Springer 1969.

MORRIS, M.W., DAVEY, F.R.: Immunologic and cytochemical properties of histiocytic and mixed histiocytic-lymphocytic lymphomas. Amer. J. clin. Path. **63**, 403–414 (1975).

NAEIM, F., GOSSETT, T., WALFORD, R.L.: Reactivity of the merrit B-cell alloantiserum with hairy cells. [Letter to the Editor.] New Engl. J. Med. **296**, 882 (1977).

NANBA, K., JAFFE, E.S., BRAYLAN, R.C., SOBAN, E.J., BERARD, C.W.: Alkaline phosphatase-positive malignant lymphoma. A subtype of B-cell lymphomas. Amer. J. clin. Path. **68**, 535–542 (1977).

NARDO, J.M., NORTON, W.L.: Chronic lymphocytosis with lymphocyte inclusions. Ann. int. Med. **76**, 265–268 (1972).

NIES, K.M., OBERLIN, M.A., BROWN, J.C., HALPERN, M.S.: Immunoglobulin biosynthesis by normal and leukemic human peripheral blood lymphocytes. J. Immunol. **111**, 1236–1242 (1973).

NOSSAL, G.J.V., WARNER, N.L., LEWIS, H., SPRENT, J.: Quantitative features of a sandwich radioimmunolabeling technique for lymphocyte surface receptors. J. exp. Med. **135**, 405–428 (1972).

O'CONOR, G.T.: Significant aspects of childhood lymphoma in Africa. Cancer Res. **23**, 1514–1518 (1963).

O'CONOR, G.T., RAPPAPORT, H., SMITH, E.B.: Childhood lymphoma resembling "Burkitt tumor" in the United States. Cancer (Philad.) **18**, 411–417 (1965).

OLDSTONE, M.B.A., THEOFILOPOULOS, A.N., GUNVEN, P., KLEIN, G.: Immune complexes associated with neoplasia: Presence of Epstein-Barr virus antigen-antibody complexes in Burkitt's lymphoma. Intervirology **4**, 292–302 (1976).

ORNSTEIN, L.: Disc electrophoresis. I. Background and theory. Ann. N.Y. Acad. Sci. **121**, 321–349 (1964).

OSSERMAN, E.F., TAKATSUKI, K.: Plasma-cell myeloma: Gamma-globulin synthesis and structure. Medicine (Baltimore) **42**, 357–384 (1963).

PAGANO, J.S., HUANG, C.H., LEVINE, P.: Absence of Epstein-Barr viral DNA in American Burkitt's lymphoma. New Engl. J. Med. **289**, 1395–1399 (1973).

PANIJEL, J., DELAMETTE, F., LENEVEN, M.: Cellular and subcellular study of the in vitro immune response. Europ. J. Immunol. **1**, 87–97 (1971).

PAPAMICHAIL, M., BROWN, J.C., HOLBOROW, E.J.: Immunoglobulins on the surface of human lymphocytes. Lancet 1971, II, pp. 850–852.

PAPAMICHAIL, M., HOLBOROW, E.J., KEITH, H.I., CURREY, H.L.F.: Subpopulations of human peripheral blood lymphocytes distinguished by combined rosette formation and membrane immunofluorescence. Lancet 1972, II, pp. 64–66.

PARASKEVAS, F., LEE, S.-T., ISRAELS, L.G.: Absence of $\gamma$-globulin receptors on mouse plasmacytoma cells. Nature **227**, 395–397 (1970).

PARKER, J.W., TAYLOR, C.R., PATTENGALE, P., ROYSTON, I., TINDLE, B.H., CAIN, M.J., LUKES, R.J.: A morphological and cytochemical comparison of human T and B lymphoblastoid cell lines: Light and electron microscopy. 1977, in press.

PARKHOUSE, R.M.E., ASKONAS, B.A.: Immunoglobulin M biosynthesis. Intracellular accumulation of 7s subunits. Biochem. J. **115**, 163–169 (1969).

Parrott, D.M.V., de Sousa, M.A.B., East, J.: Thymus-dependent areas in the lymphoid organs of neonatally thymectomized mice. J. exp. Med. **123**, 191–204 (1966).
du Pasquier, L., Weiss, N., Loor, F.: Direct evidence for immunoglobulins on the surface of thymus lymphocytes of amphibian larvae. Eur. J. Immunol. **2**, 366–370 (1972).
Pepys, M.B.: Role of complement in induction of the allergic response. Nature [New Biol.] **237**, 157–159 (1972).
Perlmann, P.: K cells. VIIth Immunopathology Symposium, Bad Schachen, Western Germany, June 1976.
Perlmann, P., Perlmann, H.: Contactual lysis of antibody-coated chicken erythrocytes by purified lymphocytes. Cell. Immunol. **1**, 300–315 (1970).
Perlmann, P., Perlmann, H., Biberfeld, P.: Specifically cytotoxic lymphocytes produced by preincubation with antibody-complexed target cells. J. Immunol. **108**, 558–561 (1972).
Pernis, B., Brouet, J.C., Seligmann, M.: IgD and IgM on the membrane of lymphoid cells in macroglobulinemia. Evidence for identity of membrane IgD and IgM antibody activity in a case with anti-IgG receptors. Europ. J. Immunol. **4**, 776–778 (1974).
Pernis, B., Forni, L., Amante, L.: Immunoglobulin spots on the surface of rabbit lymphocytes. J. exp. Med. **132**, 1001–1018 (1970).
Pernis, B., Forni, L., Amante, L.: Immunoglobulins as cell receptors. Ann. N.Y. Acad. Sci. **190**, 420–429 (1971).
Pichler, W.J., Knapp, W.: Chronic lymphatic leukemia cells bear IgM receptors. In: Immunological Diagnosis of Leukemias and Lymphomas. Haematology and Blood Transfusion, Vol. 20, pp. 163–167. Thierfelder, S., Rodt, H., Thiel, E., Eds. Berlin-Heidelberg-New York: Springer 1977.
Pierce, C.W., Asofsky, R., Solliday, S.M.: Immunoglobulin receptors on B lymphocytes: shifts in immunoglobulin class during immune responses. Fed. Proc. **32**, 41–43 (1973).
Piessens, W.F., Schur, P.H., Moloney, W.C., Churchill, W.H.: Lymphocyte surface immunoglobulins: Distribution and frequency in lymphoproliferative diseases. New Engl. J. Med. **288**, 176–180 (1973).
Potter, V.R.: Tissue homogenates. In: Methods in Enzymology, Vol. 1, pp. 10–15. Colowick, S.P., Kaplan, N.O., Eds. New York: Academic Press 1955.
Preud'Homme, J.L., Brouet, J.C., Clauvel, J.P., Seligmann, M.: Surface IgD in immunoproliferative disorders. Scand. J. Immunol. **3**, 853–858 (1974).
Preud'Homme, J.L., Hurez, D., Seligmann, M.: Immunofluorescence studies in Waldenström's macroglobulinemia. Rev. europ. Étud. clin. biol. **15**, 1127–1131 (1970).
Preud'Homme, J.L., Seligmann, M.: Surface bound immunoglobulins as a cell marker in human lymphoproliferative diseases. Blood **40**, 777–794 (1972a).
Preud'Homme, J.L., Seligmann, M.: Anti-human immunoglobulin G activity of membrane-bound monoclonal immunoglobulin M in lymphoproliferative disorders. Proc. nat. Acad. Sci. (Wash.) **69**, 2132–2135 (1972b).
Preud'Homme, J.-L., Seligmann, M.: Immunoglobulins on the surface of lymphoid cells in Waldenström's macroglobulinemia. J. clin. Invest. **51**, 701–705 (1972c).
Rabellino, E., Colon, S., Grey, H.M., Unanue, E.R.: Immunoglobulins on the surface of lymphocytes. I. Distribution and quantitation. J. exp. Med. **133**, 156–167 (1971).
Raff, M.C.: Two distinct populations of peripheral lymphocytes in mice distinguishable by immunofluorescence. Immunology **19**, 637–650 (1970).
Raff, M.C.: T and B lymphocytes and immune responses. Nature **242**, 19–23 (1973).
Raff, M.C., Sternberg, M., Taylor, R.B.: Immunoglobulin determinants on the surface of mouse lymphoid cells. Nature **225**, 553–554 (1970).
Ralph, P., Moore, M.A.S., Nilsson, K.: Lysozyme synthesis by established human and murine histiocytic lymphoma cell lines. J. exp. Med. **143**, 1528–1533 (1976).
Rappaport, H.: Tumors of the Hematopoietic System. Atlas of Tumor Pathology, Sect. 3, Fasc. 8. Washington, D.C.: Armed Forces Institute of Pathology 1966.
Rappaport, H., Winter, W.J., Hicks, E.B.: Follicular lymphoma. A re-evaluation of its position in the scheme of malignant lymphoma, based on a survey of 253 cases. Cancer (Philad.) **9**, 792–821 (1956).
Reedman, B.M., Klein, G.: Cellular localization of an Epstein-Barr virus (EBV) associated complement-fixing antigen in producer and non-producer lymphoblastoid cell lines. Int. J. Cancer **11**, 499–520 (1973).

REIF, A.E., ALLEN, J.M.V.: The AKR thymic antigen and its distribution in leukemias and nervous tissues. J. exp. Med. **120**, 413–433 (1964).

RIEBER, E.P., v. HEYDEN, H.W., LINKE, R.P., SAAL, J.G., RIETHMÜLLER, G., WALLER, H.D.: Haarzell-Leukämie. Charakterisierung der leukämischen Zelle: Oberflächenimmunglobuline, Fc-Rezeptoren und Stimulation durch Mitogene. Klin. Wschr. **54**, 1011–1019 (1976).

RIEBER, E.P., LINKE, R.P., HADAM, M., SAAL, J.G., RIETHMÜLLER, G., v.HEYDEN, H.W., WALLER, H.D., SCHWARZ, H.: Hairy cell leukemia: Simultaneous demonstration of autochthonous surface-Ig and monocytic functions of hairy cells. In: Immunological Diagnosis of Leukemias and Lymphomas. Haematology and Blood Transfusion, Vol. 20, pp. 157–161. THIERFELDER, S., RODT, H., THIEL, E., Eds. Berlin-Heidelberg-New York: Springer 1977.

RODT, H., THIERFELDER, S., THIEL, E., GÖTZE, D., NETZEL, B., HUHN, D., EULITZ, M.: Identification and quantitation of human T-cell antigen by antisera purified from antibodies crossreacting with hemopoietic progenitors and other blood cells. Immunogenetics **2**, 411–430 (1975).

ROHR, K.: Das menschliche Knochenmark. 3. Ed. Stuttgart: G. Thieme 1960.

ROSS, G.D., POLLEY, M.J.: Specificity of human lymphocyte complement receptors. J. exp. Med. **141**, 1163–1180 (1975).

ROSS, G.D., POLLEY, M.J., RABELLINO, E.M., GREY, H.M.: Two different complement receptors on human lymphocytes. One specific for C3b and one specific for C3b inactivator-cleaved C3b. J. exp. Med. **138**, 798–811 (1973).

ROSS, G.D., RABELLINO, E.M., POLLEY, M.J., GREY, H.M.: Combined studies of complement receptor and surface immunoglobulin bearing cells and sheep erythrocyte rosette forming cells in normal and leukemic human lymphocytes. J. clin. Invest. **52**, 377–385 (1973).

ROTHER, K., TILL, G.: Biologische Funktionen und Pathologie. In: Komplement. Biochemie und Pathologie, pp. 94–277. ROTHER, K., Ed. Darmstadt: Steinkopff 1974.

ROWE, D.S., HUG, K., FAULK, W.P., MCCORMICK, J.N., GERBER, H.: IgD on the surface of peripheral blood lymphocytes of the human newborn. Nature [New Biol.] **242**, 155–157 (1973).

ROWE, D.S., HUG, K., FORNI, L., PERNIS, B.: Immunoglobulin D as a lymphocyte receptor. J. exp. Med. **138**, 965–972 (1973).

RUBIN, A.D., DOUGLAS, S.D., CHESSIN, L.N., GLADE, P.R., DAMESHEK, W.: Chronic reticulolymphocytic leukemia. Reclassification of "leukemic reticuloendotheliosis" through functional characterization of the circulating mononuclear cells. Amer. J. Med. **47**, 149–162 (1969).

RUDDY, S., AUSTEN, K.F.: C3b inactivator of man. II. Fragments produced by C3b inactivator cleavage of cell-bound or fluid phase C3b. J. Immunol. **107**, 742–750 (1971).

SALSANO, F., FRØLAND, S.S., NATVIG, J.B., MICHAELSEN, T.E.: Same idiotype of B-lymphocyte membrane IgD and IgM. Formal evidence for monoclonality of chronic lymphocytic leucemia cells. Scand. J. Immunol. **3**, 841–846 (1974).

SANDILANDS, G.P., GRAY, K., COONEY, A., BROWNING, J.D., GRANT, R.M., ANDERSON, J.R.: Lymphocytes with T and B cell properties in a lymphoproliferative disorder. Lancet 1974, I, pp. 903–904.

SARIN, P.S., ANDERSON, P.N., GALLO, R.C.: Terminal deoxynucleotidyl transferase activities in human blood leukocytes and lymphoblast cell lines: High levels in lymphoblast cell lines and in blast cells of some patients with chronic myelogenous leukemia in acute phase. Blood **47**, 11–20 (1976).

SARIN, P.S., GALLO, R.C.: Terminal deoxynucleotidyltransferase in chronic myelogenous leukemia. J. biol. Chem. **249**, 8051–8053 (1974).

SARIN, P.S., GALLO, R.C.: Terminal deoxynucleotidyl transferase as a biological marker for human leukemia. In: Modern Trends in Human Leukemia II. Hämatologie und Bluttransfusion, Bd. 19, pp. 491–502. NETH, R., GALLO, R.C., MANNWEILER, K., MOLONEY, W.C., Eds. München: Lehmanns 1976.

SCHAMAUN, M.: Zur pathologischen Anatomie der sog. Makroglobulinaemie Waldenstroem. Schweiz. Z. allg. Path. **17**, 25–46 (1954).

SCHEINBERG, M., BRENNER, A.I., SULLIVAN, A.L., CATHCART, E.S., KATAYAMA, I.: The heterogeneity of leukemic reticuloendotheliosis, "hairy cell leukemia". Evidence for its monocytic origin. Cancer (Philad.) **37**, 1302–1307 (1976).

SCHLOSSMAN, S.F., CHESS, L., HUMPHREYS, R.E., STROMINGER, J.L.: Distribution of Ia-like molecules on the surface of normal and leukemic human cells. Proc. nat. Acad. Sci. (Wash.) **73**, 1288–1292 (1976).

SCHREK, R., DONNELLY, W.J.: "Hairy" cells in blood in lymphoreticular neoplastic disease and "flagellated" cells of normal lymph nodes. Blood **27**, 199–211 (1966).

SCHWENK, H.U.: Immunological cell markers on lymphoblasts of patients with acute lymphatic leukemia. Z. Kinderheilk. **118**, 87–95 (1974).

SEILER, F.R., SEDLACEK, H.H., KANZY, E.J., LANG, W.: Über die Brauchbarkeit immunologischer Nachweismethoden zur Differenzierung funktionell verschiedener Lymphozyten: Spontanrosetten, Komplementreceptor-Rosetten und Immunoglobulinrezeptoren. Behring Inst. Mitt. **52**, 26–72 (1972).

SELIGMANN, M., BROUET, J.-C., PREUD'HOMME, J.-L.: The immunological diagnosis of human leukemias and lymphomas: an overview. In: Immunological Diagnosis of Leukemias and Lymphomas. Haematology and Blood Transfusion, Vol. 20, pp. 1–15. THIERFELDER, S., RODT, H., THIEL, E., Eds. Berlin-Heidelberg-New York: Springer 1977.

SELIGMANN, M., PREUD'HOMME, J.-L., BROUET, J.-C.: B and T cell markers in human proliferative blood diseases and primary immunodeficiencies, with special reference to membrane bound immunoglobulins. Transplant. Rev. **16**, 85–113 (1973).

SELL, S., GELL, P.G.H.: Studies on rabbit lymphocytes in vitro. I. Stimulation of blast transformation with an antiallotype serum. J. exp. Med. **122**, 423–440 (1965).

SEN, L., BORELLA, L.: Clinical importance of lymphoblasts with T markers in childhood acute leukemia. New Engl. J. Med. **292**, 828–832 (1975).

SEN, L., MILLS, B., BORELLA, L.: Erythrocyte receptors and thymus-associated antigens on human thymocytes, mitogen-induced blasts, and acute leukemia blasts. Cancer Res. **36**, 2436–2441 (1976).

SHERR, C.J., UHR, J.W.: Immunoglobulin synthesis and secretion. VI. Synthesis and intracellular transport of immunoglobulin in nonsecretory lymphoma cells. J. exp. Med. **133**, 901–920 (1971).

SHEVACH, E., EDELSON, R., FRANK, M., LUTZNER, M., GREEN, I.: A human leukemia cell with both B and T cell surface receptors. Proc. nat. Acad. Sci. (Wash.) **71**, 863–866 (1974).

SHEVACH, E.M., JAFFE, E.S., GREEN, I.: Receptors for complement and immunoglobulin on human and animal lymphoid cells. Transplant. Rev. **16**, 3–28 (1973).

SILBERMAN, S., SCHREK, R.: Surface immunoglobulins of lymphocytes in chronic lymphocytic leukemia and disseminated lympho-sarcoma. Exp. mol. Path. **20**, 33–39 (1974).

SILVERSTONE, A.E., CANTOR, H., GOLDSTEIN, G., BALTIMORE, D.: Terminal deoxynucleotidyl transferase is found in protyhmocytes. J. exp. Med. **144**, 543–548 (1976).

SMITH, J.L., COWLING, D.C., BARKER, C.R.: Response of lymphocytes in chronic lymphocytic leucaemia to plant mitogens. Lancet 1972, I, pp. 229–233.

SMITH, J.L., HAEGERT, D.: B- and T-lymphocyte markers on transformed lymphocytes from mitogen-stimulated cultures of normal and CLL lymphocytes and on tonsil blasts. Clin. exp. Immunol. **17**, 547–560 (1974).

SMITH, R.W., TERRY, W.D., BUELL, D.N., SELL, K.W.: An antigenic marker for human thymic lymphocytes. J. Immunol. **110**, 884–887 (1973).

SMITH, W.I., LADOULIS, C.T., MISRA, D.N., GILL III, T.J., BAZIN, H.: Lymphocyte plasma membranes. III. Composition of lymphocyte plasma membranes from normal and immunized rats. Biochim. biophys. Acta (Amst.) **382**, 506–525 (1975).

SOLOMON, A., FAHEY, J.L., MALMGREN, R.A.: Immunohistologic localization of gamma-1-macroglobulins, beta-2A-myeloma proteins, 6.6S gamma-myeloma proteins and Bence Jones proteins. Blood **21**, 403–423 (1963).

STATHOPOULOS, G., ELLIOT, E.V.: Formation of mouse or sheep red-blood-cell rosettes by lymphocytes from normal and leukaemic individuals. Lancet 1974, I, pp. 600–601.

STEIN, H.: Zur Charakterisierung maligner Lymphome. Morphologie und immunologische Untersuchungen. Habil.-Schrift, Kiel 1975a.

STEIN, H.: Immunologische und immunchemische Techniken und ihre Bedeutung für die Klassifikation lymphatischer Neoplasien. Verh. dtsch. Ges. Path. **59**, 510–522 (1975b)

STEIN, H.: Immunchemische und immunzytologische Befunde bei Non-Hodgkin-Lymphomen. In: Maligne Lymphome und monoklonale Gammopathien. Hämatologie und Bluttransfusion, Bd. 18, pp. 167–183. LÖFFLER, H., Ed. München: Lehmanns 1976a.

STEIN, H.: Klassifikation der malignen Non-Hodgkin-Lymphome aufgrund gemeinsamer morphologischer und immunologischer Merkmale zwischen normalen und neoplastischen lymphatischen Zellen. Immun. Infekt. **4**, 52–69 u. 95–109 (1976b).

STEIN, H., BARTELS, H., WIEMER, E., KAISERLING, E.: Das Vorkommen von Immunglobulinen der Klassen D und E in malignen Lymphomen. Verh. dtsch. Ges. inn. Med. **81**, 1586–1591 (1975).

STEIN, H., BOUMAN, H., LENNERT, K., FUCHS, J., HAVSTEEN, B.: Isoelectric focusing pattern of IgM and surface markers in non-Hodkin's lymphomas. In: Immunological Diagnosis of Leukemias and Lymphomas. Haematology and Blood Transfusion, Vol. 20, pp. 315–326. THIERFELDER, S., RODT, H., THIEL, E., Eds. Berlin-Heidelberg-New York: Springer 1977.

STEIN, H., DRESCHER, S.: Darstellung von Oberflächen-IgM an Blutlymphozyten mit der Immuno-Peroxydase-Methode. Blut **26**, 35–42 (1973).

STEIN, H., KAISERLING, E.: Myeloma producing nonsecretory IgM and secretory IgG. Scand. J. Haemat. **12**, 274–283 (1974a).

STEIN, H., KAISERLING, E.: Surface immunoglobulins and lymphocyte-specific surface antigens on leukaemic reticuloendotheliosis cells. Clin. exp. Immunol. **18**, 63–71 (1974b).

STEIN, H., KAISERLING, E., LENNERT, K.: Neue Gesichtspunkte zur Systematik maligner Lymphome auf dem Boden immunchemischer Analysen. In: Leukämien und maligne Lymphome, pp. 195–201. STACHER, A., Ed. München-Berlin-Wien: Urban & Schwarzenberg 1973.

STEIN, H., KAISERLING, E., LENNERT, K.: Immunoglobulin-production and surface-bound immunoglobulins in chronic lymphocytic leukemia, lymphosarcoma, and so-called reticulum cell sarcoma. In: Modern Trends in Human Leukemia, Hämatologie und Bluttransfusion, Vol. 14, pp. 97–106. NETH, R., GALLO, R.C., SPIEGELMAN, S., STOHLMAN, JR., F., Eds. München: J.F. Lehmanns 1974a.

STEIN, H., KAISERLING, E., LENNERT, K.: Evidence for B-cell origin of reticulum cell sarcoma. Virchows Arch. A. **364**, 51–67 (1974b).

STEIN, H., KAISERLING, E., LENNERT, K.: Lympho-plasmocytoid immunocytoma—a new entity of human non-Hodgkin's lymphoma. [Lecture.] 10. Int. Congr. Int. Acad. Path., Hamburg 1974c. Abstract Book p. 58, No. 122.

STEIN, H., KAISERLING, E., LENNERT, K.: Lympho-plasmacytoid immunocytoma—a distinct entity of non-Hodgkin's lymphoma. 3rd Meeting of European & African Division of International Society of Haematology, London, August 24–28, 1975. Abstract Book 2, No. 19:05.

STEIN, H., KAISERLING, E., LENNERT, K., PARWARESCH, M.R.: Makroglobulinbildende chronische lymphatische Leukämie ohne Makroglobulinämie. Klin. Wschr. **51**, 389–396 (1973).

STEIN, H., LENNERT, K., PARWARESCH, M.R.: Malignant lymphomas of B-cell type. Lancet 1972, II, pp. 855–857.

STEIN, H., MÜLLER-HERMELINK, H.K.: Simultaneous presence of receptors for complement and sheep red blood cells on human fetal thymocytes. Brit. J. Haemat. **36**, 227–233 (1977).

STEIN, H., PAPADIMITRIOU, C.S., BOUMAN, H., LENNERT, K., FUCHS, J.: Demonstration of immunoglobulin production by tumor cells in non-Hodgkin's and Hodgkin's malignant lymphomas and its significance for their classification. 1978, in press.

STEIN, H., PARWARESCH, M.R.: Lokalisation der IgM-Fraktion in diskontinuierlichen Polyacrylamid-Elektrophoresesäulen. Blut **23**, 104–112 (1971).

STEIN, H., PARWARESCH, M.R., KAPER, G., MÄDER, C.: Elektrophoretische Darstellung von 19 S IgM in diskontinuierlichen Polyacrylamid-Säulen. Klin. Wschr. **51**, 1050–1058 (1973).

STEIN, H., PETERSEN, N., GAEDICKE, G., LENNERT, K., LANDBECK, G.: Lymphoblastic lymphoma of convoluted or acid phosphatase type—a tumor of T precursor cells. Int. J. Cancer **17**, 292–295 (1976).

STEIN, H., SIEMSSEN, U., LENNERT, K.: Complement receptor subtypes (C3b and C3d) in lymphatic tissue and follicular lymphoma. 1978, in press.

STERNBERGER, L.A., HARDY, JR., P.H., CUCULIS, J.J., MEYER, H.G.: The unlabeled antibody enzyme methof of immunohistochemistry. Preparation and properties of soluble antigen-antibody complex (horseradish peroxidase-antihorseradish peroxidase) and its use in identification of spirochetes. J. Histochem. Cytochem. **18**, 315–333 (1970).

STOECKENIUS, JR., W., NAUMANN, P.: Elektronenmikroskopische Untersuchungen zur Antikörperbildung in der Milz. Verh. des 6. Kongr. der Eurp. Ges. f. Haematol., pp. 4–9. Basel-New York: Karger 1958.

STRAUS, W.: Localization of antibody to horseradish peroxidase in popliteal lymph nodes of rabbits during the primary and early secondary response. J. Histochem. Cytochem. **18**, 120–130 (1970).

TAYLOR, C.R.: The nature of Reed-Sternberg cells and other malignant "reticulum" cells. Lancet 1974, II, pp. 802–807.

TAYLOR, C.R.: An immunohistological study of follicular lymphoma, reticulum cell sarcoma and Hodgkin's disease. Europ. J. Cancer **12**, 61–75 (1976).
TAYLOR, C.R., BURNS, J.: The demonstration of plasma cells and other immunoglobulin-containing cells in formalin-fixed, paraffin-embedded tissues using peroxidase-labelled antibody. J. clin. Path. **27**, 14–20 (1974).
TERNYNCK, T., DIGHIERO, G., FOLLEZOU, J., BINET, J.-L.: Comparison of normal and CLL lymphocyte surface Ig determinants using peroxidase-labeled antibodies. I. Detection and quantitation of light chain determinants. Blood **43**, 789–795 (1974).
THEOFILOPOULOS, A.N., BOKISCH, V.A., DIXON, F.J.: Receptor for soluble C3 and C3b on human lymphoblastoid (Raji) cells. Properties and biological significance. J. exp. Med. **139**, 696–711 (1974).
THIEL, E., DÖRMER, P., RODT, H., HUHN, D., BAUCHINGER, M., KLEY, H.P., THIERFELDER, S.: Quantitation of T-antigenic sites and Ig-determinants on leukemic cells by microphotometric immunoradiography. Proof of the clonal origin of thymus-derived lymphocytic leukemias. In: Immunological Diagnosis of Leukemias and Lymphomas. Haematology and Blood Transfusion, Vol. 20, pp. 131–144. THIERFELDER, S., RODT, H., THIEL, E., Eds. Berlin-Heidelberg-New York: Springer 1977.
THIEL, E., RODT, H., HUHN, D., THIERFELDER, S.: Decrease and altered distribution of human T antigen on chronic lymphatic leukemia cells of T type, suggesting a clonal origin. Blood **47**, 723–736 (1976).
THIELE, H.G., STARK, R.: Antigenic relationship between thymocytes and brain tissue in rats. Lancet 1971, II, p. 878.
TÖNDER, M.O., THUNOLD, S., SOLHAUG, J.H.: Properties of Fcγ receptors in normal and malignant human tissues. Scand. J. Immunol. **5**, 361–368 (1976).
TRUBOWITZ, S., MASEK, B., FRASCA, J.M.: Leukemic reticuloendotheliosis. Blood **38**, 288–298 (1971).
VADAS, M.A., MILLER, J.F.A.P., MCKENZIE, I.F.C., CHISM, S.E., SHEN, F.-W., BOYSE, E.A., GAMBLE, J.R., WHITELAW, A.M.: Ly and Ia antigen phenotypes of T cells involved in delayed-type hypersensitivity and in suppression. J. exp. Med. **114**, 10–19 (1976).
VELDMAN, J.E.: Histophysiology and electron microscopy of the immune response. Thesis, Univ. of Groningen 1970.
VITETTA, E.S., BIANCO, C., NUSSENZWEIG, V., UHR, J.W.: Cell surface immunoglobulin. IV. Distribution among thymocytes, bone marrow cells, and their derived populations. J. exp. Med. **136**, 81–93 (1972).
VOSSEN, J.: The development of the B immune system in man. In: Proefschrift, Rotterdam 1975.
WARNER, N.L., SZENBERG, A., BURNET, F.M.: The immunological role of different lymphoid organs in the chicken. I. Dissociation of immunological responsiveness. Aust. J. exp. Biol. med. Sci. **40**, 373–384 (1962).
WEINER, M.S., BIANCO, C., NUSSENZWEIG, V.: Enhanced binding of neuraminidase-treated sheep erythrocytes to human T lymphocytes. Blood **42**, 939–946 (1973).
WERNET, P., SCHUNTER, F., WILMS, K., WALLER, H.D.: New aspects in the classification of leukemic cell types by Ia alloantigens and complement receptors. In: Immunological Diagnosis of Leukemias and Lymphomas. Haematology and Blood Transfusion, Vol. 20, pp. 333–338. THIERFELDER, S., RODT, H., THIEL, E., Eds. Berlin-Heidelberg-New York: Springer 1977.
WEST, W., HERBERMAN, R.B.: A human lymphoid cell line with receptors for both sheep red blood cells and complement. Cell. Immunol. **14**, 139–145 (1974).
WHITE, A., DOUGERTHY, T.F.: Role of lymphocytes in normal and immunoglobulin production and mode of release of globulin from lymphocytes. Ann. N.Y. Acad. Sci. **46**, 859–882 (1946).
WHITE, R.G.: The relation of the cellular responses in germinal or lymphocytopoietic centers of lymph nodes to the production of antibody. In: Mechanisms of Antibody Formation, pp. 25–29. HOLUB, M., JAROŠKOVÁ, L., Eds. Prague: Publishing House Czech. Acad. Sci. 1960 (Distrib., New York: Academic Press).
WHITTINGHAM, S., MACKAY, I.R.: Rosette formation by human thymocytes. Cell. Immunol. **6**, 362–367 (1973).
WILLIAMS, JR., R.C., DEBOARD, J.R., MELLBYE, O.J., MESSNER, R.P., LINDSTRÖM, F.D.: Studies of T- and B-lymphocytes in patients with connective tissue diseases. J. clin. Invest. **52**, 283–295 (1973).

WILSON, J.D., NOSSAL, G.J.V.: Identification of human T and B lymphocytes in normal peripheral blood and in chronic lymphocytic leukaemia. Lancet 1971, II, 788–791.

WINCHESTER, R.J., FU, S.M., HOFFMAN, T., KUNKEL, H.G.: IgG on lymphocyte surfaces; technical problems and the significance of a third cell population. J. Immunol. **114**, 1210–1212 (1975).

WINCHESTER, R.J., FU, S.M., WERNET, P., KUNKEL, H.G., DUPONT, B., JERSILD, C.: Recognition by pregnancy serums of non-HL-A alloantigens selectively expressed on B lymphocytes. J. exp. Med. **141**, 924–929 (1975).

WINCHESTER, R.J., WINFIELD, J.B., SIEGAL, F., WERNET, P., BENTWICH, Z., KUNKEL, H.G.: Analyses of lymphocytes from patients with rheumatoid arthritis and systemic lupus erythematosus. Occurrence of interfering cold-reactive antilymphocyte antibodies. J. clin. Invest. **54**, 1082–1092 (1974).

WORTIS, H.H., COOPER, A.G., BROWN, M.C.: Inhibition of human lymphocyte rosetting by anti-T sera. Nature [New Biol.] **243**, 109–111 (1973).

YAM, L.T., CASTOLDI, G.L., GARVEY, M.B., MITUS, W.J.: Functional cytogenetic and cytochemical study of the leucemic reticulum cells. Blood **32**, 90–101 (1968).

YEFENOF, E., KLEIN, G., JONDAL, M., OLDSTONE, M.B.A.: Surface markers on human B- and T-lymphocytes. IX. Two-color immunofluorescence studies on the association between EBV receptors and complement receptors on the surface of lymphoid cell lines. Int. J. Cancer **17**, 693–700 (1976).

YOSHIDA, T.O., ANDERSSON, B.: Evidence for a receptor recognizing antigen complexed immunoglobulin on the surface of activated mouse thymus lymphocytes. Scand. J. Immunol. **1**, 401–408 (1972).

ZOLLINGER, H.U.: Die pathologische Anatomie der Makroglobulinämie Waldenström. Helv. med. Acta **25**, 153–183 (1958).

ZUCKER-FRANKLIN, D.: Properties of the Sezary lymphoid cell. An ultrastructural analysis. Mayo Clin. Proc. **49**, 567–574 (1974).

ZUCKER-FRANKLIN, D., MELTON III, J.W., QUAGLIATA, F.: Ultrastructural, immunologic, and functional studies on Sézary cells: A neoplastic variant of thymus-derived (T) lymphocytes. Proc. nat. Acad. Sci. (Wash.) **71**, 1877–1881 (1974).

# Author Index

# Subject Index

# Recent Results in Cancer Research

Fortschritte der Krebsforschung
Progrès dans les recherches sur le cancer
Editor in Chief: P. Rentchnick

Volume 54
**Malignant Bone Tumors**
6th International Symposium of the "Gesellschaft zur Bekämpfung der Krebskrankheiten Nordrhein-Westfalen e.V."
Düsseldorf, October 17/18, 1974
Editor: E. Grundmann
1976. 116 figures, 68 tables.
VIII, 279 pages
ISBN 3-540-07519-4

Volume 55
G. Mathé
**Cancer Active Immunotherapy**
Immunoprophylaxis and Immunorestoration
An Introduction
1976. 123 figures, 87 tables. XV, 405 pages
ISBN 3-540-07601-8

Volume 56
**Lymphocytes, Macrophages, and Cancer**
Editors: G. Mathé, I. Florentin, M.-C. Simmler
1976. 53 figures. IX, 160 pages
ISBN 3-540-07902-5

Volume 58
B.S. Schoenberg
**Multiple Primary Malignant Neoplasms**
The Connecticut Experience, 1935–1964
1977. 139 tables. IX, 173 pages
ISBN 3-540-07948-3

Volume 59
**Selective Heat Sensitivity of Cancer Cells**
Editors: A. Rossi-Fanelli, R. Cavaliere, B. Mondovi, G. Moricca
1977. 99 figures, 24 tables. XII, 189 pages
ISBN 3-540-07973-4

Volume 60
**Tumors of the Male Genital System**
VII International Symposium of the "Gesellschaft zur Bekämpfung der Krebskrankheiten Nordrhein-Westfalen e.V."
Düsseldorf 24/25 October 1965
Editors: E. Grundmann, W. Vahlensieck
1977. 123 figures, 63 tables. XII, 268 pages
ISBN 3-540-08029-5

Volume 61
D. Metcalf
**Hemopoietic Colonies**
In Vitro Cloning of Normal and Leukemic Cells
1977. 54 figures, 28 tables. IX, 227 pages
ISBN 3-540-08232-8

Volume 62
**Tactics and Strategy in Cancer Treatment**
Editor: G. Mathé
1977. 75 figures, 92 tables. XV, 219 pages
ISBN 3-540-08415-0

Volume 63
**Antitumor Antibiotics**
Editors: S.K. Carter, H. Umezawa, J. Douros, Y. Sakurai
1978. 111 figures, 198 tables.
Approx. 320 pages
ISBN 3-540-08624-2

Springer-Verlag
Berlin
Heidelberg
New York

GPSR Compliance

*The European Union's (EU) General Product Safety Regulation (GPSR) is a set of rules that requires consumer products to be safe and our obligations to ensure this.*

*If you have any concerns about our products, you can contact us on ProductSafety@springernature.com*

In case Publisher is established outside the EU, the EU authorized representative is:

Springer Nature Customer Service Center GmbH
Europaplatz 3
69115 Heidelberg, Germany

**Batch number: 10838053**

Printed by Printforce, the Netherlands